Contents

Pathology and Therapeutics for Pharmacists

A basis for clinical pharmacy practice

THIRD EDITION

Russell J Greene
BPharm MSc PhD MRPharmS
Senior Lecturer in Clinical Pharmacy
Former Head, Pharmacy Practice Group
Department of Pharmacy
King's College London
University of London
UK

Norman D Harris
BPharm PhD DIC
Emeritus Reader in Pharmaceutics
Department of Pharmacy
King's College London
University of London
UK

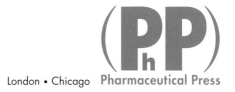

London • Chicago Pharmaceutical Press

Published by the Pharmaceutical Press
An imprint of RPS Publishing

1 Lambeth High Street, London SE1 7JN, UK
100 South Atkinson Road, Suite 200, Greyslake, IL 60030-7820, USA

© Russell J Greene and Norman D Harris 1993, 2000, 2008

(**P.P**) is a trade mark of RPS Publishing
RPS Publishing is the publishing organisation of the Royal Pharmaceutical Society of Great Britain

First edition published by Chapman & Hall 1993
First published in paperback 1994
Reprinted 1995
Reprinted by the Pharmaceutical Press 1996, 1997, 1998
Second edition published 2000
Reprinted by the Pharmaceutical Press 2003, 2006
Third edition published 2008

Typeset by J&L Composition, Filey, North Yorkshire
Printed in Great Britain by Cambridge University Press,
Cambridge

ISBN 978 0 85369 690 2

A catalogue record for this book is available from the British Library.

1 0054198858T

Disclaimer

The drug selections and doses given in this book are for illustration only. The authors and publishers take no responsibility for any actions consequent upon following the contents of this book without first checking current sources of reference.

All doses mentioned are checked carefully. However, no stated dose should be relied on as the basis for prescription writing, advising or monitoring. Recommendations change constantly, and a current copy of an official formulary, such as the *British National Formulary* or the Summary of Product Characteristics, should always be consulted. Similarly, therapeutic selections and profiles of therapeutic and adverse activities are based upon the authors' interpretation of official recommendations and the literature at the time of publication. The most current literature must always be consulted.

Dedication and acknowledgements

WE DEDICATE this book to Odilian and Minnie, whose support, patience and forbearance over many years and three editions made the travails of authorship bearable, and to all our student readers, to whom we wish good fortune in their studies, and who we hope will find this book useful.

We must also record our gratitude to the numerous people whose invaluable help made this book possible, notably the clinicians and clinical pharmacists who kindly reviewed different parts of this book at different times and provided many invaluable suggestions. For the first edition they were mostly clinicians from the former Riverside Health Authority and the NW Thames Health Region, namely Drs T. Cantopher, J. Curtis, M. Gore, J.M. Hunt, D. Jarrett, M. Johnson, A.C. Keat, S. Neill, R.J. Playford, P. Wise and D Anderson. Several pharmaceutical companies kindly supplied us with reference material or illustrations, for which we express our gratitude.

For the second edition reviewers were experienced clinical pharmacists primarily from London teaching hospitals, namely Jo Coleman, Care of the Elderly Pharmacist, Royal Free Hospital; Jatinder Harchowal, Senior Pharmacist, renal services, King's College Hospital, King's Healthcare; Alison Hole, Drug Information and Audit Pharmacist, Royal Marsden NHS Trust, Sutton, Surrey; Barry Jubraj, Teacher Practitioner and Training Pharmacist, King's College London and Chelsea and Westminster Hospital; Andrzej Kostrzewski, Principal Pharmacist for education and training, Guy's and St Thomas's Hospital Trust; Julie Mycroft, Principal Pharmacist for clinical services, Royal Marsden NHS Trust; Duncan McRobbie, Principal Clinical Pharmacist, Guy's and St Thomas's Hospital Trust; Jonathan Simms, Senior Clinical Pharmacist, Chelsea and Westminster Hospital; Tamsin Stevenson, Teacher Practitioner and Senior Pharmacist for education and training, King's College London and Basildon and Thurrock General Hospitals Trust, Essex; David Taylor, Chief Pharmacist, Maudsley Hospital and Honorary Senior Lecturer, Institute of Psychiatry.

For the third edition our reviewers were experienced specialist clinical pharmacists from various parts of the UK, with a particular expertise in the section they have reviewed. These are:

Chapter 3 Gastroenterology	Caroline Broadbent	Principal Pharmacist, Surgery	Guy's & St. Thomas' NHS Foundation Trust, London
Chapter 4 Cardiovascular	Duncan McRobbie	Principal clinical pharmacist	Guy's & St. Thomas' NHS Foundation Trust, London
Chapter 5 Respiratory	Dr Anne Boyter	Senior lecturer	Department of Pharmaceutical Sciences, University of Strathclyde

Chapter 6 Psychiatry	Stephen Bazire	Chief pharmacist	Norfolk and Waveney Mental Health Partnership NHS Trust, Norwich
Chapter 6 Neurology	Stuart Richardson	Pharmacy Clinical Team Leader	King's College Hospital, London
Chapter 7 Pain	Janet Trundle	Macmillan Specialist Pharmacist in Palliative Care	NHS Argyll & Clyde, Paisley
Chapter 8 Infection	Dr. Hayley Wickens	Senior Microbiology Pharmacist	St Mary's NHS Trust, London
Chapter 9 Diabetes	Elizabeth Hackett	Principal Pharmacist	Guy's & St. Thomas' NHS Foundation Trust, London
Chapter 9 Thyroid disease	Kathryn Forster	Lecturer – Practitioner	Kings College London/ Guy's & St. Thomas' NHS Foundation Trust
Chapter 10 Neoplasia	Simon Rivers	Formerly – Principal Pharmacist, Oncology	Guy's & St. Thomas' NHS Foundation Trust, London
Chapter 11 Haematology	Sarah Mahmoud	Haematology Oncology Pharmacist	St Mary's NHS Trust, London
Chapter 12 Arthropathy	Carole A Callaghan	Principal Pharmacist	Western General Hospital, Edinburgh
Chapter 13 Dermatology	Samuel Bundu-Kamara	Principal Pharmacist, Dermatology	St. John's Institute of Dermatology Guy's & St. Thomas' NHS Foundation Trust, London
Chapter 14 Renal	Caroline Ashley	Principal Pharmacist Renal Services	Royal Free Hospital, London

We greatly value their advice, which has enormously helped in the preparation of this edition, but of course we take complete responsibility for the opinions and judgements expressed throughout the book.

Many other individuals and companies have assisted in providing information, illustrations or permission to reproduce material and are specifically acknowledged as appropriate. We also thank the staff of the Pharmaceutical Press, notably Christina Debono, Louise McIndoe and Linda Paulus who all worked hard on this updating.

Finally, we must not forget the generations of pharmacy students who have passed through the Chelsea and later King's College Department of Pharmacy. They have provided us with much useful feedback on the suitability of our treatment of the material. Through their interest, enthusiasm and hard work in the face of a very full and difficult course, they have kept alive our faith in the importance and relevance of the subject throughout the writing and updating of this book.

Plate acknowledgements

Plates 1, 3, 4, 5, 8, 9, 11, 14 and 16 are reproduced with permission from Dr J.J.R. Almeyda, Enfield Health District, London, UK.

Plates 2, 6, 7, 12, 13 and 15 are reproduced with permission from Dr J.W. Woodward, Sidcup Health Centre, Kent, UK.

Plate 10 is reproduced with permission from the Photographic Library, St John's Hospital for Diseases of the Skin, London, UK.

Note on drug nomenclature

WE HAVE USED **recommended international non-proprietary names (rINN)** throughout for drugs. However, certain substances are referred to primarily in their physiological or pharmacological role, especially *adrenaline* and *noradrenaline*. There has been no move towards changing the physiological terms such as *adrenergic*, and so to reduce confusion the names *epinephrine* (for adrenaline) and *norepinephrine* (for noradrenaline) have not been adopted as primary names in this edition.

Preface to the third edition

THE RESPONSE TO the previous editions of this text have been favourable, and it has clearly fulfilled a need of our target audience. Consequently, we were delighted that the Pharmaceutical Press, who steered us so capably through the second edition and its several reprints, asked us to produce this third edition.

Since our last edition the important changes that have transformed pharmacotherapy are the rise of evidence based medicine (EBM) and the firm establishment of national and international therapeutic guidelines, usually based on careful meta-analyses of randomized controlled trials. These have frequently been issued by disease-specific organizations such as the British Hypertension Society, or generic bodies such as the National Institute for Health and Clinical Excellence (NICE) and the National Prescribing Centre in the UK. These guidelines have been incorporated into this edition wherever available, and have been a main focus of the update. However, as before, the overall intention remains to demonstrate how knowledge of the biomedical sciences of physiology, pathology and pharmacology underpins understanding of the rationale behind these recommendations.

The major advance in therapy has been the long awaited and much heralded advent of specifically designed 'biological treatments'. These agents, fruits of the dramatic increase in our understanding of molecular biology and genetics, and the application of combinatorial methods in drug design, are finally starting to transform many areas of therapeutics, notably cancer and inflammatory disease.

Other changes are transforming the organization and delivery of clinical pharmacy. In the UK, in secondary care the role of consultant pharmacist is developing, while in primary care it is hoped the pharmacist prescribing and a new community pharmacist contract will give impetus to far greater involvement of pharmacists in patient care and management.

We have retained the format of the second edition, but the text has been extensively reworked to improve clarity, coherence and uniformity. We have significantly reorganized and harmonized the sections and headings to improve consistency in structure and comprehension. These changes, together with a more detailed index, have enabled us to use an improved internal cross-referencing system. Where there are cross-references within a chapter, the reader is directed to a closely-associated block of text or, if the reference is more remote, the page number is given. Cross-references outside a chapter give the chapter number, which together with the index should enable the material to be located quickly. In similar vein, the book has been divided into two sections. **Part 1** (Chapters 1 and 2) covers essential introductory material. **Part 2** (Chapters 3 to 14) deals with the various body systems and their diseases, arranged in the same order as the *British National Formulary* (BNF) wherever possible. We have added coverage of Thyroid disease in the Endocrine chapter, and a new chapter on Haematological disease. The use of drugs in renal impairment has been expanded in the Renal chapter. Evidence based therapeutic guidelines have been emphasized throughout.

As before we have included only those advances in pathology that have become accepted enhancements of our understanding of disease states, but we also indicate potential growth areas of research. We also continue to restrict coverage of adverse drug reactions mainly to the most common or the most serious, particularly in relation to their presumed mechanisms, rather than simply reproducing exhaustive lists of side-effects and interactions that can be readily obtained elsewhere.

The References and further reading lists have been updated and rINNs are used throughout for drug nomenclature, following the BNF wherever possible. The BNF style in the use of hyphenation, spelling, etc. has been adopted. Many figures have been added or redrawn, and we have continued to summarize salient points in frequent tables.

Because of the pace of change we have to accept that inevitably some of our information will have become dated between the proofs leaving our desks and the finished book leaving the publisher. We emphasize that readers must check routinely in a current reference source such as the BNF or the pharmaceutical industry's Summary of Product Characteristics when considering prescribing, monitoring or advising in specific situations. All doses mentioned are checked carefully and therapeutic selections and profiles of therapeutic and adverse activities are based upon the authors' interpretation of official recommendations and the literature at the time of publication. However, the drug selections and doses given are for illustration only. The authors and publishers take no responsibility for any actions consequent upon following the contents of this book without first checking an official reference. The reader's attention is drawn to the Disclaimer (see p. iv).

We trust that pharmaceutical manufacturers will appreciate our need to restrict ourselves to broad generalizations. The omission of a drug or product does not imply ineffectiveness or unsuitability, nor does the mention of one constitute a recommendation. The listing of generic adverse effects does not imply that every member of that class of medicines causes them. Listings of cautions, side-effects and interactions are not comprehensive.

We have retained the term 'clinical pharmacy' to describe the overall scope of this book. We believe that despite the development of areas such as pharmaceutical care, medicines management and clinical governance, in essence this encompasses, for pharmacy, no more than what clinical pharmacy in its widest, original sense always did.

We were pleased that sales of the earlier editions extended beyond the undergraduate pharmacist audience originally targeted, and also far beyond the UK, with sales in over 50 countries. We hope the new edition will be as useful as the first two evidently have, and that it will continue to interest practitioners of disciplines outside the confines of pharmacy, reflecting the multidisciplinary nature of modern healthcare.

Russell J. Greene
Norman D. Harris

Department of Pharmacy
King's College London

August 2007

Extract from preface to the first edition

CLINICAL PHARMACY has been defined in many different ways, according to the interests and outlook of the practitioner. We take a very broad definition, encompassing all aspects of the use of medicines in patients and of responding to patients' concerns about their health. It is thus an essential component of the practice of virtually all pharmacists, whether working in the community, in hospital or in industry, and must be based on a sound knowledge of the mechanisms of disease and the principles of drug selection. It has been a principle of our teaching that clinical pharmacy practice requires an understanding of the medical process and of the nature of serious diseases and their treatment. This must underlie any involvement of pharmacists in contributing to the management of patients, or in the diagnosis and management of minor illness. Since pharmacists have to work with clinicians, and there are well established intellectual disciplines in medicine for diagnosis and management, aspiring clinical pharmacists need to understand the way in which doctors approach the diagnosis of disease and the treatment of patients.

Since starting clinical teaching, we have always lacked a suitable single basic text. Existing textbooks stress diagnosis, drug treatment or the pharmacist–patient interaction, but are often too detailed or cumbersome in some areas, whilst lacking sufficient detail about the pathophysiological origin of the abnormalities and the ways in which this knowledge leads to correct diagnosis and, finally, to management and treatment. Thus it has been necessary to refer students to a variety of texts on pathology, immunology, clinical medicine, clinical pharmacology and therapeutics.

Hence the present book. Our ideas were first collated as a series of lecture notes for Chelsea students. This text represents a considerable expansion of these notes, intended to serve as a basis from which clinical pharmacy practice can be developed, both for students and as a basic introduction for all practising pharmacists. We also hope that many other groups of healthcare professionals, including nurses and doctors, will find the book useful.

This book is not intended to be a textbook of clinical pharmacy, nor is it intended to replace basic biomedical science texts. We assume that the reader will have an understanding of the principles of physiology and pharmacology, and the concepts of clinical pharmacology. We are not trying to compete with detailed texts on drug therapy and so have omitted prescribing detail, about proprietary forms, precise doses, etc., unless it is necessary to an understanding of drug selection or drug use. Similarly, we have not usually included any formal consideration of the mechanisms of adverse drug reactions or interactions, but deal with these as they arise as one of several factors which constrain the prescribing and use of a drug.

Our aim is to show the rationale and role of drug therapy in the management of some common diseases through a consideration of the mechanisms of disease processes in relation to normal function. Most chapters concern a single body system, e.g. the renal system or the gastrointestinal tract. Occasionally, we felt it necessary to depart from this pattern, and to consider a single disease group (e.g. infections), or a particularly important symptom (e.g. pain). The normal physiology of the whole system is first reviewed briefly, sufficient anatomy being included to give an appreciation of where symptoms arise. This is followed by a comparative discussion of the mechanisms and measurement of the principal malfunctions (aetiology, pathology, pathogenesis and investigation), and the relationship between the pathology and the resulting signs and symptoms. Each disease is described in sufficient detail to give an understanding of what it means to the patient and how it affects their lifestyle. Finally, there is an outline of management, stressing the aims and general strategy and showing the role of drugs as one of the therapeutic options, with an emphasis on the rationale and criteria for medicine selection, including biopharmaceutic and qualitative pharmacokinetic considerations.

Although, as pharmacists, we are convinced of the value of drugs and medicines, we are conscious of the fact that medicines are often used empirically and may provide only symptomatic relief. Although cure is often impossible, medicines can usually provide relief from suffering, and a good quality of life, while the normal processes of repair and recovery proceed. Further, social change, e.g. in nutrition, education and wealth, may have contributed more to the conquest of diseases such as tuberculosis than has medical practice. We believe this book provides, in a single compact volume, succinct, integrated information about major diseases and the principles of their management, either as a primer or as a quick refresher, without the need to refer to several different texts.

About the authors

Dr Russell Greene gained his BPharm from Nottingham University in 1967 and did his pre-reg in Elizabeth Garrett Anderson hospital in London.

After working in hospital and community pharmacy in the UK and abroad he gained an MSc by research from Bath University in 1973 for a thesis on Drug administration in psychiatric hospitals.

Following a further spell abroad, including a year setting up a pharmacy training course at the University of the South Pacific in Fiji, in 1978 he became the Principal pharmacist for Education and training for the NWThames Regional Health Authority.

He joined Chelsea College in 1980 to teach clinical pharmacy and moved with it to King's College in 1987. He gained his PhD in 1993 for a thesis on Prescription monitoring by community pharmacists and the role of medication records. He became senior lecturer in 1995 and head of the Pharmacy Practice group in 1998. He was the MPharm Programme director until 2006, and his principal teaching responsibility has been organizing courses in pathology and therapeutics.

Dr Norman Harris entered Pharmacy in 1947 following National Service, having been an industrial chemist in metal processing and the food industry.

As apprentice at a very traditional London pharmacy, which dispensed for nearby embassies, he learned full-range extemporaneous dispensing, including suppositories, pessaries and silvered pills from prescriptions written in 1910!

At Chelsea School of Pharmacy he acquired the Chemist and Druggist and Pharmaceutical Chemist Diplomas, a BPharm degree, and won the Pharmaceutical Society's Pereira Medal. A spell at Imperial College led to a PhD in Microbiology and the Imperial College Diploma and Fellowship of the Pharmaceutical Society followed in 1954.

On the staff at Chelsea, he taught Pharmacognosy (briefly), Pharmaceutics (Dispensing, Microbiology, Radiopharmacy), becoming Reader in Pharmaceutics and Head of Clinical Pharmacy, Honorary Pharmacist at Hammersmith Hospital and Chairman of the Oxford Region Pharmacy Advisory Committee. He was Post-graduate Tutor for the North-West Thames Region for many years and retired in 1984.

Recommended reference sources

WE LIST BELOW some of the major tertiary reference sources in pathology and therapeutics for the reader who needs to delve deeper. Many are becoming available electronically. These general sources will provide detail on all of the topics covered in this book. Further specific reading (usually websites, textbooks or recent reviews) is suggested at the end of each chapter, which represent a consensus view of the topic. Clinical pharmacists will also need to refer elsewhere for detailed information on responding to symptoms, counter-prescribing, counselling, the interpretation of pharmacokinetic parameters, and the many other specialisms that comprise modern pharmacy practice. Basic up-to-date information for the day-to-day use of medicines is available in the *British National Formulary* (BNF) published biannually and the *BNF for Children*, published annually. These are joint publications of the BMJ Publishing Group Ltd and RPS Publishing, on which we have relied extensively.

Baxter K, ed. *Stockley's Drug Interactions*, 8th edn. London: Pharmaceutical Press, 2007.

A comprehensive review of most specific interactions, evaluated for clinical significance.

Berkow R (ed.). *The Merck Manual of Diagnosis and Therapy*, 18th edn. Rahway, NJ: Merck & Co. Inc., 2006.

A comprehensive, fact-packed and inexpensive general medical practitioners' handbook, especially useful for understanding American practice.

Govan ADT, Macfarlane PS. *Pathology Illustrated*, 5th edn. Edinburgh, Churchill Livingstone, 2004.

Guyton AC, Hall JE. *Textbook of Medical Physiology*, 11th edn. Philadelphia, PA: Saunders, 2005.

The seminal work relating normal to abnormal physiology, still important despite Guyton's death.

Katzung BG. *Basic and Clinical Pharmacology*, 10th edn. Stamford, CT: Lange, 2006.

Up-to-date and largely successful attempt to correlate a basic pharmacological approach with the clinical.

Kumar PJ, Clark M (eds). *Clinical Medicine*, 6th edn, London: Balliere Tindall, 2005.

An inexpensive but very clearly written basic medical text.

Kumar V, Abbas A, Fausto N. *Robbins and Cotran's Pathologic Basis of Disease*, 7th edn. Philadelphia, PA: Elsevier, 1999.

An extremely thorough, comprehensive and well illustrated tome.

Ledingham JGG, Warrell DA, eds. *Concise Oxford Textbook of Medicine*. Oxford, Oxford University Press, 2000.

A condensed version of the three-volume *Oxford Textbook of Medicine* (see Weatherall DJ, Ledingham JGG, Warrell DA, eds. (1996)) that is adequate for most purposes.

Male D, Brostoff J, Roth D, Roitt I. *Immunology*, 7th edn. Mosby, Elsevier, 2007.

A well illustrated account of medical immunology.

Schmidt RF, Thews GH. *Human Physiology*. Berlin: Springer Verlag, 1989.

An excellent, thorough, basic physiology book, with splendid graphics.

Speight TM, Holford NHG, eds *Avery's Drug Treatment*, 4th edn. Oxford: Blackwell, 1997.

A prime source of information on drug usage.

Sweetman SC, ed. *Martindale: the Complete Drug Reference*, 35th edn. London: The Pharmaceutical Press, 2007.

The most comprehensive single reference source on drugs and preparations.

Taussig P. *Processes in Pathology and Microbiology*, 3rd edn, Oxford: Blackwell, 1995.

Although a little dated now, this is a very systematic and readable book on the biology of disease.

Toghill PJ, ed. *Examining Patients. An Introduction to Clinical Medicine*, 2nd edn. London: Edward Arnold, 1994.

A simple introduction to basic medical techniques.

Walker R, Whittlesea C, eds. *Clinical Pharmacy and Therapeutics*, 4th edn. London: Churchill Livingstone, 2007.

A comprehensive multi-authored British clinical pharmacy textbook.

Warrell DA, Cox TM, Firth JD, Benz EJ eds. *The Oxford Textbook of Medicine*, 4th edn. Oxford: Oxford University Press, 2006.

One of the most thorough and authoritative general medical texts.

In addition, the following journals and bulletins are recommended for up-to-date comparative discussions of disease and drug selection.

Drugs. Adis Press.

In effect, a monthly update of the comparative therapeutics found in *Avery's Drug Treatment*. It also gives detailed reviews of new drugs and retrospective evaluations of older ones.

MeRec Bulletin. Medicines Resource Centre.

Regular reviews of comparative therapeutics produced by the NHS.

Medicine. The Medicine Group.

Regularly updated on a 3- to 4-year cycle, this reviews, with excellent graphics, advances in all fields of medicine, using clinical grouping similar to that of this book.

Some essential websites

www.prodigy.nhs.uk/ClinicalGuidance
www.clinicalevidence.com
www.mhra.gov.uk
www.pharmj.com
www.pharm-line.nhs.uk/home/default.aspx
www.pjonline.com
www.nice.org.uk
www.sign.ac.uk
www.bmj.com
www.rpsgb.org.uk
www.druginfozone.org/

Abbreviations

μg	microgram
AAC	antibiotic-associated colitis
AAT	alpha$_1$-antitrypsin
ACE(I)	angiotensin-converting enzyme (inhibitor)
ACS	acute coronary syndrome
ADH	antidiuretic hormone
AED	antiepileptic drug
AFP	alpha-fetoprotein
AIDS	autoimmune deficiency syndrome
ALP	serum alkaline phosphatase
ALT	alanine aminotransferase
ANA, ANF	fluorescent antinuclear antibody test
ANP	atrial natriuretic peptide
APC	antigen-presenting cells
APN	acute pyelonephritis
APTT	activated partial thromboplastin time
ARA	angiotensin receptor antagonist
ARF	acute renal failure
ARhF	acute rheumatic fever
AS	ankylosing spondylitis
ASO	anti-streptolysin antibody
AST	aspartate aminotransferase
ATN	acute tubular necrosis/nephropathy
ATP	adenosine triphosphate
BCSH	British Committee for Standards in Haematology
BDA	British Diabetic Association
BDP	beclometasone dipropionate
BG	basal ganglia
BMI	body mass index
BNP	brain natriuretic peptide
BNF	*British National Formulary*
BTS	British Thoracic Society
CABG	coronary artery bypass graft
CAPD	continuous ambulatory peritoneal dialysis
CAT	*see* CT
CAVH	continuous arteriovenous haemofiltration
CAV-HD	continuous arteriovenous haemodiafiltration
CCB	calcium-channel blocker
CCK	cholecystokinin

CCP	cyclic citrullinated peptide
CCU	coronary care unit
CD	Crohn's disease
CEA	carcinoembryonic antigen
CFTR	cystic fibrosis transmembrane conductance regulator
CHM	Commission on Human Medicines
CHMP	Committee for Medical Products for Human Use
CK	creatine kinase
CMI	cell-mediated immunity
CML	chronic myeloid leukaemia
CNS	central nervous system
COAD	chronic obstructive airways disease
COMT	catechol *O*-methyl transferase
COPD	chronic obstructive pulmonary disease
CPK	*see* CK
CRF	chronic renal failure
CRP	C-reactive protein
CRhF	chronic rheumatic fever
CRTZ	*see* CTZ
CSF	cerebrospinal fluid
CSM	Committee on Safety of Medicines (UK)
cSSTI	complex skin and soft tissue infection
CT	computed tomography (formerly 'computerized axial tomography')
CTZ	chemoreceptor trigger zone
CVD	cardiovascular disease
CVP	central venous pressure
CV(S)	cardiovascular (system)
CXR	chest X-ray
Da	Daltons
DAGT	direct antiglobulin test, direct Coomb's test
DBP	diastolic blood pressure
DDC	diverticular disease of the colon
DHP	dihydropyridine
DNA	deoxyribonucleic acid
DPI	dry powder inhaler
DSM IV	Diagnostic and Statistical Manual of Mental Disease, 4th edn
DVT	deep-vein thrombosis
Dx	diagnosis
EAA	essential amino acid
ECF	extracellular fluid
ECG	electrocardiogram
ECT	electroconvulsive therapy
EDP	end-diastolic pressure
EDRF	endothelium-derived relaxing factor
EDV	end-diastolic volume
EEG	electroencephalogram
EF	ejection fraction
EFA	essential fatty acid

EGF	epidermal growth factor
EHEC	enterohaemorrhagic *E. coli*
EIEC	enteroinvasive *E. coli*
EPS	extrapyramidal syndromes, symptoms
ERCP	endoscopic retrograde cholangiopancreatography
ESBL	extended-spectrum beta-lactamase
ESR	erythrocyte sedimentation rate
ESRD	end-stage renal disease
ESWL	extracorporeal shock-wave lithotripsy
ETEC	enterotoxigenic *E. coli*
Fab	antigen-binding fragment of immunoglobulin
FANA	*see* ANA
FBC	full blood count
Fc	crystallizable fragment of immunoglobulin
FEV_1	forced expiratory volume from the lungs in 1 second
FEV_1/FVC	forced expiratory ratio of the lungs
FFA	free fatty acid
FFP	fresh frozen plasma
fMRI	functional magnetic resonance imaging
Fr	factor, especially blood clotting factors FrI-FrXIII. Suffix 'a' indicates an activated factor
FVC	forced vital capacity (of the lungs)
GABA	gamma-aminobutyric acid
G-CSF	granulocyte colony stimulating factor
GFR	glomerular filtration rate
GHb	*see* HbA_{1c}
GIT	gastrointestinal tract
GM-CSF	granulocyte-macrophage colony stimulating factor
GORD	gastro-oesophageal reflux disease
GnRH	gonadotrophin-releasing hormone, gonadorelin
GP	general practitioner
β_2GP1	Beta$_2$-glycoprotein$_1$, apolipoprotein H
GGT	gammaglutamyl transpeptidase
GTN	glyceryl trinitrate
GTP	guanosine triphosphate
h	hour/hours
H_2-RA	histamine$_2$-receptor antagonist
HAART	highly active antiretroviral therapy
HACEK	*Haemophilus, Actinobacillus, Cardiobacterium, Eikenella* and *Kingella* (bacterial species)
Hb	haemoglobin (deoxyhaemoglobin)
HbA_{1c}	glycosylated haemoglobin
HbO_2	oxyhaemoglobin
2HBSS	2-hour blood sugar screen
HD	haemodialysis
HDL	high-density lipoprotein
HDN	haemolytic disease of the newborn

HF	heart failure
5-HIAA	5-hydroxyindole acetic acid
HIT	heparin-induced thrombocytopenia
HIV	human immunodeficiency virus
HLA	human leucocyte antigen (four loci, A, B, C, D)
HMG CoA	3-hydroxy-3-methylglutaryl co-enzyme A reductase (inhibitor = statin)
HS	hereditary spherocytosis
HSV	highly selective vagotomy
5-HT	5-hydroxytryptamine, serotonin
IBD	inflammatory bowel disease
IBS	irritable bowel syndrome
IC	immune complex, inspiratory capacity of the lungs
ICD	International Classification of Diseases
ICF	intracellular fluid
IDDM	insulin-dependent diabetes mellitus
Ig	immunoglobulin
IgA	immunoglobulin A, secretory immunoglobulin
IgE	immunoglobulin E, reaginic antibody
IgG	gamma-globulin
IgM	macroglobulin
IHD	ischaemic heart disease
IL	interleukin, plus number
IM	intramuscular
INR	international normalized ratio (for blood clotting)
IPD	intermittent peritoneal dialysis
ITU	intensive therapy unit
IV	intravenous
IVU	intravenous excretory urogram
Ix	investigation(s)
JCA	juvenile chronic arthritis
JGA	juxtaglomerular apparatus
JVP	jugular venous pressure
K cells	T-lymphocyte killer cells
kcal	kilocalorie
kJ	kilojoule
K, K$^+$	potassium (ion)
L	litre
LABA	long-acting beta-agonist
LDH	lactic dehydrogenase
LDL	low-density lipoprotein
L-dopa	L-dihydroxyphenylalanine, levodopa
LMWH	low molecular weight heparin
LOS	lower oesophageal spincter
LST	lateral spinothalamic tract of the spinal cord
LT	leukotriene (plus type number)
LTRA	leukotriene receptor antagonist

LVEDP	left ventricular end-diastolic pressure
LVF	left ventricular failure
MAF	macrophage activating factor
MAOI	monoamine oxidase inhibitor
MBC	minimum bactericidal concentration
mg	milligram
MHC	major histocompatibility complex
MHPG	3-methoxy-4-hydroxy-phenylethyleneglycol
MI	myocardial infarction
MIC	minimum inhibitory concentration
min	minute
mL	millilitre
MPTP	methylphenyltetrahydropyridine
MRI	(nuclear) magnetic resonance imaging, see also fMRI
MRSA	methicillin-resistant *Staphylococcus aureus*, multi-resistant *Staph. aureus*
MTX	methotrexate
NA	noradrenaline (norepinephrine)
NAC	*N*-acetylcysteine
NAD(H)	nicotinamide adenine dinucleotide (reduced form)
NADP(H)	nicotinamide adenine dinucleotide phosphate (reduced form)
NICE	National Institute for Health and Clinical Excellence (UK)
NIDDM	non-insulin-dependent diabetes mellitus
nm	nanometre(s)
NMR	*see* MRI
NO	nitric oxide
NP	natriuretic peptide
NPSA	National Patient Safety Agency
NRT	nicotine replacement therapy
NSAID	non-steroidal anti-inflammatory drug
NUD	non-ulcer dyspepsia
NYHA	New York Heart Association (USA)
OA	osteoarthritis
OAD	oral antidiabetic drug
OPAT	out-patient antibiotic treatment
OTC	over-the-counter
OT	occupational therapy
p.	page
P_aCO_2, P_ACO_2	partial arterial/alveolar pressure of carbon dioxide
PAF	platelet activating factor
PAH	para-amino hippuric acid
PAN	polyarteritis nodosa
P_aO_2, P_AO_2	partial arterial/alveolar pressure of oxygen
PCI	percutaneous coronary intervention (includes angiography and angioplasty)
PCO_2	partial pressure of carbon dioxide
PCV	packed cell volume, haematrocrit

PD	peritoneal dialysis
PDGF	platelet-derived growth factor
PEF	peak expiratory flow
PEG	percutaneous enteral gastroscopy
pg	picogram(s)
PG	prostaglandin (plus type letter and number)
PID	prolapsed intervertebral disc
pm	picomol(s)
pMDI	pressurized metered-dose inhalers
PMH	past medical history
PND	paroxysmal nocturnal dyspnoea
PO_2	partial pressure of oxygen
POM	prescription-only medicine
pp.	pages
PPI	proton pump inhibitor
PR	peripheral resistance (to blood flow)
PRF	peptide regulatory factors
PSE	portosystemic encephalopathy
PT	prothrombin time; physiotherapy
PTCA	percutaneous transluminal coronary angioplasty
PTH	parathyroid hormone
PUVA	psoralen plus ultraviolet radiation therapy
RA	rheumatoid arthritis
RAAS	renin-angiotensin-aldosterone system
RAP	right atrial pressure
RAS	reticular activating system
RAST	radioallergosorbent test
RBC	red blood cell
RCT	randomized controlled trial
RF	renal failure, rheumatoid factor(s)
Rh	rhesus
RhD	rhesus D antigen
RLD	restrictive lung disease
RP	Raynaud's phenomenon
RR	relative risk
rtPA	recombinant tissue-type plasminogen activator, alteplase
RV	residual volume (of the lungs)
RVF	right ventricular failure
Rx	treatment(s)
s	second(s)
SAA	serum amyloid-association protein
SABA	short-acting $beta_2$-agonist
SAD	seasonal affective disorder
SBE	subacute bacterial endocarditis
SBP	systolic blood pressure
SC	subcutaneous
SCI	stem cell inhibitor
SG	substantia gelatinosa of the posterior horn of the spinal cord

SGOT	serum glutamic-oxaloacetic transaminase, see AST
SGPT	serum glutamic-pyruvic transaminase, see ALT
SIGN	Scottish Intercollegiate Guidelines Network (UK)
SLE	systemic lupus erythematosus
sp(p).	species (plural)
SRS-A	slow reacting substance of anaphylaxis
SSRI	selective serotonin re-uptake inhibitor
SSx	symptoms and signs
SSZ	sulfasalazine
TB	tuberculosis
TBW	total body water
Tc	cytotoxic T (cell(s))
TD	tardive dyskinesia
TENS	transcutaneous electrical nerve stimulation
TFrPI	transfer factor pathway inhibitor (in blood coagulation)
TH	T helper (cell(s))
TIA	transient ischaemic attack
TIBC	total iron-binding capacity
TLC	total lung capacity
TNF	tumour necrosis factor
Ts	T suppressor (cell(s))
TSH	thyroid-stimulating hormone, thyrotropin
TV	tidal volume of the lungs
Tx	thromboxane (plus type letter and number)
UC	ulcerative colitis
UGPD	University Group Diabetes Programme
UV	ultraviolet radiation
UVA	longer wavelength ultraviolet radiation, 320–400 nm
UVB	shorter wavelength ultraviolet radiation, 290–320 nm
VC	vital capacity
VLDL	very-low-density lipoprotein
VPR	ventilation-perfusion ratio
VRE	vancomycin-resistant enterococci
VTE	venous thromboembolism
WBC	white blood cell (leucocyte)
WCC	white blood cell count
WHO	World Health Organization

Part 1

Basic strategy and introduction to pathology

1

Therapeutics: general strategy

This book is about the rationale of therapeutic decision making, and in particular the logic of drug selection. Thus, it must start with an account of where **pharmacotherapy** (drug therapy) fits into the overall management of a patient, and the factors that govern the selection of a drug regimen. The **medical process** starts with the case history, which includes examination, investigation and diagnosis, and culminates in a decision about management. A similar if less elaborate process must be followed by a pharmacist to respond to symptoms presented by a patient. All this information is gathered together to provide a systematic classification of information about a patient.

However, before considering the case history, the terminology and systematic description of disease must be introduced. Pharmacists are familiar with classifying knowledge about a drug into such categories as 'indications' and 'side-effects'. This enables the comparison of similar drugs, and facilitates learning about a new drug and anticipating its properties by assigning it to an existing class. In an analogous way, knowledge about disease is systematically described using specific categories, and this enables similar diseases to be distinguished by certain features, and helps learning about a newly encountered disease.

The medical process and the systematic description of disease form the framework for the discussion of specific conditions and disease groups in subsequent chapters.

Terminology of disease

Definition

An account of a disease starts with a description of its general nature, including the organ system affected and important features that differentiate it from similar conditions. The following are two examples:

- *Essential hypertension is a chronic slowly progressive cardiovascular condition in which the mean blood pressure is consistently above the population normal range for the patient's age, but below 130 mmHg and not rising rapidly.*
- *Rheumatoid arthritis is a severe chronic progressive inflammatory erosive polyarthropathy, primarily articular synovitis, but with systemic features.*

Aetiology and pathology

These categories are sometimes difficult to distinguish, especially when the cause of a disease is uncertain. **Aetiology** is concerned with general causes of a disease and the circumstances ('risk factors') that predispose an individual to suffer from its effects: it may be thought of as answering the question, 'why?' (see Table 1.1). Aetiology makes no assumptions or assertions about the processes by which these factors bring about the condition. Thus, the aetiology of tuberculosis (TB) involves poor public and domestic hygiene, reduced patient immune status and the mycobacterium; that of cancer may include genetic predisposition, viral infection and environmental toxins; that of essential hypertension involves obesity, salt intake and stress, etc.

Pathology is concerned with the mechanisms of the disease process, what the disease does, and how it does so. It answers the question, 'how did it cause the observed symptoms?' Ideally it will explain the steps by which the aetiological risk factors lead to the malfunction. It then describes the changes caused in body function resulting from the disease and the body's response to this. The **pathophysiology** of a disease relates its effects to the disruption of normal physiological functions, e.g. the pathophysiology of essential hypertension involves a raised peripheral vas-

cular resistance and possibly an expansion of the intravascular fluid volume. **Pathogenesis** describes the development or progression of the disease process. Thus, the pathogenesis of rheumatoid arthritis (RA) involves synovial hyperplasia followed by inflammatory cell infiltration, then articular erosion. Where immunological processes are known to be involved in the disease, e.g. the autoimmune pancreatic destruction in type 1 diabetes mellitus, the term **immunopathology** is used.

There are a few general pathogenic mechanisms, such as **inflammation** and **ischaemia**, that occur as fundamental bodily responses to very many diseases. These are described in Chapter 2.

Epidemiology

It is important to know how common a condition is, and whether any particular population group is more susceptible by virtue of birth or environment. It answers the question, 'who?' There may also be significant differences in disease occurrence between the sexes, different ethnic groups and different age groups. The **incidence** is the number of new cases of the disease; it is usually expressed as per million of a population per year. The lifetime incidence is the proportion of the population likely to suffer from the disease at some time in their life, e.g. the lifetime incidence of duodenal ulcer among British males is about 1 in 10.

Prevalence refers to the number of active cases of a disease at any one time, e.g. the overall prevalence of Parkinson's disease is about 1 in 1000, affecting men and women equally, but is 1 in 200 among those over 70 years of age. The term **morbidity** is sometimes used more loosely to describe the prevalence of a disease; thus heart disease has a relatively high morbidity, renal cancer a low morbidity. **Comorbidity** refers to any other disease the patient has.

The relationship between incidence and prevalence depends on the natural history (usual course) of the condition. Although the annual incidence of the common cold may be up to 1 in 2 in the UK, the prevalence at any given time will vary between perhaps 10 million and

Table 1.1   Terminology used in disease and its management

Term used		Description
Definition		Brief summary
Aetiology	*Why?*	Causes; risk factors
Epidemiology	*Who?*	In population as whole, and in specially susceptible groups
Incidence		Frequency of new cases
Prevalence		Number of sufferers at any time
Pathology	*How? What?*	Mechanisms of malfunction
Pathogenesis		Underlying disease process
Pathophysiology		Disorder of normal function
Clinical features (presentation)		
Symptoms		Features noticed by patient: Subjective ('complains of')
Signs		Features noted by clinician: Objective ('on examination')
Investigations		Most appropriate methods
Natural history (course)	*When?*	Onset, progression, duration, resolution
		Severity
		Complications
		Mortality
Management		
Aims		Symptomatic relief
		Slow or arrest disease
		Reverse disease (cure)
		Prevent disease
Duration		Acute, chronic
		Maintenance (continuation)
		Prophylaxis
Treatment modes		Medication
		Nursing care
		Surgery
		Occupational therapy
		Radiotherapy
		Physiotherapy
		Social support, etc.
Monitoring		Progress of disease
		Benefits of treatment
		Side-effects of treatment
Prognosis		Probable outcomes

merely several hundred thousand, depending on the season, as colds are acute in onset and short-lived. On the other hand, the prevalence of chronic renal failure depends on the annual incidence and the average survival time following diagnosis.

Knowledge about the epidemiology of a disease may provide clues about its aetiology. For example, the incidence of stomach cancer is higher in Japan than the USA, but the prevalence among Japanese immigrants to the USA is similar to that of Americans. This strongly suggests that environmental factors such as diet are more important than genetic ones.

Clinical features

Signs and symptoms, often thought to be synonymous, are distinct terms. **Symptoms** are subjective; they are noticed by the patient and either reported – the things a patient complains of – or elicited on questioning. **Signs** are usually found objectively on examination by the clinician, although occasionally may be noticed by the patient. Both are important: the former emphasise what are likely to be the patient's major concerns; the latter aid precise diagnosis.

The typical pattern of clinical features caused by a disease is called its **presentation**. Many diseases have such consistent presentations as to be almost diagnostic, e.g. a spiking fever, stiff neck and photophobia in meningitis; such definitive features are called **pathognomonic**. A well-defined group of clinical features that commonly occur together is sometimes called a **syndrome**, e.g. proteinuria, hypoproteinaemia and oedema together are known as the 'nephrotic syndrome'.

Investigations

In describing a disease it is helpful to include the tests or procedures used to confirm a diagnosis, distinguishing between closely related conditions (the **differential diagnosis**) or monitoring progress. For example, although the measurement of urinary glucose is a poor method of assessing control in a patient with diabetes

mellitus, it is quite useful for screening large groups for possible diabetes.

Natural history

Knowledge of the usual course of a disease from its onset and pretreatment phase through to its final outcome is important for several reasons. It enables predictions to be made about a patient's likely recovery or degree of eventual disability, i.e. the **prognosis**. It also helps in judging whether improvements in a patient's condition are due to treatment or to natural remission. Many chronic diseases progress by a series of exacerbations, remissions and relapses, and improvements cannot with certainty be ascribed to any treatment that is being given. The patient may have improved even without the treatment.

Different disease subgroups may be differentiated by different natural histories. For example, RA typically has an insidious onset, but if there is a sudden onset of multi-joint inflammation the prognosis is better. Furthermore, some two-thirds of RA patients will have such a slowly progressive disease that they can expect little disablement within a normal lifespan.

Knowing the average duration of the disease and its pattern of activity is important. Some diseases start with a period of characteristic warning signs, known as the **prodromal** phase. **Acute** illness starts suddenly (acute onset) and resolves either of its own accord or following treatment. A **chronic** disease usually starts insidiously, and continues for a long time, possibly lifelong. For chronic disease in particular we also need the answers to several important questions. Does it remain stable or tend to deteriorate steadily (**progressive** disease) and if so, at what rate? Is there any residual disability after the disease has resolved, or can it be cured? Does it follow a continuous or a fluctuating course, with remissions and relapses or exacerbations? Many diseases also have typical secondary complications, e.g. haemorrhage in peptic ulceration. What is the prevalence of complications, especially in different age or sex groups?

The likelihood of a fatal outcome (the **mortality**) is usually expressed as the proportion of patients expected to die within a specified time. Conversely, **survival** is the proportion of patients alive at a specified time after diagnosis. Both are commonly cited as medians, e.g. a 3-year median survival means that half of patients are expected to be still alive after 3 years. For example, the median survival of severe heart failure is 1 year. Alternatively, we might speak of, for example, mortality at 5 years being x%, or an annual mortality rate of y%. It is important to distinguish between the mortality and morbidity of a particular disease, in order to compare the suitability of different treatments. Thus, skin diseases generally have a high morbidity but very low mortality, so toxic therapy is rarely indicated. However, malignant melanoma, while having a low morbidity, has a very high mortality, so aggressive therapy is warranted.

Management and treatment

Management embraces all the decisions made to deal with the patient's complaint; it describes the strategy. Its first task is to decide realistic aims, based on a knowledge of the presentation, investigations and natural history. Within the broad area of management, **treatment** comprises the range of interventions, like drugs, surgery or physiotherapy, that can be used to achieve these aims. Of course, this can include doing very little if the condition is self-limiting. On the other hand, in very advanced or incurable disease, management might involve no more than symptom control, nursing care, simple reassurance and appropriate counselling, i.e. **palliative care**.

The assessment of the balance of harms and benefits of different treatments (the **risk-to-benefit** or harm-to-benefit ratio) must be based on knowledge of the severity and mortality of the condition, the risks of not treating and the toxicity of the treatment.

Aims

The various possible general aims of management may be set in a hierarchy (Table 1.1). In complex diseases several aims may be legitimate, for different aspects of the disease and its complications. Prevention may be the ultimate aim of medicine, but symptomatic relief is frequently all that can be offered. Only by having clearly defined aims can it be judged to what extent the treatment has been successful, and thus whether such treatment should be continued or changed.

Prophylaxis
This can only follow from an understanding of the aetiology and pathology, but that alone is not always sufficient. Some infectious diseases have been almost completely eliminated in some countries by a systematic combination of public health measures and vaccination, e.g. diphtheria. Smallpox is the only disease that has been completely eradicated worldwide, and poliomyelitis is close to eradication. Yet although much is known about the causes of chronic obstructive pulmonary disease (COPD) and ischaemic heart disease, prevention here probably resides more in the domains of education and social and economic policy than in medicine. On the other hand, there is at present little hope of preventing most cases of chronic renal failure or cancer because so little is understood of their aetiology.

Reversal
Prevention has clearly failed if a patient presents with symptoms. Some diseases are intrinsically temporary, self-limiting and reversible, such as minor gastric upset. For others, the ideal would be to reverse the disease process and leave the recuperative powers of the body to restore health completely. This amounts to a **cure**, and it is sobering to reflect that there are few important diseases for which this is a realistic aim. When patients have recovered from an infection, they are usually physiologically just as they were before their illness. In almost all other common serious chronic diseases the sad truth is that we do not do a very good job, for example in heart disease and cancer, which together account for over 50% of all premature deaths in the West. This is not to obscure the fact that immense good is done by modern medicine, and medicines, in the relief of the misery associated with serious illness, in particular the damaging effects of acute exacerbations of chronic diseases.

Transplantation is a growing area, and can reverse some diseases (although immunosuppressant therapy prevents completely normal life). In the future, gene therapy promises tremendous advances in this area.

Arrest progress

Many measures may slow, arrest or stabilise a condition, preventing deterioration and minimising exacerbations or relapses. Thus in COPD, stopping smoking will avoid further lung damage, and prompt antibiotic treatment will minimise infective exacerbations. Anticonvulsant drugs will prevent most epilepsy seizures but will not rectify the underlying disease process. Replacement therapy in endocrine deficiency diseases such as diabetes will restore normal function, although it cannot restore the original organ. In many chronic diseases, by the time a diagnosis is made there is often fixed, irreversible organ damage.

Symptomatic relief and palliation

Included in this category are the many interventions that pharmacists make in minor self-limiting conditions, where advice and symptomatic over-the-counter (OTC) medication are all that is needed.

Of course, under some circumstances there is no prospect of influencing the disease process, and all that can be done is to treat the symptoms as they arise, and more generally make the patient feel better. Terminal cancer is the prime example. Analgesics, parenteral nutrition and surgery to relieve obstruction or nerve pressure may all be directed at improving the patient's quality of life, not at controlling the disease.

Some would claim that many medical and pharmaceutical efforts do no more than meet this aim: for example, do antidepressants or anti-inflammatory drugs really do more than suppress symptoms? Yet the relief of suffering and improvement in the quality of life are surely worthwhile benefits in themselves.

Duration

Treatment can be **acute**, to manage a short-term condition, or may need to be continued long term as **maintenance**, in order to keep the disease under control. In other cases treatment can be **prophylactic**, to prevent further illness. For example in anxiety, drug therapy should be used only for acute management; diabetes requires lifelong maintenance; and atherosclerotic cardiac disease usually requires prophylaxis with antiplatelet and lipid-lowering medicines.

Modes

Having decided on a realistic aim, it is necessary to make appropriate selections from the many available modes of treatment. Thus serious joint disease may need social and economic help, as well as support from a multidisciplinary team including clinicians, nurses, pharmacists and social workers, to alleviate the condition. Treatment may involve surgery, and nearly always physiotherapy, to achieve or maintain joint mobility. Nursing skills are of paramount importance, both in hospital and in the home, if the rheumatoid patient is to return as quickly as possible to their normal activities. And of course drug therapy is essential.

Medicines play an important part in the management of many diseases, but they must be seen as only one part of the patient's whole treatment. When individual diseases are discussed in later chapters, the role of drug therapy – and its limitations – will be emphasised in relation to the other important modes of therapy.

Monitoring

Decisions about aims are incomplete unless ways of determining to what extent they are being achieved are also specified. The type of monitoring will depend on the nature of the abnormality (e.g. blood glucose level in diabetes, blood pressure in hypertension) and the aims of therapy (e.g. symptom control or tumour size in cancer). Similarly, certain treatments carry with them the obligation to watch for adverse effects (e.g. regular blood counts in cytotoxic chemotherapy). Pharmacists are playing an increasing role in these monitoring processes.

Case history

A case history is a systematic account of the progress of a patient's disease, including the information and reasoning behind diagnosis and management decisions. It is the core of the medical process and provides a central database for all concerned with the care of the patient. Taking a history and making a coherent record of it are two of the most fundamental skills of medicine, and they are being increasingly adapted for use by paramedical professions such as nursing and pharmacy.

Taking a 'good history' involves more than simply obtaining information and examining the patient. It is a subtle mixture of comprehensive clinical knowledge, detective work, lateral thinking, and communication skills such as listening and questioning. Unless the results are systematically recorded in a standardised way, its purpose may be largely defeated.

The way that these data fit into the general flow of information gathering is shown in Figure 1.1. The categories of information reported in a case history will be considered next. This will introduce some further essential medical terminology and should help the pharmacist to understand case reports in the medical literature (Table 1.2).

Although in some cases the complete work-up will not seem immediately appropriate – the accident victim admitted through the Accident and Emergency Unit need not be questioned about childhood illnesses – but a thorough history prevents important facts such as a drug allergy possibly being missed, or less obvious diagnoses being overlooked.

Patient details

A case history report is conventionally prefaced by a brief description of the patient and their complaint. This serves to orientate the reader

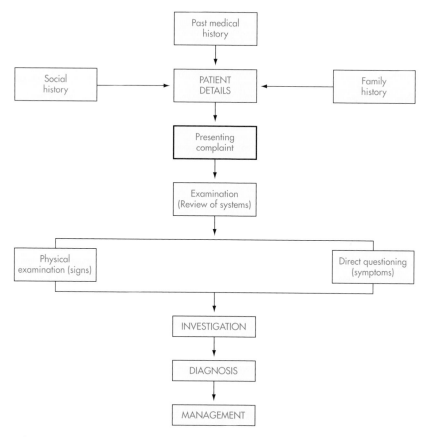

Figure 1.1   Case history. Inter-relationship of the various data recorded.

Table 1.2   Format of typical case history report, including common abbreviations

Patient details	Age, sex, occupation Race, ethnic group Place of normal residence; recent travel Build, weight Route of admission Main complaint General appearance
Past medical history (PMH)	Illnesses since childhood (including current chronic conditions)
Medication history	Current medication (prescription, OTC) – effectiveness and adverse effects Past medication problems
Family history (FH)	Relatives' (living and dead) medical history
Social history (SH)	Social drug use Domestic and financial situation Mobility How is patient coping (home, work and leisure)?
History of presenting complaint (HPC, 'complains of')	Onset, nature and intensity of symptoms Changes; provoking and relieving factors Referrals and outcomes Medication
Systematic examination (review of systems)	Directed questioning: each body system Physical examination: each body system
Investigations (Ix)	Blood, urine analysis Radiography Etc.
Diagnosis (Dx)	Differential, provisional or confirmed

Management (Rx)	For each current problem
	    Aims
	    Modes
	    Monitoring
	    Outcome(s)

and also to summarize data that will subsequently be important for both diagnosis and treatment.

Age, sex, ethnic origin and occupation are recorded because certain diseases are more prevalent in particular groups (e.g. type 2 diabetes in the elderly, haemoglobinopathies in people of Mediterranean origin), and numerous diseases are occupationally related. Exotic disease might be suggested by the ethnic group or recent travel: in the UK, fever in a non-travelling Londoner would be regarded differently to that in a newly arrived African or Asian immigrant. Decisions about

treatment may also be affected by such data, e.g. pharmacogenetic differences in drug handling and religious or ethnic dietary preferences.

It is usual to note how the patient came to medical attention and with what complaint; this gives an idea of the urgency of the problem and how it is perceived by the patient. An experienced clinician can also tell a lot from the patient's general appearance. The section might include circumstantial observations such as a walking stick or medication at the bedside, or nicotine-stained fingers. Thus, a case history might start:

Mr M, a 45-year-old slightly obese Caucasian businessman, was admitted 3 days ago through casualty after collapsing at work, complaining of a crushing chest pain of 3 h duration. On admission he appeared pale, anxious and in great pain.

Past medical history

Certain childhood diseases, and recent or current chronic illnesses, may have a bearing on the present illness. For example, rheumatic fever often causes heart disease in later life, chickenpox may manifest itself later as shingles, and asthma suggests an allergic predisposition. After using open questions, e.g. 'tell me about any serious illnesses you have had', the patient will be asked specifically about the more common chronic conditions such as epilepsy, asthma, hypertension, diabetes, jaundice and TB.

Medication history

A medication history should ideally comprise a list of current medication and recent medication used for the presenting complaint, including self-medication bought OTC and remedies recommended by a pharmacist. Sources for this information include the patient's recollection, medication list or medication bag, and their GP or community pharmacist's records. The effectiveness of each medication and any adverse effects encountered, including allergy or sensitivity, need to be recorded. Patients may need prompting, especially for self-medication, because even certain prescription items are frequently not regarded as medicines, e.g. oral contraceptives, nasal sprays, ophthalmic preparations, etc. Patients also tend to be rather unreliable or imprecise on adverse effects, e.g. the term 'allergy' may be used colloquially to describe almost any adverse effect, even mild dyspepsia. Unfortunately, an accurate and complete record is seldom easy to obtain, even when there is access to medical notes.

There is evidence that pharmacists can obtain more complete medication histories than clinicians, perhaps because of their wider product knowledge.

Family history

Because many diseases have a significant genetic basis, a knowledge of any chronic illness in siblings and parents, and the causes of death if appropriate, may provide vital clues. The connection may be direct, e.g. type 2 diabetes, or indirect, e.g. hay fever in the sibling of someone with dermatitis or a wheeze, implying a familial allergic (atopic) predisposition.

Social history

Enquiries about a patient's circumstances and way of life ('lifestyle') have a number of aims. Clearly, (anti-)social habits such as smoking, drinking and illicit drug use have a bearing on illness, although patients seldom give a reliable estimate (as a general rule, double the number of drinks or cigarettes admitted to). Excessive tea or coffee consumption may also be significant. Special dietary habits are important, especially with ethnic minorities, vegans, obsessive slimmers, etc.

Equally important is information about a patient's financial and domestic circumstances. Can they afford to be ill? Are they the sole breadwinner, or a single parent? What will be the economic impact of hospital admission, or attendance at a clinic? Is unemployment a factor? Are their living conditions contributing to their illness? What can be done for a patient with heart failure living on the tenth floor and with unreliable lifts? Who does the shopping?

If a patient has a chronic condition, how are they coping? It is also necessary to ascertain whether the patient is psychologically and intellectually able to comprehend the diagnosis and treatment, and to give genuinely informed consent to surgery or other invasive procedures.

History of presenting complaint

So far, little has been said about the patient's actual problem, but a comprehensive picture has been built up which will be useful both for the diagnosis of the current condition and for future reference. There is now an opportunity for the patient to relate their 'story'. Patients should, as far as possible, be allowed to express themselves at their own pace and in their own words, although occasionally some pertinent prompting or 'constructive interruption' is required. The aim is to discover how the symptoms arose, what they are like, how they have developed, and what has been done so far.

Consider pain, for example. The nature and intensity of pain are often significant, such as the difference between crushing cardiac chest pain and the burning retrosternal pain of gastrointestinal origin. How did it start? Is the pain constant, short-lived, episodic or persistent? Is it predictable? What makes it better or worse, e.g. warmth, cold, a particular posture? Has the patient already consulted a relative, pharmacist, NHS Direct or GP, and what was their advice? Has any treatment been tried, and if so, to what effect?

Note that the clinician need not yet have actually seen the patient. Indeed, much of the history so far could have been obtained by an assistant or a computer; in fact, trials using computers are sometimes quite effective. It is estimated that up to 75% of diagnoses in primary care can be made correctly using the data obtained by this stage, so consistent is the presentation of most illness. This explains how some doctors are sometimes able temporarily to 'diagnose' and prescribe by telephone, although it is hardly the technique of choice.

Systematic examination (review of systems)

The next stage is to look in detail at each body system. Although it is impossible to avoid this examination being influenced by information obtained so far, ideally it should be objective and complete, so that nothing obscure or unusual is overlooked and the data can be used later for reference. The examination usually starts with general observations of the patient's appearance and condition, in particular his or her coloration, body surface markings, etc. Traditionally, the presence or absence of jaundice, anaemia, cyanosis, clubbing and oedema are noted.

The details relevant to each body system will be discussed as appropriate in the following chapters. For each there are five stages:

1. Directed questioning (functional enquiry) about symptoms likely to follow malfunction of that system.
2. Observation and examination for physical signs.
3. Palpation (feeling).
4. Auscultation (listening with a stethoscope).
5. Percussion (tapping an area and listening to the sound).

Thus, for the cardiovascular system the patient will be asked about tiredness, swelling, palpitations and shortness of breath, especially at night. He or she will then be observed for objective signs such as exercise tolerance, gasping and oedema (ankles, abdomen). The pulses will be felt at different parts of the body, and the extent of any peripheral oedema estimated by local pressure. Auscultation uses a stethoscope to check cardiac rhythm and valve sounds. Percussion of the chest shows the extent of pulmonary oedema.

Obviously, history and examination must be guided by urgency and the presence of obvious symptoms or signs: a road traffic accident victim with head and chest injury is not asked about their bowel habit or the presence of athlete's foot. Nevertheless, a full review of systems would always be performed at some stage after hospital admission, as part of the clerking process.

Investigations

By this stage, a further 20% of diagnoses will have been made. This leaves perhaps 5% that require further investigation. Simple investigations may be done in a GP's surgery, e.g. ophthalmoscopy, peak respiratory flow and blood pressure measurement, and urine dipstick tests. Many practices now have electrocardiogram (ECG) equipment. Blood biochemistry and microbiology samples are collected in the surgery and usually sent to a local laboratory. The most common test for which the patient will be referred to a hospital (in the UK) is simple X-ray imaging.

If the diagnosis is still in doubt, investigations of increasing sophistication and expense are gradually employed, so that an ever greater complexity of test is used to diagnose an ever diminishing proportion of cases.

Diagnosis

A definitive diagnosis is usually clear by this stage – or it may be provisional, awaiting confirmation from investigations. If several possible diagnoses seem to fit the history, this differential diagnosis will be resolved by further investigations. Sometimes, the diagnosis remains provisional. If the patient recovers, there may be no benefit in subjecting them to invasive, uncomfortable and possibly dangerous further investigation if the result will not affect subsequent management.

Management

Each history should conclude with a management plan, which summarises the aims and the modes prescribed to meet them, monitoring and expected outcomes. In the **problem-orientated** approach, the record of management starts with a summary of all the patient's present problems, which appears at the front of the patient's notes. The summary includes:

- The current complaint (an 'active problem', e.g. hypertension).
- Important past medical history (either active, e.g. peptic ulcer disease, or inactive, e.g. a past myocardial infarction).
- Behaviour that requires modification (e.g. smoking, poor diet).
- Possibly, psychological and social problems.

A plan is outlined for each active problem. This includes any further investigations required for diagnostic confirmation or assessment of severity, the aim of management, the recommended treatment, the means of monitoring and the period of follow-up, e.g. a further appointment in so many weeks. Progress reports recorded in the patient's notes will then be based on this management plan, dealing with each problem for which treatment has been recommended, and the management strategy may be modified according to the patient's response to treatment. This systematic approach is also sometimes known by the acronym SOAP:

- **S**ubjective: patients reported or perceived problems.
- **O**bjective: data recorded by clinician or obtained from investigations.
- **A**ssessment of problems.
- **P**lan of action.

Whether or not such a formal approach is explicitly used, the history always includes progress notes. The outcome or progress of each management aim is recorded and the reasoning behind any changes in treatment explained, e.g. adverse drug effects.

For a hospital admission, the final component is the discharge summary, usually in the form of a letter to the patient's GP.

Drug disposition

Before considering the factors guiding drug choice, the basic concepts of clinical pharmacology will be briefly reviewed. These concepts underpin the drug selection decision-making process. Included are the principles of absorption, distribution, metabolism and excretion, and a brief summary of how these affect dosing and drug interactions. For details, the reader is referred to the References and further reading section.

Absorption and first-pass metabolism

The administration of a drug is the first stage of the process that eventually results in the drug acting on a receptor to produce the desired clinical action. Before it reaches the receptor it has a number of barriers to surmount, because the body has evolved very effective mechanisms to defend itself against foreign chemicals. This process is represented in Figure 1.2. Following oral administration, the first barrier is the gastrointestinal epithelium, which favours at least partially lipophilic compounds. If successfully absorbed, the drug is carried directly to the liver via the portal vein, where it is exposed to metabolising enzymes, e.g. cytochromes. Many drugs are at least partly deactivated at this stage, so-called first-pass metabolism.

Distribution

If not extracted by first-pass metabolism, the drug reaches the general circulation. Some drugs will then become bound to some extent to plasma protein. This process is reversible but bound drug, as opposed to free drug, is unavailable for clinical action, further metabolism or renal excretion.

From the plasma (where only a few drugs have their primary action, e.g. antiplatelets), the drug can potentially diffuse into all body tissues. This wide distribution is responsible for many drug side-effects, as a result of action at sites other than those intended. The extent of distribution depends on the drug's plasma level, and the areas to which it is distributed depend largely on its hydrophilic–lipophilic balance; e.g. only very lipophilic drugs can cross the blood–brain barrier. Eventually, if the administered dose raises the plasma level above a threshold value, the concentration at the intended receptor is sufficient to elicit a pharmacological response. Although we can rarely measure the drug concentration at the receptor site, plasma concentration is an acceptable substitute because it is usually proportional to the concentration at the receptor.

Clearance

Clearance refers to the (rate of) removal of active drug from the body. Drugs may be cleared by chemical modification (**metabolism**), usually in the liver, or by physical **excretion** from the body, usually by the kidney. Hydrophilic drugs

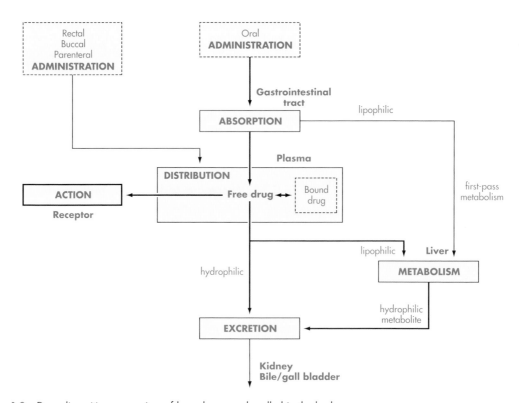

Figure 1.2   Drug disposition – overview of how drugs are handled in the body.

are easily cleared renally but a lipophilic drug filtered at the glomerulus is likely to be reabsorbed in the tubule, so clearance is very inefficient. Thus the main function of hepatic metabolism is not, as is sometimes believed, to 'detoxify' the drug, but to chemically convert it to a more hydrophilic form for renal excretion. That this process often reduces or eliminates the drug's pharmacological action is incidental; indeed, some drugs are actually activated or potentiated this way, e.g. *codeine* to *morphine*.

Figure 1.2 also shows how some alternative methods of administration can circumvent first-pass metabolism to enhance bioavailability (e.g. buccal absorption of *glyceryl trinitrate*; can evade possible destruction by stomach acid (e.g. injected insulin); or can permit faster action or target the dose (e.g. inhaled *salbutamol*, rectal steroid).

Drug selection

This introduction concludes with a general review of the factors that determine or influence the choice of drug therapy following diagnosis. The following chapters demonstrate the way these principles are applied in common diseases.

The decision process

The typical sequence is illustrated in Figure 1.3. Clinical findings may suggest several appropriate groups of drugs (or that none at all is needed). This must then be progressively narrowed down to one group, then a particular member of that group; finally a route of administration and dose must be chosen.

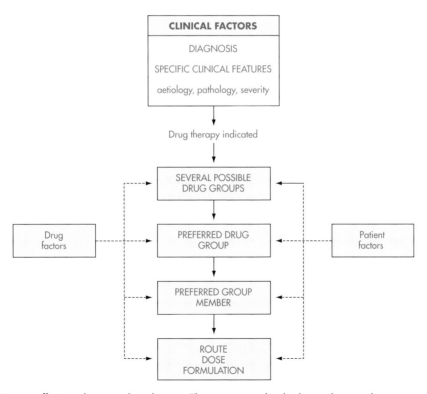

Figure 1.3 Factors affecting choice in drug therapy. This is a generalised scheme showing the sequence of decisions taken when pharmacotherapy is decided following diagnosis.

Consider, for example, managing hypertension. Precise diagnosis of the condition may suggest a particular drug group: quite different strategies will be needed depending on whether the condition is primary benign (essential) hypertension or secondary to some other disease state, e.g. renovascular disease or adrenal tumour. Clinical findings will also indicate the urgency of treatment. In primary hypertension the first choice would be from among the thiazides, the angiotensin-converting enzyme inhibitors (ACEIs) or the calcium-channel blockers (CCBs); in high renin disease an ACEI may be indicated; in the third case, surgery might be feasible. In a patient with essential hypertension and concurrent ischaemic heart disease, beta-blockers may be indicated, but should the beta-blocker be selective or non-selective, short- or long-acting, lipophilic or non-lipophilic? Finally, having selected the most appropriate drug entity, what should be the preferred route of administration, dose and formulation?

In making these decisions, clinical factors such as precise diagnostic class, drug factors such as mode of action and half-life, and patient factors such as age and renal function, are all important. The choice from among the various drugs indicated at each stage is determined initially by **drug factors** (i.e. the drugs of choice for the particular disease, independent of the particular patient). Early in the decision process the considerations are principally pharmacodynamic (i.e. pharmacological, including toxicological). As the choice becomes more focused, biopharmaceutical and pharmacokinetic factors become more relevant. Thus for essential hypertension there are several types of drugs indicated, related to their pharmacological effect on blood pressure. Once a drug group has been decided upon, selecting a particular member must take account of the spectrum of pharmacokinetic properties of the group, or the formulations available.

At each stage the selection based on drug factors may then be modified or constrained by **patient factors**, such as the patient's response to the agent (pharmacodynamics), their handling of it (pharmacokinetics), or possibly concurrent disease or drug therapy. Thus the choice of a renally cleared drug might have to be changed in a patient with renal impairment; a patient with compliance problems might benefit from a modified-release preparation; a patient with diabetes should avoid thiazides. Finally, one should not forget cost: from a number of comparably efficacious and safe drugs the most economic one must always be first choice.

There are also **prescriber factors**, i.e. the clinician's own preference, exercised on the basis of familiarity and experience, and these may be as good a guide as any when choosing from among a range of very similar preparations. On the other hand this may occasionally be based on unsystematic anecdotal evidence or outdated habits. In their role as pharmaceutical advisers, pharmacists are now helping GPs to make evidence-based choices and construct rational formularies to facilitate drug selection. Increasingly, they also prescribe independently.

Drug factors

Pharmacodynamics and toxicity

These are the primary criteria. Occasionally the diagnosis will indicate a unique drug group or even one specific drug, e.g. *levothyroxine* in hypothyroidism, but usually there are a number of approximately equivalent strategies available at this stage. Precise pharmacological properties then become important, the choice depending on the clinical presentation. For example, an arterial vasodilator may be more useful than a venodilator in certain types of heart failure; a cough suppressant rather than a decongestant may be preferred for a cough unproductive of mucus. Receptor subtype specificity may also be relevant, e.g. cardioselectivity of beta-blockers, selective amine re-uptake blockade in antidepressants.

A drug's therapeutic index must also be considered: what is the risk-to-benefit ratio of treatment? The severity of the condition may justify using a more potent but more toxic agent, but can the plasma level or adverse effects be easily monitored? Does the plasma level correlate with the concentration at the presumed site of action or the therapeutic benefit, or with the intensity of adverse effects?

Biopharmaceutics

The formulation of a medicine is important in selection for a number of reasons, e.g. for IV preparations, where stability and pharmaceutical compatibility are crucial, and dermatological preparations, where penetration, skin hydration, miscibility, etc. can influence effectiveness. Formulation can also affect bioavailability, which is particularly important for drugs with a narrow therapeutic index used to stabilize serious chronic conditions, e.g. *phenytoin* in epilepsy or *theophylline* in asthma, where changes in formulation might compromise disease control or cause toxicity.

Some drugs are unsuitable for certain routes, e.g. *benzylpenicillin* is destroyed by gastrointestinal enzymes and so is unsuitable for oral administration, *aminophylline* requires too high a dose mass for aerosolization, and *phenytoin* is too irritant for IM use.

Pharmacokinetics

A drug's physicochemical properties (especially its hydrophilic/lipophilic balance, pKa and molecular size) affect its absorption, distribution to the required site of action, mode and rate of clearance and route of elimination.

Hydrophilic/lipophilic balance

The characteristics conferred by predominant hydrophilic or lipophilic properties (summarized in Table 1.3) are particularly noticeable within a series of otherwise similar drugs, e.g. the beta-blockers (see below). Most drugs need both properties: lipophilic to cross membranes; hydrophilic to enable transport in and distribution by body fluids. For lipophilicity the drugs will need some non-polar groups in their structure and, if such drugs are ionic, they will exist to a significant extent in unionized form at body pH, i.e. their pKa should be near 7.4. Strongly hydrophilic drugs are often highly polar, and those that are ionic have pKa values significantly greater or less than 7.4.

Membrane permeability, which determines many biological properties, is highly dependent on polarity. Lipophilic drugs (e.g. most general anaesthetics), pass biological membranes easily, whereas ionized molecules (e.g. *aminoglycoside* antibiotics) generally penetrate membranes

Table 1.3   Effects of hydrophilic and lipophilic tendencies on the biological properties of drugs

Predominantly lipophilic	Predominantly hydrophilic
Good membrane penetration	Poor membrane penetration
Good absorption after oral administration	Poor absorption after oral administration
Distributed in body fat	Distributed in body water
Cross blood–brain barrier	Does not cross blood–brain barrier
Hepatic metabolism	Cleared renally unchanged
Longer half-life	Shorter half-life
First-pass effect possible	
Clearance dependent on liver function and release from fat storage sites	Clearance dependent on renal function
Biliary excretion of hydrophilic metabolites (molecular weight >400 Dalton)	Increased plasma protein binding
Possible interaction with other hepatically metabolized drugs	Possible interaction with other protein-bound drugs

poorly in the absence of specific transmembrane pumps.

Taken orally, lipophilic drugs are more likely to undergo first-pass hepatic metabolism, with consequent reduced bioavailability, e.g. *propranolol*. Highly lipophilic drugs partition into body fat, and so may have a high volume of distribution and prolonged half-life, e.g. *diazepam*. If the metabolite of a lipophilic drug is also active, the activity will be further prolonged, e.g. *carbamazepine*.

Hydrophilic drugs such as *atenolol* are cleared mainly by renal excretion, which often tends to give them a shorter half-life, especially if they undergo tubular secretion. Lipophilic drugs such as *propranolol* are likely to be metabolized rapidly by the liver to produce a more hydrophilic molecule that can then be more easily excreted by the kidney.

Although lipophilic molecules are freely filtered at the renal glomerulus, they are equally freely reabsorbed from the tubules, so their net renal clearance is inherently low. In contrast, hydrophilic molecules are less efficiently reabsorbed and are more likely to pass out in the urine.

pKa

Acidic drugs (e.g. *aspirin*) are generally more highly bound to plasma albumin, giving a lower volume of distribution, i.e. they tend to stay in the plasma rather than distribute to the tissues (Table 1.4). Basic drugs (including many CNS-acting agents such as *phenothiazines*) are theoretically more prone to binding to acid glycoprotein, an acute phase inflammatory plasma protein; however, albumin also has binding sites for basic drugs. Acidic drugs tend to interact by displacement from protein binding. Plasma protein binding reduces the free (unbound) drug plasma concentration, and thus both drug activity and clearance, because it is this fraction that is available equally for pharmacodynamic effect, and also for hepatic extraction and renal excretion.

Interactions may occur intrarenally owing to competition for the special tubular secretory transport mechanisms that exist for weak acids and bases. The pH of the urine can affect clearance: a more acid urine promotes the clearance of basic drugs, and vice versa. This is the basis of forced acid or alkaline diuresis to treat poisoning, e.g. urinary alkalinization for barbiturate or *aspirin* overdose.

Molecular size

Membrane permeability is also affected by molecular size. Ionized or highly polar molecules greater than 100 Da do not cross membranes. Hydrophilic hepatic metabolites greater than 400 Da are likely to be excreted in the bile, while smaller molecules are excreted renally.

Overall effect

The sum of all the pharmacokinetic properties of a drug will determine important parameters of its use:

* The half-life.
* The time a single oral dose will take to reach peak concentration, which affects the usefulness in an emergency and the best timing of plasma level sampling.
* The time to reach steady state, which may in turn affect the time to initial onset of useful action, and the minimum advisable interval between dose changes.
* Peak and trough plasma levels: the former determines toxicity, the latter clinical effect.
* The frequency of dosage, which may affect compliance.

Physicochemical factors may also influence **toxicity**, e.g. the more lipophilic beta-blockers read-

Table 1.4 Effects of pKa on the biological properties of ionizable drugs

pKa	Effect
<7.4	Hydrophilic; acidic Absorbed in stomach (fastest) Bound to plasma albumin Reduced solubility in normal urine
About 7.4	Lipophilic
>7.4	Hydrophilic; basic Absorbed in ileum (delayed) Bound to plasma acid glycoprotein Increased solubility in normal urine

ily cross the blood–brain barrier and may cause adverse central nervous system (CNS) effects.

As an example of how these factors affect choice, consider a drug for the oral prophylaxis of recurrent urinary-tract infection. To be effective it must be well absorbed, should not be significantly deactivated by the liver and should be excreted in antimicrobially significant concentrations in the urine. Because prophylactic therapy is often associated with compliance problems, a long-acting drug or formulation with a once-daily dosage regimen would be preferred.

Patient factors

There is often a wide interpatient variation in response, both therapeutic and toxic, to a standard dose of a drug. Thus, despite careful attention to all the above factors, there is still a need to carefully review the choice of drug and dose for an individual patient. This variation arises because of a combination of differing pharmacodynamics (Table 1.5) and differing pharmacokinetics (Table 1.6).

Response

Drug response varies with **age**. The elderly and the very young may have atypical responses to many drugs. These may be due to anomalous or exaggerated sensitivity, especially to drugs acting on the CNS, e.g. aggression in some elderly patients taking benzodiazepines. Alternatively, there may be impaired physiological or homeo-static mechanisms, e.g. among the elderly, an exaggerated hypotensive effect with vasodila-

Table 1.5   Reasons for variation in patient response

Age
Race
Compliance
Concurrent disease
Concurrent medication
Pregnancy, breastfeeding
Tolerance, hypersensitivity
Renal and hepatic function
Genetic variability in metabolic enzymes

Table 1.6   Variations and constraints in drug handling

Absorption	Interactions with diet or other drugs
	Site of absorption:
	– gastrointestinal disease
	– regional perfusion
	– airways patency
	– etc.
	Parenteral:
	– fluid volume
	– venous access
	– local perfusion
Distribution	Age
	Weight/build/body composition
	Fluid and electrolyte balance/hydration
	Systemic/regional perfusion
	Internal barriers
	Plasma protein level
	Interactions with other drugs
Elimination	Renal and hepatic function:
	– age
	– race
	– disease
	Interactions with other drugs

tors, or hyponatraemia with diuretics. In some cases there are **genetic** or **racial** differences in drug response, e.g. thiazide diuretics are much more effective antihypertensives in people with a dark skin, who respond less favourably than people with a white skin to beta-blockers.

If there are unexpected responses, particularly apparent ineffectiveness, the possibility of patient **non-compliance** should always be borne in mind. There are many possible reasons for non-compliance and pharmacists have an important role in detecting it and improving the situation. In some cases a change in drug or formulation may encourage better compliance, e.g. a long-acting, once-daily form for essential hypertension. In other cases, an inappropriate dose or exaggerated sensitivity to adverse effects may be to blame. Sensitive enquiry of the patient will often uncover an innocent or perfectly reasonable explanation, frequently deriving from poor communication or imperfect patient understanding. The recommended ideal is to develop a **concordance** between prescriber and patient, i.e. mutual confidence, mutually agreed objectives and constraints and mutually agreed treatment.

Concurrent diseases may increase the patient's sensitivity to some drugs; for example, the myocardium is more sensitive to *digoxin* after infarction, or in thyroid imbalance. Other diseases may indirectly make a patient less tolerant of the drug, e.g. beta-blockers are contra-indicated in asthma. The patient's biochemical and physiological status is often important, e.g. *digoxin* toxicity is greatly increased in the presence of hypokalaemia.

Previous or sustained exposure to a drug may produce an unexpected **tolerance** to either the therapeutic effect (e.g. prophylactic nitrates in ischaemic heart disease) or an adverse effect (e.g. anticholinergics). The patient may be taking **interacting** drugs, which may be antagonistic (e.g. corticosteroids and thiazides both antagonize oral hypogly-caemic drugs), or additive or synergistic, such as a sedative OTC antihistamine taken with an anxiolytic.

For reasons that are poorly understood, some patients have anomalous or **idiosyncratic** adverse reactions to certain drugs, the penicillins being the best example. These are often immunologically-based, non-dose-dependent type B adverse effects.

Finally, in women, the possibility of the drug having an effect on conception, pregnancy or breastfeeding requires special consideration.

Handling

Interpatient variation in pharmacokinetic para-meters may be inborn or acquired, and is partic-ularly important in dosage and route selection, but also sometimes affects which drug group is selected.

Absorption

Many diseases can affect oral absorption. Disease of the gut itself may of course affect absorption (e.g. vomiting, diarrhoea, inflammatory bowel disease), but so too can cardiovascular disease, which may compromise gastrointestinal perfu-sion. The elderly are more prone to such diseases, especially heart failure. Oral absorption

is only affected by extreme age. Oral intolerance, e.g. gastric upset, is a common adverse effect and a reason for both non-compliance and potentially serious morbidity.

There may be unwanted interactions with the patient's diet or other drug therapy, e.g. *tetracy-cline* absorption is impaired by concurrent milk or antacid consumption.

Absorption from any site depends on an adequate blood supply. SC or IM injections may be ineffective if the circulation is compromised, because blood is redirected to the core visceral circulation. Thus *morphine* must always be given intravenously following myocardial infarction. Diabetics should understand that insulin absorp-tion from a limb injection site is more variable than from an abdominal one, because limb perfusion depends on physical activity.

There may be other barriers to absorption. Bronchodilators will not easily penetrate constricted airways, and transdermal absorption will vary according to the skin thickness of the area to which a dermatological or transdermal preparation is applied and to the local blood flow (which, for example, is increased in inflammation).

If IV infusion is planned, the condition of the patient's veins must be considered, and whether the patient can tolerate the fluid load of the vehicle or any associated ions, e.g. sodium or potassium with *penicillin*.

Distribution

Distribution is affected by the proportion of adipose tissue to lean body mass (which is aqueous), and by the plasma protein level (which may affect the free drug plasma level, depending on its kinetics). This can affect both the overall volume of distribution, the distribution between different compartments, and access to the organs of elimination, chiefly the liver and kidney.

The elderly have a lower lean body mass and so a relatively smaller aqueous compartment than middle-aged adults, and the very young have a higher proportion of body water. Both the elderly and the very young have reduced plasma albumin, which reduces drug binding. The patient's nutritional state and hydration will similarly affect drug distribution between various compartments, as will a large volume of oedema fluid. A large volume of distribution will result in lower plasma levels.

Delivery to the target site is dependent primarily on the regional blood perfusion. This may be seriously impaired in heart failure, shock, peripheral vascular disease or diabetic blood vessel disease. For example, it is difficult to treat an infection in a diabetic's foot with systemic antibiotics.

Distribution may be further modified by the body's internal barriers. For example, the blood–brain barrier impedes polar molecules, but this effect is much reduced if it is inflamed, e.g. in meningitis. Pus is poorly penetrated by some antibiotics, and sputum concentrations of antibiotics are frequently far lower than plasma concentrations.

Other drugs that a patient may be taking might compete for plasma protein binding sites, causing an increase in the free drug levels of the one displaced. However, despite the many theoretical possibilities of such interactions, relatively few are clinically significant and only a small number are serious. A drug will only cause a significant elevation in the free concentration of another by displacement if both are avidly bound to the same site, are in high concentration in the plasma, and have a low volume of distribution, i.e. most of the drug in the body is in the plasma.

Moreover, clearance of the displaced drug may be increased, and this tends to counteract any rise in plasma level. Only certain drugs are likely to cause clinically significant problems by this mechanism: these include potentially toxic drugs with a narrow therapeutic index, and those whose doses are carefully titrated to stabilize a chronic condition, e.g. antiepileptics, oral hypoglycaemics and anticoagulants.

Concurrent disease may also influence binding. Endogenous metabolites such as bilirubin, which is elevated in jaundice, may compete for binding sites. A high blood urea level, e.g. in renal failure, impairs protein binding, and hypoproteinaemia in liver failure, malabsorption and the nephrotic syndrome, will reduce available sites.

Clearance and elimination
The function of either of the main organs of clearance may be impaired by disease, age or concurrent drug therapy. A knowledge of the patient's renal and hepatic function, their medication history and the mode(s) of elimination of the drug to be used, are essential when selecting therapy. The use of drugs in hepatic impairment is considered in Chapter 3 (p. 159) and in renal impairment in Chapter 14 (p. 914).

Evidence-based medicine

Patient management is moving rapidly away from being derived from observational studies and expert opinion to evidence based on critical and objective comparison of the clinical outcomes of different treatment strategies. The favoured technique is **meta-analysis**, whereby objective data from as many comparable **randomized controlled trials** (RCTs) as possible are pooled and aggregated. Obviously the skill here lies not least in ensuring comparability. Meta-analysis can increase the statistical power and therefore the reliability of the conclusions, making the recommendations far stronger than if they had been based on any individual component trial, each with far smaller patient numbers. Failing meta-analysis, less rigorous **systematic reviews** of RCTs can be used, but with less confidence. If RCTs are not available, **case-control** or **cohort** studies can be used. Least reliable are individual case reports or expert opinion.

This produces a hierarchy of **levels of evidence** upon which recommendations can be based, with the higher levels subdivided according to the quality of the analysis. These can be summarized as:

- **Level 1** (1++, 1+ or 1): meta-analyses or systematic review of RCTs.
- **Level 2** (2++, 2+ or 2): systematic reviews of case-control or cohort studies.
- **Level 3**: non-systematic studies, e.g. case reports or case series.
- **Level 4**: expert opinion.

As a result a management **guideline** for the condition being treated is devised. The recommendations in guidelines are normally graded for strength or reliability according to the level of evidence on which they are based:

- **Grade A**: level 1 meta-analysis directly applicable to the target population of the guidance.
- **Grade B**: level 2 evidence directly applicable to the target population of the guidance, or evidence extrapolated from level 1 evidence.
- **Grade C**: level 2+ evidence directly applicable to the target population of the guidance, or evidence extrapolated from level 2++ evidence.
- **Grade D**: level 3 or 4, or extrapolation from level 2+ evidence.

This is a simplification of a subtle and rigorous statistical process. The key point is that such an approach to drug selection does not need to consider directly many of the factors discussed above. These would all have been part of the original design of the RCTs. The evidence-based medicine approach is simply, 'does it work, and at what cost of adverse effects?'. This is partly what the National Institute for Health and Clinical Excellence (NICE) does, although it also has to consider the economic cost.

To this extent, evidence-based medicine guidelines may be seen as relieving the prescriber of making some of the decisions discussed in this chapter. However, no guideline can anticipate all possible combinations of circumstances, and clinical judgement will always need to be exercised, even if it ultimately supports following the guideline. Moreover, a professional practitioner is obliged not just to blindly follow guidelines, but to understand the rationale behind the recommendations.

Pharmaceutical care

As stated in the Preface, this is not a textbook of clinical pharmacy. However, it is relevant to note at this point the involvement of pharmacists in patient care. Pharmacists are increasingly taking more responsibility for the management and optimization of the entire spectrum of a patient's pharmacotherapy. This has extended the concept of clinical pharmacy beyond validating indications and screening contra-indications, interactions and dosage regimens. Pharmacists now have a commitment to anticipate or identify all possible drug-related problems. Pharmaceutical care involves devising an appropriate pharmaceutical care plan and specifying how this will be implemented and monitored for success and adverse events. Pharmacist prescribing is extending this process significantly.

References and further reading

Graeme-Smith D G, Aronson J K (2002). *Oxford Textbook of Clinical Pharmacology and Drug Treatment*, 3rd edn. Oxford: Oxford University Press.

Longmore J M, Wilkinson I B, Rajagopalan S (2004). *Oxford Handbook of Clinical Medicine (Oxford Handbooks)*, 6th edn. Chapter 3: Clinical skills. Oxford: Oxford University Press, 32–63.

National Prescribing Centre (2006). National Institute for Health and Clinical Excellence. *MeReC Bulletin* **16**(2): 5–8.

Speight T M, ed. (1997). *Avery's Drug Treatment*, 4th edn. Section I: Clinical pharmacology. Auckland: Adis Press.

Thompson A (2004). Back to basics: pharmacokinetics. *Pharm J* **272**: 769–771.

Thompson A (2004). Variability in drug dosage requirements. *Pharm J* **272**: 806–808.

Thompson A (2004). Examples of dosage regime design. *Pharm J* **273**: 188–190.

Toghill P J (1994). *Examining Patients: An Introduction to Cinical Medicine*, 2nd edn. London: Edward Arnold.

Various authors (1997). A pharmacist's guide to evidence-based medicine: special feature. *Pharm J* **258**: 510–522.

See also **Recommended reference sources** on p. xxi.

2

Major pathological processes in disease

Just as physiology is the study of the way in which the body works, pathology is the scientific study of abnormal physiology, i.e. disease.

There are many ways in which physiological processes can be upset, and knowledge of the aetiology of a disease may give valuable clues to diagnosis and management. The physician will rely on the signs and symptoms resulting from the derangement of normal physiology to reach these decisions. In this chapter we will examine how physiological processes common to all body systems are altered by disease. Aspects of pathology specific to individual diseases are dealt with in Part 2, in the chapters dealing with the various disease states.

Introduction

Physiological processes are delicately balanced to maintain a stable internal body environment, a process known as **homeostasis**. This includes, for instance, maintaining a constant temperature and blood pressure, ensuring that the body is properly hydrated and adjusting levels of electrolytes and blood cells. Homeostasis is a dynamic system involving complex inter-related positive and negative feedback signals. It is the mechanism by which the body defends itself against a changing and sometimes hostile environment. A knowledge of homeostatic mechanisms is key to understanding pathology.

One reason why physiology becomes abnormal is that the various homeostatic mechanisms have been overwhelmed, e.g. a severe infection may swamp all of the various physiological responses to injury, including the immune system. However, this explains only a relatively small number of diseases. Most appear to be due to excessive defective adaptive mechanisms (defensive or homeostatic) that, instead of maintaining stability, actually disrupt normal function. Table 2.1 lists some general causes of disease and how they can give rise to four major pathological processes: inflammation, degeneration, neoplastic change and inherited disease. Running through each of these is the recurrent theme of failure in adaptive mechanisms (**maladaptation**). For example, in infection or allergy, it is the response of the body in trying to eliminate the foreign agent rather than its presence that may cause the major problem. Immunological processes themselves can sometimes be more harmful than beneficial, e.g. a severe allergic reaction. In **autoimmune disease** antibodies and cells of the immune system attack the body's own tissues.

However a tissue is damaged, the body attempts to remove the source of the injury and repair damaged tissue. The fundamental tissue response to injury is **inflammation** (p. 46), but if that response is excessive it may do more damage than the original injury. The consequences of inflammation are far-reaching and underlie many different disease states. Consequently much of this chapter is devoted to a consideration of inflammation and the closely related **immunological** processes.

Degeneration is another major pathological process and represents a cellular response to injury. Toxins, infections, immunological reactions, ischaemia and radiation may all lead to cellular damage, degeneration and eventually tissue death (**necrosis**). In some circumstances, e.g. exposure to tumour necrosis factor alpha (TNFα) and irreparable DNA damage by radiation and cytotoxic drugs (see Chapter 10), cells can initiate programmed self-destruction, a process called **apoptosis**.

Unlike necrosis, which causes local inflammation by releasing intercellular enzymes, apoptosis is a normal physiological function that is integral to growth and development and so is not proinflammatory. The 26S proteasome is a multienzyme organelle that catabolizes proteins that are involved in regulating cell growth and reproduction. Abnormal enzymes that promote uncontrolled reproduction of tumour cells, e.g. tyrosine kinase, belong to an enzyme group called the Janus kinases, which underlie some monoclonal diseases that are characterized by uncontrolled haemopoietic stem cell prolifera-

---

Table 2.1   Classification of pathological processes

Pathological process	Aetiology	Examples of results

Inflammation (tissue response)	Infection
	Immunological
	Physical
	  • trauma
	  • toxins
	  • radiation
		Any '-itis'
		Fibrosis

Degeneration (cellular response)	As for inflammation
	Ischaemia
		Cell/tissue destruction
		  • myocardial infarction
		  • renal failure
		  • stroke

Neoplastic change	Predisposing factors Oncogenes, carcinogens (see Chapter 10)	Tumours

Inherited disease	Faulty genetic codes	Disease with strong family history
		  • organ malfunction
		  • malformation
		  • inborn errors of metabolism
		  • some cancers

tion. The name comes from the Roman god Janus, represented as having two faces, one looking back and one forward – the gatekeeper, and hence January. The enzyme Janus kinase 2 (**JAK2**) is a signal transducer for a range of cytokines, i.e. mostly small proteins that are produced by effector cells to signal other cells to respond (see Table 2.2), and causes chronic myeloid leukaemia (CML) and other haemopoietic neoplasms. Thus digestion of JAK2 by the 26S proteasome inhibits abnormal cell proliferation and may abort such diseases. The monoclonal antibody *imatinib* is a JAK2 inhibitor that has revolutionized CML treatment in patients who are unsuitable for bone marrow transplantation, in whom other treatments have failed or whose disease is in an aggressive state. Conversely, inhibition of the proteasome by the new monoclonal agent, *bortezomib*, induces apoptosis of the abnormal proliferating cells. The combination of *bortezomib* with corticosteroids produces synergism and is reported to double the response rate to corticosteroids alone in the treatment of refractory myeloma.

JAK3 deficiency is involved in the severe combined immunodeficiency syndrome, which affects both B and T cell lines (see below).

Many conditions are caused by cardiovascular problems, e.g. if blood loss is very severe, circulatory collapse (**shock**) may result. Conversely, if a **thrombus** (blood clot) is large enough to impede the circulation or block a vessel completely, this can be viewed as a defect in the homeostatic mechanisms that normally prevent blood loss. The results of thrombosis, shock and related phenomena can all lead to a reduction in blood flow to an area of tissue, i.e. **ischaemia** (literally 'blocking blood'), which may cause degeneration or necrosis of the tissue supplied (ischaemia is discussed on p. 58).

In some cases a combination of disease processes may lead to further damage, e.g. the inflammatory response evoked by a widespread burn will lead to a large exudation of protein-rich fluid from the bloodstream, causing a fall in the oncotic pressure of the plasma and a flow of fluid into the tissues, producing **oedema**. Further, the resulting low blood pressure (shock) may cause kidney ischaemia leading to degeneration of kidney nephrons and, if the number of func-

tioning nephrons falls below a critical level, renal failure will follow. Shock will also have more generalized effects throughout the body – the heart, lungs and CNS being especially vulnerable.

Immunology

Specific and non-specific (innate) immunity

There are three general lines of defence against a hostile environment:

- The simple mechanical barriers provided by the skin and mucous membranes.
- The complex but non-specific innate defence mechanisms, including the inflammatory reaction, the functions of the white cells and the **complement** system of the blood.
- The specific acquired immune defence mechanisms.

We concentrate here on the last two of these, using the theme of microbial infection to illustrate how they work together.

Following exposure to infection, a reaction will develop against the organism concerned and the chance of re-infection with the same species is usually slight. This reaction is known as **specific acquired immunity**, which may be due to circulating antibodies (**humoral immunity**) or to specific sensitized cells (CMI, **cell-mediated immunity**) or both. A similar reaction occurs when other foreign compounds or tissues, e.g. some drugs, or a transplant, comes into contact with the blood.

There are also systems of innate **non-specific immunity**, which do not depend on contact with a foreign organism, protein, etc. The key cells here are certain white blood cells (WBCs, leucocytes), especially the **neutrophils** and **macrophages**, which engulf and digest any microbe or foreign material with which they come into contact, regardless of whether or not it has previously encountered the immune system. However, the action of these cell types is greatly enhanced if the body has developed acquired immunity to the organism or material. Additionally, the complement system (p. 35) provides non-specific defence and also acts to potentiate acquired specific immunity.

It is becoming clear that **cell adhesion molecules** are important in the function of many cell–cell and cell–membrane interactions, which may be important in normal physiological processes and pathological ones. These include, for example, beta-1 integrin, which is essential to the correct morphogenesis and differentiation of mammary glands, and blood platelet surface receptors, e.g. glycoprotein 1a, which enable platelet binding to collagen, and glycoprotein 1b, which binds to von Willebrand factor, both essential in blood clotting (see Chapter 11). Bacterial pili contain surface **lectins** that recognize specific sugar residues in cell walls and this explains the selectivity of certain bacterial strains or species for specific tissues, e.g. the strains of *Escherichia coli* that produce intestinal and urinary-tract infections are demonstrably different.

Antigens and immunoglobulins

An antigen is any foreign substance, of whatever origin, that is capable of initiating the production of a specific blood protein called an **immunoglobulin** (Ig, older term is antibody) that will act against it. The Igs so formed will react specifically with that particular antigen, neutralizing its biological effect. Thus antigens are sometimes referred to as immunogens. However, other antigens possessing a sufficiently similar chemical structure may cross-react with the Ig because antigen–antibody reactions involve close intermolecular binding and depend on a 'lock and key' steric fit, similar to the binding of drugs to receptors and enzymes to substrates. We sometimes make use of this ability to cross-react, e.g. in the old Wasserman test for syphilis antibody, an indicator of past or current infection, but now replaced by an enzyme immunoassay. The Wasserman reaction does not use *Treponema pallidum* spirochaetes, which are difficult to grow and manipulate, but an artificial antigen prepared from beef hearts that reacts similarly.

Most antigens are proteins. Once these have been recognized by the immune system as 'non-self' (foreign), an immune response is initiated.

Microorganisms always express several antigenic groupings (determinants, epitopes) on their surface, so a number of different Igs may be produced against a particular organism. A vast number of non-microbial proteins are capable of stimulating antibody production, including the numerous substances to which allergies are developed. Macromolecules other than proteins can also lead to the production of antibodies, e.g. lipopolysaccharides. Smaller molecules or ions, e.g. penicillins and heavy metals, may act as antigenic determinants if they combine with 'self' (non-antigenic) proteins or cells in an individual, causing the modified protein or cell surface to be recognized as foreign by that person's immune system. These small molecules or ions, which cannot themselves elicit the production of an Ig but will react with it when it has been formed in response to the protein–small molecule complex, or a similar cell complex, are termed **haptens**.

Cell types involved in the immune system

The chief components of the immune system are three classes of leucocytes (Figure 2.1), i.e. lymphocytes, monocytes and neutrophils. All of these are derived from common precursor pluripotent stem cells in the bone marrow, which have the capacity to replicate indefinitely and are the precursors of all blood cells.

Two lineages of leucocytes are derived via intermediate lymphoid and myeloid stem cells. The lymphoid intermediate stem cells give rise to the lymphocytes (**B cells** and **T cells**) and the myeloid stem cells to the **granulocytes**, the cytoplasm of which contains numerous granules. The granulocytes comprise the neutrophils, eosinophils and basophils, which are recognized by the staining character of their granules and the shapes of their nuclei.

B-lymphocytes (B cells)

Mature B cells produce Igs and so are responsible for humoral immunity. They originate in the bone marrow and, after activation by contact with antigen, undergo clonal expansion and mature into **plasma cells**, which produce an Ig

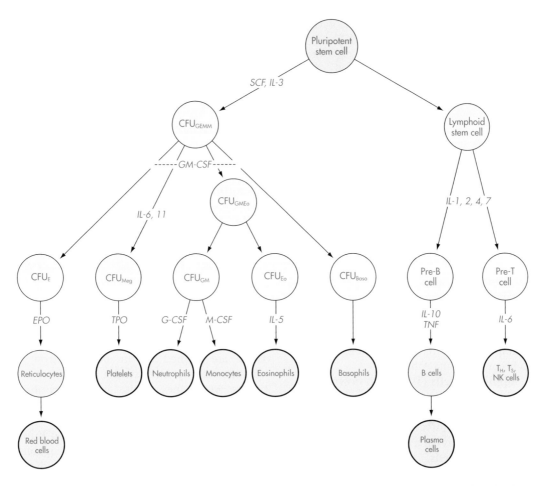

Figure 2.1 Outline of normal haemopoiesis, showing roles of growth and differentiation factors. Cell lines bold; Baso, basophil; CFU, colony-forming unit; CSF, colony-stimulating factor; Eo, eosinophil; E, erythroid; EPO, erythropoietin; G, granulocyte; GEMM, mixed erythroid–granulocyte–megakaryocyte–monocyte; GM, granulocyte–monocyte; IL, interleukin; M, monocyte; Meg, megakaryocyte; NK, natural killer (cells); SCF, stem cell (Steel) factor; TH, T helper cells; TNF, tumour necrosis factor; TPO, thrombopoietin; TS, T suppressor cells.

that will react specifically with the same priming antigen. They are capable of producing Igs only when mature. The plasma cells are stored mainly in the cortical regions of lymph nodes (Figure 2.2), only about 0.1% of B cells being found in the bloodstream. Plasma cells are terminally differentiated, i.e. each clone can carry out only the single function of producing one Ig, and have a short half-life of about 5 days. However, a small number of activated B cells do not differentiate to produce Ig, but are processed in germinal centres in lymph nodes (see Figure 2.2) to become memory cells able to respond rapidly

to a subsequent challenge with the same antigen. This memory function is a crucial property of the immune system because it protects against infection, perhaps many decades after an initial infection, e.g. second attacks of measles and whooping cough are rare.

T-lymphocytes (T cells, thymocytes)

These mature within the thymus gland, located behind the upper sternum, and are stored in the paracortical areas of lymph nodes. They have two important roles: **cell-mediated immunity**

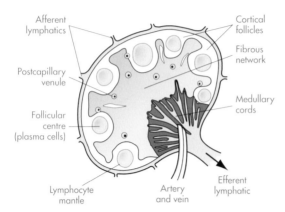

Figure 2.2   Structure of a lymph node.

(CMI), directed against certain types of micro-organisms and organ grafts, and regulation of the activity of B cells. There are four important classes of T cells:

- **T helper cells** (TH), which up-regulate B cells to become plasma cells.
- **T suppressor cells** (Ts), which down-regulate the immune system.
- **Cytotoxic T cells** (TC), which identify and eliminate virus-infected host cells, malignant cells and certain bacteria.
- **Memory T cells**, which are primed to respond rapidly when the priming antigen is re-encountered.

Undifferentiated TH cells are designated TH0. These are stimulated to differentiate into one of two subclasses by their **cytokine** environment (see Table 2.2). If interferon gamma (IFN gamma) predominates, the TH0 cells become TH1 cells, whereas if interleukin-4 (IL-4) predominates, they become TH2 cells. TH cells are CD4+ (see below and p. 33) able to recruit TC cells, and they can also stimulate B cells to form antibodies. TH cells also perform these functions through the production of cytokines, some of which are stimulatory and others inhibitory to lymphocytes. The T suppressor cells (Ts) are CD8+ and have a general inhibitory function.

Different types of T cell can be distinguished by the use of monoclonal antibodies (p. 33) to distinguish specific groups of cell surface antigens, identified by their cluster of differentiation

(CD) number. The CD antigens are specified by genes of the **major histocompatibility complex** (MHC, p. 44). All T cells have CD3 and a T cell receptor surface molecule. TC cells are CD8+ and are able to bind with MHC class I molecules, thus identifying cells that have been infected by a virus, and TH cells (CD4+) are able to bind to MHC class II molecules on the surface of **antigen-presenting cells** (APCs). Over 30 CD antigen clusters have been identified on a wide variety of cells from platelets to macrophages.

A further type of cell is the **natural killer (NK) cell**; these are CD34+ and are produced from CD3+ T precursor cells. They are non-specific cells that are neither B nor T cells. They recognize Igs that have reacted with foreign cell surfaces and cells that do not have the MHC class I molecules (see below) that characterize all 'self' cells and are thus 'seen' as foreign.

Monocytes

These are formed in the bone marrow and migrate via the bloodstream to various body tissues, where they mature into **macrophages**. Some macrophages have specific names according to the particular tissue they inhabit, e.g. macrophages in the liver are called **Kupffer cells**. Macrophages are scavengers, capable of phagocytosing (engulfing) a wide variety of 'foreign' matter, e.g. microorganisms, damaged cells and cell debris. A particle or organism is taken up by the macrophage in a **phagosome**, a cytoplasmic inclusion formed from the plasma membrane of the macrophage as it surrounds and ingests the foreign material. The phagosome then fuses with a **lysosome**, thus exposing it to the action of lysosomal enzymes and to superoxides and oxidizing free radicals, formed in a burst of respiration, which together destroy the engulfed material. The phagolysosome provides an environment that protects the rest of the cell from its highly active interior. However, some microorganisms, notably *Mycobacterium tuberculosis*, some fungi and helminths, are able to withstand the normally lethal action of the phagolysosome and may survive for long periods within macrophages, which may then aggregate to form **granulomas** (see Figure 2.16) as part of the inflammatory process (see p. 57).

Table 2.2   Some cytokines

Type	Cellular origin	Main action
Interleukins		
IL-1	APCs/macrophages	Clonal proliferation of TH cells, pyrogenic
IL-2, IL-15	TH cells	Activation of B cells, NK cells and other T cells
IL-3	Stem cells	Stimulates lymphocyte growth in marrow
IL-4	TH cells	B cell growth and differentiation
IL-5	TH cells	Recruitment and activation of eosinophils
Il-6	Macrophages	Inflammation (prostaglandin synthesis), pyrogenic, controls platelet production
IL-7	Marrow and thymus	Stimulates B and T cell growth and maturation
IL-8	Macrophages	Attracts neutrophils
IL-9	T cells	Lymphocyte growth factor, proliferation of mast cells
IL-10	TH cells	Inhibits the action of other cytokines
IL-11	Kidney, liver	Stimulates platelet production
IL-12	B cells	Stimulates T and NK cells
IL-13	T cells	Stimulates B cells
Interferons		
IFNα	Macrophages ⎱	Modulate the immune response to viral infection
IFNβ	Fibroblasts ⎰	
IFNγ	T cells	Blocks viral mRNA transcription, activates and inhibits TH cells
Tumour factors		
TNFα	Macrophages	Immune activation, pro-inflammatory
TNFβ	Lymphocytes	Immune activation, vascular shock
TGFβ	Platelets	Stimulates tumour and blood vessel production and fibrosis. Inhibits the immune response
Colony-stimulating factors		
GM-CSF (G-CSF, M-CSF)	Monocytes and T cells	Granulocyte/macrophage production
Erythropoietin	Kidney, liver	Erythrocyte production, haemopoiesis
Thrombopoietin	Kidney, liver	Controls platelet production

APC, antigen-presenting cell; G-CSF, granulocyte colony-stimulating factor; GM-CSF, granulocyte–macrophage colony-stimulating factor; IL, interleukin; NK, natural killer; M-CSF, macrophage colony-stimulating factor; TGF, transforming growth factor; TH, T helper; TNF, tumour necrosis factor.

There has been great interest in the secretory function of macrophages, particularly of the interleukin (IL) group of cytokines (Table 2.2). IL-1 and IL-6 are believed to play an important part in some of the generalized symptoms of systemic inflammatory reactions, e.g. fever and septic shock (p. 61). Also, the role of macrophages as APCs (see above) is partly facilitated by the action of interleukins. Many other substances are secreted by macrophages, some of which have an important role in chronic inflammation (p. 56).

Granulocytes

Neutrophils

Neutrophils (polymorphonuclear leucocytes, polymorphs) are so named because their large nuclei have two to five lobes and have a very variable appearance, even resembling a string of beads.

Their prime function is phagocytosis. Some common causes of acquired neutrophil deficiency (**neutropenia**), i.e. $<1.5 \times 10^9$/L, are given in Table 2.3, which shows that this is an important indicator of infection. Neutrophils are much shorter-lived than macrophages and persist in the peripheral blood for only 6–8 h. However, like macrophages they will readily ingest microbial cells that have been **opsonized**, i.e. coated with Igs and complement components (see Figure 2.6) that facilitate microbial attachment to phagocytic leucocytes, which then engulf and destroy them. Neutrophils are important in acute rather than chronic inflammation and play no part in CMI.

Eosinophils

These usually have two-lobed nuclei and their cationic cytoplasmic granules stain bright red with eosin dye. They play a key role in the clearance of damaged cells and in allergic reactions (p. 39) and are involved in defence against bacterial, fungal, helminth (worms) and protozoal infections.

Basophils

Unlike other leucocytes, basophils are non-phagocytic. Their cytoplasmic granules contain histamine, heparin and myeloperoxidases. Because they have high-affinity IgE receptors they play a role in anaphylactic-type allergic reactions (p. 39) and probably in anticoagulation, due to the presence of heparin granules, in responding to parasitic diseases and in immunoregulation. Basophils will not be considered further here.

Intercellular messengers: the cytokine network

The ways in which the various cells involved in the immune system are controlled and interact is currently of great interest. The principal cellular messengers involved comprise the cytokine network, which is being intensively researched to provide immunological treatments for a wide range of diseases.

Cytokines are produced by a range of leucocytes and mediate signalling between cells. Those produced by T cells are referred to as **lymphokines**, those by monocytes as **monokines**. Those cytokines that have the particular property of inducing **chemotaxis**, the attraction of leucocytes to sites of inflammation, are sometimes called **chemokines**.

The numerous cytokines have a number of overlapping actions, and their exact roles in the immunological response are not easy to define, often depending on the initial reason for stimulation. For instance, some cytokines produced by Tн cells to stimulate macrophages will, in other circumstances, also inhibit B cell function. The most important cytokines are the **interleukins**, **interferons**, **colony-stimulating factors** and **tumour necrosis factors**, some of which are listed in Table 2.2 with their cells of origin and range of actions. Some cytokines and cytokine inhibitors are already used in clinical practice:

- Both *aldesleukin* (rh-interleukin-2) and *IFN alfa* are used in the management of some neoplastic diseases (see Chapter 10).

Table 2.3   Some causes of acquired neutropenia

Severe infection
    Viral, e.g. AIDS; some fungal, e.g. *Pneumocystis* pneumonia
    Bacterial, causing overwhelming septicaemia, e.g. enteric fevers, mycoplasmas, tuberculosis
Neoplastic disease, e.g. acute leukaemia, Hodgkin's lymphoma
Multisystem diseases (see Chapter 12), e.g. Felty's syndrome, systemic lupus erythematosus
Drugs, e.g. cytotoxic chemotherapy (see Chapter 10), immunosuppressants
Radiotherapy
Excessive destruction, e.g. hypersplenism

- *Peginterferon alfa-2a* and *-2b* are licensed for the treatment of chronic hepatitis C (see Chapter 3).
- The immunosuppressive effects of *IFN beta* are utilized in multiple sclerosis to reduce the incidence of acute attacks in the relapsing/remitting form of the disease.
- *Filgrastim* (granulocyte-colony stimulating factor, rhG-CSF), *lenograstim* (glycosylated rhG-CSF) and *pegfilgrastim* (pegylated rhG-CSF) have been used to treat neutropenia and related conditions, especially as adjuncts to chemotherapy, to stimulate leucocyte production after treatment with myelosuppressive (antineoplastic and bone marrow suppressive) agents (see Chapter 10). Granulocyte-macrophage colony-stimulating factor (rhGM-CSF) is used similarly.
- Inhibitors of interleukins and tumour necrosis factor are also being used in the management of a variety of inflammatory autoimmune diseases, e.g. RA and ankylosing spondylitis (see Chapter 12), psoriasis (see Chapter 13) and inflammatory bowel disease (see Chapter 3). This group of apparently unrelated diseases share a common final inflammatory pathway and have been called the **immune-mediated inflammatory disorders** (IMIDs).

Humoral immunity: antibody production

When antigens first appear in the body they are taken up by B cells, monocytes/macrophages, and Langerhans cells in the skin (see Chapter 13) and the antigens are processed and their epitopes expressed on their surfaces. All of these cells are then APCs. There may be several epitopes (antigenic determinants) with complex antigens, e.g. bacteria and other cellular antigens. The epitopes of immunogens on the surfaces of APCs, in combination with MHC class II molecules (see p. 44), can then be recognized by complementary TH cells. These in turn produce interleukins, which stimulate the appropriate B cell clone to mature and produce Igs (Table 2.4 and Figure 2.3). Although most antigenic responses require this involvement of TH cells, some bacterial antigens, notably wall polysaccharides, are T cell-independent and can stimulate B cell clones directly to produce the IgM type of Ig (see Table 2.4 and p. 35).

A single B cell cannot produce all the varieties of Ig that may ever be required. At an early stage of human embryonic development, precursor B cells undergo extensive genetic rearrangement. There are three genetic regions: a **variable region** (V, between 25 and 100 genes), a **diversity region** (D, 10 genes) and a **junctional region** (J, 5–6

Table 2.4   The principal properties of the immunoglobulins

Immunoglobulin	Proportion of total pool	Function	Action
IgG	73%	Most antibody responses	Opsonization Antimicrobial Antitoxins
IgM	7% (mostly in blood)	Early antibody responses	Opsonization Bacterial agglutination
IgA	20% (mainly in epithelial secretions, e.g. intestines, lung)	Protects mucosae from infection	Antitoxin Prevents adherence of bacteria and viruses to mucosae
IgE	0.001%	Opposes helminth infection Binds to mast cells and allergens, releasing mediators	Allergy
IgD	0.02% (on surfaces of B cells)	Unknown	–

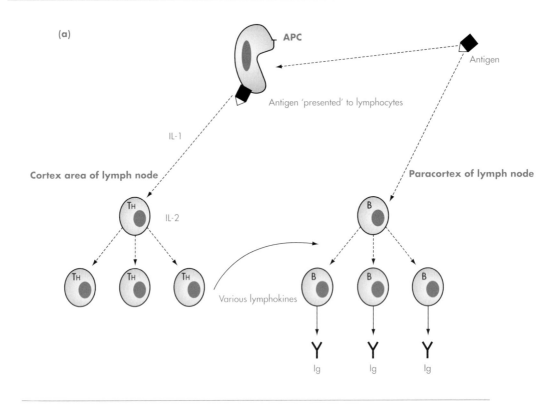

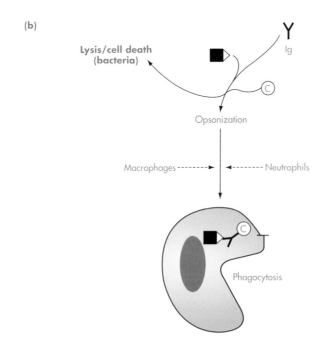

Figure 2.3 Aspects of humoral immunity. (a) Production of immunoglobulins (b) Combined actions of antigen, immunoglobulin and complement lead to opsonization and to lysis or phagocytosis of foreign antigens. APC, antigen-presenting cell; B, B lymphocytes; C, complement; Ig, immunoglobulin; IL, interleukin; TH, T helper cell.

genes). Because genes from each region can be spliced to any genes from the other regions, there is a huge number of possible VDJ combinations capable of producing different Igs. These are sufficient to meet a lifetime challenge of up to 10^9 environmental antigens. The plasma cells so produced are terminally committed, being capable of producing only a single Ig. This antigenic stimulation causes the correct complementary type of B cell to undergo clonal expansion under the influence of IL-4, IL-5 and IL-6 to produce a reservoir of **plasma cells**, all of which are capable of producing the same Ig against one antigenic determinant.

When the antigen is presented to B cells belonging to the correct clone, the B cells multiply and mature into plasma cells, which produce the appropriate Ig. Cells belonging to a particular clone can recognize the specific antigen, owing to the presence on the cell surface of the Ig that it will eventually synthesize, i.e. the Ig acts as a surface receptor, in addition to free circulation in the blood. Reaction between antigen and the Ig receptor acts as a signal for the clone to proliferate under the influence of a cytokine. A microorganism may activate a number of clones, but a specific epitope of an antigen will only stimulate a single clone, to produce **monoclonal antibodies**. Purified preparations of the latter are an important research tool, e.g. as reagents for identifying microorganisms, proteins, types of cancer cell, etc. They also have useful clinical applications, such as immunosuppression to prevent graft rejection, where the monoclonal humanized antibodies *basiliximab* and *daclizumab* (antilymphocyte globulins) have been raised against the T-lymphocytes causing graft rejection. The same principle is being investigated for the treatment of a variety of autoimmune diseases by using monoclonal antibodies against CD4 molecules, which are antigenic, to inhibit TH cell function.

The monoclonal antibodies *rituximab* and *alemtuzumab*, which cause B cell lysis, are used to treat some forms of **lymphoma** (B cell malignancies) and **leukaemia**, respectively. Further, the anti-interleukin 1 monoclonal antibody *anakinra* is being evaluated for the treatment of refractory RA (see Chapter 12), in association with *methotrexate*.

Fab fragments (see Figure 2.4 and below) of monoclonal antibodies that can complex *digoxin*, e.g. *Digibind*, have been used for some time to treat overdoses of this drug. The use of Fab fragments in the treatment of cancer has been less successful, because penetration of the antibody fragment into the tumour mass appears to be a limiting factor.

Ig production is modulated by TH and TS cells, which respectively promote and suppress Ig production. This introduces the concept of **immune tolerance**, i.e. when potentially antigenic material fails to elicit an immune response. Natural tolerance to host (self) tissues is acquired during fetal development. The mechanisms by which the immune system distinguishes between 'self' and 'non-self' depend on the recognition of 'self'-defining CD clusters, which are HLA class I molecules (see p. 44). Failure of the body to recognize self-antigens causes a variety of **autoimmune diseases**. An acquired tolerance to other antigens can also be induced later in life if the body is subjected to carefully graded, progressively larger doses of antigen. This is the basis of **hyposensitization therapy** for allergic diseases, although this technique has limited therapeutic application because it is potentially hazardous. Hyposensitization therapy should be undertaken only when full resuscitation facilities, including *adrenaline* (epinephrine) injection, are

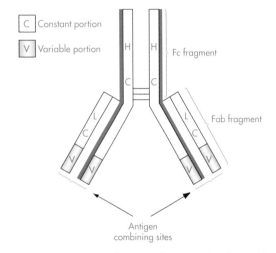

Figure 2.4   Structural diagram of gamma-globulin (IgG). C, constant region (the same in all IgGs); H, heavy chain; L, light chain; V, variable region (different in each IgG).

available, although new, less hazardous approaches are being explored.

Unfortunately, tolerance to non-genetically identical organ transplants is never acquired, so recipients require life-long immunosuppression.

Active and passive immunity

Antigenic material can make contact with the host defence system wherever lymphocytes are found, i.e. the bloodstream, lymphatic system and in epithelial tissues. Igs can be detected approximately 2 weeks after the first exposure to an antigen, corresponding to the time required for the B cells to multiply, differentiate into plasma cells and produce sufficient Ig to be capable of detection. This is the **primary response** (Figure 2.5(a)). On subsequent contact with the same antigen, a **secondary response** occurs. Now the memory B cells are triggered to synthesize Igs almost immediately and in far higher concentrations than during the primary response, thus conferring immunity. This is **active immunity** and provides the best form of

prophylaxis against infection, primarily because of the memory functions of B and T cells. Active immunization is given to those at special risk from significant infections, e.g. elderly people (influenza and pneumonia), and healthcare workers who are likely to encounter infected patients.

However, if there is no time to provide active immunization in a non-immune person, **passive immunization** may be appropriate (Figure 2.5(b)). This involves giving preformed Igs against the potential risk. This is less satisfactory than active immunization because the protection lasts only about 30 days before they are eliminated, and there is no memory effect: another contact with the corresponding antigen or microorganism elicits only a primary response.

Thus recently pregnant women who have not had German measles (rubella) as a child, or who have not been immunized against German measles, and have been in contact with a case, would be given (human) *normal immunoglubulin*. This is derived from pooled plasma and

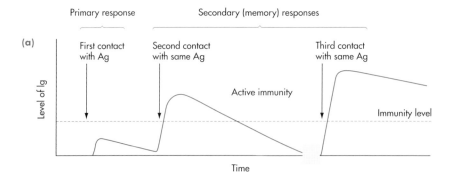

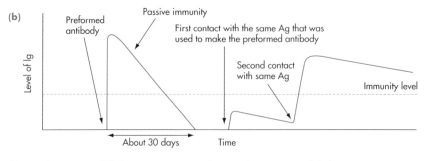

Figure 2.5 Humoral immunity. (a) Active, primary and secondary immunoglobulin responses to antigen, producing long-term memory. (b) Passive, no memory function. Ag, antigen; Ig, immunoglobulin.

contains a range of Igs. Nowadays, routine MMR vaccination should avoid this situation. People bitten by a suspected rabid animal are given *rabies immunoglobulin* immediately, to cover the period required for Ig production, and a course of *rabies vaccine* is started simultaneously. Other Igs available include tetanus, hepatitis B, cytomegalovirus (a herpes virus) and varicella-zoster, the chickenpox and shingles virus.

Passive immunization may also be indicated in immunocompromized individuals. Newborn infants are naturally passively protected by maternal Igs that cross the placenta or are secreted in their mother's milk, thus conferring resistance to infections until their immune systems are sufficiently developed to produce their own active response.

The basic structure of Igs comprises two molecules of two types of polypeptide chain (heavy and light), which together comprise a **crystallizable fragment** (Fc) and an **antigen binding fragment** (Fab). There are five groups of Igs (IgA, IgD, IgE, IgG and IgM), distinguished by the type of heavy chain. The general structure of IgG (also called gamma-globulin), of which there are at least 45 subclasses, is illustrated in Figure 2.4. The Fc portion is responsible for non-specific binding to macrophages or polymorphs and for binding **complement** (see below). The Fab fragment binds to specific antigens and has the highly variable structure responsible for the specificity of Igs. Each Fab fragment is a particular 'lock' that matches just one antigen 'key'. Because there are two Fab fragments in each Ig molecule, each Ig molecule can crosslink common antigens, e.g. the haemagglutinins or neuraminidases of influenza virus (see Chapter 8), neutralizing them, or between two red blood cells, causing clumping.

Igs combine with the antigens, and possibly complement components (see below), a process that **opsonizes** (coats) the antigen, so that phagocytosis can take place more readily. Some antibodies are also directly toxic to cells after subsequent combination with complement. The properties of the Igs are compared in Table 2.4.

All Igs, except IgM, have a similar basic structure to IgG. IgM is a pentamer of IgG, five molecules of which are linked by joining chains. IgM is the first type of Ig to be formed after stimulation and is believed to represent the most primitive form. Because of its large size and multiple Fab sites it is very efficient at causing the clumping (agglutination) of bacteria and other foreign cells, e.g. erythrocytes.

The complement system

This system has already been mentioned in connection with opsonization and will also be encountered later in connection with inflammation. The complement system is part of the innate non-specific immune mechanisms (see above), and a similar process occurs regardless of the type of stimulus.

Some 20–30 different, naturally-occurring plasma proteins make up this system and a simplified outline of the steps involved following its activation is given in Figure 2.6. In practice, the individual complement components, which are mostly enzymes, interact or combine with each other at various stages of the cascade. Note that the components are numbered in the order of their discovery, not in the order in which they react.

C1 is activated by the presence of an immune complex, and then acts as an esterase to cleave C4 into C4a plus C4b, and C2 into C2a plus C2b. The C4b and C2a fragments then combine and cleave C3, which in turn cleaves C5, and the cascade continues as shown. Finally, C8 and C9 bind with C5b67 to form a **membrane attack complex**, which forms an annular transmembrane pore, allowing cell contents to leak from the cell, thus producing cell lysis. This sequence of events is known as the **classical pathway** for complement activation.

Another initiator for the classical pathway is the interaction of mannose-binding lectin with mannose groups on bacterial surfaces. In certain situations, e.g. in some viral infections, the **alternate pathway** may be invoked and C3 can be activated directly without the production of C3a and C3b by the C4b2a convertase.

Two important aspects of the complement system should be noted. First, sequential activation results in amplification of the system. Thus one bimolecule of C3 convertase will produce

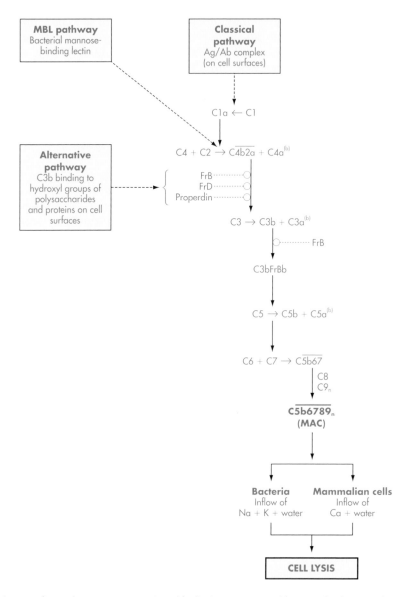

Figure 2.6   Pathways of complement activation (simplified). Ag = antigen, Ab = antibody. 'a' indicates an activated form. [b] These are anaphylatoxins that activate leucocytes and are pro-inflammatory. MAC, membrane attack complex. The C5b678 complex penetrates the plasma membrane and the addition of several molecules of C9 ($C9_n$) forms a pore in it, permitting uncontrolled influx of ions and water, and uncontrolled efflux of cell contents. The bar above the component numbers indicates an active complex, usually enzymic. FrB, FrD, factors B and D ○⋯⋯, promotes or activates.

many C3b molecules, and one molecule of C8 can bind up to six molecules of C9.

Also, many of the individual components of the system have intrinsic immunological and inflammatory properties in their own right.

Overall view of humoral immunity

We can now complete the picture of humoral immunity. After production by plasma cells, an Ig links to its specific antigen via the variable end of the Fab moiety. These **immune complexes** then bind strongly to Fc receptors on the surfaces of phagocytic cells and are then easily drawn into the cell where they can be destroyed in a phago-lysosome.

Antigenic determinants on the cell surfaces of bacteria and other small foreign cells also bind Igs. Complement then binds to the Fc fragments of the Igs, triggering the complement cascade. C3d fragments then become attached to the microbial surface and the microbe is now opsonized. This enables the Fc and C3d fragments to unite with their receptors on phagocytic cells, again facilitating engulfment and destruction.

Although opsonization is the primary mode of action of Igs, they can also act directly on bacteria and foreign erythrocytes, etc. by causing them to clump together (**agglutinate**), especially IgMs. Additionally, certain Igs (antitoxins) can neutralize bacterial toxins.

The overall series of events is illustrated in Figures 2.3 and 2.5.

Cell-mediated immunity

Bacterial, fungal and viral infections may also be combated via CMI, but it is slower-acting than humoral immunity. Even the secondary response (due to memory T cells) may take days to appear. The cells chiefly responsible for CMI are T cells and macrophages. CMI is complementary to humoral immunity. Whether one mechanism comes into play, or both, depends on the precise nature of the stimulus.

Initial contact between a lymphocyte and a cellular antigen causes the proliferation of a clone of sensitized T-lymphocytes similar to the process seen with B cells. Extremely long-lived **memory T cells** are also produced, ensuring that sensitized T cells are available on subsequent exposure to the same antigen. The initial recognition of antigens by T$_H$ cells is achieved by expression of the antigen by an APC, as previously described. CD8+ T cells interact with MHC class I molecules (see p. 45) on APCs and CD4+ T cells with MHC class II molecules. Bacteria eliciting a CMI response are generally the larger ones, e.g. *Mycobacterium tuberculosis*, which tends to form filaments. Fungi such as *Candida albicans*

are also dealt with via CMI. The process in summarized in Figure 2.8(a).

CMI can also combat viral infections if the virus has altered the surface of the cell it has invaded, so as to confer new antigenic properties on the cell. This commonly occurs because the viral genome directs the production of new viral compounds that migrate to the plasma membrane of the host cell, affecting its surface structures. The infected cell is then recognized as foreign via antigen-specific T cells interacting with MHC class I molecules on the infected host cell surface (Figure 2.8(b)) and is attacked by T$_C$ cells. Some cancer cells may be prevented similarly from proliferation, or may be eliminated at a very early stage, if the neoplastic change renders them recognizable as 'foreign' by the immune system (see Chapter 10).

Interleukins also play an important part in the process of stimulating the various cell types involved in CMI. For instance, IL-1 is released from APCs to stimulate T$_H$ cells to produce IL-2, which in turn stimulates T$_C$ cells. Furthermore, some cytokines produced by T$_H$ cells are able to stimulate and attract macrophages.

Potential problems with the immune system (immunopathology)

If part of the immune system simply fails to work (immunodeficiency), the consequences may be disastrous. In rare cases, the failure is the result of a hereditary lack of a particular immunological process or component. In **hypogammaglobulinaemia** the patient fails to produce adequate levels of Igs because of B cell defects, so children with this condition will suffer recurrent bacterial and other infections. A more dramatic example of hereditary immuno-deficiency is the **severe combined immuno-deficiency syndrome**. There are several variants, e.g. adenosine deaminase deficiency, purine nucleoside phosphorylase deficiency and the production of a common abnormal receptor for interleukins. Children born with these serious forms will fail to thrive. Although Igs can be given, the main problem is with the cell-mediated arm of the immune system because T-lymphocytes fail to

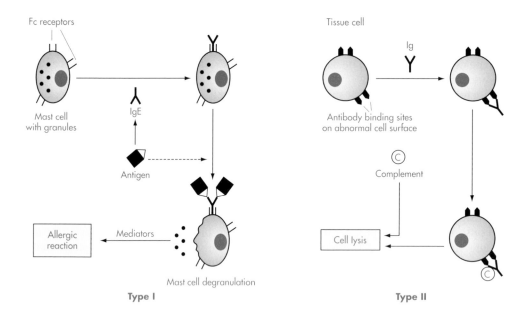

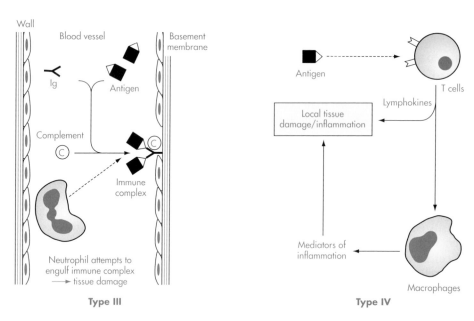

Figure 2.7   Types of hypersensitivity. For type V see text. Fc, crystallizable fragment of immunoglobulin; Ig, immunoglobulin; IgE, immunoglobulin E.

produce cytokines, or respond to them and APCs. The only remedy is to maintain the child until it is capable of undergoing bone marrow transplantation.

Most drugs used to treat cancer suppress tumour growth by inhibiting cell division. An unfortunate side-effect of this is the suppression of the immune system by similarly affecting the bone marrow. This leaves the patient very susceptible to serious infections, often by organisms that are not normally pathogenic, e.g. *Pseudomonas*, *Candida* or *Pneumocystis* (see Chapter 8). Some diseases may also cause immune suppression. The clinical consequences of HIV infection are not only potentially fatal infections but also the occurrence of certain uncommon tumours, e.g. Kaposi's sarcoma, or infections, e.g. *Pneumocystis jiroveci* (formerly known as *P. carinii*). This emphasizes the importance of T cells in limiting the growth of malignancies.

Much of immunopathology is concerned with an inappropriate or maladaptive immune response. For convenience, these have usually been divided into five classes, summarized in Figure 2.7. In each class, humoral or CMI responses (or both) that have already been described are involved, but the responses are often out of proportion to the stimulus eliciting them. Such **hypersensitivity reactions** will result in inflammation, as they all involve some tissue damage, and other symptoms.

Although hypersensitivity is sometimes described as an inappropriate or exaggerated response by the immune system, it is more correctly regarded as a normal immune reaction that happens to damage body tissue. The five classes of hypersensitivity are described below. However, a reaction to a particular stimulus may involve more than one of these, e.g. serum sickness can involve both type I and type II reactions.

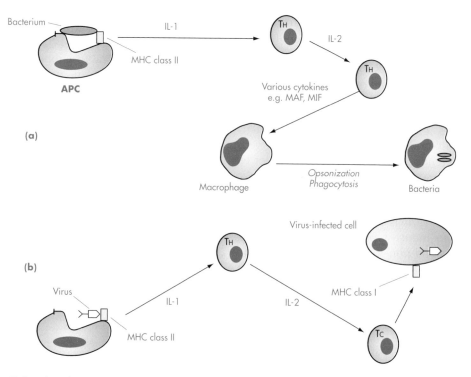

Figure 2.8   Cell-mediated immunity (CMI). (a) Bacteria. (b) Viruses. APC, antigen-presenting cell; IL, interleukin; MAF, macrophage-activating factor; MIF, macrophage migration inhibitory factor; TC, cytotoxic T cell; TH, T helper cell.

Type I: (anaphylactoid) hypersensitivity

Many **allergic** reactions involve the excessive formation of IgE, produced in response to primary contact with an antigen, called in this case an **allergen**. This IgE response by plasma cells is driven by the secretion of IL-4 by TH2 cells. The IgE binds strongly to mast cells by the Fc portion. Subsequent contact with the same allergen results in a reaction between the allergen and bound IgE on the cell surface. The crosslinking of IgE molecules by the allergen destabilizes the mast cell membrane and causes the release of **histamine** and other mediators from preformed granules within its cytoplasm and the production of **bradykinin**. These mediators play an important part in the process of inflammation (see p. 46 and Table 2.7). The consequences of this mediator release can vary from very mild reactions to life-threatening ones. The most extreme form is **anaphylactic shock**, with acute bronchoconstriction, rash, gastrointestinal disturbance, profound hypotension and collapse. Less dramatic anaphylactoid (anaphylactic-type) reactions are asthma, hayfever and eczema. However, the link between these conditions and mast cell degranulation is not always clear.

Children sometimes experience one or more different anaphylactoid reactions, and such individuals are said to be **atopic** (out of place). There is usually a family history of other anaphylactoid conditions, e.g. hayfever and allergic eczema, and positive skin tests to a variety of allergens. Both the tendency to produce high levels of IgE and the presentation of symptoms are genetically determined. Many different allergens trigger this type of reaction, notably pollens and house dust mites. Various classes of drugs also act as haptens to induce type I hypersensitivity, e.g. penicillins and non-steroidal anti-inflammatory drugs (NSAIDs).

Type II: (cytotoxic) hypersensitivity

In this type of reaction, antigens become attached to or are part of cell surfaces. Subsequently, Igs react with the antigens and activate complement, which then causes cell lysis. Complement components (C3a, C5a) may also attract phagocytes, which are unable to engulf the large cells of the body, and so release enzymes that cause much of the damage. In addition, the **NK (natural killer) cells** may have a cytotoxic action on tissue cells. NK cells belong to a group of lymphocytes that are non-phagocytic and neither T nor B type, whose immunological role is to induce lysis or apoptosis (programmed cell death) of virus-infected or otherwise abnormal cells, e.g. cells undergoing neoplastic change.

If the reaction involves red blood cells (RBCs), autoantibodies directed against the red cell surface may cause a **haemolytic anaemia** (see Chapter 11), possibly due to the binding of a foreign molecule to the RBC surface, conferring new antigenic properties on it. *Methyldopa* is well known to be likely to cause the formation of such autoantibodies, which can be detected, although a positive test for these does not always mean that haemolytic anaemia will occur.

Transfusion reactions

These are one form of type II reaction. All RBCs carry A, B or both antigens on their surfaces and the alternative natural anti-B or anti-A antibodies are in the plasma (see Table 2.5). Unusually for immunological reactions, the Igs against blood group antigens are present from birth, even though individuals have not been previously exposed to the foreign blood group, so a reaction will occur on a first transfusion. If a type A individual were to be transfused with whole blood from a type B or type O donor, the anti-A antibodies in the donated blood would haemolyse some of the recipient's red cells. More importantly, *all* the donor red cells would be haemolysed by the anti-B antibodies in the much larger volume of recipient's serum.

Table 2.5   ABO system blood groups

Group	Antigens on erythrocytes	Antibodies in serum	Frequency (UK %)
A	A	Anti-B	45
B	B	Anti-A	8
AB	A + B	None	3
O	None	Anti-A + anti-B	44

Because the objective of transfusing whole blood is to make up for the loss of oxygen-carrying capacity in the recipient, this renders the transfusion ineffective. Rectification of simple volume depletion does not require transfusion of whole blood unless there is also major loss of red cells.

However, the ABO system is not the only one to be considered when matching blood for transfusion. An individual's **Rhesus status** and certain other antigens are also important. The Rhesus system, first discovered in Rhesus monkeys, depends on three pairs of allelic genes, C and c, D and d, E and e, which are inherited as triplets, e.g. CDE or cDe, and code for the corresponding erythrocyte antigens. However, the 'd' antigen does not exist, i.e. d is a null gene, and the most important consideration is whether the D antigen is present or absent, giving RhD+ or RhD− groups. **Haemolytic disease of the newborn** (HDN) occurs when a Rhesus-negative (RhD−) mother has a child by a Rhesus-positive man. The child will always be Rhesus-positive because the D allele is unopposed (and dominant). When the child's RBCs come in contact with the mother's circulation, as happens during birth, the mother will produce anti-RhD antibodies. The child of the first pregnancy will usually be unaffected, but in subsequent pregnancies the mother's anti-RhD Igs cross the placenta to cause fetal or neonatal red cell destruction in the Rhesus-positive child. If no action is taken the fetus is aborted or the child stillborn. This may be prevented by the use of an antiserum containing anti-RhD antibodies, which is administered prophylactically to the mother within 72 h of the first birth. This causes the destruction of any Rhesus-positive fetal erythrocytes reaching the mother's bloodstream so that they cannot stimulate the production of anti-RhD antibodies in the mother. A subsequent pregnancy will then occur normally, similar to a first pregnancy, but anti-RhD serum will be needed after the birth of each child from an RhD+ father.

When blood transfusion is necessary, the potential recipient's ABO and RhD status is determined. Normally, the patient's plasma or serum is tested against the erythrocytes from two or more group O donors. If there is a positive reaction (10% of patients), a comprehensive panel of specific, typed erythrocytes is tested against the patient's plama or serum, to determine the exact cause of the reaction. Full cross-matching involves testing the recipient's serum or plasma directly against the selected donor's erythrocytes, looking for IgMs that cause agglutination, and an indirect Coomb's test (see Chapter 11), to detect IgGs that may cause haemolysis of donor erythrocytes. Occasionally, erythrocyte antigens of the Kell or other uncommon groups give problems.

In an emergency, group O RhD− blood can be used while the recipient's blood group is determined.

Organ transplants, of which blood transfusion is a simple form, can also initiate a type II reaction. Antibodies directed against a transplanted organ and pre-existing in the recipient's blood, possibly due to prior blood transfusions, may contribute to a **hyperacute graft rejection** almost immediately after transplantation (see Chapter 14).

Type III: (immune complex) hypersensitivity

When an antigen combines with an antibody an immune complex is always formed, which is normally cleared by the reticuloendothelial system. Complement may make small complexes soluble within the bloodstream, whereas the larger immune complexes are removed by phagocytes. Small complexes tend to be formed if the antigen is in excess, whereas antibody excess produces larger complexes. Under certain circumstances, relating to the size and number of these complexes, the clearance mechanisms are overwhelmed and circulating levels of immune complexes may increase. These become trapped in body tissues and often penetrate blood vessel walls and attach to the basement membrane that separates the endothelial cells from the other tissues of the vessel wall.

Subsequent complement activation causes recruitment and activation of neutrophils which release enzymes that cause collateral damage to the vessel wall and inflammation. In addition, platelets adhere to the inflamed site and initiate the clotting cascade, sometimes causing complete occlusion of smaller vessels.

A similar situation may occur in the skin if an antigen is injected intradermally. The resulting localized inflammation, known as an Arthus reaction, reaches its peak after 4–10 h. Its intensity is greatest when antigen and antibody are present in approximately equivalent amounts. The Arthus reaction is made use of in the skin test for tubercular antigens (Mantoux test; see below).

In the kidney, antigenic material from streptococcal infections is responsible for some forms of **glomerulonephritis** (see Chapter 14), in which the immune complexes lodge in the basement membranes of the glomeruli. Immune complex tissue deposition is also involved in some autoimmune diseases, e.g. **systemic lupus erythematosus** (SLE, see Chapter 12) and **rheumatoid arthritis** (RA, see Chapter 12), which explains the multisystem damage seen in these conditions.

In the early days of immunotherapy, large doses of antiserum (antitoxin) produced in immunized horses were used to treat infections such as diphtheria and tetanus. However, horse Igs are antigenic in humans and induce antibody formation. The resultant immune complex of horse antitoxin and human antibody led to the development of a systemic type III reaction known as **serum sickness**. Consequently, antisera produced in horses are now used only rarely. Instead, human or humanized Igs are used, with a much lower risk of an anaphylactoid reaction. Human normal immunoglobulin (HNIG), which contains a range of Igs, is used to protect non-immune contacts of patients with hepatitis A, measles and rubella. Other specific Igs are also used (see above). These carry a far lower risk of serum sickness but there is always the possibility of transmitting unsuspected viruses, although precautions are taken against this.

When antigenic material is inhaled, immune complexes may form in the lung alveoli. Thus in farmer's lung and bird fancier's lung (see Chapter 5) spores from mouldy hay, and feather and bird droppings and feather dust respectively, form immune complexes with IgGs in the alveoli, causing **extrinsic allergic alveolitis** with a delayed (about 8 h) allergic type of response to antigen inhalation. Repeated episodes lead eventually to a form of irreversible **restrictive airways disease** (see Chapter 5).

Type IV: cell-mediated (delayed) hypersensitivity

Antibody production plays the major role in all of the three types of hypersensitivity so far described. These reactions occur fairly rapidly, often within minutes to a few hours after contact with the antigen.

However, in some manifestations of hypersensitivity, symptoms may not occur for days or even weeks after antigenic exposure. This is seen quite frequently in **allergic contact dermatitis** (see Chapter 13) where the allergen, such as a metal earring or a watch-strap, may have been in contact with the skin for some time before any inflammation is observed. This type of reaction also plays a role in pulmonary TB and leprosy, both caused by *Mycobacterium* species. The process is similar to that discussed under CMI (Figure 2.8). The production of sensitized cytotoxic T cells plays a central role, but as they take more than 12 h to appear in the bloodstream the term **delayed hypersensitivity** is often used to describe this type of reaction. The lymphokines released by the sensitized T cells contribute directly to the overall tissue damage and recruit macrophages, which release lysosomal products and enzymes, causing further tissue damage. The result is **chronic inflammation**, often leading to the formation of scar tissue to repair the damaged area (p. 56).

TB exemplifies the link between this class of hypersensitivity and chronic inflammation. The actual tissue damage in the lung and formation of the tubercle (a granuloma) are not caused directly by the bacteria but by the body's attempts to deal with it via CMI. In the Mantoux test, a purified protein extract of tubercle bacilli (tuberculin) is injected intradermally. In individuals previously sensitized to the mycobacterium by infection or immunization, a CMI hypersensitivity reaction causes inflammation at the injection site, the result being read 72 h after injection. The induration and red weal sometimes persist for up to a year. Because of this hypersensitivity a Mantoux test should always be performed before Bacillus Calmette–Guérin (BCG) vaccination, because immunization of tuberculin-positive subjects would result in an extensive, deforming, local inflammatory reaction. However, no licensed tuberculin product is currently available in the UK.

Other stimuli eliciting this type of hypersensitivity include insect bites, fungal infections and certain chemical haptens.

Type V: (stimulating/blocking) hypersensitivity

The mechanism of this is completely different from those of the previous forms of hyper-sensitivity. In the best-known example, **Graves' disease** (see Chapter 9), the reaction is autoimmune, IgG being raised against the thyroid-stimulating hormone (TSH) receptors in the thyroid gland. The IgG has a similar effect to TSH, stimulating the thyroid cells to secrete excessive amounts of thyroid hormones, resulting in hyperthyroidism and causing the pathognomonic sign of 'staring eyes' (exophthalmos). The latter is the result of inflammation of the oculomotor muscles, caused by a cross-reaction between the anti-receptor IgG and a component in the muscles.

Because some bacteria, e.g. *Escherichia coli*, possess surface structures mimicking the TSH receptor, it is possible that the initiating event is infective. *E. coli* is ubiquitous and this may explain why Graves' disease is the commonest cause of thyrotoxicosis.

In other situations, uptake of Ig on receptors may block the normal response to receptor activity.

Autoimmune disease

In this most extreme form of maladaptation, the body turns its immunological defences against its own tissues. This can involve any of the types of hypersensitivity reaction described above and causes a wide variety of diseases. However, the immunopathological mechanisms for many of the autoimmune diseases are not well understood, and may involve more than one type of immune response. In general, autoimmune diseases may be associated with a number of different underlying abnormalities.

Sometimes, as in **allergic contact dermatitis** (see Chapter 13), normal proteins may be altered and rendered antigenic by reaction with haptens. The attachment of drugs such as *methyldopa* to RBCs may induce the formation of autoantibodies by altering red cell surface proteins. Similarly, virus infections may alter the expression of surface proteins of the cells they infect, leading to a failure of self-recognition, although their exact role in autoimmunity is still uncertain. The **autoimmune haemolytic anaemias** (see Chapter 11) may be due to hypersensitivity, but the condition often accompanies other autoimmune diseases.

If a protein is normally sequestered within a cell or tissue, and thus not exposed to the immune system, it follows that tolerance cannot develop and if such cells subsequently encounter the immune system, they will be recognized as 'non-self'. Spermatozoa are one example, and **mumps orchitis** (inflammation of the testes caused by the mumps virus) may result in the abnormal contact between spermatozoa and the immune system, leading to testicular inflammation and infertility. Similarly, trauma to one eye that breaches the circulation sometimes results in **sympathetic ophthalmitis** and destruction of the other eye.

Antibodies produced against a pathogen may occasionally cross-react with normal healthy tissue. The organisms most often associated with this type of problem are certain types of streptococci, especially in **rheumatic fever** (see Chapters 4 and 12). Although this disease is less common since the introduction of penicillin and with improved living conditions, the late complications are still sometimes encountered among the older population. The intense pain and inflammation of the joints experienced after an untreated streptococcal sore throat result from the formation of an antibody that is active against both the organism and synovial membranes. Presumably the surface proteins of the streptococci bear some resemblance to those of certain human tissues. A more serious and long-term problem is the damage caused to cardiac tissues by these Igs. The effects on heart valves will eventually lead to impairment of cardiac function that may become apparent only in later life.

By far the largest group of autoimmune diseases is caused by a breakdown in self-tolerance. In many diseases of uncertain aetiology the immune system has failed to recognize certain tissues as 'self'. We have seen that the immune system normally distinguishes 'self' from 'non-self' by the nature of the cell surface, because surface proteins, principally MHC type I molecules (see below), determine a cell's antigenic properties. There are two possible broad mechanisms for developing a lack of tolerance: the immune system may fail to recognize these surface proteins as being 'self' or, owing to an intrinsic property of the surface proteins, there is a tendency for them to become antigenic under certain circumstances. The reasons for the development of autoimmunity in any particular disease are usually unknown, so they are described as **idiopathic**. An understanding of the human leucocyte antigen (HLA) system, described below, goes some way towards clarifying the problem. If failure of self-recognition is responsible, subsequent defects in T cell regulation may give rise to an autoimmune reaction, e.g. in **SLE** (see Chapter 12), which is characterized by the development of autoantibodies to nucleoproteins.

There are other examples in which autoantibodies, possibly resulting from defective T cell regulation, play a major role. **Hashimoto's thyroiditis** (see Chapter 9) is a well-known autoimmune disease in which the antibodies produced attack both thyroid cells and thyroglobulin, causing hypothyroidism (see Chapter 9). Similarly, almost all patients with **pernicious anaemia** (see Chapter 11) possess anti-parietal cell autoantibodies and 50% also have antibodies against intrinsic factor.

The role of Igs is less certain in other autoimmune diseases. RA is often associated with the production of IgMs, known collectively as **rheumatoid factor**. These do not attack the synovial membrane directly but combine with IgG to form immune complexes that subsequently trigger the complement cascade and cause joint inflammation. The monoclonal antibody *infliximab*, a TNFα inhibitor, and other similar agents are used in severe rheumatoid disease (see Chapter 12).

Although **inflammatory bowel disease** (see Chapter 3) and the **seronegative arthropathies** (see Chapter 12) have a possible autoimmune aetiology, no autoantibodies have been identified, although *infliximab* may also be valuable in these conditions, which possess strong associations with certain HLA types (see below). **Insulin-dependent (Type 1) diabetes** (see Chapter 9), **myasthenia gravis** and **multiple sclerosis** also have an autoimmune basis.

Increasing numbers of diseases are thought to involve autoimmunity, and our understanding of the mechanisms involved, although imperfect, is improving. With greater knowledge of the immune mechanisms and the various trigger factors involved, prophylactic measures and better treatments are gradually becoming available.

The Major Histocompatibility Complex and the HLA system

The limiting factor in organ transplantation is the phenomenon of **rejection**. The transplanted organ is recognized as 'non-self' and the immune system is activated to attack it. However, transplantation between identical twins never causes rejection, although problems may still arise due to adverse technical factors, e.g. infection, leakage of the donor ureter to recipient bladder anastomosis in renal transplantation (see Chapter 14). The chances of success are reduced in inverse relation to the closeness of the relationship between donor and recipient. If the recipient is a sibling, the success rate may be as high as 80–90%, but this falls to 60% or less between unrelated individuals, even though strenuous efforts are made to find a suitable match. This is because there are surface antigens on the cells of transplanted organs that are genetically determined and can be recognized by the immune system of the recipient (host) as foreign. There must be a finite, but large, variety of these groups of antigens because transplants between unrelated individuals do not always lead to rejection.

These surface antigens are described as histocompatibility antigens, determined by the **major**

histocompatibility complex (MHC), a cluster of genes found on chromosome 6 in man. These specify surface antigen clusters that are unique to each individual and are present on all nucleated cells of the body. They are termed **human leucocyte antigens** (HLAs) because they were originally discovered on the surfaces of human leucocytes, and the antigens themselves are trans-plasma membrane glycoproteins with the physiological role of enabling the immune system to recognize them as 'self', thus not mounting an immune reaction against them. All nucleated cells possess class I MHC molecules (see below); class II molecules are found only on B-lymphocytes and APCs.

Unfortunately, the terminology is rather confusing. The MHC complex is composed of **gene clusters**. MHC gene products are the **HLA antigens**. However, **MHC molecules** are not the genes, which would be logical, but are the same as **HLA antigens**. Further, some textbooks refer to **HLA genes**, which are synonymous with MHC genes. To avoid confusion with other texts the HLA surface antigens are described here as **MHC molecules**, which has the widest use. Apart from this usage, MHC refers to genes and HLA to antigens in this text.

There are six important MHC gene loci. Any individual may possess two of a number of possible gene types (alleles) from each locus, each gene expressing a particular MHC molecule. The A, B and C regions code for **MHC class I molecules** and the three D region genes (DP, DQ and DR) code for MHC class II molecules. A third region codes for certain complement factors, sometimes referred to as class III molecules. Each gene locus is therefore identified by a letter, and the individual alleles within each series are given a number, e.g. A1–A41, although these numbers are not necessarily consecutive. New genes (and therefore antigens) are constantly being discovered and are at first given the letter W, e.g. Dw3, to denote that their existence has yet to be officially recognized. It is also common for certain antigens to occur together, a phenomenon known as **linkage disequilibrium**. Thus DR3 and B8 will occur together more frequently than might be expected from chance alone. Also some types are more common in certain races, e.g. A1 is less common in black-skinned Africans, and Bw6 is only found in mongoloid races.

MHC class I molecules play an important part in the recognition of cells that have been affected by viruses, as such cells express viral antigens on their surface. These are attacked by T cells only in the presence of an MHC molecule, possibly because T cell binding sites are not occupied by free viral antigens, maximizing the T cell potential for attacking infected cells. Class II molecules are important in the recognition by T cells of antigens taken up by APCs.

The HLA system therefore explains transplant rejection and some blood (leucocyte) groups. Only transplants between individuals with identical HLA antigens can be performed without recourse to immunosuppressive therapy. A high degree of HLA matching, short of identity but permitting a good chance of transplant success, is likely to occur only between close relatives. Most transplants are matched for A, B and DR antigens, but a single mismatch, i.e. MHC molecules not possessed by the recipient but possessed by the donor, may have to be accepted (see Chapter 14).

The link between the HLA system and disease, in particular autoimmune disease, has a wider significance. Some known associations between the occurrence of certain HLA types and various diseases are listed in Table 2.6. However, with the exception of narcolepsy, this represents only an increased risk of developing the disease, e.g. there is a strong link between HLA-B27 and **ankylosing spondylitis** (see Chapter 12), and those individuals who carry the B27 gene have a higher risk of developing this disease than those without it. Whether or not they do so depends on other factors, such as contact with an exogenous trigger, e.g. infection or a dietary toxin.

HLA antigens are also associated with some adverse drug reactions, e.g. HLA DR4 with SLE (see Chapter 12) due to *hydralazine*, a drug that is used occasionally for treating hypertension.

Some differences in **drug handling** are also specified by autosomal genes, i.e. there are two alternative genes (alleles), one from each parent, coded for at the same chromosomal locus. The gene for **fast acetylation** is dominant to that for **slow acetylation**, so slow acetylators are homozygous for the recessive

Table 2.6   Some associations between HLA and disease

Disease	Gene coding for antigen	Relative risk (%)
Narcolepsy[a]	DR2	100
Ankylosing spondylitis	B27	87.8
Reiter's disease	B27	35.9
Rheumatoid arthritis	DRw4	4.0
Multiple sclerosis[a]	A3	1.8
	B7	2.0
	Bw2	1.9
	DRw2	3.8
Myasthenia gravis[a]	B8	3.4
	DRw3	3.0
Psoriasis	A1	2.1
	B13	8.7
	Bw37	8.1
	Cw6	4.3
Addison's disease[a]	Dw3	8.8
Graves' disease	B8	2.5
	Bw35	5.0
	Dw3	5.5
Coeliac disease	B8	8.6
	Dw3	73.0
Autoimmune hepatitis	B8	9.2
	DR3	4.6

[a] These conditions are not described in this text.

gene whereas fast acetylators may be either homozygous for the dominant, fast acetylation gene, or heterozygous.

The link between HLA antigens and autoimmunity could involve cross-reactions between 'self' antigens and a microorganism or an environmental antigen, resulting in immunological activity directed against body tissues. It is known that there is a cross-reaction between HLA groups and certain *Escherichia coli* and other bacterial antigens and this is a possible, though unproven, explanation for some autoimmune diseases, e.g. Graves' disease, type 1 diabetes mellitus (see Chapter 9) and SLE. Several other explanations have been proposed, although a single cohesive theory has yet to be established. It has been suggested that some HLA groups may bind antigens more avidly than others, resulting in a more intense reaction, or that possession of a particular HLA group may involve an increased immunological response to a particular antigen. It has also been proposed that in some cases there may be an inappropriate expression of MHC class II molecules on tissues where they are not normally found.

Inflammation

Definition

This important pathological process is defined as the 'reaction of the living microcirculation and its contents to injury'. The term **microcirculation** describes the system of small vessels (arterioles, venules and capillaries) supplying the tissues with blood, within which are the various classes of leucocytes important in the inflammatory process. The injury can be any sort of damage to tissues, i.e. traumatic, heat, radiation, immunological or infectious (Figure 2.9).

The function of an inflammatory reaction is to limit and eventually resolve any such injury. In physical injury, direct damage to vascular tissue initiates the reaction. Following infection, the immune system is responsible for detecting the invader and initiating the inflammatory process, but the growth of microorganisms within tissues may also cause some physical damage, e.g. necrosis. Sometimes, inappropriate stimulation of the immune system initiates the reaction, as in autoimmune disease, or hypersensitivity reactions, e.g. to pollen in hayfever. An important function of the vascular responses in inflammation is to facilitate the access of blood-borne defence mechanisms to the site of injury. In physical injury these defences may simply function to prevent blood loss by clotting, followed by healing and repair. With infection, Igs or T-lymphocytes in the blood must gain access to enable them to deal with the infection, before healing can take place.

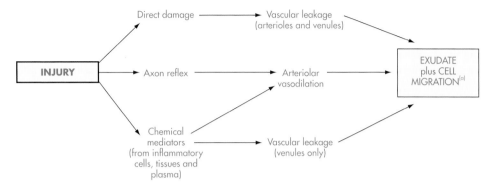

Figure 2.9   Effects of injury on the microcirculation. [a]See Figures 2.10 and 2.11.

Acute inflammation

The stages and processes involved in acute inflammation are readily seen if the forearm is scratched with some force. Almost immediately, a narrow red line will be seen on the skin along the line of the scratch. This is quickly followed by a more diffuse reddening around the line of injury and the red area will later become slightly raised. This sequence of events is the **Lewis triple response**, the three components of which are flush (central red area), flare (more diffuse red area) and weal (raised area). Furthermore, the inflamed area is somewhat warmer than the surrounding skin and, if the scratch was too vigorous, pain will also be experienced. This skin reaction displays the four so-called cardinal signs of inflammation, i.e. redness, heat, swelling and pain, described by Celsus in the first century AD. If the injury has been excessive a fifth sign, loss of function, may occur. Two important points should be noted: the same sequence of events occurs no matter what the cause of the injury, and the reaction is similar whatever the precise nature of the damage and which tissue is involved. However, the nature of any functional impairment would clearly depend on the organ involved.

The triple response resolves completely in a few hours and is therefore a simple example of **acute inflammation**, the major pathological features of which are hyperaemia, exudation and leucocyte migration. If the inflammation is inappropriate, particularly when the cause is immunological, or the reaction is out of proportion to the damage caused by the stimulus or persists when the stimulus is removed, it becomes maladaptive and pathological. Because tissue damage plays a large part in many disease processes it is not surprising that many diseases have an underlying inflammatory pathology. Such conditions or diseases are normally suffixed with 'itis', e.g. dermatitis is inflammation of the skin, arthritis is inflammation of the joints.

Hyperaemia

An essential function of inflammation is to provide an increased blood flow to the damaged area, facilitating the transport of agents involved in defence or repair. After a brief reflex vasoconstriction, and possibly also clotting to minimize local bleeding, the local arterioles dilate, flushing the capillary network with blood (Figure 2.9). Substance P may be the neuropeptide transmitter released from nerve endings to initiate this part of the response. This involvement of the nervous system may partly explain the emotional link often observed with exacerbations of certain inflammatory conditions, e.g. eczema and ulcerative colitis. A more diffuse and prolonged vasodilatation is achieved by the release of chemical mediators. Table 2.2 lists some common cytokines and it is clear that their effects explain the redness and heat associated with inflammation: the rise in local temperature is partly the result of an increase in local blood flow and partly of a higher metabolic rate in the inflamed area.

Exudation

The swelling observed is caused by leakage of blood plasma through the vessel wall into the tissue interstitial space, causing oedema (see Figures 2.10 and 4.9). In normal capillaries the hydrostatic pressure of the blood forces fluid into the interstitial space. This pressure is partly offset by the **oncotic pressure** exerted by plasma proteins, which are too large to pass through normal capillary walls and so are retained in the bloodstream. In inflammation this balance is upset. Arterial vasodilatation results in an increased capillary hydrostatic pressure and hence an increased volume of interstitial fluid.

In addition, the endothelial junctions of the capillary walls become leaky and allow some plasma proteins to enter the tissue space, thus increasing tissue oncotic pressure and further facilitating the movement of fluid from the blood to the interstitial space. A more diffuse vascular leakage from venules distant from the site of injury, adding to the exudate volume, is caused by chemical mediators. The exudation, which results in tissue swelling, is offset by an increase in lymphatic drainage, which returns the exudates to the blood via the lymph nodes and the lymphatic ducts. However, if micro-organisms are the inflammatory trigger, the infection can spread into the lymphatic system resulting in **lymphangitis** (inflamed lymph vessels) and **lymphadenopathy** (swollen, possibly tender, lymph nodes). A more general

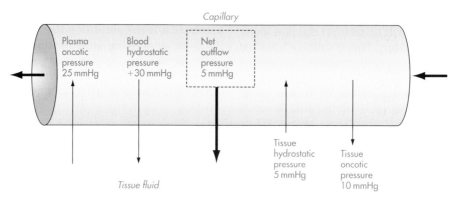

Normal: net outflow pressure to tissues about 5 mmHg

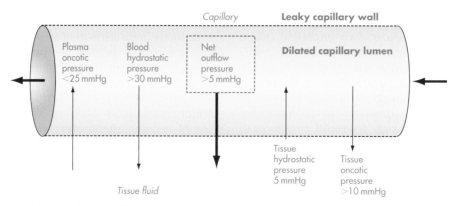

Inflammation: net outflow pressure to tissues increased

Figure 2.10   Exudation from capillaries.

account of oedema is given in Chapter 4 and Figure 4.9.

Some of the pain experienced in local inflammation may also be due to swelling, which stretches capillary walls and associated nerves.

The increased blood flow to the region and the exudation bring antibodies to the site of infection and dilutes any bacterial or other toxins. Exudation may also carry fibrinogen into the tissues that, on conversion to insoluble fibrin by the action of thrombin, stabilizes any blood clots (see Chapter 11).

Although blood clotting is essential if physical trauma has resulted in haemorrhage, fibrin deposition in other circumstances may cause more problems than it resolves. The initial exudate is a clear, cell-free fluid but eventually WBCs will appear in the exudate, attracted to the site by chemokines, particularly in the presence of infection.

Various forms of exudation can occur that may have important consequences should the inflammation fail to resolve quickly. The clear exudate seen under a blister is known as **serous exudate**, whereas the thick, protein-rich exudate from mucous membranes, e.g. a runny nose, is termed **mucinous**. If WBCs enter the exudate, as described below, it is described as **purulent**. Often a mixed picture is seen, with microorganisms, leucocytes and damaged tissue fragments producing a **mucopurulent** exudate (pus).

Leucocyte migration

Humoral and cell-mediated immunity are not the only mechanisms of defence against microorganisms; WBCs of all classes are also involved. The **neutrophils (polymorphonuclear leucocytes)** are responsible for engulfing and digesting microorganisms. These migrate from the bloodstream to the site of inflammation (Figure 2.11) and are the first to appear in an acutely inflamed area.

Loss of fluid from the bloodstream as a result of exudation increases blood viscosity locally and reduces its flow rate. The leucocytes, which are normally distributed evenly throughout the blood, then tend to collect along the endothelium outside the central axial stream (**margination**), where they adhere and, by mechanisms

not fully understood, squeeze through the junctions between endothelial cells and enter the tissue space. This movement of leucocytes is known as **diapedesis**.

Leucocytes are attracted to the site of inflammation by chemotaxins, some of which are components of the complement system (C3a, C5a). Certain bacteria, e.g. staphylococci and *Klebsiella*, also seem to exert a highly chemotactic effect, attracting very large numbers of neutrophils to the site of infection. Neutrophils then engulf and digest the microorganisms, particles of tissue debris, etc. During phagocytosis, proteolytic enzymes may be released from the lysosomes within WBCs, causing further local damage. After a day or so the number of neutrophils falls, to be replaced by macrophages.

Systemic inflammation

The preceding discussion has considered examples of local inflammation. The acute inflammatory response does not normally involve general activation of the immune system and is restricted to a specific organ or tissue. In systemic inflammation the reaction is more widespread and involves stimulation of the immune system. This is seen especially if an infection reaches the general circulation, i.e. **septicaemia**. RA is a good example of systemic inflammatory disease: the main problem for the patient may be with the joints, but there is a general inflammatory process involving many other parts of the body remote from the affected joints (see Chapter 12).

The clinical features usually accompanying systemic inflammation include:

- a raised neutrophil count (neutrophil leucocytosis);
- raised body temperature (pyrexia, fever);
- lethargy and tiredness;
- anaemia, seen especially in the more chronic systemic inflammatory conditions such as RA, SLE and **polmyalgia rheumatica** (Chapter 12).

The acute phase response involves the hepatic production of increased amounts of large proteins, e.g. fibrinogen, alpha$_1$-antitrypsin (see Chapter 5), C-reactive protein, and serum amyloid-associated protein (SAA). There is also increased synthesis of Igs, the shift from normal

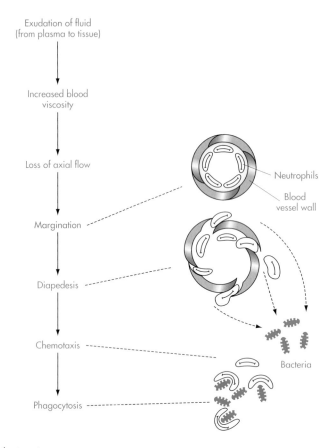

Figure 2.11   Neutrophil migration.

hepatic protein synthesis of albumin to Igs being mediated by IL-6, activated by IL-1.

This change in blood proteins causes changes in the physicochemical properties of the RBCs and the plasma, raising the **erythrocyte sedimentation rate (ESR)**. If anticoagulated blood is placed in a glass tube, the RBCs tend to clump and sediment to the bottom. The greater the clumping the faster the sedimentation; the length of the column of clear supernatant plasma remaining after 1 h (in mm) gives the ESR, normally <20 mm/h. This is therefore a non-specific sign of systemic inflammation and/or immune stimulation, which can be determined at the bedside if necessary. However, the rate of sedimentation is also affected by the haemoglobin (Hb) concentration, age and sex, being higher in females. An alternative is to measure the plasma viscosity, which is a more direct measure of the concentration of acute

phase proteins and can be determined within 15 min of taking the sample.

An alternative to the ESR is to measure C-reactive protein (CRP), the level of which is increased by the action of IL-1 on the liver. This is measured by an automated immunoassay and is less affected by variables than the ESR. It rises rapidly, within less than 6 h of the onset of fever, inflammation and in trauma, but is less useful than the ESR for monitoring chronic inflammatory conditions.

Inflammatory mediators

The list of chemical mediators believed to be involved in the various stages of inflammation increases inexorably. The following is a brief review (see also Table 2.7 and the References and further reading section, p. 63).

Table 2.7   Some mediators involved in inflammation

Mediator	Source	Effect
Vasoactive amines		
• histamine	Mast cells	Vascular dilatation
• serotonin	Platelets	Vascular leakage
Platelet activating factor	Various WBCs	Chemotaxis
IL 8	Monocytes Lymphocytes	Chemotaxis
CRP (an 'acute phase protein')	Liver	Opsonization
Prostaglandins and leukotrienes	Phospholipid membranes of tissue cells	Vascular leakage Chemotaxis Pain Anti-inflammatory
Vasoactive polypeptides	Plasma	Vascular dilatation Vascular leakage Pain
Complement	Plasma	Chemotaxis Vascular leakage Cell lysis Opsonization

IL, Interleukin; CRP, C-reactive protein; WBC, white blood cell.

Mediators can be classified according to whether they are derived from tissue or plasma. The principal tissue-derived mediators are the **prostaglandins (PGs)** and **vasoactive amines** (histamine and serotonin). Histamine is widely distributed in the body, particularly in specialized white cells resident in tissue called **mast cells**. Release of preformed histamine from cytoplasmic granules in mast cells is important in type I hypersensitivity reactions. Platelet activation by **platelet activating factor (PAF)** causes the release of serotonin, ADP and thromboxane A2 (Tx A$_2$). ADP release causes a conformational change in the platelet fibrinogen receptor, the glycoprotein GPIIb-IIIa complex, enabling platelets to bind to fibrinogen, leading eventually to the formation of a stable fibrin plug. This effect is complemented by the action of TX A$_2$, a potent vasoconstrictor, causing reduced blood flow and reduced blood loss (see Chapter 11).

There are many types of PGs, which are derived from the action of cyclo-oxygenase enzymes on arachidonic acid formed from membrane phospholipids (see Chapter 12). The most important PGs involved in inflammation are PGE$_2$ and PGI$_2$. Together with the **thromboxanes**, also derived from arachidonic acid, these constitute the class of mediators known as the **acidic lipids** (see Chapter 12).

A further group of mediators, derived from arachidonic acid via the 5-lipoxygenase pathway, are the **leukotrienes (LTs)**: the previously termed Slow Reacting Substance of Anaphylaxis (SRSA) is a mixture of LT mediators. Two leukotriene receptor antagonists (LTRAs), *montelukast* and *zafirlukast*, have been developed for the treatment of asthma (see Chapter 5).

The other two major classes of mediators, the **vasoactive polypeptides** (e.g. **bradykinins**, Figure 2.12) and complement, are both derived from plasma. The complement system (Figure 2.6) is most commonly activated by infection. The C3a and C5a fragments seem to be the most active in the inflammatory process, and the C5a

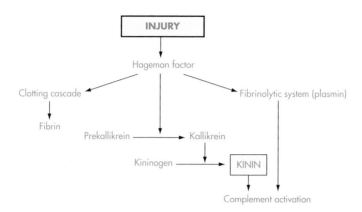

Figure 2.12   Vasoactive polypeptides and their relationship to the blood clotting/fibrinolytic system (see Chapter 11).

fragment also appears to initiate histamine release. The actions of both kinins and histamine are potentiated by PGs.

There is thus a highly sophisticated system of interactions that enable the body to initiate and maintain the inflammatory reaction long enough to deal adequately with the original injury and also to switch it off when the response is no longer required. Histamine and serotonin are responsible for the initial reaction, but their effect is short-lived, about 2 h. The reaction is then maintained by the kinins. PGs may extend the reaction still further, although their main role is probably to control the extent and intensity of the process, because certain classes of PGs have been shown to be anti-inflammatory. Lysosomal enzymes released from neutrophils may further help to maintain the reaction. The close links between the inflammatory and immunological processes ensure that invading microorganisms and environmental antigens are usually dealt with effectively. The blood clotting/fibrinolytic system also aids in the healing process.

The relative importance of particular mediators may vary between tissues. Thus, rhinitis and hayfever seem largely, but not entirely, mediated by histamine, but this plays only a minor role in asthma.

The therapeutic agents employed to modify the inflammatory process usually interfere with the action of the chemical mediators. The **anti-histamines** have a limited, and in many cases short-lived, activity. Two widely used classes of anti-inflammatory agents act by inhibition of PG production. These are the **corticosteroids**, which inhibit the conversion of phospholipids to arachidonic acid, and the **NSAIDs** (see Chapter 12), which inhibit cyclo-oxygenase activity. The corticosteroids are the most potent anti-inflammatory drugs available and are effective in controlling most types of inflammation, although they have a delayed onset of action. The NSAIDs have been used extensively to treat rheumatoid diseases (see Chapter 12) and as analgesics, but are reported to increase the risk of myocardial infarction (see Chapter 4). At the time of writing the precise role of NSAIDs, one of the most widely used group of drugs over many years, awaits clarification.

Sequels to inflammation

Acute inflammatory reactions are usually beneficial and do not always lead to major medical problems. There may be serious problems when organ function is severely compromised, e.g. in meningitis, hepatitis and asthma, but these reactions also usually subside quickly and the inflammation is unlikely to cause permanent damage if the cause is treated promptly. It is the sequels to inflammation, i.e. the resolution and healing processes, which may sometimes cause permanent damage (Figure 2.13).

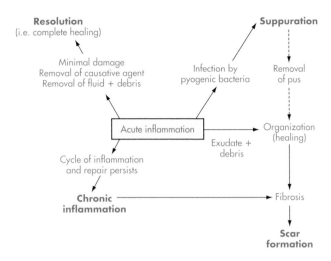

Figure 2.13   Sequels to inflammation.

Resolution

The most favourable outcome to inflammation would be the complete removal of the causative agent without any residual deleterious effects. However, complete resolution is possible only if there has been very little tissue damage and minimal cell death (necrosis). In the examples of a simple triple response or minor skin damage, these criteria are obviously fulfilled.

If the cause of inflammation is an infection, the offending organism needs to be dealt with quickly. Prompt treatment of an infection of a vital organ using antibiotics will prevent inappropriate resolution (see below) and the potential loss of function of that organ. For example, in kidney infection (**pyelonephritis**), prompt effective treatment prevents **fibrosis** of kidney tubules, **renal papillary necrosis** and eventual renal failure (see Chapter 14).

In addition to elimination of the initial trigger, exudate and dead cells must also be removed promptly, because delay may result in fibrosis. To do this efficiently the inflamed area needs to be well supplied with capillary and lymphatic vessels. In pneumonia (infection and inflammation of the lung alveoli, see Chapters 5 and 8), there may be no lasting damage once the causative organism has been dealt with, providing the initial infection is not too severe. The alveoli themselves have a very good blood supply and any fibrin that has been laid down and subsequently dissolved by plasmin can be readily removed via the circulation. The remaining debris is cleared by lung macrophages and the tissue then usually reverts to its normal state. In more serious bacterial infections, or if effective antibiotic treatment is not available, there may be pus formation, necrosis and permanent tissue damage, e.g. **bronchiectasis**, though this is rare nowadays.

Organization, healing and fibrosis

If there is an excessive amount of exudate that cannot be removed easily, or if a large amount of necrotic tissue is present, organization or 'healing' of the damaged tissue may take place. The result may be the formation of **scar tissue**.

Exudation carries fibrinogen into the inflamed area where it will eventually be converted into insoluble fibrin (see Chapter 11). Capillary buds then begin to grow into the area of dead tissue (angiogenesis) and inflammatory debris as part of the healing process, and these further facilitate the migration of macrophages and fibroblasts into the area. The fibroblasts then lay down connective fibrous tissue (collagen), which gradually replaces the fibrin. This immature fibrovascular tissue is **granulation tissue**, and the process by which it is formed is known as

organization. The formation of excessive amounts of abnormal connective tissue, leading to the production of **scar tissue** and impaired tissue or organ function, is the process of **fibrosis**.

A good example of this is that when exudate forms in the pleural cavity, e.g. following pneumonia, it tends to clear slowly, because the blood supply to this area is poor. Consequently, granulation tissue may form an **adhesion** between the two pleural surfaces. The lungs then become less compliant (see Chapter 5), making breathing painful and difficult, a condition known as **pleurisy**. Progressive fibrosis may then lead to severe restrictive lung disease. Adhesions may complicate the healing process in many tissues, e.g. they may cause considerable pain and discomfort if they form following abdominal surgery, because the gut is continually mobile.

Fibrosis and scarring are important pathological processes in a wide variety of disease states (Figure 2.14). For example, if scarring occurs in the pyloric sphincter (between the stomach and duodenum) as a result of the chronic inflammation associated with peptic ulceration (see Chapter 3), the sphincter may become incompetent, allowing large amounts of acid to be lost from the stomach. A further possible complication of fibrosis following peptic ulceration is shrinkage of the scarred area, or **cicatrization**, causing **pyloric stenosis**. This can grossly affect the transit of food through the stomach and duodenum. A similar process may cause an oesophageal stricture, leading to problems with swallowing (see Chapter 3).

Following myocardial infarction, part of the ischaemic area dies and is replaced by scar tissue. The normal elasticity and contractility of the myocardium is lost, possibly leading to heart failure (see Chapter 4). Arrhythmias will ensue if the damage is in the conducting tissue of the heart.

Therefore in a vital organ, such as the heart, brain, kidney or liver, the development of scar tissue may be serious, even fatal in some circumstances, whereas in others, e.g. a joint, the result will be loss of function.

Wound healing

The degree of scarring following organization depends on the extent of previous damage and inflammation. This is particularly true of wound healing, which is a special case of organization. Although a wound can be inflicted on any tissue, wound healing commonly refers to repair of the skin.

Following injury or laceration of the skin, blood vessels are damaged and a clot forms, consisting of coagulated blood and other debris, including microorganisms. The healing that follows a clean cut, or when the edges have been brought together promptly by suturing or after a ragged wound, is similar in all cases. The final

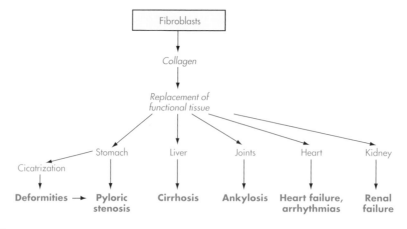

Figure 2.14 Fibrosis.

difference between these situations is merely that a ragged wound produces a larger scar, but the following sequence of events takes place in all of these (Figure 2.15):

- Initially, macrophages enter the wound area, to ingest and digest the debris.

- New blood vessels start to grow inwards from the edges of the wound, initially as solid cords of cells but soon becoming canalized, allowing blood to flow through them.
- The ingrowing blood vessels eventually join within the wound forming 'loops and arcades'.

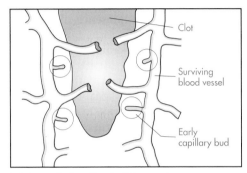

(a) Ingrowth of capillary buds in wound

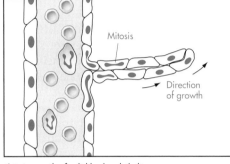

(b) Ingrowth of solid bud endothelium

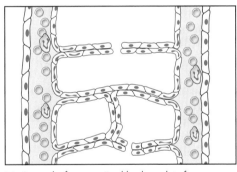

(c) Ingrowth of regenerating blood vessels to form arcades and loops

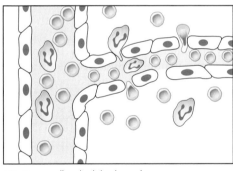

(d) New capillary bud develops a lumen

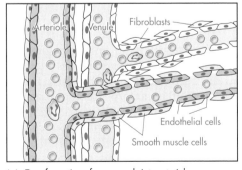

(e) Transformation of new vessels into arterioles and venules

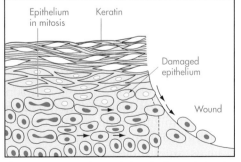

(f) Regenerating surface epithelium dividing and migrating to cover wounded surface

Figure 2.15 Wound healing. (Reproduced with permission from Spector TD, Axford JS. *An Introduction to General Pathology*, 4th edn; published by Churchill Livingstone, 1999.)

- The young vessels are leaky, allowing both blood cells and plasma to seep out. This is the serous exudate often seen in healing wounds.
- The new capillaries differentiate into arterioles and venules.
- Fibroblasts appear in the serous fluid, and lay down connective tissue.
- This mixture of newly formed blood vessels, connective tissue and serous fluid forms granulation tissue, usually heralding good wound healing.
- After the laying down of granulation tissue and removal of any remaining debris, the epithelium begins to regenerate. This is achieved by mitosis of the epithelial cells surrounding the wound, which gradually migrate to cover the wound surface.

If the wound is small, the underlying scar tissue is eventually replaced, merging with surrounding tissues, but in larger wounds scarring may become permanent. Wound healing is indistinguishable from the other forms of fibrosis and organization discussed earlier, except that it is visible when it occurs in the skin.

It has become apparent recently that wound healing is partly under the control of oestrogens. This is not as surprising as it may appear, because there has to be a mechanism of preventing excessive blood loss and promoting tissue repair following ovulation and menstruation. There is a delicate balance in wound healing between an inflammatory response, which removes tissue debris and minimizes infection, and the deposition of the collagen/proteoglycan matrix that closes the wound and underlies tissue repair. If inflammation predominates, the pro-inflammatory cells (neutrophils and macophages) that accumulate at the site release matrix-dissolving enzymes. It appears that the reaction of oestrogen and its ER-beta-receptor (ERβ) inhibits expression of the cytokine macrophage migration inhibitory factor, so the attraction of pro-inflammatory cells into the wound is reduced and matrix production and repair are maximized. If oestrogen levels are low, or the interaction with ERβ is impaired, the reverse situation holds. Thus males heal more slowly than females. Giving oestrogen to young males, and combined HRT in postmenopausal females, promotes rapid wound healing. However, elderly males are likely to require anti-androgen treatment. These findings have important implications for the management of chronic venous ulcers in the elderly.

Suppuration

The bacterium *Staphylococcus aureus*, implicated in many types of infection in man, is **pyogenic** (pus-producing). The presence of pus can also lead to fibrosis and the formation of scar tissue. The most common example of suppuration is seen in boil formation, usually caused by *Staph. aureus* and related bacteria. Although leucocytes are attracted into the area to deal with the organism in the usual way, in this case they are initially largely unsuccessful and die at the site of infection. The creamy pus so formed is a mixture of dead leucocytes, bacteria, lipid, exudate and necrotic tissue. *Staph. aureus* also produces a coagulase that leads to the formation of a 'capsule' composed of partially organized coagulated plasma which surrounds the area of suppuration. This prevents the bacteria from spreading throughout the body, but incidentally prevents the access of antibiotics to the site. Thus antibiotics, whether systemic or topical, are usually ineffective in treating large boils or abscesses, unless they are first drained surgically. When the infection has eventually cleared, this connective tissue remains and, depending on the size of the boil, scar tissue may be visible and permanent.

Chronic inflammation

The persistence of an inflammatory reaction for months or even years implies that its cause has not been removed or that there is a continuing pro-inflammatory stimulus (see above). Chronic inflammation may or may not be preceded by an acute phase. By convention, inflammation lasting more than 6 months is described as chronic, but this does not imply anything about its severity. Commonly acute inflammation is the precursor of the chronic condition, but this progression does not always occur (see below).

Features

Apart from its duration, two main features distinguish chronic from acute inflammation: the leucocytes involved and the occurrence of fibrosis.

The most important class of leucocyte involved in chronic inflammation is the **macrophage**, which soon replaces the neutrophils recruited in the early stages of acute inflammation. Macrophages are not only longer-lived than neutrophils, but are also extremely robust. Even if bacteria that have been engulfed by macrophages are not killed outright, the macrophage itself may remain unharmed or even allow the organism to multiply within the cell, as in TB. In this way a microorganism can persist for years at the site of infection. Furthermore, macrophages have the ability to change in character: they can become **epithelioid** cells, or they can combine to form multinucleate **giant cells**, both of which are present in granulomas (Figure 2.16).

If the reaction is prolonged, healing and repair will often accompany the inflammation, rather than follow it. Thus **fibroblasts** have an important role in chronic inflammation, and **fibrosis** is the main cause of residual damage, as in organization and repair. The laying down of connective tissue may be a lengthy process, with years elapsing before any loss of organ function is noted, as in **hepatic cirrhosis**. There may also be alternating cycles of inflammation and repair, e.g. in **peptic ulcer**, and again damage may not be apparent until many cycles have occurred (see below).

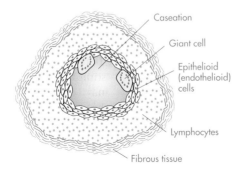

Figure 2.16   Structure of a tubercle (an example of a granuloma).

Caseation

Giant cell

Epithelioid (endothelioid) cells

Lymphocytes

Fibrous tissue

Chronic inflammation following acute inflammation

There is considerable overlap in the various sequels to inflammation. If suppuration and abscess formation predominate this is sometimes termed **chronic suppurative inflammation**, whereas the organization and repair (resulting in fibrosis) described earlier is termed **chronic fibrous inflammation**. A further example of chronic suppurative inflammation is encountered following staphylococcal bone infection (**osteomyelitis**), in which some bone may be destroyed by the bacteria during the initial acute phase. This necrotic tissue is poorly penetrated by blood, and so protects the surviving bacteria from the body's defence mechanisms. Thus the infection becomes chronic and large numbers of macrophages and fibroblasts continue to migrate into the area, which becomes chronically inflamed.

Certain other types of tissue seem prone to chronic inflammatory changes following an acute phase, the classic example being **peptic ulceration** (see Chapter 3). Small acute erosions in the duodenum or stomach may be visible after slight trauma, e.g. ingestion of alcohol. It is only if the mucosal protection mechanisms are deficient, or if the trauma is prolonged or repeated frequently, that a chronic sequel occurs. The connective tissue subsequently formed results in a weakening of the stomach wall, with the danger of gastric bleeds or even perforation during a subsequent acute episode. Other parts of the gastrointestinal tract can be similarly affected.

Cholangitis (inflammation of the bile ducts) may result from the presence of bile stones, often precipitated by infection or aggravated by it. If the stones are not removed, repeated episodes of infection and possibly acute **cholestasis** (see Chapter 3) may eventually lead to chronic inflammation and atrophy of the bile ducts.

Chronic inflammation without previous acute inflammation

In both biliary tract disease and peptic ulceration there is a discernible phase of acute inflammation, and prolongation of the acute phase may eventually lead to chronic changes. However, there is frequently no evidence of an initial acute reaction and inflammation is chronic from the outset. Even in conditions such as RA, where an 'attack' exhibits all the signs of acute inflammation, the underlying process is chronic in character, although of variable severity. Sometimes no acute phase is seen but a dense mass of tissue known as a **granuloma** is often formed (Figure 2.16), which should be distinguished from the granulation tissue in wound healing described earlier. A granuloma may be produced by an infection or aseptic foreign bodies such as asbestos, or may be of unknown origin, as in **sarcoidosis**.

The classical example of granulomatous chronic inflammation is **tuberculosis** (TB, see also Chapter 8). The bacillus is able to survive within macrophages, thus providing a focus for granuloma formation, known in this case as a tubercle. At the centre of the tubercle is an area of caseated ('cheese-like') necrotic tissue. Surrounding this are epithelioid and giant cells derived from macrophages. The structure is enclosed in a layer of T-lymphocytes. Granu-

lomas are also seen in Crohn's disease (see Chapter 3), sarcoidosis and RA (as rheumatoid nodules, see Chapter 12).

Cell-mediated immunity (CMI) is often associated with chronic granulomatous inflammation because of the sensitizing or stimulatory effect that T cells have on macrophages. Because TB invokes a CMI response, it is not surprising that chronic inflammation plays such a large part in its pathology.

Ischaemia

Causes

Ischaemia is a deficiency of blood supply to tissues. If the deficiency is sufficiently severe and prolonged, the tissue eventually dies (**necrosis**). The most common general cause is a failure of blood flow resulting from obstruction or cardiovascular insufficiency. Tables 2.8 and 2.9 classify the general causes of ischaemia, with examples

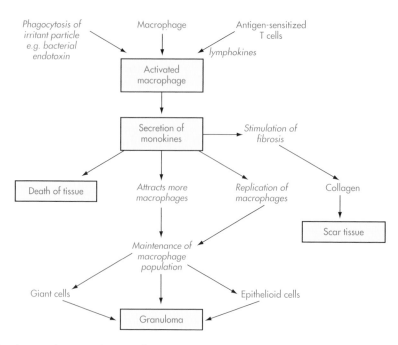

Figure 2.17   Role of macrophages in chronic inflammation.

Table 2.8   Causes and consequences of ischaemia

General cause	Examples of associated diseases or conditions
Local vascular obstruction	
Inflammation (vasculitis)	Collagen-vascular diseases
Vasoconstriction	Variant angina[a]
	Transient ischaemic attack[a]
	Raynaud's disease
Atherosclerosis	Diabetes mellitus
	Hyperlipidaemia
	Hypertension
Arteriosclerosis	Diabetes mellitus
	Hypertension
Embolism	
Fat	Bone fracture
Air	Faulty IV administration
	Diver's decompression sickness (bends)
Thrombotic	Venous stasis
	Atheroma
Hypoperfusion	
Systemic – reduced cardiac output	Chronic heart failure
	Shock:
	• cardiogenic
	• hypovolaemic
	• septic
Local – haemorrhage or thrombosis	Stroke[a]
	Myocardial infarction[a]
	Renal artery occlusion

[a] Consequences of ischaemia, all others are causes.

of resulting clinical conditions. These various conditions are discussed in the appropriate chapters.

When arteries are chronically inflamed (**arteritis**), the artery wall may be permanently damaged by the neutrophil infiltration and necrosis. If this involves small arteries, the entire arterial wall is affected and complete occlusion of the lumen may occur. If a larger artery is affected, only part of the wall may be damaged and blood is still able to pass. Healing subsequently occurs with the formation of scar tissue, which may weaken the artery wall and produce an **aneurysm** (bulge) that may eventually rupture.

A common cause of vascular obstruction is **atherosclerosis** (see Chapter 4), which affects the **intimal** lining of the artery wall, particularly in medium to large arteries. Atheromatous **plaques** are laid down that partially occlude the lumen and become sites for thrombus formation. In contrast, **arteriosclerosis** affects the **media** of the arterial wall, which becomes hard and inelastic. Once again, small arterioles may become occluded. The distinction between these two conditions is discussed in Chapter 4 (pp. 235–236).

A **thrombus** (blood clot) may be formed over the site of an atheromatous plaque in an artery. Thrombi may also form in large veins, usually in the region of valves, owing to stasis of blood. If a venous thrombus in the leg (**deep-vein thrombosis**), or a fragment of it, breaks away from its site of formation, it will travel downstream through veins of increasing diameter, through

Table 2.9   Effects of ischaemia on some organ systems

Organ/tissue	Significance	Clinical effects of:	
		Ischaemia[a]	Anoxia[b]/infarction
Less important			
Limbs/periphery	• Non-vital function • Many collaterals • Bone has a low oxygen demand • Muscle regenerates readily	• Poor healing • Local cyanosis • Cold • Pain (cramp)	• Gangrene
Lungs	• Dual circulation (bronchial + pulmonary) • Direct O_2 supply • Low intrinsic oxygen demand • Spare capacity	• Pulmonary congestion • Systemic hypoxia • Pulmonary hypertension	• Respiratory failure
More important – vital organ involved			
Brain	• No collaterals • Acutely sensitive to hypoxia • No regeneration	• Cognitive impairment (acute or chronic) • Loss of consciousness • Coma	• Stroke (acute) • Dementia (chronic)
Kidney	• Acutely sensitive to hypoxia (angiotensin/renin release)	• Fluid retention • Electrolyte disturbances • Heart failure • Hypertension	• Renal failure
Heart	• Few collaterals • Only perfused during diastole • High O_2 demand • Hypoxia sensitive • Little regeneration • Functions as integrated organ	• Angina pectoris • Heart failure • Arrhythmias	• Myocardial infarction • Cardiogenic shock (heart failure, arrhythmias)

[a] Ischaemia, relative lack of oxygen.

[b] Anoxia, complete absence of oxygen.

the heart and into the pulmonary tree, until it lodges in a small artery. This obstruction to the circulation is known as an **embolus**, i.e. a clot or clot fragment derived from a blood clot formed at one site, which lodges in another. Because it is often impossible to distinguish between an embolus and a thrombus, and because it does not affect treatment, it is usual to speak of **thromboembolic disease**. The site of formation of the original clot determines the organ eventually affected, which may be predicted on the basis of the anatomy of the vascular tree. We have just seen one example of this, with pulmonary embolism (see Chapter 5), which

may result in rapidly fatal respiratory failure if it is sufficiently large. Emboli can also be due to air introduced into the bloodstream inadvertently during IV therapy (**air embolus**) or may be the result of deep diving, causing nitrogen emboli if the diver rises to the surface too rapidly, causing the divers' syndrome known as the bends. Fat droplets released from the site of a fracture (**fat embolus**) do not cause an infarction as such, but can result in a severe interruption of gas exchange if deposited in the lung.

Thrombosis in a coronary artery may itself cause a **myocardial infarction** (see Chapter 4) or may throw off an embolus that travels further into the coronary arterial tree to obstruct a smaller vessel and so affect a smaller area of heart muscle. Emboli formed on damaged heart valves can reach the retina, affecting sight, whereas those resulting from atrial fibrillation tend to cause **strokes** by occluding a cerebral artery.

Small thromboemboli are quite quickly dissolved by natural clot-dissolving factors derived from blood plasminogen (plasmin), red cells and vessel walls, e.g. tissue-type plasminogen activator (t-PA; see Chapter 11). Temporary interruptions of CNS function, known as **transient ischaemic attacks (TIAs)**, are common and usually last less than 15 min, but may persist for up to 24 h. Circulatory brain obstructions of longer duration are classed as strokes. Acute MI is treated in the early stage with fibrinolytic (thrombolytic) drugs, e.g. *alteplase* (rt-PA), *reteplase*, *tenectoplase* and *streptokinase*, and the latter is also used in several other thromboembolic situations. All of these are unsuitable for use in early stroke unless it is certain that the stroke has not been caused by a **cerebral haemorrhage**, which would be exacerbated by clot dissolution.

Constriction of the vascular smooth muscle (**vasospasm**) may occur in coronary arteries, as in **variant angina** (see Chapter 4), and in peripheral arteries, causing **Raynaud's disease** (see Chapter 12).

Poor perfusion of tissue may also arise from circulatory insufficiency. If cardiac output is low, e.g. because of heart failure or arrhythmia (see Chapter 4), the blood supply to many tissues will be reduced. This may also occur if the blood volume is low, perhaps following severe blood loss, causing shock.

Shock

Shock is a syndrome of severely compromised peripheral blood flow with very low cardiac output and blood pressure. Severe blood loss causes a fall in blood pressure and **haemorrhagic (hypovolaemic) shock**. Other forms of shock include a sudden fall in cardiac output due to cardiac damage (**cardiogenic shock**; see Chapter 4) and the production of certain bacte-

rial endotoxins that cause profound vasodilatation (**septic shock**).

In severe sepsis causing shock, widespread clotting results in **disseminated intravascular coagulation** and large amounts of clotting factors and platelets are consumed. The resultant failure of blood clotting may result in haemorrhage, an apparently paradoxical situation in which widespread clotting gives rise to bleeding, which exacerbates the hypotension and shock.

However it is caused, a precipitate fall in blood pressure invokes homeostatic mechanisms to conserve blood flow to vital organs such as the heart, lungs, kidney and brain, which would be irreversibly damaged by even short periods of ischaemia. This **central conservation** may be at the expense of other organs or tissues, when vasoconstriction, mediated by sympathetic stimulation, diverts blood away from the periphery. This restricts blood flow to skeletal muscle, liver, skin and intestines, etc. **Renal ischaemia** may cause serious long-term problems.

The clinical features of shock include severe hypotension, increased heart rate, cold extremities and a pale appearance, fever or hypothermia. The patient may also feel disorientated and/or lose consciousness. **Respiratory distress syndrome**, with breathlessness, hyperventilation and tachypnoea, from stimulation of the respiratory centre caused by a metabolic acidosis and **hypoxaemia**, possibly central cyanosis, may further add to the patient's overall state of distress. The exact combination of signs and symptoms will depend on the severity and cause of the shock, the degree to which the compensatory mechanisms have been an effective response and the organs most affected.

In severe shock, the patient may present as cardiac arrest or collapse. The heart, lungs and brain may eventually succumb to the effects of ischaemia. When coronary perfusion is compromised, cardiac output is further reduced, adding to the vicious cycle of shock.

Other serious problems may occur in the lungs, resulting in a dramatic reduction in lung function (sometimes called **shock lung**). This is probably caused by changes in the capillaries and alveoli resulting from a combination of poor perfusion and the consequent release of PGs or other mediators. The result is a form of **alveolitis** (see Chapter 5), with exudate flooding the air sacs, causing pulmonary oedema and congestion, impairing gas exchange and increasing hypoxaemia, which aggravates ischaemia, and an increased risk of infection, i.e. pneumonia.

Treatment of shock

The most important initial requirement is immediate resuscitation, i.e. maintain a patent airway and restoration of breathing and blood flow. *Oxygen* and artificial respiratory support are usual.

Blood and samples from any identifiable, accessible source of infection are required for urgent laboratory investigation, and empirical antimicrobial treatment (see Chapter 8) is commenced until the laboratory results are available. Careful patient monitoring for early detection and treatment of abnormalities of acid-base balance, cardiac function, blood gases, respiratory rate, body temperature, kidney function, mental state, etc. and any infection.

Infusion of colloid solutions, e.g. polygelatin, hydroxyethyl starch or dextran, is required to restore cardiac preload and so effective heart action (see Chapter 4). This also corrects fluid loss in haemorrhage. Some clinicians prefer simple crystalloid infusions. Volume replenishment is often followed by the use of inotropes and vasopressors, e.g. *dopamine* infusion, plus *adrenaline* if hypotension persists, to give bridging support until the patient is stabilized.

The associated loss of RBCs is best managed with *oxygen* and respiratory support, but if the Hb level is very low, whole blood transfusion is indicated.

Transfusion of whole blood is expensive and the correct blood group may not be available in an emergency. Further, stored blood is deficient in platelets, calcium and oxygen-carrying capacity, and is hyperkalaemic. In normovolaemic patients, whole blood transfusion will lead to fluid overload, increased blood viscosity and hypertension, especially in the elderly. The best strategy seems to be the careful use of a colloid solution for any fluid replacement and of packed red cells to give a slightly lower than normal packed cell volume. Platelets are required in haemorrhagic states.

An inhibitor of TNFα, i.e. *adalimumab, etanercept* or *infliximab* (see Chapter 12), has been shown to give some benefit and inhibition of other pro-inflammatory agents may also help. Activated protein C, which is involved in the clotting cascade (see Chapter 11), significantly improves survival.

Shock, especially due to sepsis, high blood loss and myocardial damage has a high mortality.

Effects of ischaemia on body tissues

It will now be clear that the significance of local ischaemia will depend on the physiological importance of the organ affected and the extent of the damage caused. Provided that blood flow is not completely obstructed, the tissue may survive, although its function may be compromised. When the blood supply is so reduced that necrosis occurs, permanent damage or failure of the organ results. An area of necrosis of an organ resulting from ischaemia is termed an **infarct**, which may occur in almost any organ or tissue. The extent of ischaemic damage depends on a number of factors. Highly vascular tissues and those that can draw blood from other sites may have, or can develop, a **collateral blood supply**, which bypasses the obstruction, and so survive periods of ischaemia more readily than poorly vascularized ones. Extensive damage results if a major vessel is obstructed or if the obstruction is of long duration.

Furthermore, some tissues are more sensitive to the effects of hypoxia, e.g. the brain and kidney, and others have a limited ability to regenerate after infarction. Highly integrated organs, e.g. the heart and brain, may lose their ability to function properly, even if only partially damaged. An infarcted area, e.g. in the feet, has a poor blood supply and the resultant inability to mount a local immunological or phagocytic response may result in the tissue necrosis known as **gangrene**, which may or may not be exacerbated by infection, especially anaerobes. How these factors apply to various organs and the clinical consequences of hypoxia and infarction are shown in Tables 2.8 and 2.9.

Ischaemia in any muscle results in anaerobic metabolism to maintain energy supply. The lactic and other hydroxyacids so formed lead to the symptoms of **cramp**, and **angina pectoris** can be considered to be a form of myocardial cramp. For the reasons listed in Table 2.9, periods of hypoxia in skeletal muscle are unlikely to result in any serious permanent damage. The opposite is true of the myocardium where, if the patient survives the initial event, formation of scar tissue can result in arrhythmias and congestive heart failure (see Chapter 4). However, the general clinical effects of a poor peripheral circulation are reduced wound healing and the persistence of infections. In extreme circumstances this can lead to gangrene and loss of digits or even limbs, as in diabetes mellitus, in which abnormal lipid metabolism ultimately affects the circulation severely.

Obstruction of pulmonary arteries will not necessarily lead to infarction, but a large embolus may occasionally obstruct blood flow to a large area of lung tissue and greatly compromise lung function.

The brain is particularly sensitive to a reduction in blood flow and hypoxia because it has no reserves of either oxygen or glucose. Fainting (**syncope**), resulting from temporary cerebral hypoxia, is often remedied by simply placing the head between the knees or lying down with the legs raised to increase blood flow to the head. Unfortunately, the consequences of a cerebral infarct cannot be as easily resolved because nerve cells have very little capacity for regeneration. Thus necrosis can occur after only 5 min of hypoxia and even small infarcts (**strokes**) can cause paralysis or permanent cognitive impairment.

We have noted that the kidney is also very sensitive to ischaemia and both acute and chronic renal ischaemia can lead to renal failure. Furthermore, any reduction in blood flow to the kidney will tend to activate the renin/ angiotensin system, resulting in renal vasoconstriction and further ischaemia (see Chapter 14).

The treatment of thromboembolic disease, e.g. myocardial infarction, is dealt with in Chapters 4 and 11 and that of pulmonary embolism in Chapter 5. Anti-inflammatory drugs are covered in Chapters 5 (asthma, etc.), 12 (arthritis, etc.) and 13 (eczema, psoriasis, etc.).

References and further reading

Ashcroft G S, Mills S J, Lei K, *et al.* (2003). Estrogen modulates cutaneous wound healing by downregulating macrophage migration inhibitory factor. *J Clin Invest*; **111**: 1309–1318.

Govan A D, MacFarlane P S, Callander R (1995). *Pathology Illustrated*, 4th edn. Edinburgh: Churchill Livingstone.

Griffin G E, Harrison T S, eds (2001) Infections. Medicine; 29 Parts 1–3: 1–129.

McClelland D B L, ed. (2001). *Handbook of Transfusion Medicine*, 3rd edn. Norwich: The Stationery Office.

O'Connor D J (2002). *Pathology*, 2nd edn. Philadelphia, PA: Mosby (Elsevier).

Playfair J H L (1996). *Immunology at a Glance*, 6th edn. Oxford: Blackwell Scientific Publications.

Price S A, McCarty-Wilson L (1997). *Clinical Concepts of Disease Processes*, 4th edn. St Louis, MO: Mosby.

Roitt I, Brostoff J, Male D (1998). *Immunology*, 5th edn. London: Mosby.

Spector W G, Axford A S (1999). *An Introduction to General Pathology*, 4th edn. Edinburgh: Churchill Livingstone.

Underwood J C E (2004). *General and Systematic Pathology*, 4th edn. Edinburgh: Churchill Livingstone.

Part 2

Body systems and their principal diseases

3

Gastrointestinal and liver diseases

Gastrointestinal problems are a frequent cause of GP consultations and comprise about 15–20% of the primary care workload. In the West, refined diets and food additives have been implicated in many gastrointestinal and systemic diseases, problems that are exacerbated by the increasing consumption of manufactured and convenience foods. Repeated health scares have led to a proliferation of diets that are often faddist and of dubious nutritional value, and there is a plethora of sometimes conflicting and confusing dietary advice. Intensive farming and increasing technology in the kitchen, e.g. frozen foods, refrigeration and microwave ovens, have combined with a generally poor understanding of basic food hygiene to produce an apparently inexorable rise in the incidence of 'food poisoning' in the UK.

Meanwhile in the Third World, poverty, population increase, crop failure, poor hygiene, political instability and wars have caused massive malnutrition and starvation and led to refugee problems. These factors have created the conditions for epidemics of gastrointestinal diseases. Underlying all of this are the endemic helminth, protozoal, bacterial and viral infections that are already responsible for many intractable public health problems.

Gastrointestinal anatomy and physiology

Overall review

This chapter reviews briefly the anatomy of the digestive tract to help associate symptoms with organs. This leads to a synopsis of gastrointestinal physiology as a basis for appreciating the pathophysiology underlying the principal diseases and disorders, and so to their management. More detail about particular organs and their physiology is provided later, in the sections dealing with diseases of the individual organs.

The gastrointestinal tract (GIT, alimentary tract, gut; Figure 3.1) consists of an irregular tube some 6 m long, extending from the mouth to the anus. Accessory organs include the teeth, the tongue, the salivary, gastric and intestinal glands, the liver and gallbladder, and the pancreas.

For the purposes of this text, we will distinguish three groups of organs:

- The **upper GIT**, which includes the mouth, oesophagus and stomach.
- The **lower GIT**, which comprises the duodenum, jejunum, ileum, colon, rectum and anus.
- The **liver**, **gallbladder and pancreas** (the accessory organs).

Upper gastrointestinal tract

Food taken into the mouth is mixed with saliva to form a plastic mass. The salivary glands secrete about 1 L of fluid daily; this contains a lubricant (mucin) and the polysaccharidase enzyme, salivary amylase.

The food bolus is then swallowed and transferred rapidly via the **oesophagus** into the **stomach**. The stomach is joined to the oesophagus at the **gastro-oesophageal junction**, where there is a poorly defined **lower oesophageal sphincter (LOS)**.

The stomach is a highly distensible J-shaped organ that varies enormously in size and shape depending on its food content. The stomach secretes a **gastric juice** containing hydrochloric acid and pepsinogen, plus small amounts of gastric lipase. The acid converts pepsinogen into the proteolytic enzyme **pepsin**, provides the low pH suitable for its action and has a direct digestive function by hydrolysing some foods. The lipase splits short-chain triglycerides into glycerol and fatty acids. Infants, but not adults, also secrete the enzyme **rennin** (not to be confused with the renal enzyme, renin), which coagulates milk and so prevents too rapid a passage of liquid milk out of the stomach.

Gastric secretion is under complex nervous and hormonal control (see below). There are three phases of acid secretion:

- **Cephalic**, arising centrally and mediated by vagal stimulation (appetite arousal).
- **Gastric**, which occurs when food stretches the stomach and stimulates the stretch receptors and chemoreceptors in the gastric walls. The latter respond to the rise in pH when food enters the stomach.
- **Intestinal**, initiated by the passage of acid chyme (see below) into the duodenum, which provokes intestinal (local) gastrin release.

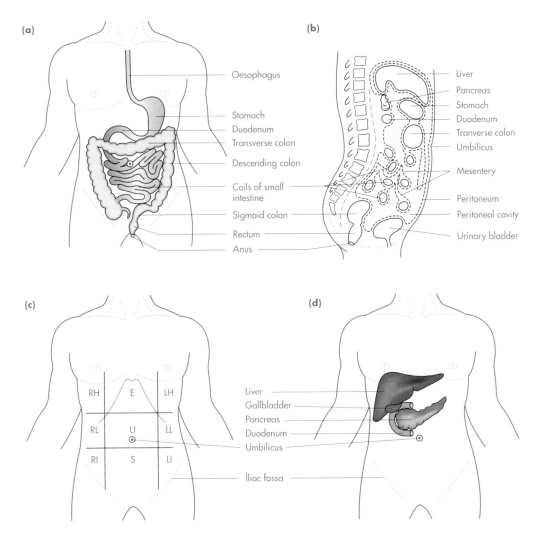

(a)

Oesophagus

Stomach
Duodenum
Transverse colon
Descending colon

Coils of small
intestine

Sigmoid colon

Rectum

Anus

(b)

Liver
Pancreas
Stomach
Duodenum
Tranverse colon
Umbilicus

Mesentery

Peritoneum
Peritoneal cavity

Urinary bladder

(c)

RH	E	LH
RL	U	LL
RI	S	LI

(d)

Liver
Gallbladder
Pancreas
Duodenum
Umbilicus

Iliac fossa

Figure 3.1   The human gastrointestinal tract. (a) General anatomy. (b) The abdomen in sagittal section. (c) Regions of the abdomen: E, epigastrium; RH, LH, right and left hypochondrium; RI, LI, right and left iliac; RL, LL, right and left lumbar (= lateral or loin); S, suprapubic (= hypogastric); U, umbilical. (d) Surface projections of the major associated organs.

The presence of food in the small intestine additionally provokes a nervous (enterogastric) reflex via the vagus nerve, which inhibits gastric secretion, and a further moderate inhibiting effect is produced by small bowel secretion of **secretin** and **cholecystokinin (CCK)**. The purposes of these mechanisms are probably to delay further gastric emptying into an already full small intestine and to inhibit unnecessary gastric secretion and digestion, once digestion is focused on the intestinal phase.

Between meals, the stomach normally secretes only a few millilitres per hour of slightly alkaline mucus (which protects the gastric mucosa from the acid and pepsin), although this is insufficient to neutralize residual gastric acid, so the basal pH remains acidic. Strong emotional stimuli may cause secretion of about 50 mL/h of gastric juice containing acid and pepsin, in the absence of food, via the cephalic mechanism.

Peristaltic waves ripple along the walls of the stomach every 15–30 s, macerating the food and mixing it with the gastric juice, finally producing a fluid called **chyme**. The presence of caffeine and partially digested protein stimulates the G cells in the pyloric antrum, the region of the stomach just before the **pyloric sphincter**, to liberate the hormone **gastrin**. Gastrin is carried via the blood and causes contraction of the LOS and the production of more gastric juice.

Over some 2–6 h, the entire content of the stomach is gradually emptied into the **duodenum** via the **pyloric sphincter**. The gastric residence time depends on several factors, including the nature of the stomach contents, being shortest for meals rich in carbohydrate and longest for those rich in fats. Gastric emptying depends on peristaltic waves, more powerful than those that mix the stomach contents, which begin in the middle of the stomach and create a relatively high pressure, overcoming the resistance of the pyloric sphincter and forcing out about 5 mL of chyme with each wave. Emptying is also influenced by feedback from the duodenum: in particular, fats in the duodenum delay gastric emptying. Little nutrient absorption occurs from the stomach, but salts, alcohol and some acidic drugs, being unionized in the acid environment and so lipophilic, may be absorbed there.

Lower gastrointestinal tract

The chyme is discharged into the first part of the **small intestine**, the duodenum, a tube about 25 cm long that curves around the head of the pancreas to merge into the **jejunum**. The duodenal mucosa secretes alkaline mucus that starts to neutralize the acid chyme and release a different set of digestive enzymes. The duodenum also receives about 1.5 L daily of pancreatic juice, and bile from the gallbladder, via the common bile duct and the **ampulla of Vater** (Figure 3.3). Chyme also stimulates the production of the hormone **secretin**, which stimulates the production of alkali in the pancreatic juice. The production of pancreatic amylase, lipase, deoxyribonuclease and ribonuclease, and proteolytic enzymes, is stimulated by signals from the vagus nerve and the small intestinal release of CCK, due to the presence of partially digested fats and proteins. The CCK stimulates

the release of an enzyme-rich pancreatic juice and of bile from the gallbladder.

The jejunum is about 1.5 m long and merges with the final part of the small intestine, the **ileum** (3 m), which joins the **large intestine (colon)** (1.5 m) at the **ileocaecal 'valve'**, although it is unclear whether any histological structure or effective valve actually exists at this location. The walls of the small intestine are covered with numerous small villi: finger-like projections, each about 1 mm long, that enormously increase the surface area of the small intestine (Figure 3.2(c)) and thus facilitate the absorption of nutrients and drugs.

Rhythmic contractions of the small intestine mix the chyme with the intestinal digestive secretions, and peristaltic waves gradually propel the mixture through the intestinal length.

Up to 3 L of intestinal juice is secreted daily. This contains mucus, digestive enzymes and bicarbonate, giving a pH of about 7.6. To this is added about 1.5 L daily of an alkaline, enzyme-laden pancreatic juice that is discharged into the duodenum via the **pancreatic duct** (Figure 3.3). The enzymes in the pancreatic juice convert proteins and protein fragments, fats, carbohydrate residues and nucleic acids into smaller, absorbable molecules.

The **large intestine** comprises the caecum and colon, and terminates with the rectum and anal canal. The **caecum** is a 6 cm pouch located in the right iliac region (Figure 3.1(c)), to which the **vermiform appendix** is attached. The latter is an 8-cm blind tube for which no proven function exists, though it may have some protective lymphoid role. Infection of the appendix (**appendicitis**) is the most common surgical emergency. The caecum merges into the **ascending colon** (15 cm long), which turns sharply downwards and to the left at the **right colic flexure** to form the **transverse colon** (50 cm), which is concave upwards and ends at the **left colic (splenic) flexure** where it turns down sharply to form the **descending colon** (25 cm).

The final part of the colon consists of two S-shaped tubes: the **sigmoid colon**, which is a loop (40 cm) in the left iliac region, merging into the **rectum** (12 cm). The latter is curved, at first backwards and upwards and then finally downwards and forwards. At its end, the rectum narrows to

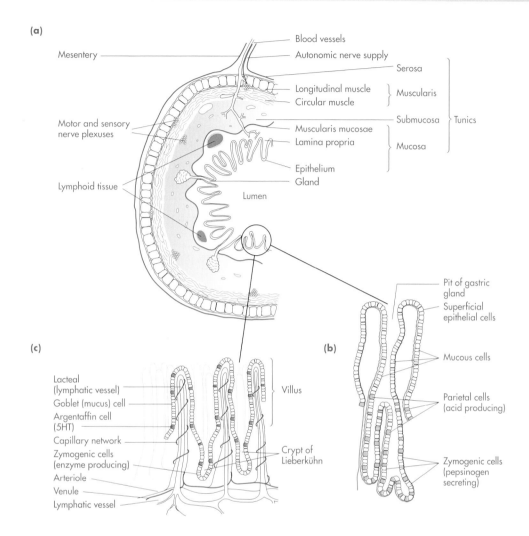

(a)

Blood vessels

Autonomic nerve supply

Mesentery

Serosa

Longitudinal muscle } Muscularis
Circular muscle

Submucosa } Tunics

Motor and sensory
nerve plexuses

Muscularis mucosae
Lamina propria } Mucosa

Epithelium
Gland

Lymphoid tissue

Lumen

Pit of gastric
gland
Superficial
epithelial cells

(b)

Mucous cells

(c)

Lacteal
(lymphatic vessel)
Goblet (mucus) cell
Argentaffin cell
(5HT)
Capillary network
Zymogenic cells
(enzyme producing)
Arteriole
Venule
Lymphatic vessel

Villus

Crypt of
Lieberkühn

Parietal cells
(acid producing)

Zymogenic cells
(pepsinogen
secreting)

Figure 3.2   The histology of the gastrointestinal tract. (a) General cross-section. (b) Gastric epithelium. (c) Epithelium of the jejunum and proximal ileum.

join the **anal canal** (3.5 cm). The upper part of the anal canal has up to 10 longitudinal folds (the **anal columns**), and is surrounded by the muscles of the **internal anal sphincter**, which hold the anal columns together very tightly in order to prevent faecal leakage. The terminal part of the anal canal, the **anus**, blends into normal skin. For greater security and control, the entire length of the anal canal is enclosed by the **external anal sphincter**: this consists of striated muscle that is under voluntary control, unlike the internal

sphincter, which is composed of involuntary circular smooth muscle.

Regions of the abdomen

The abdominal surface is thought of as being divided into nine regions, to make it easy to describe the location of organs or symptoms (Figure 3.1(c)). Comparing Figures 3.1(a), (c) and (d) shows the regions under which the various

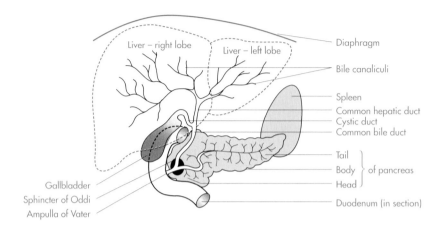

Figure 3.3   The anatomical relationships of the liver, gallbladder, pancreas, and related structures.

organs lie, and these locations are further outlined in Table 3.1.

General histology of the gastrointestinal tract

The whole of the GIT, apart from the mouth, has a similar basic tissue arrangement. A generalized cross-section of the gut is illustrated in Figure 3.2(a), which shows that there are four basic layers (**tunics**).

Tunics

The most important of these tunics, from the point of view of digestion, is the inner lining, the **mucosa**, which itself consists of three layers. The **epithelium** is in contact with the gut contents, has a protective function, and changes somewhat in character in the different areas of the gut. Although continuous with the epidermis (see Chapter 13) at both ends, the epithelium is not keratinized, and permits a variable degree of absorption of foods and drugs to occur, depending on the precise site and local conditions. The **lamina propria** contains glandular epithelium that secretes digestive enzymes and adjuncts. It also contains the blood vessels and lymphatics, bound by loose connective tissue, that carry absorbed substances into the circulation and are distributed to the tissues.

There are also lymph nodes that provide foci for protection against infective agents (see Chapter 2). The **muscularis mucosae** contains visceral smooth muscle, the tone of which throws the mucosa into small folds, providing for the considerable changes in volume that are required to respond to food intake while maintaining a large surface area for digestion and absorption.

The **submucosa** consists mostly of loose connective tissue, but has a rich blood supply and also contains glands, and nerve plexuses that provide the autonomic nerve supply to the muscularis mucosae.

The **muscularis** throughout most of the gut consists of an inner, transverse circular layer of smooth muscle and an outer longitudinal layer. Contraction of these muscles tends to break down the food masses, and causes the food to mix with the digestive juices, after which it is propelled by peristalsis along the GIT. The mouth, pharynx and oesophagus have a more complex, partly striated, musculature.

Within the abdomen, the gut is surrounded by the folds of the **peritoneum**, which form the outer layer of the gut, the **serosa**. These folds support the viscera, hold the organs in relation to each other and to the abdominal wall, and carry the blood, nerve and lymphatic supplies to the gut. Where these supplies enter the gut wall the tunics are structurally weakened, and this may result in pouches (**diverticula**, p. 124) being formed under pressure from within the lumen.

Table 3.1   Locations of the principal abdominal organs

Organ	Abdominal region[a]
Stomach	Epigastric (E, left side) and left hypochondrial (LH, right side)
Duodenum	Epigastric (E, lower right) and umbilical (U, upper right)
Caecum, appendix	(RI)
Colon	
• ascending	Right iliac (RI) and right lumbar (RL)
• transverse	Right lumbar (RL), umbilical (U), and left lumbar (LL)
• descending	Left lumbar (LL) and left iliac (LI)
• sigmoid	Left iliac (LI) and suprapubic (S, left side)
Liver	
• right lobe	Right hypochondrial (RH) and epigastric (E, right upper)
• left lobe	Epigastric (E, left upper)
Gallbladder	Right hypochondrial (RH, lower)
Pancreas	
• head	Umbilical (U, right upper)
• tail	Umbilical (U, left upper) and left hypochondrial (LH, right lower)
Kidneys	Around junctions of epigastric (E), umbilical (U), hypochondrial (RH and LH) and lumbar regions (RL and LL)
Spleen	Left hypochondrial (LH)

[a] See also Figure 3.1(c).

The part of the peritoneum that supports the small intestine is the **mesentery**, the **mesocolon** similarly supporting the large intestine. Other important peritoneal folds are the **falciform ligament** that attaches the liver to the abdominal wall and the diaphragm, the **lesser omentum** that suspends the stomach and duodenum from the liver, and the **greater omentum**, a large fold of tissue that hangs like an apron in front of the intestines. The greater omentum contains numerous lymph nodes and is the principal repository of abdominal fat. The large surface area and rich blood supply of the peritoneum make it valuable for **peritoneal dialysis** in renal failure (see Chapter 14). Peritoneal infection (**peritonitis**) is always extremely dangerous because the peritoneum is in contact with all the abdominal organs, which may be infected secondarily, and because it has a large surface area for the absorption of microbial toxins.

Stomach

The mucosa of the stomach is highly specialized. It contains many minute openings, which are the apertures of the gastric glands (Figure 3.2(b)). These glands are lined with four types of secretory cells. The **zymogenic** (chief) cells secrete **pepsinogen**, which is converted into pepsin by the hydrochloric acid produced by the **parietal** cells. The parietal cells also secrete **intrinsic factor**, a glycoprotein that binds vitamin B_{12} (**extrinsic factor**) from the food and transports it to specific ileal mucosal receptors, where it is liberated into the cells. The intrinsic factor remains in the gut lumen and is recycled. The **mucous cells** secrete an alkaline, bicarbonate-laden mucus which, together with other factors (see Figures 3.8 and 3.10), protects the mucosa from the acid and pepsin and also further moistens and lubricates the food.

Small intestine

The mucosa of the small intestine (Figure 3.2(c)) has many circular folds and numerous villi, which carry many more minute **microvilli** projecting from their surface. This arrangement produces an enormous surface area for the secretion of digestive enzymes and the absorption of food. The core of each villus contains specialized lymphatic vessels (**lacteals**) surrounded by a network of arterioles and venules. Between the bases of the villi are the **crypts of Lieberkühn**, which contain zymogenic (enzyme-producing) cells. The epithelial cells are formed at the bases of the crypts and migrate upwards over a period of about 3–4 days, after which they are shed. Thus, the epithelium is being continuously regenerated, so that any acute pathological process affecting it, e.g. inflammation or infection, is inherently self-limiting unless the damage is severe or becomes prolonged. However, this rapid cell turnover makes the gut highly sensitive to radiotherapy and cytotoxic chemotherapy, which may cause significant damage.

In addition to the lymphatic vessels, the lamina propria of the small intestine contains numerous immunologically active cells, e.g. plasma cells, lymphocytes, macrophages, mast cells, etc., solitary lymph nodes and **Peyer's patches** (aggregates of lymphatic nodules). These are concerned with the immunological defence of the gut and are more numerous in the ileum than in other regions. Specialized **microfold cells (M cells)** above the Peyer's patches permit the ready localization of antigens that stimulate the local cloning of B cells (see Chapter 2). The latter secrete IgA (secretory Ig) into the gut lumen, providing surface protection against orally ingested infective agents that are not killed by the acid gastric juice, the alkaline pancreatic juice duodenum and the surface activity of the bile.

Large intestine

The colon wall differs from that of the small intestine. It has no villi, and so little nutrient-absorbing function, although some amino acids and vitamins are absorbed there. It also has pits, which are the openings of tubular glands that extend the full mucosal thickness. The surface of the mucosa is comprised of simple columnar epithelium that extends into the glands. However, the glandular epithelium contains numerous mucus-secreting goblet cells. There are isolated lymphatic nodules, which form part of the immune system. The colon has five principal functions:

- To complete the digestion of residual foodstuff. Although the colon does not secrete enzymes, it harbours bacteria that ferment carbohydrate, convert amino acids to indole and skatole (which give faeces its characteristic odour) and **bilirubin** to urobilinogen. Bacterial activity also produces some of our daily intake of B vitamins and vitamin K and breaks down some prodrugs, e.g. *sulfasalazine* and *olsalazine* (p. 121).
- To secrete mucus, which lubricates faecal passage and protects the mucosa.
- To convert the fluid ileal contents into faecal paste by mixing and the reabsorption of water and electrolytes.
- To absorb water, electrolytes and vitamins.
- To store the faeces until defecation is convenient.

Nutrient breakdown and absorption

Proteins

The digestion of protein begins in the stomach where pepsin (under acidic conditions) converts proteins into peptides, which then stimulate the pyloric antrum to secrete **gastrin**. The gastrin enhances the secretion of **histamine**, and so of acid, from the parietal cells, and of bicarbonate-laden mucus. Discharge of the acid chyme into the duodenum stimulates further gastrin release, which in turn promotes the release of bile (by relaxing the sphincter of Oddi), and stimulates the pancreas to secrete bicarbonate.

The presence of dietary fats in the small intestine triggers the secretion of **CCK** (pancreozymin, cholecystokinin), leading to pancreatic pro-enzyme release, e.g. trypsinogen, and bile ejection from the gallbladder. Vagal acetylcholine is also involved. The trypsinogen is converted into active **trypsin**, which in turn converts other pancreatic pro-enzymes into active proteolytic enzymes. These produce absorbable dipeptides and free amino acids, and longer-chain peptides. These longer peptides are finally converted into amino acids by specific peptidases in the cells of the microvilli or the epithelium, before their systemic absorption via specific active transport mechanisms.

Thus there is a complex hormonal and neuronal positive feedback mechanism, which responds to the presence of food in the gut, and which controls the secretion and activation of appropriate enzymes (see Figure 3.8).

Carbohydrates

The digestion of carbohydrates starts in the mouth with **salivary amylase**, which continues to act until stopped by the low gastric pH. However, carbohydrates are mostly digested to monosaccharides in the upper small intestine, first by **pancreatic amylase** and finally by intestinal **saccharidases**. The resultant glucose, fructose and galactose are absorbed into the villi by sodium-dependent active transport systems. Deficiencies of maltase, sucrase and lactase enzymes cause accumulation of the corresponding disaccharides, which pass unabsorbed to the colon, producing an osmotic diarrhoea. Such deficiency may be congenital or may temporarily follow severe, prolonged diarrhoea. Also, nucleic acids are converted into nucleotides and nucleosides by cleavage of their pentose-phosphate chains.

Fats

Dietary lipids consist principally of triglycerides, plus small amounts of cholesterol and its esters and phospholipids. Lipid digestion occurs predominantly in the small intestine after emulsification by **bile salts**. The resultant fat globules are hydrolysed, primarily by **pancreatic lipase** and, being insoluble in water, can be hydrolysed only at the globule surface: emulsification is essential to provide an adequate surface area for hydrolysis to proceed effectively. Bile salts are also required for the absorption of fat-soluble vitamins (A, D, E, K) and to enhance vitamin uptake.

Pancreatic lipase hydrolyses triglycerides to monoglycerides plus fatty acids. All of these lipoid materials are solubilized and emulsified by the bile salts before they are absorbed into the villi.

Following hydrolysis, the resultant monoglycerides and free fatty acids, which are solubilized in micelles, partition into the lipid membranes of the microvilli and are readily absorbed. The bile salts are recycled by enterohepatic circulation and reused. Cholesterol esters are similarly solubilized, and are then hydrolysed by **cholesterol esterase**: without bile salt solubilization no cholesterol whatsoever is absorbed. Thus, diseases reducing gallbladder and pancreatic activity may result in only 30–50% of dietary fat being absorbed. The resultant fatty stools are pale, soft and particularly foul-smelling (**steatorrhoea**). Very short gut transit times can cause similar effects.

After absorption, the monoglycerides and fatty acids are reconstituted into triglycerides in the mucosa. Globules of these, plus cholesterol and phospholipids, are coated with protein to yield **chylomicrons**, which pass into the central lacteals of the villi (Figures 3.2(c) and 3.4) and into the general circulation via the portal vein and thoracic duct. A lipoprotein lipase produced by capillary endothelial cells completes digestion of the chylomicrons. The glycerol is metabolised and the fatty acids are absorbed into the liver and fat cells of adipose tissue, where they combine with glycerol produced in the cells to reform triglycerides.

Bile salts are highly conserved, 95% being reabsorbed in the distal ileum; thus ileal diseases, e.g. Crohn's disease (p. 114), may lead to a failure to reabsorb bile salts. Bile salts are highly irritant, and when they reach the colon are partly responsible for the severe diarrhoea of this condition. Indeed, bile salts used to be used as laxatives.

Fluid and electrolyte absorption and conservation

Sodium

Each day, about 25 g of sodium is secreted into the gut, and a further 5 g is ingested with food: this total of 30 g represents about 15% of the total body sodium. Active sodium resorption occurs in the upper jejunum, where it is associated with

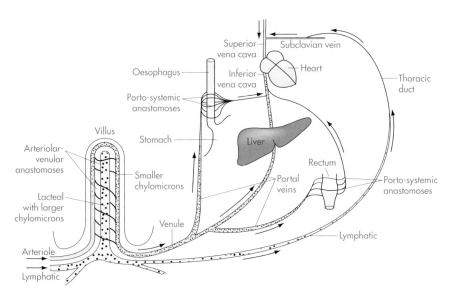

Figure 3.4   Portal and associated circulations (arrows indicate directions of flow).

monosaccharide and amino acid absorption, and in the ileum and ascending colon. Sodium transport is usually accompanied by water, except in the kidney (see Chapter 14), so almost complete water resorption also occurs, especially in the distal ileum and in passage through the colon (Table 3.2). This means that only about 100 mL of water is lost daily in the faeces.

Because the absorption of sodium from the small intestine must be accompanied by water,

this mechanism is used to treat dehydration by oral rehydration. Sodium absorption is enhanced by glucose (facilitated active transport), so water absorption is also enhanced. This is the rationale behind the use of oral rehydration salts (containing glucose) and similar proprietary products for the treatment of fluid loss caused by severe diarrhoea and vomiting.

The ileal discharge into the caecum is always fluid or semi-fluid (about 1 L/day), compared

Table 3.2   Fluid balance in the gastrointestinal tract

Process		Approx. daily volume (L)	
Fluid intake from diet		1.5	
Excretion into the gut	Saliva	1.0	
	Gastric juice	2.5	
	Bile	0.5	
	Pancreatic juice	0.7	
	Small intestine	2.8	
	Total flow into the gut		9.0
Resorption from the gut	Small intestine	7.5	
	Colon	1.4	
	Total resorption from the gut		8.9
Excreted in the faeces			0.1

with the semi-solid stools in the colon, and these differences have implications for the management of patients with stomas (p. 133).

Calcium

Absorption of calcium occurs in the small intestine, being dependent on the presence of the active form of vitamin D (1,25-dihydroxychole-calciferol, *calcitriol*) and a specific calcium-binding protein. Although still described as a vitamin, 1,25-dihydroxycholecalciferol (see Figure 3.21) is actually a hormone that controls calcium homeostasis, primarily in association with parathyroid hormone (PTH). Vitamin D synthesis and calcium absorption are regulated principally by PTH, although other hormones (i.e. calcitonin and glucocorticoids), and sex, growth and thyroid hormones are also involved.

Iron

In the UK, the average daily intake of iron is about 20 mg, only 2 mg of which is absorbed (in the duodenum and jejunum), although absorption increases in iron-deficiency states. The average daily requirement of iron for erythropoiesis is about 20 mg. Because there is a daily faecal iron loss of about 750 µg (plus about 2.5 mg/month in menstruation), it is clear that the iron content of the body is finely regulated, absorption being linked closely to needs. Most of the iron liberated by the breakdown of Hb and other molecules is conserved. Some factors that affect iron absorption are given in Chapter 11 (Table 11.2).

Potassium

The average dietary intake of potassium is about 80 mmol/day, and a further 40 mmol is excreted into the small intestine in the intestinal juice. As only about 10 mmol/day is lost in the faeces, about 110 mmol/day is absorbed in the ileum and colon. Diarrhoea and vomiting may cause substantial losses of potassium (and sodium), so fluid and electrolyte replacement is vital if these conditions are severe or prolonged. Although some degree of potassium loss occurs with long-term diuretic use, especially with thiazide diuretics, oral potassium repletion is rarely indicated (see Chapters 4 and 14).

Absorption sites for nutrients and drugs

Some 90% of nutrients are absorbed in the small intestine, the remainder being absorbed in the stomach and large intestine. Absorption may be by processes of **active transport** (e.g. amino acids, sodium, potassium, calcium and iron), or of **diffusion** (e.g. water, chloride and fats). Fructose and some other nutrients are absorbed by the energy-independent process of **facilitated diffusion**, which is faster than simple diffusion. The transport of amino acids, glucose and galactose is linked to that of sodium, the membrane transporter having binding sites for both sodium and the substance: this is **secondary active transport**. Water absorption nearly always accompanies that of solutes, as a 'carrier', and it moves freely, following osmotic gradients.

Whether or not substances (including drugs) are absorbed may depend crucially on their lipophilicity and, for some, on their ionizability (pKa). Generally, lipophilic substances will dissolve in the lipoid villus membrane and then be released inside the cell, but the pKa of an ionizable substance and the local pH will determine whether that substance is absorbed or not.

Thus, for example, *aspirin* is unionized (lipophilic) in the acid gastric juice and so will be absorbed into the gastric mucosa. Once inside the cells (internal pH about 7.4) it ionizes and is unable to diffuse out, and so is concentrated there. This property accounts in part for the ulcerogenic property of *aspirin* and related NSAIDs.

Water-soluble substances and small chylomicrons enter the mucosal blood and then the portal vein and so are delivered direct to the liver (Figure 3.4), where they are processed before discharge into the systemic circulation. This, together with any transformation that occurs during absorption, is **presystemic (first-pass) metabolism**. Although this occurs with many types of absorbed compounds, the term is usually applied to drugs and the process may be very important with some of them, reducing or enhancing their bioavailability. Thus with organic nitrates (e.g. *GTN*) and *propranolol*, high oral doses must be given to allow for that lost in presystemic metabolism, while the dopa-decarboxylase inhibitors *benserazide* or *carbidopa* are co-administered with *levodopa* specifically to prevent its mucosal and hepatic metabolism.

Because presystemic metabolism is reduced in the elderly and in liver disease, doses of drugs that have a high 'first-pass extraction rate' (i.e. are extensively metabolized in their first pass through the liver) may have to be reduced in such patients. For example, with *propranolol* the plasma concentration may be doubled in the elderly if the dose is not reduced. An alternative procedure is to avoid the portal circulation, and so bypass presystemic metabolism, by giving the drug buccally (e.g. *GTN*), transdermally (e.g. *GTN*, *hyoscine* (scopolamine) and sex hormones), or parenterally, if that is practicable or desirable. When drugs are formulated as prodrugs to enhance absorption, we depend on metabolism to liberate the active form.

The larger chylomicrons are unable to enter the bloodstream directly and are carried in the lymphatic circulation via the thoracic duct, discharging into the blood at the subclavian vein (Figure 3.4).

Investigation

Only the common general investigations are described here. More specific tests are dealt with under the diseases to which they apply.

History

As usual, it is important to obtain a good history and to listen to patients and observe their appearance and behaviour carefully. Food and the GIT are powerfully associated with emotional and social attitudes, and public misconceptions are common. Attention to these aspects may provide important clues to patient understanding, to social attitudes and emotional state, all of which may have a bearing on the interpretation of the information obtained.

It has been demonstrated that it takes only 5 min to obtain a good gastrointestinal history and, following this and an examination, a clinician will have about 80% of the information required for a probable diagnosis. The principal points to note are outlined in Table 3.3.

It is important for community pharmacists to be able to identify the signs and symptoms that may indicate the more serious gastrointestinal diseases, and to determine the urgency of treatment or referral, because they are often asked to advise on the treatment of conditions causing apparently minor symptoms. Specific symptoms and signs will be discussed under the various organs and diseases.

Imaging

Radiology

Plain X-rays of the abdomen are of little value in investigating most gastrointestinal diseases. However, they can be useful in investigating acute conditions, when they will show accumulation of air, toxic dilatation of the intestine and the presence of accumulated fluid (see Figure 3.15).

Barium contrast studies

Using fine suspensions of radio-opaque barium sulphate, these were the mainstay of investigation for many years, including the following:

- **Barium swallow**, to visualize the oesophagus or to demonstrate refluxing of gastric contents.
- **Barium meal**, to examine the stomach and duodenum. This is often combined with a small-bowel investigation, i.e. 'barium meal and follow-through', to visualize the gross anatomy of the small intestine, particularly the terminal ileum.
- **Barium enemas**. Barium sulphate is introduced into the empty large bowel rectally. This permits visualization of the entire colon and, usually, the terminal ileum, but not the rectum. A small-bowel enema uses a large volume of dilute barium suspension, introduced directly into the duodenum via an oral catheter. It provides more detailed information on areas of the small bowel that are suspicious on the follow-through.
- **Double-contrast techniques** are usually required for satisfactory visualization of the stomach, duodenum and large bowel. A

Table 3.3   The principal information to be obtained in a gastrointestinal history[a]

History of symptoms	
Duration	• intermittent, continuous, progressive, recurrent (if so, are the symptoms the same or different from the last episode?)
Site and radiation	• initial, subsequent, now
Relationship to:	• time of day • food intake • bowel motions • menstrual cycle • life events, e.g. bereavements, divorce, etc.
Relieving factors	• alkalis used • food and fluid intake • posture • local warmth, cold, etc.
Aggravating factors	• activity, work, stress, plus as in 'relieving factors' • appetite, taste, diet
Recent changes in	• weight (significant change without apparent cause) • salivation • bowel action (frequency, consistency, colour, odour)
Pain/discomfort, including any change	• site, radiation (initial, subsequent, now) • severity • quality: sharp, dull, stabbing, colicky • dysphagia (possibly serious), dyspepsia, heartburn or flatulence (wind)
Family history	
Nausea and vomiting	

Other information
Recent travel (if so, where?) Skin rashes, allergies, intercurrent diseases and medications Previous treatments (especially abdominal or surgical)

[a] See also Chapter 1.

barium meal is followed by introducing a gas (carbon dioxide in the stomach, by giving bicarbonate; air in the colon) to distend the organ and push the barium sulphate into and around lesions of the wall (see Figures 3.12 and 3.15).

Fluoroscopy

Direct real-time inspection of an X-ray image on a sensitive screen (nowadays a video monitor fed from an image intensifier to reduce the radiation dose to the radiologist) is especially useful for investigating disordered gut motility. The occurrence of gastro-oesophageal reflux (p. 82) can be observed directly.

Computed tomography (CT scanning)

This is a computer-enhanced X-ray technique that provides views of a succession of thin 'slices' of tissue, but with much greater detail and contrast than conventional radiography. Its principal use in gastroenterology is to examine organs outside the gut, e.g. the liver and pancreas. The radiation dose from CT is relatively high but is less with the newer technique of 'spiral CT scanning', in which patients are moved longitudinally while the X-ray tube is rotated around them.

Nuclear magnetic resonance imaging (MRI)

The MRI scan is a newer technique than CT scanning and depends on atomic excitation by powerful magnets to produce images. It is capable of producing images of great detail and clarity, similar to CT though often superior to it. Both investigations are expensive, especially MRI, but have the advantage of being completely non-invasive. Problems with current MRI machines are the need to confine patients in a small tunnel for some time, during which they must be absolutely still, and the very noisy environment. Some find this intolerable, but the newer machines are less claustrophobic.

Endoscopy

Endoscopes permit direct viewing of organs and structures within the body. The older type is a rigid tube containing a plastic 'light pipe' that connects the objective and eyepiece lenses. A channel is provided for powerful illumination of the object to be visualized. This type of instrument is now used only for proctoscopy and sigmoidoscopy (inspection of the rectum and terminal part of the sigmoid colon, respectively) and sometimes for the removal of obstructions from the oesophagus, e.g. fish bones.

The **fibre-optic endoscope** (Figure 3.5) is much more useful, and has revolutionized hospital gastroenterological practice. The light pipe and illumination channel consist of a flexible glass fibre-optic bundle that transmits light very efficiently and is completely steerable through the gut. **Gastroscopes** permit visualization of the oesophagus, stomach and duodenum, while **colonoscopes** provide views of the rectum, the whole of the colon, and the terminal ileum.

There is an increasing trend for **interventional endoscopy**, in which instruments are

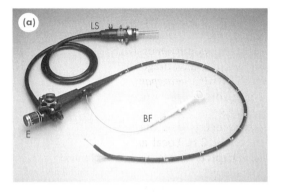

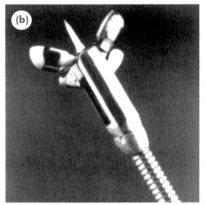

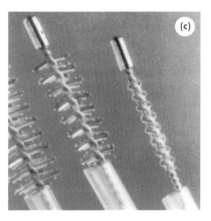

Figure 3.5   The fibre-optic endoscope. (a) Olympus gastroscope and attached high-power light source conductor (LS) and biopsy forceps (BF) inserted. E, eyepiece. (b) Biopsy forceps. (c) Brushes for surface cytology. (b) and (c) are instruments for insertion through the endoscope. (Reproduced with permission from KeyMed-Medical and Industrial Equipment Ltd, Southend-on-Sea, UK.)

inserted through the tube and used to take biopsy samples and to carry out minor surgery. These include the removal of foreign bodies, gallstones and colonic polyps, and cautery or injection of sclerosant to arrest bleeding. Patients are first sedated with a benzodiazepine (e.g. *diazepam, lorazepam, midazolam* or *temazepam*), a procedure that has the advantage of producing amnesia, especially with *lorazepam*, so patients have little recollection of an uncomfortable procedure. *Temazepam* has a rapid onset of action and gives rapid recovery, patients being reasonably alert after about 2 h. Local anaesthetic throat sprays (see Chapter 7) are used occasionally before gastroscopy.

Endoscopy is more invasive and uncomfortable than radiographic imaging and cannot be used for certain purposes (e.g. investigating refluxing), though it can show its effect on the oesophagus. Which technique is used will depend on patient suitability and the availability of facilities and local expertise.

Wireless capsule endoscopy uses a single-use miniaturized capsule, about the size of a large tablet, containing a light source, camera, wireless transmitter and battery. It is swallowed with water and transmits two images every second to a portable data recorder over an 8-h period. These are correlated with positional information from external abdominal sensors.

Capsule endoscopy gives good results in locating the source of obscure intestinal bleeding and has been shown to be superior to flexible enteroscopy and radiography in the diagnosis of small bowel pathology. Although it does not provide any interventional capability, unlike flexible enteroscopy, it is non-invasive and so is useful as an early diagnostic tool that can avoid extensive investigation and point to the most appropriate treatment. However, it is rather expensive.

Ultrasound

This technique, which uses computer analysis of ultrasonic reflections from internal organs, is completely non-invasive and non-stressful and is now used extensively. It can be used to visualize a variety of abdominal structures, especially the liver, gallbladder and biliary tree.

Stool examination

Stools are examined to look for:

- The passage of blood. Large amounts in the upper gut (>100 mL) become obvious as **melaena** (i.e. black, tarry stools), or on microscopy, while smaller amounts not apparent visually are detected by the **faecal occult blood test**, but this is of limited value because it yields a high proportion of false-positives.
- Excessive fat (steatorrhoea) or undigested food in suspected malabsorption syndromes (p. 111).
- Pathogens, by microscopy (especially protozoa, see Chapter 8), or stool culture.

Other investigations

The standard investigations provide valuable information about the possible origins of symptoms, as well as on the condition of patients and their progress. In cases of uncertainty the tests ordered should depend on the provisional diagnosis, because specialized tests are usually expensive and may not be readily available. Further, the best yield of information comes from carefully targeted tests ordered on the basis of sound clinical evidence from the history and examination. Capsule endoscopy (see above) falls into this class, and examples of a few other specialized gastroenterological tests are given below.

In developed countries, nutritional deficiency is rare and vitamin assays are unusual. However, vitamin assays may be carried out, for example in pregnancy (folate), strict vegans (vitamins B_{12}, D), anorexia (folate), liver and gallbladder disease (vitamins A, D), renal failure (vitamin D), alcoholism (B vitamins) and malabsorption syndromes.

Examples of other specialized tests in gastroenterology are oesophageal manometry in achalasia (p. 87), jejunal biopsy in malabsorption (Figure 3.14), oral *sodium amidotrizoate* to locate fast gastrointestinal bleeds, and radiolabelled erythrocytes, to locate slow bleeds. Radiolabelled leucocytes are used to locate foci of inflammation.

Disorders of the upper gastrointestinal tract

Oesophageal disorders

Introduction

The principal oesophageal disorders are **gastro-oesophageal reflux disease**, **dysphagia** (difficulty in swallowing), **pain on swallowing** and **bleeding**. These may caused by:

- local problems within the oesophagus, e.g. infection, inflammation, stricture, ulceration and malignancy;
- a manifestation of generalized disease, e.g. oesophageal varices consequent on hepatic disease, e.g. cirrhosis (p. 156), systemic sclerosis (see Chapter 12) and diabetes mellitus (see Chapter 9);
- neuromuscular dysfunction, e.g. achalasia, spasm, myasthenia gravis;
- pressure from neighbouring organs, e.g. goitre, left atrial enlargement due to hypertension;
- anatomic changes, e.g. pregnancy or hiatus hernia (see below), causing refluxing of stomach contents into the oesophagus.

Gastro-oesophageal reflux disease

Definition and aetiology

Gastro-oesophageal reflux disease (GORD, GERD in North America) is caused by refluxing of stomach contents (occasionally with some bile, i.e. **reflux oesophagitis**), into the oesophagus, causing **heartburn**, which occurs in about 75% of cases. Heartburn is a retrosternal burning pain of variable severity that accounts for about 30% of all cases of dyspepsia, but refluxing can occur without producing symptoms. The oesophageal mucosa has little or no protection against the acidity and proteolytic activity of the gastric juice. A number of factors may reduce the competence of the LOS, and so predispose to refluxing. These include:

- fatty foods, including chocolate, which lubricate the mucosa of the LOS and so facilitate the reverse passage of stomach contents;
- excessive caffeine (coffee) consumption and anticholinergic drugs, which relax the smooth muscle of the LOS;
- excessive intra-abdominal pressure caused by, for example, poor posture, obesity, pregnancy;
- hiatus hernia (see below).

It is reported that the incidence of GORD is rising, and this is accompanied by a rapid, worrying increase in the incidence of oesophageal cancer. Up to 25% of duodenal ulcer patients from whom *Helicobacter pylori* has been eradicated (see below) may develop GORD.

About 50% of pregnant women suffer from heartburn caused by raised intra-abdominal pressure, reduced sphincter tone or a temporary **hiatus hernia** (a protrusion of the stomach through the muscular diaphragm, Figure 3.6). Because the stomach is then subjected to abnormal pressure differentials, and the muscles of the diaphragm no longer aid the sphincter action, this condition predisposes to refluxing, especially on bending forward.

A **permanent hiatus hernia** may be congenital or occur in early infancy, but is more usual in the middle-aged and elderly. Although many patients with demonstrable hiatus hernia are asymptomatic, or show symptoms other than heartburn, the presence of a hiatus hernia may aggravate refluxing. Similar symptoms may also occur in normal subjects without demonstrable refluxing and with an undamaged oesophageal mucosa, resulting from an abnormality of oesophageal motility.

Causes of oesophageal damage other than refluxing

Oesophageal damage may also be caused by excessive alcohol (spirits) consumption and candidiasis. Candidal infection may result from depressed immunity (e.g. by drugs, including

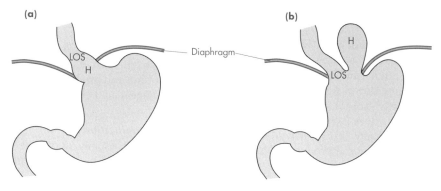

Figure 3.6   Types of hiatus hernia. (a) 'Sliding'. (b) Para-oesophageal ('rolling'). H, herniated portion of stomach projecting through the diaphragm; LOS, lower oesophageal sphincter.

inhaled corticosteroids, or malignancy), or broad-spectrum antibiotic treatment, especially in debilitated or immunosuppressed patients. Taking tablets or capsules while lying down, or without adequate fluid, may result in the medication being retained in the oesophagus and release of the drug there, causing local irritation or ulceration. This is a particular problem in elderly patients and with drugs such as *potassium chloride, aspirin, indometacin* and other NSAIDs, bisphosphonates (notably *alendronic acid* and *ibandronic acid*), and some antibiotics.

It is not known precisely why **smoking** aggravates symptoms, because it has several pharmacological effects that might be involved, but increased gastric acid production, gastric and oesophageal stasis and local irritation may all be implicated.

People with an abnormality that restricts the oesophageal lumen (e.g. oesophageal stricture), and enlargement of organs in the mediastinum (e.g. aortic aneurysm, bronchial carcinoma or an enlarged left atrium consequent on mitral valve disease), are also at risk. The left main bronchus, the heart and the aortic arch are in close proximity to the oesophagus and may indent it or cause its deviation. Disease of mediastinal organs may thus increase the risk of oesophageal restriction.

The relationship between oesophageal reflux, hiatus hernia and the occurrence of symptoms is illustrated diagrammatically in Figure 3.7.

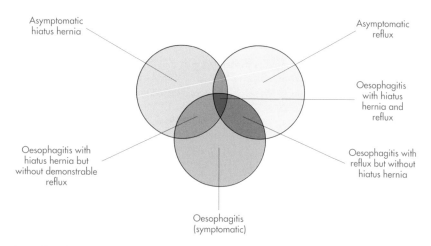

Figure 3.7   Relationships between oesophageal reflux, hiatus hernia and symptomatic oesophagitis.

Clinical features and diagnosis

The pain often occurs after food, which induces the secretion of gastric acid. An alcoholic or other 'nightcap' often causes nocturnal symptoms because lying down promotes refluxing from a consequently full, acid-laden stomach. However, refluxing does not usually disturb sleep. Exertion, especially lifting heavy objects, or bending forward, may also produce refluxing. Occasionally the pain may be so severe as to mimic that of angina pectoris or myocardial infarction (see Chapter 4). There is an association between refluxing and asthma, because reflux causes vagally mediated bronchoconstriction in about 50% of asthmatics, making asthma diagnosis more difficult. The symptoms that may be associated with refluxing are outlined in Table 3.4.

Diagnosis is based on the clinical features and endoscopy, although there is a poor correlation between the severity of symptoms and endoscopy findings of mucosal damage or altered epithelial morphology. Negative endoscopy findings do not eliminate a diagnosis of GORD if the symptoms strongly suggest refluxing. The most appropriate diagnostic category in this situation is endoscopically negative reflux disease. GORD is the likely diagnosis if heartburn occurs on 2 days a week or more. It is also probable if upper abdominal or lower retrosternal symptoms are reliably relieved by antacids. Therapeutic trial of a high-dose proton pump inhibitor (PPI; p. 86) is useful diagnostically.

However, other investigations that have been used widely in the past, e.g. fluoroscopic demonstration of reflux and production of symptoms on 24-h oesophageal acid exposure, are unreliable.

Long-term complications

Although GORD usually occurs as a relatively brief acute attack of heartburn, repeated insult may cause oesophageal damage and chronic, persistent problems. Complications of chronic mucosal damage include:

- pain on swallowing;
- ulceration;
- haemorrhage;
- oesophageal stricture causing dysphagia;
- perforation or malignancy (both are rare).

However, only about 5% of new patients with presumptive GORD are likely to experience significant local complications.

Management: general aspects

The principal aim is to prevent reflux occurring and so prevent damage to the oesophageal mucosa and the development of complications. Drugs may also be used secondarily to relieve symptoms by reducing the acidity and irritancy of the refluxed gastric contents, and to improve

---

Table 3.4 Symptoms and conditions that may be associated with a hiatus hernia

Common conditions	Uncommon conditions[a]
Heartburn, especially postural (70%)	Dysphagia
Regurgitation of food, acid in throat (60%)	Gastric ulceration
Wind, bloating (45%)	Anaemia, haematemesis, melaena
Nausea (35%)	Severe upper abdominal pain
Sharp chest pain (35%)	
Epigastric pain/discomfort (25%)	
Breathing problems (20%, especially asthmatics)	
Aspiration pneumonitis	

(a) These require extensive investigation as they usually have some other cause. Severe pain may be caused by strangulation, i.e. ischaemia of the hernia due to pressure from the muscles of the diaphragm and other organs.

the competence of the LOS. Drug treatment is primarily with PPIs. Antacids, H_2-receptor antagonists (H_2-RAs) and sphincter 'strengtheners' are also used but are less effective. General measures involving lifestyle modification, notably weight reduction to reduce intra-abdominal pressure, and raising the head of the bed by 15 cm to reduce the tendency to regurgitate stomach residues, are often recommended but there is little evidence of benefit. However, they may be useful as adjuncts to effective pharmacotherapy.

All treatments, especially the antisecretory agents, may mask the presence of gastric malignancy, so it is essential to exclude this possibility in middle-aged or elderly patients with alarm symptoms (p. 100) by gastroscopy, before initiating treatment aimed at the reduction of significant pain or if a trial of therapy is unsuccessful.

General measures

In the absence of good research-based evidence it seems sensible to avoid factors likely to precipitate symptoms, i.e.:

- take alcohol and caffeine-containing products only in moderation.
- avoid:
  - large meals (especially at night), acid foods, alcohol;
  - a fatty diet and chocolate;
  - tight clothing or belts;
  - stooping and heavy lifting (bend the knees with the back straight);
  - drugs that may reduce LOS pressure, e.g. *diazepam, nifedipine, theophylline* and antimuscarinics, including tricyclic antidepressants;
- stopping smoking may help some patients.

Feed thickeners improve symptoms in infants, as does sodium alginate in children under 2 years. Left lateral and prone positioning may help to reduce symptoms in infants under 6 months of age, but both of these positions increase the risk of sudden infant death relative to supine positioning.

These alone may be adequate in mild GORD, but good evidence for this approach is lacking. In view of this, patients should not attempt lifestyle modifications that impose excessive burdens.

Management: pharmacotherapy

The properties of the drugs discussed here are described under 'peptic ulcer' (p. 96), but aspects relevant to GORD are discussed below.

Antacids

Simple, infrequent, uncomplicated reflux oesophagitis should be treated symptomatically, using antacids as symptoms occur. Suspensions are more effective than tablets but, for convenience and prompt availability, the latter should be carried and sucked or chewed at the first sign of symptoms to minimize mucosal damage. They may also be sucked frequently between meals if symptoms tend to persist.

Alginate-antacid preparations. These depend on the reaction between alginate, sodium bicarbonate and gastric acid to form a foam, stabilized with viscous alginate gel. An alkaline 'raft' of foamed alginate then floats on top of the gastric contents and may tend to inhibit reflux. The raft will also be the first part of the gastric contents to be pushed into the oesophagus if reflux occurs, where it will form a protective alkaline coating. However, there is little evidence that this translates into significant clinical benefit compared with simple antacids, although some patients prefer them.

Most of the preparations in this class contain relatively large quantities of sodium, and so are unsuitable for patients with cardiovascular disease. Some preparations are now being marketed in which some of the sodium is replaced by potassium, but this may still cause a problem if patients are taking potassium-sparing diuretics.

If symptoms are not controlled within 6 weeks, the patient should be investigated by X-ray (barium swallow) or endoscopy.

The strength of the alginate gel is reduced by aluminium and magnesium ions, so antacids containing these should not be used concurrently with alginates. Conversely, the addition of calcium ions is probably beneficial, because they react to produce a stronger calcium alginate gel, twice as much of which is retained in the stomach after 2 h. Anything that reduces interfacial tension, e.g. *liquid paraffin* and *simeticone*, and so breaks the foam, is incompatible with alginate-antacid preparations.

Antisecretory agents

Confirmed refluxing or oesophageal damage is an indication for adding an inhibitor of acid secretion.

The drugs of choice, especially for resistant cases and if stricture or oesophageal erosion occurs, are the **PPIs**, i.e. *esomeprazole, lansoprazole, omeprazole, pantoprazole* and *rabeprazole sodium*. These are much more potent inhibitors of gastric acid secretion than the H$_2$-RAs (see below). *Pantoprazole* may have fewer side-effects than the others, but all are similarly effective: most experience is with *omeprazole*. Initial treatment is usually for 4–8 weeks. Fears were originally expressed that prolonged suppression of acid secretion may predispose to malignancy, but experience has shown that this is not a significant problem.

Patients who require long-term maintenance treatment should first be stabilized on a PPI. Those with severe oesophagitis will continue to need full PPI doses. Patients with less serious disease should be stepped down to the least expensive regimen that controls their symptoms effectively, with short-term increases for exacerbations.

H$_2$-RAs, i.e. *ranitidine, cimetidine, famotidine* or *nizatidine*, are less effective than the PPIs and relieve symptoms in about 25% of patients, but higher than normal doses may be required.

Sphincter 'strengtheners'

Metoclopramide is a *dopamine* antagonist that increases the tone of the LOS and may be added if symptoms persist. Once symptoms have been relieved, the regimen should be continued for at least 2 months, after which the dose may be carefully reduced, titrating the dosage against symptoms for individual patients. Although not licensed for this indication in the UK, the antiemetic agent *domperidone* is another dopamine antagonist that may be helpful (in the short term, because it is not recommended for chronic use). Because of their mode of action, both of these antagonize the effects of anti-Parkinson drugs, with an increased risk of extrapyramidal symptoms (EPS; see Chapter 6), and of some cardiac stimulants, e.g. *dopamine* and *dobutamine*, but

these are used rarely. Because *domperidone* does not pass the blood–brain barrier it rarely causes EPS and does not interact with *levodopa* centrally. There is also an increased risk of extrapyramidal effects and neurotoxicity with *lithium*.

Motility stimulants

Metoclopramide and *domperidone*, referred to above, also help by hastening gastric emptying, thus reducing the amount of acid gastric contents and so the possibility and adverse effects of refluxing.

Other drugs

Mucosal protectants (e.g. *tripotassium dicitratobismuthate* and *sucralfate*), have been used (unlicensed indications), but are only moderately successful. *Sucralfate* is most frequently used: the tablets are readily dispersed in water and for treating oesophageal reflux this mode of administration appears preferable to swallowing the tablets whole.

Carbenoxolone is rarely used now in the UK, because of its limited effectiveness and corticosteroid-like side-effects, e.g. hypertension, heart failure and hepatic and renal impairment.

Management: surgery

If symptoms persist despite an adequate trial of drugs, surgery may occasionally be indicated to repair a hernia or to refashion the cardia to minimize refluxing. Severe, prolonged oesophageal irritation may result in haemorrhage, with or without perforation. This is an emergency situation, the management of which is discussed below. It is now possible to repair oesophageal perforation by laparoscopic surgery.

Dysphagia

Difficulty in swallowing food or pain on swallowing may have many causes, including motility and nerve disorders, local trauma and malignancy. It is an occasional symptom of diabetes mellitus, due to autonomic neuropathy (see Chapter 9), and of Crohn's disease (p. 114). Dysphagia is always a serious symptom that merits urgent investigation.

Globus syndrome is an apparent dysphagia characterized by a 'lump in the throat' with no demonstrated physical cause, and is usually experienced by anxious or depressed patients who can nevertheless swallow food. Once investigations have ruled out significant pathology, the only treatment is reassurance, although extensive investigations may be needed to achieve this end.

Achalasia, i.e. inability to swallow solids and liquids, is caused by a failure of oesophageal peristalsis and/or of the LOS to open on swallowing. Oesophageal manometry will help to decide which of these is causative. The characteristic symptoms are a long history of central chest pain, progressive dysphagia and a tendency to regurgitate food, especially if the patient lies down after a meal. Achalasia often occurs in young patients, who sometimes experience severe pain caused by ineffective oesophageal contractions. Treatment is usually surgical, by dilatation of the LOS, or occasionally more radical surgery, but reflux oesophagitis tends to recur after both procedures. Injections of *botulinum A toxin*, which paralyses the neuromuscular junction and so relaxes the cardia, have also been used successfully.

Systemic sclerosis is characterized by widespread, diffuse tissue fibrosis, and is usually the province of the rheumatologist (see Chapter 12). In the oesophagus, systemic sclerosis causes a functional disability, with symptoms of dysphagia and heartburn. Treatment is symptomatic, because there is no adequate specific therapy.

Oesophageal bleeding

Aetiology

Bleeding usually occurs from **oesophageal varices**, which are distended anastomoses between the portal and systemic circulations. These occur around the lower part of the oesophagus (Figure 3.4) and are a consequence of portal hypertension, which is usually caused by restriction of blood flow through the liver as a result of alcoholic cirrhosis (p. 155). Changes in intravascular pressure and local trauma may cause massive haemorrhage from the varices, with a 30–50% mortality rate. Any significant haemorrhage will cause haematemesis (vomiting of blood), while less serious bleeding will cause melaena (tarry, black, blood-laden stools). The risk of bleeding is related to the severity of the underlying liver disease. In endemic areas of the tropics, **schistosomiasis** (bilharzia) is a common cause, because the parasites invade the liver and block the hepatic circulation.

Management

Bleeding varices are a medical emergency. Emergency treatment is with blood transfusions or plasma expanders. Applying direct pressure with a special balloon catheter in the oesophagus usually controls bleeding.

Terlipressin or *vasopressin* (antidiuretic hormone), which cause constriction of the splanchnic blood vessels and so reduce portal venous pressure, may be given as a temporary emergency measure. However, about 50% of patients fail to respond, even when these are combined with *GTN* to promote portal vein dilatation. *Terlipressin* is the better tolerated drug and has a longer half-life, but is considerably more expensive.

Once haemorrhage has been controlled (or occasionally as a first choice), **elastic band ligation** of the bleeding veins is preferred because it is probably more effective and leads to fewer complications. Alternatively, injecting a venous irritant (i.e. **sclerotherapy**), using *ethanolamine oleate* or *sodium tetradecyl sulphate* or *adrenaline* (epinephrine) via an endoscope, either to obliterate the vein or to constrict it, is more than 90% effective. Both of these treatments may need to be repeated until all identifiable bleeding sites have been treated, but bleeds may still recur.

Octreotide, a long-acting octapeptide analogue of *somatostatin*, has also been injected intravenously to cause venoconstriction (presumably *lanreotide* acts similarly), but this is an unlicensed indication. *Octreotide* appears superior to *somatostatin* and is safer and cheaper than *terlipressin*.

Very rarely, patients may require surgical intervention to fashion a portosystemic shunt, which diverts blood away from the varices. In severe cirrhosis, liver transplantation may be indicated, but is rare.

In the longer term a negatively chronotropic antihypertensive, usually *propranolol* (see Chapter 4), may prevent recurrence.

Helicobacter infection and gastroduodenal disease

Organism and epidemiology

Helicobacter pylori was first identified in the early 1980s. It is implicated in chronic active **gastritis**, **non-ulcer dyspepsia**, **peptic ulcer**, **gastric cancer** and a rare low-grade lymphoma (MALT [mucosa-associated lymphoid tissue] lymphoma). It is a Gram-negative, multiflagellate, spiral, microaerophilic bacterium, which appears to be an obligate parasite of gastric epithelium. *H. pylori* has been found only on gastric epithelium under the mucus layer and on areas of gastric-type epithelium that sometimes occur in the duodenum, but not elsewhere in the gut. It has powerful flagellae that help it to penetrate the mucus, and survives in the hostile gastric environment partly because of the bicarbonate-laden mucus and partly by the action of bacterial urease to produce ammonia.

Two strains are distinguished on the basis of cytotoxin production, a virulence factor that determines duodenal ulcerogenicity, i.e. cagA+ (cytotoxic antigen positive), and cagA–. Both strains occur in Western countries, so typing for this may become a routine aid to determine whether eradication treatment is required. In developing countries, most isolates are cagA+, so typing is not helpful there.

Serology is an unreliable indicator of infection because of the high carrier rate of *H. pylori* in the general population: 20% of people are carriers by the age of 30, and 50% by the age of 60. Much higher carrier rates occur in patients with active gastritis and duodenal ulcer (about 95%) and with gastric ulcer (75%). These prevalence rates are falling in the UK, probably because of improving hygiene. The high rate of gastric cancer in Peru is associated with a 50% prevalence of *H. pylori* in infants from poor families, and 60% of children by age 10 years, whereas juvenile infection is uncommon in the UK and the gastric cancer rate is much lower.

Investigation

H. pylori is urease-positive, i.e. it breaks down urea to carbon dioxide and ammonia, and this property is used to detect its presence. The patient takes an oral preparation of carbon-13 urea, and the presence of labelled carbon dioxide in the breath is detected. Detection of ^{13}C requires samples to be sent to a laboratory with a mass spectrometer. The test is very sensitive and specific. Endoscopic biopsy samples can also be examined for the organism microscopically and by culture: these samples are rapidly checked for urease by incubating in a medium containing urea, the production of ammonia being detected by the colour change of an indicator (CLO test). Both the isotopic and CLO tests have about 95% specificity, but the former is less invasive. PPIs and bismuth inhibit the bacterial urease and so should be stopped for at least 2 weeks before urease testing. Recent antibiotic use, i.e. within 4 weeks, may also give false-negative results.

An immunoassay for *Helicobacter* antigen in stool samples is widely available and can be used for diagnosis and for monitoring the eradication process.

Infection and epigastric symptoms

Although *Helicobacter* infection has not been proven unequivocally to be the prime cause of gastritis and gastroduodenal ulceration, the circumstantial evidence is very strong:

• Gastritis developed in two early research workers with previously normal gastric mucosa after deliberate self-infection.
• The presence of the organism in 95% of symptomatic patients.
• Resolution of symptoms when the organism is eradicated.
• Eradication of the organism results in longer remissions (up to 4 years in duodenal ulcer disease), than does simple suppression of acid production.

- The presence of mucosal changes in asymptomatic carriers, and association with a series of premalignant gastric changes.
- *H. pylori* causes:
  - local cytokine release, e.g. IL-6 and IL-8, and so recruitment of inflammatory cells;
  - suppression of somatostatin release and stimulation of histamine levels. The sum of these effects causes increased acid production, which produces gastric metaplasia in the duodenum, duodenal colonization with *H. pylori*, and duodenal ulcer.

There appear to be two sites of gastritis from *Helicobacter* infection: in the pyloric antrum and in the body of the stomach. Infection of the pyloric antrum seems to be associated with increased acid production and duodenal ulcer, but a low risk of gastric cancer. A minority of patients have infection of the body of the stomach and this is accompanied by reduced acid secretion and so protection against GORD: this may reflect colonization by the non-pathogenic (cagA–, commensal) strain or a genetic predisposition. Thus elimination of *Helicobacter* infection from the gastric body, which allows a variable recovery in gastric acid production, may be the cause of an observed increased incidence of GORD (see below).

Unfortunately, infection of the body of the stomach predisposes to gastric mucosal atrophy and, in some patients, to gastric cancer. This may possibly be caused by suppression of ascorbic acid secretion into the stomach or to the prolonged inflammation of mucosal cells, because ascorbic acid inactivates potentially carcinogenic nitroso-compounds and scavenges oxidizing free radicals. There is limited evidence from Japan that elimination of *H. pylori* infection reduces the incidence of new gastric cancers in those who had undergone surgery for earlier gastric neoplasms. Although it may be prudent to eradicate *H. pylori* in patients who need long-term acid suppression for peptic ulcer, and so prevent gastric cancer, the possibility of exacerbating GORD should be anticipated and patients warned to report any increased frequency or severity of symptoms, or any new symptoms.

Because chronic infection with *H. pylori* causes increased fibrinogen levels, it has been suggested that such infection may also be implicated in myocardial infarction (see Chapter 4).

Pharmacotherapy

Specific treatment should be used when *H. pylori* is found in association with peptic ulcer, especially duodenal ulcer. Some clinicians treat prophylactically if *Helicobacter* is found, even in the absence of symptoms. However, if the preliminary observations reported above are substantiated, we may need to be much more selective in the treatment of patients with proven or suspected *Helicobacter* infection.

Eradication of *H. pylori*

This is usually achieved using **triple therapy** with a PPI plus antibiotics, or bismuth chelate plus antibiotics. There are six different, though similar, regimens but none has been proved superior. Some that have been used successfully (about 90% eradication) are given in Table 3.5. It is unclear why a PPI is included as there have been reports of success with antibiotics alone. However, it may minimize further damage to a pre-existing ulcer and provide superior conditions for ulcer healing. Dual therapy regimens comprising a PPI and a single antibiotic are not recommended, because resistance is common.

One week of triple therapy is usually adequate, but 2 weeks' treatment has eliminated the bacteria in 91% of patients in one trial, with no relapse within a year. However, these longer regimens are often associated with more side-effect and compliance problems. Other trials have demonstrated protection against relapse in duodenal ulcer for up to 4 years. It is not known whether this represents a 'cure'. Although re-infection is unusual, ulcer recurrence may be expected if recolonization occurs.

Amoxicillin, nitroimidazole and *clarithromycin* resistance has been reported, and this is transmissible to other bacteria. Regimens using *amoxicillin* plus either *clarithromycin* or *metronidazole* (some clinicians use *tinidazole*) are suitable for use in the community, but those combining *clarithromycin* or *metronidazole* without *amoxicillin* are best managed by hospital consultants

Table 3.5 Drug regimens for *Helicobacter pylori* eradication

Treatment for 1–2 weeks with any of the triple regimens given below

Antisecretory		Antibiotic combination
Esomeprazole or Pantoprazole or Rabeprazole	PLUS	Amoxicillin + clarithromycin or Clarithromycin + metronidazole
Lansoprazole or Omeprazole or Ranitidine bismuth citrate	PLUS	Amoxicillin + clarithromycin or Amoxicillin + metronidazole[a] or Clarithromycin + metronidazole

Treatment for 3 days with a quadruple regimen, e.g.

Lansoprazole + clarithromycin + metronidazole + bismuth subcitrate

[a] The combination of amoxicillin and metronidazole is slightly less effective than the others.

with testing for resistance and eradication on site. Resistance testing should preferably be done before treating: this requires endoscopy with biopsy and laboratory culture.

Mild side-effects are common with regimens containing bismuth, *metronidazole, clarithromycin* and *tinidazole*, but side-effects causing cessation of treatment are rare. Antibiotic-associated colitis (AAC, see Chapter 8) is an uncommon side-effect of triple therapy.

A 3-day **quadruple regimen**, i.e. a PPI + bismuth + two antibiotics, is reported to be as effective as 1 week of triple therapy, with fewer side-effects, and a quadruple regimen is also used if a triple regimen fails to eradicate the organism.

These regimens are recommended for patients with proven peptic ulcer disease with *H. pylori* infection and where there is frequent relapse or a history of complications. They should be considered whenever long-term treatment with antisecretory agents is contemplated.

Eradication therapy gives a high remission rate in MALT lymphoma (see Chapter 10).

NSAID-induced ulceration and H. pylori infection

The nature of the ulcerogenic interaction between *H. pylori* and NSAIDs is unclear. NSAID-induced ulcers are more likely to bleed than those caused by *H. pylori*, possibly because the organism stimulates the production of gastro-protective PGE_2, whereas NSAIDs cause inhibition of PG production (see Chapter 12). However, although *H. pylori* eradication reduces the risk of new NSAID-induced ulcers in patients who have not had previous ulceration, the situation is less clear in those with pre-existing ulceration.

One study has shown that in patients with NSAID-induced symptomatic gastric ulcers, suppression of acid production with *omeprazole* is probably adequate. However, if there is a proven history of peptic ulceration and *H. pylori* infection, eradication before initiating essential NSAID treatment may reduce the risk of new ulcers. None of this applies to patients taking low-dose *aspirin*.

A recent review has confirmed that *H. pylori* eradication is a first choice in endoscopically proven peptic ulcer and functional dyspepsia, and as one option for treating uninvestigated dyspepsia.

Dyspepsia

The general anatomy of the stomach and duodenum is illustrated in Figure 3.8 and the physiology has been outlined above.

Aetiology

A self-diagnosis of 'indigestion' is one of the most common reasons for patients to consult a doctor or pharmacist. It is estimated that 40% of the UK population have dyspeptic symptoms annually, 5% consult their doctor and one-fifth of those who do so are referred to consultants for possible endoscopy (see below).

The term 'dyspepsia' is used to describe upper abdominal discomfort, usually related to food or alcohol intake. The symptoms reflect several different pathologies, and of those who have endoscopy, 40% have functional non-ulcer dyspepsia (NUD), 40% have GORD (see above), 13% have some form of ulcer and <3% have gastric or oesophageal cancer. Symptoms in the remainder result from non-gastric causes, e.g. hepatic, pancreatic or cardiovascular. The term 'functional' indicates that function is abnormal but there is no identified lesion or cause and these are often resistant to treatment.

Mistaken ideas about digestion are very common, but there is no evidence that any particular foods are 'indigestible', except for insoluble fibrous foods, the intake of which is beneficial. True dyspepsia, i.e. failure of digestion due to inadequate acid and pepsin production, is rare, and the possible causes of symptoms are listed in Table 3.6.

Clearly the range of possible pathologies is large, so careful history taking, examination and investigation are necessary to exclude potentially serious disease. Only some of these diseases are dealt with here and the appropriate sections should be consulted.

Investigation and diagnosis

The characteristics of individual symptoms, or combinations of symptoms, have poor discriminatory ability and are an unreliable guide to their origin. An approach to investigation and management is shown on p. 101. However, over-enthusiastic medication or investigation may perpetuate false ideas of organic disease.

Medication review should be used to guide the elimination of the many agents likely to cause

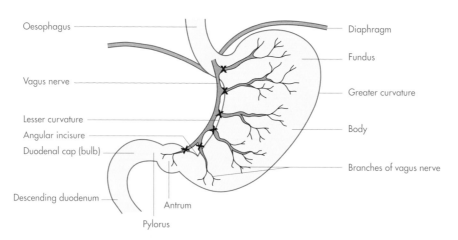

Figure 3.8   General anatomy of the stomach, duodenum and associated organs. X, points for highly selective vagotomy.

Table 3.6   Some possible origins and causes of dyspeptic symptoms

Oesophageal	Dysphagia, achalasia, reflux oesophagitis, hiatus hernia
Gastric	Gastritis, gastric ulcer, gastric carcinoma, gastric atrophy (elderly, pernicious anaemia), bile reflux, obstruction of gastric outflow, pyloric stenosis
Small bowel	Duodenitis, duodenal ulcer
Colonic	Crohn's disease, other large-bowel disease, intestinal infections
Other organs	Pancreatitis, hepatitis, gallbladder disease, hypoglycaemia, diabetes mellitus, myocardial infarction, congestive heart failure
Other conditions	Stress, inappropriate diet, pregnancy, gastrectomy, dumping syndrome[a]
Drugs[b]	Aspirin, NSAIDs, oral corticosteroids, oral iron, antimuscarinics (see Table 3.10), cigarette smoking, excessive alcohol or caffeine consumption

[a] Post-gastrectomy.

[b] Almost any oral drug may cause gastrointestinal distress in some individuals and this may even be anticipatory, e.g. with placebos. NSAIDs are the most common cause of erosive gastritis in Europe and may cause chronic or acute gastric haemorrhage.

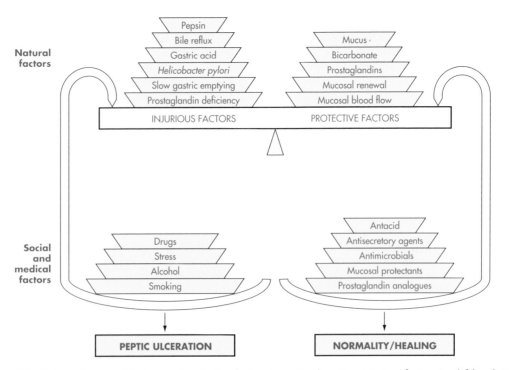

Figure 3.9   Balance between injurious and protective factors in peptic ulceration. Injurious factors (on left-hand side) guide investigations; protective factors (on lower right-hand side) indicate possible treatment.

gastric discomfort. Only one medicine at a time should be eliminated, or replaced if the treatment is essential, giving each change 1 month before concluding whether the medicine is possibly implicated. If the symptoms do not remit, that medication is clearly not implicated. However, if the symptoms do remit, the only way to be confident that that product was causing the dyspeptic symptoms is to rechallenge, i.e. reintroduce it and see whether the symptoms recur. Further, it is necessary to consider whether more than one product, or a combination of products, is causing the problem, because so many are likely to cause epigastric disturbance.

Mild symptoms in patients under 55 years of age do not need initial investigation unless there are associated **alarm symptoms**, i.e.

- dysphagia (pain or difficulty in swallowing);
- unexplained microcytic hypochromic anaemia (see Chapter 11), anorexia or weight loss;
- persistent vomiting;
- haematemesis and/or melaena;
- recent onset of progressive symptoms.

Although routine endoscopy is not recommended in the investigation of dyspepsia unless alarm symptoms are present, new dyspeptic symptoms in older patients raise the possibility of gastric or oesophageal cancer, and so a need for gastroscopy.

Patients who have not been endoscoped are classed as having **uninvestigated dyspepsia**. Endoscopy enables a distinction to be made between GORD, endoscopically negative reflux disease, NUD, peptic ulcer disease (see below) and cancer or precancerous states. **Barret's oesophagus** describes islands of columnar cells in the normal squamous cells, and is a precursor to adenocarcinoma (see Chapter 10). By the time cancer is diagnosed it is usually inoperable.

NICE has issued guidelines for specialist referral:

- Immediate (same day) – dyspepsia with significant gastrointestinal bleeding, e.g. vomiting large amounts of blood.
- Urgent (within 2 weeks) – patients of any age with dyspepsia and any of the following:
  - chronic gastrointestinal bleeding, e.g. vomiting small amounts of blood, blood in stools;

  - progressive dysphagia;
  - progressive unintentional weight loss;
  - persistent vomiting;
  - iron deficiency anaemia;
  - epigastric mass;
  - suspicious barium meal result.
- Urgent (within 2 weeks) – patients aged 55 or over if dyspepsia symptoms are:
  - recent in onset and unexplained, e.g. by NSAID consumption;
  - persistent, i.e. continuing for more than 4–6 weeks, dependent on severity.

Pharmacotherapy

Lifestyle advice (e.g. diet, smoking, drinking and weight reduction if overweight) should be given, but it is often difficult for patients to change longstanding habits.

NICE has issued guidelines on the management of simple (uninvestigated) dyspepsia (see References and further reading, p. 162).

Antacids

Self-medication with antacids is widespread and may be acceptable in patients under 40 years of age, provided that symptoms are not too severe and do not recur frequently.

The occurrence of drug-induced gastritis indicates a need to review whether this treatment should be continued. If it is essential, then an alternative formulation that is less irritant may be available. Alternatively, the concurrent administration of a PPI, H_2RA, PG or *sucralfate* is probably appropriate.

Antacids are available in a large variety of preparations (Table 3.7). Soluble antacids (i.e. simple sodium, calcium and magnesium salts), are unsuitable for anything other than short-term use, because they may cause bowel upsets, aggravate fluid retention and heart failure, or produce metabolic disturbance. Patients who drink a lot of milk to obtain relief and take calcium concurrently are particularly liable to develop hypercalcaemia (the 'milk–alkali syndrome'). However, some patients like to take sodium bicarbonate, which aids eructation of wind and may provide relief, but this should not be taken regularly and is contra-indicated in those on a salt-restricted diet and in heart failure. The types of antacids in use are summarized in Table 3.7 and their side-effects in Table 3.8.

The most desirable types of antacids are mixtures or complexes of aluminium and magnesium. Aluminium compounds alone tend to cause constipation, and magnesium alone can cause diarrhoea. Combinations of the two in appropriate proportions tend not to upset bowel habits. Suspensions are more effective than tablets, but less convenient for patients with frequent symptoms. For unknown reasons, the pain relief is unrelated to neutralizing capacity, relief being obtained with doses (e.g. 10–20 mL of a commonly used suspension such as *co-magaldrox*), that do not markedly raise gastric pH. Antacids may have some mucosal protective effect by forming a coating on damaged tissue, and some may adsorb acid as well as neutralizing it. It is reasonable to start with a product of low to moderate neutralizing capacity and to change to one of higher capacity (Table 3.9) if relief is inadequate. However, patient preference is the best guide to antacid selection. Antacids should be taken regularly to be effective.

Very high doses of antacids (about 200 mL per day) are required to neutralize acid effectively: this abolishes peptic activity and assists ulcer healing. However, these high doses are usually unacceptable to patients, especially as they obtain satisfactory symptomatic relief with much lower doses. Further, the prolonged use of high doses of insoluble antacids is particularly likely to produce adverse reactions. If gastric acid is a problem, an antisecretory agent is preferable (see below).

The basal (unstimulated) gastric acid output is about 3 mEq/h, and this is increased by about 30 mEq per main meal, plus smaller amounts for snacks. Accordingly, it has been suggested that doses sufficient to neutralize 200 mEq of hydrochloric acid per day are effective in most patients. Further, buffering capacity is important, and that of some OTC products may be too high, though the relevance of this is not clear.

There is little evidence to suggest that products containing *simeticone* are of special benefit unless wind is a problem or patients find such products particularly useful. Equally, there does not appear to be a role for products containing alginates unless there is proven reflux oesophagitis. Despite this, these relatively expensive products are frequently prescribed routinely as antacids. These latter two classes of product should not be used together because they are physicochemically incompatible.

Table 3.7 Some types of antacids in common use

Simple antacids

Soluble (more than about 10% of the dose is absorbed) — e.g. calcium carbonate, chalk; sodium bicarbonate

Insoluble (less than 5% of the dose is absorbed) — e.g. aluminium hydroxide; magnesium trisilicate; magnesium carbonate; aluminium–magnesium mixtures (co-magaldrox); aluminium–magnesium complexes, e.g. almasilate, hydrotalcite

Additional ingredients

Alginates: for reflux oesophagitis; usually contain considerable amounts of sodium or potassium bicarbonate; physicochemically incompatible with products containing simeticone

Simeticone[a]: for wind; physicochemically incompatible with products containing alginates

Antispasmodics[b], e.g. antimuscarinics (see Table 3.10); for griping or colicky pains; should be avoided in patients with reflux oesophagitis or paralytic ileus

Surface (mucosal) anaesthetics[a]: oxetacaine, for additional pain relief

[a] Of doubtful benefit, but some patients appear to find it helpful.
[b] May be useful in a few patients.

Antisecretory agents

Proton pump inhibitors (PPIs) should be used at full dosage for 1 month, because these are more effective than an H_2RA or antacids. There is no evidence of which of these is preferred, so choice usually falls on the cheapest product, usually generic *omeprazole*.

If this fails to produce adequate benefit, the patient should be tested for *H. pylori* and, if positive, this should be eradicated (Table 3.5). Although some consultants have advocated testing for *H. pylori* as the first choice, it is probably not cost-effective, because of the low yield in younger patients and because many patients are

Table 3.8 Some side-effects and interactions of antacid products[a]

Side-effects	Examples
Constipation	Aluminium (obstruction with high doses), calcium
Acid rebound	Calcium, sodium bicarbonate
Diarrhoea or loose motions	Calcium, magnesium
Wind	Carbonates, bicarbonates
Nausea and vomiting	Aluminium
Electrolyte disturbances:	
• hypercalcaemia[b]	Calcium, especially with milk
• hypermagnesaemia	Magnesium
• hypophosphataemia[c]	Aluminium, magnesium, calcium
• impaired iron absorption	All
Fluid retention	
Aggravation of hypertension	Sodium bicarbonate[b]
Metabolic alkalosis	
Renal calculi	Calcium
Encephalopathy	Bismuth[b] chelate, salicylate or subnitrate
Interference with diabetic control	
Dental caries	Sugar-containing antacids (some tablets)[b]
Antimuscarinic	See Table 3.11
Aggravation of coeliac disease	Tablets containing wheat gluten (p. 112)

Interactions Effect	Drug affected
Absorption reduced	Many drugs, e.g. Antimicrobials: ciprofloxacin, pivampicillin, rifampicin, tetracyclines, itraconazole, ketoconazole
	Chloroquine, hydroxychloroquine
	Iron
	Penicillamine
	Phenothiazines
Renal excretion	
• reduced	Flecainide, mexiletine, quinidine
• increased	Aspirin, lithium
Effect reduced	Bismuth chelate, sucralfate
Physicochemical incompatibility	Simeticone with alginates

[a] Where a cation is given this refers to all compounds of it unless otherwise stated.

[b] Effects occur only with excessive intake or in renal impairment.

[c] With frequent, chronic use: osteomalacia has been reported in extreme situations.

Table 3.9   Some common liquid antacid preparations in approximately decreasing order of neutralizing capacity[a]

Aludrox, Asilone suspension, Mucaine
Aluminium Hydroxide Oral Suspension BP
Magnesium Hydroxide Mixture BP
Maalox
Magnesium Trisilicate Mixture BP
Magnesium Carbonate Mixture BPC
Asilone Gel
Kolanticon
Gelusil
Gaviscon

[a] The most active products have about eight times the neutralizing capacity of the least active

infected without it being the cause of the symptoms.

Failure to respond to these measures should prompt a 1-month trial of an H$_2$RA, e.g. *famotidine, nizatidine* or *ranitidine*, to reduce acid production, or a prokinetic agent, i.e. *metoclopramide* or *domperidone*, to hasten gastric emptying. The H$_2$RA *cimetidine* is also used, but it inhibits cytochrome P450 hepatic oxidation and so interferes with the clearance of many drugs, enhancing their activity. Because the H$_2$RAs are less effective than the PPIs, their use has declined.

It should be remembered that all of these agents may cause gastrointestinal disturbance, so exacerbation of dyspepsia or apparent relapse after improvement may be due to the antidyspeptic product.

Figure 3.10 summarizes the factors influencing the release of gastric acid and the sites of action of antisecretory drugs and antacids.

Peptic ulcer disease

Definition

A peptic ulcer is an abnormal area of mucosa that has been damaged by the pepsin and hydrochloric acid of gastric juice, with consequent inflammation of the underlying and surrounding tissue. Erosion may subsequently occur into the lamina propria and submucosa to cause bleeding (see Figure 3.2).

Most peptic ulcers occur either in the duodenum or in the stomach, where the pH is sufficiently low for peptic action, although ulcers may also occur in the lower oesophagus, as a result of refluxing of gastric contents, and rarely in certain areas of the small intestine. Colonic ulcers are not included in this category.

Epidemiology

Dyspepsia (p. 91) is frequently thought of by patients (erroneously), as being caused by ulceration, but it usually denotes benign and transient inflammation. Nevertheless, peptic ulcers are common: it has been estimated that up to 10% of the population has an ulcer at some time, though many of these are asymptomatic, the annual incidence of symptomatic peptic ulcer being about 0.3%.

Duodenal ulcers are four times as common as gastric ulcers and occur mainly in the duodenal cap (the first part of the duodenum, Figure 3.8); among duodenal ulcers, half occur on the anterior wall.

Gastric ulcers occur mostly on the lesser curvature of the stomach, often near the angular incisure. These are usually benign, whereas an appreciable minority (5%) of tumours in the fundus and body of the stomach and the pyloric antrum are malignant. Most gastric carcinomas occur in the pyloric antrum, but it is rare for these to spread to the duodenum or for duodenal ulcers to be malignant. Gastric malignancy is

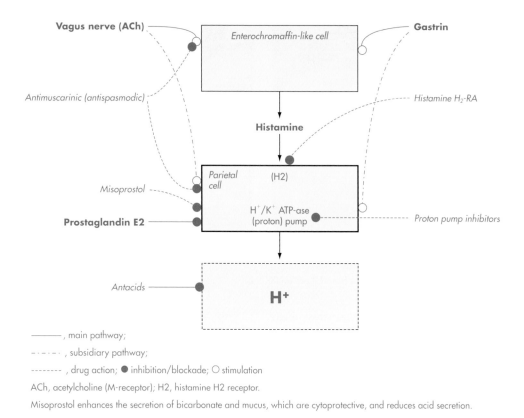

ACh, acetylcholine (M-receptor); H2, histamine H2 receptor.

Misoprostol enhances the secretion of bicarbonate and mucus, which are cytoprotective, and reduces acid secretion.

Figure 3.10   Summary of mediators affecting the release of gastric acid and the sites of action of antisecretory drugs and antacids.

much more common in Japan, Chile, Finland and Iceland than in the UK, the difference probably being a result of environmental factors, especially diet. Fortunately, the incidence of gastric carcinoma is declining fairly rapidly in the West, but it remains the third most common cause of death from malignancy in the UK and has a poor prognosis (10% survival at 5 years).

Aetiology

The aetiology of peptic ulcer disease is multifactorial, the mechanisms normally operating to protect the mucosa from self-digestion by the acid and pepsin of gastric juice either failing or being overcome by a combination of injurious factors (Figure 3.9). The most common causes of peptic ulcer in the UK are *H. pylori* infection and NSAID ingestion. The old hypothesis that ulceration is caused simply by hyperacidity is not tenable, because about 70% of gastric ulcers and 50% of duodenal ulcers (i.e. about 55% of all ulcers) are not associated with abnormally high acid production. However, gastric ulcers occurring near the pylorus may be associated with combined *H. pylori* infection plus hyperacidity, as are many duodenal ulcers.

Heredity is also important: the development of duodenal ulcer at an early age tends to run in families. Ulcers are also more common in blood group O subjects and in those who do not secrete blood group antibodies into gastric secretions, but the reasons for this are obscure.

Added to these naturally-occurring factors are a number of social and environmental ones, the most important being smoking. The ingestion of some drugs, especially NSAIDs and alcohol, also promotes acute ulceration. Spicy foods do not cause ulceration, but may aggravate symptoms.

'Stress ulcers' occur in seriously ill patients, and are common in patients in intensive care

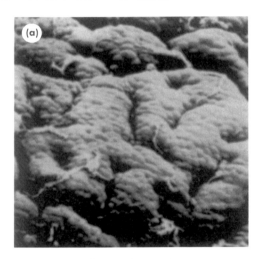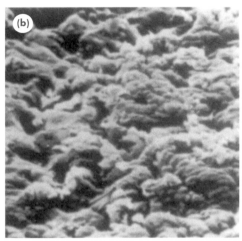

Figure 3.11   Effect of bile reflux on the gastric mucosa. (a) Normal antral mucosa. (b) After bile reflux from the duodenum. (Reproduced with permission from GlaxoSmithKline.)

units. Whether sustained emotional stress leads to chronic ulceration is unclear, although it undoubtedly triggers gastrointestinal discomfort and may aggravate symptoms. Hyperacidity, dyspepsia, and occasionally ulceration, are common psychosomatic features of psychiatric illness (see Chapter 6).

Balance between protective and erosive factors

Much more attention is now focused on the factors responsible for the maintenance of mucosal integrity. These include the secretion of bicarbonate-laden mucus and the turnover of mucosal cells every 36–48 h, factors that depend on an adequate blood supply. These are opposed by several factors that either promote erosion or facilitate it, including bile reflux, chronic gastritis (from gastric stasis, diet or alcohol), local ischaemia and hyperacidity (40%). This balance is illustrated in Figure 3.9.

The damage caused to the mucosa by reflux of bile through an incompetent pyloric sphincter (Figure 3.11) possibly accounts for the high incidence of ulcers in the pyloric antrum. The role of *H. pylori* has been discussed above, but there has also been considerable interest in the role of PGs and their synthesizing enzymes (cyclo-oxygenases; see Chapter 12), and small doses of PGs have been shown to inhibit acid secretion, promote the repair of damaged gastric mucosa, and to stimulate gastric blood flow in animal studies. PGs have therefore been described as 'cytoprotective agents', though there is considerable debate as to whether this description is justified. This partly explains why NSAIDs, which inhibit PG synthesis, are ulcerogenic.

Clinical features

Pain is the outstanding feature, varying from 'discomfort' to 'severe'. It is usually felt in the epigastric region (Figure 3.1(c)), although in longstanding, severe cases in which the ulcer penetrates into other organs, the patient may complain of backache or lower abdominal pain. The pain is often described as 'burning' or 'gnawing'. Sometimes a patient points with one finger to a spot in the epigastric region (the 'pointing sign'), and this tends to indicate an ulcer rather than simple gastritis. The occurrence of pain in either the left or right hypochondrium is an unreliable guide to the site of ulceration.

Spontaneous night pain, which may be relieved by milk or antacid ingestion, may wake the patient regularly at about 2 a.m. and tends to be more common with duodenal ulcer, although it is not known why. Generally foods – or particular items of food – do not cause pain, but strong

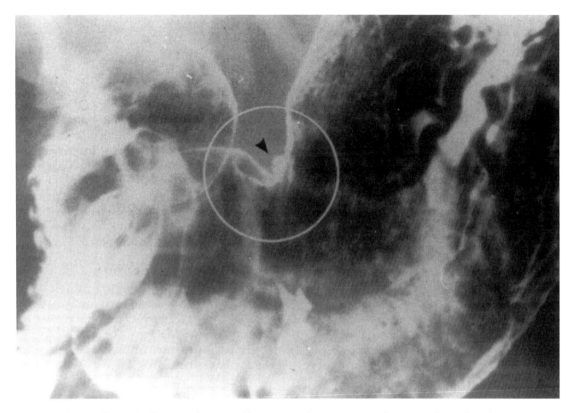

Figure 3.12 X-radiograph of peptic ulceration. The arrow indicates an irregularity in outline where barium contrast medium has filled an ulcer crater on the lesser curve of the stomach. (Reproduced with permission from GlaxoSmithKline.)

coffee or tea should be taken in moderation. Although it has been said that gastric ulcer patients may complain of pain about 2 h after eating, whereas those with duodenal ulcer may find that food or milk relieves pain, this varies considerably between patients.

The pain may sometimes be ascribed to angina or myocardial infarction (see Chapter 4), but the pain from these tends to be constricting/crushing in character. Further, none of these symptoms or signs is diagnostic, and gastric and duodenal ulcers cannot be differentiated on clinical grounds. All peptic ulcers tend to give periodic symptoms, the recurrence having no obvious cause, and the symptom-free intervals decrease with time in the absence of effective treatment. The most significant features are:

- waking from sleep with epigastric pain;
- periodicity of symptoms;
- a family history of peptic ulcer.

Investigation and diagnosis

History

The discriminatory value of a history alone is poor, because it has been shown that symptoms such as postprandial pain and nausea occur with similar frequency (in about 40% of patients) in NUD, peptic ulcer disease, irritable bowel syndrome (IBS), gallbladder disease and gastric carcinoma, although episodic pain is very uncommon with the last two of these conditions. However, history taking must not be omitted (see Table 3.3), not least because the information is obtained quickly and easily.

Patients requiring special investigation are those with complications (e.g. haematemesis, gastrointestinal haemorrhage or suspected pyloric stenosis), those who fail to respond to treatment, and patients taking NSAIDs whose symptoms fail to remit when the drug is stopped.

Investigation

The principal concern when a patient presents with symptoms suggestive of peptic ulcer is not to miss gastric cancer, but we have noted that the predictive value of the history is poor. The most significant factor for cancer is age, and any patient aged over 45 years with new persistent dyspeptic symptoms that have no obvious cause, should be investigated urgently. Additional indicators of possible malignancy are:

- male sex;
- smoking;
- a family history of gastric cancer;
- severe pain;
- dysphagia, especially with vomiting;
- unexplained weight loss;
- microcytic, hypochromic anaemia (i.e. iron deficiency anaemia due to chronic bleeding), also causing melaena (black, tarry faeces caused by the presence of partially digested blood);
- epigastric mass detected by palpation or ultrasound;
- progressive symptoms.

In the UK, the average delay from the onset of symptoms to surgery for gastric cancer is about 7 months. This is far too long, because studies in Japan, where the disease is more common, have shown that early diagnosis and treatment improves the prospects enormously. In Japan, the average overall 5-year survival rate is about 90%, whereas it averages about 10% in the UK.

Fibre-optic endoscopy is the most accurate investigation for the diagnosis of peptic ulcer and gastric cancer, and also permits biopsies and brush cytology (the removal of superficial cells for examination). If this technique is not readily available, or is contra-indicated in a particular patient because of the possibility of oesophageal or gastric perforation, a barium meal radiograph (Figure 3.12) gives good results. However, up to 20% of duodenal ulcers may be missed with this technique, especially if they are below the duodenal cap. The diagnostic yield from gastroscopy in most Western countries is poor and routine gastroscopy is not done, so early diagnosis is unusual, unlike in Japan, where they screen with mobile X-ray units.

Gastric secretion tests are of limited value and are now used only in special circumstances.

Complications

One of the most common of these is **bleeding**, which may vary from minor chronic blood loss that would eventually cause **anaemia**, to moderate bleeding causing melaena or haematemesis. The stomach is rather intolerant of blood: if the amount is small and the bleeding point is inactive, the blood may be partly digested and appear brownish in vomit, resembling coffee grounds. If bleeding is active and significant, then fresh blood will be vomited, and this is an alarming symptom.

A haemorrhage, from the invasion of the arterial bed underlying an ulcer, may occasionally be life-threatening. Therapeutic endoscopy, using rubber band ligation, laser coagulation, electro-coagulation, injection with *adrenaline* (epinephrine) or sclerotherapy, significantly reduces the need for emergency surgery.

Unobstructed **perforation** into the abdomen may occur and this is an emergency requiring surgery and broad-spectrum antibiotics. **Penetration** into adjacent organs (e.g. liver or pancreas), produces severe continuous pain, and **pancreatitis** may ensue.

Recurrent damage may result in scarring and the consequent contraction may cause gastric or duodenal stricture and obstruction. This tends to be more common with duodenal ulcer. The symptoms of this are a feeling of fullness after modest meals, nausea and vomiting. A barium meal may show an 'hour-glass' stomach, or food trapping and gastric distension. Surgery is usually required.

If **gastric carcinoma** occurs it is usually present at the outset, but a benign chronic ulcer may undergo malignant change, although this is rare.

Management

The objectives of management are to:

- relieve pain and discomfort;
- accelerate healing;
- prevent recurrence and complications.

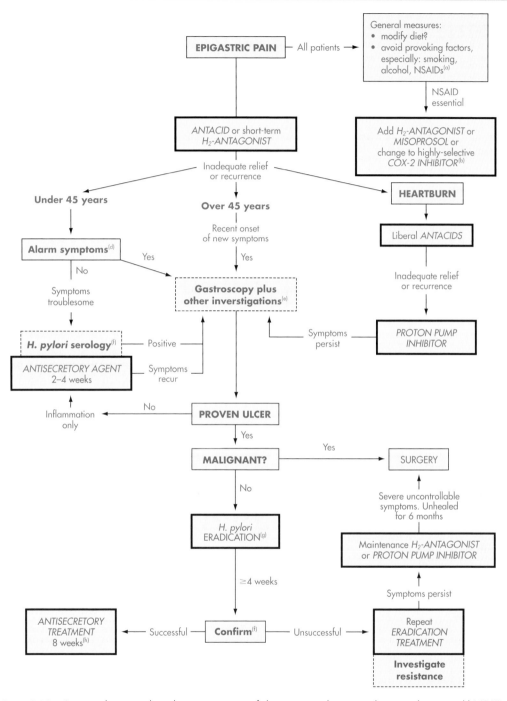

Figure 3.13   A general approach to the management of dyspepsia and suspected peptic ulceration. [a] NSAID. [b] See Chapter 12, p. 775. [c] This cut-off age will miss <3% of gastric cancers. [d] Symptoms suggestive of malignancy; see p. 100. [e] Other investigations may include full blood count, abdominal X-ray or ultrasound (to confirm perforation), etc. [f] Serology is suitable for initial screening but cannot be used to confirm eradication (because antibodies persist). See p. 88. [g] Triple therapy (Table 3.5). [h] Improves rate of ulcer healing. The figure should be read together with text on Dyspepsia (p. 91) and Peptic ulcer disease (p. 96). BOLD CAPITALS, thin line boxes, indicate diseases or conditions; ITALIC CAPITALS, thick line boxes, indicate pharmacotherapy; Bold normal text, broken line boxes, indicate examinations and tests.

Approaches are usually based on patient age. Malignancy is rare below 45 years of age, so **initially** these patients may be treated conservatively. This may miss up to 3% of gastric cancers but gives a reasonable compromise between risk and workload. Those patients aged under 45 with neoplasms should be identified fairly quickly by their lack of response to treatment and/or early relapse.

General measures

Regular small meals are advisable, and alcohol, strong coffee or tea should be taken only in moderation, because they are strong stimulants of acid secretion. Late snacks are best avoided, because they stimulate nocturnal gastric secretion. Apart from this, there is no evidence that any special diet is beneficial, although it seems likely that some dietary factor is likely to be implicated in causation, but this may differ between patients. Clearly, patients will avoid any foods that they believe provoke or aggravate their symptoms. Rigorous dietary restriction is stressful for the patient and may be counterproductive, but smoking and alcohol, which are known risk factors, should be strongly discouraged and patients should be warned against taking any medication, especially *aspirin* and NSAIDs, which is liable to cause gastrointestinal distress.

Anxiety and stress should be reduced if possible, by the adoption of a more tranquil lifestyle and the cultivation of hobbies, but this is difficult to achieve. Bedrest may be a useful adjunct in the short-term relief of severe symptoms, but has no advantage over modern drug treatment.

Pharmacotherapy

Aims

The aims of pharmacotherapy are to:

- relieve symptoms, by neutralizing acid or reducing acid secretion;
- promote healing, by enhancing mucosal resistance, eliminating bacterial gastric infection and reducing acid secretion.

Ulcers are intrinsically self-healing if the imbalance between erosive and protective fac-tors can be corrected. Healed ulcers are often found at postmortem examination in individuals with no prior ulcer history. With the exception of *sucralfate* and *bismuth chelate*, 'ulcer-healing' drugs do not actually heal or stimulate repair, but correct the imbalance and so promote natural healing. About one-third of ulcers remit spontaneously.

Antacids

These are indicated as sole therapy in young patients (under 40 years) and those with chronic, stable, mild symptoms.

Antisecretory agents

These include the PPIs and H$_2$RAs (Figure 3.9).

Proton pump inhibitors. *Omeprazole, pantoprazole* and the more recent agents *esomeprazole, lansoprazole* and *rabeprazole*, powerfully inhibit H$^+$/K$^+$-ATPase, the final common pathway for hydrogen ion (proton) secretion (hence the 'proton pump'), that is present uniquely in parietal cells. They are more effective antisecretory agents than the H$_2$RAs, and are usually the drugs of first choice.

They are enteric-coated prodrugs that are activated in the liver and bind irreversibly to the extracellular (luminal) domain of the transmembrane H$^+$/K$^+$-ATPase in the gastric pits, to produce almost complete achlorhydria following a single dose. *Omeprazole* was the first of this group, and has a plasma half-life of only 1 h, but because it produces irreversible enzyme inhibition its duration of action is at least 24 h. A single daily dose gives a peak effect after about 5 days of continuous dosing. After a single dose, or when treatment has ceased, inhibition of acid secretion persists until new enzyme synthesis occurs. The other agents are used similarly. *Esomeprazole* is more effective than *omeprazole*, but all of the PPIs appear to be similarly effective at comparable dosage.

PPIs produce more rapid healing of duodenal ulcers than H$_2$RAs, but healing rates with gastric ulcers, and the relapse rates following cessation of treatment, appear to be similar.

Side-effects and interactions. The list of common side-effects is rather long (diarrhoea or constipation, headache, rashes, pruritus and dizziness, nausea and vomiting, abdominal discomfort, bronchospasm, muscle and joint pain, depression, blurred vision and dry mouth), but these are usually mild and well-tolerated and rarely cause cessation of treatment. Although hepatic dysfunction occurs only rarely, it is prudent to monitor liver function before and during treatment, especially if prolonged treatment is likely.

In elderly males, *lansoprazole* and *omeprazole* may rarely cause gynaecomastia, i.e. breast enlargement. This needs careful investigation to exclude serious underlying pathology, e.g. bronchial carcinoma and testicular tumours. If obtrusive, mastectomy may be required, but this is rare.

Fears about possible carcinogenesis, which delayed licensing, are no longer believed to be significant. *Omeprazole* has been used for several years in some patients without untoward effects. However, it somewhat inhibits the hepatic microsomal metabolism of some drugs, increasing plasma levels, whereas *lansoprazole* is only a mild inducer. Caution is required with PPIs if patients have liver disease, are pregnant, or are breastfeeding.

Use of PPIs. Symptomatic *H. pylori*-positive patients should have eradication therapy (Table 3.5), all but one of which use a PPI. In *H. pylori*-negative patients, most PPIs give effective short-term treatment of peptic and gastric ulcer. However, *esomeprazole* is used only for GORD, NSAID-associated gastric ulcer and for the prophylaxis of gastroduodenal ulceration in those who need to continue NSAID treatment.

Generally, duodenal ulcers heal in 4 weeks and gastric ulcers in 8 weeks, but *rabeprazole* takes rather longer (6 and 12 weeks, respectively). GORD requires higher doses and longer treatment, e.g. 4–8 weeks' initial treatment and possibly indefinite maintenance treatment at a lower dose.

H2-RAs. These act by blocking histamine-mediated acid secretion via the H_2 receptors of parietal cells, and have gained wide acceptance as effective, safe drugs, having initially revolutionized the treatment of peptic ulcer before the introduction of PPIs. There are now four drugs of

this class available in the UK: *ranitidine, cimetidine, famotidine* and *nizatidine*. The first two of these have gained widespread acceptance, but all seem to be similarly effective at therapeutic dosage and are well tolerated. *Famotidine, nizatidine* and *ranitidine* do not appear to share the adverse hormonal reactions and interactions of *cimetidine*.

Dosing in acute attacks. H. *pylori*-negative patients normally use a dosage regimen consisting of a single night-time or twice-daily dose, though gastric ulcers may need larger doses and more prolonged treatment than duodenal ulcers. There is some evidence that dosing after the evening meal gives superior results to bedtime dosage. These doses provide healing in about 70% of gastric ulcer patients after 1 month and in about 80% after a further 2–4 weeks, but treatment may need to be extended to 12 weeks. Results for duodenal ulcer are somewhat better, and healing occurs in about 80% and 90% after 4 and 8 weeks, respectively. If patients are *H. pylori*-positive, then eradication therapy (Table 3.5) should be used.

Failure of therapy must always be investigated, to ensure that malignant change has not occurred and to exclude the unlikely possibility of **Zollinger–Ellison syndrome** (see below). Antacids may be needed additionally to obtain rapid symptomatic relief at the start of H_2RA therapy.

Side-effects and interactions. There are gastrointestinal side-effects, and occasional CNS confusion also occurs, especially in the elderly. Very ill and older patients are also liable to suffer the rarer side-effects of acute pancreatitis, bradycardia or AV block (see Chapter 4), depression and hallucinations. The doses of all of these drugs may need to be reduced in renal and hepatic impairment.

Cimetidine, uniquely among the H_2-RAs, potentiates the actions of *warfarin, theophylline, phenytoin*, beta-blockers and many other drugs, by inhibiting cytochrome P450-mediated liver metabolism. It should be avoided in patients taking these agents. *Cimetidine* also has anti-androgenic properties and may occasionally cause gynaecomastia and loss of libido.

However, these drugs have proved very safe and *ranitidine*, *cimetidine* and *famotidine* etc. are licensed for short-term OTC use in the UK. Although it may be reasonable to use these drugs to treat undiagnosed dyspepsia in patients under about 40 years of age, patients should always be investigated if there are prolonged (>14 days), severe symptoms, or associated systemic disturbance. A definitive diagnosis must always be made in older patients, to exclude the possibility of gastric malignancy.

Other indications. Ranitidine, cimetidine and *famotidine*, but not *ranitidine bismuth citrate*, are licensed in the UK for the treatment of patients with Zollinger–Ellison syndrome, a rare, slow-growing, gastrin-secreting pancreatic tumour that causes massive hypersecretion of acid and multiple large duodenal and ileal ulcers. However, a PPI is preferred for this condition. H$_2$-RAs are also used to reduce gastric acid secretion, and so acid aspiration into the lungs, during surgical and obstetric procedures.

H$_2$-RAs are also used for the prophylaxis of **stress ulcers** in intensive care units. However, patients with nasogastric tubes may develop pneumonia, so *sucralfate* is often preferred, provided that the patient does not have renal impairment and is not being fed enterally.

Cimetidine is used to reduce the breakdown of pancreatic enzyme supplements in cystic fibrosis patients and in those with **short bowel syndrome** after extensive bowel surgery.

Mucosal protectants
These include:

* *ranitidine bismuth citrate (ranitidine bismutrex)*, a bismuth/H$_2$RA compound;
* *tripotassium dicitratobismuthate*, a bismuth complex;
* *sucralfate*, a sucrose–aluminium complex;
* *misoprostol*, a synthetic analogue of PGE$_1$.

Apart from *misoprostol*, these form a protective sludge that binds to the ulcer crater, protecting it against further acid and pepsin attack. They are currently of great interest, because there is evidence that remissions are longer with these than with H$_2$RAs.

*Bismuth chelate (tripotassium dicitratobis-*muthate*)* is probably the preferred agent, because it has also been shown to be active against *H. pylori*, to increase mucosal PG levels, and to reduce pepsin secretion. If *H. pylori* is eradicated, the relapse rate is reduced to about one-third of that which occurs if the organism persists (80%/year).

Patients should be warned that the tablets cause blackening of the stools (and, occasionally, of the tongue), due to bismuth compound breakdown. The tablets should be swallowed with a glass of water (not milk), on an empty stomach: food, milk and antacids interfere with the coating of the ulcer by the drug, so none of these should be taken within 30 min of taking a dose. *Bismuth chelate* is not currently recommended for continuous maintenance therapy, as bismuth absorption and toxicity may conceivably occur. Although reversible bismuth encephalopathy has been reported in patients taking normal doses of bismuth salts, notably in Australia and France, this side-effect has not been reported with *bismuth chelate*. The current UK licence for *bismuth chelate* allows for a 28-day dosing period, repeated if necessary. If symptoms persist, there should be a gap of 1 month before a further repeat.

Other bismuth salts, e.g. carbonate, phosphate, salicylate and subnitrate, have been widely used as antacids and are used in some OTC products, but chronic use should be discouraged because of possible bismuth absorption, and patients referred to their doctor for investigation.

Sucralfate is also physicochemically protective and may additionally stimulate PG synthesis and the secretion of mucus. It is also used in intensive care (see above).

Although many patients take these products four times daily, there is evidence that twice-daily dosing is equally effective, and aids compliance.

Liquorice derivatives also have some mucosal-protecting properties and were popular before the advent of the H$_2$RAs. However, they are not now used for ulcer treatment in the UK, because they have mineralocorticoid properties and cause electrolyte imbalances, water retention and hypertension. Deglycyrrhinized liquorice products are of doubtful efficacy, but make useful placebos.

Other drugs

Antimuscarinics (antispasmodics, sometimes referred to less accurately as anticholinergics), which block the acid secretion produced by vagal activity, have a long history, originating from galenicals derived from belladonna and hyoscyamus. They still have a limited use today, but these and similar drugs (Table 3.10) are restricted in their use because they have a low therapeutic index and cause frequent and significant antimuscarinic side-effects. They may occasionally be useful at night, when their side-effects are less obtrusive, to reduce gastric motility and so retain antacids in the stomach. However, they are used primarily as adjuncts to antacids in the treatment of NUD if spasm is possibly implicated. Because spasm is rarely, if ever, confirmed objectively, this application is questionable.

Pirenzepine binds selectively to gastric M_2-muscarinic receptors to reduce the secretion of both acid and pepsin. It has no advantages over the H_2-RAs and has been discontinued in the UK.

Prostaglandins. Animal experiments have indicated that PGs of the E series (PGE) have

Table 3.10 Some antimuscarinics ('antispasmodics') used occasionally for the treatment of dyspepsia and peptic ulcer, their side-effects, interactions and contra-indications

Drugs[a]

Atropine, ambutonium[b], dicycloverine, glycopyrronium[b], hyoscine (scopolamine), mepenzolate[b], pipenzolate[b], piperidolate[b], poldine[b], propantheline

Side-effects[c]

Dry mouth, thirst
Dilated pupils, photosensitivity, poor visual accommodation, glaucoma
Flushing, dry skin, rashes (occasionally)
Difficulties in micturition, urinary retention in the elderly
Tachycardia, arrhythmias
Confusion (in the elderly)

Interactions

Drug affected	Mechanism
Glyceryl trinitrate	Tablets may not dissolve sublingually and not be absorbed, owing to dry mouth
Metoclopramide	Antagonism of effect
Tricyclic antidepressants	Increased antimuscarinic side-effects
Amantadine	
Ketoconazole, levodopa	Reduced absorption

Cautions and contra-indications

Elderly patients
Breastfeeding, infants under 6 months (especially dicycloverine)
Urinary retention, prostatic enlargement
Cardiac problems
Oesophageal reflux, i.e. hiatus hernia, heartburn
Paralytic ileus, i.e. obstruction due to a non-motile bowel
Ulcerative colitis

[a] Anions have been omitted.

[b] No longer used in the UK and all antimuscarinics are undesirable.

[c] This list is not exhaustive and generalizations have been made for the sake of brevity. The BNF and suitable texts should be consulted for full details.

acid-inhibiting and cytoprotective properties. Among various PGE analogues, *misoprostol*, *arbaprostil* and *enprostil* have been tested fairly extensively, but to date only *misoprostol* has been marketed in the UK. The last two of these have been shown to inhibit both gastric secretion and gastrin release, whereas *misoprostol* only inhibits secretion. However, the PGs appear to be less effective healing agents than the H_2-RAs and provide less pain relief. The PGs also cause diarrhoea and abdominal pain, side-effects that may be severe enough to require withdrawal.

The clinical value of PGs remains to be assessed, though this is clearly an important research area. Their use is contra-indicated in pregnancy, because they increase uterine tone.

Misoprostol reduces ulceration caused by NSAIDs, but does not abolish it. It is probably more effective than H_2-RAs for the **prophylaxis** of NSAID-induced gastric ulcer, but has a similar activity against NSAID-induced duodenal ulcer. *Misoprostol* is marketed in the UK in combination with *diclofenac* and *naproxen*, to minimize the risk of ulceration from the NSAIDs. Its most appropriate use is in elderly and very frail patients in whom continued NSAID use is regarded as essential, though NSAID use in this age group is undesirable. However, it is probably less effective than an antisecretory agent once ulceration has occurred.

Eradication of *H. pylori* is dealt with on p. 89.

If NSAID treatment continues to be required, NSAID-associated ulcers are best managed with continuous antisecretory treatment as long as this treatment continues.

Drug selection and maintenance therapy

Uncomplicated disease

The correct approach to maintenance in peptic ulcer uncomplicated by *H. pylori* infection or bleeding is controversial, because relapse is common. The question is whether to stop when remission occurs, or to continue with prophylactic medication.

In younger patients who have infrequent recurrences (up to two per year), the usual approach is to use a PPI and discontinue this after 6–8 weeks and give further short courses when symptoms recur.

If relapse is more frequent, or attacks are severe, the patient should be investigated for gastric cancer. However, if this is not confirmed, low-dose PPI maintenance prophylaxis may be continued for long periods, though some patients may need to continue with full doses. Maintenance prophylaxis is also indicated in debilitated or elderly patients who are unfit for surgery.

It has been suggested that the prolonged hypochlorhydria produced by maintenance antisecretory therapy may be undesirable, because the raised gastric pH reduces gastric digestion, and bacterial overgrowth, possibly resulting in nitrite-induced cancer (although there is no evidence for this). Nitrate in preserved meats may cause tumours.

Complicated peptic ulcer disease

Peptic ulcer accompanied by *H. pylori* infection or haemorrhage usually responds to one of the *H. pylori* eradication regimens listed in Table 3.5. If symptoms recur, despite confirmed eradication, retesting for *H. pylori* is indicated and a further eradication course prescribed if necessary, possibly quadruple therapy (Table 3.5). The re-infection rate is low (1–2% in Western adults). Uncomplicated peptic ulcer disease responds to PPI medication.

It is important to realize that some peptic ulcer patients may develop refluxing (p. 82) after eradication and the GORD symptoms may be misinterpreted as a recurrence of peptic ulcer disease.

Symptoms that do not respond to these measures require investigation by gastroscopy and biopsy. Perforation of the ulcer into other viscera or the peritoneal cavity requires emergency surgery.

A flow chart for the management of dyspepsia and peptic ulcer is given in Figure 3.13.

Surgery

Surgery is much less common now that effective medical management is available, but must be considered if:

• patients fail to respond adequately to drugs;
• malignancy is confirmed: all non-responding

gastric ulcer patients should be reinvestigated to confirm complete healing and the absence of neoplastic change;
• relapse and rebleeding occur frequently;
• complications occur, e.g. bleeding or perforation.

The most common procedure is highly selective vagotomy (HSV), which is less invasive than partial or sub-total gastrectomy, but rarely used now because modern medical management is very effective. HSV involves cutting selectively only those branches of the vagus nerve that supply the gastric body and fundus where acid secretion occurs (Figure 3.8), so preserving motility in the antrum. Clearly, however, stricture or malignancy may dictate the removal of a variable mass of the stomach and the duodenum. HSV is a safe procedure with relatively few complications, but it gives a higher recurrence rate (10%) and inci-

dence of diarrhoea (20%) than does partial gastrectomy (recurrence and diarrhoea about 3%). The more extensive operations leave some patients with distressing complications. These complications and their management are outlined in Table 3.11.

Nausea and vomiting

Definition and aetiology

Nausea is a prodromal symptom, i.e. it is the conscious recognition that the vomiting centre has been stimulated. **Vomiting** (emesis) is the forcible ejection of stomach contents through the mouth.

Vomiting is a common, usually benign, occasional, self-limiting condition, frequently

Table 3.11   Some possible complications arising from partial gastrectomy for gastric ulcer or tumour and their management

Complication	Causes and comments	Management
Early after surgery		
Ulcer recurrence	Up to 10%	Antisecretory agents; sucralfate (mucosal protectant); avoid smoking and NSAIDs
Diarrhoea	5%, mostly in the first month, due to a reduced intestinal transit time	Small frequent meals; antidiarrhoeals; cholestyramine (for poor bile salt reabsorption); antibiotics (metronidazole?, for bacterial overgrowth due to low gastric acid)
Dumping	Faintness or giddiness up to 2 h after a meal. A 5-HT-mediated component is involved	Eat dry meals (minimum fluid), lie down after eating Sugar if hypoglycaemic Methysergide (5-HT antagonist)
Vomiting	Uncommon: • reduced gastric motility • emotional factors • obstruction	Anti-emetics, especially prokinetic agents, e.g. metoclopramide, domperidone Surgery for obstruction
Late after surgery		
Malnutrition	May lead to anaemia, weight loss, hypocalcaemia	Symptomatic, e.g. vitamins, mineral supplements
Malignancy	Incidence at about 20 years increased fourfold[a]	Reoperation

5-HT, 5-hydroxytryptamine (serotonin); NSAID, non-steroidal anti-inflammatory drug.
[a] Compared with the general population.

with an obvious cause. When it occurs with diarrhoea, the cause is usually 'food poisoning', i.e. it is consequent on the ingestion of food or drink contaminated with bacteria, bacterial toxins, viruses or, occasionally, protozoa. Migraine, pregnancy and the over-consumption of alcohol or food account for many other cases. If there are no associated symptoms, especially systemic ones, the origin may be psychogenic, e.g. bulimia nervosa or stress. However, vomiting may occasionally be a result of more serious disease (Table 3.12).

Vertigo is an extreme, distressing form of dizziness in which the patient (or their surroundings), appear to be spinning. Unless of very brief duration, vertigo causes vomiting.

The vomiting centre in the brain consists of two areas, located symmetrically in the medulla, which coordinate the sequence of muscular contractions involved. Additionally, the **chemoreceptor trigger zone (CTZ)**, which consists of twin areas in the floor of the fourth ventricle, partially outside the blood–brain barrier, detects noxious ingested chemical stimuli and may be stimulated directly by parenteral drugs.

Central and afferent signalling involves serotonin at 5-HT$_3$ receptors, dopamine at D$_2$ receptors, acetylcholine at muscarinic receptors and histamine at H$_1$-receptors, hence the large range of anti-emetic drugs in use:

- Specific 5-HT$_3$ antagonists: e.g. *dolasetron, granisetron, ondansetron, tropisetron.*

- D$_2$ antagonists:
  - Phenothiazines, e.g. *chlorpromazine, prochlorperazine, thiethylperazine.*
  - Butyrophenones, e.g. *droperidol, haloperidol.*
  - Benzimidazoles, e.g. *domperidone.*
  - Substituted benzamides (*trimethobenzamide*, not UK-licensed).
- D$_2$/5-HT$_3$ antagonists, e.g. *metoclopramide.*
- Cannabinoids: *dronabinol, nabilone.*
- Antimuscarinics: *hyoscine* (scopolamine).
- Antihistamines: e.g. *cinnarizine, cyclizine, dimenhydrinate, meclozine* and *promethazine.*
- Corticosteroids, e.g. *dexamethasone.*

Management

General considerations

The occasional episode requires no treatment except rest, abstinence from food or alcohol and frequent small amounts of carbonated drinks, as seems appropriate.

In persistent nausea and vomiting of unknown origin it is essential to find the underlying cause and to treat that appropriately. The use of anti-emetics in the absence of a definitive diagnosis may mask symptoms and result in a failure to recognize serious disease. However, many patients demand anti-emetics to avoid discomfort or social embarrassment, but this should not preclude prior investigation.

Table 3.12   Possible causes of nausea and vomiting

Dietary indiscretion, food 'poisoning', alcohol excess

Fever, systemic infection

Organic disease: e.g. renal failure (uraemia), diabetic ketoacidosis, hypercalcaemia, myocardial infarction, COPD

Gastrointestinal disease: e.g. peptic ulcer, appendicitis, peritonitis, obstruction, gastric carcinoma, gastric surgery

Pregnancy

Central nervous system disease: e.g. migraine, meningitis, vestibular disease (Ménière's), abscesses and tumours, motion sickness

Psychogenic

Drugs: e.g. opioids, cytotoxic chemotherapy, digoxin overdose

It is always preferable to give medication in anticipation of symptoms, if that is possible, rather than to treat established vomiting. Anticipatory medication is especially important in the management of iatrogenic vomiting, notably from cancer treatment. Once vomiting has started, particularly if it is moderate or severe, the oral route clearly cannot be used, and rectal (suppositories), buccal or parenteral administration is needed. Doses adequate to control the vomiting are essential, otherwise the patient's confidence in their carers and their treatment will be undermined.

Acupuncture or **transcutaneous electrical nerve stimulation** (TENS; see Chapter 7) of the P6 anti-emetic point may be a useful adjunct to pharmacotherapy in some patients.

The neurokinin 1 receptor antagonist *aprepitant* has been introduced fairly recently for the management of nausea cause by *cisplatin*-based chemotherapy resistant to other treatments, used as an adjunct to *dexamethasone* and a 5-HT$_3$ antagonist. It has numerous gastrointestinal, cardiac and CNS side-effects.

Vestibular disorders

Motion sickness

This is best controlled with drugs that act at the vomiting centre, notably *hyoscine* (scopolamine). *Hyoscine* is available as tablets, slow-release tablets and a transdermal formulation. The latter two formulations may help to minimize the antimuscarinic side-effects of *hyoscine*, i.e. drowsiness, blurred vision, dry mouth and urinary retention, and confusion in the elderly, by avoiding the peak concentrations that occur with repeated oral dosing. *Hyoscine* is contra-indicated in patients with closed-angle glaucoma and should be used with caution in elderly patients and in patients with cardiovascular disease, urinary retention, gastrointestinal obstruction and renal or hepatic impairment.

In these patients, or if the side-effects cannot be tolerated, one of the sedating **antihistamines** (H$_1$-antagonists such as *cinnarizine, cyclizine* and *promethazine*), are less likely to cause side-effects (apart from drowsiness), but are less effective. The first dose should be taken 30 min before the journey commences (2 h for *cinnarizine*).

Promethazine is very sedating and should not be used if this might create problems, e.g. if driving, though sedation may be useful in some cases, e.g. with children or at night. Other anti-emetics act selectively on the CTZ and are ineffective in motion sickness. Alcohol potentiates the sedative effects of all the drugs used for motion sickness.

The *hyoscine* patches are applied to non-hairy skin behind the ear 5–6 h before starting a journey. The patches need replacing after 72 h and the sedation lasts for up to 24 h after removal, so patients must be warned against driving soon after removing a patch. It is essential to wash hands thoroughly after handling a patch, to avoid accidental eye contamination with *hyoscine*, which can cause fixed dilatation of the pupil and paralysis of visual accommodation.

Ménière's disease

This is associated with idiopathic dilatation of the endolymph system of the inner ear. It causes recurrent attacks of vertigo, deafness and **tinnitus** (a subjective sensation of noise generated within the auditory system), associated with nausea and vomiting. Over a period of years the disease progresses to permanent deafness, and the vertigo remits.

Betahistine reduces endolymph pressure in the inner ear and so is used in treatment, with variable benefit. A diuretic, with or without salt restriction, may be helpful and could be used as a basis for other treatments, but is of doubtful value.

In an acute attack, the antihistamine *cyclizine* or the phenothiazine, *chlorpromazine*, which can be given rectally or by IM injection, may be useful. However, the latter may cause prolonged sedation and should not be used if this is likely to be a problem. Other phenothiazines that may help include *perphenazine, prochlorperazine* and *trifluoperazine*.

Other drugs, e.g. *cinnarizine* and *hyoscine*, may also be beneficial. If the symptoms are distressing and refractory to treatment, surgical ablation of the auditory apparatus is sometimes done. This may relieve the vertigo, but it clearly causes deafness on the affected side and tinnitus often remains, and may be severe.

Vomiting in pregnancy

Generally, nausea and vomiting in the first trimester can be tolerated and drug treatment is usually contra-indicated because of the risk of teratogenicity. In common with other drugs, anti-emetics should be avoided in pregnancy, especially in the 3rd to 11th weeks, but in rare cases of severe vomiting *promethazine*, or occasionally *metoclopramide* or *prochlorperazine*, may be used in the short term (24–48 h), although they should preferably be used under specialist obstetric supervision.

Iatrogenic vomiting

This is most commonly associated with cancer chemotherapy and Parkinson's disease. Patients vary considerably in susceptibility to potentially emetogenic drugs. Emesis tends to increase with repeated exposure, though whether this is due to psychological factors, e.g. reinforcement of the unpleasant experience, or intrinsically increased sensitivity, is unclear.

The *British National Formulary* (BNF) lists three classes of potentially emetogenic antineoplastic drugs and procedures but this depends on dosage and patient factors (see Chapter 10):

- Highly emetogenic: *cisplatin, dacarbazine,* high-dose *cyclophosphamide.*
- Moderately emetogenic: *doxorubicin,* low to moderate doses of *cyclophosphamide,* high-dose *methotrexate* (0.1–0.2 g/m²), *mitoxantrone* (mitozantrone).
- Mildly emetogenic: *etoposide, fluorouracil, methotrexate* (<0.1 g/m²), vinca alkaloids, abdominal radiotherapy.

Anticipatory vomiting is best managed by prevention of **acute vomiting** during treatment, e.g. pretreatment with a phenothiazine or *domperidone,* continued for up to 24 h afterwards. For more susceptible patients, *dexamethasone* and *lorazepam* can be added beforehand. The latter has sedating, anxiolytic and amnesic properties, so patients have no memory of the unpleasant treatment. High-risk patients will need a **5-HT$_3$ antagonist** (see below).

Delayed vomiting, occurring more than 24 h after treatment has ceased, is best managed with *dexamethasone,* with or without *metoclopramide* or *prochlorperazine.*

The neurokinin 1 receptor antagonist, *aprepitant,* is licensed for the management of acute and delayed vomiting associated with *cisplatin* cytotoxic chemotherapy.

Drugs used to treat Parkinson's disease (see Chapter 6), e.g. *levodopa* and dopamine agonists (such as *apomorphine, bromocriptine, lisuride* and *ropinirole*) are very liable to cause vomiting. *Selegiline,* which increases the level of dopamine by inhibiting monoamine oxidase-B, has similar effects. The treatments outlined above are appropriate.

Metoclopramide has a wide spectrum of activity, and part of its usefulness derives from its enhancement of gastric motility, so hastening gastric emptying: an empty stomach reduces the volume of vomit, even if it does not abolish the reflex. High doses (maximum in 24 h, 20 times normal) are used in the short term to prevent vomiting induced by cytotoxic chemotherapy. The side-effects of *metoclopramide* resemble those of phenothiazines such as *prochlorperazine,* especially extrapyramidal symptoms, i.e. those due to dopamine blockade, but are usually less severe. Prolonged administration is undesirable, as it may cause tardive dyskinesia and hyperprolactinaemia, the latter causing sterility.

Domperidone has similar uses but does not readily cross the blood–brain barrier, although it acts at the CTZ, and so is less likely than the phenothiazines to cause central effects, such as sedation and extrapyramidal symptoms. It is useful in treating nausea and vomiting caused by *levodopa,* without antagonizing its anti-parkinsonian effect.

Nabilone, a synthetic cannabinoid, is reported to be superior to *prochlorperazine,* but is more likely to cause side-effects, e.g. hypertension, heart disease and psychiatric disorder, so treatment with it is best confined to hospitals. Because it may be neurotoxic, repeated or chronic use may be inadvisable. *Nabilone* may be used for intractable vomiting unresponsive to other anti-emetics. The related compound *dronabinol* is used in the USA.

The **5-HT$_3$ receptor-blocking drugs,** *dolasetron, granisetron, ondansetron* and *tropisetron,* are a relatively new group of anti-emetics. They are used for the control of post-operative nausea and vomiting and that caused by cytotoxic chemotherapy and radiotherapy, and are the most effective agents for this purpose. *Palonosetron* is licensed only for the treatment of vomiting caused by moderately or highly emetogenic cytotoxic therapy. Because of their specificity for 5-HT$_3$ receptors this group has a relatively good adverse effect profile, the principal side-effects being headache, constipation and rashes, though hypersensitivity reactions have occurred. A combination of *ondansetron* with *dexamethasone* has been shown to be more than twice as effective as *ondansetron* alone in controlling severe vomiting induced by *cisplatin*. Nevertheless, single agents are preferred in moderate emesis.

All of these 5-HT$_3$ receptor blockers are considerably more expensive than other agents and are used as first-line drugs only in oncology and intractable vomiting.

Corticosteroids

Dexamethasone (see above) has been reported to be as effective as *ondansetron* in controlling the acute emesis caused by moderately emetogenic cytotoxic chemotherapy, and is the drug of choice for preventing delayed vomiting. However, the basis for this, and the most effective dose and route, are unclear, though it may have actions at both D$_2$ and 5-HT$_3$ receptors. Moderately high IV doses are often used by infusion in cancer chemotherapy because an IV line is often already set up to ensure good hydration and renal drug clearance.

Anti-emetic adjuncts

Benzodiazepines, e.g. *lorazepam*, are useful for the management of cytotoxic drug-induced emesis, because they have sedative, anxiolytic and amnesic effects (see above).

Problems of the small and large intestine

Malabsorption

Definition

This is a syndrome of numerous diverse origins resulting in failure to absorb dietary nutrients. The term is usually used to describe a global failure of absorption, and is not usually applied to a failure to absorb specific substances, e.g. vitamin B$_{12}$.

Common causes are **gluten enteropathy** (see below), **Crohn's disease** of the small intestine (p. 114), bacterial overgrowth and gastric or small-bowel surgery. Less commonly, pancreatic, hepatic or biliary disease, or chronic *Giardia intestinalis* (formerly *G. lamblia*) or other infections (see Chapter 8), may be responsible. However, any condition causing chronic diarrhoea may lead to malabsorption.

Malabsorption may also be drug-induced. The lipid-regulating drugs *colestyramine* and *colestipol* bind bile salts and so may cause a failure to absorb dietary lipids. If these anion exchange resins are continued long term there may be an associated failure to absorb fat-soluble vitamins, so supplements of vitamin A, D and K may be required. *Orlistat* also reduces lipid absorption, with similar potential consequences. Some broad-spectrum antibiotics, notably those that cause **antibiotic-associated colitis** (pseudomembranous colitis, AAC; see Chapter 8), may also cause metabolic disturbances.

Clinical features

Generalized malabsorption commonly presents as **chronic diarrhoea**, often with **steatorrhoea**,

Table 3.13 Some symptoms of malabsorption

Deficiency	Symptoms
Calorie, protein	Weakness, weight loss, oedema, hypotension. Both together causes abdominal distension
Iron, folate, vitamin B_{12}	Anaemia, glossitis (sore tongue)
Vitamin D, calcium	Rickets (children), osteomalacia (adults), tetany (rarely)
Vitamin K	Bleeding tendency, haemorrhage
Vitamin B complex	Rashes, neuropsychiatric problems
Electrolytes	Widespread effects (see Chapter 14)
Fat absorption from diet	Diarrhoea, steatorrhoea

because failure of absorption increases the concentration of the bowel contents and so causes an osmotic diarrhoea (p. 129). Other gastrointestinal symptoms are abdominal cramps, borborygmi (bowel noises), flatulence, bloating and a swollen abdomen. However, nutritional symptoms may predominate (Table 3.13).

Gluten enteropathy (coeliac disease)

Epidemiology and aetiology

This is the most common cause of malabsorption in the UK (prevalence about 0.5–1/1000). It is about twice as common in Ireland but very rare in Africa, possibly related to the high-fibre diet there.

Patients are hypersensitive to the **alpha-gliadin** fraction of gluten, the protein in wheat, barley and rye flour that confers the physico-chemical properties that make dough suitable for bread-making. Gluten enteropathy appears to be the result of an inherited hypersensitivity state, there being an association with hyperthyroidism, insulin-dependent diabetes mellitus and dermatitis herpetiformis (see below). The jejunal plasma cells are IgA-deficient, there is an association with the MHC antigens HLA-B8, DR3 and DQW2 (see Chapter 2), and splenic lymphoid tissue degeneration occurs.

Coeliac disease may mimic many other diseases, and a diagnosis may sometimes be reached only after a long period of progressive elimination of dietary components and unsuccessful treatment for other suspected conditions.

Clinical features and histopathology

Administration of alpha-gliadin or gluten challenges to predisposed individuals results in shortening and eventual atrophy of the jejunal villi (Figure 3.14). This effect commences about 4 h after ingestion, the mucosal damage being evident within 24 h. This time course and other factors point to a type III hypersensitivity reaction.

In susceptible infants the disease usually appears as soon as cereals are introduced into the diet, causing abnormal stools, failure to thrive and occasionally vomiting. If the disease presents in later life, the diagnostic problems are considerable, e.g. adults may present with breathlessness and fatigue, consequent on anaemia. A definitive diagnosis can only be made by:

* Demonstrating the presence of IgA antibodies against gliadin, transglutaminases in tissues (tTG), and the endomysium, the thin network of fibrils surrounding all muscle fibres, and reticulin;
* jejunal or duodenal biopsy;
* remission of symptoms with gluten exclusion and relapse on challenge with its reintroduction.

Management

Management requires lifelong abstinence from gluten consumption. This is more difficult than may appear, because many processed foods contain gluten, or wheat or rye flour, as texture

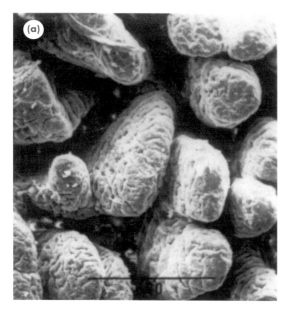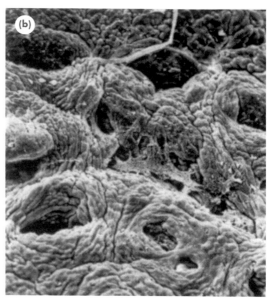

Figure 3.14 Scanning electron micrographs of the jejunal mucosa in coeliac disease. (a) Normal, showing well-developed villi. (b) After exposure to gluten: the mucosa is flat and has numerous pits and no villi. (Reproduced with permission from Dr MN Marsh, Hope Hospital, University of Manchester, UK.)

improvers. Gluten-free diets are prescribable in the UK through the NHS, and malabsorption is one of the rare indications for multivitamin therapy plus minerals. Following diagnosis, patients may need to persist with the diet for at least 3–6 months before symptoms remit, though most respond more quickly.

Some 20% of patients fail to respond satisfactorily, because of:

- exquisite sensitivity to residual traces of gluten in the diet;
- poor compliance to the severe dietary restriction involved;
- very extensive small-bowel involvement;
- pancreatic disease;
- malignancy.

Some of these problems may improve with corticosteroid therapy.

Complication: dermatitis herpetiformis

This is a rare, intensely itchy, burning, blistering sub-epidermal condition in which 70% of affected patients have associated gluten enteropathy. Malabsorption and the changes in the jejunal mucosa are usually less severe than in primary gluten enteropathy without skin involvement. The condition mostly affects adults aged 30 to 50, men more so than women, and follows a chronic, sometimes relapsing course.

Lifelong gluten avoidance is usually indicated, and this benefits both the skin condition and the malabsorption, though skin improvement may not be seen for 6 months or more. The rash is associated with the deposition of antigen–IgA complexes in the skin and responds to *dapsone*, which stimulates neutrophil and lymphocyte activity. Because patients with glucose-6-phosphate dehydrogenase (G6PD) deficiency develop haemolytic anaemia with *dapsone* and patients are often anaemic due to malabsorption, any anaemia or blood dyscrasia should be treated before starting *dapsone* treatment. Gluten avoidance spares the dose of *dapsone* required.

Topical steroids are of no benefit alone, but combinations with antimicrobial agents may be a useful adjunct to prevent secondary infection of intensely itchy scratch sites. *Colestyramine* may also help, possibly by binding IgA in the gut, but is likely to exacerbate intestinal symptoms.

Saccharide intolerance

Most patients in this group suffer from **disaccharidase deficiency**, so lactose (milk and milk products), sucrose, maltose or iso-maltose in the diet are not absorbed in the small bowel and high concentrations of these occur in the colon. This causes an osmotic diarrhoea (p. 129), with distension and flatulence. Treatment involves lifelong abstinence from contact with the disaccharides and the use of glucose or fructose.

Monosaccharide intolerance is rare and requires lifelong avoidance of glucose, galactose or fructose, and substances that yield these on digestion, e.g. sucrose and lactose, as appropriate.

Some nutritional deficiencies

Vitamin D deficiency

Simple **vitamin D** deficiency is usually caused by inadequate exposure to sunlight and is treated with small doses of *ergocalciferol*, e.g. 20 µg (800 units) daily. This is normally in the form of calcium and ergocalciferol chewable tablets, up to two daily.

However, malabsorption may cause excessive losses of the fat-soluble vitamin D and, because vitamin D is essential for the uptake and utilization of calcium, defective bone mineralization and deformity may occur, i.e. **rickets** in children, **osteomalacia** in adults. Provided that the patient has normal kidney function and an adequate dietary calcium intake, high-dose *ergocalciferol*, i.e. up to 1.25 mg (50 000 units) daily may be needed. In cases of severe deficiency an oily IM injection is available. Patients taking these high doses should have their plasma calcium levels monitored regularly, to avoid hypercalcaemia. The early signs of this are nausea and vomiting, but central nervous, cardiovascular and renal symptoms and bone pain may ensue. Because vitamin D is excreted in milk, pregnant and breastfeeding women should not indulge in the casual consumption of calcium and vitamin D, which may cause hypercalcaemia in infants.

People eating diets high in unprocessed bran may become hypocalcaemic due to calcium phosphate binding by phytic acid.

Iron and folic acid deficiencies, and anaemia, are discussed in Chapter 11.

Inflammatory bowel disease

Inflammatory bowel disease (IBD) comprises two distinct diseases: **Crohn's disease (CD)** and **ulcerative colitis (UC)**. Because the former can occur anywhere in localized sites in the GIT, from the mouth to the anus, the term 'regional enteritis' has been used. UC is confined to the large bowel and may be difficult to distinguish from CD restricted to the colon, except by biopsy. Although quite different, these conditions share many features and are considered together here, emphasizing important distinctions.

Three further conditions are now recognized: microscopic UC, microscopic collagenous colitis and microscopic lymphocytic colitis. These are diagnosed on sigmoid biopsy. They present with a mild episodic or chronic diarrhoea and, in very general terms, are treated similarly to CD and UC. They will not be discussed further here.

Aetiology

The causes of both CD and UC are unknown. Infective, immunological, dietary and psychosomatic causes have been suggested, but until recently there has been no evidence for any of these.

A possible association has been found with *Mycobacterium paratuberculosis*, measles and mumps infections: children who contract both of the latter in the same year appear to be up to seven times more likely to develop IBD some 20 years later. A causal link has not been demonstrated, but there is ongoing research into the association between *M. paratuberculosis* (see below) and measles. The research was related to natural infection with wild viruses and not to vaccination with measles/mumps/rubella vaccine, which is safe.

There is an inherited predisposition to an abnormal response to environmental agents, especially in CD, as there is familial clustering. The association between IBD, ankylosing spondylitis and the histocompatibility antigen HLA-B27 suggests some autoimmune component. Known associations in first-degree relatives are:

- About 50% concordance rate in monozygotic twins, but this implies an environmental trigger.
- The relative risk of occurrence of CD in first-degree relatives compared with more distant relatives is about 12, and in UC is about 8. The lower figure for UC implies that environmental factors are more important than in CD. There is also an influence on the type of IBD that occurs, i.e.
  - similar clinical course;
  - sites of CD in the gut.

Additional known genetic associations are:

- Between CD and genes on chromosomes 7, 12 and 16.
- Between UC and HLA-DR1*103.
- In Japanese patients, between UC and HLA-DR2.
- Between cytoplasmic antineutrophil antibodies (cANCA) and 70% of patients with UC and granulomatous vasculitis in CD.

In addition, environmental factors that may be implicated are:

- Infection: viruses and bacteria (including bacterial L-forms). Apart from the measles and mumps viruses reported above, the most promising candidate is *M. paratuberculosis*, which causes Johne's disease in sheep and cattle, involving inflammation of the distal ileum. It is interesting that these animals only develop Johne's disease if they are infected by the mycobacteria as juveniles, though symptoms occur only in fully-grown adults. This could account for the inability to isolate the organism from human CD patients. Further, some patients improve after antitubercular therapy.
- Consumption of refined sugar and diets high in fibre.
- Smoking: CD occurs more commonly in smokers, whereas UC, curiously, is often associated with smoking cessation and is twice as common in non-smokers. Further, nicotine is effective in treating UC.

The basic question to be answered is the mechanism by which an initial infection or other insult is translated into a continuing autoimmune reaction after an interval of some 20 years. This problem relates to diseases other than IBD, e.g. RA (Chapter 12).

Recent genetic studies have significantly advanced our understanding of the basis of CD and provide a link to the infective theory of causation. About 15% of patients have homozygous mutations of one of two genes (CARD15 and NOD2), which are often associated with fibrostenotic ileal disease (see 'string sign' below).

The NOD2 gene is expressed in cells in the intestinal crypts, macrophages and other phagocytic cells. Its product is involved in the innate immune system (see Chapter 2) and detects microbial components, triggering pro-inflammatory cytokine secretion and recruiting phagocytic leucocytes to promote their removal. The precise mechanisn by which the genetic defect is translated into continuing inflammation is unclear. There may be reduced microbial clearance, an impaired intestinal barrier to infection or reduced leucocyte chemotaxis to the inflamed sites. An increased sensitivity to microorganisms or their metabolic products may also occur, predisposing to enhanced inflammation.

However, not all individuals with NOD2 mutations develop CD, so other predisposing genetic factors are likely to be involved. Nevertheless, ongoing genetic research promises major advances in our knowledge of the aetiology of IBD and consequent improvements in treatment.

Epidemiology

Both CD and UC occur throughout the world, and affect all races and both sexes. However, the incidence is generally higher in developed countries, especially in Northern Europe. Although we have noted an interaction between genetic and environmental influences, possibly diet, attempts to link IBD with a lack of dietary fibre have been disappointing. The true incidence in the subtropics and tropics is unknown, because IBD may be difficult to distinguish from infective diarrhoeas, including bowel TB. Thus a trial of antitubercular therapy may be appropriate if laboratory investigation of biopsies is not readily available. Jews of central European origin seem to be about twice as liable as the general population to suffer from IBD, especially CD.

CD has a UK annual incidence of about 6/100 000, with a prevalence of about 50–100/100 000, the figures for UC being about twice as high. There was a rapid increase in the incidence of CD between 1955 and 1975, but this may have stabilized. The reasons for this are unknown, but an increase in the consumption of processed foods may have been responsible.

CD often occurs initially at a mean age of about 26 years, and is a little more common in females, whereas UC usually commences at about 34 years and is equally common in both sexes. The 15- to 40-year age group is mainly affected and there is a second peak with UC at 55–70 years, but both diseases can occur at any age.

Pathology

CD usually affects the terminal ileum and ascending colon (70% of cases). The inflammation is transmural (i.e. affects the whole thickness of the bowel wall), and often involves the mesentery and lymph nodes, causing adhesions between loops of bowel. Epithelial ulceration is discontinuous and ulcerated areas are separated by patches of oedematous or apparently normal tissue, producing a 'cobblestone' appearance of the gut lining. This gives rise to what are known as 'skip lesions' (Figure 3.15). The affected bowel is hard, rubbery and narrowed, with a small lumen (the 'string sign') and eventually becomes fibrosed.

The rectum is involved in over 90% of cases of UC, and inflammation may spread to involve the sigmoid and descending colon and, in severe cases, the whole of the colon (pancolitis). It may also affect the terminal few centimetres of ileum, though this is unusual. Unlike CD, only the mucosa and submucosa are affected, and continuously with no skips along the infected area. Severe disease is usually chronic, rather than episodic, and may result in toxic dilatation of the colon and perforation.

Clinical features

These will clearly depend on the site, extent and severity of active disease. The outstanding symptoms of both diseases (Table 3.14) are diarrhoea, unless UC is confined to the rectum or CD affects only the upper GIT. Fever, abdominal pain, malaise, lethargy and weight loss also occur. In UC, the diarrhoea is bloody and contains mucus. Acute attacks may be triggered by infections, the use of NSAIDs and severe stress.

Crohn's disease

Because CD can affect any part of the GIT, the symptoms largely reflect dysfunction of the affected region. Some patients may have only mild discomfort or may even present with general malaise, unaccompanied by gastrointestinal symptoms. About 80% of patients have diarrhoea. Onset may be acute or insidious. Severe malabsorption, leading to hypoalbuminaemia and consequent peripheral oedema, may occur when the ileum is affected and cause growth retardation in children. Recurrences are common (50% in 10 years), although the relapse rate decreases the longer the disease-free interval.

Many patients present with an 'acute abdomen' resembling appendicitis, with pain in the right iliac region.

Complications

A unique feature of CD is the tendency to cause adhesions, including perforation, and fistula formation may occur (a fistula is an abnormal connection between internal organs or between an internal organ and the skin surface); perianal abscesses may precede the onset of more general symptoms by some years.

Fistulae are especially troublesome in small bowel and perianal disease. The occurrence of prodromal perianal abscesses has already been mentioned, and rectal and anal lesions cause considerable distress, as do fistulae into the bladder or vagina. Failure of bile salt resorption may exacerbate diarrhoea and cause cholesterol gallstones and oxalate kidney stones.

Extragastrointestinal features are common and include mouth ulcers, rashes, finger clubbing

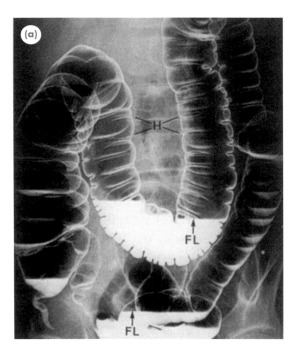
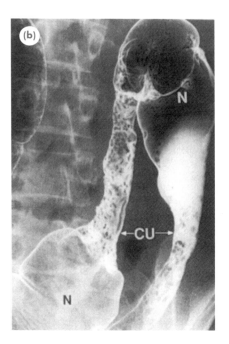
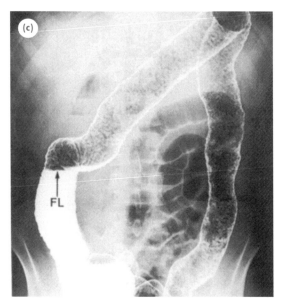

Figure 3.15   Radiological features in IBD. (a) Normal double-contrast barium enema showing a distensible colon with well-marked haustrations (segmentations, H), and fluid levels of pools of contrast medium (FL). (b) CD of the colon showing discontinuous ulceration, abrupt transition from normal areas (N) to diseased ones, good distensibility of normal (but not diseased) colon, 'cobblestone' ulceration and 'hosepipe' strictures (CU). (c) Advanced UC showing lack of distensibility, continuous ulceration of the whole colon (pancolitis) and loss of haustrations. There is a pool of contrast medium in the ascending colon, showing the fluid level. (Reproduced with permission from Pharmacia Ltd.)

Table 3.14   Principal features of the inflammatory bowel diseases

Feature	Crohn's disease	Ulcerative colitis
Diarrhoea	Mild to severe	Mild to very severe
Stools	Steatorrhoea (small intestine affected), visible or occult blood (sigmoid colon or rectal disease) Occasionally constipation, usually due to obstruction	Blood, mucus, pus
Usual site	Mostly terminal ileum and ascending colon but possible anywhere in the gut	Colon only, rectum is usually involved
Sigmoid colon	Normal, or patchy ulceration	Always diffusely inflamed or ulcerated
Gut wall	Full thickness involvement	Mucosa and submucosa only
Extra-intestinal abdominal features	Yes; fatty liver, renal stones, adhesions	No
Fistulae	Common	No
Onset	Insidious or acute	Usually insidious, occasionally sudden and severe
Pain	Colicky, may mimic appendicitis	Lower abdominal discomfort. Moderate to severe attack is accompanied by systemic symptoms, e.g. fever, tachycardia
Oral aphthous ulceration	Common	Occasionally
Peri-anal abscesses	Yes	No
ESR raised	Yes	Yes
Anaemia	Yes	Yes
Complications • abdominal • extra-intestinal	• Gallstones, perianal and internal fistulas • Eyes, joints, skin, spine, fatty liver disease, renal stones, adhesions	As for Crohn's disease, but no gallstones, fistulas or renal stones

(see Chapter 5), eye problems (7% of patients), joint pain (14%), inflammatory arthritis (10%) or ankylosing spondylitis (9%), gallstones (up to 30%), kidney stones (in patients with small bowel disease) and skin rashes (5%). Rare complications include toxic megacolon, bowel perforation, renal and liver disease and amyloid disease (see Chapter 12). Many patients have several of these complications. Obstruction may accompany ileocaecal disease.

There is a slightly increased risk of colon cancer if the colon is markedly involved, but this is very much less than in UC (see below).

Complications are frequently associated with exacerbations of the gastrointestinal symptoms. Despite this long catalogue of possible symptoms,

Table 3.15   Differential diagnosis of inflammatory bowel disease

Antibiotic-associated colitis (see Chapter 8)
Appendicitis
Bowel cancer
Coeliac disease (p. 112)
Diverticular disease (p. 124)
Irritable bowel syndrome (p. 132)
Ischaemic colitis
Lymphomas (see Chapter 10)
Infections: *Campylobacter, Yersinia, Salmonella, Shigella,* tuberculosis, sexually transmitted proctitis, giardiasis,
        amoebic dysentery, schistosomiasis

patients sometimes present with unexplained weight loss as the sole symptom.

Ulcerative colitis

Diarrhoea in acute UC may be very severe, with 10–20 watery, bloody motions with mucus occurring throughout a 24-h period. However, disease confined to the rectum may cause severe constipation. The disease may present with mild symptoms, especially if restricted to the rectum and the sigmoid colon, but severe cases may be life-threatening.

Complications

Severe diarrhoea may cause dehydration and malabsorption with hypokalaemia, metabolic acidosis, anaemia, weight loss, hypoalbuminaemia and oedema. Skin lesions, large joint inflammatory arthritis, toxic megacolon and biliary tract disease, including carcinoma, may occur. Patients with long-standing disease (10 years), and those in whom a pancolitis has ever occurred, have a greatly increased risk of bowel perforation and carcinoma of the colon.

Diagnosis

This requires a careful history and examination. Investigations include a full blood count, ESR, electrolytes, barium meal and follow-through, double-contrast barium enema, sigmoidoscopy and/or colonoscopy and biopsy, and stool cultures. CD patients may show characteristic changes in the sigmoid colon even if it is not apparently involved.

Both diseases may be difficult to diagnose and distinguish from other causes of chronic diarrhoea, unless there is a high index of suspicion, or the patient's condition is severe and characteristic. Some diseases that may be confused with IBD are given in Table 3.15.

Management

Aims

The aims of management include:

- rapid symptom relief and prompt control of acute attacks;
- correction of metabolic disturbances;
- prevention of serious complications;
- long-term immunosuppressive and/or anti-inflammatory, prophylactic or maintenance therapy (for some patients);
- anticipation of the need for surgery and, if possible, avoidance of emergency procedures.

Both diseases are treated somewhat similarly. Because there is considerable variation in presentation and the severity of their symptoms, only very general guidelines can be given here.

The precise approach will depend on the condition and response of each patient, and the likelihood of serious complications.

Clearly, any aspects of diet or medication that may exacerbate the diarrhoea should be rectified.

Nutritional support plus correction of fluid and electrolyte imbalance. Corticosteroids (see below) may be sufficient for occasional acute attacks and exacerbations. More intensive pharmacotherapy is required for those who suffer frequent exacerbations or chronic symptoms.

General measures

Patient education about the nature of their disease and its treatment is essential. They need to participate actively with their doctors in therapeutic modifications to manage unpredictable variations in disease activity. Patients should be in the care of a specialized clinic and those with moderate to severe disease treated in hospital.

Bedrest may be helpful in debilitated patients. CD patients should stop smoking. Stress reduction is frequently advised, but difficult to follow. It is not clear whether stress is a trigger factor for exacerbations of the disease or a consequence of the symptoms.

In the absence of precise knowledge of the aetiology of IBD, anti-inflammatory and immunosuppressive drugs are the mainstay of therapy. These include corticosteroids, immunosuppressants, aminosalicylates, biological agents (monoclonal antibodies, cytokine inhibitors). Antibiotics may be required in CD with perineal disease.

Acute attacks and exacerbations

Supportive therapies

A highly nutritious, low-residue fluid ('elemental') diet, enteral nutrition (i.e. by nasogastric tube), or percutaneous enteral gastroscopy (PEG) if there is mouth or oesophageal involvement in CD. This is also needed if a bowel stricture is present and obstruction is possible. Vitamin supplementation may be required, especially vitamin B_{12} and folate in CD that causes malabsorption (see Chapter 11 and p. 111). A low-fat, low linoleic acid diet is helpful if there is steatorrhoea in CD.

'Bowel rest' does not seem to be beneficial and the concept does not appear to be valid.

Anaemia will usually respond to control of the disease, but oral or parenteral iron, or blood transfusion may sometimes be needed.

Pharmacotherapy

Antidiarrhoeal agents, e.g. *loperamide* or *codeine*, may be needed to control florid symptoms, but should be used sparingly because the resultant slower clearance of faecal residues may encourage the accumulation of pro-inflammatory agents, with symptom aggravation and even **toxic megacolon**. However, patients need relief from frequent defecation, so a balance has to be struck between symptom relief and toxic risk.

Corticosteroids are the most effective agents and should be used to bring symptoms under control promptly in CD, the response rate being 60–90% depending on disease severity and location. Patients with moderate to severe disease lose confidence in their physician if they have to suffer miserably during trials of less effective drugs.

Steroids, used intravenously in severe attacks, may be combined with aminosalicylates (see below) or, if the patient has been admitted in the previous 2–3 years with moderate to severe attacks, *azathioprine*.

Oral *prednisolone* 30–60 mg daily, reducing over 6–8 weeks, is widely used, with or without *azathioprine* or its metabolite, *6-mercaptopurine* (see below). In severe cases IV *hydrocortisone* or *methylprednisolone* therapy is used, e.g. up to 100 mg *hydrocortisone* 6-hourly.

Corticosteroid retention enemas are useful in CD only for rectal or distal colonic disease. Mild to moderate CD confined to the ileum and ascending colon may get adequate benefit from oral modified-release *budesonide*. This has high topical potency and undergoes extensive first-pass metabolism, so adverse effects are less common and severe than with other corticosteroids.

In UC, corticosteroids are used to obtain remission in moderate to severe attacks or as an adjunct to aminosalicylates (see below). Corticosteroid retention enemas or rectal foams are used routinely for UC and spare the systemic corticosteroid dose.

Immunosuppressants. *Azathioprine*, or its metabolite *mercaptopurine*, is used, especially in CD and moderate to severe UC for its steroid-sparing effect. It is ineffective as sole therapy in active disease and should be given promptly in severe disease, e.g. pancolitis (affecting the whole colon), as it takes several weeks to exert its effect. They are suitable for long-term maintenance therapy, but there is a high relapse rate on discontinuation.

Methotrexate and IV *ciclosporin*, a calcineurin inhibitor, have been used to manage disease resistant to steroids and other immunosuppressants. They are effective in producing remission but not for maintenance therapy. *Mycophenolate mofetil*, given intravenously only, has been used similarly (unlicensed indication). It is effective in severe, steroid-resistant UC, being used initially as an IV infusion, transferring to oral use for maintenance. It may avoid the need for surgery or give time for surgery to be planned as an elective procedure, but this must be weighed against the risks of serious complications occurring as a result of delay.

Aminosalicylates. These include *sulfasalazine (SSZ)*, the original member of this group, which is a salt formed between sulfapyridine (SP) and 5-aminosalicylic acid (5-ASA); *olsalazine* (a dimer of 5-ASA); *mesalazine* (modified-release 5-ASA); and *balsalazide* (5-ASA linked by a diazo bond to 4-aminobenzoyl-beta-alanine, a carrier that has no pharmacological effect, unlike SP).

SSZ is not absorbed in the small intestine, and the SP acts as a carrier to deliver 5-ASA to the colon, where the *SSZ* is split by bacterial action, though the validity of this assumption has been questioned. The SP and some 5-ASA are subsequently absorbed, but about 50% of the 5-ASA remains in the colon to exert a local anti-inflammatory effect. *SSZ* is less widely used now than other aminosalicylates because of its poorer side-effect profile, due to the absorbed SP (see below).

Oral *mesalazine* is specially formulated for large bowel release, in an attempt to avoid absorption of 5-ASA from the small intestine. However, the time to reach the ileocaecal junction and the ileal residence time are very variable, due to disease activity, both between individuals and in the same patient at different times, so the extent to which 5-ASA release is confined to the large bowel is unpredictable. This may explain some failures of therapy. It is licensed for the oral treatment of mild to moderate UC and to maintain remission.

Olsalazine is similarly split by colonic bacteria to yield only 5-ASA and is licensed to treat mild UC and maintain remission. *Balsalazide* is a pro-drug of 5-ASA and resembles *SSZ* in drug delivery.

The aminosalicylates are used primarily to induce and maintain remission in UC (see below), and for maintenance in CD. *Olsalazine* is licensed for use in mild UC, *balsalazide* and *mesalazine* for mild to moderate UC. Any of this group may be adequate alone in mild attacks of UC, but moderate disease may also need corticosteroids.

SSZ is the only member of this group licensed for all severities of UC and for active CD, and also has a steroid-sparing effect. However, it has a limited place in the treatment of severe attacks, possibly because its hydrolysis to release 5-ASA is unpredictable in the diseased colon. Because of its poorer side-effect profile it is being used less often than the other aminosalicylates. *SSZ* may occasionally be used to treat active CD confined to the distal colon.

Biological agents. Only one of these, *infliximab*, is currently used in IBD. It is a chimeric murine/human monoclonal antibody against the potent pro-inflammatory TNFalpha (see Chapter 2). It is used in severe active CD, especially if there is fistulation, and spares the corticosteroid dose. It is also licensed for moderate to severe UC. However, it is antigenic and the development of antibodies limits its usefulness. Limitations on its use are the need to give it by IV infusion and that it may cause severe anaphylactic reactions, so full resuscitation facilities must be immediately available. It must not be used in patients with active TB, which must be treated for at least 2 months before initiating *infliximab* treatment. It may also trigger reactivation from dormant tubercles (see Chapter 8). Patients require careful monitoring for TB and other infections, which may be severe.

Recent trials have confirmed that *infliximab* is effective in UC. It produces about a 60% response rate at 8 weeks and about a 45% remission rate at 30 weeks. There is also significant mucosal healing and a steroid-sparing effect. Consequently, *infliximab* is likely to be especially beneficial in patients who are unresponsive to corticosteroids or are steroid-dependent, and in those who do not tolerate conventional immunosuppressive treatment.

Adalimumab is a fully human anti-TNF antibody that is currently licensed only for use in rheumatoid disease (see Chapter 12), but the licence is likely to be extended shortly for use in CD. It has been shown to produce remission in active disease. The most effective regimen, a loading dose of 160 mg followed by 80 mg 2 weeks later, gives a remission rate of about 36% at 4 weeks. These doses are much larger than those used for RA. It appears to be effective in those who are not responding adequately to *infliximab*, but it is still antigenic. It has the advantage over *infliximab* that it is given by SC injection rather than by IV infusion, but has the same restrictions regarding infections.

Certolizumab is a new, as yet unlicensed, humanised pegylated Fab fragment (see Chapter 2) of anti-TNF antibody. Given by monthly SC injection it has achieved a 53% response rate at 10 weeks in one study and a 63% response rate over 26 weeks in another, in which about 48% were in remission. This result was not affected by previous treatment or the initial level of inflammation, as measured by CRP measurement.

Another new monoclonal antibody, *natalizumab*, is directed against alpha$_4$-integrin, an adhesion molecule expressed on lymphocytes. It prevents lymphocyte adhesion to the endothelium of the inflamed intestinal microvasculature and so infiltration of lymphocytes into the intestinal lumen. Early trials showed an impressive response in CD patients. It has been withdrawn for further safety evaluation following the occurrence of progressive multifocal leucoencephalopathy in two multiple sclerosis patients, a serious viral demyelinating CNS disease leading to paralysis and death. Despite this, *natalizumab* indicates a new and promising potential mode of treatment. Because of its novel mode of action it should be effective in patients in whom anti-TNF therapies have failed.

Antibiotics.   *Metronidazole* or *tinidazole* may be useful if there is bacterial overgrowth in the bowel or if septic complications occur, because anaerobes are often involved. Bowel perforation may lead to peritonitis and septicaemia, with an urgent need for surgery and parenteral antibiotics, after the identification of microbial sensitivities. *Co-trimoxazole* (trimethoprim plus sulfamethoxazole) has been used but is now appropriate only for infections of known sensitivity that are unresponsive to other agents.

Continuing diarrhoea in well-treated patients is not necessarily due to infection, but may be due to failure of the diseased small bowel to reabsorb bile salts (see Chapter 3). Treatment with the anion exchange resin *colestyramine* is then indicated.

Topical rectal treatment.   *SSZ* and *mesalazine* are available as suppositories. *Mesalazine* is also produced as retention enemas. Some patients find the large volume (100 mL) of retention enemas difficult to use, but *mesalazine* is also available as a small volume foam enema that is lighter and better tolerated. These products are useful for mild to moderate UC and for CD confined to the distal colon and rectum. They may spare the steroid dose. The oral and rectal preparations are sometimes used together.

Side-effects.   If the SP moiety in *SSZ* causes unacceptable side-effects, and this is more likely in slow acetylators, *olsalazine*, *balsalazide* or *mesalazine* may prove more suitable. However, 5-ASA also causes side-effects, e.g. nausea, headache, rash, and even diarrhoea and occasional exacerbation of colitis. *SSZ* causes a reversible oligospermia and so is unsuitable in men wishing to raise a family. The monitoring of *SSZ* treatment is dealt with in Chapter 12.

There have also been occasional reports of nephrotoxicity with all aminosalicylates, which should be used cautiously in renal impairment and during pregnancy and breastfeeding. This is due to the absorption of 5-ASA, and *mesalazine* produces higher serum concentrations of 5-ASA than the azo-bonded products (*SSZ*, *olsalazine* and *balsalazide*). It is not clear whether this nephrotoxicity is due to 5-ASA or to its acetyl metabolite, but it seems prudent to reserve *mesalazine* for mild to moderate UC affecting the distal small bowel and colon.

All aminosalicylates may cause blood dyscrasias, e.g. agranulocytosis, aplastic anaemia, leucopenia, neutropenia and thrombocytopenia. Patients should be advised to report any unexplained bruising, bleeding, sore throat, fever or malaise. If any of these occur the drug should be stopped and a full blood count done. *SSZ* may also cause a lupus-like syndrome (see Chapter 12). They occasionally cause hypersensitivity reactions in patients hypersensitive to *aspirin* and other salicylates. However, many patients use these drugs without significant problems.

Antidiarrhoeals. *Codeine* or *loperamide* may be used cautiously, to relieve discomfort. However, they should be avoided as far as possible because they tend to cause pooling of fluid in the bowel and may aggravate or prolong symptoms. In particular, they may induce obstruction in CD and toxic megacolon. They are not used in severe attacks: it is preferable to control diarrhoea by controlling the disease process with corticosteroids etc. (i.e. treat the disease and not the symptom).

Experimental agents. Infusion of IL-10 has been used as rescue therapy and helps about 70% of patients with steroid-resistant disease. It is expensive and not yet generally available, but may point the way to potentially important developments in therapy.

Maintenance therapy

This is standard practice for both diseases, to reduce recurrence. Prophylaxis follows the general lines of the management of acute attacks, modified suitably according to disease activity and the severity of symptoms. In UC, maintenance therapy reduces the untreated recurrence rate of 80% at 1 year by about three-quarters.

Because CD often follows an unpredictable relapsing-remitting course with symptom-free intervals of several years, it has been common practice not to give maintenance therapy unless symptoms recurred. However, success with high doses of the newer aminosalicylates,

especially *mesalazine*, has changed this picture. The principal differences are outlined below.

Diet
In contrast to the management of acute episodes, a high-residue diet is preferred unless there is a possibility of bowel obstruction, e.g. as the result of stricture formation. A high-carbohydrate, high-protein diet minimizes the possibility of nutritional deficiency due to chronic diarrhoea. Vitamin and mineral supplementation, especially iron, is often given. Avoiding milk or milk products may occasionally be useful in some patients, especially those with small-bowel CD (p. 131).

Aminosalicylates
SSZ, or one of the alternatives mentioned above, are the mainstay of maintenance in UC. They reduce the relapse rate by about 75% and should be continued for life. Aminosalicylates (2 g/day, or more if tolerated) are beneficial in those with small-bowel or colonic CD. *Mesalazine* is preferred because it is released in the distal small bowel and should be started about 2 months after surgery or relapse, as soon as recovery permits. *Lactulose* and *lactitol* should not be used with enteric-coated and modified-release preparations because they acidify the bowel and prevent drug release. However, these combinations are rare. Enemas and suppositories are used for rectal and sigmoid disease and may spare the oral dose. Although *SSZ* frequently causes gastric distress, and enteric-coated tablets are available, it is doubtful whether these are beneficial.

Corticosteroids
Retention enemas and rectal foams, and sometimes suppositories, are used for rectal and distal colonic disease.

Chronic small-bowel involvement in CD is controlled with minimal oral doses, and intelligent patients should be counselled on judicious increases in dose to control exacerbations as soon as they occur: enemas may spare the oral dose required if CD is confined to the distal ileum or colon. However, patients should seek medical advice for anything other than mild exacerbations.

Oral corticosteroids do not influence the relapse rate in UC and should be tapered off and stopped completely when symptoms remit, to minimize side-effects. However, some patients are steroid-dependent and relapse as soon as dose reduction is attempted. They are normally treated with *azathioprine* or *methotrexate* (see above) to permit the corticosteroid dose to be reduced to the minimum consistent with adequate control. *Budesonide* may be preferred in ileal and ascending colonic involvement.

Immunosuppressants

Azathioprine has a limited role in maintenance therapy for UC. However, it halves the relapse rate in CD and may enable substantial withdrawal of corticosteroids. If tolerated it should be continued for at least 5 years.

Antibiotics

These should be used promptly for the treatment of any systemic infections, as there is evidence that infections may trigger exacerbations.

Surgery

Surgery is indicated if medical management fails, for the treatment of complications, e.g. toxic megacolon, perforation, obstruction, malignancy, and the repair of abscesses or fistulae. A further indication in children is retardation of growth and development despite intensive medical management.

In UC, colectomy is curative, ileoanal anastomosis with formation of a pouch to contain the faeces being the preferred procedure. However, a permanent ileostomy (p. 134) may be necessary at some stage and is the procedure of choice in older patients. Colectomy is also carried out as an elective procedure in patients who have had extensive UC for more than 10 years, or if they have ever had a pancolitis, to pre-empt possible malignancy.

However, surgery is avoided as far as possible in CD, because relapse is common (30% in 5 years, 50% in 10 years) and repeated surgery is debilitating and carries a relatively high cumulative mortality. Thus only minimal surgery to deal with complications, e.g. fistula repair, is carried out unless there are frequent severe exacerba-tions. Patients with ileocaecal disease are more likely to need surgery than those with colonic or other involvement. However, about 80% of patients with CD have surgery at some time.

Prognosis

Nearly all CD patients have chronic or recurrent disease, with at least one serious relapse. The probability of recurrence is greater if there was extensive initial disease, if perianal ulceration has occurred, or if an ileocolonic anastomosis has been formed at surgery. The mortality rate now approaches that for the population generally, with most deaths being associated with extensive severe small-bowel disease, onset in the third decade of life and emergency surgery.

In UC, some patients have only a single attack, but many have mild disease, with proctitis only, and the outlook is correspondingly good, the overall mortality being near normal. About 10% of patients have chronic symptoms, and a further 10% have severe attacks requiring surgery. Although prompt surgery may be life-saving, severe attacks are associated with only about 1% mortality if managed in specialist centres (5% elsewhere).

Other colonic and rectal disorders

Diverticular disease

Definition

A **diverticulum** is a pouch projecting from the wall of the gut. Diverticula can occur almost anywhere from the oesophagus to the rectum and may be congenital, e.g. Meckel's diverticulum in the ileum. Those in the small intestine tend to be either asymptomatic or cause only vague dyspeptic symptoms, and complications are unusual. However, diverticular disease of the colon (DDC) occurs frequently, often in the sigmoid colon where the wall is weakest.

Diverticulosis is the presence of diverticula, which may be asymptomatic or produce only mild, non-specific abdominal symptoms. **Diverticulitis** is the result of infection and inflammation of the diverticula, causing moderate to severe symptoms.

Aetiology

DDC is believed to result from a lifelong lack of dietary fibre, because the disease is common in Western countries but is unusual in rural Africa. In the absence of adequate bulk, intense contractions of bowel segments produce high local intraluminal pressures and the mucosa and submucosa become ballooned out and herniate through the overlying muscle layers at points of weakness, usually where blood vessels and nerves enter the intestinal wall.

The average age at diagnosis is 55 years and the incidence increases directly with age, being dependent on the loss of colonic muscle strength and the duration of the bowel insult. Consequently, some degree of diverticulosis is present in some 50% of people aged over 60 years.

Clinical features and diagnosis

Although diverticulosis is usually asymptomatic, it is so common that it may be blamed for symptoms caused by other diseases. However, if the diverticula become filled with stagnant faecal residues, infection and inflammation may cause diverticulitis. The most prominent symptom is spasmodic or constant pain, usually in the lower abdomen, and especially in the left iliac region. Flatulence and constipation are common, though diarrhoea may also occur. Pain may follow meals and is relieved by defecation or passing wind (flatus). In severe cases, with numerous large infected diverticula, colonic obstruction or abscess formation may cause severe localized pain (so-called 'left-sided appendicitis'). Perforation of the bowel may cause peritonitis and septicaemia. Intermittent haemorrhage may cause rectal bleeding and a misdiagnosis of haemorrhoids.

Diagnosis is by barium enema and ultrasound, but fibre-optic endoscopy may be needed in difficult cases.

Management

A **high-fibre diet**, possibly supplemented with a bulking agent (e.g. bran or *ispaghula*), is recommended to reduce intracolonic pressures and to prevent faecal stagnation and constipation, which aggravates the condition due to straining. **Antispasmodics** (e.g. *alverine, dicycloverine, mebeverine, propantheline* or *peppermint oil*) may be useful for colic. **Antibiotics**, e.g. a cephalosporin, with or without *metronidazole*, help with infection. If severely ill, the combination of *gentamicin* plus *metronidazole* is often used. Italian trials have found that the combination of a rifamycin plus increased dietary fibre was effective, about 75% of patients being symptom-free after 1 year. The equivalent UK-licensed drugs would be *rifampicin* 300–450 mg plus 3.5 g of ispaghula husk, both twice daily.

If pain is very severe, **analgesia** may be provided with *pethidine*. *Morphine* is contra-indicated because it reduces gastrointestinal motility, and so aggravates constipation and increases intraluminal pressure. Related anti-motility drugs (e.g. *codeine, loperamide*) may similarly aggravate symptoms and are also contra-indicated.

Surgery is occasionally necessary to remove large, isolated diverticula or a badly affected section of bowel, or to deal with complications, e.g. perforation.

Constipation

Definition and aetiology

Constipation may be defined as a reduced frequency of defecation, i.e. less frequently than is normal for the individual concerned, accompanied by difficulty in passing hardened stools. There may also be sensations of incomplete defecation and that the rectum remains loaded with faeces.

Some possible causes are listed in Table 3.16. Defecation is a highly variable function and normality may range from three motions per day to one in 3 days. One of the most common causes of constipation is a low-residue, low-fluid diet. This may be compounded by poor toilet facilities or a stressful busy life, resulting in an

Table 3.16 Some possible causes of constipation

Simple	Diet: unusual (holidays), low fibre, low fluid intake Lack of exercise, ignoring the call to stool, stress
Secondary	Inactive colon ⎫ Poor muscle tone ⎬ especially in elderly patients, after surgery, or febrile illness Pregnancy Irritable bowel syndrome (p. 132) Disease causing painful defecation: proctitis, anal fissure or stricture, haemorrhoids Metabolic disease (diabetes mellitus, hypothyroidism), obstruction (usually occurring acutely) Crohn's disease (rarely), carcinoma, sigmoid diverticular disease (p. 124), volvulus, gallstones (occasionally), intussusception (usually in infants) Spinal lesions: loss of transmission of sensation or sphincter control
Iatrogenic	Most drugs can cause constipation in some patients. The following are commonly implicated: antimuscarinics, amantadine, antacids (aluminium, calcium), antidiarrhoeals, benzodiazepines, codeine and other opioids, diuretics, iron, phenothiazines, antidepressants, chronic laxative abuse
Psychogenic	Anxiety, depression, stress, disruption of routine (holidays, hospital admission)

unwillingness to defecate or an inability to do so at adequate leisure.

In the elderly, poor muscle tone in the intestine and abdominal wall, perhaps associated with a lack of activity, depression and a low food and fluid intake, often leads to **faecal impaction**. The patient may complain of a hard mass in the left iliac region, or it may be detected on examination.

In young children, constipation may be due to inappropriate diet or to congenital defects, although the latter would be detected by the paediatrician or health visitor at an early age. However, it is more often the result of emotional conflict with (usually) the mother. If an attempt is made to toilet-train children before they are ready to accept it, or if the parent becomes anxious or obsessive about the problem, the child may see the withholding of defecation as a strategy for manipulating the parent. A 2-year-old often behaves negatively and a 4-year-old aggressively. Either behaviour pattern can result in a vicious cycle if the parent responds inappropriately, leading to the regular withholding of bowel motions and the start of chronic constipation.

Another common pattern is the reaction to a clinging, fearful child with over-permissiveness and over-indulgence. Moreover, if parents have incorrect ideas about what constitutes 'proper'

bowel function, children may learn unsuitable behaviour, for example that 'tummyache' leads to illness and headache – symptoms that may be rewarded with over-protectiveness, presents and time off school. All these childhood behaviour patterns can persist into adult life.

Clearly, any condition that leads to pain on defecation, notably **haemorrhoids**, will lead to reluctance to evacuate the bowel and thus to constipation. Also, the passage of a large, hard stool may tear the anus, leading to further pain and reluctance to defecate, thus greatly aggravating the problem. It is perhaps surprising that these tears rarely become infected and usually heal well.

Occasionally, constipation may be a symptom of serious disease. Large gallstones discharged into the duodenum may sometimes cause small-bowel obstruction, usually at the ileocaecal junction, with an acute onset of symptoms, whereas colonic obstruction is more often insidious in onset. Obstruction in infants may occasionally be due to **intussusception** (the bowel folding in on itself). In adults, it tends to be associated with a benign or malignant tumour. Acute obstruction may result from DDC (see above) or **volvulus**, i.e. twisting of the gut. Fortunately, most of these organic or functional conditions are uncommon, though they must be considered if there is no history of chronic or sporadic problems or if simple measures fail, particularly in middle-aged or elderly patients.

Psychogenic constipation, some aspects of which were discussed above, is common. Irrational beliefs about the optimal frequency for defecation, or the consistency and colour of faeces, are widespread, and anxiety about the need to rid the body of 'unclean' wastes may develop in individuals with obsessional, perfectionist personality styles. Such ideas may result in laxative abuse and chronic laxative use may cause the bowel to fail to respond to normal stimuli: this is self-inflicted constipation.

Iatrogenic constipation is a common adverse reaction to medication and some of the drugs that produce this effect most frequently are listed in Table 3.16.

Finally, **drug abuse** with opioids (including *codeine*) must be considered as a possible cause, especially in teenagers and young adults: constipation may be the first indication of a drug abuse problem.

Clinical features

It is important to establish exactly what a patient means when they complain of constipation, as misconceptions and misdescriptions are common.

The usual symptoms are difficult and infrequent or irregular defecation, which may be accompanied by malaise, headache, tiredness and anorexia, possibly of emotional origin.

Abdominal distension may also occur, with pain in the left iliac fossa or felt diffusely. These symptoms are accompanied by hard stools, because the long residence time in the colon causes excessive water resorption.

In elderly patients, faecal impaction may be accompanied by restlessness, confusion and overflow. The latter is a spurious diarrhoea resulting from the forcing of semi-fluid intestinal contents around the immobile mass, together with mucus, which may be secreted into the bowel as a lubricant. Impaction may also occur after prolonged bedrest and, rarely, in IBS (p. 132).

Management

Aims and strategy

Significant pathology must first be excluded. If constipation is of recent onset it is important to exclude secondary causes (Table 3.16), especially in patients over 40 years of age. The objectives are then to:

- relieve any immediate distress;
- remove any trigger factors and treat any underlying disease;
- promote normal bowel function by:
  - re-educating the patient about correct bowel habits, diet and exercise;
  - appropriate medication if the problem persists, i.e. faecal softeners, bulking agents, or osmotic or stimulant laxatives (Table 3.17).

Table 3.17   Some drugs commonly used to treat constipation

Bulking agents	Ispaghula, psyllium, methylcellulose, sterculia, (bran)
Stimulants	Bisacodyl, sodium picosulphate, sennosides (standardized[a]), dantron[b]
Lubricants and softening agents	Arachis oil enemas, docusate sodium, sodium lauryl sulphate, liquid paraffin[c]
Osmotic agents	Lactulose, lactitol, magnesium salts[c], glycerol suppositories, sodium phosphate enemas, macrogols
Motility stimulants[d]	Bethanechol, distigmine, neostigmine, pyridostigmine

[a] Unstandardized preparations of senna, and preparations of aloin, bile salts, cascara, colocynth, frangula, jalap, podophyllum and rhubarb have drastic and unpredictable effects and are best avoided.

[b] Mutagenic in animals: for the management of constipation in terminally ill patients only.

[c] Suitable for occasional use only.

[d] Exceptional use only.

General measures

In **simple constipation** the patient should be counselled on the value of a correct diet (wholemeal and bran products, fruit and vegetables are valuable), regular exercise and an adequate fluid intake. Defecation with the thighs raised towards the abdomen helps by increasing intra-abdominal pressure, so a low toilet or a 'squat box' to raise the thighs may be useful. Regular, unhurried toilet habits should be encouraged.

The regular use of laxatives should be strongly discouraged. However, laxative avoidance may be very difficult in older patients who have been chronic laxative users. Advice to the elderly to abandon their accustomed laxative in favour of bulking agents and a high-fibre diet is unlikely to succeed. The best that can usually be achieved is some improvement in bulk intake and a reduction in laxative use.

Acute relief

For the occasional simple constipation (e.g. in travellers whose normal diet and lifestyle are temporarily disrupted), **micro-enemas** (10 g) based on *docusate sodium* (dioctyl sodium sulphosuccinate), or **suppositories** (*glycerol* or *bisacodyl*) are useful as relatively fast-acting, single-dose products. Large-volume (100 mL) hypertonic sodium phosphate enemas are also suitable.

In more severe cases, products containing oral **stimulant (irritant) laxatives**, e.g. *senna, bisacodyl* or *sodium picosulphate*, may be needed. If the faeces are very hard, especially if they are impacted or the patient has haemorrhoids or an anal tear, these may need supplementation with a **softening agent** such as an *arachis oil enema*. Liquid paraffin is undesirable (see below).

Straining at stool should be avoided in patients with angina pectoris, heart failure and myocardial infarction and moderate to severe low back pain, because it aggravates symptoms: laxatives are then indicated.

Dantron was withdrawn from general use in the UK because of fears that it could cause bowel and liver tumours. However, it is an invaluable agent that has been reintroduced for the management of constipation produced by opioid analgesics in terminal care. It is sometimes used in combination with *docusate* or *poloxamer 188* (known as *co-danthrusate* and *co-danthramer*

respectively in the UK). It is licensed in the UK only for use in terminally ill patients of all ages. Patients should be warned that it may colour the urine red because they may otherwise interpret this as bleeding.

Oral **osmotic laxatives**, e.g. *magnesium sulphate* (Epsom salts) and *macrogols*, are also suitable for occasional use. An adequate fluid intake should be maintained. *Lactulose* and *lactitol* are semi-synthetic non-absorbable disaccharides that are hydrolysed by colonic bacteria to lactic acid, producing osmotic and mildly irritant effects. Although they take up to 48 h to act, they are useful agents with very wide applicability. Because they have a sweet taste they are useful in young children who might otherwise reject medication. Some patients may find *lactitol* less likely to cause cramps, wind and minor bowel disturbances. If there is an anal tear, *lidocaine ointment* is a useful local anaesthetic, but it may cause skin sensitization. Alternatively, any of the OTC haemorrhoidal ointments may help. A thin smear of soft paraffin will similarly lubricate the anal canal and ease the passage of hard stools. These, too, should be used sparingly because they will cause water retention in the perianal skin, possibly leading to skin maceration and infection.

Prophylaxis

The most suitable measures are the general ones outlined above. However, patients often find it difficult to modify their lifestyle and **bulking agents**, e.g. bran, *ispaghula husk, psyllium, sterculia* or *methylcellulose*, may be needed. However, patients react very variably to these, and any of them, including the 'natural' ones like bran, may cause discomfort, griping and flatus. Bulking agents swell when added to water and must be taken with ample fluids, to increase the volume of the colonic contents and so stimulate peristalsis and defecation. The need to drink large volumes of fluid may pose a problem with the frail elderly patient who cannot drink large volumes quickly or who has dentures.

Bulking agents should not be used if faecal obstruction or impaction is suspected, because they add to bulk and may aggravate the situation. Nor should they be taken immediately before retiring at night. All take several days to act.

Provided that a correct diagnosis has been made, bulking agents are also useful for improving the consistency of bowel contents in:

- stomatherapy (p. 133);
- patients with chronic diarrhoea associated with DDC (see above), IBS (p. 132) and UC (p. 114);
- haemorrhoids.

Older laxatives and their side-effects

Products containing *liquid paraffin* may occasionally be useful to lubricate and soften a hard faecal mass, especially if defecation is painful due to haemorrhoids or anal tears. However, in the very young and elderly there is a risk of aspiration pneumonitis (see Chapter 5) and anal leakage. If used long term, *liquid paraffin* reduces the absorption of oil-soluble vitamins, especially in the elderly. Thus, it is unsuitable for use in children under 3 years of age, or for prolonged or repeated use, and should be employed only in exceptional circumstances. In faecal impaction, an *arachis oil enema* produces softening and lubrication, and is preferable to oral *liquid paraffin*.

Although phenolphthalein has been very widely used in some proprietary medicines, it may cause skin rashes, albuminuria and haemoglobinuria. It may also cause colic and vomiting in young children and has been withdrawn in the UK.

The old herbal cathartics, e.g. aloin, cascara, castor oil, colocynth and jalap, have a very drastic action and are likely to cause severe colic, so they have largely been superseded by less drastic agents.

Laxatives must not be used if there is a suspicion of appendicitis, as they increase the risk of perforation and peritonitis. Contrary to general belief, the first sign of appendicitis is not pain in the right iliac region (see Figure 3.1), but a vague pain in the umbilical region that becomes localized to the right iliac region after some hours. Fever is usual and nausea and vomiting may occur. Prompt diagnosis by ultrasound will eliminate the possibility of other abdominal pathology, e.g. ileocaecal CD: about 50% of women have a normal appendix removed. Early appendicectomy is carried out if the diagnosis is secure or if there is any doubt, to pre-empt the possibility of appendix rupture and peritonitis.

Bowel cleansing

'Bowel prep' is used with a low-residue diet to clear the bowel of solids in preparation for colonoscopy, radiology or surgery. The drugs used include high concentrations of salts, e.g. *magnesium citrate*, *sodium dihydrogen phosphate*, macrogols plus salts and *sodium picosulphate*. None of these is suitable as a routine laxative.

Motility stimulants

These agents are rarely used gastrointestinally but may help patients with colonic atony (non-motile bowel) in initial adaptation to new laxatives. They are used about 30 min before attempting defecation. Motility stimulants are either direct-acting parasympathomimetic compounds (e.g. *bethanechol*), or anticholinesterases (e.g. *distigmine*, *neostigmine* and *pyridostigmine*), so they can have widespread side-effects such as sweating, salivation, intestinal cramps, diarrhoea, flushing, difficulty in breathing and hypotension. They are therefore contra-indicated in elderly patients.

Acute diarrhoea

Definition, aetiology and pathology

Acute diarrhoea is an increased volume or frequency of bowel movement, relative to that normal for an individual, associated with greater fluidity of the motions. As with constipation, it is essential to establish just what a patient means by the term 'diarrhoea'.

Diarrhoea may be classified according to clinical criteria (i.e. **acute** or **chronic**), although there are many possible aetiologies (Table 3.18), some of which are dealt with in this chapter and for which the appropriate sections should be consulted. Alternatively, a **pathophysiological classification** can be used:

- **Malabsorptive**, owing to a failure to absorb nutrients, causing an osmotic diarrhoea, e.g. gluten enteropathy (p. 111).
- **Osmotic**, in which hypertonic conditions prevent colonic water resorption, e.g.

Table 3.18   Some possible causes of diarrhoea

Acute	Gastroenteritis ('food poisoning'): e.g. bacterial infections, especially *Salmonella typhimurium* and other *Salmonella* spp., *Campylobacter jejuni*, *Listeria monocytogenes*, enteropathogenic *Escherichia coli* (infants), typhoid and paratyphoid fevers, dysentery (*Shigella* spp.) Toxins: bacterial (staphylococcal, clostridial); plant (mushrooms, aflatoxins) Viral infections: rotaviruses (infants), coxsackie, ECHO, norovirus Protozoal infections: *Giardia intestinalis* (formerly *G. lamblia*), *Entamoeba histolytica*
Chronic	Organic disease: Crohn's disease, ulcerative colitis, diverticular disease, irritable bowel syndrome, diabetes, biliary problems, malabsorption syndromes, pancreatic disease, cystic fibrosis, cancer Food-induced: food allergies, inappropriate diet Psychogenic: anxiety, depression
Iatrogenic	Almost all drugs can cause diarrhoea in some patients. The following are commonly implicated: • antibiotics: clindamycin, lincomycin, tetracyclines, nalidixic acid, erythromycin, rifampicin • antacids: magnesium compounds (also 'health salts') • cardiac drugs: digoxin overdose Non-drug causes: abdominal radiotherapy

disaccharidase deficiency (p. 114), saline purgatives.

- **Hypersecretory**, with massive secretion of water and electrolytes from the mucosa, e.g. cholera, verocytotoxin-producing *Escherichia coli* O157 (see Chapter 8).
- **Exudative**, in which protein, blood and fluids leak from an inflamed or damaged mucosa, e.g. IBD, protozoal infection, and bacterial toxins.
- **Neuromuscular**, i.e. overactivity leading to a shortened gut transit time and inadequate water and nutrient absorption, e.g. diabetic neuropathy, thyrotoxicosis.

The commonest causes of acute diarrhoea are contaminated food or drinks (**gastroenteritis**; see Chapter 8), especially from recent travel abroad, and medicines.

Complications
Both chronic and severe acute diarrhoea may cause:

- Dehydration, with hypovolaemia, low blood pressure and tachycardia.
- Hypokalaemia and low bicarbonate, giving metabolic acidosis. However, these abnormal-ities are not usually so great as to require active therapy, unless diarrhoea is severe and prolonged.
- Small-bowel lactase depletion.

Chronic diarrhoea may also cause anaemia, which may be microcytic or macrocytic, with low Hb, iron and folate levels (see Chapter 11).

Management

Aims

The aims of management are to:

- relieve symptoms, without prolonging the condition;
- prevent dehydration and electrolyte deficiencies, and to correct existing metabolic abnormality in severe disease;
- treat any underlying disease or, if there is no effective treatment, give symptomatic relief.

These aims are achieved by:

- removing any trigger substances, e.g. with adsorbents;

- administering:
  - glucose-electrolyte solutions;
  - antidiarrhoeal drugs to reduce gastrointestinal motility;
  - bulking agents, to improve faecal consistency;
- investigating persistent symptoms (>2 weeks' duration) and patients with severe constitutional upset;
- using antibiotics (sometimes), if there is major systemic upset and a demonstrated pathogen of proven susceptibility.

General management

The treatment of **chronic diarrhoea** depends on controlling the underlying disease (Table 3.18).

Acute diarrhoea. Any medication that may be causing the condition (Table 3.18) or aggravating its metabolic consequences (e.g. diuretics), should be stopped and, if essential, a temporary or permanent alternative found.

Most cases of gastroenteritis are self-limiting (see Chapter 8), the most important aspect of treatment being the prevention of fluid and electrolyte depletion, or their adequate replacement using oral rehydration salts or a proprietary equivalent. The glucose, or other carbohydrate yielding it, is an energy source for electrolyte absorption and improves nutrition somewhat. This is especially important in infants and young children, who can become dehydrated very rapidly, or in frail or elderly patients. Restlessness and fretfulness in an infant may be misinterpreted as a requirement for more food, and deaths have occurred from giving excessively concentrated feeds or feeds supplemented with glucose. If a baby is unwell, the safest course is to use fluid and electrolyte replacement at the recommended concentration until proper medical advice can be obtained. A properly nourished child will not come to harm if food is withheld for 24 h, but may do if fed excessively.

A short period of diarrhoea (<48 h) will not cause electrolyte depletion except in infants and the frail elderly, or unless the diarrhoea is very severe, so taking ample fluids such as water, fruit juices or commercial drinks containing glucose should be adequate. If diarrhoea is prolonged, the use of oral rehydration salts or a proprietary equivalent is appropriate, but every effort should be made to identify a cause and treat the underlying condition.

It is difficult to identify dehydration clinically, but symptoms of diarrhoea (especially with vomiting), plus recent weight loss (especially in infants), or loss of skin turgor (in well-nourished teenagers and adults up to age 50 years) is significant. Skin turgor can be roughly assessed by pinching and lifting a skinfold on the back of the hand and releasing it; the skin should return briskly to normal. If it relaxes slowly, this may indicate fluid loss. This test is inapplicable in young children, because of their high fluid levels, and in older patients, because loss of SC and elastic tissue causes a normally slow relaxation.

Milk or milk products should be reintroduced cautiously after a prolonged period of diarrhoea, as the gut mucosa may be temporarily depleted of lactase and other saccharidases, causing inadequate lactose absorption and a consequent **osmotic diarrhoea**.

Antimotility drugs. These are opioids and include *loperamide* and *codeine*. They may be necessary in the short term for social reasons, or to permit the maintenance of some semblance of normality by a mother or busy worker who cannot afford to take time off. *Loperamide* is preferable, as it does not have central or addictive properties. These agents should be avoided if possible, because they are alleged to cause the retention of potentially inflammatory and toxic products in the bowel, thus prolonging symptoms. However, this is not an important consideration in most acute diarrhoeas, which are short, self-limiting conditions. Excessive use may lead to constipation.

Antimuscarinics (antispasmodics). Examples are *dicycloverine*, *hyoscine* and *propantheline*, which do little to improve diarrhoea, but may help to relieve bowel cramps. They should not be used with antidiarrhoeals because the effects are additive. *Alverine*, *mebeverine* and *peppermint oil* are rarely used in this context.

Adsorbents and bulking agents. Examples are *kaolin* and *methylcellulose*; these serve primarily to modify stool consistency, but may aggravate symptoms by increasing stool weight. They may play a minor role if a known toxin is involved, but the formerly ubiquitous 'kaolin and morphine mixture' is primarily a placebo.

Antibiotics. These are rarely indicated in uncomplicated diarrhoea, even if an infection is likely. *Ciprofloxacin* is sometimes used for the prophylaxis of travellers' diarrhoea, but this is undesirable. The best prophylactic measures are awareness of potential sources of infection, sensible eating and drinking, and good food and personal hygiene. However, antibiotics may be required to treat properly diagnosed enteric infections, e.g. severe *Campolybacter jejuni* (*erythromycin* or *ciprofloxacin*) and *Salmomella typhimurium* infections, typhoid fever, dysentery and AAC (see Chapter 8), but multiple antibiotic resistance is now common.

Other agents. There is a recent report that *nitazoxazide* (licensed in the USA, not in the UK) significantly reduces the duration of the symptoms of severe rotavirus disease in children, without causing significant adverse reactions.

Irritable bowel syndrome

Definition and clinical features

Irritable bowel syndrome (IBS) is one form of **functional bowel disease**, i.e. function is abnormal without any demonstrable organic pathology and with a poor response to treatment. It is a diagnosis of exclusion, i.e. other possible causes of the symptoms cannot be found.

Clinical features
These include:

- recurrent or chronic mild to moderate left-sided or more general abdominal pain or discomfort, commonly in the iliac fossa, often relieved by defecation or passing wind;
- constipation with abnormal pellet-like or ribbon stools, or occasionally diarrhoea;
- frequent small amounts of stool;
- a frequent feeling of bloating or incomplete evacuation.

IBS accounts for more than half of all gastrointestinal consultations, and is a difficult problem for the gastroenterologist because extensive investigations may be needed, all of which are likely to be negative.

Aetiology

The aetiology of IBS is obscure, but may include:

- a low-fibre diet;
- sequel to severe bowel infection;
- excessive colonic contractions, as part of a generalized disorder of smooth muscle function;
- laxative abuse.

Although neurotic features (see Chapter 6) are present in two-thirds of patients, they are not causative. However, they will determine how well the patient tolerates the symptoms, whether they seek medical advice and their presentation of symptoms to their GP, and a tricyclic antidepessant may help in the short term. However, the antimuscarinic action of tricyclic antidepressants will aggravate any tendency to constipation.

Management

In the absence of organic disease and because the aetiology is obscure, treatment of IBS is symptomatic and empirical. It includes:

- Explanation and reassurance to allay fears of serious pathology.
- A tricyclic antidepressant may be effective whether there is any underlying anxiety or depression or not.
- A high-fibre diet or bulking agents to restore normal faecal bulk and consistency, although it is uncertain whether they produce significant improvement.
- Bulking agents probably improve symptoms.
- Antidiarrhoeals may be indicated.
- Activated charcoal as an antiflatulant.
- Antispasmodics, e.g. *alverine* or *mebeverine*, specific gastrointestinal musculotropic agents that reduce spasm without affecting colonic motility. Enteric-coated *peppermint oil* capsules may help. The antispasmodic (antimuscarinic) agents *dicycloverine*, *hyoscine* and *propantheline* have also been used, but are of doubtful

efficacy in IBD and have undesirable anti-cholinergic side-effects, especially in older patients.

Other antispasmodics, e.g. 5-HT$_3$ and 5-HT$_4$ agonists have been investigated, with equivocal results.

Stomatherapy

Definition

Stomas are artificial openings formed surgically between the internal organs and the skin. They are described according to the internal organ to which they are connected, e.g. **colostomy** (colon), **ileostomy** (ileum). Although **ureterostomy** is possible in some cases, an alternative procedure, a **urinary diversion**, is normally done (see below). The indications for these operations are given in Table 3.19.

Other types of stoma may be formed, e.g. tracheostomy for artificial ventilation, and PEG (p. 120) for enteral feeding when a nasogastric tube is inappropriate, but these will not be considered here.

Location

It is important for the stoma to be sited correctly in order to ensure that the patient can manage it properly. The stoma is always formed separately from the main operative incision, because the

scar causes skin irregularities and is particularly susceptible to damage by enzymes and irritants in bowel fluids that may leak from the stoma. It must be placed in an area away from skin creases, which tend to cause leakage (Figure 3.16(a)). Other sites that should be avoided include old operation scars and areas where the skin surface is uneven or covered by breasts or skin folds, especially when seated. Patients who have stomas are known as '**ostomists**'.

Types of stoma

Colostomies

Depending on the extent of disease, the colostomy may connect with the **ascending**, **transverse** or **descending** colon. The colon is turned back on itself to project about 1 cm above the skin surface to minimize skin soiling (Figure 3.16(b)), and is stitched to the skin. The projecting stump of colon is moist and bright pink, like normal gastrointestinal mucosa. Although initially oedematous, the stump shrinks somewhat over the first few months, and this may cause leakage from an initially well-fitting appliance. Occasionally retraction, prolapse or stenosis of the stoma may occur, or hernias may develop around it, necessitating surgical repair.

Because the colon progressively absorbs residual water from the faeces, the consistency of the discharge will vary with the length of bowel removed: the less that is removed, the more

Table 3.19   Indications for stomatherapy

Colostomy	Ileostomy	Urinary diversion
Carcinoma of the rectum or colon	Extensive ulcerative colitis Familial polyposis coli	Carcinoma of the bladder
Severe diverticulitis	Severe diverticulitis	Congenital or acquired neurological failure of bladder control
Uncontrolled ulcerative colitis or Crohn's colitis	Uncontrolled Crohn's disease	
Traumatic abdominal injury		

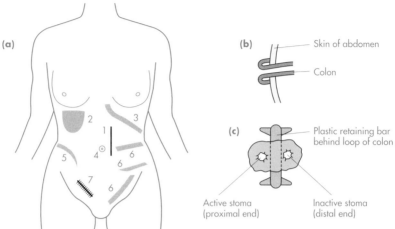

Figure 3.16 Location and formation of stomas. (a) Site of proposed main operative incision (1) and areas to avoid: 2, area under breasts; 3, margin of ribcage; 4, umbilicus; 5, iliac crest; 6, skin creases; 7, scars of old operations. (b) Formation (permanent colostomy): the cut end of colon is brought to the skin away from the main operative incision, reflexed and stitched down to form a 'spout'. (c) Temporary colostomy. [(a) is modified from a drawing supplied by Convatec Ltd.]

normal the stools. However, the discharge is always fluid initially because of inflammation, though this usually settles after a few months into a more formed stool, with a reasonably regular pattern of motions.

Colostomies are the commonest stomas that are formed. Although stomas are usually permanent, temporary colostomies may be formed to rest the distal section of bowel, following trauma or obstruction. This post-operative resting of damaged bowel to allow post-traumatic healing should be distinguished from resting of inflamed, intact bowel in IBD, which is not helpful (see above). Bowel continuity is restored after 2–3 months. Thus temporary colostomies are mostly seen in the hospital setting. Other types of stoma are managed in the community, following surgery and initial hospital treatment.

Temporary colostomies are usually 'loops', i.e. the colon is not completely divided and the partially separated ends are brought out through the skin, a plastic rod being used behind the loop of bowel to prevent retraction into the abdomen. There is thus a proximal, active end and a distal, inactive end of bowel (Figure 3.16(c)), the former discharging faeces and the latter mucus.

An interesting development is the 'continent colostomy plug', which is inserted into the stoma and then absorbs water and expands to fill the aperture, effectively blocking the passage of faeces. There is a built-in filter and valve, so that wind can usually be passed without noise or odour. The device is unobtrusive and overcomes many of the psychosocial problems of ostomists, but it is not suitable for all patients.

Ileostomies

These are formed following total colectomy and are usually permanent, though occasionally the rectum and anus can be preserved and an ileo-rectal or ileoanal anastomosis (reconnection) performed later.

The stoma is similar to that in colostomy, except that the ileum is brought to the surface. Because normal ileal contents are always fluid and rather irritant, owing to the presence of digestive enzymes, the stoma is usually formed to project further from the skin than is done with colostomies, to form a 'spout' and so minimize the possibility of skin soiling and damage immediately around the stoma.

A variant sometimes used is **Kock's continent ileostomy**, in which a reservoir (pouch) is formed in the abdomen from the terminal ileum. The stoma aperture is formed into a 'valve' to prevent leakage, and the reservoir emptied with a catheter several times a day. A variation on this is to form an anastomosis between the pouch and the anus, preserving near-normal function. The inevitable loss of fluid, due to the absence of colonic water resorption, must be compensated for in the diet.

Urinary diversions

These are usually formed as an **ileal conduit**. A segment of ileum is first removed with its blood supply, and the cut ends of the ileum are rejoined. The removed segment is closed at one end, into which the ureters are transplanted, the other end being used to form the urinary stoma. Because urinary output is continuous and liquid, the urinary stoma is always fashioned as a 2-cm 'spout' to carry urine away from the skin surface.

Management

Appliances

Unless a temporary stoma is formed, or a subsequent anal anastomosis is possible for colonic or ileal stomas, patients need to wear an appliance for the rest of their lives, to collect the stomal discharge. There are many different types available. Initially, the choice will depend on the preference of the stoma care specialist, a drainable appliance being needed until the post-operative trauma to the tissues subsides. However, modifications are necessary as recovery proceeds, and the final choice depends on the needs and preferences of the patient. The general criteria for selection are:

- **Comfort**. There should be a reasonably close fit, without damaging the stoma. The gap around the stoma should be about 5 mm: if the clearance is significantly greater than this the skin may become damaged, creating considerable problems.
- **Security**. The patient should be able to have complete confidence that the appliance will not come off or be socially embarrassing. It should be:
  - **leak-proof**: to avoid odour and skin damage;
  - **odour-proof**: fear of odour and social embarrassment is a major patient concern

and deodorants are a poor substitute; a valve with an activated charcoal filter is usual to vent wind.
- **Convenience**. Light and unobtrusive, easy to apply and change, easy to empty, or discard if disposable.

Most types of appliance in current use are disposable, though non-disposable types are still used occasionally for patients who live in areas where disposable appliances are difficult to obtain or are very expensive. Most appliances consist of two pieces (Figure 3.17), a self-adhesive base with an integral circular plastic gasket to which the bag is attached. The base remains on the skin for several days and enables easy, secure changing of the disposable bags. The advantages are that removal of the adhesive base is performed relatively infrequently, so skin trauma is minimized. Also, there is no fixed bag covering the stoma, so the skin immediately around the stoma is readily accessible between bag changes and can easily be covered with protective pastes. With one-piece appliances, the adhesive gasket and the bag must be renewed more frequently as an integral unit and filler pastes applied first. In either case, the base must fit the stoma closely in order to minimize skin soiling, yet cause minimal trauma to the stoma itself. **Protective pastes**, e.g. Stomaseal and karaya paste, are essential to protect the skin and fill in awkward creases and scars, thus minimizing leakage.

Urostomy bags have an attachment for a **night drainage** tube and bag, to avoid wetting of the bed from accidental pressure on a full bag.

A high level of skin care and hygiene is essential. Cleansing routines must be gentle, and local hair should be removed only with an electric razor. Barrier and other skin products must not interfere with gasket adhesion. The key to skin care is a well-fitting appliance: it is better to prevent skin damage than to have to treat it, however successfully.

Medication and the ostomist

Because a variable length of bowel has been removed, previously suitable medicines may become unsuitable. Further, because the excreta

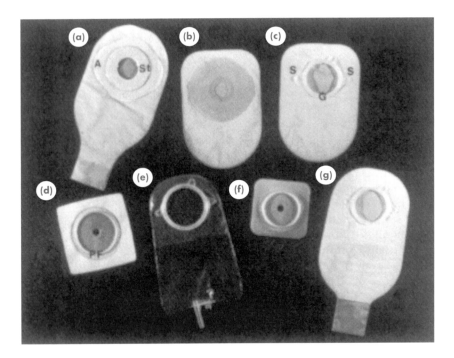

Figure 3.17   Some types of stoma appliance. (a) One-piece drainable ileostomy bag with Stomahesive seal (St) and adhesive patch (A). (b) Small one-piece non-drainable (closed) bag. This incorporates a flatus filter (not seen in this view because it is on the underside, though the bulge it creates is just visible in the top left-hand corner of the body. (c) Small two-piece closed bag with plastic gasket (G), incorporating belt supports (S). (d) Adhesive base for two-piece appliances with large plastic flange (PF) to suit bags (c) and (e). (e) Two-piece urostomy bag with large gasket and tap for drainage and attachment of night drainage bag (tap shown in open position). (f) Adhesive (Stomahesive) base with flange to suit bag (g). (g) Drainable two-piece ileostomy bag. The ends of bags (a) and (g) are sealed with a plastic clip in use. The apertures in the bases (d) and (f) are cut slightly larger than the stomas and, after application, the Stomahesive is moulded to fit closely around the stoma to protect the skin. (Reproduced with permission from Convatec Ltd.)

are discharged into bags that show their contents, or have to be emptied, patients are especially aware of changes in the colours of urine and faeces. Pharmacists should therefore avoid dispensing products that cause problems, if possible, and should counsel patients appropriately. A list of drugs that may discolour urine and faeces is given in Table 3.20, and of dosage forms that may cause problems in Table 3.21.

Generally, drug absorption is not significantly impaired, because most absorption occurs either in the stomach or in the duodenum and jejunum, unless the intestinal transit time is shortened, e.g. due to inflammation. However, ostomists should be monitored carefully in the post-operative period until any inflammation has subsided, to ensure drug efficacy.

Diet

Diet is not usually a problem, and no specific restrictions are required for urostomy patients. Colostomists have very individual requirements, but problems such as odour, fluidity and wind occur most often with salads, biscuits, tomatoes, onions, nuts and beer (Table 3.22). Odour is most frequently associated with baked beans,

Table 3.20   Some drugs that may discolour urine and faeces

Colour produced	Drug or drug class
Urine	
Blue or green	Amitriptyline, indometacin, sulphonamides, triamterene (in acid urine under fluorescent light)
Yellow or brownish	Chloroquine, metronidazole, nitrofurantoin, senna (acid urine)
Pink, red or reddish/brown	Cascara, dantron, levodopa, methyldopa, phenindione, phenothiazines, phenolphthalein (alkaline urine), senna (alkaline urine), rifabutin, rifampicin
Darkening	Ferrous salts, senna (if urine is allowed to stand)
Faeces	
Whitish or speckled	Insoluble antacids
Black	Bismuth salts, charcoal, iron salts
Pink or red to black[a]	Anticoagulants, aspirin and salicylates, NSAIDs
Greenish or greyish	Antibiotics, indometacin

[a] 'Tarry' faeces may indicate gastrointestinal bleeding.

Table 3.21   Possible effects of dosage forms on ostomists

Drug or drug class	Type of patient[a]	Effects produced
Antibiotics	C, I	Diarrhoea, bacterial overgrowth
Antimuscarinics[b]	C, I	Constipation
Antacids, beta-blockers	C, I, U	Constipation or diarrhoea
Methyldopa	C, I, U	Diarrhoea
Opioid analgesics	C, I, U	Constipation
Sulphonamides	U	Crystalluria
Modified-release preparations	C, I	May be ineffective due to impaired absorption
Diuretics	I	May cause impaired fluid and electrolyte balance
	U	Increased urine volumes in bags

[a] C, colostomy; I, ileostomy; U, urinary diversion. Ostomists are particularly susceptible to the side-effects of drugs and react very variably. (See also Table 3.20.)
[b] Includes antihistamines, antispasmodics, tricyclic antidepressants, phenothiazines.

eggs, cabbage, cheese, fish and beer. It is clearly a matter for each patient to learn to avoid those items that cause them problems. If a major part of the colon is removed, *methylcellulose* may help to give firmer motions.

Ileostomy involves similar considerations, except that the discharge is always fluid and the larger volume of water lost with it must be replaced; thus patients need to drink up to 1.5 L extra daily, sometimes with added electrolytes.

Rehabilitation

Full physical and mental rehabilitation is the aim of stomatherapy, and many patients live full and normal lives. However, despite the enormous advances in the design of appliances in recent years, and corresponding improvements in support systems for patient care, some patients (and/or their families), fail to come to terms with their stomas.

Table 3.22   Dietary guidelines for colostomists and ileostomists[a]

General advice for achieving a consistent stoma output
- Eat regularly, three times a day, in moderation
- Identify and avoid foods and drinks that cause problems, or reduce their intake
- Eat wind-producing foods sparingly. Do not: eat too fast, talk while eating, or wash food down with drinks, especially fizzy drinks
- Balance intake of foods causing constipation or loose motions to produce a neutral effect

Some foods that may cause problems
- *Odour*: asparagus; beans, peas and other pulses; cabbage, brussels sprouts and other brassicas; coleslaw; cheese; eggs; fish; onions
- *Wind*: beans, peas and other pulses; cabbage, brussels sprouts and other brassicas; coleslaw; cucumber; fatty, rich foods; fizzy drinks; onions; radishes
- *Constipation*: beansprouts; celery; chocolate; coleslaw; coconut and other nuts; eggs; fried foods; grapefruit; high-fibre foods; nuts; macaroons; popcorn and sweetcorn; raisins and dried fruits; rice and tapioca; seeds; skins of fruits and vegetables
- *Diarrhoea*: alcoholic drinks, especially beer; green beans; broccoli and calabrese; fruit juices and raw fruit; mangetout; spinach; very spicy food

[a] The reactions of ostomists are highly individual.

The operations are major, emotionally traumatic, and are often performed at very short notice or as an emergency. When time allows, expert preoperative counselling of patients and their families is essential, as is skilled and sympathetic post-operative support. Contact with one of the self-help groups is invaluable, and pharmacists can help greatly by dealing sympathetically with patients' problems and by ensuring the prompt supply of appliances and ancillary products. Good records ensure that the correct type of appliance is always supplied, because prescriptions are often incomplete or incorrect. Most districts have a specialist stoma care nurse, and it is very helpful for community pharmacists to establish a working relationship with them. Appliance manufacturers also employ nurse advisers who will provide technical advice by telephone and visit patients in their homes, with a varying degree of commerciality.

Liver diseases

Because the liver is the largest single organ in the body and carries out vital metabolic functions (Table 3.23), liver diseases cause profound and widespread effects.

Many diverse pathological processes may cause liver dysfunction. This short section deals briefly with jaundice and some common liver diseases, notably those that may be caused by drugs. The reader is referred to the References and further reading section for further information.

Clinical physiology of the liver

Anatomy and histology

The liver is usually totally enclosed within the right lower rib cage, below the diaphragm (see Figures 3.1(d) and 3.3). It receives only 25% of its blood supply (but 50% of its oxygen) from the hepatic artery, the remainder being derived

Table 3.23   Principal functions of the liver

Type of function	Examples
Anabolic and synthetic	Conversion of surplus glucose to glycogen and fat
	Manufacture of proteins, e.g. albumin, transferrin, lipoprotein (VLDLs, HDLs)
	Synthesis of coagulation factors, e.g. prothrombin; fibrinogen; factors V, VII, IX, X, XIII
	Production of heparin
	25-Hydroxylation of vitamin D_3
Storage	Energy (glycogen, fat)
	Vitamins A, B_{12}, D, E, K
	Minerals, e.g. Fe, Cu
	Non-metabolizable toxins, e.g. DDT
Catabolic	Breakdown of a wide range of compounds, e.g.
	• Hormones, e.g. insulin, glucagon, glucocorticoids, oestrogens, growth hormone
	• Conversion of:
	– nitrogen residues to urea
	– glycogen, fat and protein to glucose
	– haemoglobin to bilirubin with recirculation of iron
Detoxification	Bilirubin (to its glucuronide), drugs[a], alcohol, antigens
Scavenging and protective	Phagocytosis of blood-borne microorganisms and effete erythrocytes by Kupffer cells

[a] The liver is the main site of drug metabolism. Hepatic 'detoxification' usually increases the water solubility of lipophilic drugs, thus enabling renal excretion.
HDL, high-density lipoprotein; VLDL, very-low-density lipoprotein.

from the portal vein, which drains the circulation of the GIT and the spleen (see Figure 3.4).

The liver has a modular structure, being divided into approximately polyhedral functional units, the **lobules** (Figure 3.18), at the angles of which are branches of the portal vein and hepatic artery. The blood flows from these through irregularly shaped **sinusoids** into a **central vein**, and from there to the hepatic vein and the inferior vena cava. Between the sinusoids are cords of hepatic cells that carry out the crucial metabolic functions. Although most of the products of metabolism are secreted into the hepatic vein or are stored in the liver, the **bile** produced does not normally enter the blood. It is secreted into tiny non-vascular capillaries (**canaliculi**) situated between the cells. These drain into small ducts and then into the **right** and **left hepatic ducts**, which in turn unite to form the **common hepatic duct** that finally joins with the outflow from the gallbladder to form the **common bile duct**. The common bile duct is joined by the

pancreatic duct just before it terminates at the duodenum, into which it discharges via the **sphincter of Oddi** at the **ampulla of Vater**. This sphincter closes the ducts when the duodenum is empty, and bile is then diverted into the gallbladder where it is stored and concentrated until required. There is an accessory duct that drains the head of the pancreas and discharges separately, above the ampulla of Vater.

Chronic liver damage, usually caused by excessive alcohol ingestion or viral hepatitis, leads to **hepatic cirrhosis** with loss of the characteristic liver histology. The lobules initially show fatty degeneration, progressing to areas of dead cells with islands of regenerating tissue, surrounded by dense fibrosis. The damage is irreversible when the fibrotic phase is established, but frequent alcohol-free 'holidays' in the early stages may permit regeneration of the liver tissue, with normal liver function tests. Later, cessation of alcohol consumption and treatment of any underlying disease will prevent further

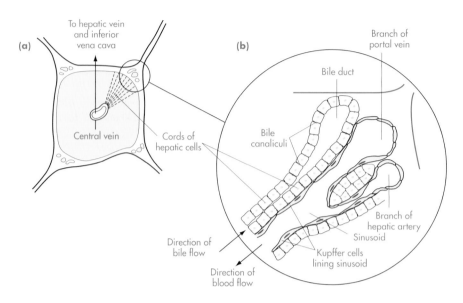

Figure 3.18   Liver histology (diagrammatic). (a) A lobule. (b) Arrangement of blood vessels and bile ducts.

deterioration. This emphasizes the importance of early testing in those who admit to heavy alcohol consumption.

Investigation

Imaging

Plain abdominal **X-rays** are of limited value, but do indicate the sizes of the liver and spleen and may show gas in the biliary tract, opaque gallstones, gallbladder and liver calcification, and ascites. An oral **cholecystogram** or IV **cholangiogram**, performed with an iodine-based contrast agent, visualizes both radiolucent and radio-opaque gallstones. However, these traditional methods have largely been replaced by ultrasound, CT and MRI scanning and endoscopic retrograde cholangiopancreatography (ERCP; see below).

Ultrasound scanning is now used routinely to define the size and shape of the liver and to detect intrahepatic lesions (e.g. cysts, tumours), ascites, abnormalities of the biliary tract and gallstones. This can be done during open surgery, a sterile probe being used to guide the surgeon. **Doppler ultrasound** will measure blood flow. **Endoscopic ultrasonography** is being used increasingly in specialist centres to visualize the biliary tree, pancreas and portal vein, and to obtain biopsy specimens.

CT scanning can also delineate organ size, and can detect internal lesions and the presence of fat and excess iron. The development of **spiral CT scanning** enables information on arterial and portal blood flow and hepatic lesions to be obtained rapidly. The use of contrast media enhances CT visualization of liver metastases (see Chapter 10) and the biliary tree, but the agents used are rather toxic and allergenic.

MRI is increasingly used because it can provide superior results to CT (with no radiation dose), and is less invasive than endoscopy.

Numerous compounds labelled with technetium-99m are used for **scintiscanning**. The procedure is more invasive, but can be used to define the shape and size of the liver and spleen, and to detect internal lesions. It also gives a direct semi-quantitative assessment of reticuloendothelial function, because the Kupffer cells preferentially take up colloidal formulations. Radiopharmaceuticals can also be used to visualize the biliary tract and cystic duct and estimate biliary function. **Positron emission tomography** has been used to detect both primary and secondary tumours.

Visualization of the biliary tract may be done by X-ray following the injection of a radio-opaque dye into an intrahepatic bile duct (**percutaneous transhepatic cholangiography**), with antibiotic cover. There is a small but significant risk to the patient, so alternative, non-invasive ultrasound examination is used increasingly. Oral and IV dye administration carries the risk of major allergic and other adverse reactions, though these are less likely following the introduction of new radio-contrast agents with lower iodine concentrations and nonionic compounds.

ERCP (endoscopic retrograde cholangiopancreatography) can be used to visualize the common bile duct and biliary tract and the pancreatic duct. In this technique, the papilla of Vater is cannulated via an endoscope and contrast medium is injected to visualize gallstones, the pancreatic duct and other anatomical features. The endoscope can also be used to remove stones that block the common bile duct. ERCP may also provide valuable further information on the aetiology of biliary obstruction, e.g. pancreatic carcinoma, or of its consequences, e.g. pancreatitis.

Blood (plasma) and urine tests

'Liver function tests' are only indirect indicators of hepatic function. The estimation of plasma proteins, i.e. albumin and prothrombin (via clotting tests; see below and Chapter 11), which are synthesized in the liver, are more direct. Further, finding normal values does not exclude appreciable liver damage, because 20% of patients with stable, chronic cirrhosis have normal values.

Serum proteins

Because their synthesis occurs only in the liver, reduced levels of serum proteins (especially albumin) are a useful general indicator of hepatic disease.

Prothrombin (clotting factor II) is not measured directly but as **prothrombin time (PT)**, i.e. the time taken for a fibrin clot to be produced in plasma under standard conditions. The test is always done in comparison with a normal sample of pooled plasma. In general, PT abnormalities are caused by liver malfunction, indicating either defective prothrombin synthesis (liver disease) or vitamin K deficiency due to obstructive jaundice (see below). Inadequate bile function may cause failure to absorb fat-soluble **vitamin K_1** (phytomenadione) from the diet. However, deficiency of vitamin K can also be due to malabsorption (p. 111) or oral anticoagulant therapy (see Chapter 11). These possibilities can be eliminated by repeating the PT test 24 h after a single IM injection of vitamin K, because PT does not respond to this in liver disease whereas it does in vitamin K deficiency. PT is probably the single most useful indicator for monitoring patient progress in most liver disease, being sensitive, specific to the liver (apart from vitamin K deficiency and anticoagulant therapy), and easily performed.

There are also unusually high Ig levels in alcoholic liver disease (IgA), chronic autoimmune hepatitis (IgG) and primary biliary cirrhosis (IgM), but these indicate possible causes of liver disease rather than the consequences, because they are not synthesized in the liver.

Other blood tests

Many other tests are used, e.g. transaminases (alanine aminotransferase, ALT; aspartate aminotransferase, AST), serum alkaline phosphatase (ALP) and gamma-glutamyl transpeptidase (GGT), which reflect cholestasis, ammonia (p. 148), bilirubin (p. 143) and lactate dehydrogenase (LDH), but these may be useful only if targeted to carefully selected patients. The interpretations of the most common tests are outlined in Table 3.24.

Numerous other biochemical tests are carried out to detect specific abnormalities, e.g. serology for viral hepatitis (A, B, C, etc.), autoantibodies (antimitochondrial, antimicrosomal) and alpha-fetoprotein (a tumour marker; see Chapter 10), but the reader is referred to the References and further reading section for accounts of these.

Urine testing

This has been a conventional part of screening for liver disease, but is now less important with the introduction of improved serum biochemistry methods.

Table 3.24   Serum, blood and urine tests of liver function and their interpretations

Test and abbreviation	Notes and implications of results
Serum tests	
Bilirubin	>17 µmol/L (>1 mg/dL) + 80% unconjugated = haemolytic jaundice or congestive heart failure <80% unconjugated = hepatitis or metastatic liver disease
Alkaline phosphatase (ALP)	Non-specific. Raised levels = hepatic obstruction, or bone or pancreatic disease
Gamma-glutamyl transpeptidase (GGT)	Raised GGT with normal ALP = alcohol consumption Raised GGT plus raised ALP = cholestasis
Aminotransferases • aspartate (AST, SGOT[a]) • alanine (ALT, SGPT[a])	For monitoring disease progression and the effects of therapy Levels normally parallel each other: • both very high = acute viral hepatitis • both high = myocardial infarction or shock • AST high, ALT normal = alcoholic liver disease
Albumin	Useful indicator of chronic liver disease ($t_{1/2}$ = 20 days)
Whole-blood tests	
Prothrombin time	2–3 s > normal or more = liver disease, vitamin K deficiency or anticoagulant therapy
Urine tests	
Bilirubin	Excess (dark urine on standing) = hepatic obstruction
Urobilinogen	Total absence = cholestasis (also gives pale stools) High = haemolysis, chronic liver disease or portosystemic shunting of blood (e.g. due to alcoholic cirrhosis)

[a] SGOT and SGPT are former abbreviations that are no longer used.

The 'equals' symbol is used here to mean 'implies'.

Dynamic tests. The blood and plasma tests outlined above are static tests, i.e. they give a snapshot at the time of sampling, but little idea of liver processes. The excretion of certain drugs, e.g. *sulphobromophthalein sodium* (bromsulphthalein) and *lidocaine* (lignocaine) are used in research and in specific cases to assess liver damage. These drugs have a high first-pass extraction, e.g. <5–7% of bromsulphthalein normally remains in the plasma 45 min after injection, and their clearance is a measure of liver blood flow. However, these tests are done only infrequently nowadays.

The clearance of drugs with a low first-pass extraction, e.g. *phenazone* (antipyrine) and *aminophenazone* (amidopyrine, aminopyrine), is virtually independent of liver blood flow and is a better measure of liver function.

Other investigations

Invasive investigations, which may carry a significant risk, may also be undertaken. **Liver biopsy** may be needed to confirm a diagnosis, establish prognosis, monitor progress, and to diagnose certain systemic diseases, e.g. sarcoidosis, TB and brucellosis. Samples are taken percutaneously with a special biopsy needle, preferably under ultrasound or CT guidance. There should not be a significant bleeding (clotting) problem, but cross-matched blood or at least cross-matching facilities must be available, especially if the PT is prolonged. In skilled hands the procedure can be done as a day case, but overnight observation may be required.

Biopsy is not usually done in suspected malignancy because of the risk of seeding of malignant cells along the needle track. Non-invasive investigations are preferred, e.g. ultrasound will show the presence of space-occupying lesions. Primary liver tumours and metastases (most common; see Chapter 10) are visualised very well by MRI. These investigations, considered together with clinical features, normally give the diagnosis, but a blood test for **serum alpha-fetoprotein** will detect 70% of hepatocellular carcinoma.

When occasionally the diagnosis is dubious, **laparoscopy** (examination of the abdominal organs with a percutaneous fibre-optic endoscope), or open **laparotomy** (surgical incision of the abdomen to permit examination) may be undertaken.

Clinical features of hepatic disease

General symptoms and signs

Many non-specific symptoms accompany early liver disease, e.g. malaise, anorexia, nausea and vomiting, and arthropathies. Fever is common, being mild to moderate in alcoholic hepatitis, though high fever with rigors may precede jaundice in acute viral hepatitis. **Steatorrhoea** (pale, bulky, fatty, abnormally foul-smelling stools) is a common feature in acute hepatitis, though less common in chronic disease, and the failure of fat absorption may contribute to weight loss.

Dupuytren's contracture (tendon contraction causing permanent flexure of one or more fingers) and **parotid gland enlargement** tend to occur most commonly in alcoholic liver disease. Palmar tendon contracture may be the first sign of liver disease in people following sedentary occupations, but may be occupationally acquired in manual workers.

Specific features of hepatic malfunction will be discussed first, before considering the causes, consequences and treatment of global liver failure.

Jaundice (icterus)

Definition

This most common symptom of liver disease is seen as a yellow coloration of the skin and sclera of the eyes, caused by **hyperbilirubinaemia**. Skin and scleral discoloration become visually evident at about two to three times the normal serum bilirubin levels (normal = $<20\ \mu mol/L$, $<1.0\ mg/dL$). Although jaundice is always the result of a high bilirubin level, it will not occur if the bilirubin level is only slightly raised. A spurious jaundice may result from excessive ingestion of carotene (in 'health diets'), or drugs (e.g. *mepacrine* and *busulfan*), but in these cases only the skin is coloured, and not the eyes.

The formation and excretion of bilirubin is summarized schematically in Figure 3.19, which shows that there are two forms of bilirubin. These appear differently in the urine and faeces in health and disease.

Excess **unconjugated bilirubin** is found in the serum when there is impaired hepatic removal and conjugation of bilirubin, e.g. in congenital glucuronidase deficiency (Gilbert's syndrome), or when excessive production of bilirubin overwhelms the capacity of the conjugation system, e.g. in haemolytic anaemias. Under these circumstances, bilirubin (water-insoluble) is absent from the urine, but urinary **urobilinogen** levels are raised to an extent that depends on the underlying cause and its severity. Although urobilinogen is colourless, the urine may darken on standing, as oxidation produces urobilin.

Excess **conjugated bilirubin** is present in the serum when there is **obstruction of the biliary tree**, e.g. due to gallstones or carcinoma. In this situation, bilirubin appears in the urine, because the glucuronide is water-soluble, but urinary levels of urobilinogen are reduced, or absent if obstruction is complete. If bilirubin is not discharged into the duodenum, urobilinogen and faecal bile pigments are not produced, so the faeces are pale and the urine is dark.

Classification

Jaundice may be classified according to its origin (see Figure 3.19):

- **Prehepatic**, arising from the blood before it enters the liver, e.g. due to haemolysis (see Chapter 11; serum total bilirubin 5–17 µmol/L, 0.3–1.0 mg/dL).
- **Intrahepatic**, due to disease of the liver parenchyma, e.g. viral hepatitis or alcoholic cirrhosis (serum total bilirubin 50–350 µmol/L, 0.3–20 mg/dL).
- **Post-hepatic**, the result of obstruction of the biliary tree outside the liver, e.g. by gallstones or carcinoma (serum total bilirubin 100–750 µmol/L, 0.6–45 mg/dL).

However, mixed types of jaundice are common, especially in the last two of these. Thus **cholestatic jaundice**, formerly called obstructive jaundice, may be due to inflammation of either the small bile canaliculi and ductules within the liver, or of the hepatic and common bile ducts outside it.

Obstruction of bile outflow causes a conjugated hyperbilirubinaemia and high concentrations of bile salts in the skin, often causing intense pruritus (itching). Pruritus may also be caused by increased endogenous opioid production (see

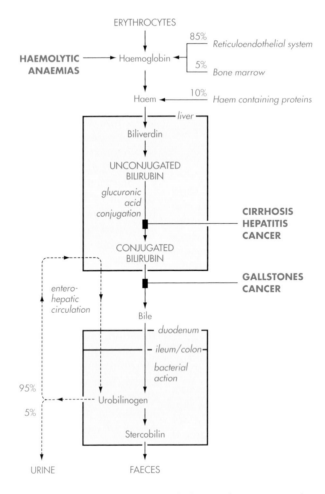

Figure 3.19 Formation and excretion of bilirubin and its metabolites, and some causes of jaundice. Causes of jaundice in bold capitals, sources of bilirubin and processes in italics (percentages are of bilirubin from the source indicated).

Chapter 7) and consequent abnormal neuro-transmission or neuromodulation of sensory nerves in the skin.

Aetiology

Jaundice is a symptom or sign and not a disease, so a cause must always be sought, especially because some are eminently treatable. The principal causes of jaundice are summarized in Table 3.25 and, in particular, the possibility of a drug aetiology must always be considered (Table 3.26).

Haemolytic anaemias and haemoglobinopathies may be inherited or acquired and these conditions and their management are discussed in Chapter 11.

Management

Because jaundice is a symptom, management depends on treatment of the underlying disease.

Table 3.25   Some causes of jaundice

Site of origin	Mechanism	Examples of causes
Prehepatic	Increased haem liberation	Haemolytic anaemias, malaria, reduced red cell lifespan
Intrahepatic	Defective liver metabolism	Congenital enzyme defects, iron storage disease, reduced hepatic bilirubin uptake
	Obstruction of small bile ducts	Alcoholic cirrhosis, autoimmune liver disease, drugs[a] and environmental chemicals, hepatic tumours, pregnancy, viral or other infections, gallstones (depends on diet), primary biliary cirrhosis
Post-hepatic	Obstruction of large bile ducts	Infection or inflammation of the biliary tree; gallstones, carcinoma of the pancreas, gallbladder, bile ducts and ampulla of Vater; pancreatitis; drugs[a]

[a] See Table 3.26 and Figure 3.19.

Table 3.26   Some drugs that may cause jaundice

Action	Examples[a]
Dose-dependent hepatocellular damage	Paracetamol (acetaminophen), salicylates, high-dose tetracyclines
Dose-independent hepatocellular damage	Desflurane[b], isoflurane[c] and sevoflurane[c] Dantrolene, ketoconazole, antidepressants, aminosalicylic acid, isoniazid, pyrazinamide, ethambutol
Haemolysis	Methyldopa, mefenamic acid
Cholestasis	Carbimazole, chlorpromazine, chlorpropamide, erythromycin estolate, oral contraceptives, sodium aurothiomalate, synthetic anabolic steroids

[a] This list is not comprehensive. Many drugs are capable of causing jaundice, but this is usually reversible on stopping the drug.
[b] Unlikely to cause hepatocellular damage
[c] Less likely than halothane (now withdrawn) to cause hepatocellular damage

Any drug that may precipitate jaundice (Table 3.26) should be stopped.

Neonatal jaundice is common, and occurs in all preterm babies because liver glucuronyl transferase is poorly developed in neonates, especially if premature. The condition usually disappears spontaneously within 2 weeks, as liver function matures. However, moderate bilirubin levels (up to about 250 µmol/L, 14 mg/dL) can be dealt with by exposure to blue light (phototherapy), which promotes bilirubin breakdown in the skin. Dangerously high bilirubin levels (>300 µmol/L, >17 mg/dL) may require exchange blood transfusion to prevent **kernicterus** (i.e. deposition of bilirubin in the brain, the neonatal blood–brain barrier being permeable to bilirubin) and permanent brain damage.

Inherited **glucose-6-phosphate dehydrogenase (G6PD) deficiency** (see Chapter 11) affects millions of people (mostly males) in the Mediterranean region, the Middle East, Africa and South-East Asia. G6PD deficiency renders red cell membranes liable to oxidation. The erythrocytes are then sensitive to a variety of minor insults, causing haemolysis. Thus haemolysis may be precipitated by drugs, especially oxidizing agents (see Chapter 11) and acute illnesses, e.g. infections and diabetic ketoacidosis.

Skin signs

Generalized pruritus is widespread itching of the skin. Patients with hepatic disease often present with severe, persistent itching of apparently normal skin, probably caused by the epidermal deposition of bile salts. The accumulation of bile salts and bilirubin are not necessarily related, so pruritus can occur without jaundice, especially in early disease. Because itching may have several other causes (see Chapter 13), the diagnosis of intractable pruritus in the absence of jaundice may require extensive investigation.

Spider naevi (spider telangiectases) are a frequent sign of liver disease, the naevi appearing as red spots on the upper trunk, above the nipple line. The naevi consist of a small central spiral arteriole with smaller vessels radiating from it. Central pressure with a finger or stylus causes blanching, showing that all the vessels are fed from the central arteriole. The pathogenesis of spider naevi is not fully understood, but they are probably caused by excessive oestrogen levels, a consequence of failing hepatic catabolism, causing vessel overgrowth. Isolated spider naevi may occur in healthy individuals, especially in pregnant women or those on oestrogen therapy, but multiple spider naevi strongly suggest liver disease.

Raised oestrogen levels also cause body hair loss (including pubic and axillary hair), testicular atrophy and gynaecomastia (breast enlargement in men).

Palmar erythema occurs when there is increased blood flow through the skin as a result of blood being diverted by obstruction of the portal circulation. *Leuconychia* (white nails) is a reflection of impaired liver protein synthesis.

Abdominal signs

Pain

The liver parenchyma has no sensory nerve supply, so pain is not a marked feature of liver disease unless the **capsule** is damaged or stretched or other organs are involved. However, right hypochondrial pain is a common feature of acute alcoholic liver disease.

Ascites

Ascites is the accumulation of an abnormal volume of fluid in the peritoneal cavity. In liver disease the causes are hypoproteinaemia, hepatic venous obstruction and failure of hepatic metabolism (Figure 3.20). Ascites produces a tense, painfully distended abdomen, though clinical signs are not apparent unless the volume exceeds about 2 L, depending on the patient's stature. Peripheral (ankle) oedema may also occur in liver disease, though this is secondary to ascites rather than being a primary event, as it is in heart or kidney failure (see Chapters 4 and 14). Ascites of hepatic origin is usually due to cirrhosis (see below), but there can also be non-hepatic causes, e.g. advanced congestive heart failure, nephrotic syndrome, malignancy and TB.

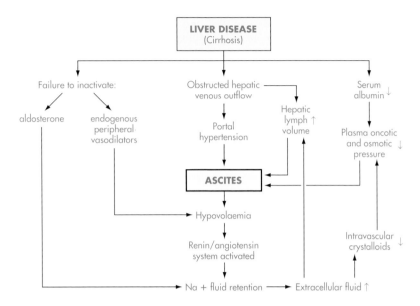

Figure 3.20   Mechanisms of ascites formation in hepatic disease (it may also have intestinal, renal and cardiac origins).

Similarly to the formation of oedema fluid (see Chapter 4), the principal initial event is that intravascular hydrostatic pressure (in this case in the portal vein) greatly exceeds the plasma oncotic pressure. This pressure difference is greater than usual in liver cirrhosis, because the portal pressure is increased owing to restricted flow through a fibrosed liver, while the oncotic pressure is reduced due to a failure of protein synthesis. These two conditions combine to give increased outflow of fluid from the portal vein into the peritoneal cavity.

Complications

Ascites is frequently accompanied by the general complications of hepatic failure, including:

* Consequences of the increased volume of intra-abdominal fluid, e.g. restricted mobility and respiratory distress due to reduced diaphragm function.
* Spontaneous bacterial peritonitis, owing to the failure of the reticuloendothelial protection mechanisms of the liver.
* Hepatorenal syndrome (renal failure secondary to hepatic failure), which may be due to hypovolaemia causing pre-renal failure and an abnormality of tubular sodium handling. It may be precipitated by certain

drugs, e.g. diuretics, NSAIDs, ACE inhibitors and aminoglycosides.
* Encephalopathy (see below).
* Clotting defects.
* Increased volume of distribution of hydrophilic drugs.

Management

Management is primarily supportive and symptomatic. Bedrest may improve hepatic blood flow and function.

Paracentesis and drainage, i.e. the removal of a limited volume of fluid (1–2 L) via a fine needle inserted through the abdominal wall, provides fluid for diagnostic purposes and improves patient comfort. The rapid drainage of large volumes of fluid by this means may prove fatal unless a plasma expander (i.e. low-salt human albumin) is given proportionately to the drained volume. Other plasma expanders, e.g. polymerized gelatin, dextran or etherified starch solutions, are unsuitable. If the plasma oncotic pressure is not increased the ascites volume is rapidly replaced, so the patient suffers further fluid and protein depletion, and the shift of further fluid from the blood into the abdomen causes hypovolaemia, hepatorenal syndrome and shock. However, up to 15 L, at a rate of 0.5–1.0 L/day, may be removed in total.

Salt and fluid restriction is a useful adjunctive therapy, but fluid restriction is only appropriate if the patient is hyponatraemic.

Potassium-sparing **diuretics** are used. *Spironolactone* is preferred initially, for several reasons: patients tend to be hypokalaemic, any hyperaldosteronism is counteracted, and its action is slow. Slow action is beneficial as the rapid mobilization of fluid and electrolytes causes harmful imbalances. Careful monitoring of serum electrolytes is essential to avoid hyperkalaemia and hyponatraemia. If gynaecomastia is a problem with *spironolactone, triamterene* or *amiloride* are suitable alternatives. If these give inadequate fluid loss, it is usual to add a low dose of a loop diuretic, e.g. *furosemide*, rather than use high doses of potassium-sparing agents, but this increases the risk of hepatorenal syndrome, due to excessive fluid depletion.

Under certain circumstances, diuretics should be avoided:

- In hyponatraemia, to avoid further sodium depletion.
- If renal function is impaired; serum creatinine is the best guide, as liver failure results in failure of urea formation.
- If there is evidence of encephalopathy (see below). Diuretics may aggravate encephalopathy or precipitate it, by causing further disturbances of electrolyte and fluid distribution.

In refractory chronic ascites, fluid can be shunted from the peritoneal cavity into the internal jugular vein through a subcutaneously implanted catheter (transjugular intrahepatic portocaval shunt [TIPS]). Alternatively, ascites fluid may be pumped from the abdomen, treated by ultrafiltration and the protein-enriched fluid returned to the circulation through a peripheral vein. Both techniques provide symptomatic relief, but carry the hazards of bacterial peritonitis and cardiovascular problems.

Encephalopathy

This complex neuromuscular/neuropsychiatric syndrome occurs in severe liver disease, either late in chronic disease or as a presenting symptom of acute hepatic failure (see below). It is characterized by changes in mood and behaviour, confusion, disordered sleep rhythm, drowsiness and, eventually, delirium and coma. There is a strong similarity to senile dementia, and it is important to distinguish between them as encephalopathy is potentially correctable.

Liver flap (asterixis) is an irregular, coarse, rapid flapping movement of the hand(s), occurring when the arm is extended or the fist is clenched. It reflects metabolic disturbance, but the precise origin is unclear. It may occur in the absence of overt central nervous symptoms and is often the earliest sign.

The term **portosystemic encephalopathy (PSE)** describes the aetiology, i.e. it is triggered by substances that are shunted from the portal vein into the systemic circulation, escaping hepatic detoxification. The syndrome has been attributed to:

- The action of gamma-aminobutyric acid (GABA), benzodiazepine receptor agonists and a GABA-ergic neurosteroid. The levels of these are enhanced by ammonia produced by colonic bacteria.
- A changed branched-chain amino acid/aromatic amine ratio in the CNS, causing the production of false neurotransmitters, e.g. octopamine, phenylethanolamine, and serotonin.
- Fatty acids, mercaptans and other substances that may also act as false neurotransmitters.

High blood levels of ammonia occur in 90% of patients, but this does not wholly account for the syndrome. Some potential precipitants of PSE are given in Table 3.27.

In acute liver failure, if there is a short interval between the appearance of jaundice and the onset of PSE, e.g. progression from mild to severe in 1–2 h, there is a high risk of potentially fatal cerebral oedema. In contrast, PSE complicating cirrhosis or a portosystemic shunt rarely causes cerebral oedema, so it is clearly important to distinguish these situations.

Management

Management of encephalopathy involves:

Table 3.27   Some precipitants of portosystemic encephalopathy

Mechanism	Examples of precipitants
Increased absorption of ammonia and other nitrogenous metabolites	GI bleeding (extra GI protein), especially from bleeding oesophageal varices (p. 87), excessive dietary protein, constipation (prolonged colonic residence times), uraemia
Increased levels of monoamine neurotransmitters in the CNS	MAOIs, tricyclic antidepressants
CNS depression	Sedatives, acidosis, uraemia
CNS excitation	Febrile infections, alkalosis
Decreased cerebral, renal and hepatic perfusion	Hyponatraemia, diuretics, heart failure, myocardial infarction, hypovolaemia, shock Drugs (see Table 3.31)
Liver damage	Diseases: e.g. viral hepatitis, Wilson's disease, malignancy

- withdrawal of precipitants, e.g. alcohol and drugs;
- control of infection, hypotension and renal impairment;
- correction of metabolic abnormalities;
- a prophylactic antisecretory agent (e.g. a PPI, p. 102), to reduce the risk of haemorrhage from gastric erosions;
- suppression of colonic bacterial metabolism;
- removal of toxic nitrogenous substances from the gut, including ammonia.

Pharmacotherapies used to achieve the last two of these objectives include the following:

- Purging with *phosphate enemas*. Magnesium enemas are sometimes recommended, but absorption may cause electrolyte disturbance.
- *Lactulose* or *lactitol* to maintain bowel evacuation, and to acidify the colon, so inhibiting bacterial metabolism and minimizing the production and absorption of ammonia and nitrogenous bases. This is sometimes used with antibiotics, the effects possibly being additive.
- An oral antibiotic (e.g. *neomycin*, occasionally *metronidazole* or *vancomycin*) is sometimes used to 'sterilize' the bowel. Because of poten-

tial antibiotic toxicities, it is more usual to rely on *lactulose* or *lactitol*.
- IV infusion of *ornithine aspartate* in fructose decreases blood ammonia concentration, but causes nausea and vomiting.
- *Flumazenil*, a benzodiazepine receptor antagonist, gives rapid improvement if encephalopathy was induced by benzodiazepines or other GABA-ergic drugs.

The restriction of dietary protein has been widely advocated, based on the ammonia–aromatic amine–amino acid theory of PSE aetiology. However, there is no evidence of clinical benefit for this. The 1997 guidelines of the European Society for Parenteral and Enteral Nutrition recommend a daily protein intake of 1–1.5 g/kg body weight for patients with liver disease, if tolerated. Those intolerant of this should have 0.5 g/kg/day of protein initially, plus amino acids to make up the deficit, possibly as branched-chain amino acids, although this last point is unclear. The protein intake should be sufficient to maintain nitrogen balance. Aggressive nutritional support has been demonstrated to be beneficial for patients with alcoholic liver disease and may apply to all those with severe hepatic disease. Expert dietetic involvement is desirable.

Vitamin D deficiency

The functions of vitamin D are outlined on p. 77, and its formation is illustrated in Figure 3.21, from which it is clear that both hepatic and renal failure can lead to vitamin D deficiency, in addition to poor nutrition and lack of sunlight.

Vitamin D deficiency caused by malabsorption or hepatic failure is treated with *ergocalciferol* (calciferol, vitamin D_2) or *colecalciferol* (vitamin D_3) whereas 1-alpha-hydroxycholecalciferol (*alfacalcidol*) or 1,25-dihydroxycholecalciferol (*calcitriol*) is used in renal failure. Although expensive, *alfacalcidol* and *calcitriol* have a shorter duration of action than the older vitamin D derivatives and are less likely to cause hypercalcaemia, so they are safer in use. The most potent compound is *calcitriol*, which can be given either orally or intravenously.

Gallstones (cholelithiasis)

Epidemiology

Gallstones are common, with some 10–15% of adults in Western countries having stones that can be demonstrated by ultrasonography, although only about one-third of these are symptomatic. About 50 000 cholecystectomies (gallbladder removals) are carried out each year in the UK. Gallstones can occur at any age, although they are rare under the age of 10 years and most common at 50–60 years in both sexes. Women are more prone to develop gallstones than men, the M : F ratio rising from 0.25–0.50 at under 40 to about 0.66 at over 80 years.

Relatively high prevalences occur in Italians and Swedes, Mexican women and North American Pima Indians. Black women are less likely to have stones than Caucasians, and Asians less likely than Europeans. These differences are real, having allowed for predisposing factors. The typical patient has been described as '5Fs', i.e. Female, Fair, Fat, Fertile and (approaching) Forty.

Aetiology and pathology

Most gallstones are composed of cholesterol and bile pigments in varying proportions. They are usually calcified to some extent. It is not known why only a minority cause symptoms.

The pathology is uncertain, but several factors are implicated in producing bile supersaturated with cholesterol:

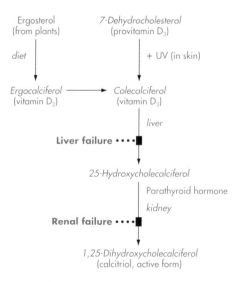

Figure 3.21   Formation of the active form of vitamin D.

- reduced low-density lipoprotein (LDL) uptake by the liver;
- up-regulation of HMG-CoA reductase, thus increasing cholesterol synthesis;
- down-regulation of bile acid synthesis, causing reduced cholesterol solubilization in the gut;
- distal ileal disease, causing reduced reabsorption and recycling of bile acids (another risk factor because these surfactants are needed to solubilize bilirubin and calcium);
- gallbladder stasis causing reduced emptying.

It has also been suggested that a defect of **cholecystokinin** release (or of gallbladder response to it), causing delayed gallbladder emptying, is a precursor to gallstone formation. Supersaturation depends on the balance between solubilizing and procrystallizing factors.

Predisposing factors for **cholesterol stones** include:

- obesity;
- age over 30 years;
- female sex, pregnancy and increased sex hormone levels (oral contraceptives increase cholesterol saturation of the bile);
- Western diet (rich in saturated fats);
- diabetes mellitus, which causes hyperlipidaemia;
- iatrogenic: drugs (*clofibrate*, *octreotide*); parenteral nutrition (which reduces the need for bile salts and so gallbladder emptying); and ileal surgery (by reducing recycling of bile salts).

Pigment stones are brown/black in colour and relatively radio-opaque. They are associated with liver cirrhosis (see above) and haemolytic anaemia (Chapter 11), both of which cause increased bilirubin and calcium excretion.

Clinical features and diagnosis

About 1% of individuals with asymptomatic, demonstrable stones in the gallbladder present annually with a gradual onset of non-specific symptoms, i.e. mild to severe right hypochondrial or epigastric pain, often referred to the right scapula, accompanied by a varying degree of anorexia and nausea. Acute onset also occurs, usually due to impaction of stones in the cystic duct. Diagnosis is by:

- Ultrasonography: this is sensitive, but cannot distinguish between types of stone.
- Radiography: plain X-rays detect only the calcified stones (20%), but oral radiocontrast medium enables the detection of radiolucent stones and gallbladder anatomy and contraction. Small stones are poorly visualized.
- CT scanning is better for detecting radiolucent stones.
- ERCP for complications, e.g. common bile duct stones. The technique also permits intervention for removal of small stones and stone fragments (see below).
- Liver function tests: serum conjugated bilirubin, ALP and ALT may be raised.

If the diagnosis is in doubt, high serum amylase levels will indicate pancreatitis and exclude salivary gland disease and bowel perforation or infarction. High serum lipase levels are more specific for pancreatitis.

A patient's description of symptoms such as 'biliousness', and the commonly held erroneous belief that symptoms are associated with fatty meals, are of no diagnostic value.

Complications

Common complications of gallstones include the following:

- Biliary colic (i.e. spasm of the inflamed gallbladder and/or bile duct) causes moderate to severe pain in the epigastrium or right hypochondrium, with excruciating exacerbations lasting for a few hours against a background of constant pain.
- Acute cholecystitis and cholangitis (i.e. inflammation of the gallbladder and common bile duct respectively), associated with the presence of stones or obstruction by a stone. These are usually followed by infection with intestinal bacteria that requires antibiotics and cholecystectomy.
- Acute pancreatitis, caused by reflux of bile up the pancreatic duct, produces moderate to severe pain in the epigastrium. The pain penetrates to the back, usually causing vomiting. This is a potentially serious condition, occasionally causing acute respiratory or renal failure.

• Cholestatic jaundice (p. 144), usually fluctuating in character.

Upper abdominal pain with nausea, vomiting and wind has frequently been ascribed to cholecystitis, but there is no evidence that these symptoms represent a recognizable clinical entity.

Management

Treatment of gallstones may be either medical or surgical.

Pharmacotherapy

A bile acid, e.g. *ursodeoxycholic acid*, is suitable for patients with a normal gallbladder function, and small or medium-sized radiolucent (cholesterol) stones in whom other treatments have failed or are inappropriate. The drug is taken for up to 2 years in order to dissolve radiolucent stones, as cholesterol is about 2×10^5 times more soluble in bile salt solutions than in water. However, bile acid treatment may not be successful, or stones may recur, so this approach is usually reserved for patients who are unfit for surgery and as an adjunct to **extracorporeal shock-wave lithotripsy** (ESWL, see below). Some patients find that symptoms are relieved very rapidly, well before stones could be dissolved, possibly because gallbladder and bile duct spasm are reduced.

Surgery and interventional endoscopy

Surgery nowadays is conducted almost exclusively by **laparoscopic cholecystectomy**, i.e. gallbladder removal with endoscope guidance via a small incision in the abdominal wall. This technique is much less traumatic than conventional open surgery, requires less analgesia and recovery is quicker. However, conversion to open surgery is necessary with patients:

• in whom bleeding cannot be controlled;
• in whom laparoscopic cholecystectomy risks damage to surrounding viscera;
• who have a fistula between the gallbladder and the bile duct or the intestines;

• who have perforation into the liver, with abscess formation.

Patients with a few non-calcified gallstones can have these dispersed ultrasonically (using ESWL), although endoscopic removal of residual fragments may be necessary. Other techniques include percutaneous lithotomy (removal of stones via a catheter inserted through the skin) and endoscopic laser fragmentation of stones, the endoscope being manoeuvred into the bile duct.

The biliary system can also be intubated surgically and flushed with *monoctanoin*, a monoglyceride, to dissolve cholesterol stones in the bile duct, but this is effective in only 50% of cases.

Patients unfit for surgery are treated with a low-fat diet, prophylactic antibiotics and possibly the endoscopic insertion of a cannula into the bile duct, to improve drainage of bile and permit the passage of gallstones. Surgery can follow later, when the patient is fit.

Liver failure

Acute failure

Classification

There are three types of acute hepatic failure:

• **Fulminant (hyperacute) hepatic failure (FHF)** is a syndrome of abrupt onset (fulminant = explosive), characterized by progressively severe encephalopathy occurring within 7–14 days of the onset of jaundice. FHF is the result of massive hepatocellular necrosis, i.e. death of the liver parenchyma, or other severe functional impairment.
• In **acute hepatic failure** encephalopathy occurs within 14–28 days of the onset of jaundice.
• **Subacute hepatic failure** is defined as acute failure occurring in patients without pre-existing liver disease, in whom the signs of encephalopathy develop more than 8 weeks after the onset of illness. These patients are generally older than those with FHF and tend not to have viral hepatitis. Survivors may have **autoimmune hepatitis** (p. 155).

Acute-on-chronic hepatocellular failure occurs as a result of decompensation in patients with chronic liver disease. This may result from protein overload due to diet, substantial gastrointestinal bleeding, sepsis, or intervention with drugs or surgery.

Aetiology of FHF

In the UK, *paracetamol* (acetaminophen) poisoning is the most common cause. Many other drugs may cause FHF (see below), anaesthesia with *halothane* being a well-recognized cause, but monoamine oxidase inhibitors (MAOIs), antiepileptics and antimicrobial agents may also be involved. FHF may also occur in Wilson's disease, Reye's syndrome (see below and Chapter 12) and pregnancy and following solvent ingestion or 'glue sniffing'. About 1% of patients with viral hepatitis develop fulminant disease.

Clinical features

The symptoms and signs are similar for all types of acute hepatic failure. Because of the numerous functions of the liver, the initial signs are widespread and non-specific. Any of those outlined on pp. 143–150 may be present.

Jaundice may be absent, mild or obvious. Asterixis is virtually always present and **hepatic fetor**, an offensive breath odour of methyl mercaptan, is common. The liver size may be normal, enlarged, or small and hard. The presence of a small, hard liver, and the early onset of ascites, implies a very poor prognosis.

Management

Apart from general supportive measures, and the elimination of any precipitants, only limited treatments are available. A listing of some of the available measures is given in Table 3.28. Generally, the prognosis depends on the severity of the failure and the regenerative ability of the liver.

In the case of FHF due to *paracetamol* (acetaminophen) overdose, gastric aspiration and absorption with activated charcoal is carried out if ingestion occurred within 2 h of hospital admission. IV infusion of *N-acetylcysteine (NAC)* in 5% glucose is the antidote of choice and is started immediately, but oral *methionine* is also used if appropriate facilities for infusion are not available, e.g. in remote areas. *Methionine* must be used with care in patients with known hepatic impairment, because it may precipitate coma.

NAC should be given within 10–12 h of *paracetamol* (acetaminophen) ingestion to be optimally effective, but administration up to 36 h reduces mortality and limits the severity of symptoms. The need for *NAC* treatment is assessed by nomogram, using the *paracetamol* (acetaminophen) plasma concentration determined on a sample taken not less than 4 h after ingestion, i.e. after complete absorption of the drug. *NAC* must be used cautiously in asthmatic patients.

NAC protects the liver against the depletion of glutathione by the reactive metabolite N-acetyl-benzoquinoneimine (NBQ). If *NAC* is not used, hepatic glutathione is exhausted and the NBQ then reacts with hepatic intracellular protein sulphydryl groups, causing hepatocellular necrosis. *NAC* also acts as a cardiac inotrope, increasing peripheral blood flow and oxygen extraction, and may potentiate vasodilatation due to endothelium-derived relaxing factor (EDRF, nitric oxide), thus increasing hepatic and cerebral blood flow.

Prophylactic parenteral H_2-RAs reduce the incidence of gastro-oesophageal bleeding, but regrettably have little influence on mortality.

It is usual to establish a central venous line to facilitate **total parenteral nutrition**, if required, and to avoid repeated venepuncture for blood sampling in patients who often have coagulation defects.

Liver damage is maximal 3–4 days after ingestion, and reports exist of death occurring after ingestion of only 10–15 g of *paracetamol* (acetaminophen) (20–30 tablets). Over-dosage with the popular combination analgesic *co-proxamol* (*paracetamol + dextropropoxyphene*) poses a greater risk than does plain *paracetamol*, because *dextropropoxyphene* causes CNS depression and inhibition of liver enzymes. *Dextropropoxyphene* is a mild opioid, so *naloxone* is required as an opioid antidote in addition to *NAC*, and ventilatory support may be needed.

Because of this and the facts that *co-proxamol* is not a superior analgesic to plain *paracetamol* and

Table 3.28   Management of hepatic failure

Problem	Aetiology or pathology	Treatment
Ascites	Malignancy, hypoproteinaemia, cirrhosis	See p. 156 (cirrhosis)
Portosystemic encephalopathy	Ammonia?, other blood 'toxins'	See p. 148
Cerebral oedema	Uncertain: metabolic stress?, toxic amines → false neurotransmitters?	Mannitol IV, dexamethasone?, N-acetylcysteine? Haemofiltration, surgical decompression
Hypoglycaemia, hyperglycaemia	Inability to mobilize carbohydrate or control blood glucose	Check blood glucose hourly Glucose IV (in hypoglycaemia) IV insulin (in hyperglycaemia; + KCl in acidosis)
Electrolyte imbalance	Failure of regulation } Vomiting/diarrhoea } Fluid retention	Correct ion levels, restrict sodium, calcium gluconate IV, ion exchange resins, fluid replacement? Use of diuretics is controversial
Respiratory failure	Fluid retention, restriction of diaphragm due to ascites	Ventilate; monitor blood gases Use of diuretics is controversial
Infections	Impaired reticuloendothelial function Renal impairment causing uraemia[a]	Specific antibiotics
Anaemia, coagulation disorders	Haemorrhage Bone marrow depression Reduced prothrombin level	Blood, plasma (platelet?) transfusion, vitamin K H_2-blocker IV (prophylaxis of gastric bleeding)
Hepatocellular necrosis	Paracetamol (acetaminophen) overdose	N-acetylcysteine/methionine
General considerations		Identify and treat any precipitating cause Low-protein, high-carbohydrate diet Barrier nursing of infections Central venous line for total parenteral nutrition, manometry and blood sampling Purgation if constipated No sedatives or potentially hepatotoxic substances Transplantation?

[a] Urea increases membrane permeability and facilitates microbial tissue invasion.
KCl, potassium chloride; IV, intravenous.

is a common suicide agent, this combination is being withdrawn in the UK.

Numerous attempts have been made at more specific therapies, with variable and limited success. Corticosteroids are often used, although there is little rational basis for this. Many abortive attempts have been made to remove postulated blood toxins, e.g. by exchange

Table 3.29   Some causes of chronic liver disease

Aetiology	Examples
Alcohol abuse	
Drugs	See p. 159 and Tables 3.31 and 3.32
Infection	Infections: amoebic dysentery, helminths, TB, brucellosis
	Sequel to viral hepatitis (HBV, HCV)
	Secondary to biliary obstruction, diverticulitis, appendicitis or malignancy
Genetic	Abnormal copper metabolism (Wilson's disease) or iron metabolism
	Autoimmunity to hepatic nuclear, smooth muscle or microsomal antigens
	Inflammatory bowel disease
Iron overload	Repeated blood transfusion or excessive iron intake, abnormal iron metabolism, alcoholic liver disease

HBV, HCV, hepatitis B and C viruses.

transfusion. Haemodialysis, using a polyacrylonitrile membrane to remove small molecules (<5000 Da), is promising, but unproven. **Liver transplantation** is rarely possible because a suitably matched donor organ is unlikely to be available at short notice. However, artificial livers have been developed and may offer support until a suitable donor organ becomes available, similarly to renal dialysis.

Chronic liver failure

Aetiology

Chronic liver failure may be the consequence of any chronic liver disease (Table 3.29). However, some patients show evidence of raised serum transaminases or persistent viral hepatitis (HBV, see below), discovered by chance during investigations (e.g. when donating blood), without ever showing symptoms or progressing to liver failure.

Chronic progressive liver disease always leads to portal hypertension, resulting in ascites or bleeding oesophageal varices (p. 87), and encephalopathy. Cirrhosis (see below) frequently develops insidiously.

Management

The liver has great powers of regeneration so apart from the withdrawal of precipitants, which leads to recovery if the liver damage is not too severe, management is again largely supportive and symptomatic.

However, there is some specific pharmacotherapy. *Penicillamine* is effective in Wilson's disease, an inherited abnormality of copper metabolism, and *desferrioxamine* in iron overload. Immunosuppression with a combination of corticosteroids and *azathioprine* is beneficial in some forms of chronic hepatitis.

Liver transplantation is the only satisfactory treatment for established severe failure, but the results depend on its aetiology. The 5-year survival rate is currently about 85% in primary biliary cirrhosis, with most problems occurring in the first year. If the cause of cirrhosis is unknown, the 5-year survival rate falls to about 65%.

Autoimmune hepatitis

This is normally a chronic progressive disease of unknown aetiology, although it may also have an acute presentation resembling that of acute viral hepatitis. Because of this, the earlier description of 'chronic active hepatitis' has been abandoned.

Autoimmune hepatitis can affect both sexes at any age, the onset being most common in women aged 20–40 years. The condition is characterized by:

- serum autoantibodies;
- hyperglobulinaemia;
- an association with other autoimmune diseases, e.g. RA and sicca syndrome (see Chapter 12), renal tubular acidosis, Hashimoto's thyroiditis and UC.

Prompt diagnosis of autoimmune hepatitis, to distinguish it from conditions such as chronic viral hepatitis (see below), Wilson's disease and other causes of liver cirrhosis, is essential to ensure appropriate treatment.

Pharmacotherapy is aggressive because severe disease has an untreated mortality of 30%. The mainstay of treatment is high-dose *prednisolone*, with or without *azathioprine*, depending on severity. *Ciclosporin* is used for those intolerant of *azathioprine*, and may be added to the *prednisolone + azathioprine* regimen for non-responders.

Liver transplantation is used for end-stage disease.

Cirrhosis

Cirrhosis is a chronic, irreversible degeneration of liver cells followed by scarring and infiltration of the tissues with dense fibrotic strands. This leads to a progressive loss of liver function and circulatory obstruction, the latter causing portal hypertension. The diagnosis can be made only by biopsy and histology.

Aetiology

Common causes include prolonged alcoholism and viral hepatitis (B, B+D, or C; see below). Less common causes include:

- primary biliary cirrhosis, i.e. progressive idiopathic bile duct destruction, mostly in middle-aged females;
- autoimmune hepatitis;
- haemochromatosis (iron overload caused by, for example, repeated blood transfusions), genetic mutations, haemorrhagic conditions, impaired erythropoiesis, excessive oral iron intake;
- Wilson's disease;

- schistosomiasis;
- drugs and toxins.

Clinical features

The clinical features of cirrhosis are numerous and varied, and depend on both liver failure and past patient history. The initial symptoms are non-specific and common to many liver diseases (see above). Generalized **pruritus** may precede jaundice by some years. **Ascites** and **encephalopathy** occur inevitably in the later stages. Management is similar to that for liver failure generally (see Table 3.28).

Viral and other infective hepatitis

Aetiology

Viral hepatitis is caused by one of several different viruses: hepatitis A virus (HAV), HBV, HCV, HDV, HEV, HGV and possibly other species.

Other viral infections may present with symptoms of liver disease, but these are not normally classified as viral hepatitis. These include the Epstein–Barr virus, which causes **infectious mononucleosis** (glandular fever), **cytomegalovirus** (usually in the immunocompromised), herpes virus, yellow fever, and such exotica as Lassa fever and Ebola and Marburg virus infections. Protozoa, helminths and to a lesser extent bacteria and fungi also cause liver inflammation.

Thus, **Weil's disease**, caused by *Leptospira interrogans* var. *icterohaemorrhagiae*, is a potentially severe infection contracted from infected rodents, usually after participating in inland water sports in water contaminated with rat urine. The incidence of Weil's disease (about 30 cases/year in the UK) is increasing because of the growing interest in water sports. In severe infections, the leptospirae cause jaundice, haemorrhage and renal and hepatic impairment, and 50% of cases also have meningism (see Chapter 8). Mild cases can be treated with *doxycycline*, but more severe infection requires parenteral *penicillin* or *erythromycin* and intensive support.

In patients from tropical areas, amoebic dysentery, malaria, schistosomiasis and liver fluke infections may also be involved. The following account is confined to the hepatitis viruses.

Although these viruses are grouped together because they cause human hepatitis, they are structurally and taxonomically diverse:

- HAV, HEV and HGV are non-enveloped, single-stranded RNA viruses.
- HBV is an enveloped, polyhedral, double-stranded DNA virus.
- HCV is an enveloped, polyhedral, single-stranded RNA virus, related to the rubella (German measles) virus.
- HDV is an unusual circular RNA, incomplete virus, unable to replicate on its own. It is coated with the HBV surface antigen and requires co-infection with HBV for transmission. Its genome resembles that of some plant viruses.
- HEV is an RNA virus, spread similarly to Weil's disease (see above).

About 15% of isolates cannot be typed by current techniques, so other viruses exist, but these are thought not to cause significant human disease.

Both HAV and HEV cause **infective hepatitis**, the most common form, which is responsible for some 40% of overt disease in the UK.

Clinical features

The diseases may be asymptomatic, e.g. about 50% of UK adults have antibodies against HAV, although there are relatively few identified cases. However, there is a complete spectrum of severity, from subclinical up to fulminant, life-threatening disease. The symptoms and signs are similar in all forms. There is initially a prodromal **anicteric** phase, i.e. no jaundice, with nausea, vomiting, headache, malaise, and a varying degree of fever. In moderate to severe disease this is followed by the **icteric** phase, with jaundice, dark urine and pale faeces (caused by intrahepatic cholestasis), abdominal discomfort, hepatomegaly and enlargement, sometimes splenomegaly and tenderness.

With HBV, the immunological response of the host causes a syndrome resembling serum sickness, sometimes with rashes and polyarthritis.

Prognosis

Nearly all patients with HAV and HEV, about 95% with HBV, and about 60% with HCV have a self-limiting illness, followed by complete recovery. Fulminant hepatitis has a high mortality but is fortunately uncommon, occurring in about 1% of cases. Infection with HBV and HCV confers an increased risk of primary liver cancer. HGV is common in the USA and causes an apparently benign long-lasting viraemia.

There are few specific treatments, and full recovery may take several months. Infection due to HBV and HCV may cause chronic disease, a carrier state and cirrhosis (see below). Further, chronic HBV infection may cause hepatocellular carcinoma.

Hepatitis A and E

HAV and HEV have a faecal–oral route of transmission, causing infections that may be asymptomatic or acute. The incubation periods are prolonged, about 14–50 days, and symptoms start to resolve after about 3 weeks. Infections by HAV and HEV cannot be distinguished clinically. There are no chronic carriers.

HAV infection occurs worldwide, often in autumnal epidemics spread by faecally contaminated food (especially shellfish), and water, and primarily under poor living conditions. Man is the only known host, so spread is person-to-person.

HEV was one of the viruses described as causing 'Non-A Non-B hepatitis'. It is responsible for most hepatitis outbreaks in endemic regions in Africa, Asia, Central America and the Middle East, but causes only about 1% of cases of acute hepatitis elsewhere. In endemic regions, HEV has been found in sheep and pigs.

The prognosis for HAV infection is usually excellent, though a few patients may have more severe disease. However, there is a fatality rate of about 2.5% in patients aged 50 or over. Although patients feel debilitated for many months, neither chronic disease nor a carrier state occurs.

HEV infection poses a special risk in pregnancy. In the third trimester there is a high maternal mortality rate (20–25%) and a high fetal risk. Treatment is symptomatic and supportive because neither diet nor drugs influence the course of the disease. Alcohol is best avoided, especially in the severe phase. The most effective prophylactic measure is good hygiene, especially after defecation.

Passive immunoprophylaxis against HAV is conferred by normal Ig and lasts for 2–6 months, but is not possible for HEV, because antibody levels in pooled human plasma are too low. However, a safe vaccine is now available for HAV, which confers rapid, long-term active immunity. Booster doses of the vaccine are required after 12 months. An effective bivalent vaccine against HAV and HBV is available.

Because there is currently no suitable cell culture system for HEV, it is not possible to produce a vaccine against HEV comparable to that for HAV. However, trials are being done with a non-pathogenic virus, genetically modified to express HEV capsid protein. Immunity to HEV following infection is short-lived, so any vaccine may need to be given annually.

Hepatitis B and D

Hepatitis B virus

HBV used to be called 'Australia antigen', because of its discovery in the blood of an Australian aboriginal. It occurs worldwide and is solely a human parasite, persisting in a human carrier reservoir. In Western countries the carrier rate is 0.1%, but some 12% may be carriers in Africa and the Far East. Spread is by infected blood, e.g. 'main-line' drug addicts, unhygienic tattooing and acupuncture, or by sexual contact, especially homosexual. In the Far East, mother-to-fetus transmission is common.

The course of HBV infection is very variable: there is an acute phase, followed by a slow elimination of virus, apparent recovery and then a second acute phase. About 5–10% of patients become chronic asymptomatic carriers, especially if they are male, immunosuppressed, are on long-term haemodialysis, or are long-term mental inpatients with poor hygiene. Neonatal exposure also predisposes to chronic infection. Some 3% of patients develop **autoimmune hepatitis**, probably owing to a chronic immunological reaction.

Chronic HBV infection may be treated with:

- **Antivirals**, e.g. *famciclovir*, *lamivudine* and *adefovir* (licensed in the UK; *lobucavir* is under trial).
- **Cytokines**, e.g. interferons and *interleukin-2 + IFN alfa* for 3 months being the most successful, leading to eradication of the virus in about 40% of cases.

Prophylaxis is provided by an effective monovalent vaccine produced by recombinant DNA technology. Because of the risks of cirrhosis and hepatocellular carcinoma associated with HBV infection, the vaccine is used very widely, especially for those at special risk, e.g. medical and paramedical workers, staff and patients in residential homes, patients with chronic renal failure and undergoing renal dialysis, partners and spouses of HBV-positive patients, and homosexual or bisexual individuals. Short-term travellers to endemic regions do not normally require vaccination unless they are likely to engage in risky behaviour, but needs to be commenced at least 6 months before travel. The initial course consists of three doses, usually given over 6 months, during which period effective protection should develop. The deltoid muscle is the preferred site: injection into the buttock reduces efficacy.

The divalent HAV + HBV vaccine is not recommended for accidental occupational exposure, e.g. needle-stick injuries and ocular contamination by aerosols, etc. In these circumstances, simultaneous use of monovalent HBV vaccine and specific HBV Ig is recommended.

The initial course may be given over 2 months with a booster dose at 1 year, for more rapid protection. Some 10% of individuals respond poorly and need additional booster doses or revaccination. The duration of protection is uncertain, but a further booster dose is recommended after 5 years. Improved vaccines are under active investigation, and offer the hope of universal cheap immunization.

Hepatitis D virus (delta virus)

As noted above, HDV depends on HBV for its replication. It may occur simultaneously with HBV infection, or as an opportunistic infection in HBV carriers.

HBV + HDV usually causes severe infections, being implicated in about 50% of patients with fulminant hepatitis, and is likely to cause hepatic cirrhosis (see below). Prophylaxis against HBV also protects against HDV.

Hepatitis C

Before characterization, this was the principal cause of 'Non-A Non-B hepatitis'. HCV causes an acute infective hepatitis, with an incubation period of 6–12 weeks. Only about 25% of patients are jaundiced. Most chronic cases follow overt acute infection and the disease may last for several decades. Infection at an older age, concurrent infection and other illnesses may cause progressive cirrhosis and occasionally hepatocellular carcinoma.

It is believed to be responsible for up to 90% of cases occurring after unsafe blood transfusion. UK transfusion practice excludes blood donation from members of high-risk groups. Blood products, e.g. clotting factor concentrates, are treated with solvents, detergents and heat. Organ transplant patients and those receiving haemodialysis are also at risk. IV drug abusers comprise 40% of patients, and high-risk sexual activity accounts for a further 10%.

There is no vaccine, but immunization with the **HAV + HBV vaccine** may prevent severe complications. A combination of *ribavirin* (tribavirin) and *peginterferon-alfa* is used for chronic infection, under NICE guidelines in the UK (see References and further reading). Most other antivirals, including *ribavirin* alone, have not given a sustained benefit. *Peginterferon-alfa* is superior to non-pegylated IFN alfa. The early use of IFN alfa in acute HCV infection

may prevent chronic infection (unlicensed indication).

Drugs and the liver

The relationship between the liver and drugs is important for three reasons:

- The liver is the principal site for drug metabolism. Consequently, while liver disease may impair hepatic drug-metabolizing activity, the drugs themselves may reduce or enhance these processes. This consideration applies primarily to lipophilic drugs, which are normally metabolized to hydrophilic compounds for urinary excretion.
- Liver impairment has other physiological effects, which affect drug handling and disposition, for example:
  - increased volume of distribution of hydrophilic drugs in ascites (p. 146);
  - reduced plasma binding of acidic drugs by low plasma protein levels;
  - reduced biliary excretion (cholestasis) causes hyperbilirubinaemia and reduced excretion, e.g. of *rifampicin* and *fusidic acid*;
  - *morphine* and overenthusiastic diuretic therapy may precipitate hepatic encephalopathy (p. 148) in patients with cirrhosis.
- Drugs may cause liver damage, e.g. *paracetamol* (acetaminophen) and antidepressants.

The bioavailability of drugs may be influenced by patient factors that are unconnected with liver disease: only those connected with the liver will be discussed here.

The liver and drug metabolism

A full discussion of this complex subject is out of place here, although some specific aspects are outlined below. A brief treatment of drugs to be used with caution in liver disease is given in Appendix 2 to the BNF and readers are referred to Chapter 1 and the References and further reading section of this chapter (p. 162).

Biological (patient) factors influencing drug availability

Pharmacogenetic factors
Two points are relevant here:

* Slow acetylators are more likely to experience toxic reactions with normal doses of drugs than fast acetylators.
* Oxidative drug metabolism varies substantially (20-fold) between patients, so some patients fail to respond to doses of drugs that cause unacceptable side-effects in others.

Disease state
Although diseases that compromise the blood supply to the liver may be expected to impair drug metabolism, the data are conflicting, and it is difficult to draw satisfactory conclusions. It is probable that liver function needs to be considerably impaired before significant effects are seen. The effects of liver disease are complex because several factors change simultaneously, e.g. metabolism, protein binding, volume of distribution and elimination in the bile. The greatest effects are seen when metabolism, espe-cially first-pass metabolism, is high and protein binding is low, because the free plasma concentration is then markedly increased. Conversely, the plasma levels of drugs that undergo little first-pass metabolism and are highly protein-bound will be little changed. These effects are listed in Table 3.30.

Age
The decline in hepatic function with age leads to reduced levels of serum albumin and decreased hepatic metabolism, and these combine with other age-related changes to influence the availability of many drugs (see Chapter 1). Interacting factors and interindividual variation make it difficult to predict what the effect will be in a particular patient.

Drugs and liver enzyme activity

The metabolism of many drugs may be either increased or decreased by the effects of other drugs on microsomal mixed function oxidase, of which the cytochrome P450 family of enzymes provide the terminal stage. Table 3.31 lists the more important drugs that are known to induce or inhibit hepatic microsomal enzymes.

Generally, **enzyme induction** will reduce the biological availability of drugs and their activity.

Table 3.30   Some effects of liver disease on the availability of drugs with different pharmacokinetic properties

Drug		Effect of liver disease on availability	Examples
Hepatic extraction[a]	Protein binding		
Low	High	Nil	Diazepam, indometacin, phenytoin[b], rifampicin, theophylline, tolbutamide, warfarin
Moderate	Moderate	Increased	Chlorpromazine, isoniazid, pethidine (meperidine), metoprolol, nortriptyline, paracetamol (acetaminophen), quinidine
High	Moderate	Greatly increased	Labetalol, lidocaine (lignocaine), morphine, pentazocine, dextropropoxyphene (propoxyphene), propranolol, verapamil

[a] First-pass metabolism.
[b] Phenytoin clearance may be increased in the elderly.

However, this is clinically significant only with drugs having a narrow therapeutic window and when loss of activity severely compromises the patient, e.g. *warfarin*, with which loss of activity may result in thrombosis, stroke or death, and the oral contraceptive pill, as enhanced metabolism of oestrogen may cause an unwanted pregnancy.

There are some drugs whose toxicity may be enhanced by metabolism, because the metabolite causes the damage, e.g. *paracetamol* (acetaminophen) and *isoniazid*.

Enzyme inhibition increases drug activity, if other factors do not change. Again, it is those drugs with a low therapeutic index that are important, e.g. *warfarin*, which may provoke severe spontaneous haemorrhage. *Phenytoin* has a non-linear dose–response curve, and small increases in plasma levels may give rise to acute toxic reactions, e.g. nausea, vomiting, dizziness, tremor, ataxia and blurred vision, if the steady-state level is near the top of the therapeutic range. With a hypnotic or sedative, enzyme induction only impairs the level of sedation, but enzyme inhibition might result in over-sedation, confusion and serious falls in the elderly.

While inhibition occurs rapidly, enzyme induction depends on new synthesis, so the effects take some time to become apparent. Some of the drugs most likely to be affected by changes in liver enzyme activity are also listed in Table 3.31.

In addition, some drugs inhibit a specific enzyme, leading to higher levels of another drug that is metabolized by the same enzyme, e.g. *allopurinol* inhibits xanthine oxidase and may cause unacceptable toxicity with *azathioprine* and *mercaptopurine*.

Hepatotoxicity

As in other situations, side-effects may be either toxic (type A, predictable) or **idiosyncratic** (type B, unpredictable). Table 3.32 lists some drugs that may produce these effects in the liver, though such adverse reactions are uncommon.

The principal risk factors for hepatic drug injury are given in Table 3.33, together with the mechanisms involved.

Among these effects, *paracetamol* poisoning is the principal cause of acute hepatic failure in the UK (p. 152).

Halothane and its congeners are generally very safe general anaesthetics. However, a small proportion of patients experience an unexplained fever, with mild signs of liver involvement. Exposure after a patient has been sensitized to *halothane* or to desflurane, isoflurane and sevoflurane, should be avoided in such patients, as it may cause acute, often fatal, liver failure, usually in obese, elderly females.

Reye's syndrome follows febrile illness in young children, although fortunately only rarely. Affected patients develop signs of liver disease with severe encephalopathy, and there is severe fatty degeneration of the liver. Because there is a high probability that the syndrome can be triggered by *aspirin*, this is contra-indicated in children under 16 years of age. The mortality rate is about 50%, usually from cerebral oedema.

Table 3.31 Some drugs which affect hepatic drug metabolism

Enzyme inducers
Alcohol, aminoglutethimide, barbiturates, carbamazepine, chlorpromazine, griseofulvin, phenytoin, primidone, rifampicin

Enzyme inhibitors
Amiodarone, chloramphenicol, cimetidine, clofibrate, indometacin, omeprazole, sodium valproate, sulphonamides, tolbutamide

Drugs with which the clinical effects may be significant
Carbamazepine, clomethiazole, diazepam, phenytoin, theophylline, tolbutamide, warfarin, oral contraceptives

Table 3.32   Some hepatotoxic drug effects

Type of reaction	Examples
Toxicity	
Hepatocellular necrosis	Paracetamol (acetaminophen)
Gallstone production	Clofibrate, oestrogens
Sensitivity (idiosyncrasy)	
Cholestasis	Chlorpromazine, co-amoxiclav[a], erythromycin estolate, fusidic acid, glibenclamide, phenothiazines, sodium valproate
Hepatic dysfunction/failure	Methotrexate
Hepatitis	Amiodarone, azathioprine, dantrolene[b], halothane, isoniazid, MOAIs, methyldopa[b], nitrofurantoin[b], novobiocin, rifampicin, salicylates, sulfasalazine, sodium valproate
Granuloma formation (see Chapter 2)	Allopurinol, hydralazine, phenylbutazone[c], sulphonamides and sulfasalazine
Reye's syndrome	Aspirin, sodium valproate, high-dose tetracycline
Neoplastic disease	
Benign	Oral contraceptives, other steroids
Malignant[c]	Arsenic, thorotrast, plasticizers, benzene, toluene

[a] Amoxicillin plus clavulanic acid.

[b] May cause chronic hepatitis.

[c] Unusual, non-UK or discontinued drug. All these malignancies are due to environmental or industrial chemicals.

MAOI, monoamine oxidase inhibitor.

Table 3.33   Some risk factors for hepatic drug injury and side-effects in liver disease

Risk factor	Mechanism involved
Liver disease (e.g. cirrhosis)	Reduced blood flow gives reduced oxidative metabolism
	Fluid retention causing changed volume of distribution
	Increased cerebral sensitivity
Age and sex	Hepatotoxicity rare in children (except with sodium valproate)
	Females more susceptible
Genetics	Impaired or absent enzyme activity, e.g. slow acetylators, glucose-6-phosphate dehydrogenase deficiency

References and further reading

Aspinall R, Robinson S T (1997). *Gastroenterology: A Color Atlas and Text*. London: Mosby.

Delaney B C. Who benefits from *Helicobacter pylori* eradication? *BMJ* 2006; **332**: 187–188.

Dent J, Brun J, Fendrick A M, *et al.* (1999). An evidence-based appraisal of reflux disease management – the Genval Workshop Report. *Gut* **44** (Suppl. 2): S1–S16.

Farrell G C (1997). Drug induced hepatic injury. *J Gastroenterol Hepatol* **12**: S242–S250.

Farthing M J G, Ballinger A, eds (2000). *Drug Therapy for Gastrointestinal Disease*. London: Martin Dunitz.

Fitzgerald R, Parkes M, eds. (2007). Gastroenterology: Medicine 35 (Parts 3–6).

Fox C, Lombard M (2004). *Gastroenterology*, 2nd edn. Edinburgh: Mosby (Elsevier).

Irvine E J, Hart R H, eds (2001). *Evidence-Based Gastroenterology*. Hamilton, Ontario: B C Decker.

Marks D J B, Harbord M W N, MacAllister R, *et al.* (2006). Defective acute inflammation in Crohn's disease: a clinical investigation. *Lancet* **367**: 668–670.

Morgan D J, McLean A J (1995). Clinical pharmacokinetic and pharmacodynamic considerations in patients with liver disease: an update. *Clin Pharmacokinet* **29**: 370–391.

Moayyedi P, Talley N J (2006). Gastro-eosophageal reflux disease. *Lancet* **367**: 2086–2100.

National Prescribing Centre (2006). The initial management of dyspepsia in primary care. *MeReC Bulletin* **16**(3): 9–12.

National Institute for Clinical Excellence (2004). Hepatitis C – pegylated interferons, ribavirin and alfa interferon. Technical Appraisal 75. http://www.nice.org.uk/TA075 (accessed 21 August 2007).

Sherlock S, Dooley J (1997). *Disease of the Liver and Biliary System*, 10th edn. Oxford: Blackwell Science.

Sleisenger M A, Fordtran J S (1997). *Gastrointestinal and Liver Disease: Pathology, Diagnosis and Management*. Philadelphia, PA: W B Saunders.

Travis S P L, Taylor R H, Misiewicz J J (1998). *Gastroenterology: Pocket Consultant Series*. Oxford: Blackwell Science.

Zuckerman A J, Thomas H C, eds (1998). *Viral Hepatitis. Scientific Basis and Clinical Management*, 2nd edn. Edinburgh: Churchill Livingstone.

4

Cardiovascular system

In the West, cardiovascular disease is the most common cause of premature death in men, and a frequent cause of disability. Factors such as smoking and diet are strongly implicated, so much of this illness is preventable. If health professionals understand the mechanisms of the various disease processes it is easier for them to help patients avoid or cope with these illnesses.

Cardiovascular disease (CVD) and its treatment frequently causes considerable confusion because there are a number of closely related conditions and a wide range of drugs, many of which can be used in more than one condition. It is the aim of this chapter to explain how an understanding of the principles of haemodynamics in particular can clarify not only the relationship between various cardiovascular diseases but also common threads running through their pharmacotherapy.

The first section discusses some important general principles of the normal function of the cardiovascular system. We will first consider the cardiovascular system simply as a closed system of pump, tubes and fluid designed to perfuse the tissues. We then discuss energy handling in cardiac muscle, its oxygen demand and its oxygen supply. The physiology of the vascular endothelium and the neurohormonal control of cardiovascular function must also be considered. This approach allows predictions to be made about how the cardiovascular system responds to normal and abnormal circumstances, and how drugs can affect its function.

Physiological principles of the cardiovascular system

This section assumes a basic understanding of the physiology of the CVS. Appropriate background material for revision of the anatomy, physiology and pharmacology of the CVS is suggested in the References and further reading section.

Haemodynamics

Haemodynamics is the term used to describe the interactions of the physiological parameters that govern the behaviour of the CVS.

Blood flow and blood pressure

The purpose of the CVS is to provide an adequate perfusion of blood to all body tissues in response to a wide variety of sometimes swiftly changing demands. The ability of the heart to act as a pump to maintain this perfusion may be called the **pump performance**, usually expressed as **cardiac output**.

Fluid flow through a rigid tube depends on the pressure gradient and inversely on the resistance to flow:

$$\text{Flow} \propto \frac{\text{Pressure gradient}}{\text{Resistance}} \quad (4.1)$$

Because blood vessels are not strictly rigid this relationship does not precisely describe blood flow, but it is a useful approximation. The pressure gradient is generated by the heart during contraction, i.e. when doing work and using energy. It is equivalent to the blood pressure, or more precisely the **mean arterial pressure**, which is approximately equal to diastolic pressure plus one-third of the systolic–diastolic pressure difference. Note that pressure is merely a means to an end: the goal is output.

Blood pressure is required to overcome the **peripheral resistance**, which depends predominantly on the radius of the blood vessels (r) and the viscosity of the blood (Poiseuille's law):

$$\text{Resistance} \propto \frac{\text{Viscosity}}{r^4} \quad (4.2)$$

Blood viscosity is approximately constant, although it may be altered pathologically, e.g. by increased RBC mass or acute dehydration. Thus variations in resistance usually reflect changes in the calibre of blood vessels. Not all vessels contribute equally. The arterioles are the main resistance vessels; together with the arteries they represent about 70% of the peripheral resistance.

Thus changes in systemic blood pressure, or perfusion of any particular region of the body, are readily achieved by altering the calibre of the resistance vessels, especially because the resistance depends on the fourth power of the vessel radius. From Equations 4.1 and 4.2:

$$\text{Flow} \propto \text{pressure} \times r^4 \quad (4.3)$$

Thus very small changes in vessel diameter will produce large changes in flow if pressure is unaltered. For example, a small sustained constriction of all the body's resistance vessels will mean that a considerable increase in blood pressure is required if the same flow is to be maintained. This may be relevant to the aetiology of hypertension. Conversely, vasodilatation will permit increased flow.

Regional control of resistance and flow: autoregulation

The CVS exploits the flow/resistance relationship to increase the perfusion of specific areas temporarily at no extra cost in cardiac work. Blood is diverted from areas of lesser need, such as the skin, to those of greater need, such as muscle, by constricting vessels in the former and dilating those in the latter. Because the overall peripheral resistance does not change, cardiac output and blood pressure also remain unchanged and there is no requirement for extra cardiac work.

How are these adjustments made? When activity in a tissue or organ increases, more oxygen is required. Initially blood flow does not increase, so oxygen demand outstrips supply and the tissue becomes hypoxic; consequently metabolic by-products, including acids and carbon dioxide, accumulate extracellularly. These have a direct dilating effect on local resistance vessels, facilitating increased perfusion. Conversely, when a tissue is receiving too much blood for its needs, the reverse mechanism mediates local vasoconstriction.

Here is an elegant example of the economy of the body, a sensitive self-regulating system that continuously monitors blood flow through all tissues and redistributes it according to need. Note that, initially at least, no interventions from the nervous or hormonal systems are required.

The lung is an important exception to this general rule of hypoxic vasodilatation. Lung arterioles constrict when hypoxic, and it is not difficult to see why. Hypoxia (low tissue oxygen) in an area of lung implies inefficiency in gas transport, possibly as a result of local disease. Blood perfusing that area will be inadequately oxygenated and thus it will dilute the total pulmonary oxygen output. Consequently, blood is directed away from damaged areas of lung by local vasoconstriction. However, this mechanism becomes counterproductive (i.e. maladaptive) when large areas of lung are involved (see Chapter 5).

Other local influences on blood vessel calibre include injury (causing constriction to limit blood loss) and numerous local hormones and mediators, including **prostaglandins** (prostacyclin is a vasodilator), **thromboxanes** (predominantly constrictor), **endothelins** and **angiotensin** (constrictor) and **nitric oxide** (NO; vasodilator). Most are released from vascular endothelial cells and some may also have a crucial influence on blood vessel growth and proliferation, which has a bearing on vascular obstructive disease (see p. 235).

Distribution of blood volume

The amount of blood contained in different components of the circulation is in inverse proportion to their resistance. Low-resistance veins and venules contain up to 75% of blood volume and are referred to as **capacitance vessels**. They have little effect on peripheral resistance but have two other important roles in circulatory regulation. Firstly, they exert a crucial influence on cardiac output (discussed below). Secondly, being both compliant and muscular, veins can dilate or constrict to accommodate sudden changes in blood volume (e.g. IV infusions, fluid depletion), buffering potentially destabilizing effects on venous return and cardiac output (p. 189).

Conversely, **resistance vessels** (arteries and arterioles) contain only a small proportion of the blood; thus changes in their calibre alter the blood volume only slightly. Their primary function is the maintenance of the blood pressure via control of the peripheral resistance.

Cardiac output and blood pressure

Equation 4.1 can be expressed more familiarly as:

$$\text{Cardiac output} = \frac{\text{Blood pressure}}{\text{Peripheral resistance}} \quad (4.4)$$

This illustrates important relationships between the main haemodynamic parameters. For example, any rise in resistance requires an increased blood pressure, generated by the heart, if cardiac output is be maintained. If this situation is sustained, the extra work required will take its toll and eventually this may lead to heart failure. An increased peripheral resistance is commonly found in most hypertensive patients, but rather than always being the cause of the condition this could be a secondary autoregulation in response to an excessive cardiac output (p. 213). Thus in treating hypetension, although reducing peripheral resistance is the most obvious therapeutic target, strategies to reduce cardiac output are equally appropriate. Indeed one of the ways that both beta-adrenergic blockers (beta-blockers) and diuretics are thought to act is by initially reducing cardiac output.

Pump performance

It is crucial to appreciate how the heart behaves as a pump. To understand the pathogenesis of heart failure in particular, and the rationale for treating CVD generally, the factors that influence cardiac performance must be considered. Three variables determine the performance of a pump: (i) its initial priming with fluid to be pumped; (ii) its intrinsic power; and (iii) the resistance it must overcome in expelling fluid. In cardiac terms these are known as **preload**, **intrinsic contractility** and **afterload** respectively.

Cardiac cycle

A brief summary of the main stages in the cardiac cycle is given in the text accompanying Figure 4.1, and will be referred to in the subsequent discussion.

Preload

The force of contraction of a muscle is proportional to the degree to which it is stretched before contracting – this is the preload. In the heart it is equivalent to the degree of distension of a chamber at the end of diastole, the **end-diastolic volume (EDV)**. This is the basis of the well-known **Starling's law**, which is often simply stated as: 'the cardiac output equals the venous return'. It may be restated more precisely as: 'the stroke volume is proportional to the EDV', where the **stroke volume** is the volume expelled in one systolic beat. Some readers may find the mechanical analogy given in Figures 4.2 and 4.3 helpful in understanding this concept (see also References and further reading).

An important implication of Starling's law is that the heart is driven by the venous return. This is another example of economical self-regulation. Consider what happens when exertion such as running is initiated. The leg muscles need extra blood immediately, and the leg arterioles rapidly dilate as the tissue becomes hypoxic. But even as this happens there will be an increased venous return, owing to the **peripheral muscle pump**. As deep-lying peripheral veins in the leg are compressed by contracting muscles, an increased blood flow is immediately delivered to the right side of the heart (one-way flow being ensured by the non-return valves in veins). Thus immediately vigorous activity starts, the preload is

increased, raising the cardiac output by the Starling mechanism.

This does not require the intervention of any hormonal or neural mechanisms, the increased venous return and cardiac output being directly proportional to the increased activity. It also explains the benefit of raising the legs of someone who has fainted (it certainly does not 'increase the blood supply to the head' directly).

Filling pressure

The preload on a cardiac chamber can also be expressed as the pressure within it at the end of diastole, the **end-diastolic pressure (EDP)**, which is approximately the **filling pressure** of the blood flowing into that chamber. A sustained rise in either of these factors implies that a normal heart is being overloaded or that an ineffective heart requires an elevated preload to maintain normal output. The right atrial pressure (RAP) and the left ventricular EDP (LVEDP), measured by cardiac catheterization via peripheral arteries, give important information about the degrees of right- and left-sided heart function respectively. The RAP also indicates whether the systemic circulatory volume is appropriate, and so can be used to monitor IV infusions and prevent the heart, and the circulation generally, becoming overloaded.

The right heart preload may be determined more conveniently and less invasively by measuring the pressure in the great veins as they enter the right atrium. The **central venous pressure (CVP)** is measured by passing an IV catheter percutaneously in the neck region so that its tip rests in the superior vena cava.

Filling is not a passive process; it is energy-dependent. This energy is derived partly from relaxation of the compressive deformation of the previous systolic contraction, elastic recoil aiding the restoration of diastolic shape. An important determinant of filling is ventricular **compliance** (distensibility, the inverse of stiffness). If it is reduced, a higher preload will be needed, possibly leading to **diastolic failure** (p. 189).

Ejection fraction

The ratio of the stroke volume to the EDV represents the effectiveness of cardiac emptying

(a)

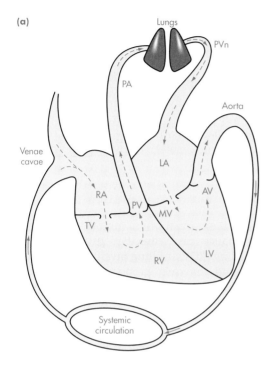

CIRCULATION (starting with return of blood to the heart from the peripheral circulation)

- Deoxygenated blood returns to the right side of the heart from venae cavae during **diastole (relaxation)**
- It enters the right atrium at a pressure of 0–10 mmHg
- Right atrial contraction increases pressure until the tricuspid valve opens
- Blood flows through the tricuspid valve into the right ventricle during diastole, partially assisted by atrial contraction (the 'atrial kick')
- As right atrial pressure rises, the tricuspid valve closes and the pulmonary valve opens
- Right ventricular **systole (contraction)** sends blood via pulmonary arteries to the lungs at a pressure of about 30 mmHg
- Blood is oxygenated in the lungs and returns to the left atrium via the pulmonary veins
- Left atrial systole increases pressure until the mitral valve opens
- Blood flows through the mitral valve into the left ventricle during diastole
- Left ventricular contraction during systole
- As pressure rises, the mitral valve closes ('lub') and the aortic valve opens
- Left ventricular contraction during systole sends blood via the aorta to the body at a maximum pressure of about 120 mmHg
- Ventricular pressure falls and the aortic valve closes ('dup')
- Blood perfuses the periphery and oxygenates tissues
- Mean pressure falls to 30 mmHg at the arterial end of capillaries and 15 mmHg at the venous end
- Deoxygenated blood returns to the heart via the veins; flow is facilitated by the peripheral muscle pump, and back flow is prevented by one-way venous valves

(b)

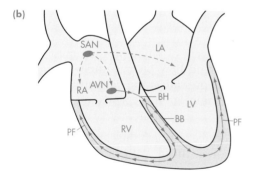

CARDIAC CYCLE (starting at end of diastole)

- Impulses originate in the sino-atrial node, which controls rhythm and causes atrial systole
- Impulses spread across the atrium to the atrioventricular node
- Impulses traverse the bundle of His and bundle branches in the septum (between Left and Right heart)
- Ventricular systole starts from the apex of the ventricles
- Intraventricular pressure rises, initially without change of size because the aortic and pulmonary valves are closed (isovolumic phase)
- Impulse spreads towards the base of the ventricles (valves) via Purkinje fibres
- Mitral and tricuspid valves close as pressure rises
- Aortic and pulmonary valves open as pressure exceeds systemic or pulmonary
- Blood propelled towards the aortic and pulmonary valves by contractile wave spreading from the apex and twisting deformation of the ventricles due to asymmetric myocardial muscle sheets (ejection phase)
- Blood flows to the lungs from the right ventricle, and to the rest of body from the left ventricle
- Pressure in the ventricles falls and the aortic and pulmonary valves close
- Blood flows from the aorta into the coronary arteries as the ventricles relax; ventricular diastole

Figure 4.1   Important components of the heart. (a) The main internal structural components of the heart. This diagram (not anatomically precise or to scale) also shows the blood flow through the different chambers, emphasizing the origins and destinations of blood on each side. (b) The main centres of electrical excitation and pathways of electrical conduction in the heart. NB All given pressures are approximate and typical of a healthy young adult. AV, aortic valve; AVN, atrioventricular node; BB, bundle branches (right and left); BH, bundle of His; LA/RA, left/right atrium; LV/RV, left/right ventricle; MV, mitral valve; PA, pulmonary artery; PF, Purkinje fibres; PV, pulmonary valve; PVn, pulmonary vein; SAN, sinoatrial node; TV, tricuspid valve.

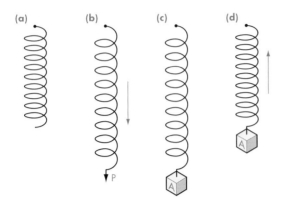

Figure 4.2   Spring model of the loading on a pump. (a) Spring in resting position. (b) Spring stretched (primed) by preload P. The degree of stretch, and therefore the energy stored for subsequent recoil, is proportional to the magnitude of preload. (c) Afterload A applied to spring. (d) Spring recoils (contracts). Resistance to recoil depends on magnitude of afterload, and force of recoil depends on physical properties of spring ('contractility').

during systole. It is thus a good index of cardiac efficiency and is used as a quantitative measure of the degree of heart failure:

$$\text{Ejection fraction} = \frac{\text{Stroke volume}}{\text{End-diastolic volume}} \quad (4.5)$$

The average ejection fraction in health, measured by echocardiography, is 60–70%.

Intrinsic contractility

The biochemical and metabolic condition of heart muscle will influence its performance regardless of preloading. Variable contractility is a property not found in other smooth muscle or in skeletal muscle. It is affected by the autonomic nervous system, systemic hormones (e.g. adrenaline [epinephrine]), and disease (e.g. ischaemia due to obstructed coronary vessels), so that the same preload may produce a greater or lesser performance. Contractility also increases with increased heart rate (the force-frequency effect). These represent further adaptive mechanisms available to the CVS.

Afterload

This is the resistance that the heart meets in contracting and doing work to drive blood through the arteries. A raised peripheral resistance will at first reduce cardiac output, although normally a reflex increase in contractility will promptly restore it, at the expense of extra cardiac work. For most purposes the afterload is approximately equivalent to the blood pressure.

Summary

Within the normal physiological range, cardiac performance is directly proportional to preloading (EDV or filling pressure) and contractility, and inversely proportional to afterload (vascular resistance). These relationships are illustrated and explained further in Figure 4.4.

Factors affecting pump performance

Preload

This, the most complex of all determinants of cardiac performance, is usually taken as equivalent to the venous return. However, the more precise concept of filling pressure must be used to understand how preload varies (Figure 4.5). The filling pressure at the right atrium is usually about 10 mmHg. It depends on three main factors:

1. The degree to which the circulatory system as a whole is 'filled' with blood, i.e. the blood volume.
2. The pressure exerted by the veins to accommodate this, i.e. the venous tone.
3. The contribution of muscular activity to venous return, i.e. the peripheral muscle pump (p. 168).

Blood volume

Fluid and electrolyte clearance by the kidney is varied to defend blood pressure. In particular, fluid is retained if renal perfusion is threatened. This is achieved through a variety of endocrine mechanisms including the renin-angiotensin-aldosterone system (RAAS),

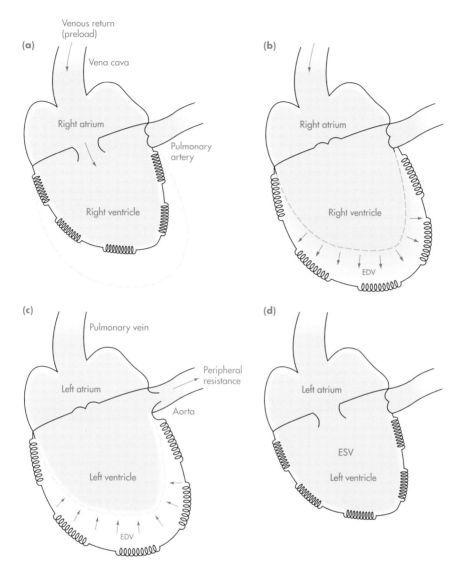

Figure 4.3   Stages in the cardiac cycle to illustrate loading, using the analogy of the spring. The effects of preload and afterload may be grasped more easily if it is imagined that there are springs in the ventricular wall that behave in a similar way to those in the previous figure. The **right** side is shown during diastole (a, b) to illustrate preload and the **left** side during systole to illustrate afterload (c, d). This is because changes in preload (systemic filling pressure) usually affect the right side, while the left side is usually affected by changes in afterload (systemic vascular resistance). However, similar considerations apply to both sides and they fill and empty simultaneously. (Volumes given below apply to average resting cardiac cycle, i.e. no exertion.) (a) Right side of heart at the end of systole (ESV, end-systolic volume; about 50 mL). Myocardial fibres are contracted ('springs' recoiled). Venous return starts to fill right atrium and then right ventricle, producing preload. (b) Right side at the end of diastole (EDV, end-diastolic volume; about 120 mL). Myocardial fibres are stretched, to a degree proportional to preloading (equivalent to volume of venous return). The potential force of subsequent contraction is proportional to the degree of myocardial stretch (equivalent to EDV). (c) Left side of heart at end of diastole. Myocardial fibres now start to contract. The afterload is equivalent to the resistance of the systemic arterioles (peripheral resistance) against which the left ventricle must eject the stroke volume (approx. 70 mL). The stroke volume will also be determined by the condition of the myocardium (contractility, perfusion, etc.). (d) Left side at end of systole; position is similar to (a). RV starting to fill. Stroke volume (SV) = EDV − ESV. Ejection fraction = SV/EDV (usually approx. 60%).

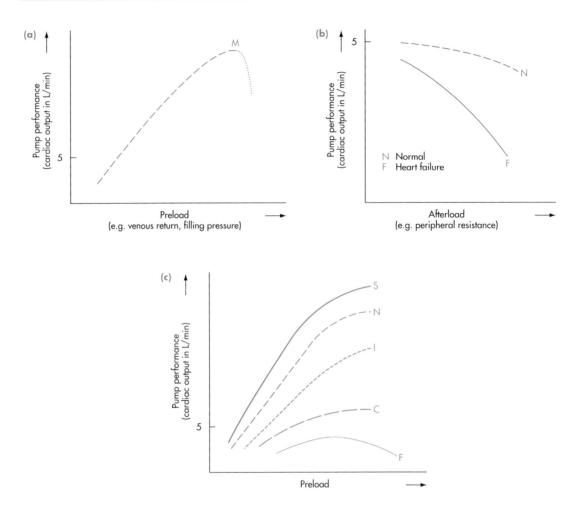

Figure 4.4 Variation of pump performance with preload, afterload and contractility. (a) **Preload**. Assuming afterload and contractility remain constant, the preload/output curve is normally steep up to a maximum M (which depends on fitness). M is seldom reached and above it performance declines steeply with increasing preload. Note that the average resting cardiac output is 5 L/min. These 'contractility curves' or Frank–Starling curves clearly show how cardiac output is driven by venous return. They are useful to illustrate variations in cardiac performance resulting from changes in other parameters. (b) **Afterload**. If contractility and preload remain constant, increases in afterload (usually peripheral resistance) reduce performance almost linearly, as shown in curve F. However, a curve such as this would only be found in heart failure. Normally, preload and contractility do not remain constant but increase reflexly to defend cardiac output (curve N), producing an almost flat relationship over a wide range. Comparison of curves F and N shows why arterial vasodilators, which reduce afterload, have little effect on output in health but can considerably improve it in failure. (c) **Contractility**. This family of contractility curves shows how different intrinsic contractilities affect the response of the heart to preload (assuming afterload is constant). Curve N is as in (a). Curve S, showing positive inotropic stimulation (e.g. sympathetic nervous system) is steeper and goes higher. Curve I shows the inhibitory effect of negative inotropic influences (e.g. parasympathetic nervous system). Curves S, N and I represent normal physiological variation. In compensated heart failure (C) the curve may barely rise above the minimum resting output. In decompensated failure (F), output actually falls with increases in preload beyond a certain point. This explains why preload reduction in heart failure can actually improve output (see p. 199).

vasopressin/antidiuretic hormone, PGs and kinins. Urine output also varies with renal perfusion. The renal control of body fluid volume is discussed in detail in Chapter 14.

The most recently identified mediators are the **natriuretic peptide (NP)** hormones, released from a variety of tissues. The most important are **atrial natriuretic peptide (ANP)** (from the atria) and **brain natriuretic peptide (BNP)** (from brain and cardiac ventricles) and they are proving useful as markers for heart failure because they are released when the circulation is failing. They have both vasodilator and natriuretic actions, and serve as counter-regulatory influences to limit excessive cardiac dilatation, peripheral vasoconstriction and renal fluid retention, and as protection against fluid overloading.

Venous tone

The balance between the volume of fluid within blood vessels and its pressure is controlled by the tone of the vessels. If fluid volume is increased, e.g. by renal fluid retention, the pressure will tend to rise. The veins, being more compliant than arteries, will then dilate to accommodate the extra volume and hence buffer what may otherwise generate a dangerous rise in filling pressure and cardiac drive. Without this compliance the heart could rapidly be overloaded and fail. Conversely, sudden falls in blood volume, e.g. as a result of severe haemorrhage, can be partially compensated by venoconstriction.

However, venous compliance is limited and large rises in blood volume do increase filling pressure at first, although further compensatory mechanisms eventually come into play, e.g. increased renal fluid clearance.

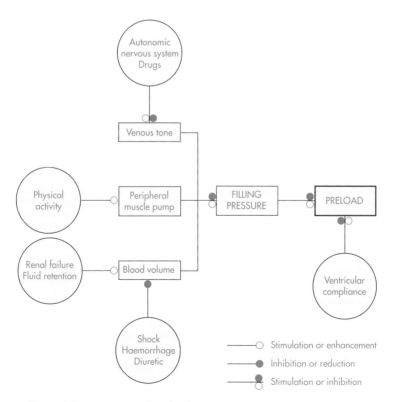

Figure 4.5 Factors affecting filling pressure and preload.

Venous tone, like arterial tone, is under autonomic control. Adrenergic drugs or stimulation of the sympathetic nervous system cause venoconstriction, which is consistent with the stress response ('fight or flight'): it increases the venous return and filling pressure and so cardiac output. Conversely, extensive venodilatation is implicated in the pathogenesis of circulatory shock because it causes a profound reduction in cardiac output and blood pressure.

Ventricular compliance

Resistance to filling is determined by the ease with which the shape and size of the ventricle are restored during diastole. The hypertrophy of ventricular muscle that accompanies hypertension, some forms of cardiomyopathy (diseased heart muscle) and the diffuse fibrosis of chronic ischaemic heart disease can produce a stiff myocardium that significantly reduces ventricular compliance, preventing adequate filling (p. 188).

Afterload

The afterload is determined mainly by arteriolar tone, which is affected by both normal physiological mechanisms and disease (Table 4.1). In health, the overall tone is kept within narrow limits because there is rarely any physiological advantage in raising afterload. In hypertension, afterload is persistently raised, so the heart must work harder to maintain normal output; the ultimate result may be left ventricular failure (LVF).

In health, blood viscosity is also constant. Persistent hypoxaemia (reduced blood oxygen level, e.g. in COPD), causes a reflex rise in RBC count (polycythaemia). The resulting increase in blood viscosity increases the afterload, which can contribute to right ventricular failure (RVF; see Chapter 5).

Contractility

Agents or circumstances that increase or decrease contractility are termed positively or negatively inotropic, respectively (Table 4.2). Small changes in perfusion demands are normally accommodated by changes in preloading and the Starling effect rather than in contractility. However, if necessary, positive inotropic effects can be activated rapidly by the sympathetic nervous system, and more slowly under hormonal influences, e.g. thyroxine.

Table 4.1   Factors affecting afterload

	Increase afterload	Reduce afterload
Peripheral resistance		
Physiological		
Autonomic nervous system via vasomotor centre	Sympathetic tone ↑	Sympathetic tone ↓
Renal system	Renin/angiotensin system	? Kinins
	Vasopressin	
Atrial endocrine function		Atrial natriuretic peptide
Local factors?	Endothelin	Nitric oxide
Drugs	Alpha-adrenergic stimulants e.g. noradrenaline (norepinephrine)	Alpha-adrenergic blocker (e.g. prazosin) Arterial dilators (e.g. hydralazine)
Pathological	Hypertension Arteriosclerosis	Shock
Blood viscosity		
Pathological	Polycythaemia	

The myocardial adrenergic receptors are mainly beta$_1$. However, the existence of a small but significant population of beta$_2$-receptors means that beta$_2$ selectivity among agonists such as the bronchodilators can never entirely free them from cardiac effects. This contrasts with highly selective beta$_1$-adrenergic blocking drugs, which will spare the lung and other beta$_2$-populated sites. The parasympathetic nervous system has negatively inotropic effects via muscarinic receptors, restricted mainly to the atria.

Among drugs, two main groups affect contractility: the beta-adrenergic agents (stimulants and blockers) act via their normal autonomic receptors, while the cardiac glycosides and other agents, e.g. the phosphodiesterase inhibitors, affect myocardial cells directly.

Myocardial pathology

Numerous conditions cause deterioration in myocardial contractility, hypoxia (low tissue oxygen level) being one of the most important. It usually results from impaired coronary perfusion, i.e. ischaemic heart disease. However, reduced blood oxygenation (hypoxaemia) will have a similar effect, e.g. severe chronic anaemia (Chapter 11) or COPD (Chapter 5).

Subtle problems can result from excessive myocardial hypertrophy. A modest increase in myocardial mass is usually a beneficial adaptive response to chronically increased cardiac loading, as in any well-exercised muscle. However, if the myocardium grows too quickly it may outpace the formation of new coronary vessels, causing relative ischaemia. In addition, a thick myocardium is less compliant (impairing filling), and the extra cardiac work required to contract it during systole will also reduce efficiency.

Overloading, e.g. excessive afterload in chronic hypertension, or excessive preload in fluid retention, can damage the myocardium by forcing it to operate beyond its ability to compensate, causing heart failure. This and the various other pathological processes that directly affect the myocardium are discussed in more detail on pp. 188–193.

Table 4.2   Factors affecting intrinsic myocardial contractility

	Contractility increased	Contractility reduced
Physiological		
Cardiovascular centre and autonomic nervous system	Sympathetic tone ↑ (atria and ventricles)	Parasympathetic tone ↑ (mainly atria)
	Heart rate ↑ (adrenaline (epinephrine))	Heart rate ↓ (acetylcholine)
Endocrine	Levothyroxine (thyroxine), adrenal hormones	
Compensation	Myocardial hypertrophy	
Drugs	Digoxin	
	Beta$_1$-adrenergic stimulants, e.g. dopamine, noradrenaline (norepinephrine)	Beta$_1$-adrenergic blockers, e.g. atenolol
Pathological		Hypoxia
		Excessive hypertrophy
		Excessive loading, etc.

Heart rate

This represents yet another compensatory option for the CVS because cardiac output can quickly be changed without necessarily changing stroke volume or intrinsic contractility:

$$\frac{\text{Cardiac}}{\text{output}} = \text{Stroke volume} \times \text{heart rate}$$

(4.6)

Heart rate is under broadly similar physiological influences to contractility. However, while the sympathetic nervous system exerts an excitatory influence on contractility, the predominant physiological control on resting rate is inhibitory parasympathetic tone via the vagus nerve, slowing the heart (i.e. negatively **chronotropic**). When the heart rate is increased the diastolic interval is reduced but the systolic time is mostly unchanged. Generally speaking, the CVS will use changes in rate only to produce rapid temporary changes in output. Medium-term output changes require altered contractility, and chronic changes involve renal compensation and possibly myocardial hypertrophy.

Summary

The relationships between the factors discussed above are summarized in Figure 4.6. This emphasizes the multifactorial nature of CVS adjustments, involving coordination of haemodynamic, neural and endocrine feedback loops and control paths.

Coronary circulation

Because the heart pumps continuously and has little reserve energy substrate (e.g. glucose), its blood supply is critical. Moreover, it has the highest oxygen extraction of any organ in the body (i.e. its coronary arteriovenous oxygen difference is greatest). This means that increases in oxygen demand need to be met mainly by increases in perfusion. Many common cardiac diseases result from impaired coronary perfusion.

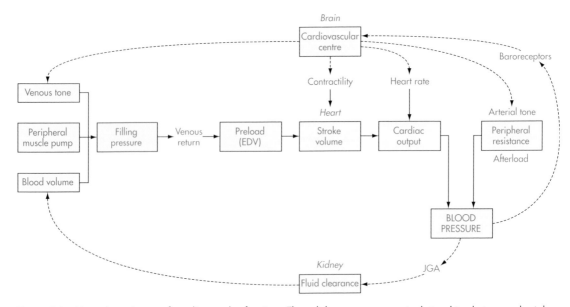

Figure 4.6 Main determinants of cardiovascular function. The solid arrows represent relationships between physiological variables. The broken arrows show hormonal or neuronal feedback loops and control paths. EDV, end-diastolic volume; JGA, juxtaglomerular apparatus.

Coronary perfusion

Flow into the coronary arteries is driven by the elastic recoil of the aorta immediately following systole, as the myocardium relaxes (Figure 4.7). Perhaps surprisingly, ventricular muscle is effectively perfused only during diastole, because myocardial contraction during systole compresses the coronary vessels, especially in the inner layer (endocardium).

The perfusion pressure driving blood into the coronary arteries is the difference between the pressure in the aorta and the pressure within the heart chamber during diastole (Equation 4.7).

$$\left\{ \begin{array}{c} \text{Coronary} \\ \text{perfusion} \\ \text{pressure} \end{array} \right\} = \left\{ \begin{array}{c} \text{Mean} \\ \text{arterial} \\ \text{pressure} \end{array} \right\} - \left\{ \begin{array}{c} \text{End-} \\ \text{diastolic} \\ \text{pressure} \end{array} \right\} \tag{4.7}$$

Thus both low blood pressure and a raised EDP, e.g. during heart failure, can compromise coronary perfusion. Note also that blood has to change direction and flow back towards the heart during diastole to enter the coronary arteries, which branch off the aorta just after the aortic valve. This tends to produce turbulence, which may be a factor in the particular sensitivity of the coronary arteries to atherosclerosis.

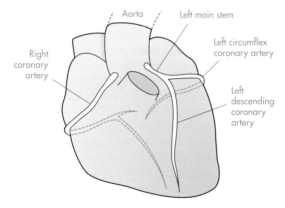

Figure 4.7 Main coronary arteries. The left main stem and right coronary arteries arise near the origin of the aorta. The left main stem coronary artery divides early; thus there are three principal coronary arteries. Atherosclerosis is commonly found in any of these arteries or their branches; disease of all three is known as 'three-vessel disease'. Myocardial infarction is commonly associated with occlusion of the left descending artery

Control and compensation

The principal physiological controls on coronary vasculature are autoregulatory, with dilatation occurring in response to increased demand as metabolic by-products accumulate in the stimulated myocardium. Autonomic control plays a minor role via alpha-adrenergic constrictor and beta$_2$-adrenergic dilator nerves. These may however play a role in coronary vasospastic diseases such as variant angina (p. 249).

The heart does not normally have a well-developed system of collateral vessels; thus it is more compromised by vascular obstruction than other tissues. Therefore atheromatous plaques that occlude coronary arteries in ischaemic heart disease (p. 236) will have a disproportionately large effect. However, regular exercise and chronic vascular obstruction both stimulate the development of coronary collaterals.

A fixed obstruction such as an atheroma (see below) not only reduces the lumen but also impairs the vessel's ability to dilate, and may abolish it completely. Furthermore, during ischaemia, autoregulated dilatation normally occurs in vessels adjacent to the obstructed one; this may actually divert blood away from the area served by the obstructed vessel if that area does not have a collateral supply. This phenomenon, known as **coronary steal**, is sometimes seen when vasodilators are used in acute angina; the pain actually increases as blood is redirected away from the ischaemic area.

Myocardial energetics

Oxygen demand

The work done by the heart is given approximately by the product cardiac output × blood pressure. Clearly, oxygen demand is related to the work done. This relationship is governed by several variables. One way of expressing it is:

$$\begin{aligned} O_2 \text{ demand} = \text{ } &\text{contractility} \\ &\times \text{myocardial wall tension} \\ &\times \text{time in tension} \end{aligned} \tag{4.8}$$

Contractility depends on the contractile state of the myocardium (p. 174), time in tension is related to heart rate, and wall tension is related to mean arterial pressure (for the left ventricle). Thus adrenaline (epinephrine), hypertension and tachycardia (increased heart rate) all increase oxygen demand if other factors remain unchanged. This is particularly important to remember when the coronary supply is compromised, because increases in such factors may precipitate acute angina.

If contractility is approximately constant, Equation 4.8 simplifies to:

$$O_2 \text{ demand} \propto \text{heart rate} \times \text{blood pressure}$$
$$(4.9)$$

This semi-quantitative approximation, known as the 'rate–pressure product', is convenient for clinical studies because the variables are easily measured. It can be used to predict the effect of various strategies or drugs on oxygen demand. In the treatment of certain conditions the aim is to reduce the rate–pressure product, e.g. in ischaemic heart disease, where oxygen supply to the myocardium is restricted.

Efficiency

This may be taken as the work the heart does in relation to its oxygen consumption. Although absolute values do not concern us here, relative changes do. A number of important consequences affecting efficiency follow from the heart being a hollow chamber.

First, 'volume work' is more efficient than 'pressure work'. That is, work done to increase cardiac output requires a smaller increase in oxygen demand than does the same amount of work done to raise blood pressure. Thus volume overloading is less harmful to the heart than sustained high blood pressure. Consequently, heart failure or angina develop far more readily from hypertension or aortic stenosis (narrowing of the aortic valve) than from fluid retention or aortic incompetence (incomplete closure of aortic valve). Conversely, strategies to reduce afterload might be expected to be more effective at reducing cardiac workload than strategies reducing preload.

A more important consequence relates to myocardial wall tension, a major determinant of oxygen demand. The ability to expel blood during systole depends on the tension generated in the ventricular wall and this is determined by the diastolic stretch imparted by preloading. However, the effect is not linear and as preload increases there are disproportionately greater increases in oxygen demand. Thus doubling the preload will require more than double the oxygen demand if output is also to be doubled.

The explanation is given by **Laplace's law**. Clearly, the walls of a hollow container need to develop (or maintain) tension in order to generate (or withstand) pressure within. Laplace's law states that this tension is proportional not only to the magnitude of the required pressure but also to the size of the container. In the cardiovascular context the 'containers' we are interested in are blood vessels and heart chambers:

$$\text{Wall tension} \propto \text{internal pressure} \times \text{radius}$$
$$(4.10)$$

This explains, among other things, why large arteries need much thicker walls than smaller ones, despite their internal pressure being similar. (Similarly, thin bicycle tyres, because of their small radius, can withstand much higher pressures than much thicker car tyres.)

Thus the larger the size from which a heart has to contract, i.e. the greater the EDV, the greater will be the wall tension required to generate the same internal pressure needed to overcome the afterload. This means an increased oxygen demand for the same output (Equation 4.8). So for a given individual, the larger the heart, the less efficient it is. 'Larger' in this context means an increase in chamber size and should be distinguished from 'hypertrophy', which is an increase in muscle mass (p. 181).

The significance of this may be gauged when we recall that cardiac enlargement by the Starling mechanism is a prime strategy for accommodating extra haemodynamic demands. Normally it causes no problem because there is sufficient cardiac reserve. However, in the failing or ischaemic heart this reduced efficiency can mean the difference between compensation (i.e. coping) and decompensation. It also explains the rationale for the use of vasodilators in heart failure, which reduce preload or afterload and therefore ventricular wall tension.

Cardiovascular reserve

The cardiovascular (cardiac) reserve is the degree to which the CVS can increase its performance to meet additional circulatory demands, or can maintain performance in the face of increased afterload or impaired contractility. Changes in cardiovascular demand are detected by a comprehensive system of receptors (Figure 4.6). Baroreceptors in the aortic arch, the carotid body, the atria and the ventricles detect changes in intravascular or intracardiac pressure and relay these to the cardiovascular/vasomotor centre in the medulla. This then mediates an appropriate response via adjustments in sympathetic and parasympathetic outflow, principally to the vasculature and myocardium, and also via antidiuretic hormone (ADH, vasopressin) secretion. Chemoreceptors in the carotid body and the aortic arch detect oxygen tension, which would fall if lung perfusion were compromised. Intracardiac baroreceptors also mediate NP secretion.

The renal juxtaglomerular apparatus is another important detector of reduced perfusion, mediating its response principally via the RAAS. In chronic situations, the kidney may increase erythropoietin secretion, expanding RBC numbers.

At rest, the average cardiac output is approximately 5 L/min. Because it depends on body size, the cardiac output is sometimes adjusted for body surface area: the resting **cardiac index** is approximately 3 L/min/m². In a fit adult, cardiac output can be increased on demand up to 20–25 L/min; there may also be a rise in blood pressure. The difference between resting and maximum cardiac output is the **cardiac reserve**. With a diseased heart, the cardiac reserve is reduced. In mild heart failure the reduction may be small and therefore only noticeable on vigorous exertion, when the patient will become unusually fatigued. As heart function deteriorates, the degree of exertion that produces the same level of fatigue becomes progressively smaller. This reduced **exercise tolerance** is a measure of diminishing cardiac reserve.

As long as the patient can maintain an adequate cardiac output at rest the heart failure is **compensated**. However, as the condition dete-riorates the patient will eventually be unable to sustain an adequate cardiac output for normal activity, or may even be breathless at rest; this is **decompensation**.

The various haemodynamic, neural and endocrine mechanisms and strategies of cardiovascular compensation are summarized in Table 4.3; many have already been discussed. They are classified according to the speed with which the CVS can mobilize them. Note that medium- and long-term compensation mechanisms resemble normal physiological responses to exercise training.

Acute compensation

The CVS can respond very rapidly to acutely increased demand. Cardiac output may be raised through the Starling mechanism following increased venous return and/or venoconstriction. The cardiovascular centre and sympathetic nervous system also contribute by acting on the myocardium and pacemaker, giving positive inotropic and chronotropic responses. Falls in blood pressure are also compensated by a sympathetic nervous system vasoconstrictor response.

ANP may be secreted by the right atrium when atrial baroreceptors detect an increase in atrial filling, as a counter-regulatory response to limit or buffer these actions. This counters excessive activity of the sympathetic nervous system.

Medium-term compensation

If the stress is more prolonged, many acute compensatory mechanisms may persist, but others also come into play. Renal compensation (see Chapter 14, p. 881) involves the RAAS and fluid retention to expand or maintain circulating fluid volume. There may also be secretion of ADH. More directly, if renal perfusion pressure is reduced there will be reduced urine output owing to reduced filtration and increased reabsorption.

Long-term compensation

Chronically increased demand induces myocardial hypertrophy, an increase in myocardial muscle mass that increases contractility (note

Table 4.3   Mechanisms of cardiovascular reserve

Mechanism	Effect
Acute	
Starling effect: preload ↑	End-diastolic volume ↑ (= heart size ↑)
Inotropic: – sympathetic nervous system ↑	Contractility ↑
– parasympathetic nervous system ↓	
Chronotropic: – parasympathetic nervous system ↓	Heart rate ↑
– sympathetic nervous system ↑	
Vasomotor: – sympathetic nervous system ↑	Arteriolar constriction → blood pressure ↑
	Venous constriction → preload ↑
Medium-term	
Persistence of acute mechanisms above	May become down-regulated
Renal compensation:	
• juxtaglomerular apparatus:	Fluid retention, vasoconstriction
renin/angiotensin/aldosterone ↑	
• pressure natriuresis ↓	Fluid retention
Endocrine:	
• adrenaline (epinephrine) ↑	Positively inotropic, chronotropic
• ADH (vasopressin) ↑	Fluid retention, vasoconstriction
• natriuretic peptide ↑	Diuresis, vasodilation
Long-term	
Cardiac hypertrophy	Contractility ↑
Polycythaemia	↑ O_2 to tissues
Renal compensation	As in 'medium-term'

that this differs from 'cardiac enlargement', which means an increased EDV). If there is persistent hypoxaemia as a result of poor pulmonary perfusion, an increased red cell count will eventually be induced, possibly resulting in polycythaemia. The kidneys continue to retain fluid.

Constraints on cardiac reserve

There are limits to most of these mechanisms; the CVS cannot accommodate increasing demands indefinitely (Table 4.4). Eventually these primarily beneficial haemodynamic and neuroendocrine mechanisms come to be deployed in circumstances beyond their design limits: they then become maladaptive (counterproductive). This accounts for many of the features of heart failure.

Renal/Starling

The kidneys will attempt to support a failing circulation by retaining fluid, increasing the filling pressure and thus cardiac output. However, because of the Laplace limitation (p. 178), a failing myocardium cannot benefit indefinitely from this. As the heart becomes progressively more stretched, not only does it become less oxygen efficient but the cells also become fatigued and unable to respond. There is a limit to the degree of stretch (cardiac enlargement) that the muscle fibres can tolerate, dependent at the ultracellular level on the degree of interdigitation of the actin and myosin filaments. Beyond this, fluid retention becomes maladaptive. There is also the more obvious anatomical constraint of the pericardial sac around the heart.

Table 4.4   Limitations on cardiovascular compensation (cardiac reserve)

Compensation	Limitation
Starling	Overstretch → myocardial cell damage
	Laplace-related inefficiency
Sympathetic nervous system	Overactivity → depletion of cardiac transmitter stores
	and down-regulation of cardiac beta-receptors
Vasomotor	Accommodation of baroreceptors
Heart rate	Arrhythmias: impaired filling
Endocrine	NP response blunted
Renal fluid retention	Becomes maladaptive when heart cannot respond to
	dilatation by increasing contractility
Hypertrophy	Chamber size ↓
	Coronary perfusion ↓
	Myocardial compliance ↓

NP, natriuretic peptide; although level raised, effectiveness appears to be diminished.

Sympathetic nervous system

Adrenergic receptors on myocardial or vascular smooth muscle eventually become desensitized (accommodated) to prolonged and unrelieved stimulation, and therefore less responsive, possibly through down-regulation or post-receptor un-coupling. This may induce reflex sympathetic over-activity that, among other things, produces an unsustainable increase in myocardial oxygen demand and promotes arrhythmia.

At this stage, which is found in early chronic (compensated) heart failure, a further protective mechanism is activated. Atrial and arterial baroreceptors (stretch receptors) signal the CVS centre to limit sympathetic activity and promote increased vagal activity. This reduces myocardial wall stress by reducing excessive cardiac stimulation and peripheral vasoconstriction; arrhythmias are also inhibited. Thus as cardiac function declines the heart is protected against excessive demands. As we will see below, this mechanism later becomes blunted; baroreceptor failure signals the onset of decompensation and over-whelming maladaptive stimulation of heart and arteries.

Renal/endocrine

Renin secretion may also become excessive, partly mediated by the sympathetic nervous system, and angiotensin then contributes to

the decompensation. Failure in the counter-regulatory NP and nitric oxide mechanisms exacerbates the situation. This will allow excessive fluid retention and vasoconstriction by no longer attenuating the actions of aldosterone and angiotensin.

If the heart rate increase is excessive, coordination becomes disrupted and arrhythmias develop that compromise the efficiency of ventricular ejection. The practical maximum heart rate in a young fit person is about three times the resting rate, but is reduced to double the resting rate at age 80 years. Even before this stage efficiency may be reduced because of inadequate time for complete emptying or refilling within each cardiac cycle.

Finally, myocardial hypertrophy is not without disadvantages (Figure 4.8):

- The heart becomes stiffer, i.e. less compliant, and so more work and more oxygen are required for each contraction.
- The muscle growth will be partly inwards, reducing the chamber size.
- The thicker walls will produce unequal stresses at different levels within the thickness during contraction, so more energy will be expended in deforming them.
- Muscle development may outstrip new coronary vessel growth (angiogenesis).

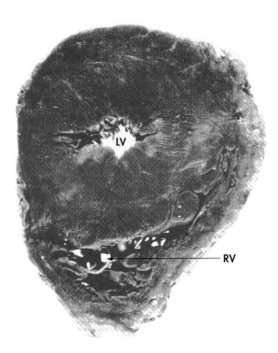

Figure 4.8 Myocardial hypertrophy. Transverse section of a hypertrophied heart showing gross thickening of the left ventricular wall. Note how the chamber size is reduced. This leads to increased stiffness and restriction of coronary perfusion. LV, left ventricle; RV, right ventricle. (Reproduced with permission from JR Anderson (ed.). *Muir's Textbook of Pathology*, 10th edn; published by Edward Arnold, 1976. © JR Anderson 1976.)

It must be remembered that the main function of the Starling mechanism is to maintain stroke volume under conditions of increased loading. Even under maximal exercise stimulation stroke volume rarely increases by more than about 25%. The increase in cardiac output during exercise is principally due to increased heart rate. The main cardiovascular effect of training is to increase resting stroke volume and EDV and reduce resting heart rate. This increases cardiac reserve by allowing greater latitude for increased heart rate and ejection fraction.

Thus although the CVS is beautifully designed to compensate most economically for wide variations in physiological demands, there are certain stresses with which it cannot cope and these can lead to CVD, particularly heart failure.

Clinical features of cardiovascular disease

Symptoms

Because the CVS supplies all organs, symptoms may arise in any one of these, and the cause may not be obviously cardiovascular, especially to a patient. Further, because most CVD is chronic, symptoms may at first be noticeable only on exertion. As the disease progresses, the point at which symptoms develop comes earlier. The severity of many acute cardiovascular symptoms can be graded empirically by applying the widely used functional scale of the New York Heart Association (NYHA):

- Grade I. Asymptomatic. No symptoms at ordinary physical activity.
- Grade II. Mild. Symptoms evident on strenuous exertion.
- Grade III. Moderate. Symptoms evident on moderate exertion.
- Grade IV. Severe. Symptoms at rest.

Fatigue

Impaired perfusion to body skeletal muscle due to reduced myocardial function (heart failure) will cause patients to tire easily. Reduced exercise tolerance can be estimated empirically by asking how far a patient can walk, climb stairs, etc. or quantified by formal exercise testing on a treadmill or exercise bicycle (with ECG monitoring). Of course, fatigue can have many other causes, both physical and mental. Common iatrogenic causes include beta-blocker therapy and, in the elderly especially, diuretic-induced sodium and potassium imbalance.

Dizziness; fainting (syncope)

Temporarily interrupted CNS perfusion (transient ischaemic attacks, TIAs) commonly result from, among other causes, sudden temporary ventricular arrhythmias or postural hypotension. It is usually reversible within a few minutes (contrast this with epilepsy, stroke, etc.). Possible iatrogenic causes of syncope are CNS depressants, vasodilator therapy or diuretic-induced hypovolaemia. Simple faints in otherwise healthy individuals are not uncommon and usually are due to increased parasympathetic activity causing transient hypotension (vaso-vagal attack).

Dyspnoea

Shortness of breath or difficulty in breathing is a subjective feeling that may or may not be associated with objectively reduced blood oxygenation. Possible causes are mainly cardio-vascular (i.e. pulmonary oedema from LVF), primary pulmonary disease (Chapter 5) and anaemia. Postural variation is common in cardiovascular dyspnoea: it is worse when supine, so that the patient breathes more easily when erect or sitting (**orthopnoea**). This is because intrathoracic pressure is increased when the patient is recumbent, raising pulmonary venous pressure and thus promoting the forma-tion of alveolar oedema (see below).

Palpitations

An abnormal awareness of the heartbeat is usually caused by an arrhythmia, particularly an extrasystole. Patients may also notice severe tachycardia or bradycardia.

Pain

Pain arising in the chest region can have many origins, including the upper GIT, the lungs and the chest wall, as well as acute anxiety. The typical cardiac ischaemic pain associated with coronary artery disease is characteristically described as 'crushing' or 'choking', but seldom as 'sharp' or 'momentary'. Patients may illustrate it by making a fist against their sternum or describing it as "like someone bear-hugging you from behind". The pain may radiate up to the jaw or down the left arm. The most important differential diagnosis for a pharmacist is dyspeptic pain from the oesophagus, or from the stomach or duodenum, which may be described as sharp ("like a knife") and patients illustrate by pointing (see Chapter 3). However, it may not be possible from the patient's description to distin-guish between cardiac pain and that of epigastric origin, and such symptoms should not be used in isolation to diagnose cardiac events.

Examination: signs and history

Pulse

Palpating the pulse indicates cardiac rate and rhythm. If vascular obstructive disease is suspected, it is customary to take the pulse at several sites on either side of the body (both wrists, elbows, ankles, knees) to check for possible impaired or asymmetric perfusion. For example, a diabetic may have normal pulses at the knee but weak ones at the ankle owing to angiopathy. The **pulse pressure**, the difference in pressure between systole and diastole, can be estimated by palpation and yields useful semi-quantitative information (e.g. both the arterial rigidity of arteriosclerosis in the aged, and an incompetent aortic valve, cause a sharp differ-ence with each beat, i.e. wide pulse pressure).

Palpation of the left chest at the fouth or fifth intercostal space, about halfway between the sternum and side of body, will reveal the **apex beat**. This is where the left ventricle impacts on the chest wall during systole, yielding informa-tion about the rhythm and strength of the heart beat. In an enlarged heart this point is shifted leftwards (away from the sternum).

Blood pressure

Measurement of **systemic arterial blood pres-sure** is discussed on pp. 214–216. The pressure is at or near systolic level for only a short part of the cardiac cycle: for most of the cycle, pressure is nearer diastolic. Thus **mean arterial pressure (MAP)**, which gives an indication of the average stress put on the arterial system, is not a simple average: it is calculated by giving greater weight to the diastolic:

$$\text{Mean arterial pressure} = \text{diastolic} + 1/3 \text{ (systolic} - \text{diastolic)} \tag{4.11}$$

In developed countries, blood pressure increases with age. Systolic pressure is affected more than diastolic, and continues rising, possibly to 180–200 mmHg at age 80 (which indicates the need for treatment) as arteriosclerosis (p. 235) reduces arterial compliance. Diastolic pressure rises less steeply to around 90 mmHg at age 60, and then flattens out. Thus, the pulse pressure widens on ageing, reflecting decreasing aortic compliance. Between the ages of 20 and 60, the approximate normal values are given by:

$$\text{Systolic blood pressure} = 100 + 2/3 \text{ age} \tag{4.12}$$

$$\text{Diastolic blood pressure} = 67 + 1/3 \text{ age} \tag{4.13}$$

Blood pressure is normally a little lower in younger women than men but tends to rise faster postmenopausally so that pressures converge, and older women have higher systolic pressures than men. In less developed and rural areas there is little change with age, but migrants from rural areas to industrialized ones tend to acquire the rising pattern, suggesting the existence of strong environmental factors.

The **central venous pressure (CVP)** is the blood pressure at the point where the great veins enter the right atrium and is normally between 0 and 10 mmHg. The CVP represents the RAP or preload and is a good index of cardiac performance, because reduced ventricular performance will cause it to rise. It may be used to monitor possible fluid overload in heart failure or IV fluid therapy. The **jugular venous pressure (JVP)** is a non-invasive external indicator, detectable by examining for possible swelling of the jugular vein in the neck. It is measured by estimating the height of this swollen portion above the line of the clavicle (with the patient sitting with their thorax at 45°). Normally it is undetectable but in right heart failure it is raised.

Cyanosis

This blue coloration of blood is caused by reduced oxygen saturation (increased deoxyhaemoglobin level). It is noticeable clinically in highly vascular areas such as lips, tongue or nailbeds. The terms central and peripheral in relation to cyanosis refer to its origin and not where it is observed – a common source of confusion. **Central cyanosis** is caused by generalized arterial **hypoxaemia**, due for example to pulmonary oedema. In **peripheral cyanosis** the arterial oxygen saturation may be normal but perfusion of a particular area (usually fingers or toes) is compromised. In heart failure this commonly occurs in the skin as vasoconstriction there diverts blood to more important areas. Local blood flow is slowed, more oxygen is extracted, the arteriovenous oxygen difference is raised, and the blood becomes abnormally deoxygenated and blue-tinged. The area will be cold, but if it is massaged to improve local perfusion then normal colour may be restored (contrast this with central cyanosis).

Oedema

The origins of oedema are complex. The conventional explanation is illustrated in Figure 4.9, although recent evidence has questioned the completeness of this. On this model the oedema of heart failure is primarily caused by a combination of raised total body water (owing to renal fluid retention) and the preferential redistribution of an abnormal amount of this water to the extravascular extracellular compartment, i.e. tissue fluid (owing to raised peripheral venous pressure). As will be discussed below, hydrostatic factors also contribute. Generally, pulmonary oedema results from left heart failure, and peripheral oedema (in ankles, sacrum, abdominal organs) from right heart failure. If the oedematous area is compressed firmly with the thumb for about 10 s (this is usually painless for the patient), the impression remains as a pit for very much longer than would be the case for normal skin – hence the term **pitting oedema**.

Investigation

Electrocardiogram

An ECG reveals to the trained eye both qualitative and quantitative information about the heart's activity and electrical conduction system. The multiplicity of leads enables localization

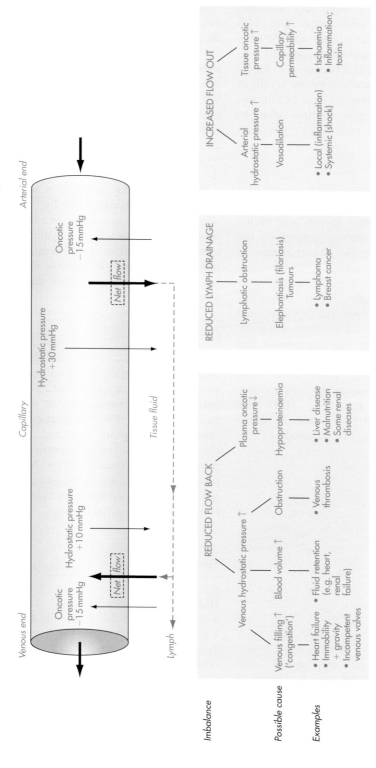

Figure 4.9 Formation of oedema. Tissue fluid is formed by ultrafiltration of plasma at the arterial end of capillaries, carrying with it nutrients and O_2. The motive force is the excess of hydrostatic pressure within the vessel forcing fluid out, over the oncotic (osmotic) pressure of the plasma proteins drawing it in. At the venous end, hydrostatic pressure has fallen but the oncotic pressure is little changed because plasma proteins do not pass out. Thus tissue fluid drains back, carrying with it metabolic waste products and CO_2. A small excess of 2.5 L daily for the whole body forms the lymph. Excess tissue fluid will accumulate if this balance is disturbed by either excess formation, impaired flow back to veins or lymphatic obstruction. The major ways in which this balance is upset are shown. Note: tissue pressures are ignored.

of certain lesions; e.g. where an infarction has occurred. Exercise provocation and 24-h recording may be useful modifications. The trace as it most commonly appears in generic ECG illustrations (similar to lead II) is shown in Figure 4.10, together with an account of the origin of each component. A number of basic ECG traces will be used in the relevant sections below to illustrate some typical abnormalities.

Imaging

A plain chest X-ray (see Figure 4.12(a)) will show the size of the heart and whether or not the lung fields are clear. Shadowing at the base of the lungs along the lower margin (defined by the diaphragm) usually indicates accumulation of fluid (i.e. pulmonary oedema).

Undoubtedly the most generally useful technique is **echocardiography**, which uses ultrasound. This is relatively inexpensive and completely non-invasive. It provides a continuous timed record of all the movements and dimensions of cardiac structures (including wall thickness, chamber size, shape and valve movements), and can measure ejection fraction. **Magnetic resonance imaging (MRI)** and **computed tomography (CT)** scanning of the thorax may also sometimes be required.

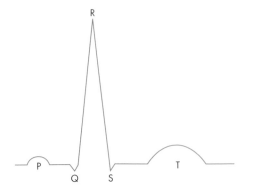

Figure 4.10 Normal ECG. The P wave represents atrial depolarization, the QRS complex ventricular depolarization, and the T wave ventricular repolarization. The PQ interval represents impulse speed between atrium and ventricle, altered in heart block. The height of the R wave represents ventricular mass, increased in hypertrophy. Myocardial ischaemia often manifests as abnormalities of the ST complex.

In **ventricular angiography**, heart movement throughout the cardiac cycle can be visualized by injecting radio-opaque material into the general circulation. In **coronary angiography**, much smaller quantities of contrast medium are precisely injected via a catheter at the root of a coronary artery to visualize possible obstructive lesions. This is becoming a standard investigation and diagnosis of cardiac ischaemic symptoms, and for deciding whether bypass or angioplasty (p. 253) is indicated, and if so where.

Nuclear imaging is used in two ways. In radionuclide ventriculography, thallium-201 taken up from coronary blood by healthy myocardial tissue leaves 'cold' spots that identify under-perfused (ischaemic) areas. Technetium-99-labelled RBCs enable visualization of the heart chambers and their movement; the ejection fraction can be measured accurately.

Catheterization

A fine plastic catheter may be introduced into the heart via a peripheral artery to access the left side of the heart or a vein (right side) so as to lie with its tip in a heart chamber or great vessel. Radiocontrast medium may then be injected, pressure at that point measured or blood withdrawn for gas analysis. It is particularly useful to measure the RAP (equivalent to CVP or preload), pressure drop across a valve, and pressure in the pulmonary vein (pulmonary 'wedge' pressure, equivalent to left atrial pressure).

Heart failure

Heart failure (cardiac failure) is not a disease but a syndrome, with many possible aetiologies and a complex pathogenesis, yet it may be simply defined as the failure of the heart to meet the normal perfusion demands of the body. Many diseases can impair cardiac performance and all are usually serious. Consequently, chronic cardiac failure has a poor prognosis, comparable with that for many forms of cancer.

Whatever the cause of failure, the clinical picture resulting from reduced contractility is similar. This is due to a combination of the consequences of impaired perfusion and the secondary consequences of maladaptive attempts by the CVS to compensate (p. 180; Table 4.3). The cardiac failure syndrome may also involve peripheral organ damage not directly caused by reduced blood supply, especially in skeletal muscle.

Terminology

Terms commonly used to describe different aspects of heart failure are given in Table 4.5. Most cases of heart failure would be classified as 'chronic compensated low-output left ventricular systolic failure'. The clinical features of left and right failure differ in certain crucial aspects, but many patients, especially the elderly, present with bilateral failure. The distinction between acute and chronic is important for management. The difference between systolic and diastolic failure is discussed below.

Epidemiology

Determining the prevalence of heart failure depends upon which grade, ejection fraction cut-off point and population are being considered. Estimates for symptomatic heart failure vary between 0.5% and 2%, but among those aged over 80 this rises to over 10%. If asymptomatic cases (Class 1) are included, overall prevalence is almost 10%. The annual incidence in the UK is approximately 0.3%, representing over 150 000 cases.

Aetiology

The causes of heart failure may be considered in two broad groups:

1. **Pump failure**, with primary reduction in myocardial contractility.
2. **Overloading**, with either excessive afterload (pressure overload) or excessive preload

---

Table 4.5   Terminology of heart failure

Term	Comment/Typical cause
Acute	Sudden onset (e.g. myocardial infarction)
Chronic	Gradual onset, usually progressive course (e.g. valve disease)
Right	Lung disease (cor pulmonale)
Left	Untreated essential hypertension
Bilateral	Almost any cause (usually chronic)
Ventricular	Failure of ventricle(s) only (the usual form)
Atrial	Failure of atria only (uncommon)
Low output	Reduced contractility – most causes (usual form)
High output	Anaemia, thyrotoxicosis – due to excessive cardiac drive
Systolic	Reduced contractility → impaired emptying (usual variety)
Diastolic	Reduced ventricular compliance → impaired filling (less common)
Compensated	Compensation prevents symptoms at rest but cardiac reserve diminished
Decompensated	Cardiac reserve exhausted
Congestive (CHF, CCF)	Imprecise traditional term describing generalized oedema; usually implies bilateral ventricular failure
Cardiogenic shock	Acute severe decompensation: very low BP and CO; poor tissue perfusion
LVF/RVF	Left/right ventricular failure

BP, blood pressure; CCF, congestive cardiac failure; CHF, congestive heart failure; CO, cardiac output.

(volume overload), which arise outside the heart and reduce contractility secondarily.

Specific causes within these groups may give rise to failure acutely or chronically and may initially affect one specific chamber or side of the heart. However, in chronic heart failure both sides are usually affected eventually. Table 4.6 shows the common causes in each group.

Despite this wide range of possible aetiologies, in industrialized countries by far the most common cause of LVF is ischaemic heart disease, causing over half of cases; the second most common is cardiomyopathy (see below) and the third is valvular disease. Untreated systemic hypertension used to be a common cause but is no longer a major factor. Valve disease secondary to childhood rheumatic fever is now uncommon as a result of improved public health and sanitation. However, in developing countries the picture is quite different, with infective and nutritional causes predominating.

Pathogenesis

Primary pump failure

Damage to the myocardium usually results in **systolic failure. Ischaemic heart disease** (IHD, restriction of the coronary blood supply) is the most common cause; it usually affects just one chamber, most often the left ventricle. Ischaemic failure may develop suddenly following **myocardial infarction (MI)**, with no prior warning signs of ischaemic chest pain over the preceding weeks or months. Alternatively there may be slowly progressive **diffuse fibrosis** with multiple minor and possibly asymptomatic infarcts, especially in the elderly. Chronic ischaemia may also induce asymptomatic **myocardial hibernation**, with progressive decline in systolic function, although potentially this is reversible by revascularization. However, it must be remembered that IHD is a separate disease entity from heart failure and

Table 4.6   Aetiology of heart failure

Haemodynamic defect	Cause	Side affected[a]	Acute or chronic
Pump failure			
Systolic failure	**Ischaemic heart disease**	L usually	Acute or chronic
	Cardiomyopathy	L ± R	Chronic
	Arrhythmias	L + R	Acute, chronic
	Infection, inflammation, alcohol	L + R	Acute, chronic
	Systemic disease (e.g. amyloidosis)	L + R	Chronic
	Diffuse fibrosis (senile, ischaemic)	L + R	Chronic
Diastolic failure	Ischaemia, cardiomyopathy, fibrosis	L + R	Chronic
Excessive afterload	**Hypertension – systemic**	L	Chronic
	– pulmonary (COPD)	R	Chronic
	Valve stenosis	L or R	Chronic
Excessive preload			
Obligatory	Vasodilatation: beri-beri, septicaemia	L + R	Chronic
Hypervolaemia	Fluid retention, e.g. renal failure, aldosteronism	R	Usually chronic
	Excess IV infusion		
	Polycythaemia		
Excessive demand	Regurgitation: valve incompetence	R or L	Chronic
	Hyperdynamic: anaemia, thyrotoxicosis	R	Chronic

Commonest causes in **bold**

[a] Initial side of heart affected (L, left; R, right); in chronic disease usually both sides eventually fail.

COPD, chronic obstructive pulmonary disease; IV, intravenous.

does not invariably lead to it. Heart failure rarely results from stable angina pectoris.

The cardiomyopathies are a miscellaneous group in which diffuse damage occurs throughout the myocardium. They are either idiopathic or secondary to conditions such as infection, toxins (e.g. alcohol), inflammation or autoimmune disease. In **dilated cardiomyopathy** the myocardium becomes thin, weak and excessively enlarged, with a raised EDV and a low ejection fraction. This may arise as a consequence of, for example, infection, thyroid disease or alcohol abuse. In **hypertrophic cardiomyopathy** there is excessive thickening of the myocardium, leading to poor ventricular filling and obstructed ejection, particularly due to structural distortion around the valves, whereas in **restrictive cardiomyopathy** there is increased ventricular stiffness but little hypertrophy.

In the ageing heart a diffuse ('senile') **fibrosis** can occur and a number of systemic diseases such as sarcoid and amyloidosis may have diffuse cardiac complications that lead to eventual failure. Arrhythmias may also cause pump failure. Interestingly, cardiac tumours are rare.

While most forms of pump failure cause reduced contractility and systolic failure, some diffuse diseases of the myocardium can lead to it becoming fibrosed and stiff, with reduced compliance. This results in difficulty in filling the heart adequately during diastole, and leads to **diastolic failure**. This has been recognized in about one-fifth of patients with symptoms of failure (i.e. low cardiac output), but a normal heart size and ejection fraction (and thus normal systolic function), and may be present in up to half of all heart failure cases. Causes include patchy ischaemic or senile fibrosis, restrictive cardiomyopathy and hypertrophic cardiomyopathy (e.g. owing to untreated hypertension).

Overloading

Both over-work and over-stretch cause structural and biochemical abnormalities in myocardial cells, such as the deposition of fibrils and impaired calcium utilization. The result is a decreased force and velocity of contraction and delayed relaxation. These effects are usually irreversible.

Excessive afterload

If the systemic vascular resistance is abnormally high, causing systemic hypertension, the raised afterload on the left ventricle may eventually cause it to fail, but the right ventricle will initially be unaffected. The heart is far more prone to damage from pressure overloading than from volume overloading, although the former is now relatively uncommon because hypertension is detected earlier and treated better. However, it is possible that failure diagnosed as ischaemic or cardiomyopathic may have been aetiologically related to chronic undetected hypertension.

Similarly, sustained rises in pulmonary vascular resistance, causing pulmonary hypertension (e.g. secondary to many chronic lung diseases), can eventually lead to RVF, known as **cor pulmonale**, although it may be secondary to many other conditions.

Theoretically, the afterload on both sides may be increased by abnormally high blood viscosity, such as in polycythaemia, but this is unlikely to cause failure in the absence of other abnormalities.

Excessive preload

This is an uncommon general cause of failure. Whether or not excessive increases in venous return lead to failure depends on the cause and other factors. The heart tolerates volume overload well, and because the output initially is high, symptoms are not at first evident. The left side of the heart receives the same volume of venous return as the right, at approximately the same preloading, because the lungs usually offer little resistance. Because the left ventricle is by far the more powerful, if decompensation is caused by raised systemic filling pressure the right side will be first to fail.

If moderate hypervolaemia develops, the initially raised output will be surplus to the perfusion needs of the body. Owing to autoregulation there will be vasoconstriction throughout the body and a rise in peripheral resistance: blood pressure will increase and output will return to normal (remember, blood pressure = cardiac output × peripheral resistance). Thus, the raised preload is converted to a raised afterload and, if not corrected, this may itself lead to failure. This could also have a bearing on the pathogenesis of essential hypertension (p. 213).

Precisely the opposite occurs in diseases where widespread vasodilatation results in a severely reduced peripheral resistance, e.g. in septicaemic shock. This produces an obligatory requirement for raised cardiac output to maintain blood pressure, leading eventually to what is known as **high-output failure** (although this is a misleading term because by definition it does not become failure until the myocardium can no longer sustain the output). Other conditions create an excessive (hyperdynamic) systemic demand for output, stimulating the heart via the usual CVS reflexes. Examples include chronic severe anaemia, low blood oxygen being the stimulus, and thyrotoxicosis, where basal metabolic rate is increased.

Although not usually primary causes of heart failure, anaemia, severe infection, fluid retention (including that from drugs such as NSAIDs and corticosteroids) or over-enthusiastic IV infusion can be causes of decompensation in patients with otherwise stable compensated heart failure.

Valve disease

Stenosis (narrowing or failure to open fully) causes an outflow obstruction, which increases afterload; thus mitral stenosis can cause left atrial failure. Alternatively, valve incompetence (failure to close fully) will permit regurgitation, which causes volume overload in the chambers both upstream and downstream of the valve: upstream, because of the back-flow and downstream because there will eventually be an abnormally large ingress as the upstream chamber overfills. On this basis we can predict the consequences of stenosis or incompetence of the mitral, tricuspid, aortic and pulmonary valves, i.e. which chamber(s) will fail and whether this is the result of excessive afterload or preload.

Pathophysiology

Haemodynamic changes

Heart failure is a dynamic process rather than a single event, even when acute. Whatever the aetiology, the process is similar and the reductions in cardiac effectiveness can be represented by pump performance curves (Figure 4.11).

As contractility falls the stroke volume is reduced; this leaves a higher EDV after ejection. This means an increased preload for the next

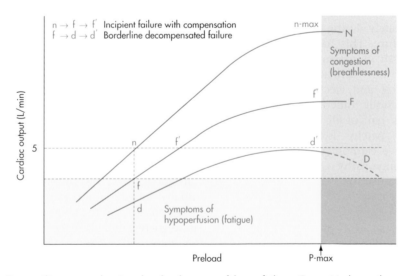

Figure 4.11 Contractility curves showing the development of heart failure. Curve N shows the pump performance (contractility) curve of the normal heart with cardiac output plotted against preload in arbitrary units (e.g. end-diastolic volume). Curve F shows compensated failure and curve D decompensated failure. P-max is maximum preload. See text for further details.

contraction so that contractility is increased appropriately (by the Starling mechanism). Consequently output is restored, but as long as the myocardium is impaired then output is being maintained only at the expense of increased diastolic size, i.e. the EDV is increased. Because the heart is now 'larger' it is less efficient, according to Laplace's law. In health this is usually insignificant, but in heart failure this compensation eventually reduces efficiency and erodes the cardiac reserve.

In Figure 4.11, curve N represents normal contractility. Point n represents the resting cardiac output of 5 L/min (that which is sufficient to maintain resting organ function and renal fluid clearance); the difference between n and n-max represents the cardiac reserve. If output falls much below 5 L/min there will be symptoms of hypoperfusion, notably fatigue. Alternatively, should perfusion demands exhaust the cardiac reserve by requiring preload to rise beyond point P-max, output will not increase and may fall. Consequently venous pressure will rise, causing congestive symptoms (i.e. oedema). On the left side of the heart this will result in pulmonary oedema and breathlessness.

Acute failure

Suppose that a patient with normal cardiac function suddenly were to suffer a moderate MI. Contractility immediately drops and output may quickly fall below the normal resting minimum, to point f on a new, less steep, contractility curve (F). The patient experiences fatigue even at rest, among other symptoms, and the CVS initiates compensation.

The heart enlarges until a new equilibrium is attained at a higher preload (point f′). The cardiac reserve is now reduced, as is the maximum output that can be reached by maximal preload (f″). At rest, the patient may be unaware of any disability but he or she will have reduced exercise tolerance, becoming breathless earlier than before the MI. This situation (n → f → f′) is termed **compensated failure**. Note that a higher preload than before is needed to sustain even resting cardiac output (f′), so the heart is permanently less efficient.

If the infarction is very severe, the output may drop precipitately to point d, putting the patient

on curve D, and they would probably collapse. After maximum compensation to point d′, normal resting output can only just be attained at maximal preload; the patient may even be beyond this, on the falling arm of the curve. There is now zero cardiac reserve and the patient will be fatigued at the slightest exertion and may be breathless even at rest: this is **decompensated failure**.

Chronic failure

A gradual reduction in cardiac contractility produces a similar pattern, except that the patient's haemodynamics would be represented by a series of progressively declining contractility curves, rather than a sudden fall.

A patient could remain in chronic compensated failure indefinitely if the disease progression is arrested or is sufficiently slow. However, a supervening severe stress (e.g. a serious infection, sudden fluid overload, excessive exertion or chronic anaemia) often drives them into decompensation.

A plain chest X-ray (CXR) dramatically visualizes severe heart failure. Figure 4.12(a) shows a normal chest: the heart shadow occupies about half the width of the thorax, i.e. the **cardiothoracic index** is 0.5. In Figure 4.12(b) (severe failure) the cardiac enlargement is easily seen; the index is nearer 0.7. The increased size is not due to cardiac hypertrophy, which does not show up on plain X-ray (the absolute increase in size in hypertrophy being relatively modest and growth predominantly inwards). What is shown is the result of an increased diastolic volume.

Compensation and consequences: decompensation

Heart failure is more than simply a reduction in cardiac output and accompanying tissue hypoperfusion. As was shown above (p. 180), when the cardiac reserve is mobilized in circumstances where its main effector system – the heart itself – cannot respond, it soon becomes maladaptive. Cardiac enlargement, driven in part by excessive fluid retention and possibly by venoconstriction, brings inefficiency and over-stretch as muscle fibres lose mutual adherence. Excessive hypertrophy interferes with ventricular filling and

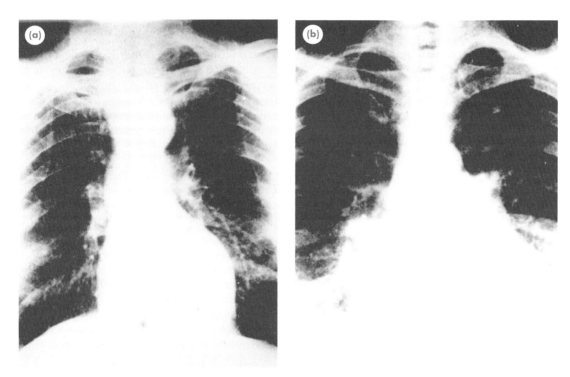

Figure 4.12   Chest X-ray in heart failure. (a) Normal pattern. (b) Patient with severe heart failure. Note the increased width of the heart shadow indicating cardiac enlargement, and the diffuse shadowing at the lung bases indicating pulmonary oedema.

ejection. The maladaptive changes in ventricular shape caused by dilatation and hypertrophy are termed **remodelling**, especially when they follow MI. Angiotensin may contribute to this process.

These changes are accompanied by the neuroendocrine mechanisms we met in discussing cardiac reserve. In heart failure these can exacerbate the situation as one or more components fail to respond satisfactorily, e.g. a failure to increase myocardial contractility following increased sympathetic nervous system activity.

The normally protective baroreceptor-mediated inhibition of sympathetic outflow becomes blunted, and unrestrained sympathetic drive results in excessive inotropic stimulation of the myocardium and widespread peripheral vasoconstriction. Both conditions place further loads on the heart. In addition, renal perfusion is reduced and atrial pressures rise. Thus circulating levels of noradrenaline (norepinephrine),

angiotensin, aldosterone, ADH (vasopressin) and NP all rise.

Decompensation follows as these mechanisms combine to reduce cardiac output, rather than to increase or even just maintain it. The heart has passed the maximum on its contractility curve (see Figure 4.4). Irreversible myocardial cell damage and necrosis follow. The sequence of events is illustrated in Figure 4.13. Clearly, treatment must target not only low cardiac output but also these maladaptive mechanisms.

Cardiogenic shock

If contractility falls below that which can sustain the resting cardiac output, producing widespread hypoperfusion, this counterproductive cycle deteriorates rapidly. Peripheral arterioles throughout the body respond to local hypoxia by autoregulatory dilatation, overcoming the centrally mediated vasoconstriction that attempts to defend blood pressure. The result is a disastrous fall in blood pressure, low venous

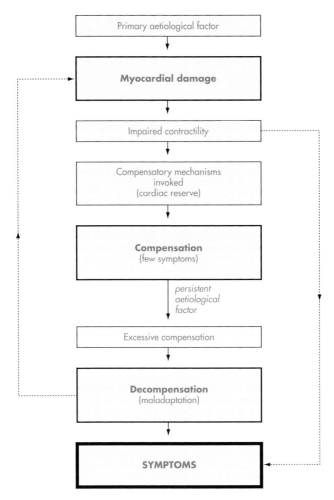

Figure 4.13   Sequence of events in heart failure.

return and poor coronary perfusion; together these result in even worse contractility and lower cardiac output. At the same time, hypoxic lung vessels constrict, thereby increasing right ventricular afterload. The entire syndrome is termed **cardiogenic shock**.

Despite the most aggressive management, the whole devastating vicious cycle can be rapidly fatal, especially if irreversible multi-organ damage occurs before circulation is restored.

Clinical features

The classical symptom triad of heart failure is exercise limitation (fatigue), shortness of breath (dyspnoea) and oedema. However, the clinical picture, although fairly consistent, is often more complex. Many of the clinical features result from impaired flow ahead of the affected chamber; this **hypoperfusion** is termed the **forward component** of heart failure. Other symptoms are caused by an increase in pressure in the veins draining into the affected chamber; this results in **congestion** or **oedema**, termed the **backward component** (Figure 4.14). Both components usually coexist – they are different aspects of failure, not different forms of it. However, the symptoms may vary according to which side of the heart is primarily affected, and the picture is further complicated by the neuroendocrine compensatory mechanisms.

A feature that commonly accompanies chronic failure is the anaemia of chronic disease, which contributes to the fatigue and also exacerbates the failure by putting an extra load on the heart owing to increased circulatory demands.

Forward component (hypoperfusion)

The effects of hypoperfusion are independent of which side of the heart fails because the outputs from either side are always equal, even when reduced. The principal feature is fatigue, but numerous other symptoms follow from poor peripheral perfusion. The extremities will be cold and pale as the CVS attempts to redirect the reduced cardiac output away from skin and muscle to the brain, heart and kidney by peripheral vasoconstriction. Reduced renal perfusion pressure will cause fluid and electrolyte retention, partly via activation of the RAAS, contributing to oedema. Over-activity of the sympathetic nervous system produces symptoms such as **tachycardia** and **tachypnoea** (increased respiratory rate).

It is possible that fatigue is not due just to skeletal muscle hypoperfusion but is part of a generalized **myopathy** secondary to heart failure. It may result from impaired energy handling and subsequent atrophy, or rises in catabolic cytokines, possibly of cardiac origin, such as TNF. Both myocardial and respiratory muscles are affected, exacerbating the cardiac problems and contributing to the breathlessness.

Backward component (congestion/oedema)

Right-sided failure. The raised pressure within the great veins draining into the right side of the heart (i.e. systemic venous congestion) will be communicated back to the venous end of systemic capillaries where it impairs the venous drainage of tissue fluid, causing peripheral oedema (p. 184). A further factor in acute failure is the haemodilution caused by expansion of the blood volume. This reduces plasma protein concentration and thus oncotic pressure, contributing to further loss of fluid from the vascular compartment.

Not all areas of the body are affected equally. The additional effect of gravity will make oedema first noticed in the ankles of erect patients, or in the sacral area of the bed-bound. The liver, being highly vascular, is affected early, causing **hepatomegaly** (enlarged liver), and the patient may then feel bloated, nauseous and anorexic. Congestion of the stomach and

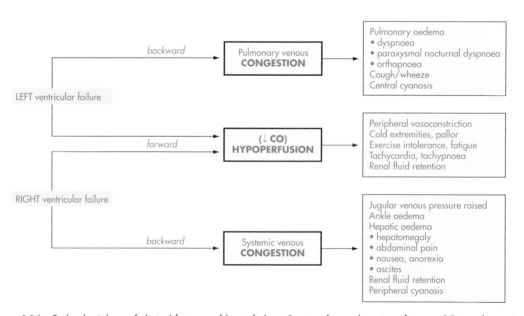

Figure 4.14   Pathophysiology of clinical features of heart failure. See text for explanation of terms. CO, cardiac output.

duodenum may impair nutrient and drug absorption. Later, **ascites** (free oedema fluid in the abdominal cavity) may develop.

A raised JVP (p. 184), seen as distension and pulsation of the external jugular veins in the neck, gives an accessible, approximate clinical index of the severity of right-heart failure. The CVP (p. 184) is a more precise indicator for monitoring the progress of severe failure, but measuring it is invasive. The raised systemic venous pressure reduces the arteriovenous pressure difference, slowing peripheral blood flow and causing **peripheral cyanosis**.

In the kidney, raised venous pressure has more far-reaching consequences. It reduces the glomerular filtration rate (owing to raised efferent arteriolar pressure; see Chapter 14) thus exacerbating the fluid and electrolyte retention. This is maladaptive because the resultant increased intravascular volume further raises venous pressures, exacerbating excessive preload and oedema.

In summary, right-sided failure causes fatigue, fluid retention, peripheral oedema, abdominal congestion and peripheral cyanosis.

Left-sided failure. This is more common and usually more serious. The rise in pulmonary venous pressure causes pulmonary congestion and **pulmonary oedema** by a similar mechanism to that causing peripheral oedema in right-sided failure. However, unlike most other tissues, lungs do not normally have any tissue fluid and the equivalent of the extravascular space is the normally dry alveolar space. Thus even a small imbalance in transcapillary pressure can allow fluid into the alveoli, which seriously interferes with gas diffusion and also reduces pulmonary compliance (thereby increasing the work of breathing). The resulting hypoxaemia causes severe breathlessness (**dyspnoea**) and **central cyanosis**. Severe pulmonary oedema can be rapidly fatal (see also Chapter 5).

The dyspnoeic effects of mild pulmonary oedema are particularly noticeable when the patient is supine because the oedema fluid then spreads throughout the lungs. When erect, i.e. sitting or standing, venous filling pressure is reduced as intravascular fluid is redistributed to lower parts of the body; this reverses the conditions that produce pulmonary oedema. This is

orthopnoea, breathing adequately only when erect. Even a moderate change in posture, such as propping a patient up in bed with pillows, promotes redistribution of the fluid, which collects at the lung bases to leave the apexes relatively clear and permitting adequate ventilation at rest. This is easily visualized by X-ray (Figure 4.12). However, in all but the mildest pulmonary oedema, changes in posture alone are insufficient and drug therapy is needed. In addition to *oxygen* and diuretics, opiates may be used in severe cases; they work in part by venodilatation, causing a rapid reduction in filling pressure.

A typical history given by patients with untreated left-heart failure is of waking breathless, wheezy and coughing after a few hours' sleep. They go to the window for a 'breath of fresh air', and quite soon feel better: not because of the air, plainly, but owing to the change in posture. This phenomenon, because it may recur throughout the night, is called **paroxysmal nocturnal dyspnoea (PND)**. It is a classical, almost pathognomonic sign of LVF. Such patients are advised to sleep with three or four cushions, or in a chair, which usually improves matters at least in the early stages.

To summarize, left-sided failure causes severe fatigue, pulmonary oedema, severe breathlessness and central cyanosis.

Predominant pathophysiological pattern

The backward and forward components can occur to different extents in the same patient. Which predominates – congestion or hypoperfusion – depends on the shape of the patient's contractility curve and the position of its maximum. Figure 4.15 shows left ventricular contractility curves in heart failure. The 'dyspnoea threshold' represents the preload above which pulmonary venous pressure is so high as to cause breathlessness. Below the 'fatigue threshold', output is so low as to cause severe tiredness.

If the maximum output attainable is below the dyspnoea threshold (curve H, hypoperfused pattern), fatigue will occur after even moderate exertion, but before breathlessness. On the other hand, the patient whose heart is on curve C will become breathless before their muscles actually become fatigued (congestive pattern).

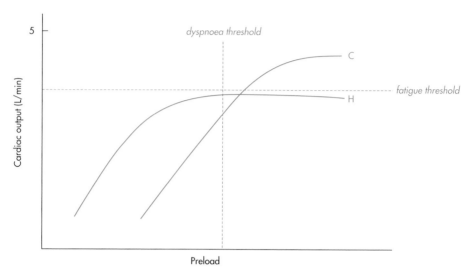

Figure 4.15   Different contractility patterns in heart failure. Hypoperfusive pattern (curve H), exercise is limited by fatigue. Congestive pattern (curve C), exercise is limited by breathlessness. See text for details.

Bilateral (biventricular) failure

Unilateral chronic failure is uncommon. Usually, patients present with bilateral failure and have mixed symptoms because failure of one side eventually compromises function on the other: this is the classical 'congestive cardiac failure'. The hypoperfusion that follows failure of either side affects the pulmonary and systemic circulations equally. Coronary hypoperfusion will ensue, leading eventually to chronic ischaemic ventricular failure on the opposite side. Following unilateral LVF, pulmonary congestion will increase the afterload on the right ventricle and if this is untreated, the result will be RVF.

Asymptomatic left ventricular dysfunction

The early stages in slowly deteriorating chronic heart failure are initially fully compensated and therefore asymptomatic (Class I on the NYHA scale; p. 197). It can only be detected by investigation, but there is evidence that early detection and treatment, before irreversible myocardial damage develops, improves prognosis.

Presentation

A few common examples of heart failure patients will serve to illustrate typical presentations. One might be an undiagnosed hypertensive male in his mid-forties, probably somewhat obese, possibly living a stressful life, perhaps starting to suffer from angina pectoris. His heart failure may be precipitated acutely by MI or may develop slowly along with ventricular hypertrophy. Another example might be an older smoker with COPD (Chapter 5), slowly developing cor pulmonale. A third example might be an elderly patient with underlying asymptomatic IHD and developing valve disease, perhaps following childhood rheumatic fever.

Most will complain at first of increasing fatigue and a reduced exercise tolerance: climbing stairs, running for a bus, working or going shopping, etc. They will find breathing particularly difficult at night and may have obvious ankle oedema after a day on their feet. They may complain of palpitations. Eventually they will see their GP, when a provisional diagnosis will usually be straightforward. However, NICE recommends definitive investigation.

Investigation and grading

Investigations are used in heart failure to confirm the diagnosis and exclude other possible diagnoses, to determine the cause and any exacerbating or precipitating factors, to grade the extent of dysfunction, and to monitor the progress of treatment. It is important to try to determine the cause of heart failure because it may be reversible or correctable.

Extensive investigation is not usually required. A CXR will show the extent of cardiac enlargement and the existence of lung congestion, i.e. pulmonary oedema. The stethoscope may reveal the characteristic sounds of valve disease or the crackles on breathing (crepitations) that are characteristic of pulmonary oedema. The pulse may indicate an arrhythmia. An ECG will reveal any cardiac hypertrophy (usually from long-standing hypertension), ischaemia, the possibility of MI and any arrhythmia.

Echocardiography is becoming mandatory as the single most useful non-invasive indicator of ventricular function and the best predictor of prognosis, through measurement of ejection fraction. Other routine investigations would include urea and electrolytes, full blood count, and liver, renal and thyroid function tests.

More sophisticated tests and instruments are available for the few cases that present diagnostic problems, including isotope imaging, cardiac catheterization and coronary angiography. These can also be used to measure the extent of myocardial damage. Except in acute severe failure, invasive haemodynamic measurements are rarely indicated.

Currently the potential of measuring a natriuretic peptide precursor, **N-terminal pro-BNP (NT proBNP)** as a diagnostic marker and index severity and progress is being evaluated. At present its use is restricted to ruling out significant heart failure if its level is low or normal.

Grading

A variety of semi-quantitative bedside methods and scales are employed for grading. The patient is asked about limitations on daily activities such as walking distance or stair climbing before the onset of fatigue or dyspnoea, or how many pillows they sleep with. These questions may be supplemented by formal exercise testing. Examination of the JVP and the extent of oedema are important.

Such observations can be used to grade the patient on the NYHA scale for heart failure, and although symptoms do not always correlate with objective functional impairment, it is useful to indicate the approximate ejection fraction (EF) of each class:

- Class I. Asymptomatic. No symptoms at ordinary physical activity (EF 40–50%).
- Class II. Mild. Breathlessness and fatigue evident on strenuous exertion (EF 35–40%).
- Class III. Moderate. Breathlessness and fatigue evident on moderate exertion (EF 30–35%).
- Class IV. Severe. Breathlessness at rest (EF <30%)

Symptomatic improvement also correlates poorly with changes in haemodynamic indices. Thus for monitoring therapy and progress generally, subjective assessments by the patient, global measures of exercise tolerance and estimations of the 'quality of life' are often the most useful methods. For patients on medication these must be supplemented by regular clinical biochemistry monitoring.

Prognosis

The seriousness of heart failure can be judged from its poor prognosis, which the advent of ACEI therapy has improved only modestly. For NYHA Class IV heart failure the median survival is only 1 year, while for Classes II and III it is 3–5 years. The annual mortality rate from asymptomatic left ventricular disease (Class I) is about 5%.

Management

The management of heart failure involves correcting the consequences of low cardiac output and congestion, and addressing the various maladaptive pathophysiological responses that have complicated the clinical picture. The general approaches will be reviewed first, before discussion of the management strategies. A fuller account of many of the drugs mentioned in this section is given on pp. 224–232 in the section on Hypertension. Only properties pertinent to heart failure are covered here.

Aims

The various aims in managing heart failure are listed below. They overlap in sequence, objectives and methods and are not in order of precedence.

- Identify and correct any causative or contributory factors.
- Improve cardiac efficiency and effectiveness.
- Reduce cardiac workload.
- Counteract maladaptive responses.
- Increase cardiac output.
- Relieve symptoms.
- Reduce progression and prolong survival.

Ideas about improving declining cardiac performance have changed. Rather than attempting to force the heart to maintain an unrealistic output while impaired and under maximal physiological stimulation, current practice favours two alternative strategies:

1. Reduce the load on the heart to match its reduced pumping ability.
2. Limit the counterproductive compensatory mechanisms.

Stimulation, unloading or cardioprotection?

The traditional treatment for heart failure has been to use inotropic agents, notably cardiac glycosides. However, there is little evidence for the benefit of this approach.

Careful trials have shown that simple **inotropic** agents do not improve prognosis, and indeed most worsen mortality. The possible exception is *digoxin*, the value of which probably rests on various actions other than its inotropic activity (see below).

Unloading is theoretically more attractive than simple stimulation because it is more physiological. If the heart cannot sustain an adequate output to meet current demands, it is appropriate to reduce those demands. Put more prosaically, in order to open a stiff door on rusty hinges, a few drops of oil are preferable to brute force. However, although this approach often produces haemodynamic improvement, it confers little survival benefit, so has now been augmented by **cardioprotection**.

Thus attention has focused on the failing myocardium and the high level of endogenous stimulation it undergoes via compensatory mechanisms. Particularly important are the neuroendocrine mechanisms involving the RAAS, the sympathetic nervous system and cardiac beta-receptors. In heart failure there is excessive sympathetic drive to which the myocardium can no longer respond, and also high renin and aldosterone levels. It has been shown that blocking these mechanisms with ACEIs and beta-blockers protects the heart against further damage, retards progression of the failure, and significantly improves prognosis.

These new insights could also explain why extra stimulation by inotropic drugs might be superfluous and possibly harmful. Moreover, increasing contractility inevitably increases oxygen demand, which is counterproductive, particularly in ischaemic failure.

Correct causative or contributory factors

Although attending to the underlying cause of the failure would seem to be a priority, it may not be immediately feasible, whether obvious (e.g. MI) or only revealed on investigation (e.g. valve disease, coronary artery disease). Both causal and potential contributory factors (e.g. hypertension, anaemia) may have to wait until the patient is stabilized before appropriate, possibly long-term, corrective measures are initiated. These might include attention to CVS risk factors, salt restriction, stopping smoking, antihypertensive therapy, weight reduction, valve replacement and haematinics.

Reduce cardiac workload

A basic form of unloading has always been practised. Rest is imposed by the exercise limitation of the condition and patients are often fatigued. Bedrest has been the traditional advice, but if excessive it can be detrimental to exercise tolerance, predisposing to muscle atrophy, deconditioning, and possibly thromboembolic complications. Moreover, moderate aerobic physical training has now been shown to improve quality of life even if it does not benefit survival. Thus it is strongly encouraged, under supervision, in all patients with stable failure in Classes II and III.

Further, our better understanding of haemodynamics now enables us to intervene positively to reduce the myocardial workload, either by reducing preload with venodilators or diuretics, or by reducing afterload with arterial dilators (Figure 4.16).

Preload reduction

Starling's law predicts that reducing preload will reduce cardiac output. If so, would reducing the preload not exacerbate the hypoperfusion (forward component) of heart failure? This would be true if the failing myocardium were not operating on the falling limb of its contractility curve (see Figure 4.3(a)) and therefore no longer governed by Starling's law. In this situation reducing preload may actually increase output, as well as decreasing oxygen demand by reducing diastolic volume (Laplace's law, p. 178).

Diuretics. Dietary sodium and fluid restriction and natriuresis are the first-line strategy in all patients with evidence of fluid retention. Diuretics have several diverse but interdependent effects. They mobilize the excess fluid retained by the kidneys, reducing intravascular fluid (i.e. blood volume), which reduces preload. Consequently, venous end-capillary pressure is lowered, an effect enhanced by the venodilator action of diuretics (Table 4.7). This reduces oedema by facilitating the return of oedema fluid to the circulation, to be cleared by the kidneys. Kidney function benefits from the improved cardiac function.

The principal danger is dehydration, especially if loop diuretics are needed, because this would further compromise cardiac and renal function. Clearly, diuretics are contra-indicated

Table 4.7   Predominant vascular sites of action of vasodilators used in heart failure

Arterioles	Arterioles and veins	Veins
Hydralazine	ACEIs, ARAs	Nitrates
CCBs	Alpha-adrenergic blockers	
Beta$_2$-adrenergic agonists	Thiazide/loop diuretics	
Dopaminergic agonists	Nitroprusside	

ACEI, angiotensin-converting enzyme inhibitor; ARB, angiotensin receptor antagonist; CCB, calcium-channel blocker.

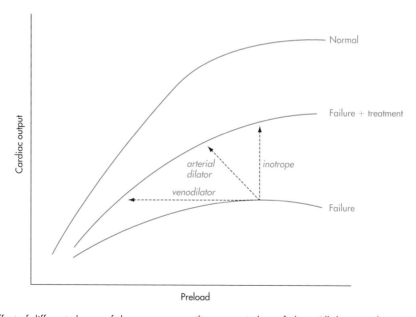

Figure 4.16   Effect of different classes of drugs on contractility curves in heart failure. All drugs act by moving heart onto a more favourable contractility curve. Venodilators reduce preload, maintaining reduced output more efficiently (before compensation). Inotropes increase output for the same preload (before compensation). Arterial dilators have an intermediate effect (after compensation; see also Figure 4.3(b)).

in hypovolaemic, low-output states. Potassium, and perhaps magnesium, plasma levels need to be monitored carefully because of the arrhythmogenic effects of hypokalaemia and hypomagnesaemia on the myocardium, especially in the presence of cardiac glycosides. (For a more detailed discussion of diuretics, see pp. 226–227.)

Venodilators. Dilating veins increases venous capacitance, which leads to reduced pressure in the venous system, lowering filling pressure and venous end-capillary pressure, as with diuretics. Either nitrates (predominantly venodilator) or venous-arteriolar dilators, e.g. alpha-adrenergic blockers, ACEIs or angiotensin receptor antagonists (ARAs) may be used. The main problems with nitrates are tolerance and acute falls in cardiac output and blood pressure causing syncope. Nitrates may be used alone or in combination with arterial dilators in both acute and chronic failure, but nowadays are most often used in acute failure.

Afterload reduction

Almost invariably, as cardiac output and blood pressure fall, the body responds by increasing sympathetic drive and renin/angiotensin levels. This may defend blood pressure, but only at the expense of raised peripheral resistance, further overloading an impaired myocardium. If the blood pressure continues to fall, attempts to restore it with vasoconstrictor drugs will have the same effect.

Although changes in peripheral resistance have little effect on the output of the normal heart (see Figure 4.3(b)) owing to reflex compensation, the performance of the diseased heart can be markedly improved by reducing afterload. Thus ideally, if afterload is reduced output will rise while blood pressure is maintained. Moreover, because pressure work is the most energy-consuming component of cardiac performance, reducing the afterload is a very effective way to reduce myocardial oxygen demand. This may be particularly important in ischaemic failure.

Balancing the benefits of reduced resistance against the possible problems of hypoperfusion of vital organs may be very difficult, and in acute severe failure this strategy is restricted to specialist units.

Arterial vasodilators (p. 225). These are a heterogeneous group (Table 4.7) that act by several different mechanisms. In theory, this group is most appropriate for patients with hypoperfusion or heart failure secondary to hypertension. However, they are often helpful in any severe or resistant failure.

Although the older sympatholytic (e.g. *prazosin*) and direct-acting (e.g. *hydralazine*) agents are still used, the ACEIs are now first-line vasodilators, having both arterial and venodilator effects as well as several other actions (p. 225). Further, the ACEIs are free from adverse effects of postural hypotension, tolerance and reflex compensation. The specific arterial and/or venodilators do not have a beneficial long-term effect, probably because of reflex activation of the RAAS, which ACEIs block. Thus combined dilator therapy (e.g. *hydralazine* plus nitrates) has been replaced by monotherapy with ACEIs unless contra-indicated. However, vasodilators may be added if severe failure is not controlled with diuretics and ACEIs.

CCBs have not been found helpful and are generally avoided, especially the negatively inotropic ones like *verapamil*. However, those with a predominant vasodilator action (dihydropyridines, DHPs, particularly *amlodipine*; Table 4.25) may be useful in ischaemic failure or where there is hypertension.

Counteract maladaptive responses

We have seen that the consequences of maladaptive neurohumoral activation include excessive sympathetic drive, vasoconstriction, raised aldosterone secretion, renal fluid retention and cardiac hypertrophy with ventricular dilatation. Several of the agents already discussed mitigate these effects; the following are directed more specifically at them.

Angiotensin-converting enzyme inhibitors

The action of angiontensin-converting enzyme inhibitors (ACEIs) is complex. Inhibition of the production of circulating angiotensin causes both venous and arterial dilatation and reduced aldosterone levels. They also reduce the local production of angiotensin in many tissues, notably the kidney, where it normally inhibits glomerular filtration, and the heart and blood vessels, where it has growth-promoting action. The action of ACEIs is not reduced by tolerance or reflex sympathetic compensation.

The renal action of ACEIs counteracts the aldosterone hypersecretion found in some heart failure patients and reduces fluid retention in most, with no risk of hypokalaemia. Indeed there is a risk of hyperkalaemia, especially when used with potassium supplements or potassium-sparing diuretics. It is also likely that reduced local tissue angiotensin production leads to reduced vascular and myocardial hypertrophy (remodelling), including that which usually follows MI.

Most importantly, several large trials such as SOLVD, CONSENSUS and V-HeFT have demonstrated that in adequate doses after careful titration ACEIs prolong survival by up to 50% even in mild heart failure. They also reduce disease progression, hospitalization and MI. (For further discussion of ACEI therapy generally, see p. 229).

Angiotensin receptor antagonists (ARAs) have a more specific pharmacological action. They provide similar but no greater benefits than ACEIs and are useful where patients cannot tolerate the cough caused by ACEIs. Combinations of ACEIs and ARAs may provide a small additional benefit, presumably owing to a more complete block, but are not currently widely used.

Beta-blockers and partial sympathetic agonists

Trials have convincingly, if rather unexpectedly, demonstrated beneficial effects of conventional beta-blockers such as *metoprolol* in most classes of heart failure. Newer beta-blockers also shown to be beneficial include *bisoprolol* and *carvedilol*; the latter also has an alpha-blocking vasodilator action. These drugs have been shown to reduce hospitalization, disease progression and symptoms, and to reduce significantly all-cause mortality. The resultant increase in survival is greater than that conferred by ACEIs and additional to it. Possible mechanisms include reduction of sympathetic stimulation, heart rate and oxygen demand, and up-regulation of receptors.

The best evidence is for use in NYHA Classes II to III failure. In chronic severe heart failure (Class IV) or acute severe decompensation the myocardium relies on sympathetic drive, so the well-known negative inotropic problem of beta-blockers in heart failure could be hazardous. However, there is even evidence of benefit in this class too. They are particularly indicated in failure associated with IHD. At present their value in the elderly, and in failure with normal systolic function, has not been demonstrated.

Beta-blockers should usually be initiated by specialists, at low doses and with great care, and there may be an initial transient worsening of symptoms. Thus at present most primary care prescribers would seek consultant cardiological opinion before starting patients on them.

The seemingly anomalous use of beta-blockers in heart failure, although it goes against conventional teaching, which has always warned of the danger in this situation, is not without precedent. Beta-blockers are indicated in hypertrophic cardiomyopathy, in which grossly thickened, fibrosed ventricular walls obstruct outflow if systolic contraction is too vigorous. Inotropic agents and venodilators exacerbate this condition.

The realization that beta-blockers can improve the prognosis of most cases of mild to moderate heart failure has changed clinical practice and heart failure management protocols significantly (see p. 206). Because both ACEIs and beta-blockers are effective only in systolic dysfunction, it is important that suspected failure is always investigated echocardiographically to confirm a reduced ejection fraction. As yet, it is unclear whether beta-receptor cardioselectivity (see p. 229) is preferable for heart failure, because myocardial beta-$_2$ receptors may be involved. Evidence of benefit has been shown by both selective (*metoprolol*) and non-selective (*carvedilol*) agents. (For a general discussion of beta-blocker therapy, see p. 227.)

Aldosterone antagonists

In addition to its role in promoting fluid clearance, aldosterone has vasoconstrictor action and promotes myocardial fibrosis. Therefore, the raised levels in heart failure could be significantly maladaptive. Both *spironolactone* and the newer *eplerenone* have been found to improve survival in large trials (RALES and EPHESUS, respectively). They are effective at low doses that have little diuretic effect and are currently third-line agents for more severe failure. Surprisingly, combination with ACEIs does not produce significant hyperkalaemia (which, like the use of beta-blockers in heart failure, is another traditional contra-indication discredited). The more expensive *eplerenone* lacks *spironolactone*'s adverse endocrine effects of gynecomastia, oligomenorrhoea and impotence, and appears to offer benefits in heart failure following MI. For both drugs, careful monitoring of serum potassium is essential, especially in renal impairment.

Digoxin

Recognition of the neuroendocrine complications in heart failure has indicated how the diverse actions of *digoxin* (Table 4.8) may contribute to its beneficial effect, independently of its inotropic action. The precise mechanisms have not been fully elucidated but an important component is the restoration of baroreceptor activity. As heart failure develops, baroreceptor responses to increased atrial and arterial pressure serve to dampen sympathetic outflow and increase parasympathetic activity, protecting the heart from excessive stimulation and loading (p. 181). However, these responses eventually become blunted due to stretch receptor damage from prolonged activation, permitting excess sympathetic activity. *Digoxin* appears to improve baroreceptor function and thus mitigate this counterproductive development. Consequently, noradrenaline (norepinephrine) levels fall, vagal activity increases, contributing to the negative chronotropic action, and myocardial wall stress and peripheral vasoconstriction are both reduced. The activity of the RAAS is also depressed, limiting fluid retention and vasoconstriction.

These observations may explain some possible actions of *digoxin*, but are not sufficient reason for increasing its role, which is still mainly directed at improving cardiac output and is covered in more detail below.

Improve effectiveness: increase cardiac output

In severe heart failure, symptoms may persist despite the measures mentioned above, especially if shock has supervened. Inotropic drugs are then needed. The three main groups, each of which acts at a different site, are the traditional cardiac glycosides, the sympathomimetic amines and the phosphodiesterase inhibitors. They have different roles, advantages and drawbacks and none is regarded as a first agent. All can improve symptoms, although only *digoxin* has been shown to reduce mortality.

Table 4.8   Actions of digoxin and other cardiac glycosides

Pharmacological action	Effect on cardiovascular function	Site or mode of action
Positive inotropic	↑ Contractility	↓ Na/K-ATPase in myocyte
Negative chronotropic	↓ Conduction velocity	Direct (AV node, etc.)
	↓ Heart rate	↑ Parasympathetic activity (vagus)
Reduced sympathetic activity (↓ noradrenaline).	↓ Excessive myocardial stimulation	Restored baroreceptor sensitivity
	Peripheral vasodilatation	• ↓ central sympathetic activity • ↓ noradrenaline (norepinephrine) level
Reduced renin secretion → angiotensin ↓	↓ Fluid retention	Kidney (juxtaglomerular apparatus)
	↓ Peripheral vasoconstriction	• ↓ sympathetic stimulation? • ↓ Na/K-ATPase reduces renin release?

Cardiac glycosides

Action. The traditional role of digitalis glycosides has been as inotropes, mediated by the action in increasing intracellular calcium through inhibition of membrane Na/K-ATPase. The observation that they improve contractility without an increase in myocardial oxygen demand is probably explained partly by their multiple other actions (Table 4.8). These actions may also account for their superiority over conventional inotropes.

Digoxin has a negative chronotropic effect, owing partly to increased vagal activity. This is invaluable when the failure is complicated by atrial fibrillation, and generally it tends to limit oxygen demand. The action on conduction is complex, and includes a negative dromotropic action (slowing conduction times). The negative chronotropic effect is distinct from the positive inotropic effect, the latter usually being observed first.

Note that by contrast the sympathomimetic amines are both positively inotropic and positively chronotropic and so almost always increase oxygen demand. For detailed accounts of the pharmacology of the cardiac glycosides, see the References and further reading section (p. 270).

Side-effects. The principal drawback of glycoside therapy is the narrow therapeutic index, with toxicity sometimes resembling the symptoms being treated, i.e. various arrhythmias (Table 4.9). This problem is compounded by the sensitivity of plasma level and receptor activity to diverse pharmacokinetic and pharmacodynamic factors (Table 4.10). Routine plasma level monitoring is not essential for safe and effective use if there is close monitoring of clinical and toxicological signs. However, it is invaluable where the response is unexpected, or when renal impairment is known or suspected.

Digitoxicity is managed by drug withdrawal and use where appropriate of:

- plasma level measurement of *digoxin*, potassium and creatinine;
- oral potassium;
- *digoxin*-specific antibody fragment (Digibind);
- oral binding agents (e.g. *cholestyramine*);
- occasionally anti-arrhythmic drugs.

Table 4.9 Adverse drug reactions of digoxin

Gastrointestinal	Nausea, anorexia, dyspepsia, vomiting, diarrhoea
Central nervous system	Blurred vision, other visual disturbances
	Confusion, drowsiness
Cardiovascular	Bradycardia, premature ectopic beats, heart block, almost any other arrhythmia

The DIG trial demonstrated that *digoxin* is safer than was previously thought, which implies that previous fears about *digoxin* toxicity were exaggerated and that the toxicity that did occur previously could have been due to inadequate monitoring, or excessive plasma levels.

Role. *Digoxin* has seemed perennially to be on the verge of popular revival, without ever quite making it. Well-organized trials (e.g. RADIANCE, DIG) have improved its image, having demonstrated significant reductions in signs and symptoms with fewer adverse effects than expected, definite deterioration when discontinued and a small reduction in heart failure deaths. However, there was no reduction in all-cause mortality.

Digoxin has a first-line indication only in heart failure associated with atrial fibrillation. Otherwise, its current role is third- or fourth-line in failure not controlled adequately with ACEIs, beta-blockers and spironolactone. Moreover, its target plasma level is now considerably lower than before (<1 ng/ml). It is of no benefit in shock or cor pulmonale (possibly because of hypoxaemia) and has been superseded in severe acute heart failure and after MI by unloading strategies.

Sympathomimetic inotropic amines

Prolonged reflex stimulation of the failing myocardium by the sympathetic nervous system may become counterproductive, resulting in depletion of catecholamines and downregulation of myocardial beta-receptors, with the paradoxical result that although beta-agonists are helpful in some situations, beta-blockers are preferred in others.

Table 4.10   Problems with digoxin therapy

Low therapeutic index – may require plasma level monitoring

Pharmacokinetics
- absorption depends on gut perfusion (may be reduced in heart failure)
- long half-life; easily accumulated but difficult to remove
- highly tissue-bound (myocardial and skeletal muscle) – high volume of distribution
- renal clearance, but renal function may be reduced in heart failure and in the elderly

Interactions, including with other drugs used in cardiac disease
Pharmacokinetic (alter plasma levels), e.g.
- absorption – cholestyramine, sulfasalazine
- non-renal clearance – some CCBs
- renal clearance – quinidine, verapamil
Pharmacodynamic (on the myocardium), e.g. anti-arrhythmics, CCBs

Toxicity
Serious cardiac toxicity
Enhanced by hypokalaemia (e.g. from diuretic treatment), hypomagnesaemia, hypercalcaemia

Myocardial sensitivity increased in:
- ischaemia, e.g. after infarction, in lung disease and cor pulmonale
- hypothyroidism (but sensitivity decreased in hyperthyroidism)
- elderly and infants

CCB, calcium-channel blocker.

Inotropic amines, usually given parenterally, have traditionally been a last resort in refractory failure and shock. They affect a variety of receptors, producing a mixed spectrum of effects (Table 4.11). This is especially true of natural mediators such as *adrenaline* (epinephrine) and *noradrenaline* (norepinephrine), which cause unwanted arterial vasoconstriction that increases afterload and reduces cardiac output. *Isoprenaline* (isoproterenol), an early synthetic agent, causes hypotension and arrhythmias. All raise heart rate and myocardial oxygen demand, sometimes excessively, although this may eventually be offset by increased efficiency.

Dopamine has dose-dependent receptor selectivity. In low doses it has a vasodilator action on dopaminergic receptors, a potentially useful property in shock. At higher doses it also stimulates inotropic beta$_1$-receptors. However, further dose increases result in alpha receptor-mediated vasoconstriction, raising blood pressure and possibly inducing regional ischaemia; it also liberates *noradrenaline* (norepinephrine). *Dobutamine* only affects beta$_1$-receptors and this pure inotropic effect is sometimes preferable. *Dopexamine* has a greater affinity for both cardiac and peripheral beta$_2$-receptors, and there is evidence that in chronic failure, although beta$_1$ myocardial receptors may be down-regulated, the beta$_2$-receptors are not. Its main action is likely to be vasodilatory.

All these agents can only be given parenterally and are limited to specialist use for severe resistant failure in a coronary care unit (CCU). Predominant beta$_2$-agonists, more commonly used in obstructive airways disease, e.g. *salbutamol*, also have peripheral vasodilator actions, which is particularly useful in cor pulmonale. These agents offer more choice in their route of administration, including oral and inhalation, which is beneficial in chronic failure. A particular risk of these drugs is hypokalaemia.

Phosphodiesterase inhibitors
Aminophylline, a methylxanthine, has traditionally been used in acute failure complicated by pulmonary oedema, where bronchoconstriction ('cardiac asthma') is common. As well as bron-

Table 4.11   Pharmacological properties of cardioactive sympathetic agonists and antagonists, including receptors affected

	Positively inotropic (β_1) ISA	Positively chronotropic (β_1) Arrhythmias	Vasodilate[a] (β_2, DA)	Vasoconstrict (α) BP ↑	Negatively inotropic (β_1 block)
Adrenaline (epinephrine)	++	++	+	++	–
Noradrenaline (norepinephrine)	+	++	–	++	–
Isoprenaline (isoproterenol)	++	+++	+	–	–
Dopamine[b]	++	+	+	++	(+)
Dobutamine	++	+	–	+	–
Dopexamine	++	–	++	–	–
Salbutamol	(+)	–	++	–	–
Pindolol	+	–	++	–	–
Carvedilol	–	–	++	–	+

[a] 'Inodilators'.

[b] Levodopa, ibopamine also used.

α, alpha-adrenergic receptor; β_1, beta$_1$-adrenergic receptor; β_2, beta$_2$-adrenergic receptor; DA, dopaminergic receptor; ISA, intrinsic sympathomimetic activity.

–, no activity; (+), minimal activity; +, minor activity; ++, substantial activity; +++, maximal activity.

chodilator activity it has inotropic, diuretic and respiratory stimulant properties. However, xanthines are also arrhythmogenic and increase oxygen demand, and are no longer used.

The bipyridines have inotropic and vasodilator action. *Milrinone, enoximone* and related agents act by a novel mechanism, increasing cardiac output and reducing peripheral resistance with little or no increase in oxygen demand. They improve symptoms and exercise tolerance but increase mortality. They can only be used parenterally and have similar roles and restriction to the sympathomimetic amines.

Calcium sensitizers

Levosimendan, not yet available in the UK, is the first in a new class of drugs that increase contractility without apparent increase in oxygen requirement, are vasodilator and are not arrhythmogenic. It is used parenterally in acute severe decompensated failure where other agents have failed.

Other methods

In severe heart failure that is resistant to drug treatment, an intra-aortic balloon pump (counterpulsation) may be temporarily placed in the thoracic aorta. Synchronized with the ECG, the balloon is inflated during diastole to improve systemic and coronary perfusion. Cardiac transplantation is being seen increasingly as a realistic option in otherwise untreatable end-stage heart failure, especially that caused by cardiomyopathy. Although a satisfactory completely artificial heart is yet to be developed, a number of sophisticated ventricular assist devices are proving useful on a temporary basis for patients awaiting transplantation. Alternatively, these may relieve the damaged heart of its workload for few months, which in some cases may enable a degree of recovery to occur.

Alternative, potentially simpler surgical procedures are currently undergoing development. In cardiac myoplasty a muscular pouch surrounding the heart is fashioned using local chest wall muscle tissue. Surprisingly, this skeletal muscle acquires the structural characteristics of cardiac muscle. Where there is gross ventricular dilatation (dilated cardiomyopathy) the Batista procedure involves remodelling (by excision of a wedge of ventricle), producing a smaller, less stressed chamber.

Another possibility is revascularization, either by bypass or angioplasty, which is becoming a viable option and has shown benefits in patients with evidence of ischaemia even in the absence of angina symptoms.

Reduce symptoms

The above strategies will usually bring about symptomatic improvement such as reduced oedema, fatigue and dyspnoea, an improved sense of well-being and quality of life, and possibly an increased exercise tolerance.

In mild failure the main aim of diuretic therapy may be simply to reduce uncomfortable or unsightly oedema.

The opioids are frequently used in pulmonary oedema, having venodilator, anxiolytic and respiratory depressant actions. This last action is useful in suppressing the inefficient, fast, shallow respiration (tachypnoea) commonly found in pulmonary oedema. In addition, a severely hypoxaemic patient will be given *oxygen*, provided care is taken in chronic pulmonary disease present (see Chapter 5, p. 338).

Reduce progression and prolong survival

Nowadays it is realistic to expect retarded disease progression and increased survival. ACEIs and beta-blockers in particular improve survival in chronic heart failure patients, and this is due in part to a cardioprotective action inhibiting further myocardial damage. Almost all patients with symptomatic heart failure should take them, in the absence of contra-indications.

Drug selection

A summary of the current consensus for drug selection in systolic failure, as recommended by the European Society of Cardiology and NICE, is given in Figure 4.17 (see References and further reading). The main criterion is severity, the strategy being gradually to increase intervention with the addition of more drugs. Few patients are managed by monotherapy. Although most chronic cases can be managed in the community, particular complications such as arrhythmias and pulmonary oedema will require specific additions, while acute failure may require

management in a specialist CCU where parenteral therapy and close haemodynamic and ECG monitoring are available.

Recent trends include the almost obligatory use of ACEIs in most cases (unless contra-indicated), the recommendation for the wider if cautious use of beta-blockers, and the use of *digoxin* in severe cases (even in sinus rhythm).

Asymptomatic (Class I)

ACEIs should be used alone where evidence of systolic dysfunction is discovered, to reduce progression. Systolic dysfunction is indicated by a dilated heart and an ejection fraction below 45% (normal >60%). ARAs can be sustituted where ACEIs are not tolerated.

Patients with atrial fibrillation should be started on *digoxin* straightaway, usually with *warfarin* to protect against stroke from an embolism originating in the atria. Ventricular or supraventricular arrhythmia may require *amiodarone*, but care must be taken with potential *digoxin/warfarin* and *digoxin/amiodarone* interactions.

Mild–moderate (Class II)

Where there are no signs of fluid retention ACEIs can be used alone, titrating the dose up to an effective target level. Oedema is more usually present and diuretics are used in combination with ACEIs. Loop diuretics are routinely used, although thiazides can be used in mild failure, and in the elderly where they are less likely to cause dehydration than loop diuretics. Because diuretics are invariably combined with ACEIs, potassium-sparing adjuncts are not required and may be harmful.

Where fluid retention is particularly resistant, possibly due to a low glomerular filtration rate with poor delivery of diuretic to the tubule, a synergistic diuretic combination may be required for a few days. A loop diuretic with the thiazide *metolazone* is often successful ('sequential nephron blockade'), although any thiazide should work as well. For pulmonary oedema, high doses of loop diuretic may be given with *morphine* and *oxygen* and the patient is nursed sitting almost erect. With high-dose and combi-

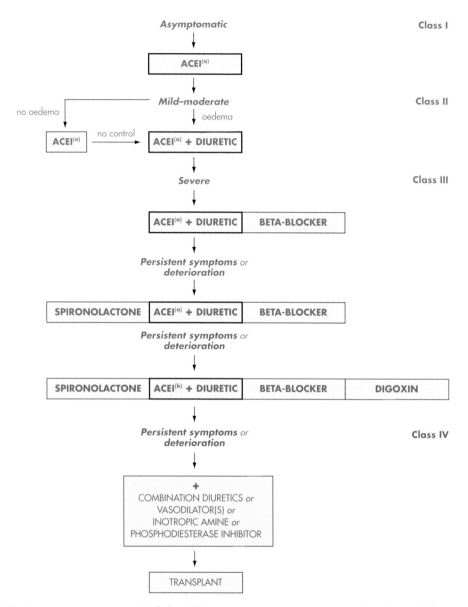

Figure 4.17   Treatment strategy in systolic failure. [a]Angiotensin receptor antagonist may be substituted if ACEI not tolerated. [b]Angiotensin receptor antagonist may be added if further control required. ACEI, angiotensin-converting enzyme inhibitor.

nation diuretics, attention should be paid to the patient's renal function and their serum potassium level, and they require close monitoring.

As the patient improves, the diuretics may be stepped down, although ACEIs should always be continued.

Severe (Class III)

If symptoms persist or the patient deteriorates, a beta-blocker is added. Subsequently, if there is no improvement an aldosterone antagonist should also be added.

Very severe (Class IV)

This stage represents irreversible myocardial damage and the only curative measure is transplantation. The prognosis is otherwise very poor, with a median survival of less than a year. Medical therapy is mainly palliative while awaiting surgery. Various schemes have been devised for the optimum combination of diuretics, arterial dilators and venodilators, based on haemodynamic parameters such as filling pressure and pulmonary venous pressures (see References and further reading).

IV sympathomimetic or dopaminergic inotropes, may be tried but their potential to increase myocardial oxygen demand must always be remembered. None is beneficial in long-term use but they may have a palliative role.

Diastolic failure

This form of heart failure is especially difficult to treat, and there is as yet no reliable trial evidence. Efforts to increase diastolic time with cardiodepressants such as beta-blockers, or with CCBs such as *verapamil*, may be tried. Drugs that reduce preload (and hence diastolic filling) need to be used with great caution: this includes nitrates and diuretics. The only agents to have shown promise are the ARAs.

Hypertension

Definition and epidemiology

For most diseases a population can usually be divided into two fairly distinct groups, 'normal' or 'ill', on the basis of a defining characteristic or measurement. You are either diabetic or not, on the basis of blood glucose; you have airways obstruction or you do not, on the basis of peak expiratory flow. Unfortunately, it is less easy to define normal or abnormal blood pressure because within a given population there is a continuous distribution of blood pressure about a single modal value, although this value varies with age, ethnic group, etc. Figure 4.18 shows

the distribution of diastolic pressure for a Western industrialized population: it is almost uniform, but is skewed towards the higher levels. Clearly, the oft-cited 'normal' levels of 120 mmHg systolic blood pressure (SBP) and 80 mmHg diastolic (DBP) are only a statistical approximation for a majority around the modal value. The majority do lie between 70 and 90 mmHg DBP, but there is a substantial minority above 90 mmHg.

A clear distinction would be invaluable in identifying those who need treatment, because untreated high blood pressure is associated with long-term morbidity and premature mortality. Although the risk to an individual cannot be precisely predicted from their blood pressure, actuarial data confirm that excessive blood pressure is harmful. We know that different population groups with different mean blood pressures have different prevalences of diseases thought to be caused by hypertension. However, these risks are also graded continuously, and the challenge is to know at which point the benefits of treatment (reduced long-term complications) outweigh the harms of treatment (adverse effects, reduced quality of life, etc.). The balance

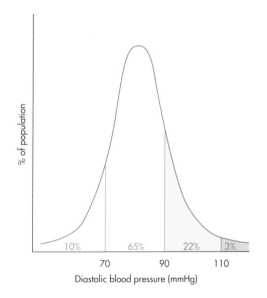

Figure 4.18 Approximate distribution of mean diastolic blood pressure in a Western urban population. The curve shows the skewed but continuous distribution of blood pressure, with a greater proportion above the modal value.

will vary between individuals according to numerous other factors including age and comorbidity (Table 4.12). Generally, the cut-off point has tended to be reduced gradually over the years as less toxic drugs have been developed that reduce the harms of treatment.

Variations in blood pressure

Variations with age and gender were discussed on pp. 183–184. Monitoring of blood pressure over 24 h shows that it varies continuously throughout the day owing to both regular diurnal variation (lower overnight and higher in the morning) and irregular physical and mental stress, as might be predicted from physiology. Thus it is important to standardize the conditions of measurement (see below) if longitudinal comparisons are to be made. Even so, large-scale epidemiological studies have shown a close correlation between single random blood pressure measurements and cardiovascular risk.

Definitions

The first important distinctions to be made are whether the cause of the hypertension is readily identifiable or not, and how elevated the pressure is.

Primary (essential) and secondary hypertension

In about 10% of cases of raised blood pressure there may be obvious reasons (Table 4.13). This is termed **secondary hypertension**; it is often associated with very high pressure and rapid progression, but appropriate therapy (possibly surgical) will often correct the problem.

Table 4.12   Risk factors and aetiological influences in hypertension

Risk factor or aetiological influence	Possible rationale and comment
Major	
Family history	Inherited tendency – probably polygenic
Dietary Na high	Fluid retention; vascular wall oedema; ion pump defect (p. 214)
Obesity	Possible artefact of measurement (problem with arm cuff)?
	Greater perfusion demands of increased body mass
	Reducing weight can reverse borderline HPT
Alcohol	Unknown mechanism; possibly 30% of HPT related to alcohol abuse
Sedentary life	Unknown mechanism; regular exercise lowers BP
Renal disease	Overt or occult renal disease often implicated: cause or effect?
Minor	
Age	See text
Stress or type A personality	Overactive sympathetic nervous system → vasoconstriction and/or raised CO
	Difficult to quantify; effect may have been exaggerated
Dietary	
Ca, K, Mg ↓	Some evidence, especially for K
Saturated fat ↑	May induce vasoconstriction via endothelial interactions
Animal products	Vegetarians may have lower BP
Glucose intolerance	Complex interaction between insulin resistance, hyperlipidaemia and HPT
Race	Increased average BP in urban Blacks: ↑ response to stress or dietary salt?
Smoking	**No** sustained effect on BP itself but greatly exacerbates atherosclerotic complications

BP, blood pressure; Ca, calcium; CO, cardiac output; HPT, hypertension; K, potassium; Mg, magnesium; Na, sodium.

However, in most cases there is usually only a mild or moderate elevation of blood pressure, for which no obvious cause can be found. Moreover, the body resists attempts to lower the pressure. It seems that part of the body's pressure control mechanism (e.g. baroreceptors) has been reset at a higher level: hence the term **essential hypertension**.

Benign and malignant hypertension

Hypertension is called **malignant** or accelerated (terms not strictly synonymous but often used so) when the DBP is above 120 mmHg and usually rising rapidly. Urgent reduction of the pressure is essential to prevent stroke, cardiac failure or renal failure. The prognosis for the 5% or so of hypertensive patients who present with or who develop this form is much poorer than for the majority with **benign** (mild or moderate) hypertension. This is a rather unfortunate, historical misnomer because no degree of hypertension can be described as benign. Malignant hypertension commonly has an underlying renal cause. Most of the following discussion concerns benign essential hypertension.

Diastolic or systolic?

Most attempts to distinguish high blood pressure from the normal range definitions of hypertension allow for the greater proportional rise in SBP than DBP and include intermediate classifications to recognize the continuous variation. Because increased risk is associated with pressures sometimes regarded as normal, an 'optimal' grade has been proposed (Table 4.14).

SBP is inversely proportional to arterial compliance, which declines with age owing to smooth muscle fibrosis and calcification (arteriosclerosis). DBP by contrast reflects the peripheral resistance, a measure of the average size of blood vessel lumens throughout the body, against which the heart has to develop and maintain a pressure.

Because the vasculature is exposed to diastolic pressure for the greater part of the cardiac cycle, it was formerly assumed that DBP was the main

Table 4.13   Causes of secondary hypertension

Possible cause or underlying disease	Raised haemodynamic parameter	
	Peripheral resistance	Cardiac output
Renal/endocrine		
Glomerular damage → ↓ GFR → fluid retention	–	+
Increased renin secretion → angiotensin ↑	+	+
(e.g. renal artery disease)		
Endocrine		
Phaeochromocytoma → adrenaline	+	+
(epinephrine) – very rare		
Cushing's disease/Conn's syndrome →	–	+
aldosterone ↑		
Vasomotor		
Increased intracranial pressure	+	–
(e.g. trauma, tumour)		
Anatomic		
Aortic coarctation (constriction)	+	–
Iatrogenic, e.g.:		
NSAIDs, corticosteroids, oral contraceptives,	+	+
sympathomimetics, MAOIs		

GFR, glomerular filtration rate; MAOI, monoamine oxidase inhibitor; NSAID, non-steroidal anti-inflammatory drug.

+, parameter raised; –, parameter not affected.

Table 4.14   Gradations of blood pressure and hypertension

		Systolic pressure (mmHg)	Diastolic pressure (mmHg)
Optimal		<120	<80
Normal		<130	<85
High normal		130–139	85–90
Mild hypertension	Grade 1	140–159	90–99
Moderate hypertension	Grade 2	160–179	100–109
Severe/Very severe hypertension	Grade 3	≥180	≥110
Isolated systolic hypertension	Grade 1	140–159	<90
Isolated systolic hypertension	Grade 2	≥160	<90

Based on British Hypertension Society Guidelines (BHS-IV), 2004.

marker for the vascular damage that is the main complication of hypertension. Thus most early trials monitored DBP and aimed to reduce it. However, following more recent trials (e.g. Syst-Eur), systolic pressure is increasingly being accepted as an equally or more important prognostic indicator. Because both tend to be elevated in hypertension this is not so important.

However, patients with **isolated systolic hypertension (ISH)** and normal DBP are increasingly recognized. Such patients are at greater risk, but also benefit more from treatment. These tend to be older patients and there was some doubt about the wisdom of aggressive treatment because resultant excessive hypotension or reduced perfusion to vital areas may increase mortality. However, the need to treat ISH is now established and it is recognized in the official classification (Table 4.14). Furthermore, the calculation of an individual's 'cardiovascular risk' (see p. 216) uses SBP not DBP.

Thus, the definition of hypertension is essentially statistical and epidemiological. All that can be done is to mark off certain pressures on either side of the median as bounding the 'normal' limits, and class all others as 'abnormal'. Exactly where this borderline is drawn has changed as understanding of the risks of untreated hypertension has grown and as more effective, less toxic treatments have been developed. Formerly, active treatment was considered only if the DBP was consistently above 100 mmHg. Now, with better and safer drugs the borderline has dropped to 90 mmHg, or even 85 mmHg for

those with several other cardiovascular risk factors, if not all patients.

Prevalence

Estimates of prevalence depend crucially on how hypertension is defined, i.e. what thresholds are assumed. Based on a definition of hypertension as a DBP above 95 mmHg or SBP above 150 mmHg, it has been estimated that there may be 4 million hypertensives in the UK. If a level of 140/90 mmHg is taken as the threshold, the figure will be nearer 20% of the population, i.e. up to 12 million. This shows the difficulty of defining a condition solely on the basis of a physiological measurement that varies continuously throughout the population. There is increasing concern over the potential labelling and 'medicalizing' of large numbers of people on the basis of probability alone, knowing many of them will never develop any complication but will have been made anxious by being diagnosed as 'ill' rather than healthy. A similar dilemma arises with falling thresholds for acceptable cholesterol levels.

Hypotension

The definitions of blood pressure in Table 4.14 imply that no harm is believed to be associated with pressures moderately below 'normal', i.e. 70–80 mmHg diastolic. This is indeed the case in the UK and the USA. In mainland Europe, however, a distinct diagnostic category of what is in effect **essential hypotension** is recognized, a condition usually treated with various drugs including inotropic and pressor agents. Interestingly, evidence is emerging of an adverse prognosis for persons with low blood pressure, with vague and subjective symptoms including depression, tiredness, etc., although as yet it is not a recognized illness in the UK.

This phenomenon must be distinguished from blood pressure low enough to affect normal function or consciousness (as in postural hypotension or shock), and it is necessary to exclude specific pathologies that cause hypotension, such as hypothyroidism or Addison's disease. Moreover hypotension needs to be considered as a potential result of over-treatment of borderline hypertension in the elderly (see below).

Course and prognosis

Hypertension is a chronic, life-long condition with a variable rate of progression and a highly variable prognosis. Being insidious in onset and initially symptomless, it may go undetected for years, and is often discovered incidentally. Yet if untreated the patient will eventually develop one or more of the complications, frequently leading to premature death.

What then are the risks of having too high a blood pressure? After all, if a person asked what blood pressure was for, you might reply that it drove blood round the body. They might then justifiably retort that surely then you could not have too much of it – the more the better. This credibility gap needs to be bridged when a diagnosis is first made, without causing undue alarm. It must be reinforced when adverse drug effects occur in a previously asymptomatic person who has now become a 'patient'.

For although hypertension is almost invariably symptomless for many years there are subtle, sinister pathological processes at work causing long-term damage to the heart and blood vessels, as well as to other vital organs, especially the kidney and eyes. A middle-aged patient with a DBP above 110 mmHg has a 1 in 5 chance of dying within 5 years; a 35-year-old patient with DBP over 105 mmHg has their life expectancy reduced by 15 years compared to a normotensive. The list of conditions from which hypertensives may ultimately suffer reads like a recitation of the ills of civilized man: MI, stroke, heart failure and renal failure. Death is usually from stroke or MI, far more commonly than in normotensives. These risks are related to the duration and severity of the elevated blood pressure. Adequate early treatment can reduce the incidence of complications by up to 50%.

Aetiology

Heredity

Hypertension occurs about equally in men and women, although younger men in particular are more prone to atherosclerotic complications. There is often a family history, but it is probably a susceptibility to hypertension that is inherited and this is only expressed if certain environmental factors are present. Immigrant populations with low mean blood pressures tend to assume the prevalence of the host country. However, certain races have a higher prevalence of hypertension even in mixed societies (e.g. African Americans in the USA), although environmental variables such as diet and response to stress may still contribute to this. There are almost certainly several genes involved.

Many factors may complicate epidemiological studies. In making cross-cultural and international comparisons it is difficult to ensure control for all environmental factors, and to reliably compare blood pressure measurements. Nor, in following the fate of migrant communities, can we always assume that the migrant population is representative of the area of origin (for example, those who choose to migrate may include a higher proportion of those with higher blood pressures). On the other hand, even prenatal influences may be environmental (e.g. maternal diet or smoking), so that a positive family history does not necessarily imply a genetic mechanism.

Environmental factors

Whatever the genetic contribution to susceptibility, environmental factors are extremely
important in the manifestation of the disease
(see Table 4.12) and these factors have to be
addressed in the assessment, management and
education of the hypertensive patient. Because
the precise pathogenesis of hypertension is still
unresolved, the way in which most aetiological
factors contribute to raised blood pressure is
usually unknown.

Controversy still surrounds the various 'salt
hypotheses'. Salt intake is difficult to measure
accurately, and a general correlation both within
and between populations is difficult to demonstrate. Dietary salt restriction, although generally
regarded as beneficial, usually produces disap-
pointingly small reductions in blood pressure.
However, some individuals and some races (e.g.
Black people) do have a 'salt-sensitive' hypertension, in which blood pressure is very responsive
to changes in sodium intake.

Other factors, particularly smoking and hyperlipidaemia, exacerbate the complications of
hypertension (especially atherosclerosis), but do
not contribute significantly to a sustained elevation in blood pressure. Hyperlipidaemia, and by
extension a high fat/cholesterol diet, has been
implicated as a minor independent causal factor
for raised blood pressure, possibly through
interaction with vascular mediators such as
endothelin at the vascular endothelium, but the
popular idea of widespread cholesterol plaques
causing a generalised arterial obstruction is
erroneous.

Certain factors contribute to both hypertension and atherosclerosis, e.g. stress and a
sedentary life. Whether glucose intolerance,
hyperinsulinaemia and insulin resistance
contribute directly to the raised blood pressure
or merely exacerbate the potential for complications is unclear (see Chapter 9, p. 600).

Obesity and lack of exercise are important
factors in modern life that have a significant
hypertensive effect. Alcohol intake, considerably
in excess of that providing the putative beneficial
effect on reducing atheroma, is a major contributor to the overall hypertensive load. Also, many
drugs are hypertensive agents (Table 4.13).

Pathophysiology

Underlying haemodynamic defect

Blood pressure can be expressed as the product
of cardiac output and peripheral resistance, so an
elevated blood pressure means that one or both
of these factors must also be raised. Attention
has traditionally focused on the peripheral resistance, and because this is almost invariably
raised in hypertension, most early theories
tried to account for this increase through an
underlying increased vascular tone.

More recently, the possibility of a raised
cardiac output as a prime cause has been
explored. Fluid retention is known to be an occasional cause of secondary hypertension. This is
readily explained in haemodynamic terms:
blood volume is increased, venous return and
preload are raised and cardiac output rises, at
least initially. However, systemic peripheral resistance would then increase, as part of the normal
autoregulation of blood flow. The aim of this is
to limit the resulting excessive, unnecessary
perfusion of the body. As the peripheral resistance rises, the cardiac output would then return
to normal. When the patient eventually
presents, these compensations will have reached
equilibrium and only a raised peripheral resistance is found.

Pathogenesis

Most theories of essential hypertension implicate
the kidney. This creates a difficulty because renal
damage is also often a consequence of prolonged
hypertension caused by damage to renal arterioles. Thus renal damage found in a patient with
hypertension of indeterminate duration could be
either a cause or a consequence. Indeed, by that
stage a vicious cycle will have been initiated:
renal damage raises blood pressure, which in turn
causes further renal damage. In early hypertension an identifiable renal lesion or functional
impairment can rarely be found, but this does not
mean that subclinical or microscopic damage has
not already occurred. Figure 4.19 illustrates one
theory of how renal damage can initiate, and
then sustain, hypertension.

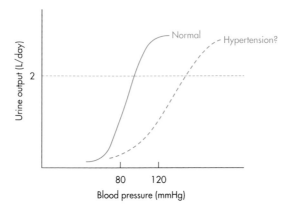

Figure 4.19   'Pressure natriuresis' theory of hypertension. In the figure, urine output is plotted against blood pressure. The solid curve represents the normal response of the kidney to changes in arterial pressure, equivalent to renal perfusion pressure. This is the prime mechanism for the maintenance of blood pressure and body water. Normal urine output assumed to be 1.5–2 L/day. The steepness of the curve around this point shows the brisk diuresis caused by a small elevation in blood pressure, and the rapid fluid retention following any fall in blood pressure. In some hypertensive patients (broken curve) there may be a renal lesion resulting in the kidney needing a higher pressure to clear the same daily fluid load. The CVS then resets barore-ceptors to maintain a sufficiently elevated pressure. In other words, the higher pressure is required for optimal renal function.

Other major theories are summarized in Table 4.15, and Figure 4.20 provides an overview of how some of these proposed mechanisms may interact to alter cardiac output or peripheral resistance. Figure 4.20 shows one possible way in which sodium is implicated, via a defect in the transmembrane sodium pump. In the kidney this defect would impair sodium and water clearance, and in blood vessel smooth muscle it could lead to calcium accumulation and vasoconstriction.

One approach to this, which is helpful for predicting response to treatment, categorizes hypertension on the basis of plasma renin levels, because this appears to correlate with the distinction discussed above between vasocon-striction and expanded blood volume. Some hypertensive patients have raised renin levels and tend to have primary **vasoconstriction**; these patients tend to respond better to drugs that block the RAAS such as ACEIs and beta-blockers. Others have low renin levels, owing possibly to inhibition of the RAAS by salt and **fluid overload**; these patients respond poorly to ACEIs and beta-blockers, and better to diuretics and CCBs. This distinction is supported by the observation that Black people generally fall into the latter category in terms of both their renin levels and their response to antihyperten-sives. As discussed below, this forms the basis is the British Hypertension Society treatment guidelines.

There may be several subgroups of hyperten-sion, in each of which a different mechanism operates. Patients with high renin levels may perhaps have silent renal damage caused by subtle intrarenal ischaemia. On the other hand, a low renin level would be an expected response to hypertension if the renal mechanisms were intact, because of feedback inhibition. It has been speculated that avid salt retention, permitted by low renin, might confer a survival advantage in hotter climates where salt loss can be a problem.

Further detail is not given here because there is still no firm evidence for the most likely mechanism. In the absence of a more defined pathogenesis, the management of essential hypertension generally, and antihypertensive drug selection specifically, remain largely empir-ical. The aim is simply to reduce pressure rather than target underlying pathologies.

Diagnosis and investigation

Measurement

Blood pressure should be measured in a consis-tent and standardized manner. Semi-automatic electronic manometers are rapidly replacing mercury manometers. These are sufficiently accurate provided they are regularly recalibrated. In all cases care must be taken to use the correct cuff size for the patient's arm girth, otherwise readings may be unreliable. The British Hyper-tension Society's recommendations for the procedure include:

- The effects of stress, anxiety, time of day, smoking, alcohol and room temperature should be minimized or standardized.

Table 4.15   Pathogenetic theories of essential hypertension

Site	Lesion	Possible consequences
CV centre	↑ Activity	SNS outflow → vasoconstriction and/or ↑ contractility Arterial baroreceptors reset
Kidney	↓ Na/water clearance	Fluid retention → ↑ CO Renin suppressed?
	(? occult malfunction)	Higher pressure set by CV centre to maintain normal fluid/electrolyte clearance (see Figure 4.19)
	↑ Renin	Vasoconstriction and fluid retention
Circulating Na pump inhibitor	↑ Intracellular [Na]	Vascular wall oedema → ↓ lumen ↑ Intracellular Ca availability and/or ↓ resting membrane potential → vasoconstriction
Endocrine	↑ Renin-angiotensin-aldosterone ↓ Bradykinin-prostaglandin ↓ Atrial natriuretic peptide ↑ ADH	Vasoconstriction and fluid retention ↓ Vasodilatation Vasoconstriction and fluid retention Fluid retention
Arterial structure	Hypertrophy (↑ growth factors?)	↓ Vascular lumen → ↑ PR → ↑ BP → further vascular damage

ADH, antidiuretic hormone; BP, blood pressure; Ca, calcium; CO, cardiac output; CV centre, cardiovascular centre in medulla; [Na], Na concentration; PR, peripheral resistance; SNS, sympathetic nervous system.

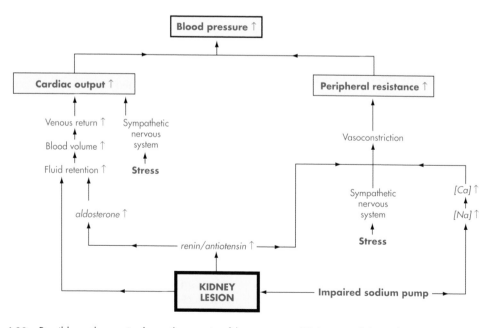

Figure 4.20   Possible pathways in the pathogenesis of hypertension. [Ca], intracellular calcium concentration; [Na], intracellular sodium concentration.

- The patient should have rested for 10 min beforehand, and the procedure should have been explained (this is rare, but obviously sensible).
- The patient may be sitting or lying, as long as the cuff is at heart height.
- The average of two or three readings at any one time should be taken.

The so-called phase 5 recording is recommended to measure DBP; i.e. when sounds completely disappear, rather than just being muffled, as there can be a 5–10 mmHg pressure difference according to the method of recording.

Unless a very high pressure is discovered (i.e. DBP >115–120 mmHg), little need be done at once, although this will depend on the patient's age. Measurements as outlined above should be repeated twice, at intervals of a few weeks. Often the pressure will settle down as the patient becomes familiar with the procedure and their 'white-coat hypertension' subsides. Simply being labelled as hypertensive is stressful, so the diagnosis should not be made lightly, and care taken when explaining it to the patient.

In certain cases where the pressure seems erratic, borderline or resistant to therapy, or when a more objective and reproducible measurement is required, it may be helpful to arrange 24-h ambulatory monitoring. A cuff is connected to a portable, battery-powered electronic manometer that samples pressure over a period of 24 h at approximately hourly intervals to determine the diurnal pattern and compute a mean.

Investigation

There are three aims in investigating a newly diagnosed hypertensive:

1. To discover any primary, perhaps treatable, cause or contributory factor.
2. To identify significant risk factors.
3. To assess the extent of end organ damage.

Clinical examination, simple blood chemistry (urea, electrolytes, glucose and lipids), urinalysis (protein, glucose, cells), CXR and ECG will suffice in most patients. A basic grading derives simply from the blood pressure itself (Table 4.14). However, a global grading that takes into account not just elevation but also duration and possible extent of potential organ damage can be made by ophthalmoscopy (fundoscopy), which assesses the degree of retinal arterial damage. A drug history is also important. These data will serve as a baseline for subsequent monitoring and also reveal clinical signs or biochemical abnormalities suggestive of secondary hypertension. In such cases more invasive investigations would then be needed, including renal function tests and excretion urography, echocardiography and additional blood analysis for corticosteroids, aldosterone, catechols and renin.

At the same time an assessment is made of risk factors both for hypertension and for arterial complications, e.g. smoking, alcohol, body weight, exercise habits, diet, diabetes, stress and family history (Table 4.16), so that an initial plan of general advice for the patient may be devised.

A formal **cardiovascular risk prediction** can then be made. This uses an algorithm that takes into account risk factors such as:

- gender;
- smoking status;
- age;
- SBP;
- ratio of total plasma cholesterol to high-density (HDL) cholesterol (p. 238).

This has been constructed on the basis of epidemiological data, largely from the USA Framingham study. A number of algorithms have been published but the one currently recommended by NICE is that published by the Joint British Societies (BHS IV, 2004). An example is included at the back of the BNF, in the form of nomograms. A person's status is usually expressed as the percentage risk of a cardiovascular event (developing angina, or suffering or dying from MI or stroke) in a specific number of years; for example, a "10–20% risk over the next 10 years". These are used for asymptomatic patients with moderately elevated blood pressure or cholesterol to guide the decision about starting drug therapy.

The aim is to move away from basing treatment decisions solely on inflexible population-based thresholds of a single parameter applicable to all patients (such as blood pressure or cholesterol level), to one where all aspects of an indi-

Table 4.16   Risk factors in hypertensive patient

	Increase risk of hypertension	Increase risk of complications, esp. atherosclerosis
Major modifiable	Na Alcohol Obesity Sedentary life	Smoking Hyperlipidaemia High dietary saturated fat
Major unmodifiable	Family history of HPT Renal impairment	Family history of vascular disease Glucose intolerance
Minor	Age Type A personality Glucose intolerance Race	

See also Table 4.12.

vidual's risk are considered. It thus avoids treating possibly very large numbers of people at perhaps very low risk. The tables also help the patient to understand their personal risk, and which aspects of their life or behaviour are affecting it. This enables them to make a more informed choice about whether or not to start drug therapy.

For patients with higher levels of blood pressure or cholesterol there will usually be a guideline that recommends mandatory primary prevention. However, the tables or charts are not to be used without consideration of the patient's full history. Patients with diabetes in particular, being at far greater risk, are not covered by this approach: any degree of hypertension in diabetics needs vigorous treatment. Also, the data on which they are based derive predominantly from Caucasians, so they are not directly applicable to other races. For example, South Asian immigrants to the UK appear to have a higher risk of CVD than natives for the same risk factor levels.

Clinical features and presentation

Moderate essential diastolic hypertension is symptomless. Complaints of nosebleeds, tiredness or vague headaches usually derive not from raised pressure but from popular misconceptions about hypertension, or possibly concern about the diagnosis itself. However, malignant hypertension certainly may cause severe headaches and other neurological phenomena, known as hypertensive encephalopathy. Consequently, essential hypertension is usually identified opportunistically during routine screening, or life insurance or employment medical examinations. Increasingly, screening by GPs is identifying cases much earlier. Any genuine presenting symptoms will usually have been caused by one of the complications of untreated hypertension (e.g. angina, visual problems). Thus all new cases of heart failure, IHD, etc. are investigated for hypertension.

Complications

The problems caused by a chronically elevated arterial pressure can be largely anticipated from a consideration of the disturbed haemodynamics (Table 4.17). In general, the extent of the damage will be proportional to the increase in pressure and its duration before detection. There are two broad groups of complications, depending on how much the pressure is raised. If pressure is greatly raised there will be direct organ or vascular damage, including heart failure, renovascular disease/malignant hypertension, hypertensive encephalopathy, retinal damage and haemorrhagic stroke. The benefits of blood pressure-reducing interventions are most easily demonstrated in this group. For more modest elevations, most problems are caused indirectly and more chronically by the promotion and acceleration of atheroma formation. These complications are significantly exacerbated by interaction with other common atherogenic risk factors, notably smoking and hyperlipidaemia.

Heart failure

Hypertension was a common cause of heart failure before safe and effective treatment became available. The persistently increased afterload on the left ventricle initially leads to compensatory hypertrophy (remodelling), often seen on the ECG of newly diagnosed hypertensive patients as a higher R-wave (see Figure 4.10). Eventually there is left ventricular dilatation and decompensation.

Arteriosclerosis

Excessive stress on the walls of resistance vessels exposed to elevated pressure stimulates the development of thicker muscular walls in order to withstand it (Laplace's law; p. 178). The resulting hypertrophy of arterial walls, especially arterioles, has several consequences:

- It encroaches on the lumen, narrowing it (remodelling), which reduces end-organ perfusion, causing ischaemia, especially in the kidney.
- Peripheral resistance is further raised (because all arteries throughout the body are affected).
- Arterial compliance falls, which increases afterload and hastens ventricular failure.
- Damaged vascular walls are more prone to aneurysm (bulging) and haemorrhage, especially cerebral vessels.

Atherosclerosis

Perfusion problems are exacerbated by an increased tendency to arterial atheroma, which is encouraged by high pressure and associated blood turbulence. In atherosclerosis (not to be confused with arteriosclerosis), there is focal deposition of lipid-rich fibrous lesions (atheromas) in the inner lining layer of certain arteries. Atheroma, atherosclerosis and thrombosis are all accelerated by hypertension.

Morbidity and mortality

Almost any organ can be affected by these problems, but the heart, brain, kidney, eyes and (particularly if the patient smokes) lower limbs

Table 4.17   Complications of untreated hypertension

Pathology	Pathogenesis	Clinical consequence
Direct effects		
↑ Peripheral resistance	Elevated LV afterload	LV failure
Arteriosclerosis	↑ Wall stress, medial hypertrophy	Renovascular disease → renal failure
		Haemorrhagic stroke, multiple infarcts
		Dementia → hypertensive encephalopathy
		Retinal damage
Indirect effects		
Atherosclerosis	Possible: ↑ fat penetration, vessel wall damage, turbulent flow	Ischaemic heart disease
		Peripheral vascular disease
		Renal failure
		Cerebrovascular disease → thrombotic stroke, multi-infarct dementia

LV, left ventricular.

are especially prone. The results may be heart failure, angina, MI, stroke, renal failure, visual problems or possibly limb amputation: the most common causes of death among hypertensives are stroke and MI. These complications can be prevented or retarded by effective antihypertensive therapy although stroke, heart failure and renal impairment seem to be far more effectively prevented than atheromatous complications such as MI. Ventricular and possibly vascular hypertrophy are partially reversible with optimal treatment.

Assessments of the effect of different treatments on prognosis have sometimes been inconclusive, perhaps because many of the complications are advanced at first diagnosis owing to the silent preclinical progression. Moreover, some antihypertensive drugs, especially beta-blockers and thiazides, may have adverse atherogenic effects.

Management

Decision to treat

In a patient with mild hypertension the most important decision to be made is at what point to initiate drug treatment. In addition to the level of the blood pressure itself, the patient's age and cardiovascular risk must be taken into account in balancing the likely benefits of intervention against the possible harms and reduced quality of life from lifelong drug therapy (Table 4.18).

Numerous protocols exist for determining the threshold for starting drug treatment, notably from the World Health Organization (WHO), the British Hypertension Society, and the American Joint National Committee. Figure 4.21 represents a consensus. At the borderlines of different grades the recommendation is that the patient should be monitored closely over 1–3 months and treatment started or amended if the pressure remains high. Protocols are frequently updated so the reader is urged to check the appropriate sources in the References and further reading section for the latest recommendations.

Table 4.18   Signs of high cardiovascular risk in hypertensive patient, indicating need for earlier drug treatment in hypertension

Risk factor for producing end-organ damage	Evidence of established end-organ damage
Hyperlipidaemia	Retinal damage
Smoking	Renal impairment
Diabetes mellitus	Cardiac enlargement or hypertrophy
Family history of CVD	Cardiac ischaemia (ECG)
Older patient	Angina/past MI
Male sex (younger patient)	Past stroke
	Peripheral vascular disease

See also Tables 4.12, 4.16

Note: there is no direct link across the columns between individual risk factors

CVD, cardiovascular disease; ECG, electrocardiogram; MI, myocardial infarction.

Severe hypertension

Very severe hypertension (i.e. above 210/120 mmHg) represents a medical emergency, with the risk of encephalopathy, renal damage or haemorrhagic stroke. Nevertheless, this is not corrected too aggressively because a rapid fall in blood pressure can compromise cerebral perfusion. Parenteral therapy is generally avoided, a smooth fall over a number of hours being preferred, and this can be attained effectively with oral therapy (e.g. *ACEI, hydralazine, labetalol*). IV *nitroprusside* is reserved for established hypertensive encephalopathy and other situations of immediate danger.

For pressures consistently above 110 mmHg diastolic and/or 180 mmHg systolic, the normal treatment protocol (see below) should always be initiated.

Moderate hypertension

A DBP of 100–110 mmHg and/or SBP of 160–180 mmHg should probably always be treated, but in the absence of risk factors observation over 4 weeks is suggested to see if the pressure can be reduced with conservative

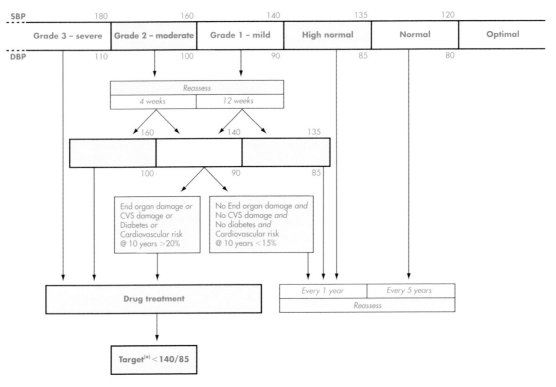

[a]If high cardiovascular risk, reduce target to 130/80

Figure 4.21   Treatment thresholds in hypertension.

general measures (see below). It must be remembered that there is clear evidence that older patients benefit as much from treatment as younger ones, especially in the reduction of stroke.

Mild hypertension

The current UK consensus (British Hypertension Society) is that a DBP of 90–100 mmHg and/or SBP of 140–160 mmHg only need immediate attention in those already showing complications or with specific risk factors, and drug treatment is rarely justified below this.

Some cardiologists caution against over-vigilance. Patients with marginal or illusory disease, especially the elderly, are perhaps being over-diagnosed and over-treated. In older patients there may be less time for the complications to become significantly limiting, and in the meantime reduced pressure might compro-

mise cerebral or coronary perfusion. Thus therapy might cause more problems immediately than it might prevent in the future, and lowering blood pressure below 80–85 mmHg may be associated with an increased mortality from IHD. There is some evidence for a J-shaped mortality curve for blood pressure, with mortality lowest around 80 mmHg diastolic and rising at pressures not only higher but also lower than this. This might explain the failure to demonstrate a reduction in IHD mortality in some hypertension trials. However, this relationship has not been conclusively demonstrated and most evidence supports similar treatment of the elderly to younger persons, with comparable benefit.

Isolated systolic hypertension

Although raised SBP without a raised DBP was formerly regarded as less dangerous, it has been shown to be associated with similarly increased mortality. In particular the Syst-Eur trial showed a significant benefit in treating SBP above 150 mmHg in the elderly, with less stroke and less dementia.

Aim and strategy

From a community perspective the management of hypertension, although improving, is still far from ideal. Detection rates are increasing but it is still estimated that up to half of cases remain undiagnosed at any given time. Of those diagnosed, half may be sub-optimally treated. Of those prescribed optimal treatment perhaps no more than half are normotensive, owing to inadequate compliance or other problems. Thus active screening and follow-up monitoring are crucial. Furthermore, pharmaceutical care is important in ensuring optimal prescribing, patient comprehension and concordance.

Strategy

NICE has issued guidance to cover the management of hypertension in primary care, and much of the following is based upon this. The general strategy in managing hypertension follows several stages:

- Ensure that blood pressure is genuinely elevated by repeat measurements.
- Decide a target for reduced pressure.
- General measures: reassurance; health education; advice on lifestyle.
- Non-drug interventions.
- Optimal drug monotherapy.
- Combined drug therapy.
- Regular monitoring.

Target blood pressure

The recommended objective for hypertension treatment has gradually been reduced as the risk–benefit ratio changes, as already noted. New studies with safer drugs, such as the HOT (Hypertension Optimal Treatment) trial, have produced greater reductions in morbidity and mortality by targeting lower pressures, with no significant increase in adverse effects. The British Hypertension Society recommends aiming for 140/85 mmHg in patients without complica-

tions and 130/80 mmHg for those with a high CVD risk or renal damage.

General measures

Because hypertension is a chronic progressive disease, lifelong monitoring and usually a progressively increasing level of intervention will be required. In such an insidious, symptomless condition the patient's cooperation and compliance are essential, and patient education is an important means of securing concordance. Ultimately the decision rests with the patient: imposed medical edicts are no longer acceptable. The initial plan should be to counsel and to educate the patient about their disease, but perhaps suggest nothing positive at first. A mildly elevated blood pressure, discovered incidentally, will often return to normal within a few months and may remain so for several years.

The notion of a general change in habits and way of life should be introduced next. Simple psychotherapy or 'brief counselling' (an informal but structured targeted session of 5–10 min) is sometimes helpful, e.g. engendering the idea of a combined effort of health workers and patient to conquer the condition. Continuous encouragement and reassurance are important. Scare tactics are almost invariably unhelpful: the history of anti-smoking propaganda teaches us this, even though the connection between smoking and its respiratory consequences is far more obvious.

Suitable advice and recommendations at this stage are summarized in Table 4.19. Measures are included to reduce both blood pressure and the risk of arterial complications. Alas, this is not a list to endear the clinician to an otherwise healthy, apparently fit and symptomless patient.

A moderate reduction in sodium intake is a realistic goal, especially if done by simply cutting down on added salt. The ideal is about 6–9 g sodium chloride daily (100–150 mmol Na). By analogy with sugar intake and the 'sweet tooth', the subjective saltiness of food may be relative, determined in part by average consumption. If intake is reduced, eventually less salt will taste equally salty as the salt content of saliva is reduced. However, very low-salt diets are unappetizing, result in poor compliance and are of arguable benefit, especially because salt reduction rarely produces blood pressure falls

Table 4.19   Non-drug measures to reduce blood pressure or hypertensive complications

	Reduce blood pressure	Reduce complications
Reduce salt intake	+	
Increase potassium intake	(+)	
Hypnosis, biofeedback	+	
Reduce stress:	+	+
relaxation techniques, yoga, meditation		
Moderate alcohol intake	+	(+)
Aim for ideal body weight	+	+
Moderate exercise	+	+
Reduce saturated fat/cholesterol intake	(+)	+
Stop smoking		+

+, definitely desirable; (+), possibly beneficial.

greater than about 5 mmHg (except in those patients with 'salt-sensitive' hypertension). An overall reduction in the salt added to processed foods might be more beneficial in reducing community hypertension prevalence than individual targeting. A moderate increase in potassium intake (e.g. in fresh fruit and vegetables) may also be helpful: the most important factor could be a lowering of the dietary Na/K ratio.

The role of calcium and magnesium supplements is dubious. Diets low in fat and cholesterol may be both anti-atherogenic and hypotensive. Achieving the ideal body weight should be encouraged. The role of pharmacists in smoking cessation is well established. Exercise is important and a very efficient method of lowering blood pressure: even modest increases can be very beneficial. As few as three half-hour sessions a week at less than 50% maximum capacity can be enough to produce sustained falls of up to 10 mmHg. Cholesterol also falls and exercise capacity increases.

Non-drug interventions

Encouraging results have been obtained with non-invasive techniques to reduce blood pressure. Some may act by reducing stress: for example, moderate routine aerobic exercise (such as walking a few miles a day), biofeedback (where the patient monitors their own blood pressure and consciously tries to lower it), relaxation therapy, hypnotherapy and meditation. The effectiveness of these approaches very much depends on patient preferences and health beliefs.

Pharmacotherapy

Despite the best efforts of clinician and patient, the above measures rarely produce more than a modest fall of about 5–10 mmHg, even when combined, and the effect is not permanent. Blood pressure eventually starts to rise again and most patients then require active treatment. Furthermore, many drug regimens, after working effectively for some time, gradually fail to control the condition. This may be because of poor compliance with drug therapy or general measures, progression of the condition, or the body's reflex (though maladaptive) defence of the abnormal pressure.

General principles. The philosophy of 'stepped care' in treating hypertension means a progressive increase in intervention to maintain control. At one time it also implied a fairly rigid sequence of specific drugs at specific stages: nowadays a more tailored approach is used. The general sequence and important general considerations are summarized in Table 4.20.

Patients are likely to be taking antihypertensive drugs for the rest of their lives so it is important to use agents with the fewest adverse effects first, at the minimum effective dose, and to monitor therapy regularly. Compliance can be increased by minimizing the number of daily doses using long-acting agents or modified-release formulations.

Table 4.20   Principles of drug therapy in hypertension

- As few drugs as possible
- As few daily doses as possible
- Start with most suitable initial drug[a]
- Increase the dose gradually until adequate effect achieved
- If primary failure, substitute another suitable drug from different group
- If effectiveness declines, add another agent rather than substitute
- Combine agents acting by different mechanisms
- Combine agents tending to reduce each other's adverse actions
- Monitor adverse reactions and patient compliance regularly

[a] No contra-indications, least toxic, best tolerated, most suitable to established organ damage; see Figure 4.25.

Any new dose level must be given for several weeks to achieve both pharmacokinetic and, more importantly, biological steady state. Some drugs, notably the thiazide diuretics and the beta-blockers, have a non-linear dose–response curve that plateaus early, so that maximum clinical effect is achieved at little above the minimum effective dose. In contrast, adverse effects are usually dose-dependent so it is counterproductive to increase the dose if adequate control with these drugs is not achieved.

Details of specific drug selection, indications and contra-indications are considered below.

Continuous cover. There is evidence that complications are lessened if the antihypertensive effect is as consistent as possible throughout the day. It is likely that variability in blood pressure contributes to end-organ damage independently of absolute pressure levels. For example, the diurnal morning surge in blood pressure is thought to be a trigger for CVS events such as MI and stroke. Thus during development of antihypertensive drugs, particularly long-acting (once daily) ones, which are known to be desirable for improved compliance, the ability of a drug to sustain its effect is evaluated. One parameter used is the trough : peak (T/P) ratio, which is the blood pressure reduction recorded before the next dose compared to the maximum blood

pressure reduction attained following the last dose. The ideal would be 1, but a minimum value of 0.5 is recommended by US FDA guidelines. Note that peak and trough in this context do not refer to plasma levels. Thus whatever dosage regimen is used, it should aim to produce a sustained reduction of blood pressure with minimal variability. This objective has not yet been incorporated into UK guidelines.

Combination therapy. Antihypertensive drugs act on many different sites or mechanisms that the body uses to maintain blood pressure (Figure 4.22). Thus, if control is not achieved by the optimal dose of one type there are several advantages to combining two or failing that even three agents:

- Additive or possibly synergistic effect.
- Reduced individual adverse effects.
- Mutual antagonism of adverse effects.

When choosing a drug to be added, one from a different group should be added to the regimen to give an additive or possibly synergistic effect, ensuring that adverse interactions are avoided (see below).

Combinations can minimize adverse effects in two ways: firstly by keeping individual doses low and secondly by specific antagonism. In hypertension the body's blood pressure control mechanisms have been reset to maintain an abnormally high pressure, so that when a drug lowers pressure by interfering with one mechanism, e.g. by dilating arterioles, the body eventually responds by recruiting another, e.g. tachycardia or fluid retention, in an attempt to raise pressure again. Thus diuretics can cause palpitations (tachycardia) and renin release, and vasodilators can cause fluid retention (with possible oedema) and tachycardia. However, diuretics will counteract oedema and beta-blockers will prevent tachycardia and renin release. Furthermore, vasodilators will counteract the peripheral vasoconstriction that occurs with beta-blockers (causing cold hands and feet). Thus the combination of all three is logical if blood pressure warrants it.

Fixed-dose proprietary combination products are indicated only occasionally, owing to the usual problems of being unable to manipulate the doses of components independently, and

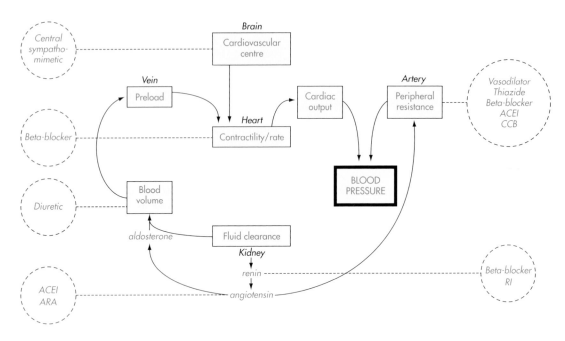

Figure 4.22   Proposed targets and haemodynamic actions of antihypertensive drugs. CCB, calcium channel blocker; ACEI, angiotensin-converting enzyme inhibitor; ARA, angiotensin-II receptor antagonist; RI, renin inhibitor. Central sympathomimetic, e.g. methyldopa.

the difficulty of ascribing adverse effects. One strategy is first to stabilize the patient on the individual components separately and then to introduce a combined product, if a suitable one is available, to aid compliance.

Monitoring

Regular follow-up is essential to monitor compliance with therapy, possible adverse drug effects and disease progression, especially complications. Pharmacists have a role in promoting and reinforcing this process, through repeat prescribing, supplementary prescribing and involvement in chronic disease management programs.

Drugs used in hypertension

This section first discusses the properties of the various groups of antihypertensive agents and concludes by reviewing the rationale for drug selection.

Mode of action

Figure 4.22 shows the possible sites of action of common antihypertensive agents; their general haemodynamic actions are summarized in Table 4.21. However, their modes of action in hypertension are often uncertain and some may act by more than one mechanism.

All antihypertensive agents, either directly or indirectly, affect cardiac output or peripheral resistance. However, cardiac output is rarely raised in essential hypertension, and long-term reduction would compromise exercise tolerance or even resting systemic perfusion. So when we reduce cardiac output we rely on subsequent reflex vascular autoregulation to dilate vessels and decrease resistance in response to the reduced perfusion, thus restoring normal output. Recall that the effect on cardiac output of reducing the afterload varies according to whether the myocardium is unimpaired or in failure (Figure 4.4).

Table 4.21   Antihypertensive drugs classified haemodynamically

Cardiac output reduced	Peripheral resistance reduced	Examples
Beta-blocker	Beta-blocker	Atenolol
Diuretics	Thiazide diuretic	Bendroflumethiazide
ACEI	ACEI	Captopril, enalapril
ARA	ARA	Losartan
RI	RI	Aliskiren
	CCB	Nifedipine, diltiazem
	Direct-acting vasodilator	Hydralazine, nitroprusside, minoxidil, diazoxide
	Alpha-blocker	Prazosin, doxazosin, labetalol, phentolamine
	Centrally acting sympathomimetic	Methyldopa, clonidine[b]
	Centrally acting selective imidazoline receptor agonist[a]	Clonidine[b], moxonidine
	Adrenergic neurone blocker[a,b]	Guanethidine

[a] Often classed as vasodilators.

[b] Rarely used now.

ACEI, angiotensin-converting enzyme inhibitor; ARA, angiotensin-II receptor antagonist; CCB, calcium-channel blocker; RI, renin inhibitor.

Diuretics

These cause a small sustained reduction in blood volume, and as a consequence also in cardiac output, but how far this contributes to their action remains unclear. They also promote vasodilatation, partly due to autoregulation. The thiazides are more effective in hypertension than the more powerful loop diuretics, partly because they have a direct vasodilator action and partly because they generally have a longer duration of action (although loop diuretics may be given twice daily).

Angiotensin-converting enzyme inhibitors and angiotensin receptor antagonists

Angiotensin-converting enzyme inhibitors (ACEIs) act at several sites crucial to blood pressure maintenance, which probably accounts for their considerable success, although doubt still surrounds the principal antihypertensive mechanism. The most likely explanation is that inhibition of angiotensin production causes both a direct reduction of arteriolar vasoconstriction and a secondary reduction of aldosterone-induced fluid retention. At least two other mechanisms may contribute. Angiotensin-converting enzyme (ACE) is also responsible for the breakdown of vasodilatory bradykinin, so kinin levels rise when ACE is inhibited (causes the cough and angio-oedema associated with ACEIs; see below). There may also be a direct vascular action inhibiting local angiotensin-induced vessel wall hypertrophy; in untreated hypertension this hypertrophy contributes to the long-term vascular complications.

Angiotensin receptor antagonists (ARAs) have very similar therapeutic actions. However, because they act directly on the angiotensin receptor rather than the converting enzyme that activates angiotensin, they do not inhibit the breakdown of bradykinin so do not cause a cough. Renin inhibitors are being evaluated.

Calcium-channel blockers

The mode of action of calcium-channel blockers (CCBs) is complex because the different calcium channels and associated receptors have not been fully characterized. There are at least two types of calcium channel, associated with different tissues: the L-type (in smooth muscle, including myocardium) and the T-type (in nodal/neuronal tissue). Existing agents block either the former only, or both.

A further distinction between target tissues is in the post-receptor excitation coupling involving calcium. In cardiac muscle cells CCBs are synergistic with beta-blockers. Normally, adrenergic stimulation of adjacent beta-adrenergic receptors opens the calcium channel, leading to an increase in intracellular calcium concentration. This promotes the Ca^{2+}-troponin C interaction that eventually leads to contraction. Thus beta-blockers and CCBs have similar, synergistic inhibitory effects; in the heart, this negative inotropism and chronotropism can lead to severe depression of contractility. By contrast, in peripheral vascular smooth muscle, intracellular calcium interacts with calmodulin to promote contraction, whereas beta-stimulation inhibits this. Thus beta-blockers cause vasoconstriction but CCBs promote relaxation; indeed, CCBs will antagonize the peripheral constriction sometimes experienced with beta-blockers.

The two main CCB groups, the dihydropyridines (or DHPs, e.g. *nifedipine, amlodipine*) and the non-DHPs (*diltiazem* and *verapamil*), bind to different receptor sites within the calcium channel. More importantly, they have different affinities for target tissues. The non-DHPs are more active on cardiac and nodal tissue, the DHPs preferentially target vascular smooth muscle.

Beta-blockers

By inhibiting the intracellular adenylate cyclase/kinase system, beta-blockers effectively prevent calcium entry into cells, so reducing sarcoplasmic calcium concentration. This inhibits both smooth muscle contraction and tissue conduction, and explains their similar spectrum of activity to CCBs. The negative inotropic action of the beta-blockers will certainly reduce cardiac output, but there are other possibilities. Thus beta-blockade reduces renin release and peripheral adrenergic (vasoconstrictor) tone and there may also be central actions. Long-term reduction in peripheral resistance is an important overall effect.

Other vasodilators

This diverse and lesser used group of drugs acts on arteriolar tone at a variety of different sites, both locally and through the autonomic nervous system (Figure 4.22 and Table 4.21). Thus vasodilators with different modes of action may be combined.

Clinical use

Diuretics

Thiazide diuretics have long been first-line drugs, owing principally to their low toxicity and the fact that they were among the first to have been convincingly shown to reduce mortality in hypertension. They have numerous potentially adverse metabolic or biochemical effects on plasma lipids, glucose, urate and potassium (Table 4.22). The contribution of these adverse effects to cardiovascular morbidity and mortality via arrhythmias, glucose intolerance and atheroma is uncertain. In addition, they can cause impotence (erectile dysfunction) in males, seriously impairing quality of life.

Nevertheless, thiazides are still recommended by many authorities (e.g. NICE and the British

Table 4.22   Advantages and disadvantages of thiazide diuretics in hypertension

Advantages	Disadvantages
Cheap	Metabolic effects – altered blood chemistry:
Effective	• ↓ K, ↓ Ca, ↓ Mg
Proven to reduce mortality	• ↑ glucose
Well tolerated	• ↑ lipid
Single daily dose	• ↑ urate
Little acute toxicity	• hyponatraemia/dehydration, especially in elderly
Suitable in:	Impotence
• Blacks	
• elderly	
• renal impairment[a]	

[a] Use loop diuretics in severe renal impairment; otherwise, thiazides usually used.

Hypertension Society) as first-line drugs for mild to moderate hypertension (for certain patients, see below). One reason is that at low doses (e.g. *bendroflumethiazide* 1.25–2.5 mg daily), they are almost equally as effective as at the originally recommended higher dose (5 mg), but cause significantly fewer adverse effects. This is because the dose–response curve for an antihypertensive effect reaches a plateau at quite low doses, whereas the dose–adverse effect curve is more linear (Figure 4.23); thus raising the dose increases the side-effects with no increase in therapeutic effect.

Potassium supplementation, which used to be routinely co-prescribed, although poorly tolerated and poorly complied with, is at this dose rarely needed. Besides, thiazides are increasingly used in combination with potassium-sparing diuretics or ACEIs. If potassium supplements are used in these circumstances the risk then is of hyperkalaemia rather than hypokalaemia.

Choice. There is little to choose between the available thiazides; *bendroflumethiazide* is among the cheapest. Most may be given once each morning. They seem particularly beneficial in Blacks, whose hypertension is often volume-dependent, and in the elderly because of their freedom from acute toxicity in low doses. In renal impairment loop diuretics are required, but these diuretics are otherwise avoided because they act briefly and so do not provide sustained control; they also lack the direct vasodilator effect of thiazides.

Beta-blockers

The generally mild and predictable adverse effects and wide choice available within this group meant that for a long time they were usually first-line therapy for newly diagnosed hypertension. However, serious doubts were first raised by the ASCOT-BPLA and ALLHAT trials and they were confirmed by subsequent meta-analysis. It was found that beta-blockers (particularly *atenolol*) were not as effective as ACEIs and CCBs in the primary prevention of cardiovascular complications, despite having comparable hypotensive potency. Moreover, beta-blockers have been shown to cause a relatively high incidence of diabetes on long-term use. This prompted NICE in 2006, in collaboration with the British Hypertension Society, to cease recommending beta-blockers as initial treatment.

Their precise role in multiple drug therapy for resistant hypertension, and whether certain beta-blockers are less acceptable than others, has yet to be decided. At present they still have an important role in hypertension associated with IHD (especially following MI) or stable heart failure. Further, patients already stabilized and well controlled on beta-blockers, experiencing no problems, should continue. On the other

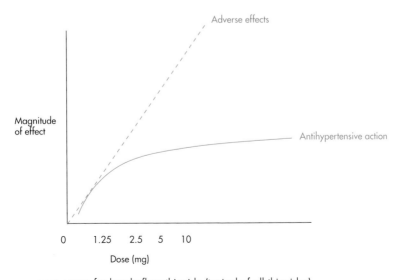

Figure 4.23   Dose–response curves for bendroflumethiazide (typical of all thiazides).

hand, patients taking beta-blockers who are not well controlled should be considered for stepping down and stopping them, converting the patient to the scheme discussed below (see Figure 4.25).

Dose. As with diuretics, recommended doses of beta-blockers have been reduced (e.g. *atenolol* 50 mg daily) with no loss of antihypertensive action, but reduced adverse effects. Once- or twice-daily dosing is usually sufficient because the effect of beta-blockade is not directly related to plasma level. For once-daily dosing, to improve compliance, drugs with a longer half-life (e.g. *atenolol*), or modified-release formulations may be used. The dose should start low and be increased gradually. Should it be necessary to stop therapy, the dose must be tapered off equally slowly, especially in those with IHD, to reduce the risk of rebound adrenergic over-stimulation causing tachycardia, ischaemia, hypertension, etc.

Side-effects, contra-indications and cautions. The well-understood dose-related and physiologically predictable adverse effects are summarized in Table 4.23. Probably as a result of a combination of these, beta-blockers can significantly reduce the quality of life of some patients. Cautions and contra-indications can be anticipated from the adverse effect profile. Beta-blockers must be used with extreme caution in obstructive airways disease, and probably not at all in asthma, although cardioselective ones can be cautiously introduced under specialist advice in mild asthma. They should also be avoided in peripheral vascular disease, Raynaud's syndrome, bradycardia and heart block. Their use in heart failure is discussed on p. 201.

In patients with diabetes given beta-blockers, early physiological responses to developing hypoglycaemia (hunger, tachycardia, etc.) and the patient's perception of these effects are dimin-

Table 4.23   Side-effects and contra-indications of the beta-adrenergic blocking drugs

Site	Side-effect	Caution or contra-indication[a]
Bronchial smooth muscle[b,c]	Bronchoconstriction	C/I in obstructive airways disease; depends on severity
Peripheral arterioles[b,c]	Vasoconstriction: cold hands and feet; muscle weakness; fatigue	C/I in peripheral vascular disease, Raynaud's syndrome; use agent with intrinsic sympathomimetic activity
Myocardium[c] • negative inotropic • negative chronotropic	Fatigue, reduced exercise tolerance Bradycardia	Use with caution in heart failure[d] C/I in bradycardia, heart block
Systemic beta-receptors[b]	Atherogenic dyslipidaemia ($\uparrow$ triglyceride; $\downarrow$ HDL) $\downarrow$ Response to hypoglycaemia	Care in dyslipidaemia Care in diabetes or impaired glucose tolerance
Pancreas[b]	Reduced insulin secretion; possible hyperglycaemia	Care in type 2 diabetes
Central nervous system[e]	Nightmares, confusion, depression, psychotic reactions Impotence and reduced libido – may reduce compliance	Avoid evening dose; avoid lipophilic agents Counsel

[a] Contra-indication (C/I) may be relative or absolute.
[b] β blockade; effect more prominent with non-selective agents.
[c] Effect offset in agents with intrinsic sympathomimetic activity.
[d] May be used in certain circumstances; see p. 201.
[e] Effects more common or severe with lipophilic agents.

ished, with potentially serious, though fortunately rare, results. In type 2 diabetes, insulin release may be inhibited, which aggravates hyperglycaemia and impairs control (see Chapter 9, p. 586). Thus in general they should be avoided in hypertensive patients with diabetes.

Choice. All beta-blockers have equivalent antihypertensive activity. Three main properties yield criteria for differentiating beta-blockers (Figure 4.24). Possible adverse effects and precautions (Table 4.23) further qualify choice.

Cardioselectivity is conferred by a greater affinity for beta$_1$-receptors, located mainly on the myocardium, compared with beta$_2$-receptors (most other beta-adrenergic sites). Cardioselectivity is relative and is less marked at higher doses. Nevertheless, selective agents are preferred in all but those few indications where information on their use is inadequate, such as hypertrophic cardiomyopathy, thyrotoxicosis, migraine and immediately after an MI. Respiratory, metabolic and peripheral vasoconstrictor effects (mediated via beta$_2$-receptors), are still seen, and even selective agents are potentially hazardous in patients with severe asthma.

Intrinsic sympathomimetic activity (ISA, partial agonist activity) may offset broncho-constriction, peripheral vasoconstriction and myocardial depression in some patients. The vasodilator action is perhaps the most useful. *Pindolol* has the greatest ISA. A similar effect is achieved in agents that have additional alpha-blocking activity (*labetalol, carvedilol*). *Celiprolol* combines highly selective beta$_1$-blocker with selective beta$_2$-stimulant activity, which also counteracts peripheral vasoconstriction. *Nebivolol* has vasodilating activity via a NO mechanism.

Lipophilic beta-blockers, as expected, cross the blood–brain barrier and require hepatic metabolism before elimination. Central beta-blockade can cause CNS disturbances, most marked with *propranolol*. Hepatic clearance means potentially low bioavailability (owing to first-pass metabolism) and a shorter half-life (unless there are active metabolites). *Pindolol* and *timolol* are cleared both renally and hepatically, making their elimination less susceptible to impairment of either system.

ACEIs

ACEIs seem to interfere with quality of life less than other antihypertensive agents, particularly important in lifelong treatment. They are now

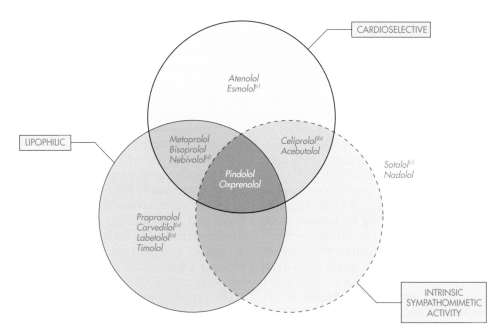

Figure 4.24 Classification of adrenergic beta-blockers. [a]Alpha- and beta-blockade. [b]Beta$_2$-agonist. [c]Mainly used as anti-arrhythmics. [d]Nitrate-like vasodilator action.

often used as first choice in moderate hypertension in combination with a diuretic, as well as in severe resistant hypertension regardless of renin levels because they effectively combat the raised renin levels induced by diuretics. Combination with CCBs or beta-blockers is also successful. ACEIs are especially useful in diabetic hypertension because they protect against nephropathy (see Chapter 9, p. 603). ACEIs have an undisputed place as sole therapy in renovascular, high-renin hypertension.

ACEIs are proving to be remarkably free of the adverse effects common with other potent antihypertensive agents, both serious (central, postural, dysrhythmic and metabolic) and simply troublesome (fatigue, sexual and mental impairment). Most, apart from *lisinopril* and *captopril*, are prodrugs activated in the liver.

Side-effects, contra-indications and precautions (Table 4.24). The main problems with ACEIs are related to their potent antihypertensive and anti-aldosterone actions. Severe first-dose hypotension may occur, particularly in volume- or salt-depleted patients such as those already on diuretic therapy. Sometimes patients are initiated on a low dose of the short-acting *captopril* given at night to test their reaction, and switched to a longer-acting preparation if successful; alternatively low initial doses of long-acting drugs such as *perindopril* or *lisinopril*, and careful titration, can minimize this problem. If possible, diuretics should be stopped a day before starting ACEI therapy, and reintroduced carefully if necessary under medical supervision. Significant hyperkalaemia may follow concomitant use of potassium-sparing diuretics or potassium supplements. Rarely, severe hypersensitivity reactions (i.e. angio-oedema, with fatal laryngeal obstruction) have occurred.

The possibility of severe renal impairment is related to hypotension, especially if there is pre-existing renal disease, owing to reduced renal perfusion pressure. A particular problem is bilateral renal artery stenosis (usually atherosclerotic in origin). In such cases the blood pressure is being kept high by elevated renin levels in order to maintain renal perfusion. Inhibition of the RAAS may then produce a disastrous fall in blood pressure, even precipitating acute pre-renal failure. In the elderly, caution is even advised

Table 4.24 Side-effects of the angiotensin-converting enzyme inhibitors

Side-effect	Comment
Hypotension	Common, especially first dose effect
	Especially if hypovolaemic, hyponatraemic, or on diuretics
Renal impairment/ failure	Especially with renal artery stenosis, pre-existing renal disease, cardiac failure or on NSAIDs
Hyperkalaemia	Avoid potassium-sparing diuretics, potassium supplements, NSAIDs
Dry cough	If persistent, change to ARA
Angio-oedema	Rare; bradykinin-related?
Neutropenia/ agranulocytosis	Rare
Proteinuria, impaired taste, skin rash	Rare; only captopril in high doses?

ARA, angiotensin receptor antagonist; NSAID, non-steroidal anti-inflammatory drug.

with ACEIs in unilateral stenosis. Peripheral vascular disease or other evidence of widespread atheroma would suggest the possibility of renal artery stenosis and indicate the need for avoidance or careful monitoring.

Persistent dry cough affects up to 20% of patients. It is probably due to excess bradykinin (which is usually metabolized by ACE), and sometimes proves intolerable, in which case an ARA can be substituted.

Initial reports of bone marrow toxicity (neutropenia) with *captopril* resulted from the use of unnecessarily high doses. Moreover, these and some other adverse effects, e.g. taste disturbance and skin rash, may be immunologically based, and related to the sulphydryl group found in *captopril* but not later ACEIs (see also *penicillamine*; Chapter 12, p. 772). Rarely, neutropenia can occur with any of the ACEIs.

The principal drug interaction of the ACEIs, apart from that with potassium-sparing diuretics, is with NSAIDs. Partly through their action on intrarenal PGs, NSAIDs used in combination with ACEIs can result in a reduced anti-hypertensive effect, increased renal toxicity and increased potassium retention.

Renin inhibitor. Recently released is *aliskiren*, a direct inhibitor of renin, which works upstream in the renin/angiotensin cascade.

Angiotensin-II receptor antagonists

At present, the only strong indication for this group is when ACEIs are not tolerated. They produce far less cough and angio-oedema. Otherwise, they are equally effective antihypertensive agents and yield equal improvements in cardiovascular morbidity and mortality. One recent analysis has suggested they may increase MI but this is not yet widely accepted.

Calcium-channel blockers

These are increasingly used as initial therapy in hypertension because they cause fewer adverse cardiovascular, bronchial and metabolic problems than the beta-blockers. Careful selection within the group is needed for specific indications (Table 4.25). Predominantly vasodilator agents are preferred in hypertension, but anti-arrhythmic and negative inotropic activity is useful in hypertensive patients with IHD. The non-cardiodepressant CCBs (the DHPs) can be usefully and safely combined with a beta-blocker.

Side-effects. Most problems, such as flushing and headaches, are minor and result from vasodilatation, particularly with the DHPs. Similarly, reflex tachycardia with possible palpitations may occur. However, this is undesirable in ischaemic patients because it increases myocardial oxygen demand so, in the absence of ventricular dysfunction, the use of a non-DHP (e.g. *verapamil*), or combination with a beta-blocker, is recommended. Peripheral oedema, usually in the ankles, is a common problem and is caused by leakage from precapillary vessels subjected to higher pressures owing to arteriolar dilatation. Because it is not caused by fluid retention, the oedema does not respond to diuretics but may respond to an ACEI. Non-DHPs have less effect on blood vessels but are cardiodepressant, with the risk of heart failure or bradycardia.

Table 4.25 Comparative properties of calcium-channel blockers

	DHPs	Non-DHP
Examples	Nifedipine Amlodipine Isradipine Felodipine, etc.	Verapamil Diltiazem
Main clinical action	Vasodilator	Anti-arrhythmic −ve inotrope (vasodilator)
Indication	Angina HPT	Supraventricular arrhythmia Angina HPT
ADR	Peripheral oedema, dizziness, palpitations, gastrointestinal problems	Peripheral oedema, dizziness, palpitations, gastrointestinal problems Bradycardia
Caution/ contra-indications	Heart failure, hypotension	Heart failure, hypotension Atrial arrhythmias, bradycardia

Drugs are grouped for clarity, but there may be detailed differences – check in reference source for individual properties.
ADR, adverse drug reaction; DHP, dihydropyridine; HPT, hypertension.

Cautions and contra-indications. Discontinuation has been associated with exacerbated ischaemic events in those with IHD, and so should be performed gradually. Combination of the negatively inotropic agents *verapamil, diltiazem* and *nifedipine* with beta-blockers is best avoided or used with great care, especially where there is left ventricular dysfunction, because it can cause heart failure or heart block. Enzyme inhibition by grapefruit juice enhances the action of most CCBs, except *amlodipine*. Different modified-release preparations of CCBs are not interchangeable and should not be prescribed or supplied generically.

Vasodilators

This large heterogeneous group (Table 4.21) has had a chequered history in hypertension treatment. Not surprisingly, the first antihypertensive agents used targeted the peripheral arterioles. Predominant arterial dilatation is preferred but this can cause postural hypotension by inhibiting natural reflex vasoconstriction. Early sympatholytic vasodilators, including ganglion blockers (e.g. *hexamethonium*) and non-specific alpha-blockers (e.g. *phentolamine*), had limited effectiveness and serious adverse effects, chiefly postural hypotension, impotence and reflex tachycardia. *Reserpine* caused severe depression. The adrenergic neurone blockers (e.g. *guanethidine*), although somewhat more successful, still have serious adverse effects and are reserved now for resistant hypertension.

Newer vasodilators cause fewer postural problems and most induce fewer lipid abnormalities than beta-blockers or thiazides. Other common vasodilator drawbacks, such as headaches, dizziness, palpitations, flushing and reflex fluid retention, are less serious. One of the miscellaneous 'reserve' group of the more toxic direct-acting vasodilators (e.g. *minoxidil*) is still sometimes needed.

Centrally acting sympatholytics (e.g. *methyldopa, clonidine*) have long been used as third- or fourth-line drugs, but now have little place owing to central effects such as impotence and depression. However, *methyldopa* remains a useful alternative in a variety of special circumstances where standard drugs are contra-indicated, e.g. in diabetes, in the hypertension of pregnancy and when postural hypotension is especially hazardous, such as in the elderly or in those with cerebrovascular disease. *Clonidine* is now known to act partly via central imidazoline receptors and has been associated with depression; the newer more specific *moxonidine* may have fewer adverse effects.

The direct-acting spasmolytic *hydralazine* lost favour owing to its tendency to precipitate a lupus-like syndrome, especially in slow acetylators. However, at doses below 100 mg daily the risk is small. The selective (post-synaptic alpha$_2$) adrenergic blockers, e.g. *prazosin, terazosin, doxazosin*, seem to cause less tachycardia and, except for the first dose, less postural hypotension.

They also reduce plasma cholesterol and produce a favourable change in the HDL/LDL ratio.

Drug selection

Diuretics, ACEIs, ARAs and CCBs have all been shown in long-term controlled trials to reduce overall mortality in hypertension. The first has long been known to be effective, but more recently the HOT trial produced evidence in support of ACEIs and CCBs. Nevertheless, after the ALLHAT trial, diuretics still emerged as the cheapest and least toxic first drugs, and they are usually recommended as effective first-line therapy by many authorities in the absence of contra-indications.

Because almost all existing antihypertensive drugs have comparable blood pressure-lowering efficacy, the optimal order of selection in an individual patient is governed primarily by adverse effects, precautions and contra-indications. Factors that modify choice in common conditions or patient groups are summarized in Table 4.26.

Numerous schemes have been devised to aid selection. The scheme favoured by the British Hypertension Society (2006) shown in Figure 4.25 represents one of the simplest and clearest. It is based on the categorization of hypertension into low-renin (fluid overloaded) and high-renin (vasoconstricted) forms, and makes the primary distinction for initial therapy based on the lesser effectiveness of ACEIs in black people, the greater suitability for or tolerance to diuretic or CCBs in older patients, and the greater likelihood of renovascular atheroma in the elderly (thus avoiding ACEIs). Younger patients who cannot tolerate ACEIs, or women of childbearing age, should be considered for beta-blockers. It may be advisable to try several different monotherapies if control is not achieved with the first, before starting dual therapy. Logical combination dual therapy is the next step. A particular combination that should be avoided is diuretic plus beta-blocker, which has an increased risk of inducing diabetes. Triple therapy is the third stage; although the evidence base for this is poor, it represents consensus advice and has

Table 4.26   Specific indications, precautions and contra-indications of antihypertensive drugs

Situation	Drugs to avoid/caution	Specific alternatives or recommendations[a]
Elderly	Sympatholytic (postural effect)	Thiazide, methyldopa
Young male	Thiazide, beta-blocker	ACEI[b], CCB
Black ethnic group	Beta-blocker, ACEI	–
Peripheral vascular disease	Beta-blocker, ? ACEI	Vasodilator
Vascular disease in elderly	ACEI	–
Angina	Vasodilator	Beta-blocker, CCB
Post-MI	–	Beta-blocker, ACEI
Heart failure, LVD	CCB esp. verapamil, diltiazem	Thiazide, ACEI, ? beta-blocker
Heart block	Beta-blocker, CCB	–
Hyperlipidaemia	Beta-blocker, thiazide[c]	ACEI, CCB, selective alpha-blocker
Diabetes (especially type 1)	Thiazide[c], beta-blocker[d]	ACEI, selective alpha-blocker
Obstructive pulmonary disease	Beta-blocker[d]	
Pregnancy	Thiazide, ACEI	Methyldopa, labetalol, furosemide
Hepatic impairment	CCB	Methyldopa
Renal impairment:		
– early	Thiazide	ACEI
– severe	ACEI	Furosemide, beta-blocker
Diabetic nephropathy		ACEI
Renal artery stenosis	ACEI	–
High renin	–	ACEI
Thyrotoxicosis	–	Beta-blocker
Depression	Lipophilic beta-blockers, methyldopa, clonidine	–
Gout, hypokalaemia	Thiazide	–
Prostatic hypertrophy	–	Alpha-blocker

[a] See also Figure 4.25.

[b] Angiotensin receptor antagonists may usually be substituted wherever ACEIs are used.

[c] Thiazides have significant effects on lipid and glucose levels only at doses higher than required in treating hypertension.

[d] Except possibly cardioselective agents, with care.

ACEI, angiotensin-converting enzyme inhibitor; CCB, calcium-channel blocker; LVD left ventricular dysfunction; MI, myocardial infarction.

sound pharmacological and pathophysiological logic.

At every stage, the cautions and contra-indications of each drug for the particular patient need to be considered. However, as the need for multiple therapy increases there is less room for manoeuvre and compromises may have to be made.

Many other combinations are possible, particularly in refractory hypertension. If a patient is not controlled on three drugs, expert advice should usually be sought. The choice of a fourth drug would be an alpha-blocker, a potassium-sparing diuretic (*amiloride*, *spironolactone*) or a beta-blocker.

Attention must also be paid to potential drug interactions of antihypertensive agents. Table 4.27 illustrates the general principles with some representative examples. Details will be found in standard texts (see References and further reading).

Additional therapy. Atherosclerosis prophylaxis with antiplatelet drugs and a statin also need to be considered for all hypertensive patients, in the light of their overall CVD risk (p. 216). For *aspirin*, the side-effect risk is not trivial and the current recommendation is first to ensure good blood pressure control then use *aspirin*, in the absence of contra-indications, i.e. for primary prevention:

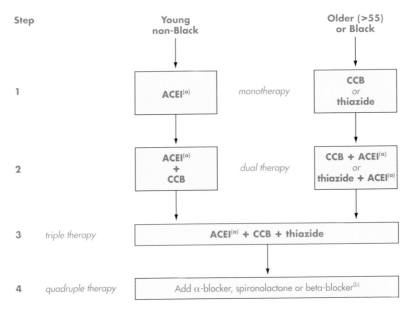

Figure 4.25   Drug selection in hypertension – recommendations of NICE and British Hypertension Society (2006). ACEI, angiotensin-converting enzyme inhibitor. [a]Angiotensin receptor antagonist may be substituted where ACEI contra-indicated or not tolerated. [b]Diuretic + beta-blocker combined has relatively higher risk of inducing diabetes – avoid if possible.

Table 4.27   Potential interactions with antihypertensive therapy[a]

Drugs that elevate blood pressure

Vasoconstrictor sympathomimetics	Oral decongestants (e.g. phenylephrine, xylometazoline), bronchodilators especially non-specific[b], amphetamines
Drugs causing fluid retention	Corticosteroids, oral contraceptives, NSAIDs

Drugs that lower blood pressure

CNS depressants	Tranquillizers, alcohol
Vasodilators	Nitrates, specific bronchodilators[b]

Specific interactions

Beta-blockers	Verapamil, diltiazem → cardiac depression, failure
Alpha-blockers	Beta-blockers, diuretics → exaggerated first-dose hypotension
ACEIs	Potassium-sparing diuretics, potassium supplements → hyperkalaemia

[a] This table only lists the overall interference with blood pressure control and mutual interactions of antihypertensives. Interactions of antihypertensive agents with other specific drugs can be found in the British National Formulary.

[b] Bronchodilators: non-specific, e.g. ephedrine; specific, e.g. salbutamol.

ACEIs, angiotensin-converting enzyme inhibitors; CNS, central nervous system; NSAID, non-steroidal anti-inflammatory drug.

- in patients over 50 years with evidence of hypertension-induced organ damage;
- where the 10-year CVD risk is >20%;
- in diabetes.

For secondary prevention, use aspirin in all cases, i.e. where there is existing ischaemic disease.

The use of statins also depends on CVD risk and is discussed in detail below (p. 247; Table 4.32), but the considerations are similar to *aspirin* without the age criterion. Thus use statins for primary prevention where the 10-year CVD risk is >20% and in all cases for secondary prevention.

Ischaemic heart disease

Ischaemia means literally 'to hold back blood'. Ischaemic heart disease (IHD) is the collective name for a number of conditions in which obstructive lesions of the coronary arteries restrict myocardial blood flow. IHD is also called 'coronary artery disease' or simply 'heart disease'. The main clinical manifestations are angina pectoris and MI, but heart failure and arrhythmias also occur. IHD is the greatest single cause of death, especially premature death, in industrialized societies. In the UK it is responsible for about a third of all male deaths and causes considerable morbidity. This is especially significant because IHD is largely preventable.

There are wide geographic, ethnic and national variations in prevalence, e.g. male mortality from IHD per 100 000 varies between 400 in Finland and 30 in Japan. However, immigrant groups tend to assume the same prevalence as their host country when fully assimilated, showing the importance of environmental risk factors. Epidemiological and pathological studies and large-scale intervention trials strongly suggest that the causes lie in the industrialised or developed way of life.

Atherosclerosis and vascular obstructive disease

The pathology and treatment of IHD can best be understood in the general context of vascular obstruction (partial block) and occlusion (complete block), and so we will review this first.

Classification

The main processes responsible for chronic arterial obstruction are arteriosclerosis and atherosclerosis. In addition, thrombosis may occur as an acute complication, in both veins and arteries (Figure 4.26).

Arteriosclerosis

Although this term is commonly used to describe all degenerative or proliferative arterial lesions, it should be reserved for the symmetrical thickening of the middle muscle layer (media) of arterioles throughout the body. It usually arises in response to hypertension, when it may be partially reversed by treatment, but it also seems to be a normal consequence of ageing. Because it is widely disseminated and invades the vessel lumen it increases peripheral resistance, thus aggravating hypertension and perpetuating a vicious circle. The media often becomes fibrosed and calcified, especially in the elderly. It is popularly known as 'hardened arteries'.

At first there may be no significant impairment of perfusion. However, in the elderly there may be chronically reduced cerebral or renal perfusion. Moreover, the stiffened, non-compliant vessels are weakened and eventually may bulge (aneurysm) and rupture, particularly in cerebral vessels where the result is acute haemorrhagic stroke.

Arteriosclerosis is described here to differentiate it from atherosclerosis. It will not be considered further and all that follows will apply specifically to atheroma/atherosclerosis.

(a)

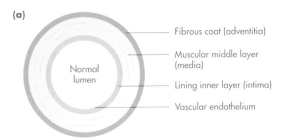

(b)

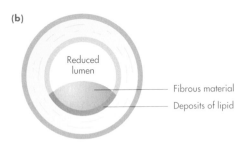

(c)

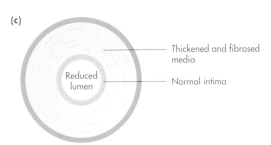

Figure 4.26 Pathology of atheroma, atherosclerosis and arteriosclerosis. A diagrammatic representation emphasizing distinctions between arteriosclerosis and atherosclerosis. (a) Normal arteriolar wall: the middle layer (media) is composed of muscle and elastic tissue. (b) Simple atheroma: an asymmetrical deposit of fat and fibrous tissue in the inner layer (intima) invades the arterial lumen. New endothelium has overgrown the lesion. Should there be further damage, with mural thrombosis, it would be termed atherosclerosis. (c) Arteriosclerosis: symmetrical thickening of the media in most arterioles, usually in response to chronically raised arterial pressure.

Atherosclerosis

In this condition, fatty-fibrous plaques or **atheromas** are deposited asymmetrically within the innermost layer (intima) of certain, but not all, arteries. Sites such as bends, branches or bifurcations seem especially prone. This patchy (focal) distribution means that there is little

effect on total peripheral resistance, but local perfusion may be crucially impaired. Atherosclerosis can occur in many different organs, the result being a wide spectrum of clinical manifestations (Figure 4.27).

Thrombosis

Thrombi result from abnormal triggering of the coagulation process within intact arteries or veins (rather than, as is normal, after damage or rupture). This causes sudden occlusion. Small particles of thrombus may break off forming **thromboemboli**, which lodge further downstream, with similar outcome. Arterial thrombi frequently form at the sites of coronary or cerebral atherosclerotic lesions, with potentially fatal consequences (Figure 4.27). For a full discussion of thrombosis, see Chapter 11.

Aetiology

Classes of contributory factors

An understanding of the formation of atheroma and thrombosis is important for both prevention and treatment. At the most general level the contributory factors may be grouped into three categories: **histological** (endothelial damage), **rheological** (abnormal blood flow) and **biochemical** (abnormal blood or tissue constituents). These may occur independently or together (Table 4.28). The response to injury theory proposes that atherosclerosis arises from a maladaptive chronic inflammatory reaction in which an attempt is made to repair the vascular wall or to limit chronic damage. This reaction persists at the expense of obstructing the vessel lumen and possibly promoting further damage.

Vascular endothelial damage
An atheroma is probably initiated by factors that breach the arterial endothelial defences, exposing underlying tissue. Constituents of tobacco smoke undoubtedly contribute to this. It is also possible that partially oxidized components of the plasma lipid particle LDL irritate the endothelium, with more significant oxidation occurring within the wall. Recent findings have

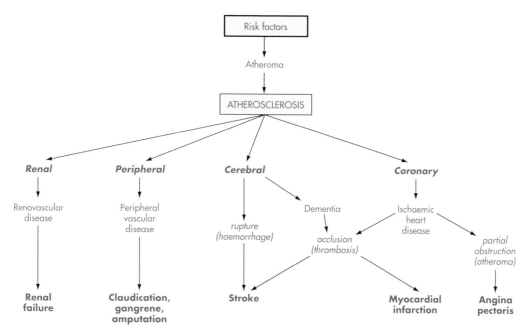

Figure 4.27   Clinical manifestations of atherosclerosis.

Table 4.28   Pathological factors initiating atheroma and thrombosis

Abnormality	Arterial atheroma	Arterial thrombosis	Venous thrombosis
Histological	Chronic inflammation (? oxidized LDL, smoking) Infection (*Chlamydia, Helicobacter*) Hypoxia (smoking)	Ruptured atheroma? Heart valve (i) inflamed (ii) vegetation (endocarditis)	Inflamed venous valve (phlebitis)
Rheological	High pressure (i.e. HPT) High wall stress (i.e. HPT) Fast turbulent flow at bends, branches	Atrial fibrillation	Venous stasis, e.g. prolonged bedrest, recumbency
Biochemical	Dyslipidaemia ($\uparrow$ LDL, $\downarrow$ HDL) Platelets (growth factors) Diabetes (dyslipidaemia) Irritants (smoking)	Clotting factors ($\uparrow$ fibrinogen) Platelets (adhesiveness, growth factors)	Clotting factors Platelets Drugs, e.g oral contraceptives

HDL, high-density lipoprotein; LDL, low-density lipoprotein; HPT, hypertension

implicated chronic inflammatory damage from systemic microbial colonization, possibly with *Chlamydia* or *Helicobacter* species. Finally, hyperlipidaemia itself may be directly damaging to the vessel wall.

A sudden rupture or ulceration of a previously stable atheromatous plaque may trigger thrombosis, with acute effects. Inflamed venous or heart valves are also foci for thrombosis.

Abnormal flow

In arteries, atheromas are most commonly found where flow is turbulent and wall shear forces high. Presumably this causes endothelial cell dysfunction; possibly this is because it interferes with shear-triggered, nitric oxide-mediated vascular relaxation, which alters LDL flow through the vessel wall, or causes enlargement of intercellular gaps allowing abnormal access of irritants. Atheromas do not usually form in veins, although they are found in the normally low pressure pulmonary arteries in cases of pulmonary hypertension.

In veins, it is abnormally sluggish flow that causes problems, e.g. prolonged bedrest or long-distance air travel predispose to venous ('deep-vein') thrombosis, usually in the leg. This is one reason why patients are mobilized rapidly after surgery. In atrial fibrillation, static pools of blood develop within the heart and may clot. In either case thrombi may be carried downstream as emboli. From the leg the path taken by emboli follows widening veins to the right heart, ultimately to lodge in a pulmonary artery. Thrombi originating from the right atrium also lodge in the lungs, while those from the left atrium lodge in the brain or coronary arteries.

Abnormal constituents

Endothelial damage can trigger platelet adhesion and aggregation or the clotting cascade, especially if there is an imbalance between platelet promoter and inhibitor factors. For example, certain PGs (e.g. prostacyclin released from vascular endothelium) tend to inhibit platelet activation and aggregation while others, notably the thromboxane series, are pro-aggregatory. Clotting factor abnormalities, e.g. high levels of fibrinogen, have been found in IHD patients. Coagulation is also disturbed following severe trauma, e.g. major surgery, and by certain drugs, e.g. oral hormonal contraceptives. Smoking may contribute by providing irritants or local hypoxia.

Risk factors

The major international INTERHEART study (2004) of 15 000 individuals from all continents identified nine modifiable risk factors that could account for 90% of all MIs (a condition that can act as a surrogate for atherosclerosis in general). Moreover five of these accounted for 80% of the risk: hyperlipidaemia (dyslipidaemia), smoking, diabetes, hypertension and abdominal obesity (Table 4.29). Dyslipidaemia is measured as the LDL/HDL ratio (see below); obesity is measured as the waist to hip ratio (found to be more closely linked to disease than the traditional body mass index); diabetes may act partly through the associated dyslipidaemia. These act synergistically, so that for example possessing any two poses more than twice the risk.

Many other less critical factors have been implicated, some of them associated with industrialized societies and modifiable by changes to lifestyle, others not modifiable (Table 4.29). A possible protective effect of moderate alcohol intake is still widely debated. There is also evidence of prenatal influences on the fetus. Maternal nutritional deprivation may cause not just low birthweight but also a predisposition in later life to atherosclerosis, hypertension and diabetes. The prevalence in younger males is about three times that in females, but the rates converge later in life because the incidence among postmenopausal women is greatly increased.

The lipid hypothesis

The lipid hypothesis of atherogenesis traces the causal links between dietary lipid, plasma lipid, atherosclerosis and IHD. An outline of the steps in the argument is given in Table 4.30. Patients with **familial hyperlipidaemia** have long been known to suffer a high incidence of premature atherosclerotic disease. A similar pattern is seen in diabetics, whose lipid metabolism is also disturbed. However, the relationship between dietary lipid and plasma lipid, especially cholesterol, and the mechanisms controlling the metabolism, transport and interconversions of lipid within the body, are incompletely understood. Note that plasma cholesterol is only part of the body pool of cholesterol, 75% of which derives from hepatic synthesis and only a quarter directly from dietary cholesterol. This is why, although dieting often helps to reduce lipid levels moderately in many patients, even the most rigorous diet may not reduce plasma lipids

Table 4.29   Risk factors for developing atherosclerosis

Primary modifiable	Secondary modifiable	Unmodifiable
Hyperlipidaemia[a]	Abdominal obesity[c]	Family history
Smoking	'Stress'[d]	Ethnic group
Diabetes[b]	Sedentary life/lack of exercise	Type A personality[d]
Hypertension	Diet poor in fresh fruit/vegetables	Age
	Excess or no alcohol	Male sex
		Female sex post-menopause
	Industrialized society	
	High sugar and low fibre intake	
	? Fetal deprivation due to maternal malnutrition	
	? Chronic infection[e]	
	? Raised plasma urate	
	? Raised plasma homocysteine	
	? Soft water	

Factors in box are the top nine modifiable factors as identified in INTERHEART study (2004), in order of attributable risk.

[a] Measured as LDL/HDL ratio (or apolipoprotein B : A ratio).
[b] Modifiable insofar as diabetes can be well controlled.
[c] Measured as waist : hip ratio.
[d] 'Psychosocial' factors: external stressors acting on striving, highly motivated individual.
[e] e.g. *Chlamydia*.

sufficiently in some. Moreover, dietary saturated fat has more influence on plasma cholesterol than dietary cholesterol itself.

Saturated fatty acids (SFA, from animal sources) raise LDL levels, partly by stimulating cholesterol synthesis, and both cholesterol and saturated fats may stimulate the synthesis of aggregatory PGs. Of course, some dietary SFA intake is nutritionally essential.

By contrast, unsaturated fats in general (mostly oils from plant sources and fish oils) appear to have a protective effect, possibly by increasing the breakdown of LDL. Polyunsaturated fatty acids (PUFA) are thought to be beneficial in both reducing LDL and increasing synthesis of antithrombotic anti-aggregatory blood factors. PUFA, however, and particularly those of the n-6 series, are prone to oxidation and in large amounts may reduce HDL. Monounsaturated fatty acids (MUFA; found especially in olive oil and rape seed oil) do not have these disadvantages. Polyunsaturates in the omega-3 series (especially fish oils) appear to be protective, probably by an antithrombotic action. It is

known that fish-eating populations such as the Eskimos and the Japanese have a low incidence of atherosclerosis.

Other factors
Regular exercise is protective, partly by raising plasma HDL levels and possibly by encouraging the development of collateral blood vessels. Both exercise and low-fat diets may reduce blood pressure, and hypertension is an independent atheroma risk factor. A large number of other substances have been implicated in the aetiology and pathogenesis of IHD, including dietary factors (e.g. folic acid, flavinoids) and other plasma constituents (e.g. lipoprotein a, homocysteine and fibrinogen), but the evidence is currently less convincing for these.

Evidence.   The lipid hypothesis is strongly supported by two important epidemiological observations. First, a correlation exists between the mean plasma cholesterol levels of different population groups (even those with relatively low mean levels) and their prevalence of

Table 4.30   Lipid hypothesis of atherosclerosis

Summary of the argument for the central role of lipids in the pathogenesis of atherosclerosis

- The risk of atheroma formation is related to total plasma ChE
- Total plasma ChE is related to (but is not dependent entirely upon) total dietary lipid, but more closely to saturated (animal) fat intake than to dietary cholesterol. It is inversely related to unsaturated (vegetable) fat intake
- ChE is transported in the blood in solubilized form as lipoprotein (along with triglyceride, phospholipid and protein)
- LDL and VLDL fractions carry ChE from the GIT or liver to the tissues; HDL carries it away from the tissues and back to the liver
- Atherogenesis is most closely correlated with VLDL/LDL levels and inversely related to HDL (i.e. high HDL is protective): the HDL/LDL ratio may be the most important parameter
- Coronary risk correlates more closely with the total plasma cholesterol:HDL ratio than any one fraction
- Triglycerides (TG) are not an independent risk factor
- Diets high in total lipids and with a high ratio of saturated to unsaturated fats raise plasma ChE levels, especially the VLDL/LDL fraction, and this favours atheroma formation
- Diets low in saturated fats and ChE and relatively high in unsaturated fats reduce atherogenic plasma lipids and this reduces an individual's susceptibility to atheroma formation
- Lowering plasma lipids (by diet or drugs) will retard or halt progression of atherosclerotic lesions
- Lowering plasma lipids will reverse atherosclerotic lesions
- Retarding or reversing lesions will reduce the mortality and morbidity from the associated clinical syndromes, including ischaemic heart disease

Terminology

Dyslipidaemia – abnormality in one or more of blood lipid fractions.

Hyperlipidaemia – elevation of one or more of blood lipid fractions.

ChE, cholesterol; GIT, gastrointestinal tract; HDL, high-density lipoprotein; LDL, low-density lipoprotein; VLDL, very-low-density lipoprotein.

atherosclerosis. Secondly, large population groups who have reduced dietary lipid intake, e.g. in the USA and Finland, have achieved a decline in heart disease.

The role of pharmacological intervention with lipid-regulating drugs in secondary prevention is now well established, even in patients with what were formerly considered 'normal' lipid levels (<5.5 mmol/L total cholesterol). Furthermore, their use in primary prevention is justified in harm/benefit terms for those with a high CVD risk. Four major intervention trials reporting from different parts of the world have provided persuasive evidence of the benefits of reducing lipid levels pharmacologically on morbidity and mortality from IHD and stroke. They have also shown that using statin lipid-regulating drugs significantly improves the outcome, with very little added harm.

The Scandinavian 4S trial targeted secondary prevention in 4400 patients with hyper-lipidaemia and existing IHD (angina or MI). The CARE trial was similar, but the 4000 patients had near-average lipid levels. The Scottish WOSCOPS trial involved primary prevention in over 6500 men with hyperlipidaemia but no ischaemic symptoms. In the Heart Protection Study (HPS), 20 000 high-risk patients with cholesterol levels that would not at the time have mandated lipid-lowering were treated. In all cases the beneficial effects were correlated with the reduction in lipid levels. A significant observation was that the degree of benefit depended more on the degree of reduction than on the initial cholesterol level. This has brought about a change in the approach to lipid lowering. Now the aim is to lower cholesterol based on overall cardiovascular risk rather than absolute lipid level.

Recently the penultimate step in the lipid hypothesis received support in the ASTEROID clinical trial, which showed a reduction in atheroma lesions after 2 years of high-dose statin therapy (*rosuvastatin*). Statins may also have a role here beyond simply lowering plasma lipid, acting on platelets or directly on the vascular endothelium. However, evidence is still awaited that such plaque reduction produces significant improvement in clinical outcomes such as ischaemic events in the long term.

Pathogenesis

The precise sequence of events leading to the development of an atheromatous plaque is complex and incompletely understood. In an evolving plaque there are chronic immuno-inflammatory cells such as T-lymphocytes, macrophages and fibroblasts, together with a wide variety of mediators and cytokines with chemotactic, cytotoxic, growth-promoting, pro-aggregatory and pro-inflammatory actions. This supports the concept of atheroma being primarily a protective mechanism. In addition, in the latest modification to the lipid hypothesis, a primary causative role is given to an abnormally oxidized form of LDL. It is uncertain exactly how and where the LDL becomes oxidized, but it is likely to be after uptake into the intima, where macrophages, endothelial cells and smooth muscle cells may be involved.

The process may result in part from an imbalance between pro-oxidant factors and natural antioxidant substances such as tocopherol (vitamin E), carotene (vitamin A) and ascorbate (vitamin C). However, no convincing benefit has yet been shown to result from regular antioxidant vitamin therapy. Similarly, although inflammation secondary to chronic low-grade infection with *Clostridia* or *Helicobacter* species has been proposed as a factor, trials of antibiotics have proved negative.

Figure 4.28 gives an overall picture of the process. It is necessarily a simplified summary of complex and poorly understood events, but will serve to identify potential targets for therapeutic intervention.

Following endothelial damage, LDL particles gain access to the intima. Here their components are oxidized by peroxidase enzyme and thereby rendered immuno-active (particularly the oxidized apoprotein component) as well as perhaps doing further direct damage. Part of the protective action of HDL may be in antagonizing this process, or removing oxidized LDL particles before they do harm. Otherwise, T-lymphocytes recognize the particles as foreign and secrete mediators that recruit other immune cells, as well as causing further local inflammatory damage. Macrophages displaying receptors for oxidized LDL scavenge it by phagocytosis, forming 'foam cells', some of which break down to release free lipid.

The process may cease at this point, resulting in relatively innocuous 'fatty streaks' of little haemodynamic consequence within arteries. Such lesions are often found in young, otherwise healthy adults, but there is still debate over whether they are early signs of clinical atherosclerosis or a separate harmless phenomenon.

If the risk factors persist, the defence mechanisms may be overwhelmed. Platelets are attracted and secrete chemotaxins and platelet-derived growth factor. This induces smooth muscle cells to migrate from the media into the intima, and fibroblasts to start producing collagen fibres. Locally produced angiotensin may also contribute to growth promotion, providing one possible prophylactic role for ACEIs. The connective tissue matrix of the developing atheroma is thus strengthened, and eventually a protective fibrous cap forms over the lipid and foam cells, which becomes overgrown by new endothelial cells. Some are almost undetectable and have been classified as 'lurking future lesions'. A stable plaque will have a high proportion of fibrous components whereas an unstable one – which is liable to rupture and promote thrombosis – has more macrophages and lipid.

Progression and outcome

Chronic vascular obstruction may follow a number of courses (Figure 4.29). The most benign outcome is repair. The atheroma remains small, and is overgrown by a tough fibrous cap. The small degree of residual obstruction is unlikely to cause symptoms. If the obstruction grows larger before it stabilizes, new blood channels may eventually be formed through it

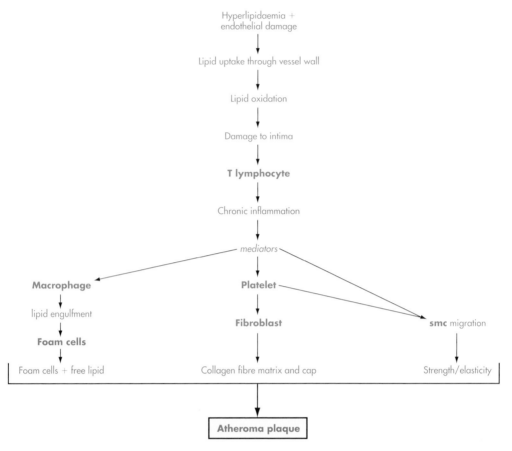

Figure 4.28   Possible pathways in pathogenesis of atheroma. Mediators have been omitted from the diagram. smc, smooth muscle cell.

(recanalization). However, slow progression of the flow restriction is more usual, with gradually worsening symptoms, e.g. angina in the heart or **intermittent claudication** in the periphery (usually the legs).

Sometimes there will be an acute complication. The plaque may rupture, followed by platelet aggregation and possibly thrombosis; or perhaps a weakened atheroma cap may split and haemorrhage. Such an event does not necessarily result from a particularly large plaque: it seems to be not the size but the stability of the plaque that is critical.

In milder cases the result is a platelet aggregate with only a small degree of thrombosis, which is reversed by the normal plasma defence processes, e.g. plasmin, which dissolves small accidental intravascular clots. This could underlie unstable angina or TIAs, and there is minimal anoxic cell death (necrosis).

In other cases there is substantial rupture and a massive irreversible thrombus develops causing complete occlusion and subsequent anoxia downstream. This commonly occurs in coronary or cerebral vessels, resulting in myocardial or cerebral infarction (MI or stroke). It is even possible that relatively innocuous 'lurking' lesions could rupture and cause a major ischaemic event, in which case the patient would not have had any prior warning – nor would conventional angiography, had it been performed, have revealed any significant abnormality.

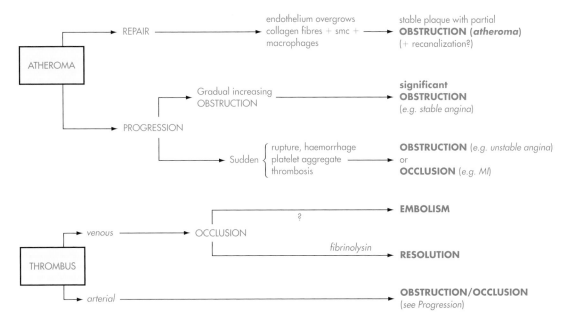

Figure 4.29   Progression of atheromas and thrombi and possible sequels. Obstruction, partial blockage; occlusion, complete blockage. MI, myocardial infarction; smc, smooth muscle cell.

Figure 4.30 shows the transverse section of an artery severely obstructed by an atherosclerotic plaque.

Myocardial ischaemia

Why the heart?

The general clinical consequences of ischaemia were discussed in Chapter 2 (p. 58). The factors that make the heart particularly sensitive are:

- The myocardium has a high O_2 demand and high O_2 extraction.
- The heart works continuously.
- There are relatively few coronary collateral vessels.
- Myocardial cells regenerate poorly after damage.
- The heart is an integrated organ.

Unlike the brain, the lung or the kidney – other important organs that are sensitive to ischaemia – the whole heart functions in an integrated manner so that malfunction of any part will have a disproportionate effect on overall effi-ciency. Because it is not composed of many identical functional subunits, the heart cannot divert function from damaged areas to healthy ones. The efficient ejection of blood requires coordinated contraction, and the process uses the whole myocardium to conduct the electrical excitation, so even small areas of ischaemia or necrosis can severely reduce pump performance.

Thus the heart is a prime target for circulatory insufficiency, and because it is such a vital organ the results are almost always serious. This is why IHD is such a problem. Furthermore, atheromas seem to be deposited preferentially in the coro-nary circulation. This may be a consequence of the anatomy, because coronary flow is retrograde (backwards towards the heart) and thus poten-tially turbulent. Because the left ventricle has the greatest oxygen demand and the most vascula-ture, coronary atherosclerosis usually affects the left ventricle.

Myocardial oxygen balance

The degree of ischaemia in a tissue depends on the balance between oxygen supply (in blood) and oxygen demand. Myocardial oxygen

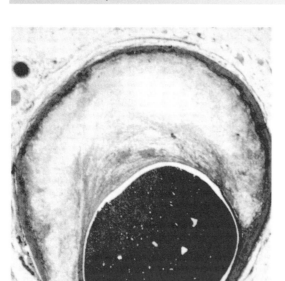

Figure 4.30 Transverse section of artery with atherosclerotic lesion. This photomicrograph shows a much thickened asymmetrical intimal lesion and considerable narrowing of the lumen. The arrow points to normal arterial wall. The dark mass within the lumen is an artefact. (Reproduced with permission from Davies (1985) *Med Int* **20**: 1.)

demand varies according to circulatory requirements. Assuming that blood is adequately oxygenated, myocardial oxygen supply is normally determined by the calibre of the coronary vessels and coronary perfusion pressure. The calibre is altered mainly by reflex autoregulation in response to local oxygen levels. The perfusion pressure is the difference between pressure in the left ventricle at the end of diastole (LVEDP) and mean aortic pressure. This balance between supply and demand can be disturbed by either excessive demand or reduced supply.

Excessive myocardial demand

The fixed lesions of atherosclerosis limit the extent of the dilatation that can be induced by autoregulation (or drugs). Thus while coronary perfusion may be adequate at rest, at some point during escalating effort blood flow will be unable to increase sufficiently to meet the rising demand. Because normally the myocardium has few collateral vessels, the area beyond a lesion will become ischaemic.

Symptoms become evident only after 75% of the lumen of a major coronary vessel has become obstructed, at first only on strenuous exertion. There will be no permanent damage to the myocardium if effort, and thus cardiac workload, is promptly reduced. The ischaemia is partial and is reversed when oxygen demand falls. This produces the typical clinical picture of acute predictable onset and rapid reversibility that is characteristic of classical angina pectoris (often called 'angina of effort').

Restricted oxygen supply

If an event such as rupture followed by thrombus formation produces complete occlusion, or greater than 90% obstruction, then myocardial anoxia occurs. The precipitating event may be unrelated to excessive effort or exertion. If this occlusion is not reversed within about 6 h the anoxic myocardial tissue will die: this is MI. Alternatively, there may be severe but transient, reversible spasm of one or more sections of either atheromatous or apparently normal coronary artery. This may account for 'variant' or Prinzmetal angina. Intermediate stages, known as the acute coronary syndrome, can also occur (see below).

Clinical consequences

Angina and MI, although similar pathologically, are two distinct clinical entities that can exist independently. MI is one extreme of a spectrum of acute conditions known collectively as **acute coronary syndrome (ACS)**. Angina is not invariably a precursor of MI and not all angina patients go on to suffer MI. Their differential pathogenesis is illustrated in Figure 4.31.

Other cardiac abnormalities may follow from myocardial ischaemia, possibly asymptomatically. Numerous small, subclinical infarcts can produce a widely disseminated patchy fibrosis of the myocardium leading to dilated cardiomyopathy and chronic heart failure, without the patient ever complaining of typical ischaemic pain. Twenty-four-hour ECG monitoring has

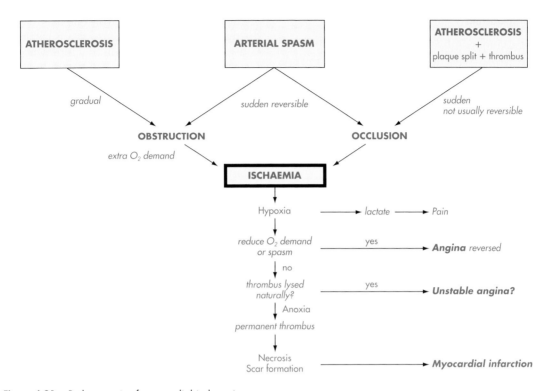

Figure 4.31   Pathogenesis of myocardial ischaemia.

shown that this so-called 'silent ischaemia' may be more common than was previously supposed. Heart failure also frequently follows frank MI.

Ischaemia may affect conducting tissue as well as cardiac muscle, either acutely (during MI), or chronically, leading to **arrhythmias**. Ventricular fibrillation may account for many cases of sudden cardiac death.

Less commonly, ischaemic symptoms may occur unassociated with any coronary obstruction, not even vasospasm. Examples include:

- excessive cardiac oxygen demand, e.g. thyrotoxicosis;
- severely reduced oxygen supply, e.g. severe anaemia;
- reduced coronary perfusion pressure, as in hypertrophic cardiomyopathy, aortic stenosis (raised LVEDP) and cardiogenic shock (inadequate aortic pressure).

Ischaemic pain is probably related to the accumulation of the products of anaerobic metabo-lism, e.g. acid or lactate. However, the picture of angina or MI pain as a type of muscle cramp, although adequate for most purposes, is probably an oversimplification.

Prevention and treatment

Primary prevention theoretically implies preventing the atherosclerotic process from starting, whereas secondary prevention means taking measures to limit or perhaps reverse damage that is discovered subsequently, or prevent symptomatic recurrence. In practice however, primary prevention is usually extended to mean preventing the appearance of signs or symptoms of ischaemia, even though clinically silent atheromas may be present. Unfortunately, most patients only discover they have athero-sclerosis when symptoms – which may not be cardiovascular, but usually are – first occur, in which case secondary prevention is the best that can be offered.

Hyperlipidaemia

The pathology of hyperlipidaemia in relation to atherosclerosis was discussed above (pp. 238 and 240). The current non-drug prophylaxis recommendations are summarized in Table 4.31, and the reader is directed to the References and further reading section for detailed reviews (p. 270).

Primary prevention

The major problem with interventions to reduce the lipid level lies in identifying the threshold of risk. As with blood pressure, total plasma cholesterol varies unimodally throughout the population (Figure 4.18), and an increased risk can be demonstrated at levels near or even below the population average (6 mmol/L for middle-aged males in the UK). Thus the same risk stratification approach to that used for managing hypertension has to be adopted (p. 216). A coronary heart disease risk evaluation looks at evidence-based treatment thresholds for hyperlipidaemic patients of different ages with various combinations of major coronary risk factors. The intervention threshold for a given patient is based not solely on their lipid level but also on the presence of other atherosclerosis risk factors and existing ischaemic symptoms, so this is balanced against the inherent risk of the intervention. However, universal lipid screening is not currently cost-effective and opportunistic screening needs to be targeted on high-risk groups (Table 4.29).

As with hypertension, the initial approach is for abnormal readings to be repeated; if hyperlipidaemia is confirmed, possible underlying primary causes must then be eliminated. Unless the cholesterol level is dangerously high (>10 mmol/L approx.), the total cholesterol: HDL ratio is >6, or there are other risk factors, the first step is to initiate non-drug methods and to try them for 3–6 months. Simple risk factor reduction (lifestyle recommendations and dietary measures) would be suitable for an asymptomatic younger non-smoking patient with normal blood pressure, no family history and a total cholesterol level below 6.5 mmol/L (7.8 mmol/L in younger women). If this fails or there are other risk factors, drug therapy is the next stage, as shown by the HPS trial. A cholesterol level >8 mmol/L will usually require drug treatment eventually in all patients. Special consideration applies to diabetic patients,

---

Table 4.31   Reducing risk factors for atherosclerosis

Recommendation	Rationale – pathological factor targeted
Stop smoking	Vascular endothelium, platelets
Reduce salt intake	Blood pressure
Reduce cholesterol intake	Cholesterol absorption
Reduce saturated fat[a]	Cholesterol synthesis
Increase unsaturated fat[a]	LDL level; also encourage anti-aggregatory mediators, etc.
Increase fibre intake[b]	Lipid absorption?
Increase fresh fruit and vegetable intake	Lipid level; also provide antioxidants
Moderate alcohol intake	BP; also protect against atheroma?
Moderate exercise	BP and lipid level; also encourage coronary collateral vessel development
Reduce sugar intake	Calorie intake/weight
'Reduce stress'	Reduce BP
	Reduce atheroma formation?
Aim for ideal body weight	Lipid level, cardiac load, blood pressure

[a] Fats to provide no more that 30% total energy intake: 10% as saturated fat, 10% as n-3 polyunsaturated fat, and 10% as mono-unsaturated fat.

[b] Non-starch polysaccharide (NSP), 'soluble fibre'.

BP, blood pressure; LDL, low-density lipoprotein.

who would normally be started earlier (see Chapter 9).

Secondary prevention

The decision is simpler if a patient already has ischaemic symptoms or has suffered an MI or stroke. There is now ample evidence of the benefits of lipid-regulating drugs in almost all patients after MI or unstable angina whether the lipid level is high (4S trial) or not (CARE trial).

The presence of disabling ischaemic symptoms would indicate the need for prompt surgical intervention (see below).

Risk factor reduction

Tables 4.29 and 4.31 indicate the general approach to identifying and addressing atherosclerotic risk factors. Of the primary modifiable risks, diabetes is discussed in Chapter 9 and hypertension in this chapter. Smoking and its cessation are discussed in Chapters 5 and 10. The focus here is on the management of hyperlipidaemia.

Targeting known risk factors through health promotion and regular screening in general can reduce the individual risk and community load of IHD in particular and atherosclerosis. Most of the advice coincides with the general recommendations for a healthy life, and is in many ways similar to specific recommendations for reducing hypertension; of course keeping blood pressure within normal limits itself reduces atherosclerosis. However, hypertension screening and medication compliance are notoriously poor. The difficulties of smoking cessation are also well known. Dietary habits too are difficult to change, although average reductions of 10–15% in serum cholesterol can be achieved in this way.

Much effort is therefore being put into attempting to change the habits of whole communities so as to reduce the prevalence of the disease and its multi-system consequences. There is still far to go in changing public perceptions and practices regarding a healthy lifestyle, but there is epidemiological evidence from the USA and Finland that population-wide changes can produce significant falls in atherosclerosis prevalence. A prolonged population reduction of no more than 0.6 mmol/L (which can be achieved by dietary means alone) has been shown to reduce the incidence of coronary disease by 30%.

Pharmacotherapy

Drug therapy is indicated in secondary prevention and for primary prevention of IHD in high-risk individuals.

Lipid-regulating therapy

The **statins** (hydroxymethyl-glutaryl-CoA reductase inhibitors; HMGIs) are the drugs of choice. By inhibiting hepatic cholesterol synthesis, they reduce cholesterol levels, causing a significantly reduced rate of coronary events and slower progression (and possibly regression) of atherosclerotic lesions. Serious adverse effects are uncommon, although liver and muscle damage are possible. Liver function should be checked before starting the drugs and after 1–3, 9 and 15 months. Patients are warned to report any muscle pain or weakness. If the pain is associated with serum creatine kinase (CK) level greater than five times normal the drug should be discontinued; if not and the pain is tolerable, it would be sensible to monitor CK levels as long as the pain persists. Statins need only be given once daily, and for the shorter-acting ones (including *simvastatin*) an evening dose is preferred because that is when most cholesterol is synthesized; for longer-acting ones (e.g. *atorvastatin*) timing is not critical.

Thresholds. The decisions as to who should receive drug therapy and at what point are always subject to debate and change. Current guidance by NICE and the Joint British Societies (JBS-2) recommends pharmacotherapy for three specific groups:

- People with a 10-year CVD risk >20% (primary prevention).
- All patients with pre-existing atherosclerotic CVD (secondary prevention).
- All patients with diabetes.

In addition, people with certain specific risks should be covered, regardless of other criteria. These are: blood pressure >160/100; total cholesterol:HDL ratio >6; and familial hyperlipidaemia.

Targets. As with hypertension, target levels have fallen as evidence accumulates of increased benefit with little increase in harm. The optimal targets are total cholesterol below 4 mmol/L and LDL cholesterol below 2 mmol/L. Alternatively, if it produces lower levels, the aim should be a 25% reduction in total cholesterol together with a 30% reduction in LDL. JBS also specify less stringent, perhaps more practical minimum targets of 5 mmol/L total and 3 mmol/L LDL. There is still debate as to how low is desirable or safe, with some authorities now recommending 3.5 mmol/L total cholesterol as optimal.

Other agents such as fibrates, nicotinic acid derivatives and bile-salt binding resins may be added if necessary. Fibrates are particularly useful for raised triglycerides. Useful adjuncts include *ezetimibe*, which impairs gastrointestinal absorption of cholesterol and is useful where lipid levels cannot be controlled by a statin alone. As target levels go down, increasing use will be made of combination lipid-regulating therapy. For the detailed pharmacotherapy of hyperlipidaemia, see the References and further reading section.

Antiplatelet therapy

Secondary prevention of MI and stroke routinely involves low-dose *aspirin* (see also Chapter 11). Recent understanding of the role of inflammation in atheroma has further validated this approach. However, less gastro-erosive platelet inhibitors have been developed. *Clopidogrel* is more effective than *aspirin*, blocking a different pathway to platelet aggregatory factor synthesis, but is more expensive. It is a useful alternative for *aspirin*-intolerant patients and is used in combination with *aspirin* in ACS. *Dipyridamole*, an older antiplatelet, may be used in combination with *aspirin* for stroke or TIAs.

The final common platelet aggregation pathway involves glycoprotein IIb/IIIa, the fibrinogen receptor on the platelet membrane, and blockers of this have been developed. Chimeric glycoprotein receptor antibody fragments such as *abciximab*, and small molecule direct inhibitors such as *eptifibatide* and *tirofiban*, are limited to specialist units because they are only available for parenteral use. These drugs are at present used in association with angioplasty and in ACS.

The use of *aspirin* as primary prevention is controversial, because of the small but significant risk of gastrointestinal haemorrhage. While some have recommended it as routine for everyone over 50, the current view is that it should only be used where there is an increased CVD risk. A comparison of primary and secondary prevention of IHD is given in Table 4.32.

Polypill

With the increasing number of medications being given to patients at even moderate CVD risk, supported by evidence of increased survival, the suggestion has been made that all people over 55 should be given a drug combination as primary prevention. The proposal is for everyone to take a low dose of a beta-blocker, an ACEI, *aspirin*, a statin, a thiazide and folic acid. The aim would be to benefit from an additive or even synergistic effect of each component. All except folate have been shown to reduce CVD risk as

Table 4.32 Primary and secondary prevention of ischaemic heart disease

Primary prevention	Secondary prevention
No ischaemic signs	Patient already has signs or symptoms of atheroma (e.g. MI, angina or stroke) or has diabetes
1. Reduce risk factors by non-drug means (see Table 4.31)	1. Reduce risk factors by non-drug means
2. Drug therapy if 10-year CHD risk >20% • statin • aspirin (>50 years of age)	2. Drug therapy • statin • aspirin
3. Antihypertensives if BP >160/100	3. Antihypertensives if BP >140/90

BP, blood pressure; CHD, coronary heart disease; MI, myocardial infarction.

secondary prevention, and some as primary prevention. Folate reduces levels of homocysteine, a minor atherosclerosis risk factor. There is no trial evidence that this combination will be effective, nor can there be any realistic calculation of the risk–benefit balance on a theoretical basis, but it remains an interesting idea.

Vascular surgery

Revascularization is indicated in secondary prevention when drug therapy fails or as emergency treatment. Coronary bypass and angioplasty will be discussed in the sections on angina and MI below.

Angina pectoris

Definition and classification

Angina is both defined and diagnosed by clinical criteria. Typical ischaemic cardiac pain is retrosternal (behind the breastbone), intense, diffuse rather than sharp, and gripping, constricting or suffocating. Patients describe the sensation of having their chest crushed by a bearhug, or they may clench their fist over their chest. Yet even when it radiates to the upper arms, neck or jaw on either side it may be difficult to distinguish from severe dyspepsia, 'heartburn' or oesophageal pain (see Chapter 3), or even pericarditis, so other signs must also be sought.

In **classical angina pectoris** pain comes on acutely following exertion, and is relieved within a few minutes by resting or by taking buccal or sublingual *GTN*. Attacks occur predictably at the same level of effort. Coronary atherosclerosis is almost invariably present. A minority (about 10%) of patients suffer from a variant (Prinzmetal) form, where attacks are unpredictable and may occur even at rest, although commonly under emotional stress. In such cases there may be no permanent coronary obstruction, the attacks being due to reversible vasospasm. This section considers mainly chronic state angina. Unstable angina and ACSs will be covered below, after discussion of MI.

Clinical features, investigation and diagnosis

Angina can be triggered by any circumstances that acutely increase cardiac workload (Table 4.33). The clinical features are highly suggestive and rapid relief with *GTN* is almost conclusive. However, in ambiguous cases an exercise ECG (e.g. on a treadmill), will usually show reversible ST segment changes typical of myocardial ischaemia (Figure 4.32). The resting ECG is usually normal but may provide evidence of a past, possibly silent MI (Figure 4.32(d)), or of myocardial hypertrophy (usually resulting from untreated hypertension), which would show as an elevated R-wave. In variant angina, ST elevation is more common but the exercise test may not cause an attack, and 24-h ambulatory ECG monitoring can be valuable.

More invasive tests are rarely justified in moderate stable disease. Angiography (Figure 4.33) or isotope scans are reserved for worsening disease, unstable angina or evaluation before surgery because their results would otherwise not affect management. Moreover, patients with little objective obstruction may have severe symptoms, while evidence of extensive atherosclerosis is sometimes found in patients who complain little. Angiography indicates objective severity and provides a baseline for assessing progress. In general, the elderly seem less likely to experience ischaemic pain, and neuropathy in diabetics can disguise it.

A functional assessment is essential – at what point does the pain occur and what does it prevent the patient doing? Angina can be graded using the NYHA functional scale:

- Grade I. Asymptomatic. No pain at ordinary physical activity.
- Grade II. Mild. Pain evident on strenuous exertion.
- Grade III. Moderate. Pain evident on moderate exertion.
- Grade IV. Severe. Pain unpredictable and unrelated to exertion.

Table 4.33   Trigger factors, symptoms and signs of an angina attack

Trigger factors
Exertion, e.g. climbing stairs, sexual intercourse
Emotion – increased heart rate
Heavy meals – diversion of blood for increased gastrointestinal perfusion
Getting into a cold bed
Going out in cold windy weather } peripheral vasoconstriction raises peripheral resistance

Symptoms
Onset: pain builds up over seconds or minutes (not instantaneous)
Crushing, constricting, dull central chest pain
Relieved by rest or glyceryl trinitrate
Radiation of pain into throat, left jaw and arm, occasionally into back and right arm
Tachycardia, sweating, anxiety
Breathlessness

Signs
ECG[a]
- between attacks   –   normal
- during attack   –   classical: ST segment depressed
                  –   variant: ST segment elevated

[a] See also Figure 4.32.

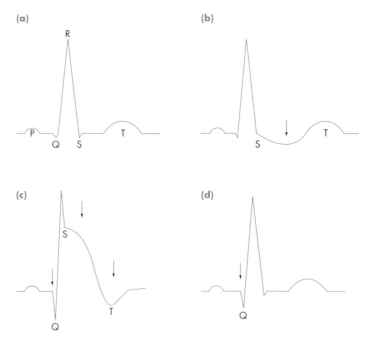

(a)   (b)   (c)   (d)

Figure 4.32   ECG changes in myocardial ischaemia. (a) Normal trace. (b) Myocardial ischaemia typical of an angina attack, the ST segment is depressed. (c) Early myocardial infarction (MI), with Q-wave depression and ST segment elevation; the latter gradually returns to normal over the course of weeks. (d) Months or years after MI; the abnormal Q wave, indicative of permanent infarct, persists after the patient has recovered from acute symptoms. Note: In myocardial hypertrophy the R-wave is increased.

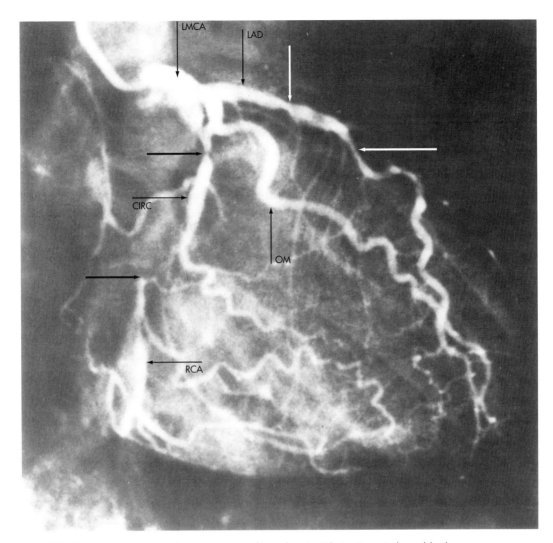

Figure 4.33 Coronary angiogram showing severe atherosclerosis. Obstructions, indicated by heavy arrows, occur on three main coronary arteries ('three-vessel disease'). Those in the left anterior descending (LAD) and circumflex (CIRC) coronary arteries reduce perfusion. The right coronary artery (RCA) shows retrograde filling distal to the obstruction, via collaterals. Also labelled are the left main (LMCA) and oblique marginal (OM) coronary arteries. (Reproduced with permission from Pfizer Inc from Gotto (1977) Atherosclerosis. Upjohn, Kalamazoo: Scope Publications.)

Course and prognosis

Many angina patients have such slowly progressive disease that it causes little disability. Nevertheless, their mortality rate is on average about four times that of those without coronary disease, some eventually dying of MI. The rate of progression depends partly on how early the disease is detected and partly on what measures are then taken to reduce risk factors, although the effectiveness of such measures once symptoms have become evident is uncertain. The 5-year mortality rate for moderate stable uncomplicated angina involving only one main coronary vessel is less than 10%, but this may be doubled if more risk factors are involved.

Some patients experience an acceleration of symptoms with a rapidly reducing exercise tolerance and unpredictable attacks, often unassociated with exercise or their accustomed trigger factors. This is **unstable angina**, part of the ACS spectrum, considered in a later section (p. 266).

Management

Aims and strategy

The overall aim in the management of angina is to minimize myocardial ischaemia. There are three objectives:

1. To abolish the symptoms of an acute attack.
2. To prevent or minimize the frequency of symptomatic or silent myocardial ischaemia.
3. To halt or reduce the progression of the underlying atherosclerosis.

In acute management and prophylaxis, the main strategy is to readjust the oxygen supply/demand balance favourably (Table 4.34). For long-term management, coronary risk factors must also be reduced.

Reducing oxygen demand

As in heart failure, drug therapy is mainly aimed at 'unloading' the heart. Thus negative inotropes such as beta-blockers and non-DHP CCBs are used, although in heart failure the former are only used with great care and the latter avoided. Arterial dilators if used alone can produce reflex tachycardia, which will increase cardiac work, and so combination with beta-blockers is preferable. A cardiodepressant (non-DHP) CCB may serve both functions. Both beta-blockers and the sinus node inhibitor *ivabradine* reduce cardiac rate.

Nitrates act indirectly, through peripheral venodilatation. By dilating the great veins they reduce venous return, thus rapidly reducing cardiac output and thus cardiac work and oxygen demand. Although they also dilate arteries, it is a common misconception that they act by coronary vasodilatation: coronary arteries obstructed by atherosclerosis are minimally dilatable.

Table 4.34   Restoring myocardial oxygen balance

Strategy	Methods	Example
Reduce oxygen demand		
Reduce cardiac workload		
Reduce perfusion demands	Rest	
	Avoid stress	
	Stop smoking	
	Reduce weight	
Reduce preload	Venodilator	Nitrate, potassium channel activator
Reduce afterload	Arterial dilator	CCB, nitrate[a], potassium channel activator
Reduce rate/contractility	Negative inotrope	Beta-blocker, CCB
Reduce rate	Sinus node inhibitor	Ivabradine
Improve cardiac efficiency	Improve fitness	Exercise, stop smoking, lose weight
Improve oxygen supply		
Increase coronary flow	Arterial dilator	CCB, nitrate[a]
	Surgery	Bypass, angioplasty
Prevent further obstruction		
Reduce progression of atherosclerosis	↓ Risk factors	Diet, stop smoking, etc.
	Antiplatelet	Aspirin
	Lipid-regulating	Statin, fibrate, etc.

[a] Nitrates are predominantly venodilators, but in chronic use also affect arteries.
CCB, calcium-channel blocker.

It is equally important to improve overall cardiovascular efficiency. Regular moderate exercise enables the best use to be made of reduced myocardial capacity. Stopping smoking improves oxygen carriage in the blood by reducing carboxyhaemoglobin levels, and this reduces cardiac output requirements. Thus despite drug treatment that apparently reduces cardiac performance, i.e. reducing preload, rate and contractility, there may be no fall in absolute exercise capacity.

Improving oxygen supply

This is more difficult medically because most angina is caused by fixed lesions. If the atheroma occupies less than about 60% of the arterial circumference (which is uncommon in symptomatic angina), arterial dilators may be beneficial by direct action on the obstructed part of the coronary vessel. However, there will usually be maximal natural autoregulatory dilatation anyway. Indeed, vessels near the diseased artery may be preferentially dilated by autoregulation or vasodilators, thereby diverting blood away from the deprived region and exacerbating symptoms (**coronary steal**).

In the rarer **variant angina**, which is caused by vasospasm, vasodilators do work, mainly by direct action on the coronary arteries. Recent angiographic studies also suggest that transient vasospasm superimposed on fixed obstructions may contribute partially to classical angina pain, thus providing a limited role for coronary vasodilatation.

In severe advanced angina, with almost complete blockage of one or more main coronary arteries, surgery becomes necessary. In **coronary artery bypass graft (CABG)** a length of vessel, taken from a leg vein or from the more conveniently located internal mammary artery, is grafted between the aorta and a site beyond the obstructing lesion (Figure 4.34). This can produce dramatic improvements in symptoms but unfortunately atherosclerosis at the same site tends to recur after 5–10 years.

Percutaneous transluminal coronary angioplasty (PCTA) is a far less invasive technique. In this method a coronary catheter is inserted via a

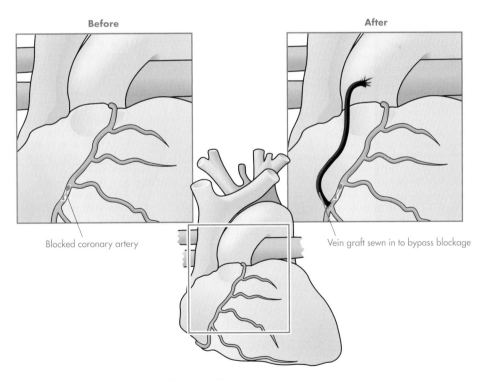

Figure 4.34   Coronary artery bypass grafting (CABG).

peripheral artery until a small balloon at its tip rests adjacent to the plaque. Inflation of the balloon breaks up the plaque, flattens or stretches it, or stretches the surrounding vessel wall (Figure 4.35). The patient is heparinized for the procedure, and it is followed by a short course of intensive antiplatelet therapy (e.g. *aspirin* + *abciximab*), then *clopidogrel* for a month and *aspirin* indefinitely. Subsequent microembolization occasionally causes further obstructions downstream (<1% of cases). Angioplasty has few other complications and avoids the need for open-heart surgery. The technique is also used for other stenosed arteries, including the femoral and renal arteries.

Recurrence of obstruction can occur in up to 60% of cases after as little as 6 months. This is not from new plaque but from initial recoil and subsequent overgrowth of endothe-lium (endothelial hypertrophy); however the procedure may be repeated. To reduce re-occlusion the standard procedure following coronary angioplasty is to place a tubular mesh supporting structure (**stent**) intra-arterially at the site of the lesion after balloon expansion. Costing around £1000, these alloy devices are up to a few centimetres long and about the diameter of the vessel being remodelled. After insertion, the stent eventually becomes overgrown with new endothelium. The use of stents has led to a significant reduction in the restenosis rate. A recent innovation is the use of **drug-eluting stents**, which are coated with an anti-proliferative agent such as *sirolimus* or *paclitaxel*. The drug is slowly eluted and inhibits local growth. There are as yet no long-term data on these expensive devices but they are recommended by NICE for very narrow or very long lesions.

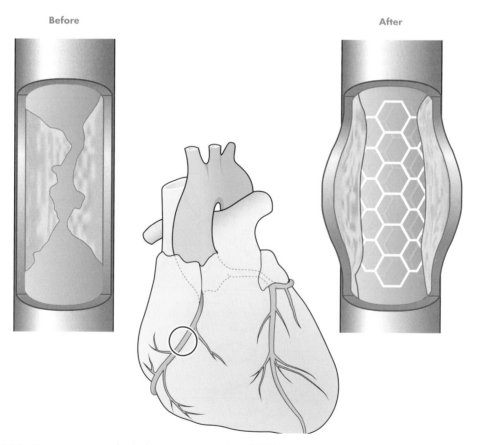

Before   **After**

Figure 4.35   Percutaneous transluminal coronary angioplasty (PTCA).

Preventing further obstruction

General measures such as stopping smoking, losing weight, keeping fit, modifying diet, etc. are an essential part of initial angina management, and are aimed at either directly inhibiting further atheroma or reducing other risk factors. The onset of angina symptoms renders the patient receptive to such advice.

As noted above (p. 247), the risk–benefit ratio at present also favours giving life-long lipid-regulating agents and *aspirin* as secondary prevention to all symptomatic angina patients. The HOPE trial has suggested that ACEIs might be beneficial for high-risk angina patients, e.g. those with diabetes, even in the absence of heart failure.

Acute attack

Glyceryl trinitrate

The traditional *GTN* has yet to be bettered for rapid symptomatic relief (Table 4.35). Patients should be encouraged to anticipate situations that will provoke an attack, and use *GTN* prophylactically immediately beforehand, which keeps the ischaemic burden to a minimum. The sublingual aerosol formulation is preferred because it has greater stability and thus a longer shelf-life after dispensing. It also has a more prompt action. Rapid falls in blood pressure may follow the dose so patients are advised to sit when taking it. Acute headache and flushing are other side-effects of the widespread vasodilatation. The absence of side-effects such as headache and flushing is a marker for either non-compliance or inactive tablets.

GTN tablets have a short shelf-life, and careful selection of the bottle closure is needed. If a patient on *GTN* tablets complains of worsening or accelerating symptoms, with declining effectiveness, poor storage rather than unstable angina may be to blame. *Isosorbide dinitrate* is also available in sublingual spray form.

Prophylaxis

Atherosclerosis prophylaxis was covered on pp. 245–249.

Table 4.35   Use of glyceryl trinitrate for acute angina attacks

Mode of action	Peripheral venodilatation → reduced preload Coronary vasodilatation?
Rapid effect	Buccal/sublingual absorption • avoids delay in absorption • effect within 1 min; lasts 30 min • may be chewed for more rapid effect • avoids hepatic first-pass metabolism • sublingual aerosol available
Side-effects (vasodilatation)	Hypotension – patients advised to sit when taking Flushing Headache (often regarded as an index of effectiveness)
Stability	Sublingual tablets are volatile, easily absorbable – use tightly sealed glass containers, with foil-lined closures To be discarded 8 weeks after dispensing Buccal modified-release and aerosol formulations more stable – longer shelf-life

Beta-blockers. These are first choice unless contra-indicated (Table 4.23). In addition to the details given on pp. 227–229, a number of specific points about the use of beta-blockers in angina should be noted:

- Their action in secondary protection following MI has been clearly demonstrated.
- They improve exercise capacity.
- They are contra-indicated in coronary spasm (e.g. variant angina), because they permit unopposed coronary alpha-constrictor tone.
- Withdrawal, if necessary, should be slow (over 4 weeks), to avoid rebound exacerbation or even MI (owing to beta-receptors having been up-regulated).
- Cardiospecific drugs are preferred.

- Drugs without intrinsic sympathomimetic activity are preferred because they have a reduced likelihood of reflex tachycardia.
- A higher dose than used for hypertension is usually required.

Formerly, a resting heart rate of about 60–70 beats/min was the therapeutic target, but a more reliable predictor of effectiveness might be the limitation of exertional tachycardia to 100 beats/min. This permits higher doses.

Calcium-channel blockers. These are often successful if beta-blocker therapy fails or is inappropriate (see p. 231) and they are the first choice for variant angina. Those with considerable negative chronotropic and negative inotropic action as well as vasodilatation, i.e the non-DHP agents such as *verapamil* and *diltiazem*, may be beneficial provided that ventricular function is adequate and they are not combined with a beta-blocker. Otherwise, a DHP (e.g. *nifedipine*) is used, although these can cause reflex tachycardia. CCBs are perhaps better tolerated than beta-blockers and are suitable for a wider variety of patients.

Nitrates. These act as in angina to reduce preload, with a lesser effect on afterload and perhaps a small effect on coronary vessels. Various formulations of organic nitrates are available to help counteract the problems of this group, which are related to systemic vasodilatation or tolerance (Tables 4.35 and 4.36). Adverse effects may prevent up to a quarter of patients from using nitrates. Preventing tolerance requires a daily 'washout' period of low plasma level, e.g. overnight, in the absence of nocturnal attacks. It occurs because sulfhydryl (-SH) groups on receptors become saturated and can no longer produce NO from the nitrate for dilatation.

Topical *GTN* patches are expensive and offer little advantage except the psychological benefit of direct application to the chest. Unless used with care they may even exacerbate tolerance,

Table 4.36 Problems with nitrates in angina prophylaxis, and possible solutions

Problems	Solutions
Poor bioavailability First-pass metabolism Variable absorption Brief action	Alternative dose forms: • sublingual tablets • sublingual metered-dose aerosol • buccal tablets • high-dose modified-release oral • percutaneous (patch) • IV injection Use mononitrate
Ready tolerance	10-h daily washout period

which is encouraged by a stable plasma level. Buccal modified-release preparations provide a combination of prompt and sustained action.

Because there is no convenient clinical index of plasma levels, such as bradycardia with beta-blockers, dose adjustment is imprecise.

Potassium channel activators. These drugs, e.g. *nicorandil*, combine nitrate-like venodilator action (due to NO production) with CCB-like arterial dilatation. Theoretically they could replace a combination of nitrate and CCB, with the potential advantage that nitrate intolerance would be masked by the arterial dilator action. The IONIA trial suggests they may have superior outcomes to nitrates.

Sinus node inhibitors. *Ivabradine* reduces cardiac rate by acting directly on the sinus node, the result being reduced oxygen consumption. Experience is limited but it seems to have fewer side-effects than beta-blockers but a similar clinical action, and so may prove to be a useful alternative in patients who cannot tolerate beta-blockers.

ACEIs. Evidence is accumulating (e.g. the HOPE (*ramipril*) and EUROPA (*perindopril*) trials) that ACEIs may be beneficial in stable angina even in the absence of heart failure. This makes their spectrum in CVD as broad as that of beta-blockers. This should not be suprising in view of their widespread unloading properties. At present they are used only for high-risk angina patients, though they are not licensed for this in the UK.

Drug selection

All patients should have regular statin and *aspirin*, and *GTN* as required. If prophylaxis is indicated, beta-blockers are the first choice if tolerated. For other drug choices see Figure 4.36, which shows most possible rational combinations. It is rare that a patient is unable to take either beta-blockers or CCBs as initial mono-therapy. If either of these alone fails, a variety of synergistic dual therapies is available. Some have particular advantages, e.g. a beta-blocker plus CCB counteracts the peripheral vasoconstriction induced by the former, and the tachycardia induced by the latter; a DHP CCB should be chosen to avoid excessive myocardial depression. The tendency to tachycardia induced by nitrates is countered by the bradycardia induced by *diltiazem* or beta-blockers. Hypotension can occur with a nitrate plus a CCB, in which case the DHPs should be avoided. The role of potassium channel activators in combinations is not yet established.

Most patients will be well controlled on dual therapy, but triple therapy is sometimes needed. Otherwise, failure of dual therapy is an indication that the patient is a candidate for angioplasty or bypass surgery.

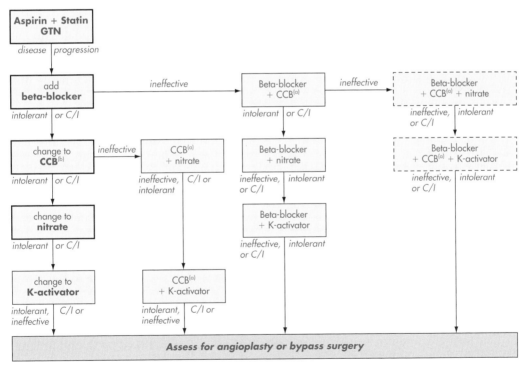

Figure 4.36   Drug selection in stable angina. First choice monotherapy shown bold. C/I, contraindication; CCB, calcium channel blocker; GTN, glyceryl trinitrate; K-activator, potassium channel activator. [a]Dihydropyridine (DHP) group. [b]Verapamil.

Myocardial infarction

Myocardial infarction (MI, 'heart attack', 'coronary thrombosis') occurs when a coronary vessel becomes occluded for more than about 6 h, whether or not the occlusion is subsequently relieved.

Angina and MI

Unlike for angina, exertion is not a trigger for MI, and although MI is frequently associated with current stress or general 'life events', the patient may be unable to recall a particular precipitating event. MI is not simply an intensification of angina: it differs in a number of crucial respects (Table 4.37). Many patients have stable angina for many years and never develop an MI. For others a fatal MI is their first and last experience of heart disease – about 50% of MIs occur without previous ischaemic symptoms.

Table 4.37   Comparison of classic angina and myocardial infarction

Angina	Myocardial infarction
Caused by atherosclerosis	Caused by atherosclerosis
Triggered by exertion	Triggers often unknown
Pain: severe, crushing, retrosternal, possibly radiating	Pain: severe, crushing, retrosternal, possibly radiating
Pain reversed on resting in a few minutes	Pain persistent
Pain relieved by glyceryl trinitrate	Pain unrelieved by glyceryl trinitrate
↑ Oxygen demand	↓ Oxygen supply
Partial obstruction	Complete occlusion
Myocardial hypoxia	Myocardial anoxia
Reversible	Irreversible

Acute coronary syndrome

Angina and MI stand at either end of a spectrum of ischaemic states referred to as acute coronary syndrome (ACS). In between are a range of increasingly severe acute conditions. Therefore MI will be discussed in detail first, because doing so will bring in most of the features of the less serious conditions. ACS will then be discussed by comparison with MI.

Pathogenesis

Initiating event

Postmortem examinations after MI almost invariably show advanced coronary atherosclerosis with a thrombotic occlusion in one vessel. 'Sudden ischaemic death' within an hour or so of the onset of symptoms, before infarction proper can develop, also occurs. This is probably due to ventricular fibrillation. However, these patients usually also have obstructive lesions.

Why should an apparently stable atheromatous plaque suddenly precipitate thrombosis and occlusion? Stress-induced acute abnormalities in both clotting factors and platelets have been proposed, but it is currently thought that a particularly lipid-rich plaque, with low amounts of smooth muscle and fibrous support, may fissure or rupture. This exposes lipid and subendothelial structures, triggering massive platelet aggregation and subsequent thrombosis.

In the few cases where no substantial atheroma is found on angiography or at postmortem examination, the cause may be severe vasospasm or a primary platelet or clotting abnormality.

Severity

The process of infarction in general was described in Chapter 2 (pp. 58–61). If a tissue undergoes a period of anoxia, then irreversible damage occurs, followed by wound healing and organization of scar tissue. Scar tissue can never fulfil the functions of the tissue it replaces. In the heart this means that as well as being non-contractile, the infarcted area is inelastic and poorly conducting. This has the following potential consequences:

- Poor contractility leads to poor ejection, i.e. systolic failure.
- Poor elasticity (reduced compliance) leads to poor filling, i.e. diastolic failure.
- Poor conductivity leads to arrhythmias.

The consequences in individual cases depend primarily on the size of the area of myocardium served by the coronary vessel that is occluded. The mildest form involves a small arteriole, resulting in a clinically silent (symptomless) infarction. Moreover, dilatation of neighbouring vessels by autoregulation may protect the area adjacent to the ischaemic core from complete anoxia, thereby limiting infarct size. However, if this is repeated over a long period it results in widespread 'patchy fibrosis' and eventual cardiac failure. Occlusion of larger arterioles will cause a classical presentation of MI, but if the area damaged is not too extensive the patient will survive, possibly with a degree of permanent cardiac failure. At its most severe an MI may involve one of the main coronary arteries, often the left anterior descending, which supplies most of the left ventricle (Figure 4.7), causing an anterior infarct. Death is likely if more than about 50% of the left ventricle is damaged.

One important factor determining outcome is how well developed the patient's collateral coronary vessels are; another is how much conducting tissue is involved. Conduction across the whole myocardium is necessary for normal coordinated contraction, and ischaemic muscle may conduct erratically. In addition, ischaemic damage to nodal tissue or nerve tracts may have a disproportionate effect because arrhythmias can compromise the function of the entire heart.

Course and prognosis

About half of all patients suffering an MI in the UK die within a month; half dying in the first hour and three-quarters within the first 24 h. Deaths occurring in the first few hours, before medical help becomes available, are usually from ventricular fibrillation. Subsequent deaths are mainly from heart failure. The 5-year survival rate among those who survive the first month is 76%, compared to people of a similar age without MI of 93%.

In the immediate post-infarction period the myocardium surrounding the developing lesion becomes hyperexcitable owing to excess sympathetic tone and the high local levels of potassium released from the damaged cells. The patient is then at great risk of a fatal arrhythmia. Some community-based 'coronary first aid' programmes have significantly reduced mortality. Lay people are instructed in elementary resuscitation, and the emergency services, e.g. ambulance staff and firemen, are taught the 'blind' use of defibrillators, parenteral antiarrhythmics and in some cases thrombolytics. Defibrillators are now being placed in public spaces such as railway stations.

The patient who survives this critical period has a reasonable prognosis: ironically, those who get to hospital include those who least need it. Many patients with uncomplicated MI require, after emergency treatment, only supportive therapy and are soon discharged. Such patients may do better at home in familiar, unthreatening surroundings rather than in a stressful high-technology CCU. However, the consensus view is that all suspected MI patients should preferably be assessed initially in a hospital. Poorer prognosis is indicated by older age, history of IHD or hypertension, and the development of heart failure or arrhythmias.

Clinical features

Some MIs may be so mild as to be dismissed by the patient, relatives and sometimes even doctors as indigestion, especially if the patient has not experienced ischaemia before. It may be some time before the persistent pain brings a patient to medical attention. Angina patients, however, will recognize an MI because although the pain is familiar it persists, tends to be more severe, and is not relieved by normal medication (i.e. *GTN*). With large areas of myocardial damage the patient may collapse from acute heart failure or cardiogenic shock.

On admission, patients are usually cold and pale (owing to central conservation of reduced cardiac output), clammy (due to sympathetic discharge), nauseated and breathless with rapid shallow breathing. Their great distress is due not only to severe pain but also to profound fear and anxiety. This heightens the perception of pain because patients are literally mortally afraid. There may be hypotension, tachycardia or profound bradycardia, and signs of pulmonary oedema (e.g. crackles heard through the stethoscope).

Investigation and diagnosis

All patients with suspected MI are closely monitored for 72 h to confirm the diagnosis and anticipate complications. Precise diagnostic criteria vary, but generally the diagnosis depends on significant findings in at least two of three crucial areas:

- Clinical presentation and history.
- Progressive ECG changes.
- Progressive serum cardiac marker changes.

In many cases the 'classical' clinical features are absent and it can be very difficult to ascribe a cardiac cause. This is especially true of milder attacks with minimal myocardial damage and no cardiac failure, and in diabetics and the elderly. Objective criteria then become important.

Electrocardiogram

Certain characteristic changes occur after a typical **transmural** MI, i.e. affecting the full myocardial thickness. The ST segment quickly becomes markedly elevated, only settling down to normal after several weeks (Figure 4.32(c)). A 'pathological' Q-wave occurs early and persists as a permanent marker of a past MI (Figure 4.32(d)). The particular ECG leads that detect these changes indicate the position of the infarct within the myocardium, while their magnitude indicates the severity of the MI. Less commonly, if the infarct does not affect the entire thickness of the cardiac wall, the Q-wave remains normal and the ST segment is depressed. This is non-Q-wave or subendocardial infarction.

In hospital, these time-dependent changes can be followed by continuous monitoring. A more important reason for such monitoring is the early detection of serious arrhythmias, an alarm sounding automatically when these occur.

Cardiac serum markers

Measurement of the serum levels of certain enzymes typically found in myocardial cells, but released on injury or death, provides additional evidence (Figure 4.37). A particular range, quantity and sequence of enzyme release is characteristic of MI, an isoform or CK being the most specific. Elevation more than 15% above the normal range is diagnostic. An even more specific serum marker of myocardial damage is cardiac **troponin-T (cTn)**. This component of cardiac muscle fibrils is detectable within minutes of an MI, peaks at 12 h and persists for about 2 weeks. Its presence during unstable angina indicates a greater likelihood of subsequent infarction.

Complications

About half the patients with MI who survive the first few hours develop one or more of the complications shown in Table 4.38, mostly within the first few days. The frequency and

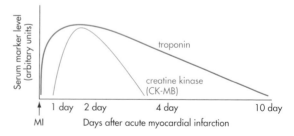

Figure 4.37   Plasma marker changes following myocardial infarction (MI). Myocardial necrosis releases a characteristic group of intracellular enzymes in a well-defined sequence over the first 2 weeks. The creatine kinase MB enzyme isoform (CK-MB) is the enzyme most specific for cardiac muscle. Even more specific markers are the cardiac troponins (see text).

Table 4.38 Complications of myocardial infarction

Complication	Comment
Early	
(Left) ventricular failure	Common
Pulmonary oedema	If LV failure severe
Cardiogenic shock	10% MI patients; if ventricular damage >33%
Arrhythmias, especially ventricular fibrillation and asystole	Potentially fatal; monitoring essential
Thromboembolism	Hypercoagulable state
• further infarct, stroke	• transmural infarcts (endocardial damage)
• deep vein thrombosis	• prolonged immobilisation
Hypotension/bradycardia	Autonomic imbalance
Late	
Pericarditis	First few days
Systolic stretch, ventricular aneurysm, ventricular remodelling	Causes ventricular failure
Ventricular rupture	
• cardiac tamponade[a]	Causes 10% of hospital MI deaths
• septal defect	Rare
Post-MI autoimmune syndrome	Pericarditis, fever, effusion

[a] Fluid within pericardium, inhibiting cardiac filling.
LV, left ventricular; MI, myocardial infarction.

severity of these are the best arguments for the existence of CCUs, where continuous monitoring and prompt attention are assured. If such complications do not develop, the patient is at less risk and may do better at home. The occurrence of heart failure is the single most accurate predictor of long-term outcome.

A transmural infarct may be overly compliant, bulging during systole (forming an aneurysm), which reduces ventricular output and thus causes heart failure. A septal infarct may rupture into the right ventricle. Rupture into the pericardial cavity is usually fatal but the risk is reduced by early beta-blockade. A ventricular aneurysm may persist after the infarction has healed. Non-Q-wave infarction is initially less serious but has a poorer prognosis: there is a likelihood of a full MI in the near future with a higher overall mortality than normal.

Ventricular remodelling by dilatation and hypertrophy gradually compensates for the loss of functional myocardium, a process that may continue for up to 6 months after the infarction. Although this may be beneficial in many patients, progressive dilatation can lead to chronic ventricular failure, and cardiac enlargement is a poor prognostic factor. Early ACEIs limit this process.

Weeks or months after an infarct, and particularly after a second or third such occurrence, an autoimmune reaction to necrotic cardiac tissue (Dressler's syndrome) may develop, which is managed with steroids.

Management

The aims in managing MI are, in sequence, to:

• act promptly to save life and reduce complications;
• treat acute symptoms;

- restore flow through the affected artery (revascularization);
- minimize subsequent infarct size;
- treat complications;
- rehabilitate;
- ensure secondary prevention of subsequent attack.

Immediate management

The emergency management of MI is primarily symptomatic and supportive (Table 4.39). The IV route is preferred because reduced peripheral perfusion delays uptake from IM sites, and frequent injections are more conveniently given via an *in situ* IV line. Early revascularization by thrombolysis or PTCA is mandatory but is not always immediately available (see below).

Opioids are invaluable as analgesics, tranquillizers and venodilators. Paradoxically, their respiratory depressant action is also useful: it reduces the ineffectual fast respiration associated with panic. In the UK, *diamorphine* (heroin) is routinely used, but *morphine* or *pethidine* (meperidine) are also suitable; an anti-emetic (e.g. *cyclizine* or *metoclopramide*) may be required. A 300-mg *aspirin* tablet (for its antiplatelet effect, not analgesia) is chewed to promote more rapid absorption. A *GTN* tablet is taken sublingually or buccally. High-concentration *oxygen* (40% or more by mask, unless the patient is known to have chronic airways disease, see Chapter 5) is often needed. Heart failure and shock are discussed below.

Myocardial salvage: reducing infarct size

It was previously thought that after an MI little could be done to prevent myocardial damage, which was assumed already to have occurred irreversibly. However, several interventions have been developed. They are best initiated within 3 h of the onset of symptoms, although evidence is emerging that the thrombotic process in some infarctions evolves continuously over the first 24 h, so that later interventions may still be beneficial. Broadly, these techniques involve methods of improving oxygen supply and methods to reduce myocardial oxygen demand that spare less severely hypoxic areas. Audit criteria for this phase include 'pain to vein' time – the time between onset of symptoms and start of treatment – and 'door to needle' time – the speed with which patients admitted to an A&E department are started on treatment, ideally <30 min.

Antithrombotics

Aspirin is given as soon as possible and continued, with the aim of preventing extension of the existing thrombus or re-thrombosis. It does not reduce the size of the culprit thrombus. There is some evidence that *clopidogrel* enhances this action, but glycoprotein IIb/IIIa inhibitors probably do not. There is no evidence to support the routine use of *heparin* except in association with angioplasty or thrombolysis.

Reperfusion: thrombolysis

The key to improving outcome in MI is to restore blood flow to the ischaemic area by opening up the occluded coronary artery as soon as possible. In some areas (especially the USA), it is possible to organize balloon angioplasty or even bypass surgery sufficiently rapidly as a primary intervention, and this is becoming more common

Table 4.39   Routine acute management of myocardial infarction symptoms

Target	Management
Pain	GTN, opioid plus anti-emetic
Distress, anxiety	Opioid
Minimize thrombus extension	Aspirin
Hypoxaemia	Oxygen
Dissolve thrombus	Thrombolytic
Heart failure	Nitrate, diuretic, ACEI
Pulmonary oedema	Diuretic, opioid

ACEI, angiotensin-converting enzyme inhibitor; GTN, glyceryl trinitrate.

in the UK. However, pharmacological **thrombolysis** (fibrinolysis) is the usual treatment. Angioplasty is also used where thrombolysis has failed (salvage angioplasty).

The natural endogenous fibrinolytic enzyme is plasmin (see Chapter 11). This lyses fibrin clots forming intermittently and accidentally within the normal circulation, or following repair of any vessel damage (Figure 4.38). It also destroys other clotting factors, inhibiting further thrombosis. Both blood and tissue factors activate its precursor, plasminogen. Normally a delicate equilibrium exists between clotting and anticlotting factors but this is overwhelmed following pathological thrombosis. Thrombolytic drugs activate plasminogen artificially (Figure 4.38 and Table 4.40).

Indication and use.   Pharmacological thrombolysis is now considered for all patients with symptoms strongly suggestive of MI and confirmed by ECG. Thrombolysis recanalizes up to 50% of patients and reduces mortality rate by 25%. Patients with anterior infarcts benefit most, the benefit being greatest for those patients treated earliest. Ideally, this should be within 2 h of onset of symptoms (i.e. usually before reaching hospital), but 4–6 h is probably more

Table 4.40   Comparison of fibrinolytic agents

	Streptokinase	Alteplase	Reteplase	Tenecteplase
Mode	Infusion	Infusion	Bolus	Bolus
Duration	1 h	3 h	30 min[a]	10 s
Antigenicity	Antigenic	Non-antigenic	Non-antigenic	Non-antigenic
Side-effect	Haemorrhagic[b]	Less haemorrhage?	Less haemorrhage?	Less haemorrhage?
Cost	Cheap	Expensive	Expensive	Expensive
Half-life	Longest half-life (25 min)	Shortest half-life (5 min)	Intermediate half-life (15 min)	Intermediate half-life (20 min)
		Better recanalization than streptokinase, but no better outcomes		

[a] Approximate value.
[b] Especially stroke.

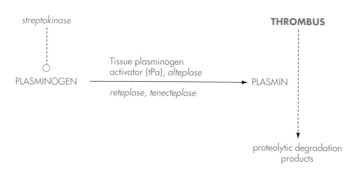

Figure 4.38   The action of fibrinolytic agents.

realistic and 12 h is the maximum for significant benefit. There are only small gains after longer delays.

Heparin is used routinely as an adjunct to *alteplase* therapy, because *alteplase* has a short half-life. It is also indicated in patients with a tendency to thrombosis, to reduce venous thrombosis and pulmonary embolism. However, there is an increased chance of bleeding and *heparin* is not recommended routinely.

Side-effects, contra-indications and precautions. Early fears that thrombolysis would cause massive haemorrhage proved unfounded, but bleeding is still the major risk. This may be at the site of injection, so that further venepuncture should be delayed and cautious. More serious is internal bleeding, especially intracerebrally (e.g. haemorrhagic stroke). Major contra-indications include recent surgery (including dental extraction), recent head injury, a history of cerebrovascular disease or if there is a risk of bleeding from a peptic ulcer. A more complete list is given in Table 4.41.

Choice. *Streptokinase (SK)* is a foreign protein and therefore antigenic; it acts directly on plasminogen anywhere in the circulation. *Alteplase*

(rt-PA) is a genetically engineered human tissue plasminogen activator that has a greater affinity than *SK* for fibrin. *Reteplase* and *tenecteplase* are similar but modified to be more clot-specific by being selective for plasminogen in the presence of fibrin. They also have a longer half-life.

SK is currently the cheapest agent. Because it is antigenic, antibodies form within 4 days. This may cause allergic reactions, but fortunately anaphylaxis is uncommon. The outstanding problem is the lack of effect if treatment is repeated after 4 days, because the antibodies bind the drugs and prevent them from acting. Another thrombolytic must be used if a patient has a second infarct after *SK* treatment.

Alteplase and *reteplase*, although more expensive, permit lower doses and hence reduce systemic bleeding by targeting the coronary clot. However, this property is generally exploited to use higher doses for a better vessel opening rate, thus vitiating the advantage. Used in this way the clot-specific agents are more likely to produce haemorrhagic stroke as a complication. Either way, the advantage of selectivity is not translated into as large an increase in survival as expected. Thus, despite the fact that *reteplase* and *tenecteplase* produce better arterial opening, neither produces a better clinical outcome.

Overall, differences in efficacy are small and of far less significance in survival terms than variations in the time between symptoms and thrombolysis or admission and thrombolysis. Thus research continues for a thrombolytic agent closer to the ideal. In the UK at present, *SK* is the drug of choice in the absence of contra-indications.

Primary angioplasty. There is increasing evidence that prompt angioplasty, if it can be arranged, produces better long-term outcomes than thrombolysis. It is indeed becoming routine in some parts of the USA. However, the facilities do not yet exist in the UK for its widespread use.

Cardiac workload reduction
Surrounding an evolving infarct there are relatively hypoxic, but not completely anoxic, areas. Reducing the oxygen deficit of these might be expected to aid their recovery, reduce the size of

Table 4.41   Contra-indications and cautions with thrombolytic therapy

Active problems
Anticoagulation therapy
Peptic ulceration
Oesophageal varices
Severe liver disease (varices)
Diabetic retinopathy
Severe systolic hypertension
Pregnancy
Severe menorrhagia

Recent history of:
General surgery
Stroke
Subarachnoid haemorrhage
Major head injury

the subsequent infarct, and thus improve prognosis. In addition this contributes to the management of any heart failure. The strategies used are similar to those in angina:

- Reduction of heart rate and contractility using beta-blockers.
- Reduction of afterload using arterial dilators, e.g. ACEIs.
- Reduction of preload using venodilators, e.g. nitrates, ACEIs.

Early IV beta-blockers have been shown to reduce infarct size, arrhythmias and cardiac rupture. Because the usual cardiac contra-indications to beta-blockers are all common after MI (especially serious heart failure, bradycardia, heart block and hypotension) many patients who might benefit would normally be excluded. However, cautious use of certain beta-blockers (e.g. *carvedilol*) in heart failure is now known to be beneficial. There is little evidence that cardioselectivity is to be preferred, but obviously non-selective agents would on theoretical grounds be expected to do more harm and those with intrinsic sympathomimetic activity, which increase heart rate, should be avoided. Therapy is continued orally for secondary prevention (see below).

Oral ACEIs started within 24 h of infarction have also been shown to improve outcome, especially when there is overt failure, impaired ventricular function or hypertension. They appear to counter the ventricular enlargement (remodelling) that occurs after infarction and worsens ventricular function and prognosis. They are particularly useful when beta-blockers are contra-indicated but may be used together with them. ACEIs are routinely used for at least 6 weeks if not contra-indicated, e.g. by hypotension, and are continued if heart failure persists. As usual, ARAs may be substituted where ACEIs are not tolerated. Neither beta-blockers nor ACEIs should be started before the patient has been stabilized haemodynamically.

Other drugs that might be started very early but for which there is either insufficient evidence or lack of experience are *eplerenone* (in severe heart failure), a statin and *clopidogrel*. There is no consensus on the routine use of early IV nitrates in the absence of ischaemic pain or heart failure, although in addition to reducing oxygen demand they will counter any primary or reflex coronary spasm. CCBs are not beneficial.

Complications

Arrhythmias

Ventricular fibrillation needs prompt electrical defibrillation. Early prophylactic *lidocaine* (lignocaine) or *procaine* enjoyed a vogue, but are not used now in the UK. Other specific arrhythmias are treated as usual when they occur. Early prophylactic magnesium infusions are not useful.

Heart failure and shock

These are managed as usual (pp. 197–208). They require careful haemodynamic monitoring because of the autonomic imbalance and unstable homeostatic control after MI.

Thromboembolic complications

These may be deep vein, pulmonary, cerebral or endocardial (mural) and are prevented by a short course of *heparin*, perhaps followed by *warfarin* for a few weeks. Long-term oral anticoagulation is not needed if *aspirin* is being given.

Rehabilitation

Patients without complications are mobilized within 2–3 days and discharged soon after. This reduces the chance of venous thrombosis, and is good for morale. Other aspects of rehabilitation are summarized in Table 4.42. Patients may eventually lead near-normal lives. Although most do eventually die of IHD, nothing indicates that a life of self-imposed semi-invalidism improves their chances and the quality of such a life is inferior. By following simple positive health recommendations, to which infarct survivors are especially receptive, by 6 months after their infarct many patients say that they feel better than for many years before.

Table 4.42   Rehabilitation   and   general   health
education after myocardial infarction

Gradual re-establishment of normal activity, including
work and sex
Counselling and reassurance
- little interference with normal activity expected
Improve general fitness
- stop smoking
- moderate routine aerobic exercise
- attain ideal body weight
- join 'post-MI' self-help group
Stress reduction?
- simple psychotherapy, relaxation therapy, group
therapy

MI, myocardial infarction.

Secondary prevention

Antiplatelet therapy

The long-term benefit of regular low-dose *aspirin*
is clear, especially following thrombolysis.
However, even large-scale trials have failed fully
to resolve uncertainty over the optimal dose:
recommendations range between 50 and 300 mg
daily but the usual dose is 75 mg. If the patient
is *aspirin* intolerant, *clopidogrel* is indicated.

Anticoagulants

Early trials of anticoagulants following MI,
usually using *warfarin*, were flawed and used
imprecise monitoring methods, and toxicity
seemed to outweigh any potential benefit.
However, despite re-analysis, more reliable
monitoring methods and even revival of the
thrombosis theory, these drugs are unlikely to be
used routinely for the majority of patients after
MI. *Warfarin* therapy is inconvenient and expensive to manage, requiring regular blood monitoring (see Chapter 11), and there are risks of
misdosing and interactions. The combination of
aspirin and *warfarin* may have a superior effect
but these problems count against its adoption.
Nevertheless, there is much research into alternative types of antithrombotic, such as the oral
ximelagatran, an oral thrombin inhibitor.

Beta-blockers

Routine   prophylactic   cardiospecific   beta-
blockade (for at least 2–5 years, and perhaps lifelong) is beneficial. Even patients with moderate
heart failure can be treated. On the other hand,
very low-risk patients seem unlikely to benefit.
Pooled data suggest an overall 25% reduction in
mortality rate.

ACE inhibitors

Regular ACEIs are recommended for all patients,
in combination with beta-blocker or alone if
beta-blockers are contra-indicated (about 25% of
patients). The optimum duration of treatment is
not yet clear, but is at least 5 years. However,
high-risk patients will probably be on them for
life.

Lipid-regulating agents

These have been clearly demonstrated to be of
benefit in all at-risk patients, which obviously
includes those post-MI, whatever the lipid level.
Targets were discussed above (p. 248).

Figure 4.39 summarizes the various treatment
options for a wide spectrum of possible presentations and clinical opinions. Note that this is not
a flow chart for management, but an overall
framework   for   comprehending   the   many
possible eventualities and remedies.

Acute coronary syndrome

Classical angina and MI are clearly defined and
diagnosed but there exist a range of intermediate
conditions where patients present with atypical
features. Their pain occurs at rest and it does not
relent on resting or with *GTN*, but the ECG and
serum marker signs do not fulfil the criteria for
full MI. These conditions have been variously
described as unstable, crescendo or pre-infarc-
tion angina, or acute coronary insufficiency, but
the preferred term is **acute coronary syndrome**
(ACS). There are a number of ways of defining
the   intermediate   stages   that   comprise   this
syndrome but all are characterized by identifying

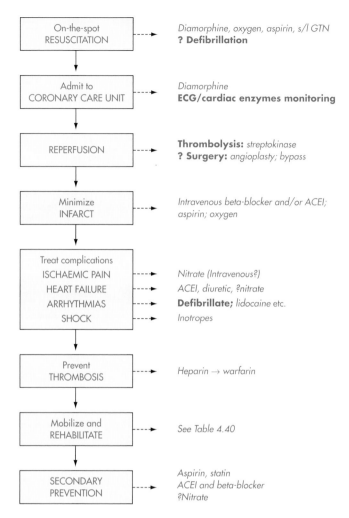

Figure 4.39 Overview of management of myocardial infarction. Precise treatment will depend on the severity of infarction and occurrence of complications. ACEI, angiotensin-converting enzyme inhibitor; GTN, glyceryl trinitrate; IV, intravenous; s/l, sublingual.

which of the criteria for full-blown MI are or are not met (p. 260). Figure 4.40 summarizes a common classification, with a summary of treatment.

The primary criterion of ACS is the typical clinical presentation of myocardial ischaemia (chest pain, etc.) but which is unprovoked and/or prolonged and/or unrelieved by resting or *GTN*. If there are neither typical ECG nor cardiac serum marker changes it is described as **unstable angina**. That description would also

apply if there were atypical 'dynamic' ECG changes, i.e. ST segment instability, associated with pain, but no consistent elevation. ECG changes typical of MI but with no serum markers is termed **ST-elevation myocardial infarction (STEMI)**, and serum markers without ECG changes is **non-ST elevation myocardial infarction (NSTEMI)**. If all three criteria (clinical features, ECG, marker changes) are met the event is termed **acute myocardial infarction (AMI)**; this may be considered the extreme end

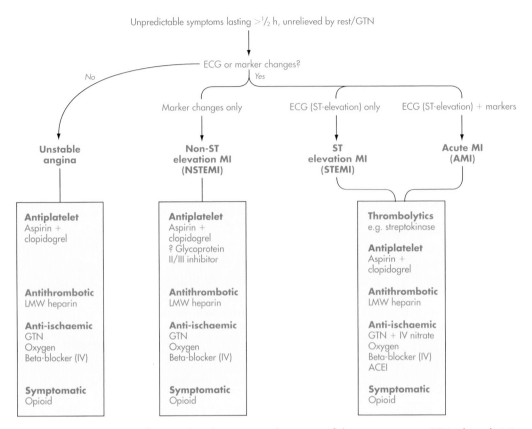

Figure 4.40   Acute coronary syndrome – clinical spectrum and summary of drug management. GTN, glyceryl trinitrate; IV, intravenous; ACEI, angiotensin-converting enzyme inhibitor.

of the ACS spectrum. There also may be an atypical AMI without Q-wave changes, i.e. non-Q-wave MI.

It is likely that all these situations start with the coronary plaque rupturing to some extent, and platelet aggregates or small thrombi (or both) forming. Except in AMI these are probably cleared naturally before infarction supervenes, but which syndrome eventually develops depends on factors such as the size of the vessel affected, the maximum degree of obstruction and the time before resolution. All cases represent a medical emergency, because without aggressive prophylaxis in a CCU, half such patients would go on to develop a full MI. Indeed, many AMIs are preceded by similar, if perhaps accelerated phenomena, and this

dynamic process continues after symptoms develop. Thus infarction is to be viewed not as a discrete event but as a process evolving over 12–24 h, so that anti-thrombotic treatment may significantly minimize thrombus extension, and fibrinolytic therapy may be beneficial over a longer period than was at first thought.

The management of the various forms of ACS varies according to the criteria outlined above and also to the patient's risk stratification. This is based on factors such as continuing pain, ventricular failure, ECG instability, age and ischaemic event history. Moreover, the patient's categorization can change quickly in the first 12–24 h.

The routine immediate management of ACS is much as for a suspected MI (Figure 4.40), involving *aspirin*, opioid, *oxygen* and *GTN*. Admission to a CCU should be rapidly arranged so that the ECG and marker status can be determined, the risk stratified and complications managed. Unstable angina and NSTEMI do not require thrombolysis, but need intensive antiplatelet and antithrombotic therapy with *aspirin*, *clopidogrel*, and LMW *heparin*. Anti-ischaemic therapy is also given, with IV beta-blockers and nitrates if there is persistent ischaemic pain or heart failure. For NSTEMI a glycoprotein IIb/IIIa inhibitor is added. All cases of STEMI are treated as for AMI, with thrombolysis. If the pain does not respond within 48 h of the onset of pain in any form of ACS, angiography with a view to revascularization by angioplasty/stenting is indicated.

Summary of cardiovascular aetiologies

CVD is potentially very confusing, with a variety of similar but distinct conditions affected by a range of overlapping but not identical risk factors, and which can affect one another. Thus IHD can lead to heart failure, but is itself accelerated by hypertension; hyperlipidaemia can directly promote IHD but not hypertension; a sedentary lifestyle can promote both hypertension and IHD. In conclusion, therefore, it may be helpful to summarize some of the main points that link the conditions covered. Figure 4.41 gives an overview of the main CVDs, the aetiological relationships between them and the various risk factors that affect them.

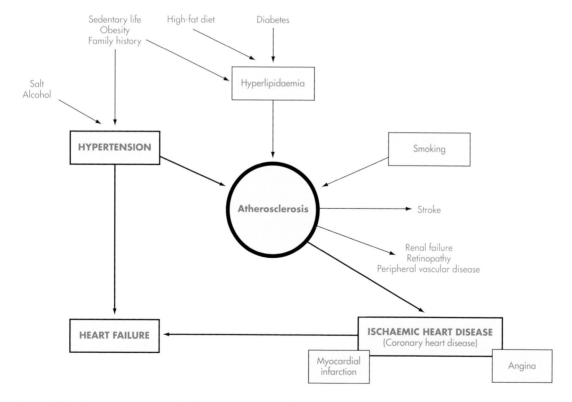

Figure 4.41   Overview of relationship between cardiovascular diseases and cardiovascular risk factors.

References and further reading

Beavers G, Lip G Y H, O'Brien E (2007). *ABC of Hypertension*, 5th edn. London: BMJ Books.

Boersma E, Mercado N, Poldermans D, *et al.* (2003). Acute myocardial infarction. *Lancet* **361**: 847–858.

British Hypertension Society (2004). Guidelines for hypertension management 2004 (BHS IV): summary. *BMJ* **325**: 634–640.

Connolly G, Lip Y H, Chin B S P (2002). Antithrombotic strategies in acute coronary syndromes. *BMJ* **325**: 1404–1407.

Dalal H, Evans P H, Campbell J C (2004). Recent developments in seconday prevention and cardiac rehabilitation after AMI. *BMJ* **328**: 963–967.

Davies R C, Davies M K, Lip G Y H (2006). *ABC of Heart Failure*, 2nd edn. London: BMJ Books.

European Society of Cardiology (2005). Guidelines for the diagnosis and treatment of chronic heart failure. *Eur Heart J* **26**: 1115–1140.

Gibbs C R, Davies K K, Yip G Y H (2000). *ABC of Heart Failure*. London: BMJ Books.

Gross Z, Reese G E, Williams H (2005). Dyslipidaemia. *Hosp Pharm* **12**: 169–181.

Hillis G S (2006). Management of stable angina and unstable angina/non-ST-elevation MI. *Medicine* **34**: 181–187.

Hobbs F D R (2006). Primary prevention of IHD. *Medicine* **34**: 178–180.

Lynch R, Williams H (2003). Hypertension. *Pharm J* **270**: 52–54.

McMurray J J V, Pfeffer M A (2005). Heart failure. *Lancet* **365**: 1877–1889.

Mohrman D E, Heller L J (1997). *Cardiovascular Physiology*, 4th edn. New York: McGraw-Hill.

NICE (2003). Chronic heart failure: Management of chronic heart failure in adults in primary and secondary care (CG5). Available from http://guidance.nice.org.uk/CG5/?c=91497 (accessed 16 August 2007).

NICE (2006). Hypertension: Management of hypertension in adults in primary care (CG34). Available from http://guidance.nice.org.uk/CG34/?c=91497 (accessed 16 August 2007).

NICE (2007). MI: secondary prevention (CG48). Available from http://guidance.nice.org.uk/CG48/niceguidance/pdf/English (accessed November 2007).

Opie L H, ed. (2005). *Drugs for the Heart*, 6th edn. Philadelphia, PA: W B Saunders.

Packer M (1992). Pathophysiology of chronic heart failure. *Lancet* 340: 88–91.

Sani M (2004). Chronic heart failure. *Hosp Pharm* **11**: 87–100.

Siva A, Noble M (1999). *Mosby's Crash Course: Cardiology*. London: Mosby.

Strange J W, Knight C J (2006). Management of acute MI. *Medicine* **34**: 1188–1195.

5

Respiratory diseases

Respiratory diseases are major worldwide causes of morbidity and mortality, especially in Third World countries and those affected by war and natural disasters. The World Health Organization estimates that tuberculosis infects one-third of the world population, causing about 1400 deaths in the UK in 2004. This imposes great health burdens and large economic costs in terms of lost productivity, and comprises a major restraint on the growth of poorer economies. Developed Western societies are also affected. Increasing asthma is the most common chronic disease in the UK and affects about 12 million North Americans. Further, acute respiratory infections are still important causes of death in the elderly.

The respiratory tract is exposed to environmental hazards to a greater extent than any organ system except the skin. Lung tissue is extremely delicate and has limited protective mechanisms, so it is easy to understand the high incidence of respiratory diseases. It is somewhat surprising that these are not more common, given the increasing airborne insults from expanding industrial activity and population growth. Respiratory infections (i.e. pneumonia and tuberculosis) are dealt with in Chapter 8.

Anatomy and clinical physiology of the respiratory system

Anatomy

The lungs are intimately connected with the heart in that they receive and process the entire cardiac output. To appreciate the effects of respiratory diseases it is essential to understand the cardiovascular system (CVS; Chapter 4). This chapter outlines the anatomy and physiology of the respiratory system as an introduction to the aetiology, pathology and management of its important diseases.

The gross anatomy of the respiratory tract is illustrated in Figure 5.1(a). The various parts have specialized functions, reflected in the types of tissue of which they are composed (Table 5.1). Most of the structures only serve to conduct gases between the air and the **acinus**, the smallest functional respiratory unit (Figure 5.2). This comprises a **terminal bronchiole** that communicates with the **respiratory bronchioles, alveolar sacs** and **alveoli**. Most of the exchange of oxygen and carbon dioxide between the inspired air and the capillary blood occurs across the walls of approximately 300 million alveoli, each about 250 µm in diameter, which together provide about 70 m^2 of membrane for gas exchange. The alveoli are not isolated units but are interconnected by pores.

Some of these structural and functional aspects (Table 5.1) are of interest here. Only

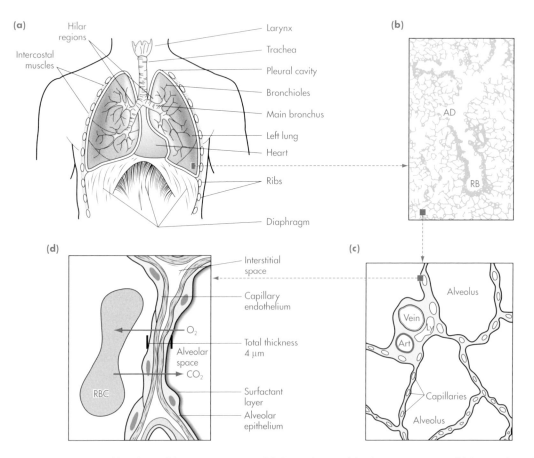

Figure 5.1   Anatomy and histology of the respiratory tract. (a) General view of the thoracic structures. (b) Section through the lung parenchyma. (c) Lung parenchyma at higher magnification. (d) Section through the alveolar wall. AD, alveolar duct; Art, arteriole; Ly, lymphatic vessel; RB, respiratory bronchiole; RBC, red blood cell.

Table 5.1   Structure, histology and function in the respiratory tract

Organ or structure	Relative cross-sectional area	Function[a]	Ciliate epithelium	Mucous and serous glands	Goblet cells	Lymphoid and phagocytic[b]	Muscle[c]	Elastic	Cartilage
Nose, etc.	1	C, O	+	+	–	A	V	–	+
Pharynx	1	C	+	+	+	T	V	+	+
Larynx	1	C	+	+	+	L	V	+	+
Trachea and bronchi	1	C	+	+	+	L	S	+	+
Bronchioles									
• larger	0.8	C	+	–	+	L	S	+	–
• terminal	1.3	C	–	–	+	(M)	S	+	–
• respiratory	3	C (E)	–	–	–	(M)	S	+	–
Alveolar									
• ducts	10	C, E	–	–	–	M	–	+	–
• sacs	2000	C, E	–	–	–	M	–	+	–

(a) C, conducting; E, gas exchange; O, olfactory; ( ), some function.

(b) A, adenoids; L, scattered lymphoid cells; M, macrophages; T, tonsils.

(c) S, smooth muscle; V, striated (voluntary) muscle.

+, present; –, absent.

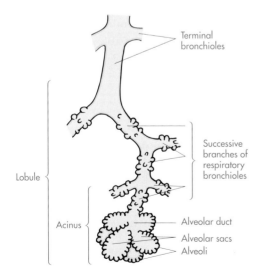

Figure 5.2   Respiratory lobule and acinus.

those conducting airways that are not substantially supported by cartilage can be reduced considerably in bore by smooth muscle spasm, so it is these small airways that are involved in asthma and, to a lesser extent, in **chronic obstructive pulmonary disease (COPD)**: supported airways can constrict to a lesser extent. Thus, bronchodilators can be beneficial only if there is smooth muscle spasm causing bronchiolar constriction and **airways obstruction**. Further, because mucous glands and goblet cells occur primarily in the larger airways, their stimulation to produce excessive amounts of mucus, as in COPD and bronchiectasis, does not affect the smallest airways and the alveoli. In these diseases it is medium-to-small airways obstruction, due to variable degrees and combinations of bronchoconstriction and mucus plugging, which causes the problems. In addition, damage to the pulmonary blood vessels occurs in COPD and bronchiectasis.

Ciliated epithelium provides an important defence mechanism. The cilia beat in organized waves, sweeping mucus (and microorganisms and other particles trapped in it), towards the larynx. The mucus and its trapped contents are usually swallowed and digested, but if large quantities are produced the sputum is coughed up.

Elastic tissue is present throughout the lungs and is especially important in the alveolar walls. The muscles of the airways and the thorax also have elastic properties. Although this elasticity produces a tendency for the expanded lungs to collapse, it accounts for only about one-third of the total recoil effect. The remainder is caused by interfacial tension within the film of fluid lining the alveoli, but this is counteracted by **surfactant lipoproteins** derived from dipalmitoyl lecithin, produced by specialized alveolar cells. These surfactants assist spreading of the fluid over the alveolar surfaces, help to keep the delicate tissues moist to provide for good gas exchange, and reduce both the tendency of the alveoli to collapse at low lung volumes and the work required to expand the lungs during inspiration. A brief increase in alveolar surface area increases the benefit of the surfactant. Hence the importance of the occasional deep breath or sigh during quiet breathing – this expands any respiratory lobules (Figure 5.2) that have collapsed under interfacial tension.

During the first 4 weeks of life, a congenital deficiency of natural surfactant results in **hyaline membrane disease** in a small proportion of neonates, especially in premature infants. If the deficiency is severe, the lungs collapse completely at the end of expiration and are difficult to re-expand. This is **respiratory distress syndrome of the newborn (RDSN)**. If neonatal artificial ventilation is unsuccessful, the infant may die in the immediate postnatal period or, depending on the extent of the deficiency, in early infancy. Some 40–50% of the complications of RDSN may be prevented by giving the mother a short course of corticosteroids at least 24 h before a premature birth, i.e. <37 weeks' gestation. This is done preferably between the 24th and 34th weeks, e.g. 20–40 mg of

betamethasone over 48 h. Artificial surfactants (e.g. *beractant* and *poractant alfa*) are available for neonatal treatment, and a liposomal formulation of prostaglandin E is in clinical trial. Other surfactants (e.g. *colfosceril palmitate* and *pumactant*) and natural respiratory surfactant are available in other countries.

RDSN should not be confused with adult respiratory distress syndrome, which is usually due to trauma or inhalation of toxic material.

Pleural membranes

Each lung is surrounded by a double membrane, the **pleura**, and is attached to the inner of these membranes. The outer membrane forms the lining of the thoracic wall, diaphragm, and the lateral aspect of the mediastinal organs (see below). The **pleural cavity** between them is filled with a few millilitres of fluid, which is normally maintained at a slight negative pressure relative to the lung tissue. This negative pressure is essential for respiration because if air enters the pleural cavity (i.e. a **pneumothorax** due to trauma or disease), the affected lung tends to collapse. The pleural fluid lubricates the membranes, permitting them to slip easily over each other during breathing. Inflammation or infection of these membranes (**pleurisy**) causes the cavity to fill with inflammatory exudate, resulting in adhesions (see Chapter 2, p. 54) between the layers of membrane and a variable degree of inspiratory pain which enforces shallow, rapid respiration.

Mediastinum

The mediastinum is the central space between the pleural sacs around each lung (Figure 5.1(a)), and contains the heart and major blood vessels, the trachea and bronchial bifurcation, important nerves (vagus, cardiac, phrenic and splanchnic), the oesophagus, lymphatic vessels and tissues (thoracic duct, lymph nodes) and the thymus gland.

Although mediastinal diseases are outside the scope of this chapter, the course of the recurrent laryngeal nerves, especially the left (which loops under the aortic arch before ascending to the larynx), has important implications for the occurrence of certain respiratory symptoms. Notably, persistent hoarseness may be produced by any condition causing pressure on these nerves, e.g. tumours or an aortic aneurysm.

Clinically relevant aspects of respiratory physiology

The lungs have three interdependent functions:

1. Conduction of inspired air to the alveoli and of expired gases to the trachea.
2. Maintenance of blood flow to and from the alveoli.
3. Exchange of oxygen and carbon dioxide between the alveolar spaces and the blood.

Regulation of respiration

Respiration consists of two phases: **inspiration** is the expansion of the lungs and the conduction of air to the alveoli (alveolar ventilation) and **expiration** is the relaxation of the expanded lungs and the expulsion of alveolar gas. A combination of chemical and nervous stimuli adjusts the alveolar ventilation almost exactly to the bodily requirements, so that the arterial partial pressures of oxygen (P_aO_2) and of carbon dioxide (P_aCO_2) in the arterial blood are relatively constant over a wide range of systemic demands.

These stimuli are derived from sensors in various organs and tissues and the principal factors that influence respiration are summarized in Table 5.2.

Central nervous reflex signals arise primarily from chemoreceptors in the cerebral ventricles, carotid bodies, aortic arch and brainstem, which

Table 5.2   Some humoral and nervous factors influencing respiration

Origin of stimulus	Factors that affect respiration	
	Increase	Decrease
Cerebral cortex	Arousal/fear Desire to exercise Fever	Sleep CNS depressants Trauma
Respiratory centre	pH[a] ↓ Salicylate poisoning Fever	pH[a] ↑ Severe hypoxaemia Sedatives
CSF	pH[a] ↓	pH[a] ↑
Carotid and aortic bodies	P_aO_2 ↓ pH[a] ↓ Blood pressure ↓	P_aO_2 ↑ (weak effects) pH[a] ↑ Blood pressure ↑

Lungs
  • parenchyma
  • bronchioles
	Relaxation
	Pulmonary embolism/oedema
	Smoking/irritants
		Stretching

Periphery	Muscle stretch ↑ Chronic pain	Acute pain
	———— Proprioreceptors in chest wall and joints ————	

[a] [H+] is the primary mechanism and reflects P_aCO_2 (see text).

CNS, central nervous system; CSF, cerebrospinal fluid.

are sensitive primarily to carbon dioxide levels in the blood, and so to pH. The cerebral cortex and the respiratory muscles (see below) also drive respiration (and heart rate) according to voluntary exercise demand. The signals from all of these are coordinated in the 'respiratory centre' in the brainstem (medulla and pons). Perhaps surprisingly for such an important function, the respiratory centre is not well defined, there being three widely separated groups of neurones located in the upper part of the brainstem that interact and send appropriate signals to the respiratory muscles.

These central mechanisms interact with peripheral ones to form a series of complex inter-relationships and feedback mechanisms. The most important peripheral input is derived from chemoreceptors that respond to blood levels of carbon dioxide, pH and oxygen, in that order of importance under normal conditions. The partial pressure of carbon dioxide in arterial blood (P_aCO_2) exerts by far the greatest influence, there being an approximately eightfold increase in respiration rate from low to high values (Figure 5.3(a)). Conversely, P_aO_2 has little influence because, as the shape of the oxygen/Hb dissociation curve shows, there is an almost complete saturation of oxygen-carrying capacity over the whole of the normal range of oxygen levels (Figure 5.3(b)), and because a change in P_aO_2 increases the sensitivity of the respiratory centre to carbon dioxide. A change in blood pH has a similar sensitizing effect on the respiratory centre and influences the oxygen-carrying capacity of Hb more than oxygen does in the normal range (Figure 5.3(b)). Further, both the P_aCO_2 and pH mechanisms react to exert a braking effect on the response to oxygen. Although the effect of pH appears to be small, if all other parameters are controlled, the principal agent acting on the respiratory centre becomes the hydrogen ion, because changes in carbon dioxide levels immediately change the pH:

$$[H^+] = K \frac{[CO_2]}{[HCO_3^-]} \qquad (5.1)$$

The hydrogen ions reach the respiratory centre primarily via the blood and to a lesser extent via the cerebrospinal fluid (CSF).

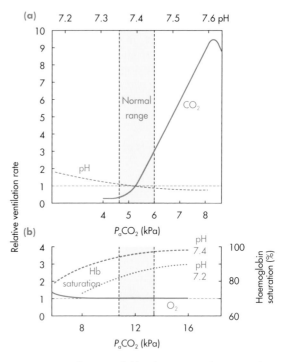

Figure 5.3   Influence of blood gases and pH on the ventilation rate. (a) Carbon dioxide and pH. (b) Oxygen and haemoglobin saturation.

Although the carbon dioxide effect is large initially, if hypercapnia (high P_aCO_2, also known as hypercarbia) is sustained, as in severe COPD, the respiratory centre becomes desensitized to the level of carbon dioxide. The patient then depends on their P_aO_2 to provide their respiratory drive. This has important implications for *oxygen* therapy in COPD (see p. 338).

Respiratory muscles

Inspiration is an active process, the principal mechanism being contraction of the **phrenic (diaphragm) muscles** and to a lesser extent of the **external intercostal (rib) muscles**. However, during quiet breathing expiration is a passive process that depends on the elastic recoil of the stretched muscles and lung tissue, and interfacial tension effects in the alveoli. The force of expiration during exercise is increased by the action of the **internal intercostal muscles**.

In severe respiratory deficit the muscles of the shoulders, chest wall and abdomen are used to increase the force applied for both inspiration and expiration, so these are known as the **accessory muscles of respiration**. Use of these can be recognized in a patient by excessive movements of the shoulders and abdomen – in very severe disability the patient will grasp the arms of a chair or other surface strongly in an attempt to increase the applied force. However, these manoeuvres may be counter-productive, because excessive respiratory force increases the intra-thoracic pressure abnormally, so that the airways tend to collapse, especially if they are weakened by disease, thus increasing the resistance to expiratory flow (see below). Thus, difficulty in expiration may often be the first sign of respiratory obstruction.

Respiratory mechanics

Airways resistance

This is measured as the pressure difference between the mouth and the alveoli per litre of gas flow. It is the result of friction between the gas molecules themselves, and between them and the walls of the airways. Quiet breathing produces laminar gas flow but rapid breathing causes turbulence, so a greater pressure difference is then required to maintain the flow. Anything that causes airways narrowing (e.g. bronchoconstriction in asthma or mucus plugging in COPD), will increase airways resistance markedly. In COPD and emphysema there is a variable combination of airways inflammation and loss of both tissue supporting the airways and the elastic recoil pressure of the lungs. This makes the airways more likely to collapse on expiration, when intrathoracic pressures increase, thus increasing resistance and making it difficult to exhale. Even small changes in airways bore make large differences to flow rate: Poiseuille's law (see also Chapter 4) states that flow through a tube is proportional to the fourth power of its radius. However, bronchoconstriction may have some beneficial physiological effects, because it reduces the dead space (p. 278), and this improves the

efficiency of ventilation when tidal volumes are low.

In normal respiration, airways resistance reduces gas flow almost to zero by the time the air reaches the entrances to the alveolar sacs, so diffusion is the final mechanism by which the gas molecules travel to and from the alveolar membranes and blood vessels.

Mechanical factors affecting gas flow

The lungs and respiratory muscles resist changes in size and shape because of tissue viscosity and elasticity.

Compliance is the term used to describe the ability of the lungs and thoracic wall to expand, and is a reflection of elasticity, the converse of stiffness. Compliance is reduced by any disease that increases lung stiffness, e.g. pulmonary fibrosis and oedema (pp. 282, 325), pneumonic consolidation and TB (Chapter 8). Compliance is increased in emphysema (p. 333), due to destruction of lung tissue, and in old age due to tissue degeneration.

However, such factors account for only about 20% of the total pulmonary resistance and become a problem only if fibrosis or oedema are extensive. When this occurs, patients often breathe shallowly but rapidly. This is a normal physiological response that minimizes the effort required, but is very inefficient (see below).

Work of breathing

The energy expended during respiration is that required to overcome airways resistance and mechanical factors (e.g. lung compliance, muscular work). During normal quiet breathing this amounts to only about 2% of the total bodily energy requirement, and is negligible. However, disease may increase this so greatly that there is insufficient oxygen available for other purposes and patients become exercise-limited (e.g. in pulmonary fibrosis), or may be exhausted on admission to hospital (e.g. severe asthma).

Figure 5.4 shows the effect of lung volume on the change in pressure required to produce a unit change in that volume. Because air trapping occurs in obstructive lung disease (p. 284), increasing the total lung capacity (TLC, Figure 5.6), patients with severe asthma and COPD have to exert a much greater effort to move air in and out of their lungs than do normal subjects, and this requires the expenditure of more energy.

Ventilation and perfusion

The composition of the alveolar gas varies markedly depending on the respiration rate, blood flow, diffusion across the alveolar membrane, Hb concentration, carbon dioxide production, etc. Further, the alveolar gas cannot be expelled completely from the lungs at expiration because about 150 mL of it is contained in the conducting airways (the **anatomical dead space**). This residual gas is the first to be washed into the alveoli during inspiration and is removed only by dilution with the inspired air. Hence shallow, rapid breathing may do little more than move this volume of gas in and out of the alveoli, and is a very inefficient mode of ventilation.

The **alveolar ventilation**, the total volume of gas exchanged in all the alveoli in unit time, is approximately 5 L/min during quiet breathing. The lungs receive the entire cardiac output, so in a normal resting adult the **pulmonary perfusion** is approximately 5 L/min. Thus, the overall resting **ventilation/perfusion ratio (VPR)** is

about 1.0. However, this overall balance masks large differences that occur throughout the respiratory cycle and regional differences within the lungs. An imbalance between ventilation and perfusion is known as **mismatching**.

The resting value of VPR is not constant throughout the lung because blood flow decreases markedly from base to apex in an upright individual, whereas ventilation is less affected. Figure 5.5 shows that ventilation/perfusion mismatching is greatest in the upper lobes, so that oxygenation of the blood is relatively poor there. Ventilation is particularly unevenly distributed at the low lung volumes that occur at the end of expiration or the beginning of inspiration, because the lungs are suspended in the chest only at the hilum, and so the weight of their upper part plus the weight and hydrostatic pressure of the blood contained in the lungs compresses the lower lobes. When we breathe in after a maximum expiration, air initially enters the upper lobes, which are less compressed, but when about 1 L has been inhaled the situation is reversed, the lower zone airways open and the lung bases are better ventilated.

The volume at which the lower airways close (**closing volume**), due to intrathoracic pressure exceeding airways pressure, increases with increasing age (due to reduced elastic recoil) until it encroaches on normal breathing. Consequently, elderly normal subjects often have poorly ventilated lungs with poor gas exchange and are exercise-limited. An increased closing volume may be a sensitive early indicator of lung disease such as smoking damage or emphysema.

The VPR is a crucial parameter affecting oxygen delivery to the tissues. The systemic P_aO_2 results from a balance between the rates of oxygen delivery to the lungs, i.e. ventilation, and its removal in the blood, due to perfusion. Thus high values of VPR lead to high values of P_aO_2, and vice versa. At the extreme limits, zero ventilation would give a P_aO_2 equal to that of venous blood, and zero oxygen uptake, whereas minimal perfusion would give a P_aO_2 equal to that of the inspired gas, but little or no oxygen would be carried to the tissues. Such conditions can occur only locally, because neither of them is compatible with life if they were to occur widely. However, very high oxygen levels in the alveoli

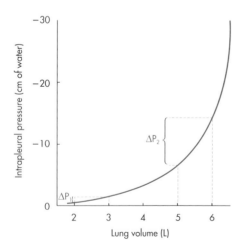

Figure 5.4 Relationship of intrapleural pressure to lung volume. ΔP_1, ΔP_2, the change in intrapleural pressure (negative, a measure of inspiratory effort) required to inspire 1 L of air at different lung volumes.

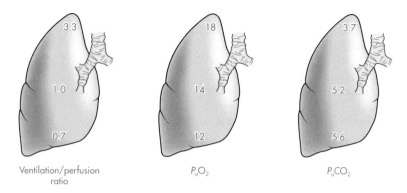

Ventilation/perfusion ratio P_aO_2 P_aCO_2

Figure 5.5   Variation of ventilation/perfusion ratios in the normal lung and its effect on arterial partial gas pressures.

give only a limited increase in the oxygen-carrying capacity of the blood, because Hb saturation is almost maximal under normal conditions (Figure 5.3), so a high VPR in one localized area of lung cannot compensate for low values elsewhere.

Although the alveolar–arterial deficit (i.e. the difference between the partial pressures of oxygen across the alveolar membrane) is negligible in the normal lung, it may be very large in disease. The body attempts to compensate for this by vasoconstriction in hypoxic areas of lung, thus diverting blood from poorly ventilated or presumably damaged areas to those that are better ventilated, and this does give some improvement. However, if lung damage is widespread this process becomes maladaptive, because the pulmonary vasoconstriction produces pulmonary hypertension and this may lead to heart failure (**cor pulmonale**, p. 285; see also Chapter 4). Nevertheless, the VPR is the key factor controlling oxygenation of the blood, and no amount of increased ventilation or circulatory diversion can compensate for ventilation–perfusion mismatch in the diseased state: exercise limitation is inevitable.

The VPR is always grossly abnormal in COPD (p. 326), due to a combination of hypoventilation and a variable degree of diffusion limitation. Additionally, beta$_2$-bronchodilators tend to reduce the P_aO_2 by about 10% in some patients with COPD and asthma because they cause non-selective pulmonary vasodilatation and so increase blood flow to unventilated alveoli. However, the favourable action of bronchodilators in reducing airways resistance, and so increasing ventilation, outweighs this. Thus this adverse effect is negligible unless the patient is grossly hypoxaemic, when the additional oxygen deficit caused by the bronchodilator may be important.

Gas transfer

The transfer of gases across the alveolar membrane depends on the functional membrane area, the membrane thickness, the concentration gradient across the membrane, and the diffusion coefficient of the gas.

The **diffusion coefficient** of a gas is proportional to its solubility in extracellular fluid and inversely proportional to the square root of its molecular weight. Thus, carbon dioxide diffuses about 20 times as rapidly as oxygen due to its high solubility, so its diffusion is not a limiting factor. Consequently, as ventilatory function deteriorates in COPD the P_aO_2 tends to fall before the P_aCO_2 rises.

The **functional membrane area** is the most important parameter controlling diffusion, and this is reduced in emphysema and by ventilation–perfusion abnormalities. The latter are also important in **concentration gradient** effects, because hypoventilation reduces the alveolar oxygen concentration. Diseases causing alveolar fibrosis or oedema produce a membrane that is up to five times thicker than normal and interferes markedly with gas exchange, primarily that of oxygen (especially if it is fibrosed).

The **transfer factor** is an overall measure of the effectiveness of diffusion, and is expressed as the rate of gas transfer per unit of partial pressure. It is determined by taking a single breath of helium/air mixture containing a small amount of carbon monoxide, which is absent from normal blood, combines readily and completely with Hb, and is easily measured: hence the term T_{CO} (transfer factor for carbon monoxide). The old term, diffusing capacity, DL_{CO}, is now out of favour, because diffusion is only one aspect of gas transfer. The use of helium enables the alveolar volume to be determined. T_{CO} is reduced in fibrosis, oedema, emphysema, pulmonary embolism, severe anaemia and in smokers, but is increased in polycythaemia, ventilation–perfusion remodelling and alveolar bleeding.

The overall effects of the ventilatory and metabolic processes are summarized in Table 5.3. There is a progressive fall in P_aO_2 from the alveoli to the tissue cells, and a converse increase in P_aCO_2. Under conditions of normal ventilation and blood flow, about 11 mmol/min of oxygen and 9 mmol/min of carbon dioxide are transported in and out of the body respectively, giving values for P_aO_2 of 10.6–13.3 kPa and for P_aCO_2 of 4.5–6.0 kPa.

Gas transport in blood

Table 5.3 also gives the relative proportions of oxygen and carbon dioxide that are transported by various mechanisms. Although most of the oxygen is carried by Hb, that dissolved in the plasma may be important in patients in whom the oxygen-carrying capacity of the blood is significantly reduced, e.g. in severe anaemia. Because Hb is almost completely saturated under normal conditions, increasing the dissolved fraction may be the only way of increasing the oxygen content of the blood.

This is one rationale for the use of hyperbaric (high-pressure) oxygen chambers. An increase in dissolved oxygen level is useful in severe carbon monoxide poisoning, in which most of the Hb is bound firmly to carbon monoxide and is not available to bind oxygen. The high oxygen

Table 5.3 Partial pressures of oxygen and carbon dioxide in the body and their transport mechanisms

Partial pressures[a] Tissue	Oxygen	Carbon dioxide
Atmosphere	21.3	0.04
Alveoli	14.0	4.5
Blood capillaries Pulmonary		
• arteriolar	5.3	6.0
• venous		
Tissue	13.3	4.5
• arteriolar		
• venous		
Tissue cells	5.3	6.0

Transport mechanism	Oxygen (%)	Carbon dioxide (%)
Dissolved in plasma	3	7
HbO₂	97	–
HCO₃⁻	–	70
HbNHCOOH	–	23

[a] kPa, approximate values only; 1 kPa = 7.5 mmHg.
HbO₂, oxygenated haemoglobin; HbNHCOOH, carbaminohaemoglobin.

concentration also assists the dissociation of carbon monoxide from Hb.

The **oxygen saturation** of arterial blood (S_aO_2) is given by the expression:

$$S_aO_2 = \frac{O_2 \text{ combined with Hb}}{\text{Total } O_2 \text{ capacity of the blood}} \times 100\% \quad (5.2)$$

the denominator being the sum of the oxygen combined with Hb and the dissolved oxygen. This is an important parameter if a patient is severely anaemic. **Cyanosis**, due to the blue-purple colour of reduced Hb, is an unreliable indicator of low oxygen saturation because its recognition varies with skin pigmentation, lighting, etc. and it is difficult to detect if the Hb concentration is low (i.e. in anaemia) and hence the need to measure arterial blood gases (e.g. in a very severe asthma attack). Conversely, in the presence of polycythaemia, i.e. an increased red cell count, cyanosis may be marked because of the high concentration of reduced Hb. This produces the 'blue bloater' of COPD (p. 331). Cyanosis is best observed under the nails or in the tongue in good lighting. Oxygen saturation is usually measured by the colour of the blood in the nail bed, which is why hospital patients are told not to use nail varnish.

Because of its high aqueous solubility, most of the carbon dioxide is carried in solution as bicarbonate, these two compounds forming an important pH buffering system. Hb is an important intermediary, picking up carbon dioxide in the tissues in exchange for oxygen.

Lung volumes and capacities

An idealized spirogram for a normal young adult male is shown in Figure 5.6. This illustrates the trace obtained when the subject is initially breathing quietly at rest, and what happens when they then inhale and exhale maximally and as rapidly as possible. The **residual volume (RV)** cannot be used for ventilation but it plays an important part in buffering against the large swings that would occur in blood gas partial pressures if there were no gases in the lungs that

could be exchanged with those in the blood at the end of expiration.

Clinical aspects of respiratory disease

Classification

It will be obvious from the preceding discussion that the respiratory process can go wrong in various ways, and these are summarized in Table 5.4. There may be one of four basic problems:

1. Obstruction of gas flow in the airways.
2. Impaired alveolar diffusion.
3. Reduced lung compliance or a restricted thoracic capacity and expansibility.
4. Impaired ventilatory drive.

Obstructive defects (p. 292, Figure 5.8) are the most common, and usually affect the smaller airways. They may be a consequence of bronchoconstriction, inflammation or excessive mucus production. However, **bronchiectasis** (chronic airways dilatation, usually resulting from infective damage, and normally associated with massive sputum production; p. 340) affects the larger and medium-sized airways. Large airways

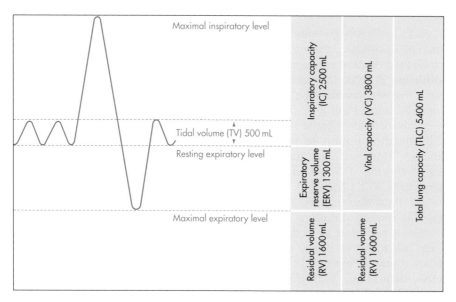

Figure 5.6 Lung volumes and capacities. Capacities are the sums of lung volumes. IC = TV + IRV; VC = TV + IRV + ERV; TLC = VC + RV.

Table 5.4   Types of respiratory disease

Type of defect	Pathological process	Some possible causes[a]
Obstructive	Obstruction or spasm of the airways	Asthma, COPD; emphysema; bronchiectasis; carcinoma; cystic fibrosis; physical obstruction, e.g. food; severe chest trauma, e.g. crushing
Diffusion	Alveolar damage	Hypersensitivity reactions, e.g. farmer's lung; emphysema; fibrosing alveolitis; iatrogenic, e.g. bleomycin, excessive oxygen concentration
	Pulmonary oedema	Left ventricular failure; lymphatic obstruction; inhalation pneumonitis
	Acute circulatory failure	Pulmonary embolism; myocardial infarction; shock
Restrictive	Pulmonary fibrosis	Hypersensitivity reactions, e.g. farmer's lung; iatrogenic, e.g. bleomycin, chest radiotherapy; environmental, e.g asbestosis, paraquat poisoning
	Rigidity of chest wall or vertebral column	Obesity; ankylosing spondylitis; systemic sclerosis; sarcoidosis; congenital deformity; systemic lupus erythematosus; tuberculosis
	Inspiratory pain	Pleurisy; trauma
	Pneumothorax	Emphysema; pneumonia; trauma
Ventilatory	Nerve damage	Stroke; trauma or infection of brain or spinal cord; paralysis of respiratory muscles, e.g. poliomyelitis
	Depressed nerve transmission	Narcotics; psychotropic drugs

[a] A disease or condition may appear in more than one heading, e.g. emphysema causes both obstruction and diffusion defects; farmer's lung causes both diffusion and restrictive defects.
COPD, chronic obstructive pulmonary disease.

may also be blocked by a foreign body: this may be inhaled food or, in children, almost any small toy or object, and is a medical emergency.

Chronic **diffusion defects**, in which there is impaired gas transfer across the alveolar membrane, usually result from a thickening of the respiratory (alveolar) membrane as a result of chronic inflammation leading to permanent fibrotic damage. However, in **pulmonary oedema**, e.g. following LVF or pulmonary thromboembolism (p. 342, Chapter 4), the accumulated alveolar fluid also acts as a physical barrier to prevent oxygen diffusion. An acute failure of pulmonary perfusion, or of the general circulation, e.g. due to MI or shock, will cause hypoxaemia and central cyanosis.

In **restrictive defects** (p. 342) there is an inability to expand the lungs adequately. Such defects may be caused by reduced lung compliance, but are often due to problems outside the lungs. Thus pleural disease, causing fibrosis, effusion or adhesions, will limit expansion of the underlying lung. A similar effect results from a **pneumothorax**, because if gas leaks into the pleural space following rupture of peripheral lung tissue (e.g. due to emphysema, infection, trauma or surgery), a lung may collapse partially or completely. Provided there is no serious underlying pathology the damaged area will heal, and fluid and gas will be reabsorbed fairly quickly by the pleural capillaries, thus restoring normality. Rib cage and spinal defects, e.g. due to congenital TB or ankylosing spondylitis (see Chapters 8 and 12), also restrict lung expansion.

Respiratory (ventilatory) failure is the result of an inadequate ventilatory drive to the respiratory muscles or inability of these to respond. A primary loss of the central drive to breathe is rare except in:

- head trauma;
- CNS disease and central depression by drugs, e.g. opioids, anaesthetics and, rarely nowadays, barbiturates;
- neuromuscular damage due to disease, e.g. Guillain-Barré syndrome, motor neurone disease, multiple sclerosis, poliomyelitis, diphtheria, severe hypokalaemia and chest trauma;
- severe airways obstruction, causing cyanosis and carbon dioxide retention;
- obesity, especially associated with rapid weight gain.

Clinical features

As in any other clinical situation an accurate history and examination are the essential first steps, and will often permit a reasonably confident diagnosis to be made before any investigations are carried out. The following symptoms and signs are characteristic of respiratory diseases.

Dyspnoea

This is a subjective, unpleasant sensation of breathlessness (**shortness of breath, SOB**) that probably results from an inappropriate effort of breathing. It does not correlate with blood P_aO_2. Objective signs, e.g. laboured breathing, rapid breathing (**tachypnoea**), breathing with pursed lips, hypoxaemia and hypercapnia, may also be present. The UK Medical Research Council has published a subjective graded dyspnoea scale (Table 5.5).

The time course for the development of breathlessness may help in diagnosis:

- Months to years: COPD, thyrotoxicosis.
- Weeks: anaemia, tumours.
- Hours to days: LVF, pneumonia.
- Minutes: acute severe asthma, major pulmonary embolism, pneumothorax.

Reduced exercise tolerance will initially present as **exertional dyspnoea** and should be defined quantitatively in terms of the patient's ability to walk on the flat or to climb stairs. However, there are many possible causes for dyspnoea apart from lung disease, e.g. cardiac disease, obesity, anaemia, anxiety and hyperthyroidism.

Orthopnoea is dyspnoea that occurs only when lying down. The symptom disappears when the patient is erect because fluid that has distributed from the legs to the lungs and interferes with oxygen absorption redistributes to the lower body, especially the ankles. It may be of cardiac origin, and is consequent on the reduced gravitational load on the circulation when the patient lies down. This produces an increased venous return and **pulmonary congestion**, i.e. an excessive volume of blood in the lungs. Redistribution of fluid throughout the lungs also occurs. If there is airways obstruction, limitation of diaphragm movement when lying down will also produce dyspnoea, especially in obese patients. These patients are also dyspnoeic on bending over.

Table 5.5   MRC dyspnoea scale

Grade[a]	Degree of breathlessness related to activity
1	Breathless only on strenuous exercise or excessive for the level of exercise
2	Short of breath when hurrying or walking up a slight hill
3	Walks slower than contemporaries on level ground, or has to stop for breath when walking at own pace
4	Stops for breath after walking about 100 m or after a few minutes on level ground
5	Too breathless to leave the house, or breathless when dressing or undressing

[a] After Fletcher CM, Elmes PC, Fairbairn MC, *et al*. The significance of symptoms and the diagnosis of chronic bronchitis in a working population. *BMJ* 1959; **2**: 257–66.

Pursed lip breathing occurs when lung compliance is increased by disease, e.g. emphysema causing loss of lung tissue (Figure 5.20), so that the airways have less support and an increased tendency to collapse on expiration. The patient then unwittingly breathes shallowly through partly closed lips to maintain a greater positive pressure than normal within the airways, thus keeping them open.

Breath sounds

Audible on examination
Wheezes (rhonchi) are sounds caused by gas flowing through airways obstructed by spasm or excessive secretions. This causes an obvious, more or less musical note that is usually more marked on expiration (see below). It is usually a symptom of obstruction but may be secondary to cardiovascular problems (so-called 'cardiac asthma').

Stridor is a harsher, inspiratory sound caused by obstruction of the larynx, trachea or other major airway.

Audible on auscultation
In the normal lung, respiration usually gives gentle, rustling sounds in the stethoscope. **Bronchial breathing** consists of higher-pitched sounds found on both inspiration and (more prolonged) on expiration. **Crackles** (crepitations, 'creps'; râles) are fine crackling noises caused by the opening of blocked, small airways at the periphery of the lung. Coarse crackles are caused by gas bubbling through copious secretions in larger airways. A **friction rub** results from friction between inflamed pleural membranes, similarly to pericardial friction. Wheezes are also heard.

The complete absence of lung sounds is a very sinister sign that indicates an inability to move air in and out of the lung, e.g. in a very severe asthma attack, severe thoracic trauma or physical obstruction of a major airway.

Cough and sputum

Coughing is usually caused by minor infection. It is abnormal when it is persistent, or associated with pain or significant sputum production. Although the nature of the cough may indicate the underlying pathology (e.g. the characteristic inspiratory 'whoop' of whooping cough or the softer, longer cough resulting from paralysis of the vocal chords), the associated features are usually more informative. A 'dry' cough (unproductive of sputum), may occur in asthma, early acute bronchitis or pneumonia. **Post-nasal drip**, the drainage of discharge from infected sinuses, etc. into the throat, also causes coughing.

A productive cough is one caused by the formation of excessive sputum. **Mucoid sputum** (white or grey) is usually produced in COPD, fibrosing alveolitis or asthma. **Purulent sputum** (green or yellow, containing pus) indicates infection, usually bacterial.

Haemoptysis (coughing up of blood or blood-streaked sputum) is an alarming symptom that is usually due to an acute lung infection (pneumonia or TB), or to an exacerbation of COPD. It may also indicate the possibility of serious disease such as pulmonary oedema (producing pink, frothy sputum), bronchial carcinoma or pulmonary embolism.

Hyperinflation

Because expiration through obstructed airways is more difficult than inspiration, severe obstructive airways disease leads to progressive **air trapping**, because not all of the inspired volume of gas in the lungs can be exhaled before the next inspiration occurs. The chest thus remains partially expanded at all times and, in extreme cases, this may eventually lead to a 'barrel chest'. There will then often be abnormally large cavities (**bullae**) in the lung parenchyma, which may be detectable by hyper-resonance on percussion. Hyperinflation tends to occur together with pursed lip breathing (see above).

Chest pain

Pain of respiratory origin may be due to **pleurisy** (i.e. pleural inflammation or infection), and a pneumothorax (i.e. air in the pleural space, usually due to trauma), may give a similar sharp pain. Acute tracheitis or bronchitis and pulmonary emboli may also give pain, particularly if embolism causes infarction, but disease in the lung parenchyma is normally painless. However, infarction is rare in lung tissue because of the excellent oxygen supply. Bronchial carcinoma may give only a vague, aching pain.

Chest pain may also be due to trauma, cardiovascular (see Chapter 4) or gastrointestinal conditions, bone tumours, herpes zoster (shingles), etc. Such pain may often be referred to the neck, back or abdomen because many major nerve tracts run in the mediastinum and may be affected secondarily. Thus, pain is a very non-specific diagnostic feature in most respiratory disease, even if linked to respiratory movements.

Finger clubbing

The cause of this sign (Figure 5.7) is unknown, but it often indicates a serious chronic chest disease that produces chronic hypoxaemia (e.g. bronchial and other tumours, bronchiectasis, advanced TB, cystic fibrosis and lung abscesses). However, it may also be due to congenital heart disease or chronic gastrointestinal disease and may even occur as a familial trait. The early changes are subtle, there being the loss of the angle between the nail and the skin at its base. Eventually there is pronounced longitudinal curvature of the nail, softening of the nail bed and 'drum-stick' fingers.

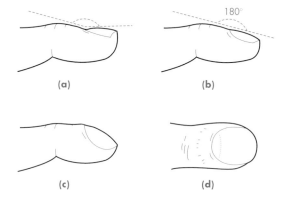

Figure 5.7 Finger clubbing. (a) Normal. (b) Early clubbing showing loss of the nail angle. (c) and (d) Late clubbing.

Heart failure due to lung disease

Right ventricular failure (RVF; see Chapter 4) secondary to lung disease is known as **cor pulmonale**. It is a consequence of **pulmonary hypertension** produced by:

- Alveolar and arterial hypoxia causing widespread pulmonary vasoconstriction and hypertrophy of pulmonary vascular smooth muscle.
- Distortion and fibrosis of the pulmonary blood vessels.
- Destruction of pulmonary arterioles and arterioles when alveoli are destroyed.
- Increased blood viscosity due to the polycythaemia resulting from chronic hypoxaemia.

The outstanding feature in these patients is fluid retention, with the usual symptoms of ankle oedema and progressive dyspnoea and exercise limitation. The increased afterload on the right ventricle, which has to work harder in order to perfuse the lungs, eventually leads to heart failure. However, in the early stages the heart may compensate for the failure by right ventricular dilatation (see Chapter 4, Figure 4.12).

Investigation

Examination

From the above review of the clinical features the following are clearly relevant:

- Observation: pattern of respiration, cough, cyanosis, finger clubbing.
- Palpation: lymph nodes, diversion of the trachea (by a mass or pneumothorax), tenderness.
- Percussion: both sides are normally equally resonant. Hyper-resonance indicates a loss of tissue (a cavity) and dullness an area of consolidation, e.g. fluid in pneumonia.
- Auscultation (listening to breath sounds, etc.).
- Cardiovascular examination.

Imaging

A plain CXR is the most valuable adjunct to the history and examination. An erect postero-anterior (PA) view, i.e. the X-rays pass from back to front, is usually preferred because there is less magnification of the image. It shows the locations and sizes of the heart and other organs as well as lung tissue abnormalities. The lung fields should be evenly translucent and without shadowing, except in the hilar regions (where the main blood vessels and bronchi enter the lungs) and from the ribs (see Figure 5.1). Excessive spacing between the ribs and a gap between the apex (bottom) of the heart and the left diaphragm indicate hyperinflation.

Complete collapse of a lung will cause a shift of the heart and other mediastinal structures into the area of collapse. Lesser degrees of collapse produce a well-defined shadow due to the increased density of the collapsed lung.

Ultrasound scanning has a limited role in investigating chest problems because currently it is possible only to visualize objects that are in contact with the chest wall with this technique. However, it is useful when guiding a needle for biopsy or aspiration of an effusion.

Computed tomography (CT) and **magnetic resonance imaging (MRI)** are widely used and provide valuable additional information. Both techniques permit accurate visualization of major organs and highlight the nature and extent of any abnormal or doubtful shadows in the CXR. Conventional CT scanning involves a high radiation dose, e.g. 40 to 250 times that of a normal CXR, but the advent of 'spiral' scanning, in which patients are moved slowly lengthwise while the X-ay beam is rotated around them, enables data to be obtained rapidly. This is less stressful to patients, reduces the X-ray dose and can provide dynamic information, e.g. visualization of pulmonary emboli by demonstrating obstruction to blood flow, using an injected venous contrast medium.

MRI involves no radiation dose, and gives detailed images of the lung parenchyma. The introduction of rapid acquisition scanning has improved patient acceptability. Another technique, **magnetic resonance angiography**, a form of **functional MRI (fMRI)**, may be used to visualize blood vessels, without having to inject contrast medium.

Fluoroscopy is an X-ray technique used to visualize dynamic events (e.g. the movements of organs, etc., such as refluxing of stomach contents into the oesophagus) that may cause chest pain (GORD; see Chapter 3), and is used only for specialized investigations. The use of image intensifiers and a television monitor display reduces the high radiation dose received formerly by radiologists, and has improved the utility of the technique. However, it has been largely replaced by **ultrasound scanning**.

Bronchoscopy and biopsy

Flexible **fibre-optic endoscopes** (see Chapter 3, Figure 3.5) are indispensable for the direct observation of the airways and the biopsy of lesions located by imaging. Bronchial brushings and washings can also be taken for cytological and bacteriological examination. Modern bronchoscopes will reach nearly all parts of the lungs, especially in the upper lobes.

Most bronchoscopies are performed to diagnose potential malignancy, infections and diffuse parenchymal disease, and to confirm uncertain diagnoses. Obstructing tumours may also be treated through the endoscope by diathermy or lasers if they are small enough. Older-type rigid bronchoscopes are still used occasionally for the removal of small inhaled foreign bodies from the trachea.

Superficial lesions and the pleura may be biopsied percutaneously using special needles, usually guided by X-ray or CT, and are less invasive. Open lung biopsy is done as an adjunct to essential surgery.

Lung function tests

These are used to determine the type of disease, its severity and the response to therapy. **Ventilatory function** is assessed using a recording spirometer, such as the Vitalograph (Figure 5.8(a)) or the Microflow, both of which work on a simple bellows principle. The patient inspires maximally and then blows as hard and as fast as possible into the mouthpiece, producing a

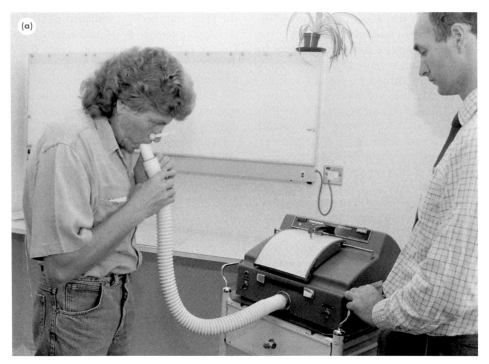

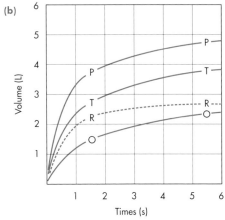

Figure 5.8 Pulmonary function testing with the Vitalograph respirometer. (a) Testing in progress, patient wearing a nose clip. (b) Traces obtained showing: O, typical obstructive pattern; T, improvement after a test dose of a beta$_2$-bronchodilator in an asthmatic patient (A; see Table), showing excellent reversibility; P, result after regular bronchodilator use in the same asthmatic patient; R, typical restrictive pattern (Patient B).

| Patient[b] | Curve | FEV$_1$ (L) | FVC (L) | FEV$_1$/FVC (%) | Type of respiratory defect | Predicted normal values[a] | | |
						FEV$_1$ (L)	FVC (L)	FEV$_1$/FVC (%)
A	O	1.2	2.4	50	Obstructive,			
	T	2.3	3.8	61	becoming	4.2	5.2	81
	P	3.3	4.8	69	normal			
B	R	2.0	2.6	77	Restrictive	3.3	3.9	85

[a] FEV$_1$, forced expiratory volume in 1s; FVC, forced vital capacity; FEV$_1$/FVC, forced expiratory ratio.

[b] Patient A, asthma, male, 43 years of age, height 180 cm.

Patient B, spinal deformity from childhood tuberculosis, female, 25 years of age, height 168 cm.

recording similar to that shown in Figure 5.8(b). Several parameters can be derived from the curve, the most useful being the **forced vital capacity (FVC)**, the maximum volume of gas that can be blown out, and the **forced expiratory volume**, usually recorded as the volume forced out in 1 second **(FEV$_1$)**. The predicted values of these for a normal subject can be estimated from nomograms that relate them to age, height and sex. These parameters are relatively independent of the force applied during expiration.

Generally, a fit young adult will have an FVC of 4–5 L and the FEV$_1$ will be at least 75% of this, i.e. the **forced expiratory ratio (FEV$_1$/FVC)** exceeds 0.75, indicating efficient ventilation. Obstruction of the airways leads to a low FVC and to forced expiratory ratios of <0.65 (curve O, Figure 5.8(b)); in severe disease it may be as low as 0.3. Restrictive patterns of disease reduce both

the FEV$_1$ and the FVC similarly, so that the ratio is normal (curve R, Figure 5.8(b); Table 5.6). Forced expiratory ratios of about 0.6 lead to dyspnoea only on severe exertion, at 0.5 there will be significant exercise limitation, and below 0.3 there is likely to be chronic disability, orthopnoea (breathlessness that occurs when lying down), hypercapnia and frequent invalidism.

Figure 5.8(b) shows that the spirometer can also be used for a diagnostic trial of drugs and to monitor the benefits of therapy objectively. If an obstructive pattern is seen, the patient inhales a dose of a bronchodilator and repeats the test after 20–30 min. Good to moderate **reversibility** (≥15% improvement) is observed in asthmatics (e.g. curve T), in whom there may be a return to a near-normal trace (curve P). There may be some reversibility in chronic bronchitics, but this rarely exceeds 5%.

Table 5.6 Changes in some common pulmonary function parameters and normal values[a] in respiratory diseases of moderate severity

Parameter	Values or changes[b]			
	Asthma	COPD	Emphysema	Restrictive lung disease
FVC	N/[↓]	N/[↓]	N/[↓]	50–60% of normal
FEV$_1$/FVC (%)	40–60	40–60	40–60	N/[↑]
Improvement with bronchodilator (%) (i.e. reversibility)	10–50	0–20	0–10	Nil
RV (% of normal)	150	150	150	75
PEF	↓/↓↓	↓/↓↓	↓/↓↓	N
TLC	N/↑	N/↑	↑	↓
Gas transfer	N	N/↓	50% of N	N/↓
P_aO_2	N/↓	↓/↓↓	[↓]	↓ (E)
P_aCO_2	N/[↑]	↑	N/[↑]	N
Lung compliance	N	N/↓	N/↑	N/↓
Dyspnoea	+/++	+/++	+/++	++

[a] Approximate normal values for adults aged 30 years; heights: males, 175 cm; females, 165 cm: FVC (L): M, 4.8; F, 3.51; FEV$_1$ (L): M, 4.0; F, 3.1; FEV$_1$/FVC (%): M, 83; F, 89; RV/TLC (%): M, 29.2; F, 26.2.

[b] Values determined at rest, unless otherwise stated: many asthma patients appear virtually normal (N) between attacks; (E), patient exercised; [ ], slight effect; +/++, present/strongly present.

COPD, chronic obstructive pulmonary disease; FEV$_1$ forced expiratory volume in 1 s; FVC, forced vital capacity; FEV$_1$/FVC, forced expiratory ratio; PEF peak expiratory flow; RV, residual volume; TLC, total lung capacity; P_aO_2, P_aCO_2, arterial partial pressures of oxygen and carbon dioxide.

The **flow–volume loop** is obtained by asking the patient to inspire maximally and to blow into the instrument as hard as possible to maximal expiration and then to inhale again to TLC. This is a sensitive test that will discriminate between asthma and other types of airways obstruction (Figure 5.9).

The **peak expiratory flow (PEF)**, the maximum expiratory flow rate in L/min measured over the first 10 msec of expiration, may be determined directly from the flow–volume loop (Figure 5.9) or calculated from the initial slope of the spirometer curve shown in Figure 5.8(b). However, PEF is much more easily determined using a peak flow meter or gauge (Figure 5.10), although this measures flow over only the first 2 ms of forced expiration. A nomogram, a simple 'slide rule' or a chart (Figure 5.11) is used to predict normal values. The PEF is a simple and sensitive indicator of the presence and severity of airways obstruction, so the determination is popular in chest clinics and general practice as a simple, rapid, cheap diagnostic and monitoring tool. However, the accuracy of the test depends on the instrument used and on the patient making a maximal inspiration and applying maximal force during expiration, whereas the FEV_1 is less energy-dependent. Further, lung function is overestimated in individuals with moderate reduction in airflow. The PEF is not diagnostically reliable because it will not distinguish between the different types of airways obstruction, unlike the flow–volume loop, but is strongly suggestive.

Peak flow gauges are particularly useful for observing rapid changes and monitoring the severity of disease and the effects of medication in an individual, especially in asthma. They are invaluable for the routine home self-monitoring of patients with significant asthma. Because the same instrument is always used, the absolute accuracy of the instrument is not important, because it will still show relative changes in lung function. If a diary is kept, patients can detect the warning signs of an impending, possibly severe, attack and take appropriate therapeutic measures (p. 311). However, one study has shown that a high proportion of patient diaries are unreliable. Furthermore, PEF measurements are less useful in those with chronic asthma (p. 309) or

COPD (p. 326), where there is significant fixed (irreversible) airways obstruction.

Other tests may be performed in specialist centres, e.g. determination of lung compliance, T_{CO}, ventilation/perfusion estimates and lung volumes and capacities.

Blood gases

Measurements of P_aO_2, P_aCO_2 and pH, done on a sample of arterial blood taken from the radial artery or the ear lobe, provide valuable information on the levels of hypoxaemia and hypercapnia, the response to oxygen and other therapy, the adequacy of ventilation, and the nature and severity of any metabolic disturbance. They are mandatory in hospital for the management of seriously ill patients. S_aO_2 is determined readily by **pulse oximetry**, which measures the level of blood oxygenation from the colour of the blood in the nail bed or the earlobe. However, this is unreliable if the peripheral circulation is impaired.

Exercise testing

It is preferable to use a treadmill or cycle ergometer because performance can be related directly to predetermined levels of effort. The speed, slope or resistance is increased progressively until the patient stops because of breathlessness, chest pain, etc., or reaches their predetermined safe heart rate. In health the heart rate should never be allowed to exceed $220 - $(age in years) beats/min and should preferably be kept below 70% of this rate. The ventilation rates, composition of the expired gas mixture and oxygen saturation of the blood are measured (preferably by pulse oximetry) and an ECG is recorded (see Chapter 4) and the S_aO_2 falls if there is ventilation–perfusion mismatch, e.g. in obstructive pulmonary disease. These parameters enable the severity of lung disease to be determined, abnormalities of ventilation or oxygen uptake to be assessed, and pulmonary or cardiac causes of disability to be distinguished.

However, simple walking tests are often done, in which the patient is asked to walk up and down a corridor for 2, 6 or 12 min. The distance walked in the time is measured, or the time or distance reached when breathlessness or pain forces cessation.

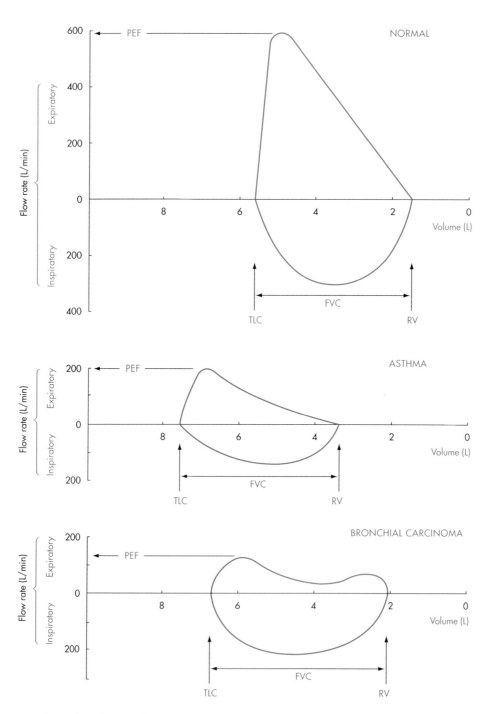

Figure 5.9   Flow–volume loops in obstructive respiratory diseases. FVC, forced vital capacity; PEF, peak expiratory flow; RV, residual volume; TLC, total lung capacity.

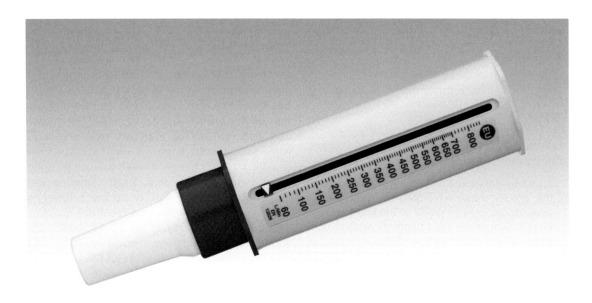

Figure 5.10   The Mini-Wright Standard-range peak flow meter (60-800 L/min), a popular model suitable for patient self-monitoring by adults and children (prescribable via the NHS in the UK).

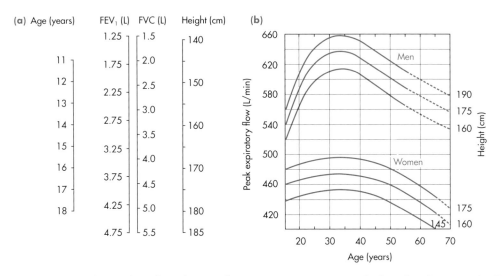

Figure 5.11   Some predictive charts for pulmonary function tests. (a) Nomogram for forced vital capacity (FVC) and forced expiratory volume in 1 s (FEV1); both sexes, 5–18 years. (b) Partial relationship for the prediction of normal peak expiratory flow (PEF) in adults. Note that the PEF for adult males is higher than that for females of the same age and height and that ventilatory function peaks at 30–35 years, rather different from that for most physical attributes. (Reproduced with permission from Vitalograph Ltd.)

Obstructive pulmonary disease

Asthma

Definition

No entirely satisfactory definition exists, although the following covers most patients:

> A chronic inflammatory disease of the airways, the precise cause of which is incompletely understood. In susceptible individuals, inflammatory symptoms are usually associated with widespread, variable airflow obstruction and an increase in airways' response to a variety of stimuli. Obstruction is usually reversible, either spontaneously or with treatment'.

This somewhat vague clinical definition reflects our lack of knowledge about the precise nature of the disease. Winsel (see References and further reading, p. 364) has proposed that asthma is probably an overlapping complex of separate, genetically defined syndromes – this could explain the imprecise definition.

Thus diagnosis depends on clinical judgement in addition to airflow measurement, provoking factors and reversibility on treatment. This is 'bronchial asthma': the term 'cardiac asthma' has been used to denote pulmonary oedema consequent on LVF (see Chapter 4) but this usage is now obsolete and 'asthma' now invariably means 'bronchial asthma'.

Epidemiology and natural history

There was an international increase in asthma prevalence from 1979 to 1990. This trend was confirmed by an 18-country study of hospital admissions for asthma. Since then, the prevalence of asthma has declined (Table 5.7). The reasons for these changes are not clear. In developed countries, the prevalence is currently about 20%, with about 10–15% of the 10–20-year age group being affected. Studies of occupational asthma indicate that up to 20% of workers may develop symptoms if they are exposed to sensitizing agents. The consulting rate for asthma doubled in the decade 1971/2 to 1981/2 but has since stabilized. Some of this increase may be due to increased awareness of the disease and expectations of effective treatment and some to improved diagnosis, but it is considered to reflect a real change. The prevalence in some developing countries (e.g. South America and Fiji) appears to be similar, but is much lower in some African and Far Eastern countries.

The incidence peaks at age 10–12 years, with about 20% of children wheezing annually, and there is a secondary peak at about 65 years (6%). These two peaks correspond to the two main clinical types of disease (Table 5.8). If triggered by identifiable external allergens in atopic individuals the condition is called **extrinsic** or **episodic asthma**. In other patients the agents, circumstances or conditions responsible for attacks are unknown or poorly defined. This latter form tends to be chronic, or becomes so after a time: this is **intrinsic** or **cryptogenic asthma**. Extrinsic asthma tends to occur in the younger age group, is usually relatively mild and is related to atopy, i.e. sufferers have a general allergic tendency and often have hay fever and eczema (see Chapter 13). In contrast, the

Table 5.7   Asthma prevalence (% of age group) in 12-year-old children in the UK

Condition	Year		
	1973	1988	2003
Asthma ever	5.5	12.0	27.3
Wheeze in last year	9.8	15.2	19.5
Wheeze ever without URTI	6.6	13.8	17.8
PEF fell by – 15% or more	6.7	7.7	4.7[a]
– 25% or more	2.0	4.1	2.4[a]

[a] Falls were due to increased use of inhaled corticosteroids.
URTI, upper respiratory tract infection.

intrinsic asthmatic is usually older, with more persistent disease. However, this distinction is of only limited value because about 30% of patients have mixed-type disease and it does not materially affect management. On average, each doctor in the UK will have about 125 asthma patients, and a community pharmacy can expect to see about twice this number.

Up to 80% of children suffer episodic symptoms of wheezing, usually associated with respiratory infections, but most of these are not regarded as asthmatics. Asthma is the most common chronic disease in the UK and the principal cause of childhood morbidity. It is the commonest cause of absence from school on medical grounds. Boys are more likely to develop asthma than girls, the relative prevalence before puberty being M : F $\geq$2 : 1. In many children, the frequency and severity of attacks declines from the age of 6–8 years, with at least 30% growing out of the condition by puberty, at which point the sex prevalence is about equal. However, a tendency to **bronchial hyper-reactivity** may persist throughout life, with a highly variable frequency of attacks or chronic wheeziness. Above the age of 20 years, more women are affected, the M : F ratio of incidence being about 1 : 1.5.

Interestingly, a high salt intake has been shown to increase bronchial hyper-responsiveness in men, but not in women. Further, an above average dietary intake of magnesium has been shown to improve the FEV_1 and to reduce hyper-reactivity and wheezing. Clearly, the role of dietary minerals needs to be explored more fully.

The increasing prevalence of asthma suggests the probable importance of environmental agents as triggers for the onset of the disease in genetically predisposed individuals, but evidence for this is equivocal. In the UK, a recent study found little urban–rural or geographical variation in prevalence. The prevalence in the unpolluted Scottish highlands was found to be similar to that in nearby urbanized areas. Further, the prevalence in New Zealand, with a favourable climate and an unpolluted atmosphere, is one of the highest in the world. However, studies in the USA have implicated outdoor, and especially indoor, air contaminants as important risk factors for the development of childhood asthma and as determinants of severity. One possible reason for this discrepancy

Table 5.8   The two clinical types of asthma

Feature	Episodic (extrinsic)	Chronic (intrinsic)
Proportion (%)[a]	20	50
Age of onset	Childhood	Usually adults
Atopic patient	Yes: family history common[b]	No
Known allergens or precipitating factors	Yes	None or URTI Often sensitive to aspirin
Skin tests	Positive	Negative
Severity	Usually episodic Often mild	Often chronic May be severe
Treatment	Effective	Moderately effective, oral corticosteroids may be required

[a] 30% have mixed type disease.

[b] There is often a personal or family history of eczema and allergic rhinitis.

URTI, upper respiratory tract infection.

may be the larger number of centrally heated, air-conditioned homes in the USA with limited fresh air exchange – conditions that favour the persistence of dust mite, animal and other airborne allergens and irritants.

The indicators of a poorer prognosis are:

- severe or early onset;
- persistent attacks;
- an atopic patient;
- a family history of atopy;
- female sex.

Asthma accounts for about 1400 deaths annually in the UK, and many of these are the result of under-diagnosis and under-treatment. A 1998 study of 12–14-year-olds found that 4% had been diagnosed as asthmatic but were poorly controlled, and a further 1–3.4% had moderate to severe symptoms but were undiagnosed and untreated. Also, patients may not appreciate the severity of an attack. The British Thoracic Society (BTS) surveyed 90 asthma deaths in north-west England in 1998 and found that only 36 of the patients had been sufficiently alarmed to see their doctors, and of those only nine were then managed appropriately, though unsuccessfully. A 1999 survey in Scotland produced similar results. All of these factors are theoretically preventable. Although the situation has improved since these reports, there is still a great deal to be done before the 2.1 million symptomatic people with asthma are treated satisfactorily and preventable asthma deaths are reduced substantially.

However, a 2006 systematic review of 19 trials (34 000 asthma patients) worldwide found that 80% of deaths were related to the use of long-acting beta$_2$-agonists (LABAs; *salmeterol* and *formoterol*; see below). The data indicate that patients taking LABAs are 3.5 times more likely to die from asthma than those taking a placebo and 2.5 times more likely to be admitted to hospital. Of particular concern is the finding that LABAs can trigger bronchial inflammation and hyper-reactivity without prior warning signs. This seems to bear out long-standing concerns about the safety of LABAs, although some respiratory physicians have some reservations, awaiting confirmation of the data.

Pathophysiology

The underlying problem is intense **airways inflammation**, leading to **bronchial hyper-reactivity**. Inflammation is present even when patients are asymptomatic. Everyone's airways will become constricted if exposed to a sufficient dose of a bronchoconstrictor, e.g. histamine or methacholine. Following viral respiratory tract infection the airways of non-asthmatics will be more sensitive than usual for up to 6 weeks as a result of mucosal damage and the exposure of receptors for physiological mediators (e.g. histamine, kinins, LTs and PAF; see Chapter 2). Asthmatics may be up to 100 times more sensitive than normal subjects and atopic individuals suffering from hay fever but not asthma form an intermediate group.

The precise cause of this hyper-reactivity is unknown, though LTs are definitely implicated, and LT receptor antagonists are used in therapy (see below). Also, **remodelling** over time causes changes in all the layers of the airway walls (e.g. goblet cell hyperplasia, shortening of smooth muscle cells and swelling of the adventitia), which contribute to hyper-reactivity, especially in chronic asthma. A number of other putative mediators have been identified and we know of many factors that may precipitate attacks (Tables 5.9 and 5.10; Figure 5.12). Although some patients are sensitive to only a single trigger factor, most are sensitive to several, so attacks may be due to the combined effects of two or more of these. Inflammation is clearly the single most significant sign. In an acute attack, the epithelium is intensely infiltrated with eosinophils, causing the release of pro-inflammatory eosinophil products (e.g. proteins and neurotoxins), which damage the epithelium.

Other inflammatory cells (mast cells, basophils, etc.) also accumulate and release a wide variety of inflammatory mediators, e.g. histamine, LTs, PGs, thromboxanes and PAF. These cause bronchiolar smooth muscle contraction and marked oedema of the bronchial mucosa, epithelial shedding and receptor exposure. The extent of the damage produced is reflected in the degree of airways hyper-responsiveness produced. Lymphocytes and

Table 5.9   Some substances and conditions that may precipitate asthmatic attacks

Environmental and medical factors	Examples
Common allergens	Pollens, especially grasses; mould spores; animal fur and dander; house dust mite (*Dermatophagoides pteronyssimus*); proteolytic enzymes, e.g. biological detergents, some foods and food additives
Foods	Milk, eggs, nuts, alcoholic drinks, tartrazine colorant, sulphur dioxide preservative
Non-specific irritants	Dusts; cigarette smoke; atmospheric pollutants, especially sulphur dioxide
Exercise	
Medical conditions	Pregnancy; menstruation; respiratory infections, especially viruses; thyrotoxicosis; levothyroxine therapy; reflux oesophagitis
Medicines	See Table 5.10

Occupational causes[a]

Metal salts, e.g. platinum, chromium, nickel; laboratory animals and insects; plastics, e.g. epoxy resins, isocyanates, PVC; microorganisms, e.g. fermentation plants, humidifiers and air-conditioning plants, mushrooms; pharmaceuticals, e.g. antibiotics, acacia gum, ethylenediamine, formaldehyde, animal products; colophony fumes, e.g. soldering fluxes; proteolytic enzymes; dyes and hairdressing solutions; fabrics, e.g. silk; plant materials, e.g. pollens, coffee beans, tobacco, tea, wood, dust, cotton, flour and grain dusts

[a] These may be legally recognized grounds for industrial injury compensation.

Table 5.10   Some drugs and medicines that may provoke asthmatic attacks

General drugs

Antimicrobials: cefaloridine, erythromycin, griseofulvin, nitrofurantoin, penicillins, streptomycin, tetracyclines
Aspirin, some non-steroidal anti-inflammatory drugs
Beta-blockers, carbamazepine, sulfasalazine, iodine-based contrast media, dextrans, pituitary snuff, preservatives and dyes used in formulation

Drugs and devices used in asthma treatment

Ipratropium bromide, methylxanthines, hydrocortisone
Dry powder inhalers, aerosol propellants, nebulized hypotonic solutions

macrophages are also abundant, but less so than eosinophils. Goblet cell hyperplasia causes hypersecretion of mucus, which may be abnormally viscous and may plug the smaller airways.

The initial step in this inflammatory process is believed to be T cell activation (see Chapter 2). Lymphokines are produced which amplify the immune response, notably by the production of IgE antibodies and their induction of allergic reactions. Allergic mechanisms are especially important in episodic asthma associated with ocupational allergens.

Bronchoconstriction may also be mediated by cholinergic action via the vagus nerve. Although there is no adrenergic innervation of the airways, alpha- and beta-receptors are present and are targets for bronchodilating drugs. Emotional upset does not normally trigger an attack but it may aggravate symptoms. However, severe stress, e.g. battle fatigue in soldiers, can exacerbate an asthmatic tendency and cause symptoms in patients with a subclinical condition.

About 80% of asthmatics suffer **nocturnal attacks**, described as 'morning dipping' (see below and Figure 5.13), during which the early morning peak flow may fall by as much as 50%. This marked diurnal variation in respiratory

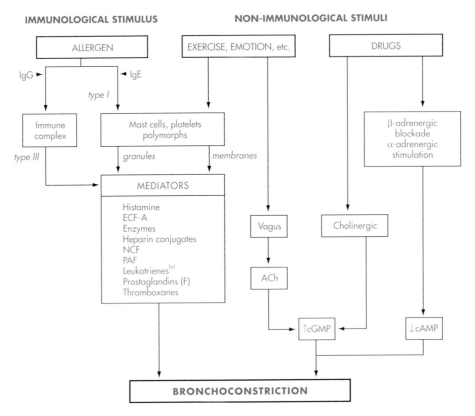

Figure 5.12   Some factors involved in producing bronchoconstriction. [a]Leukotrienes $C_4 + D_4 + E_4$ used to be known as 'slow reacting substance of anaphylaxis' (SRS-A). Reaction types I and III, Coombs and Gell classification (see Chapter 2, p. 39). ACh, acetylcholine; cAMP, cGMP, cyclic adenosine and guanosine monophosphates; ECF-A, eosinophil chemotactic factor A; NCF, neutrophil chemotactic factor; PAF, platelet activating factor; ↑, ↓, increased or decreased level.

function is much greater than is seen in normal subjects, in whom nocturnal falls are about 8%. The tendency to nocturnal attacks is exacerbated by allergen exposure, especially following a severe attack, when patients are particularly vulnerable. It is tempting to associate this with the nadir of adrenal cortical activity, which occurs at a similar time, though evidence for this is lacking. The principal factor appears to be other physiological changes that occur during sleep, e.g. lower levels of blood sympathomimetic amines, reduced sympathetic outflow, increased vagal (cholinergic) activity and reduced mucociliary clearance. Airways cooling during the night may also make a small, though significant, contribution, so it is reasonable to counsel patients not to sleep in cold rooms.

Although it has been suggested that a fish oil diet may be beneficial by promoting the formation of 5-series LTs as opposed to the 4-series compounds derived from arachidonic acid (see Chapter 12, Figure 12.9), available data indicate that they are not clinically beneficial and may even be harmful. No fish oil product is licensed for asthma treatment in the UK.

Exercise-induced asthma occurs in many patients, especially the young. The attack comes on after a short bout of vigorous exercise or during a prolonged sporting period, e.g. a football match, and may be the only symptom of asthma. The trigger seems to be the excessive cooling and drying of the airways epithelium by the increased airflow during exercise, because inhalation of cold, dry air can also provoke

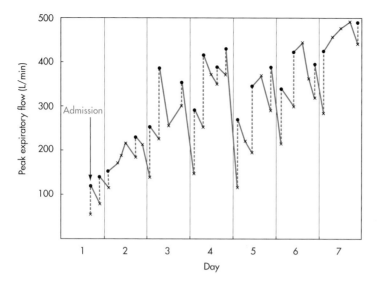

Figure 5.13   Peak flow chart of a patient recovering from a severe attack of asthma. The chart shows morning dipping and considerable variability imposed on a pattern of underlying improvement towards normality. x, readings immediately before medication; • readings 15 min after inhaling a beta$_2$-bronchodilator.

attacks, whereas swimming is the exercise least likely to do so. However, exercise-induced asthma may indicate poor asthma control, so patients who suffer such attacks should be reassessed to ensure their treatment is optimal.

The complexity of the mechanisms and mediators that appear to underlie asthma (see Figure 5.12) may reflect our limited understanding of the pathological processes concerned. However, these uncertainties may be resolved within the next 10 years by the application of new techniques from the rapidly expanding fields of genetics, immunology and molecular biology.

Occupational asthma is estimated to cause 5–10% of cases in adults aged 20–44 years in industrialized countries, notably cleaners, spray and other painters, and plastics workers. Agricultural workers also have a high risk, but it is unclear how much of this is due to modern farm chemicals and how much to exposure to fungal spores. A partial listing of possible agents is given in Table 5.9.

Clinical features

The classic symptoms of asthma are attacks of breathlessness, wheezing, 'chest tightness' and cough that start within 15 min of exposure to a trigger factor. Depending on the severity of the attack, peak flow may fall to 25–75% of that recorded between attacks, and usually recovers over a period of 60–90 min without treatment (Figure 5.14), but more promptly if a bronchodilator is used. Between attacks, patients may have an apparently normal respiratory function.

However, this pattern is shown in only about the 20% of patients showing an immediate allergic (type I) hypersensitivity reaction (see Chapter 2). About 50% of asthmatics experience delayed attacks (see below) and a further 30% suffer both immediate and delayed attacks.

Dyspnoea in asthmatics is worse in the early hours of the morning, whether they experience acute severe nocturnal attacks or not, and most asthma deaths occur at night or in the early morning.

The criteria for a diagnosis of acute severe asthma in children and adults are given in Table 5.11. In a severe attack there will be hyperventilation and hyperinflation, to the extent that patients are incapable of speaking in complete sentences, with prolonged expiration and the use of the accessory muscles of respiration. Peak flow may fall below 100 L/min. Patients are very anxious, the heart

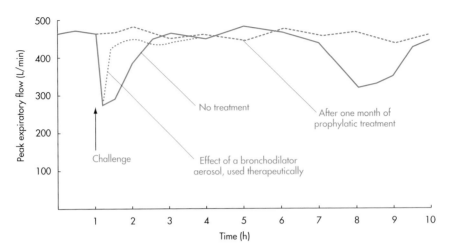

Figure 5.14   Peak flow chart of an asthmatic patient following an allergic challenge showing the effects of therapeutic and prophylactic treatment on the early and late reactions.

Table 5.11   Indicators of asthma severity

Indicator	Adults	Children over 2 years[a]	Children under 2 years[a]
Moderate exacerbation: No features of acute severe asthma			
Symptoms	Increasing[b]	Cough and/or wheeze	Cough and/or wheeze
PEF	50–75% of best or predicted (mild airflow obstruction)	Attack exercise-induced <50% of best or predicted	Attack exercise-induced N/A
Acute severe asthma			
	Any of the following:	**Any** of the following:	**Any** of the following:
Breathlessness	Cannot complete sentences in one breath	Cannot complete sentences in one breath **or** too breathless to talk or feed Rhonchi	Too breathless to talk or feed Rhonchi
Respiratory rate	≥25/min	>30/min (>5 years) >50/min (2–5 years) Use of accessory muscles of respiration	>50/min Use of accessory muscles of respiration
PEF	30–49% of best or predicted (moderate air flow airways obstruction)	≤50% of best or predicted	N/A
Heart rate	≥110/min	>120/min (>5 years) >130/min (2–5 years)	>130/min

Table 5.11   (*Continued*)

Life-threatening asthma

	Any of the following:	**Any** of the following:	**Any** of the following:
Breathlessness and central nervous signs	Feeble respiratory effort, silent chest Exhaustion, confusion, coma	Silent chest or poor respiratory effort Exhaustion, confusion, agitation, reduced consciousness or coma	Silent chest or poor respiratory effort Exhaustion, confusion, agitation, reduced consciousness or coma
PEF	<30% of best or predicted (severe air flow obstruction)	<33% of best or predicted	N/A
Oxygenation	Cyanosis SpO_2 <92%[c] P_aO_2 <8 kPa	Cyanosis	Cyanosis
Carbon dioxide	P_aCO_2 normal[d]		
Heart signs	Bradycardia (<60/min) **or** other dysrhythmia		
Blood pressure	Hypotension		

Near fatal asthma; always requires hospital admission

	Any of the symptoms/signs of life-threatening asthma **and/or** raised P_aCO_2 **and/or** requiring mechanical ventilation with raised inflation pressures	Any of the symptoms/signs of life-threatening asthma	

[a] Lung function tests cannot be used for children under 2 years.
[b] Increase in severity or frequency.
[c] By pulse oximetry at finger or ear lobe.
[d] Normal = 4.6–6.0 kPa. N/A, not applicable in this age group.

rate may exceed 120 beats/min, and there may be palpable pulsus paradoxus (see below) and peripheral cyanosis. A 'quiet chest' on auscultation, indicating very poor air flow, also indicates a severe attack.

Many patients experience a variety of non-respiratory symptoms before an attack:

- Mild to moderate **chest pain** (about 75%), the severity being unrelated to asthma severity. The pain worsens on coughing, deep inspiration and most changes in position, but 65% obtain relief by sitting erect. This may result in fruitless investigations for cardiac problems or pulmonary embolism (p. 342).

- Other symptoms include nose or throat irritation, sleepiness, dry mouth, thirst, urinary frequency, flushing, irritability and depression.

Diagnosis

This is based on the history, examination and the investigations outlined below. It must be remembered that patients with episodic asthma may appear completely normal between attacks unless provocation testing is used, but this is potentially hazardous. Those with chronic asthma will show abnormal signs at all times, depending on severity.

Moderate asthma exacerbations

The following features may be found:

- Forced expiratory ratio <0.65 (normal ≥0.75). A spirogram has the general appearance of that in Figure 5.15(b).
- PEF reduced to 50–75% of the predicted normal or best value.
- Flow–volume loop showing air trapping with increased TLC and RV (Figure 5.9).
- Blood gases are not normally measured in moderate exacerbations, but should be done for all asthmatic patients admitted to hospital.
- WBCs: eosinophils >0.5 × 10⁹/L (normal <0.4 × 10⁹/L) in extrinsic asthma and they may be present in sputum.
- Reversibility with an inhaled beta₂-agonist (Figure 5.8): a 15% increase (or more) in FEV₁ or PEF is conclusive: lesser degrees of reversibility do not distinguish between asthma and COPD (see Table 5.20). In very

severe attacks, or in chronic asthma, this reversibility may not be seen, because the airways become unresponsive.

Severe attacks

Retention of carbon dioxide in near-fatal asthma may be indicated by drowsiness, sweating and cyanosis, and a high-volume, bounding pulse. Central cyanosis is a serious sign but its absence does not preclude a life-threatening attack.

Pulsus paradoxus is a pulse that decreases markedly in pressure during inspiration and is a sign of LVF. Although it is mentioned in many texts, it is present in less than half of patients and is consequently an unreliable sign.

Other features have been described above.

Other investigations

IgE blood levels may be raised indicating atopic reactivity and are determined by the radioallergosorbent test (RAST) procedure (Figure 5.16), but this is used for patients who are difficult to diagnose (see below), as a

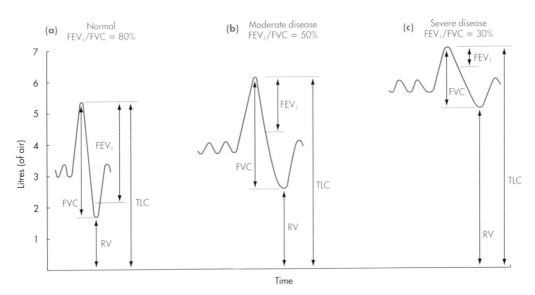

Figure 5.15 Spirograms in normal subjects and in obstructive lung disease. Expiration is slowed markedly in disease. The increase in TLC is due entirely to increased RV (unusable), the result of air trapping and, possibly, emphysema. FVC, forced vital capacity; FEV₁, forced expiratory volume in 1 s; FEV₁/FVC, forced expiratory ratio; RV, residual volume; TLC, total lung capacity.

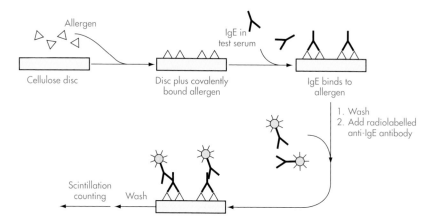

Figure 5.16 Radioallergosorbent test (RAST) procedure. IgE, immunoglobulin E (reaginic antibody). The final radio-activity on the disc is proportional to the amount of radiolabelled anti-IgE antibody that is bound to the disc by IgE bound from the test serum, i.e. the serum IgE level. The test is very sensitive because the disc carries large amounts of allergen.

research tool and to guide treatment with *omalizumab* (p. 324).

The aetiology may be ascertained by skin testing with allergens (see Chapter 13) as a guide to allergen avoidance, though it may be impracticable to avoid allergens, especially if patients react to several simultaneously. However, negative skin tests may indicate the need to investigate an alternative diagnosis. **Bronchial challenge** by inhaling suspected allergen aerosols may be conclusive, but is hazardous, with a risk of anaphylactic shock (see Chapter 2), and should not be attempted unless full resources for resuscitation are immediately available.

Exercise stress testing may also be helpful, especially in children, to assess the degree of exercise limitation and the role of exercise in inducing attacks.

Diagnostic problems

The following features may cause difficulties:

- Dry cough, sometimes with the production of small amounts of very viscid sputum. Cough, particularly troublesome at night, may be the only presenting symptom of asthma, especially in young children.

- Many infants have attacks of wheezing, possibly because they have rather small airways as a result of maternal smoking during pregnancy, but only about one-third of these go on to develop asthma. Diagnosis in very young children is clearly difficult but relief following a trial of drugs (e.g. the inhalation of a nebulized beta-agonist bronchodilator held near the nose) may be diagnostic. The likelihood of asthma is increased if wheezing is unrelated to respiratory infection or there is a family history of atopy (asthma, eczema or hay fever).

- Delayed attacks that occur some 6–8 h after provocation (Figure 5.14) and recover slowly over a period of hours without treatment. These are associated with increased bronchial hyper-reactivity and are caused by an immune complex hypersensitivity reaction (type III; see Chapter 2).

- Recurrent 'chest colds' or 'wheezy bronchitis' in children, and sometimes adults, may be due to undiagnosed asthma. A proportion of children eventually diagnosed as asthmatics have had repeated visits to their doctors with respiratory complaints (the 'wheezy baby' syndrome), for a year or more.

- Persistent airflow obstruction in an older patient with a limited degree of reversibility may be due to asthma, COPD or emphysema. It may be impossible and unnecessary to distinguish between these because they may coexist: what counts is the extent to which treatment is effective.

- Paroxysmal nocturnal dyspnoea (PND; see Chapter 4) may mimic nocturnal asthma, but is due to orthopnoea, i.e. accumulated fluid from the lower body redistributes to the lungs, causing pulmonary oedema (so-called 'cardiac asthma'). PND is often the first sign of LVF. A therapeutic trial of a bronchodilator, with or without corticosteroids, will distinguish between these conditions, because asthma will be relieved but not PND. The latter is relieved merely by standing erect, when the fluid flows back to the lower body. Moreover, pulmonary oedema will usually show characteristic X-ray, ECG and clinical signs, e.g. a raised venous pressure and the presence of a third heart sound.
- Some undiagnosed asthmatics present for the first time with cor pulmonale (see Chapter 4).
- Recurrent respiratory tract infections may cause difficulty. However, there will not be significant airflow obstruction or diurnal variation in PEF between infections.
- Large airways obstruction (outside the lungs) will usually be persistent, show inspiratory stridor rather than expiratory wheeze, and give a characteristic flow–volume loop (see Figure 5.9).
- Delayed attacks (see above and p. 297) apparently unrelated to allergen exposure.

Management

Aims

The aims of management are to:

- control symptoms, minimize anxiety and permit as normal a life as possible, including participation in sports;
- minimize the need for reliever medication and eliminate exacerbations;
- educate the patient about the disease and its treatment;
- identify and eliminate triggers, thus minimizing morbidity and preventing death.

General measures

General management measures include the following:

- **Environmental control**, as far as is possible, by:
  - Stopping smoking, in both patients and their families.
  - Removing pets, using non-allergenic bed clothing, etc. and minimizing house dust, e.g. by moist dusting and eliminating carpets. These measures are particularly important in childhood asthma. However, it is not possible or practicable to eliminate all environmental allergens, e.g. normal vacuum cleaning does not significantly reduce the concentration of house dust mite allergens in the atmosphere, although cleaners with high-efficiency particulate air (HEPA) filtered output are now available and may help some patients. However, there is little evidence to support their use.
- **Reduce stress** by effective treatment.
- **Control infections** promptly.
- **Physiotherapy**, especially supervised swimming, may help to develop respiratory function: the humid atmosphere of a swimming bath helps to avoid exercise-induced attacks and is less stressful physically.
- **Patient education** has a crucial role. There are repeated reports that patients are confused about their medication and its proper use. Patients (and their families, teachers, employers, etc.) need to understand the nature of the disease and how to prevent exacerbations and manage them effectively if they occur. Pharmacists can and should play an important part in this process: they understand the drugs and products and are readily accessible to patients. Active pharmacist counselling has been shown to reduce markedly both morbidity and the demands made on the community and hospital medical services. Additionally, there are the substantial benefits of increased patient well-being, less time off work or school and the satisfaction of patients being in control of their disease, rather than vice versa. Further, if patients are properly counselled and, for those who have moderate to severe exacerba-

tions, keep a diary, they can detect the first signs of deterioration in their condition (i.e. increasing dyspnoea, declining PEF and increasing medicines usage). They can then adjust their medication to respond to the problem immediately, hopefully aborting an attack, before seeing their doctor. Patients are reported as having a different perception of well-being from health professionals. Whereas patients see good disease control as freedom from constraints on activity, professionals use objective measures, e.g. absence of symptoms, low (or no) medicines usage. This gap can be closed by effective counselling, with improvement in patients' satisfaction with treatment.

Pharmacotherapy: general aspects

Drug treatment is often thought of in terms of either prophylaxis or the relief of symptoms. In asthma, both approaches are commonly used concurrently, and combination therapy is normal. However, effective prophylaxis should minimize exacerbations and avoid the need for rescue therapy.

General strategy

A general approach to the control of the two cardinal features of asthma, airways inflammation and bronchoconstriction, is outlined in Table 5.12.

A stepwise addition of medication is used after diagnosis, starting at the step most likely to abolish symptoms. At all steps the patient should have an inhaled, short-acting beta$_2$-agonist (SABA) bronchodilator ('reliever') available for mild infrequent attacks, but this should need to be used only occasionally. Regular use of this is no longer recommended and indicates the need for patient reassessment. Many patients are maintained with a regular inhaled corticosteroid, at appropriate dosage, plus the occasional use of a reliever (Tables 5.13 and 5.14).

However, if attacks are frequent, or moderate to severe (i.e. PEF 50–80% of predicted or best), it is preferable to gain control of symptoms promptly with greater initial intervention and to 'step down' treatment once this has been achieved. Control is usually gained with anti-

inflammatory agents, usually low-dose or high-dose inhaled corticosteroids or an LTRA. An LABA bronchodilator may be added if the asthma is still not well controlled, provided that the continuing symptoms are unacceptable to the patient and that they accept the risk of a serious cardiovascular event (see above). The LABA should be stopped if it does not give objective benefit. All of these may be used concurrently in severe cases. An SABA should also be available for rescue treatment. Additional drugs may need to be introduced at any stage as the patient's condition and progress dictate.

All changes of treatment should be validated by careful monitoring of PEF and medicines usage, or FEV$_1$ and FVC if the equipment is available in GP surgeries, with ample time for prophylactic medication to take full effect (see below). Inhaled corticosteroids, bronchodilators and LTRAs, and *nedocromil sodium* for children 5–12 years, used singly or in combination, will give excellent, safe control in most patients. Sedatives must never be used to aid sleeping or control restlessness, because they may dangerously depress an already compromised respiratory function.

The BTS and the Scottish Intercollegiate Guidelines Network (SIGN) have published evidence-based guidelines for the management of asthma, summarized in Table 5.13 for adults and schoolchildren, and Table 5.14 for younger children. More detailed information on the drugs and their delivery systems are given below, but some general points are now discussed.

Treatment in an acute attack

This is designed to promote recovery and prevent deterioration to the point when hospital treatment becomes necessary.

The techniques of inhalation therapy are discussed on pp. 348–360, but it is sufficient here to say that pressurized metered-dose inhalers (pMDIs) or dry powder inhalers (DPIs) are normally used. If higher than normal doses are necessary, a nebulizer may be required.

Occasional attacks in an adult can be treated with an inhaled selective SABA bronchodilator (p. 314). If a consistent trigger can be identified (e.g. sport, infection, drugs or visits to a home having a pet), prior use of an SABA inhaler or regular use of a corticosteroid inhaler may

Table 5.12   General approach to the treatment of target feautures in asthma

Target feature	Therapeutic aim	Drugs used	
		Class	Examples[a]
Inflammation and and bronchial hyper-reactivity	Reduce • eosinophil recruitment and activation • lymphocyte activity • toxicity to epithelial cells	Corticosteroids	Inhaled: beclometasone, budesonide, ciclesonide, fluticasone, mometasone Oral: prednisolone
	• mast cell etc. degranulation	Inhibitors of mediator release	Sodium cromoglicate?[b] Nedocromil sodium? Theophylline? Selective beta$_2$-agonists
	• cytokine activity	Leukotriene receptor antagonists	Montelukast, zafirlukast
Bronchoconstriction	Bronchodilatation: • increase sympathomimetic activity	Selective beta$_2$-agonist	Inhaled: salbutamol, terbutaline, fenoterol, reproterol, tulobuterol Long-acting Inhaled: formoterol, salmeterol Oral: bambuterol
	• block parasympathetic activity • increase cAMP levels in bronchiolar muscle cells?	Antimuscarinic Phosphodiesterase inhibitors Inhibitors of mediator release	Ipratropium Aminophylline? Theophylline? Sodium cromoglicate?[b] Nedocromil sodium?

[a] Some drugs fall into more than one class. Their precise modes of action may be unknown.

[b] Cromolyn sodium

? = possible or secondary action; cAMP, cyclic adenosine monophosphate

prevent attacks (Table 5.13, Step 2). If there are more frequent or more severe episodes, routine prophylactic treatment is added. This usually starts with an inhaled regular standard-dose corticosteroid, plus an inhaled SABA bronchodilator when required. The beta$_2$-agonists enhance the anti-inflammatory effects of the corticosteroid on cells. If a corticosteroid cannot be used an LTRA, e.g. *montelukast* or *zafirlukast*, may be substituted. There is one report that adding an LTRA in patients taking a stable dose of *budesonide* may reduce night disturbance and increase the number of asthma-free days. However, there is no clear consensus about the place of LTRAs in therapy, but a trial of LTRA

therapy is warranted in patients whose asthma is inadequately controlled on conventional treatment.

Because of fears of side-effects, especially of corticosteroids, and if they do not understand the principles of prophylaxis, patients often do not adhere to regular use of their corticosteroid inhalers, with a consequent deterioration in symptom control.

Patients should have their response to therapy, their inhaler technique and concordance reviewed regularly. Those who still have not responded adequately should have their corticosteroid dose doubled and this may avoid instituting an oral corticosteroid.

Table 5.13   Treatment of chronic asthma in adults and schoolchildren

Start at step most appropriate to initial severity[a]
Achieve early control
Maintain control by stepping up treatment in exacerbations and stepping down when good sustained control has been achieved

Step 1: Mild intermittent asthma: occasional relief bronchodilators

Inhaled short-acting beta$_2$-agonist as required (up to once daily)[b]
Note: Move up to Step 2 if needed twice weekly or more, if there are night-time symptoms more than once a week, or if there has been an exacerbation in the last 2 years requiring systemic corticosteroid or a nebulized bronchodilator.
Check adherence and inhaler technique[c]

Step 2: Regular preventer therapy: regular inhaled prophylactic therapy

Inhaled short-acting beta$_2$-agonist as required *plus*
regular standard-dose inhaled corticosteroid[d] (alternatives are considerably less effective)

Step 3: Add-on therapy: inhaled corticosteroids plus long-acting inhaled beta$_2$-agonist

Inhaled short-acting beta$_2$-agonist as required *plus*
Regular standard-dose inhaled corticosteroid[d] *plus*
Long-acting inhaled beta$_2$-agonist[f]
If asthma not controlled
Increase dose of inhaled corticosteroid up to maximum standard dose
If asthma still not controlled add **one** of: leukotriene receptor antagonist **or** modified-release oral theophylline **or** modified-release oral beta$_2$-agonist[e]

Step 4: Persistent poor control: high-dose inhaled corticosteroids plus regular bronchodilators

Inhaled short-acting beta$_2$-agonist as required *plus*
Regular high-dose inhaled corticosteroid[e] *plus*
Long-acting inhaled beta$_2$-agonist[f] *plus*
In adults a 6-week sequential trial adding one or more of: leukotriene receptor antagonist or modified-release oral theophylline or modified-release oral beta$_2$-agonist
In adults and teenagers >12 years: if still not controlled and high IgE levels consider a 12- to 16-week trial of omalizumab[g]

Step 5: Continuous or frequent use of corticosteroid tablets

Inhaled short-acting beta$_2$-agonist as required *with*
Regular high-dose inhaled corticosteroid[e] *and*
Regular long-acting inhaled beta$_2$-agonist[f] *plus*
Regular prednisolone tablets (as a single morning dose)
Consider **oral** long-acting beta$_2$-agonist[h]
Note: In addition to regular prednisolone continue high-dose inhaled corticosteroids[c] to spare the prednisolone dose: **these patients should be referred to an asthma clinic**

continued overleaf

Table 5.13   (*Continued*)

Stepping down

Review treatment every 3 months; if control is achieved, stepwise dose reduction may be possible; use the lowest dose of corticosteroid; reduce the dose of inhaled corticosteroid slowly if treatment longer than 21 days. Consider reduction every 3 months, decreasing dose by 50% each time, to the lowest dose that controls the asthma.

Notes on usage

[a] **Severity**, see Table 5.11.

[b] **This reliever inhalation** should always be available to manage an exacerbation. If required often, the patient should see their doctor for a medication review.

[c] **Adherence and inhaler technique** should be checked whenever a change in medication occurs.

[d] **Standard-dose inhaled corticosteroids** (given by pMDI) are: beclometasone dipropionate *or* budesonide 100–400 µg (child 100–200 µg) twice daily *or* fluticasone propionate 50–200 µg (child 50–100 µg) twice daily *or* ciclesonide 80–160 µg daily (child or adolescent <18 years, not recommended) *or* mometasone furoate (given through a DPI) 200 µg twice daily. The initial dose should be prescribed according to the severity of the asthma.
Alternatives to inhaled corticosteroids are a leukotriene receptor antagonist, modified-release **oral** theophylline, and **in adults** regular cromoglicate and **in children** regular nedocromil.

[e] **High dose inhaled corticosteroids**, given through a pMDI, are beclometasone dipropionate *or* budesonide 0.8–2.0 mg daily (child 100–400 µg) *or* fluticasone propionate 0.4–1.0 mg daily (child 50–200 µg) twice daily *or* ciclesonide 160 µg daily *or* mometasone furoate (given through a DPI) up to 800 µg twice daily.
Child 5–12 years: beclometasone dipropionate *or* budesonide up to 400 µg twice daily *or* fluticasone propionate up to 200 µg twice daily. **Use a large volume spacer**.

[f] **Long-acting inhaled beta₂-agonists** are formoterol fumarate, given via a DPI twice daily and salmeterol, given via a pMDI or a DPI twice daily. If there is no objective benefit after a 6-week trial the treatment should be discontinued: **but see text p. 294**.

[g] The SC dose of this monoclonal antibody against IgE is based on body weight and IgE titre (see manufacturer's literature) and should be initiated by a clinician who is experienced in managing refractory asthma.
Omalizumab is not recommended by the Scottish Medicines Consortium (May 2006).

[h] **Long-acting oral beta₂-agonists** are *bambuterol hydrochloride* and modified-release *salbutamol*. If there is no objective benefit after a 6-week trial the treatment should be discontinued: **but see text p. 294**.

Lung function measurements cannot be used to guide treatment in children under 2 years old. Guidance on usage for this group is given in Table 5.14.
pMDI, pressurised metered dose inhaler; DPI, dry powder inhaler.

Based on the recommendations of the British Thoracic Society and the Scottish Intercollegiate Guidelines Network with permission from British Medical Specialist Journals and the editors of the British National Formulary 50 (updated 20 April 2004).

Table 5.14   Management of chronic asthma in children under 5 years[a]

Start at step most appropriate to initial severity[b]

Step 1: Occasional relief bronchodilators

Short-acting beta₂-agonist as required (not more than once daily)
Move to Step 2 if needed twice a week or more, if night-time symptoms occur more than once a week or if there has been an exacerbation in the last 2 years
Use a short **'rescue course'** of *prednisolone* at **any time** or **any step**[c]

Step 2: Regular inhaled prophylactic therapy

Inhaled short-acting beta₂-agonist as required
plus regular inhaled standard paediatric dose corticosteroid[d], by pMDI or DPI via a large-volume spacer. If inhaled corticosteroid cannot be used a leukotriene receptor antagonist may be added, but is less effective
Consider (to stabilize patient) a 3- to 5-day course of soluble prednisolone tablets[c] or temporary doubling of inhaled corticosteroid dose

Table 5.14   (Continued)

Step 3: Increased-dose inhaled corticosteroids

Inhaled short-acting beta$_2$-agonist as required
plus regular inhaled standard paediatric dose corticosteroid[c]
plus leukotriene receptor antagonist
Consider: Short course of soluble prednisolone tablets[c]
Regular inhaled salmeterol (long-acting beta$_2$-agonist[e] not in children <4y) **or** regular modified-release oral theophylline/aminophylline
Note: Modified-release oral theophylline/aminophylline may be helpful (particularly for nocturnal symptoms) but has appreciable side-effects in up to one-third of children (plasma- or salivary-concentration monitoring recommended). The manufacturer's literature should be consulted about suitable dosage and ages.

Step 4: Persistent poor control

Refer child to respiratory paediatrician

Stepping down

Review need for treatment

Notes on severity and usage:

Whenever possible use inhalers with a large-volume spacer (oral dosing gives more side-effects and is often less effective).

Check frequently: adherence, inhaler technique and that the inhaler model is appropriate for the patient.

[a] A paediatric respiratory physician should be consulted if high doses or oral dosing is contemplated especially for children <2y in whom asthma is not controlled satisfactorily at step 2.

[b] **Severity:** Lung function tests cannot be used to guide treatment in young children. See Table 5.11 for the signs of acute severe asthma in this age group.

[c] Doses of soluble prednisolone tablets are: child under 2 years, 1–2 mg/kg daily; maximum 20mg daily; 2–18y, maximum 40mg daily. Rescue courses are usually for 3–5 days. IV hydrocortisone should be considered if the child cannot retain tablets.

[d] When in doubt of doses for children under 5 years, consult BNF for Children, the Drug Information Departments of the Alder Hey Children's Hospital in Liverpool or the Great Ormond Street Hospital for Children in London. See also References and further reading.

The general standard paediatric inhaled corticosteroid dose is beclometasone dipropionate or budesonide: <2y up to 100 µg twice daily; 2–5y, up to 200 µg twice daily; or fluticasone propionate, <5y, up to 200 µg daily (in divided doses); initial dose according to age, weight and severity of asthma.

The long-term treatment of children in this age group should be monitored regularly because requirements change as the child grows. Failure to thrive may be due to corticosteroid medication or unsatisfactorily controlled asthma.

Note that BNF54 and the BNF for Children do not agree on paediatric dosage.

The response should be checked after 1 month before adjusting doses; if control is not adequate consider doubling dose of inhaled corticosteroid for 1 month (alternatively give a 5-day course of soluble prednisolone tablets or consider introducing other treatments before increasing dose of inhaled corticosteroid for long periods).

High paediatric dose of inhaled corticosteroid is beclometasone dipropionate or budesonide; <2y up to 200 micrograms twice daily; 2–5y, 400 mµ twice daily or fluticasone propionate; <2y not recommended, 4–16y up to 200 micrograms twice daily; use a large-volume spacer and, if necessary, a face mask.

[e] Use of LABAs is in doubt – see text (p. 294).

Based on the recommendations of the British Thoracic Society and the Scottish Intercollegiate Guidelines Network with permission from British Medical Specialist Journals and the editors of the British National Formulary 54 (updated 20 November 2007).

Chronic management in children aged under 12 years

At all levels of management patients should have an SABA available for the control of symptoms. With frequent or moderate to severe episodes (see Table 5.13) an inhaled corticosteroid may be used, e.g. 200–400 µg of *beclometasone dipropionate (BDP)* daily, or the equivalent of another corticosteroid (see notes to Table 5.14). The starting dose should be appropriate to symptom severity. High doses carry a significant risk of serious side-effects, notably growth retardation,

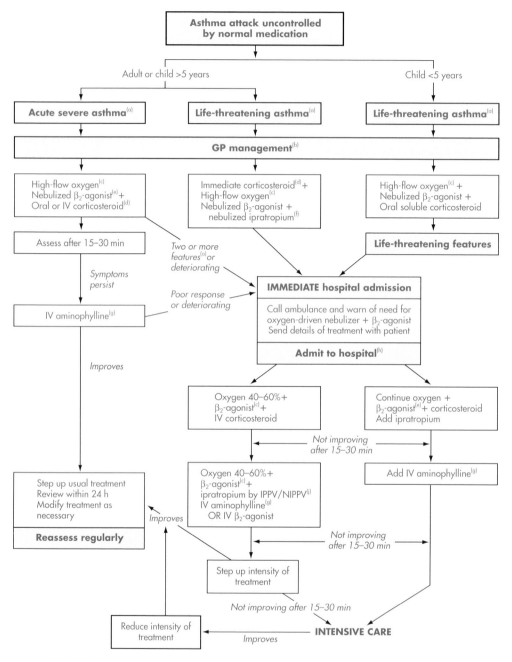

Figure 5.17   Flow chart for the management of acute severe asthma (status asthmaticus). Note that **severity** is often not appreciated by both the patient and the doctor: **peak flow rates should always be measured**, except in young children. [a] This figure should be read in consultation with the text, particularly Tables 5.13 and 5.14, and with the recommendations of the British Thoracic Society and the Scottish Intercollegiate Guidelines Network (see References and further reading), especially charts 2, 3, 4 and 8 of the latter. [b] If the GP is not available, patients should dial 999 or go to the nearest A&E department. [c] High-flow oxygen (giving 40–60% via face mask) does not depress respiration in asthmatics (pp. 360–364). It may not be available to GPs. [d] Soluble tablets are preferred: adults, 30–60 mg/day; 1–15 years, 1–2 mg/kg/day, maxima 1–5 years, 20 mg/day, 5–15 years, 40 mg/day. If very ill, oral *prednisolone* and IV *hydro-*

osteoporosis and adrenal suppression, and should be used as sparingly as possible. However, short high-dose courses are safe, and failure to control asthma symptoms may itself cause growth retardation.

If a corticosteroid cannot be used an LTRA may be tried as an alternative regular prophylactic. If this therapy is not effective, it may be necessary to double the corticosteroid dose. Similar considerations regarding inhaler technique, response and concordance to those outlined above apply here also.

If this does not achieve satisfactory control alternative prophylactic measures need to be considered. Cromones, e.g. *nedocromil sodium*, may be beneficial and modified-release *theophylline* or *aminophylline* may have to be used. Because the methylxanthines have a different mode of action, they may augment the response to other agents. Use of some *theophylline* preparations in 6-year-olds and under is not recommended (see the BNF and manufacturers' literature).

Sodium cromoglicate may help as a regular prophylactic for exercise-induced asthma in children, but this may indicate poor control and the child should be reassessed; it is of no value for acute asthma attacks. In some children aged under 5 years, *ipratropium bromide* may be useful.

Children under 2 years who are inadequately controlled with a daily use of an SABA plus up to 400 μg of *BDP* (or its equivalent) daily are best managed by a paediatric respiratory physician. This also applies if the use of an oral corticosteroid is being considered as a measure of last resort when adequate trials of the other agents fail to give satisfactory control.

It may take 3–4 weeks to establish the level of response to prophylactic inhalation therapy, so persistence is required on the part of patient, doctor and carer. This places a premium on early initial control to create patient confidence in their doctors and cooperation with them, and adherence to their prescribed medication.

Chronic adult asthma

The management of chronic asthma in adults and children over the age of 12 years is similar to that just described and is based on the use of inhaled corticosteroids. The starting dose is usually in the range 200–800 μg of *BDP* or its equivalent daily; most patients are started on 400 μg of *BDP* (or an equivalent). If the response is inadequate, an LABA may be added (but see p. 294).

With a partial but inadequate response the LABA should be continued and the corticosteroid dose increased to 800 μg of *BDP* or its equivalent daily, provided that dose is not already being used. If the LABA does not give demonstrable benefit, it should be stopped.

If control is still inadequate, a trial of an LTRA or a modified-release methylxanthine should be instituted. Persistent poor control should prompt an increase in the inhaled corticosteroid to 2000 μg of *BDP* or its equivalent daily (see below), plus an LTRA, a slow-release methylxanthine or an oral beta$_2$-agonist (see Table 5.13, steps 4 and 5).

The final step to achieve adequate control is to add an oral corticosteroid, e.g. *prednisolone*, at the lowest dose that controls symptoms. The inhaled high-dose corticosteroid and other medications that have given benefit should always be continued to minimize the oral corticosteroid dose. At this stage the patient should be in the care of a specialized respiratory team.

---

cortisone can be started together, with parenteral administration being stopped as soon as possible. Maximum daily IV dose at any age is 400 mg in 6-hourly divided doses. [e] An oxygen-driven nebulizer with a flow rate of 6–8 L/min should be used (p. 358). Some children will not tolerate a face mask, and similar doses can be given via a spacer. [f] Patients aged over 40 may respond better to *ipratropium*, which is also used if there is a poor response to bronchodilators. [g] Bolus *aminophylline* must not be given to those already taking an oral theophylline. Blood level monitoring should be used where available, especially if treatment is continued for more than 24 h, and the dose given by slow, small-volume IV infusion. Doses: adults 750–1500 mg/day; 1–15 years, loading dose 5 mg/kg over 20 min (omit if already receiving oral theophylline), then 1 mg/kg/h. [h] Treatment on admission will depend on prior GP/ambulance treatment. [i] (See p. 361). [k] Percent of predicted or best value, provided that patients are not too ill or too young (<5 years) to give reliable results.

Older adults (aged >50 years) may not respond adequately to beta$_2$-bronchodilators, probably because of a deficiency of bronchiolar beta$_2$-receptors, so the **antimuscarinic agent** *ipratropium bromide* may give better results as a reliever in these patients; however the first dose should be used under medical supervision because it may trigger paradoxical bronchospasm. If all this amounts to so many inhalations daily that adherence is compromised, *tiotropium* may be an alternative antimuscarinic, which is given via a DPI once daily and is suitable for prophylactic use only and not for the relief of acute bronchospasm. *Tiotropium* is not suitable for children and adolescents under 18 years and its use in asthma is an unlicensed indication: it is licensed for use in COPD (see below). The use of antimuscarinics in this older age group needs to be managed carefully, because they may cause or exacerbate glaucoma, difficulty in micturition, even acute urinary retention in men with an enlarged prostate gland, and tachycardia or atrial fibrillation (see Chapter 4).

High-dose inhaled corticosteroids (see the notes to Table 5.13) may avoid the need for **oral steroids** completely, or enable the dose of the latter to be reduced substantially. In the community a large-volume spacer device (see p. 352) should be used to reduce the risk of oropharyngeal thrush (see below). A nebulizer (p. 354) can be used to deliver doses higher than those readily obtained with pMDIs. The choice of drug delivery system in a hospital setting will depend on the patient's general condition, e.g. an *oxygen*-driven nebulizer, IPPV (p. 361) or parenteral medication. The dose–response curve for inhaled corticosteroids flattens at moderate doses and increasing the dose above 800 µg of *BDP* daily, or the equivalent of another corticosteroid, may give little or no further improvement but cause increased side-effects. LTRAs may be preferred because their effect is additive to that of a steroid. Clearly, there will be no further benefit if the response to existing therapy is the maximum that can be achieved in damaged lungs.

All of these agents should be given an adequate trial before using an oral steroid, the latter being a measure of last resort in patients who are poorly controlled despite standard treatment.

Morning dipping (see Figure 5.13) was traditionally managed with an oral slow-release bronchodilator (beta$_2$-agonist or a methylxanthine) taken before retiring, but an LTRA may now be preferred.

Moderate exacerbations of asthma in adults are characterized by worsening symptoms, with no features of acute severe asthma.

Appropriate treatment in the community is to step up the patient's usual treatment.

The clinical features of acute severe asthma in adults are given in Tables 5.11 and 5.13. Treatment in the community then includes:

- High-flow *oxygen* (40–60% by face mask; p. 361), if available.
- *Oxygen*-driven nebulized *salbutamol* or *terbutaline* (if available) for 15 min (or 4–6 puffs from a pMDI with a large-volume spacer, each puff taken separately. The response should be monitored 15–30 min later.
- Nebulized *ipratropium bromide*, especially for those not responding to beta$_2$-agonists.
- Hospital admission if any two of severe breathlessness, high respiratory or heart rate are present or the patient's condition persists or deteriorates.
- Oral *prednisolone* 40–50 mg daily for 5 days or until recovery. IV *hydrocortisone* 100 mg four times daily is an alternative if the patient cannot swallow tablets.
- There should be a review within 24 h, and if the patient has improved, review standard medication after stopping *prednisolone* (this short period of corticosteroid treatment does not require gradual step-down).

In **life-threatening asthma** the patient will exhibit one or more of the signs given in Table 5.11.

Immediate hospital admission is necessary if any of those above features is present or the patient's condition persists or deteriorates. Referral to an intensive care unit should be considered.

Emergency treatment in the community includes:

- High-flow *oxygen* (p. 361), if a suitable supply is available. If a patient is already using *oxygen*, they must seek immediate medical treatment and should not rely on *oxygen* to treat a severe attack.

- 100 mg IV *hydrocortisone*.
- Nebulized *salbutamol* or *terbutaline* with nebulized *ipratropium*, preferably *oxygen*-driven. The nebulized beta$_2$-agonist should still be given if a suitable *oxygen* supply (p. 358) is not available.
- The patient should be supervised by the doctor until the ambulance arrives.
- An IV infusion of 1.2–2.0 g *magnesium sulphate* (p. 293) should be given over 20 min, after consultation with a senior doctor.

We have already noted that the severity of such attacks is often not appreciated by the patients or their doctors, so many patients arrive at hospital virtually moribund. Some patients are not distressed, or the severity of symptoms may be masked by over-enthusiastic use of beta$_2$-agonists, especially with a nebulizer (p. 354). It is better to recognize that a severe attack is impending and treat the patient aggressively at the first signs to gain control and prevent deterioration, because it is more difficult to treat severe symptoms once they are established. Even large doses of beta$_2$-agonist bronchodilators and corticosteroids, given by MDIs with a large-volume spacer or nebulized, are safe in the short term. However, patients are often unresponsive to bronchodilators in severe attacks, so it may be dangerous to persist with these because they may aggravate hypoxia (p. 315). If a patient is unresponsive to a nebulized beta$_2$-agonist it may be better to use IV *aminophylline* (see below), which has a different mode of action.

The groups most at risk in an acute severe attack are patients who:

- are aged between 12 and 25 years;
- are immigrants, migrant workers or holiday-makers;
- were in hospital for asthma in the previous year;
- have a history of severe attacks;
- use three or more classes of medication;
- have initiated an emergency call or repeatedly attended an A&E department for asthma treatment.

In addition, these patients may have:

- progressive symptoms or signs (nocturnal episodes, declining or increasingly labile PEF);
- exposure to seasonal or occupational allergens;
- psychosocial problems, i.e. stress in their lives;
- denial of the severity of their condition;
- obesity, which should be addressed after the severe attack has subsided.

The general management strategy is outlined in Figure 5.17, but this is empirical and needs to be considered in light of the patient's current therapy. Thus if this already includes a nebulized beta$_2$-adrenergic bronchodilator and oral corticosteroids, it may be appropriate to give a slow IV bolus of *aminophylline*. If the patient is already taking oral *theophylline*, the initial loading IV dose should be omitted and the patient observed for cardiac arrhythmias. Emergency self-admission ('open door') schemes may be life-saving. The A&E doctor, or other admitting doctor, should be notified if the patient is already taking a methylxanthine.

Following admission, PEF or FEV$_1$ and serum electrolytes are monitored. Blood gases are measured in life-threatening and near-fatal attacks. The serum potassium level is particularly important, because there is a risk of serious hypokalaemia with beta$_2$-agonists (see below and Chapter 4) and this may be exacerbated by high-dose corticosteroid and methylxanthine use.

All patients should be educated to recognize any significant deterioration in their condition, e.g. with home monitoring of PEF, and about what action to take. These 'personal action plans' may involve:

- A protocol agreed with the patient's GP or consultant and instructions to see their doctor without delay.
- Increasing the dose of their inhaled corticosteroid, if appropriate, or using an oral corticosteroid at the first signs of significant deterioration.
- Reserve supplies of:
  - oral and high-dose inhaled corticosteroid;
  - antibiotics, if severe attacks are known to be triggered by antibiotic-sensitive infection (the routine use of antibiotics is inappropriate if there is no positive indication).

Brittle asthma. This describes the condition in a few patients who suffer sudden, severe attacks with very few or none of the warning signs described above. The peak flow charts of these patients will show a chaotic pattern. Provided that such patients are measuring and recording their PEF correctly, they need reserve supplies of drugs as described above, so that they can start intensive treatment immediately an exacerbation occurs (according to protocol; see above). They must also obtain expert assistance without delay and often have special arrangements with their local hospital. Clearly, these patients will need to have been thoroughly assessed by a specialist respiratory physician and trained in the use of the equipment (i.e. peak flow meters, inhalers and nebulizers), and their medication.

Asthma in children (see also above). Children cannot coordinate the relatively complex manoeuvres required to use an unmodified MDI (pMDIs, p. 349; see Figure 5.23) before the age of 5–7 years. A range of specially designed spacers and face masks for use with pMDIs is available for young children (Figure 5.23). For older children, breath-actuated pMDIs or DPIs are preferred. Nebulized drugs (p. 354) or oral medication may be used at any age, especially in infants and during severe attacks. Children vary enormously in their rates of mental and physical development, so the route of administration has to be tailored to their abilities and tolerance of treatment. Their parents or carers should be educated to recognize the warning signs of deterioration and to know how to respond appropriately. Regular monitoring is especially important in this age group because their requirements change rapidly with age.

Within these constraints, and with appropriate dosage, the management of childhood asthma (Tables 5.13 and 5.14) is generally similar to that in adults. However, adrenergic bronchodilators are often ineffective in young children because only a small proportion of the dose may reach the lungs. It has been shown that a beta$_2$-agonist bronchodilator used with a large-volume spacer is more effective than a nebulizer in children aged over 3 years with acute asthma. This finding requires confirmation, but provides a less costly and simpler alternative to nebulizer treatment.

First-line prophylaxis against exercise-induced bronchoconstriction includes low-dose corticosteroids and *sodium cromoglicate*, or an SABA used before anticipated activity. Higher doses of inhaled corticosteroids, administered via a spacer device (p. 352), are introduced as necessary. One study has shown that the early use of an inhaled corticosteroid may prevent the development of acute, severe airways obstruction. However, trial results are conflicting and one trial found that doubling the dose of inhaled corticosteroid did not improve symptom scores and reduced growth velocity after 1 year of treatment. This confirms the known flat response with corticosteroid dosage and emphasizes the need for objective assessment following any medication change and for regular medication review.

Oral corticosteroids must be avoided if possible, because they retard growth, even if given in alternate-day dosage, but it has been shown that nebulized *budesonide*, and presumably *BDP* also, may permit a dramatic reduction in oral corticosteroid usage. Alternate-day dosing is unsuitable in asthma because patients deteriorate on the steroid-free days. The possibility of growth retardation should always be borne in mind. One systematic review found a clear preference by children's parents for inhaled corticosteroids over placebo. As usual with severe chronic diseases, effective control comprises a sometimes difficult balance between the harmful effects of the disease and the side-effects of treatment.

Severe childhood asthma. Young children present special problems in diagnosis and treatment. The emotional response of the child (and its parents) to the knowledge that they have a potentially severe, chronic disease, and the loss of time from school, are also important, so careful counselling of the child and its parents, siblings and teachers (with the parents' permission), is essential. Features of acute severe and life-threatening asthma in children are given in Table 5.11 but children may not show obvious signs of distress.

Emergency treatment in the community may include:

• Referral to a children's hospital.
• Nebulized SABA (*oxygen*-driven if possible) or 10 puffs from an SABA pMDI via large-volume

spacer (with a face mask in the under 5s). If there is a favourable response, repeat as necessary.

- Start a short course of oral soluble *prednisolone*, e.g. daily doses of:
  - 10 mg <2 years
  - 20 mg 2–5 years
  - 30–40 mg <5 years
  - IV *hydrocortisone* should be considered if unable to take *prednisolone* tablets.
- If unresponsive or there is a relapse within 3–4 h:
  - Refer to hospital immediately.
  - High-flow *oxygen*, if available, via a face mask.
  - Nebulized SABA (*oxygen*-driven if possible) plus nebulized *ipratropium bromide* (250 µg every 20–30 min).
- Children over 12 years are treated as adults.

Immunotherapy

Hyposensitization.   Many attempts have been made to 'desensitize' patients to allergens. Because episodic asthma is often associated with high levels of IgE, it is attractive to try to prevent IgE production or to prevent the resultant hypersensitivity reaction.

In the past, this has been attempted by injecting a minute dose of an identified allergen and following this with regularly increasing doses, none of which must provoke a significant reaction. Theoretically, this should result in effective immunization with the production of sufficient IgG (so-called 'blocking antibody') to scavenge any allergen before it is able to elicit the formation of IgE.

However, it is rarely possible to achieve this effectively because, even if patients can be desensitized to a single allergen, they are usually sensitive to several allergens at first diagnosis and do not respond adequately. Further, being atopic they will later become sensitive to other allergens. Hyposensitization has largely been abandoned in the UK following a number of severe anaphylactic events and 11 deaths. The UK's Committee on Safety of Medicines (CSM) has advised that desensitizing vaccines should not be used unless full cardiorespiratory resuscitation facilities are immediately available and patients can be observed for 2 h following each injection.

Current research in this field is directed towards the minimization of major reactions during immunization by using modified allergens or immunomodulatory agents. A more fundamental approach to immunotherapy involves the control of IgE production in atopic individuals by promoting TH1 lymphocyte differentiation and suppressing TH2 responses and so the production of IL-4 (see Chapter 2). The role of immunotherapy, used in carefully selected patients under controlled conditions, requires continual reappraisal in the light of our increasing understanding of clinical immunology. There is now, current interest in this.

Immunosuppression. The term 'immunotherapy' may be stretched to include the blocking of the release or action of inflammatory eicosanoids and cytokines by lymphocytes. The first agents with such properties are the LTRAs (see below) and *omalizumab* (p. 324), a recombinant, humanized, monoclonal antibody against Ig E. The latter has been introduced recently and is licensed as additional therapy for those with a proven IgE-mediated basis to the attacks. However, it has to be given by SC injection in a dose determined by the IgE level and body weight. It should be initiated only by a physician experienced in the management of severe asthma.

In a small number of patients, who are not well controlled despite all of the above agents, conventional immunosuppressive anti-inflammatory drugs, e.g. *ciclosporin* or *methotrexate*, have been used. These agents should be prescribed by clinicians who are experienced in their use and patients supervised closely with appropriate monitoring of the blood picture and kidney function (see Chapters 10, 12, 13 and 14).

Drugs used in obstructive pulmonary disease

This section includes the treatment of both asthma and COPD. A summary of the treatment of target features was presented in Table 5.12 and the topic of inhalation therapy is dealt with separately on pp. 348–360.

Beta$_2$-agonist bronchodilators

Mode of action

These drugs interact with a membrane-bound receptor coupled to an intracellular protein with a subunit that regulates effector molecule activation in the cell, e.g. adenylcyclase, phospholipases, ion channels or transport proteins. Beta$_2$-receptors ultimately cause the opening of Ca^{2+} channels and reduce both the phosphorylation of myosin light chains and calcium-dependent actin–myosin coupling, producing smooth muscle relaxation.

Secondary effects relevant to asthma are:

- Increased mucociliary clearance from the airways, reducing obstruction.
- The reduction of bronchial reactivity to a variety of stimuli, due to:
  - decreased microvascular permeability, reducing the recruitment of inflammatory cells;
  - inhibition of phospholipase A$_2$ activity.
- Inhibition of the liberation of LTs, especially IL-4 and histamine from mast cells and other effector cells.

These secondary effects are probably less important acutely, but may contribute to the beneficial effect of the beta$_2$-agonists when they are used regularly. Because the density of beta$_2$-receptors is greatest in the smaller airways, it is there (the site of the problem in asthma) that the beta$_2$-agonists exert their major effect.

Use

The short-acting beta$_2$-agonists are the drugs of first choice in the treatment of mild asthma and are used therapeutically as 'relievers' to control occasional acute attacks and breakthrough attacks in otherwise well-controlled patients.

Short-acting agents (SABAs).   The currently available drugs, *salbutamol* and *terbutaline sulphate*, have very similar pharmacokinetic characteristics. The most widely used, *salbutamol*, has an intermediate duration of action of about 4 h and a rapid onset of action, with a peak effect about 60 min after inhalation. *Terbutaline* seems to have a slightly longer duration of

action, but the difference is not clinically relevant. Both of these are therefore used for asthma management as relievers.

Long-acting agents (LABAs).   *Bambuterol* (not in children) requires only once-daily oral dosing, while *formoterol* and *salmeterol* (in children over 6 and 4 years, respectively) are usually inhaled twice daily, enhancing convenience and patient compliance. It is important to note that these long-acting agents are not replacements for the shorter-acting drugs because they are suitable only for regular prophylaxis and not as relievers for 'rescue therapy': the shorter-acting drugs are the drugs of choice for treating the occasional acute attack.

However, a recent systematic review has concluded that LABAs are associated with increased death in severe asthma (p. 294). This needs urgent clarification, because they are otherwise valuable in those patients who show significant morning dipping, or who continue to wheeze despite using low-dose inhaled steroids and short-acting bronchodilators.

Side-effects.   It is clear from the distributions of the two types of beta-adrenoreceptors (Table 5.15) that the SABAs are without significant adverse cardiac effects at normal dosage. This selectivity is enhanced because they can be delivered directly to their sites of action in the bronchioles, where they are very effective at about one-tenth of the oral dose. They are thus very safe and have replaced the non-selective adrenergic agents (*adrenaline* (epinephrine), isoprenaline (isoproterenol), etc.), the CNS (restlessness, agitation) and cardiovascular (increased heart rate) side-effects of which are particularly harmful in patients who are stressed by a severe asthma attack. Inhaled doses of *terbutaline* eight times the normally recommended maximum have been used to achieve greater bronchodilatation, with no increase in side-effects.

The selective beta$_2$-agonists are not completely receptor-specific and so do have some predictable side-effects (e.g. central stimulation and insomnia, headache, peripheral vasodilatation and tachycardia), especially if they are inhaled excessively (e.g. with nebulisers) or taken orally. Tremors, usually a fine

Table 5.15 Beta-adrenergic receptor subtypes and some effects of their stimulation in certain tissues

Receptor type	Tissue in which present	Effect of stimulation
β_1	Heart	Increased rate, force, conduction velocity, automaticity
	Kidney	Renin secretion
	Fat tissue	Lipolysis
β_2	Smooth muscle	
	• bronchial	Bronchodilatation
	• vascular	Vasodilatation
	• intestinal	Reduced motility and tone
	• bladder	
	Skeletal muscle	Increased contractility, glycogenolysis, potassium uptake; tremor (overdose)
	Pancreas	Increased insulin secretion
	Liver	Glycogenolysis, gluconeogenesis
	Central nervous system	Nervous tension, headache, insomnia

hand tremor (caused by direct stimulation of beta$_2$-receptors in skeletal muscle), are common and are a significant problem in a minority of patients. A very small proportion of patients may experience paradoxical bronchospasm with inhaled bronchodilators, possibly due to direct bronchial irritation. Although it is very rare, perhaps as low as one in 50 million doses, this possibility should be borne in mind. Because of the adverse cardiac effects of the oral use of these drugs, inhaled forms (which use lower doses) are always preferred, especially if there is evidence of cardiac disease.

The beta$_2$-agonists, especially in high doses, are known to cause serious **hypokalaemia** by increasing cellular potassium uptake (see Chapter 4). This effect is potentiated by hypoxia and concomitant treatment with **methylxanthines, steroids** and **diuretics**. Life-threatening hypokalaemia is fortunately rare, but the potential is clearly greatest during severe exacerbations of asthma when hypoxia and the use of drug combinations occur concurrently. Serum potassium levels should always be monitored during severe episodes.

Bronchodilators should be used with caution in patients with hyperthyroidism (because they exert many of the symptoms just described), or with cardiovascular problems and in the elderly. The beta$_2$-agonists tend to aggravate hypoxaemia in severe asthma, so nebulizer therapy with *oxygen* as the driving gas may be the preferred mode of administration in this situation.

As usual, they should be used with care in pregnancy, but the benefits of good asthma control outweigh any slightly detrimental cardiovascular effects on the mother or fetus. Beta$_2$-agonists are used by inhalation (to minimize effects on the fetus), to control premature uterine contractions in the last trimester; *oxygen* must be given to counter the possibility of maternal and fetal hypoxia.

Antimuscarinic agents

Mode of action

Antimuscarinic drugs are competitive inhibitors of acetylcholine at muscarinic receptors, of which there are several subtypes. M_1 receptors are present in ganglia in the airways walls and M_3 receptors in airways smooth muscle. *Ipratropium* and *oxitropium* block the uptake of acetylcholine at both of these receptor types, reducing muscle tone and producing dilatation of both larger and small airways. They do not affect M_2 receptors, which are widespread elsewhere in the body.

Use

Although anticholinergics were used widely in the past in the form of belladonna or hyoscyamus galenicals, and more recently as *atropine*, they were largely abandoned because of widespread antimuscarinic adverse reactions. However, inhaled *ipratropium* and *tiotropium* bromides are useful because they appear to be fairly specific for lung tissue and are virtually without side-effects. This results from their poor absorption, a consequence of their highly polar, quaternary ammonium structure. Because they do not penetrate mucous membranes they do not reduce mucus secretion, although an antimuscarinic agent should theoretically do so, and there is no convincing evidence that any of these drugs, including *atropine*, affect sputum volume or viscosity. Further, they do not interfere with mucociliary clearance, so mucus is cleared normally.

The antimuscarinics seem to show some synergism with beta$_2$-adrenergic bronchodilators, enhancing and prolonging their activity, although this has been disputed. This discrepancy seems to have been resolved by a survey of schoolchildren and adolescents, which found little support for using the combination routinely and for mild to moderate exacerbations of asthma. However, the addition of multiple doses of an antimuscarinic to beta$_2$-agonist inhalations improved lung function and reduced hospital admission in severe exacerbations.

Antimuscarinics are particularly useful in older, chronic asthmatics in whom responsiveness to beta$_2$-agonists tends to decline progressively from age 40, probably owing to a reduction in the number of bronchiolar beta-receptors. They are more useful in the treatment of COPD (p. 326) and the long-acting *tiotropium* is licensed in the UK only for this purpose. However, there is a special problem in this older group of patients (see below).

Ipratropium bromide has a slightly slower onset of action (30–60 min, peak effect at 90–120 min) and a slightly longer duration of action than the beta$_2$-agonists and so is normally used three times daily, for prophylaxis only. The long-acting agent *tiotropium* is used only once daily, given by a DPI, usually for the maintenance treatment of COPD.

Side-effects

There are few significant problems. Nebulized *ipratropium bromide* occasionally causes paradoxical bronchospasm although isotonic, preservative-free formulations have been introduced to minimize this risk. Even so, this form of treatment should be initiated only in hospital with careful supervision for the first week, though this should not be a problem if it is added to a regimen comprising an SABA.

Although *ipratropium* is poorly absorbed topically, it sometimes causes dry mouth, headache and constipation and (rarely) urinary retention. It may also cause **acute angle closure glaucoma** in the elderly when used by nebulization, as a result of escape of drug aerosol and direct eye contact. This occurs especially in conjunction with *salbutamol*, and probably also with other SABAs. Thus nebulized *ipratropium bromide* should be used with care in glaucoma patients and in the elderly, and precautions must always be taken to prevent escape of aerosol from masks, which should fit closely: mouthpieces are preferable. The occasional patient may react adversely to the bromide radical.

Tiotropium has similar side-effects to *ipratropium* and may also cause candidiasis, pharyngitis and sinusitis. It is not suitable for the treatment of acute bronchospasm and is used for the treatment of moderate to severe COPD (Table 5.22).

Methylxanthine bronchodilators

Mode of action

Theophylline is the most potent of these agents. For many years it was thought to act solely as a cyclic nucleotide phosphodiesterase inhibitor (PDI), thus increasing the levels of cyclic 3',5'-adenosine monophosphate (cAMP) in cells and causing airways relaxation. However, relaxation of the airways occurs *in vitro* at concentrations that have no effect on cellular cAMP levels. Also, several PDIs that are more potent than *theophylline* provide no significant benefit in asthma.

However, *theophylline* is now known to have other actions:

- Antagonism of receptor-mediated adenosine-induced bronchospasm.

- Direct effects on intracellular Ca^{2+} concentration and indirect effects via cell membrane hyperpolarization.
- Uncoupling of intracellular Ca^{2+} concentration from muscular contraction.

Thus, despite some 150 years of use the precise mode of action of the methylxanthines remains obscure. Other possible actions have been suggested, e.g. increased mucociliary clearance, inhibition of mediator release, central stimulation of ventilation and improved contractility of the respiratory muscles. However, it is doubtful whether these can contribute materially to the observed increases in FEV_1 or PEF. Recent evidence suggests that *theophylline* also has anti-inflammatory, immunomodulatory and bronchoprotective effects that may contribute to its usefulness as an asthma prophylactic.

There is evidence that cAMP modulation of intracellular calcium levels may be a common pathway for bronchodilatation, however caused, and it is interesting that beta$_2$-agonists share this effect. The action of *theophylline* to mobilize intracellular calcium as referred to above may prove to be its principal effect.

Use

Theophylline (1,3-dimethylxanthine) itself is relatively insoluble but is well absorbed (although slowly) from solutions, capsules and uncoated tablets, with peak concentrations occurring after 1–2 h. However, clearance is very variable (see below). Thus microfined, slow-release oral formulations have been introduced that provide therapeutic blood levels which persist over approximately 12 h. These slow-release forms are used for prophylaxis and are taken once or twice daily. Because peak blood levels tend to occur after about 8 h, the evening dose should be taken at about 8 p.m. to minimize morning dipping. Methylxanthines should not be used unless the patient has failed to respond adequately to high-dose inhaled corticosteroids.

Theophylline, when combined with ethylenediamine as *aminophylline*, is much more soluble and in this form is used parenterally, preferably as a low-volume IV infusion. However, it is very irritant.

Side-effects

Theophylline can cause numerous side-effects [e.g. central nervous (headache, irritability, insomnia) and gastrointestinal (nausea and vomiting)], even when its serum levels are within the therapeutic range (10–20 mg/L). Above this level serious CNS reactions can occur, e.g. seizures, encephalopathy, coma, even death, and convulsions may occur without warning signs, especially if the patient is hypoxic, because cerebral hypoxia is exacerbated. Because the side-effects of methylxanthines and beta$_2$-agonists are additive, and both cause hypoxaemia and are frequently used together, the risk of convulsions is increased with this combination.

A similar situation occurs due to the hypokalaemic effect. Hypoxaemia, SABAs and corticosteroids all cause hypokalaemia and *theophylline* is usually added to a regimen containing these. Thus the UK's CSM advises that blood potassium levels should always be monitored in severe asthma attacks.

Theophylline has been considered suitable for use in pregnancy. However, it needs especially careful therapeutic drug level monitoring because blood levels are affected by the stage of pregnancy and by delivery.

Aminophylline is more irritant than *theophylline* by all routes. Even normal therapeutic oral doses may cause nausea and vomiting, although this is less likely with the modern modified-release products. Suppositories may cause proctitis. When given intravenously, *aminophylline* is best given as a very slow or continuous IV infusion, because venous irritation may cause phlebitis and rapid bolus injections may cause cardiac arrhythmias, profound hypotension and hypokalaemia, resembling an acute overdose situation. A very few patients may be hypersensitive to the ethylenediamine component. In emergency situations in the community, it may be given as a very slow bolus IV injection over 20 min. However, it is best given as a small-volume IV infusion, if circumstances permit.

Toxicity and therapeutic levels of *theophylline* and *aminophylline*. The therapeutic range of *theophylline* is rather narrow, and non-pulmonary side-effects may occur at plasma concentrations below 10 mg/L. Thus, it is preferable to institute treatment with plasma level monitoring, especially if the patient has been taking an oral form and receives IV treatment in an emergency or if there is any evidence of *theophylline* toxicity (see below) or hepatic impairment. Blood samples must be taken at steady state: approximately 4–6 h after the start of an infusion and 8–12 h after an oral dose of a modified-release product. *Theophylline* is primarily cleared by the liver, only 10% of a dose being excreted renally, so renal impairment should not affect blood levels significantly unless there is renal failure in a patient whose blood level is approaching toxicity. Regrettably, many patients in the community are given slow-release oral preparations on a standard dosage regimen and, because absorption may be erratic and metabolism variable, it is

not known whether levels in the therapeutic range are achieved: an appreciable proportion has sub-therapeutic blood concentrations. However, some benefit may be achieved at concentrations below 10 mg/L, so patient response must guide low-dose regimens. A summary of the factors that influence *theophylline* serum levels is given in Table 5.16.

Because of the variations in patient response to the different formulations, modified-release forms from different manufacturers should not be changed without careful clinical and blood level monitoring. The brand of product should be stated on prescriptions. In emergency admissions, hospital A&E doctors must be informed if patients are taking an oral *theophylline* product, in which case the usual parenteral loading dose of *aminophylline* should be omitted to avoid serious toxicity. In the absence of blood level

Table 5.16 Some drugs and conditions affecting theophylline and aminophylline plasma levels and activity[a]

Increased plasma level or effect

Inhibition or reduction of liver microsomal enzyme activity
Azithromycin?, cimetidine, ciprofloxacin, norfloxacin, erythromycin, isoniazid?, propranolol, combined oral contraceptives, fluvoxamine, viloxazine
Heart failure, hepatic diseases, age (neonates, old age), interferons and viral infections, immunization (possibly), high-carbohydrate/low-protein diet (vegetarians)

Competitive inhibition of xanthine metabolism[a]
Allopurinol

Reduced clearance (abnormal physiology)
Diltiazem, verapamil, mexiletine, propafenone
Late pregnancy[b]

Reduced plasma level or effect

Induction of liver microsomal enzymes
Aminoglutethimide, barbiturates, phenytoin and other anticonvulsants, rifampicin, St John's wort
Cigarette and marijuana smoking, high-protein/low-carbohydrate diet

Increased clearance
Sulfinpyrazone, furosemide[c]
Pregnancy[b]

[a] Theophylline is 1,3-dimethylxanthine, aminophylline is its water-soluble ethylenediamine derivative.

[b] The effect of pregnancy on blood levels is uncertain and varies with the stage of pregnancy, so careful therapeutic blood level monitoring is essential. Parturition results in increased blood levels.

[c] The situation with furosemide is unclear. Plasma concentrations of theophylline may be increased with concurrent IV use of both drugs: caution is necessary. Other loop and thiazide diuretics: increased risk of hypokalaemia with theophylline.

?, possible interaction.

monitoring, not more than four 250-mg doses should be given in 24 h. If therapeutic drug monitoring is available, an infusion rate of 500 µg/kg/h is appropriate for maintenance in adults. To avoid overdosage in obese patients, doses should be calculated on the basis of the ideal weight for height.

Despite their potential toxicity, methylxanthines have been widely used as the drugs of first choice in North America. However, they are used less frequently now and have been supplanted by the inhaled long-acting beta$_2$-agonists and corticosteroids. Nevertheless, there is a subgroup of patients who seem to respond better to *theophylline* than to other drugs.

Other xanthine derivatives are used in the USA and continental Europe. *Enprofylline* (3-propylxanthine) is a soluble, well-absorbed, potent compound that does not yield *theophylline* on metabolism and does not have many of its side-effects. Further, because it is excreted unchanged via the kidneys, it does not have the complex pharmacokinetics and interactions of *theophylline*. However, it tends to cause headaches. *Diprophylline* (dyphylline, dihydroxypropyltheophylline) has similar kinetic and toxic properties to *enprofylline* and is better tolerated than *theophylline* or *aminophylline*.

Glucocorticosteroids

These are the most potent anti-inflammatory drugs available and thus are used extensively in the treatment of asthma and other respiratory diseases (Table 5.17). They are life-saving in severe asthma attacks and may modify disease progression in intractable, infiltrative lung diseases, e.g. rheumatoid lung disease, SLE and polyarteritis nodosa (PAN; see Chapter 12).

Mode of action

These agents are presumed to diffuse passively into cells, bind to a specific receptor protein and finally stimulate the synthesis of **lipocortin**. The latter inhibits phospholipase A$_2$ and in turn the synthesis of PG and LT mediators from macrophages, monocytes and mast cells. The formation and release of potent inflammatory cytokines interleukin 1 (IL-1), IL-2, IL-3, IL-6, TNFα, interferon (IFN) gamma and the production of complement (C$_3$) acute phase reactants are also blocked (see Chapter 2).

Thus, steroids inhibit the production and release of a number of pro-inflammatory agents from a variety of immune and inflammatory cells, e.g. vasoactive and chemoattractive factors, lipolytic and proteolytic enzymes. Additionally, the extravasation of lymphocytes, fibrosis and production of PAF (an important inflammatory mediator) and IgE are also reduced. These actions combine to reduce inflammatory damage in the airways and hyper-reactivity.

Use

Inhalation therapy. For the treatment of asthma, corticosteroids (*beclometasone*, *budesonide* and *fluticasone*, all available in pMDIs and

Table 5.17   Some indications for the use of corticosteroids in diseases with respiratory involvement

Primary lung disease
Asthma, prophylaxis and severe attacks Allergic bronchopulmonary aspergillosis Extrinsic allergic alveolitis Interstitial lung disease

Secondary lung disease (see Chapter 12)
Granulomatous lung diseases, e.g. rheumatoid lung disease, sarcoidosis Vasculitis, e.g. systemic lupus erythematosus, polyarteritis nodosa, temporal arteritis (see Chapter 12) Autoimmune, e.g. Goodpasture's syndrome

DPIs; see p. 349) are preferably given by inhalation. *Mometasone* is available as a dry powder inhalation. *Ciclesonide* is a new long-acting agent and is given as a single daily pMDI dose. They are used prophylactically only, being particularly useful in controlling the delayed inflammatory response (see Figure 5.14).

It may take 7–14 days or more to obtain the maximal therapeutic response so a single dose will not control an attack and they cannot be used as rescue medication (but see below). Since the fundamentally inflammatory nature of asthma has been recognized, inhaled corticosteroids are introduced at an early stage, for example if:

- there are significant nocturnal symptoms, causing waking on more than one night per week;
- there are three or more wheezy episodes per week;
- short-acting bronchodilators are used more than two to three times weekly;
- there has been a moderate to severe exacerbation of asthma in the last 2 years.

However, many patients, and some doctors, are reluctant to use these valuable agents because of unjustified fears of serious side-effects, arising from experience with oral corticosteroids. The approximate relative anti-inflammatory potencies of these drugs are given in Table 5.18.

The dose requirement varies widely between patients and in any one patient over a long period. Although a high dose (e.g. 40–50 mg *prednisolone* orally daily in adults for 5 days or until symptoms have remitted) may be needed initially to control symptoms, it may be possible to reduce the dose substantially once symptoms are well controlled. Gradual step-down is not necessary after the short periods used to treat exacerbations of asthma, but is needed if treatment has lasted more than 21 days, especially in COPD. Once stabilized, short-term dose increases can be instituted by the patient (under an agreed protocol) to treat exacerbations.

Even if it is decided to give an oral corticosteroid, a high-dose corticosteroid inhalation and other anti-asthmatic medication should be continued to spare the corticosteroid dose. A *beclometasone* or *budesonide* inhaler, used with a spacer and face mask (p. 352), may be particularly suitable for young children who are unable to use a pMDI, which delivers only about one-tenth of the oral dose required to give a comparable effect, so only minor local and systemic side-effects occur (see below).

Oral use: maintenance therapy. *Prednisolone* and comparable agents (e.g. *betamethasone, deflazacort, dexamethasone, methylprednisolone,* etc.; see Table 5.18) may be taken orally as a last resort in chronic (intrinsic) asthma and may be the only practicable means of controlling symptoms adequately. However, as usual, dosage must be kept to a minimum to avoid their well-known long-term side-effects as far as possible.

Oral use: aborting exacerbations. The prompt use of glucocorticosteroids may be

Table 5.18   The approximate relative potencies[a] of corticosteroids used for the treatment of respiratory diseases

Systemic use		By inhalation	
Hydrocortisone	0.2	**Beclometasone**	**1** (2 in Qvar inhaler)
Deflazacort	0.8	Budesonide	1
Prednisolone	**1**	Ciclesonide	2.5
Methylprednisolone	1.3	Fluticasone	2
Triamcinolone	1.3	Mometasone	1.5
Dexamethasone	7		
Betamethasone	7		

[a] Relative to: prednisolone = 1 (systemic use); beclometasone = 1 (by inhalation).

Note: The two sides of the table cannot be compared as they have different bases for comparison.

invaluable in aborting a severe asthma attack that occurs against a background of worsening symptoms and decreased response to bronchodilators (see above). However, the full anti-inflammatory effects of this will not be apparent for some days and these agents should not be confused with the use of beta$_2$-agonists or other short-acting drugs used for rescue therapy. Doses equivalent to 40–50 mg or more of *prednisolone* daily (Table 5.18) may be required for about 5 days initially in adults, depending on the severity of symptoms. When the patient has been stabilized, the dose may be reduced (see Tables 5.13 and 5.14), but it is essential to continue treatment until it is clear that dose reduction does not lead to relapse. Peak flow monitoring, or FEV$_1$ if available, should be maintained during and after the treatment of exacerbations to ensure adequate control and the absence of deterioration. There is evidence that some patients are relatively steroid-resistant and that this is a reflection of a generalized tissue resistance to steroids, and is not confined to the lungs.

Alternate-day dosing, which is often used in other situations to minimize steroid side-effects, especially adrenal suppression, is usually unsuitable in asthma because patients tend to deteriorate on the corticosteroid-free day. As usual, dose reduction must always be gradual after more than 21 days of corticosteroid use to permit recovery from adrenal suppression and the resumption of adequate endogenous cortisol secretion. However, it is rare for asthma patients to require prolonged 'rescue' therapy. It is more common in COPD.

Patients on long-term corticosteroids require temporary increases in dose to cover exceptionally stressful situations (e.g. severe illness, surgery or trauma), for which the body requires higher than normal corticosteroid levels, because the normal adrenal response does not occur.

Parenteral use. In acute severe asthma, *hydrocortisone* (up to 2 g daily) or *methylprednisolone* (up to 500 mg daily) is given by slow IV infusion, with transfer to oral therapy as the patient improves (see Figure 5.17). However, it has been suggested that oral dosage of 40 mg *prednisolone* may be equally effective. Oral corticosteroids may also be useful in the occasional patient who bronchoconstricts in response to IV *hydrocortisone*.

Side-effects

Too much emphasis has been placed on the harmful side-effects of using steroids in asthma, leading to an aversion on the part of both doctors and patients, and subsequent under-use. As usual, the hazards of therapy need to be weighed against their undoubted benefits in the treatment of this potentially debilitating and occasionally life-threatening disease. It is clearly important to use minimal doses. This discussion deals primarily with the side-effects of inhaled corticosteroids. Those occurring with oral administration are discussed in connection with rheumatoid disease (see Chapter 12).

Inhaled steroids usually cause very few, minor adverse reactions, the most common being mild throat irritation and hoarseness (dysphonia). The oral deposition of drug may sometimes cause oral thrush (candidiasis). These effects can largely be prevented by twice-daily administration, which is as effective as the same total dose given four times daily, by rinsing the mouth with water (or a mouthwash if preferred) or brushing the teeth after using the inhaler, and using a spacer device (p. 352). If thrush does occur, it is readily controlled with topical *nystatin*, *amphotericin* or an imidazole, e.g. *ketoconazole* or *miconazole*. If these prove inadequate to control the candidiasis, or if topical treatments are not suitable (e.g. if saliva production is poor), a triazole (e.g. *fluconazole*) may be given orally. The triazoles are best reserved for resistant infections (see Chapter 8).

Although adverse systemic effects are unlikely unless the daily dose exceeds 1500–2000 µg of inhaled *BDP* or equivalent, osteoporosis, dermal thinning and, in children, growth retardation may occur. Toothbrushes have been reported to be reservoirs of *Candida* infection in patients using inhaled corticosteroids: patients should be advised to change their toothbrush if they develop hoarseness or a significant sore throat or mouth during treatment.

Long-term research in Scotland has shown that side-effects on the height and weight of children are significant only in those on Step 3 of the BTS's treatment protocol (see Tables 5.13 and 5.14). This effect was less than the effects of social deprivation, and independent of them. The risks are small and although there may be some retardation of growth velocity with normal doses, this does not appear to affect the ultimate adult height. However, growth is also affected by the severity of asthma and the degree of control, so it may be necessary to accept some drug-related growth retardation to prevent that arising from severe disease.

Nebulized steroids given with a face mask may cause facial eczema and, if this treatment mode is used over a long period, unacceptable skin damage may occur. This may be prevented by coating the skin under the mask with soft paraffin and washing the face thoroughly immediately after dosing. Masks should fit closely, or a mouthpiece may be preferred. Rarely, a patient may be sensitive to the drug or the propellant of a pMDI.

Chronic oral therapy may lead to the well-known side-effects of these drugs (see Chapters 12 and 13), e.g. Cushing's syndrome, growth suppression in children, hypertension, electrolyte disturbances and immunosuppression, though these should be mild if the daily dose does not exceed 7.5 mg daily of *prednisolone* or its equivalent (in adults and older children). Young children who require chronic oral corticosteroids should be supervised by a paediatric physician. A few patients may become steroid-dependent and rely on continuous therapy, relapsing whenever an attempt is made to reduce the dose.

Relative contra-indications include hypertension, obesity, diabetes mellitus, peptic ulceration, psoriasis, pregnancy, childhood and intercurrent infection (especially TB).

Anti-allergic drugs: cromones

Considerable attention has been focused on drugs that prevent the release from leucocytes and mast cells of the pharmacological mediators of bronchospasm and bronchial inflammation. These include *sodium cromoglicate (SCG)* and *nedocromil sodium (NDCS)*.

Mode of action

The mode of action of these drugs is still uncertain, despite intensive research. *SCG* has been regarded as the classic drug, alleged to stabilize mast cell membranes, preventing both immediate and delayed degranulation, and so the release of mediators of bronchoconstriction. This antagonism occurs whether the stimulus is immunological (IgE) or irritant (due to exercise, cold air or inhaled hypertonic saline). The development of bronchiolar hyper-responsiveness is also blocked by pretreatment with *SCG*. *NDCS* is a much more potent inhibitor of mediator release than is *SCG*, and also inhibits WBC, macrophage and platelet activation. However, doubts have been expressed about the importance of mast cell stabilization, and the true mode of action of these drugs in asthma remains to be elucidated.

Some stimuli, e.g. sulfur dioxide, are believed to produce bronchoconstriction via a neuronal mechanism involving the release of the peptide neurotransmitter, **substance P**, at the endings of unmyelinated C-fibres. Substance P is a potent airways constrictor, the action of which in the lungs is also blocked by *SCG* and *NDCS*: it is also involved in the transmission of pain sensation (see Chapter 7). *SCG* also affects phosphodiesterase enzyme levels and calcium influx into cells, thus influencing smooth muscle contraction.

Use

The cromones are not absorbed orally and so must be administered by inhalation. *SCG* is particularly useful in exercise-induced asthma in children, but rarely in adults. However, exercise-induced asthma may reveal that control is inadequate, so these children should be reassessed. It can only be used prophylactically and may take up to 4–6 weeks to achieve its full effect.

NDCS has similar properties to *SCG* but is a more potent anti-inflammatory agent. It appears to have a wider spectrum of clinical activity and is more effective in children aged 6–12 years, having a steroid-sparing effect, although it is difficult to predict those who will benefit. It may be useful in mild to moderate asthma and for those patients (and their parents) who are fearful of using corticosteroids. However, it is less effective than corticosteroids and should not be regarded as a replacement for them, so it is used only rarely.

Side-effects

SCG is a very safe drug, the most common adverse reaction being a transient bronchospasm from the DPI presentation, although the pMDI form avoids this problem and is cheaper. If a patient cannot use the DPI, a beta$_2$-adrenergic bronchodilator may be inhaled beforehand.

NDCS tends to cause slightly more undesirable effects than *SCG*, e.g. headache, nausea and vomiting, dyspepsia and abdominal pain, although these do not normally cause discontinuation of treatment.

Biological agents

Leukotriene receptor antagonists (LTRAs)

Mode of action. The **leukotrienes (LTs)** are straight-chain eicosanoids derived from arachidonic acid, and are potent pro-inflammatory agents. They are mostly produced from arachidonic acid by the phospholipase A$_2$ pathway (see Chapters 2 and 12). This pathway is activated by a specific protein, **5-lipoxygenase activating protein (FLAP)**, which binds the enzyme to the cell membrane.

Leukotriene B4 (LTB$_4$) is derived from the labile intermediate LTA$_4$ and is mostly produced by neutrophils. It is a potent neutrophil chemotactic agent. However, the role of neutrophils in asthma is controversial because they are only found in the lungs in appreciable numbers in patients with some types of occupational asthma. Although eosinophils are present in increased numbers in the lungs of asthmatic patients, LTB$_4$ probably plays only a minor role in eosinophil recruitment. It has only a weak effect on eosinophils, with other chemoattractants (e.g. PAF, IL-2, IL-5) being much more potent.

LTA$_4$ is also converted into the cysteinyl leukotrienes LTC$_4$, LTE$_4$ and LTF$_4$, initially by conjugation with glutathione. All of these have been implicated in asthma because they are potent bronchoconstrictors and can be produced by a range of effector cells, e.g. granulocytes and monocytes, mast cells and macrophages. The LTs have a long persistence in lung tissue and also stimulate mucus secretion, cause mucosal oedema and sensitize the airways to other spasmogens. The LTC$_4$/D$_4$/E$_4$ mixture used to be known as SRS-A (slow reacting substance of anaphylaxis).

LTs act via at least three distinct receptors, for LTB$_4$, LTC$_4$ and LTD$_4$/LTE$_4$, which are blocked by the LTRAs. The CysLT$_1$ receptor is activated by LTC$_4$/LTD$_4$/LTE$_4$ and is also blocked by the LTRAs.

There are thus two routes by which LT activity may be reduced in asthma: by preventing their formation, inhibiting phospholipase A$_2$, 5-lipoxygenase, FLAP or LT synthase, or by blocking LT receptors in the lung.

The first 5-lipoxygenase inhibitor, *zileuton*, is licensed in the USA for the prophylaxis and treatment of chronic asthma and two LTRAs, *montelukast* and *zafirlukast*, are available in the UK.

Use. These agents are useful adjuncts when existing treatment with inhaled beta-agonists and corticosteroids fails to provide adequate control. They are not substitutes for existing treatments, but may have advantages over corticosteroids because they inhibit bronchoconstriction induced by exercise and allergens, against which corticosteroids are relatively ineffective. They are well tolerated, and fit into Step 4 of the BTS and SIGN guidelines for adults and schoolchildren (see Table 5.13) and Step 2 of those for young children (see Table 5.14), i.e. as an adjunct to an inhaled beta$_2$-agonist plus an inhaled high-dose corticosteroid, or as an alternative if the latter cannot be used.

Because they are oral products they may be of special benefit to patients who have compliance problems with inhaled therapy, e.g. the elderly and mentally or physically handicapped.

Side-effects. These are usually mild and infrequent, but abdominal pain, hypersensitivity and skin reactions occur. CNS stimulation and headache have also been reported. Churg–Strauss syndrome (asthma, sinusitis, rhinitis, eosinophilia and systemic vasculitis) has occurred when they are used in combination with corticosteroids and patients should be warned to report any rashes, worsening symptoms or possible cardiac problems. They thus avoid the principal disadvantage of corticosteroids but have their own problems. Once again, a balance has to be struck between benefits and disadvantages.

Zafirlukast has the possible additional problem of severe hepatic problems (e.g. malaise, vomiting and jaundice) and patients must be warned to report any of these symptoms promptly.

Omalizumab

This recombinant, humanized, monoclonal antibody combines with IgE (see Chapter 2) and so prevents its allergenic effects.

Use. It is licensed for use as add-on prophylactic therapy in those who have severe persistent allergic asthma associated with elevated IgE levels (pp. 300, 313) and whose asthma is not controlled satisfactorily with full doses of corticosteroids plus an LABA (p. 294), though the status of the latter is in doubt.

Administration is by SC injection every 2 or 4 weeks, in a dose determined by a patient's IgE level and body weight. It is not recommended for use in children under 12 years of age.

Side-effects. *Omalizumab* should be used with caution in those who have an autoimmune disease, hepatic or renal impairment or are pregnant. Because it increases susceptibility and the immune response to helminth infections, precautions are necessary in areas where these are endemic and should be discontinued if a helminth infection does not respond to treatment. It is contra-indicated if a mother is breastfeeding.

Common side-effects include headache and injection site reactions. Gastrointestinal and CNS reactions, and rashes, pruritus, flushing, photosensitivity and influenza-like symptoms are less common.

Like all injected proteins, the possibility of severe allergic reactions on repeated administration, including anaphylaxis, must be borne in mind. There may also be a loss of effectiveness, due to the production of Igs.

Oxygen

Oxygen may be life-saving in acute severe asthma and should be given in these circumstances, even if there is no overt cyanosis. Because the pure gas causes pulmonary damage and retinal fibrosis (**retrolental fibroplasia**) it is always mixed with air. If there is no history of COPD (see below), patients may be given 35% *oxygen* while being transferred to hospital, and up to 60% may be used for short periods after admission. The hazards associated with higher concentrations mean that artificial ventilation by **intermittent positive pressure ventilation** (IPPV, p. 361) is preferable. Concentrations greater than 28% are not suitable for chronic bronchitics with type 2 respiratory failure (see p. 347).

If alveolar ventilation is inadequate in a seriously ill patient, both P_aO_2 and P_aCO_2 may be reduced initially and patients may be cyanosed even when breathing *oxygen*-enriched air. Later, the P_aO_2 may continue to fall while the P_aCO_2 rises, producing respiratory acidosis. This may occur very rapidly in children. Any increase in P_aCO_2 is a serious sign in an asthmatic patient. Blood gases should be determined initially, and if the P_aO_2 is <8 kPa, serial determinations should be made to monitor therapy. The P_aO_2 may rise only slowly in these circumstances.

High-flow *oxygen* (giving 50–60%) is normally given with a suitable mask (see Table 5.27 and p. 361), but if patients are exhausted then NIPPV may be used. The techniques of *oxygen* therapy are discussed on p. 360.

Other drugs

Immunoglobulins are sometimes used for severe asthma, e.g. in the final step in Tables 5.13 and 5.14 and Figure 5.17.

A number of **fixed drug combinations** (e.g. a non-selective sympathomimetic agent plus a methylxanthine) were used before effective asthma treatments became available, and some of these are still marketed. Most are oral formulations that are not now prescribed in the UK, but if older patients who are already using them find that they give adequate relief there is no reason to change that situation.

Non-selective bronchodilators are rarely prescribed for asthma treatment because of their undesirable cardiovascular effects. Bronchodilators combined with sedatives should be avoided because they may cause respiratory depression in patients whose ventilatory function is already compromised.

The **respiratory stimulant** *doxapram* is generally of no value in asthma and may be harmful: it should be used only under expert supervision in hospital. In situations where it might be considered necessary, artificial ventilation is preferred, but it may have a limited role in community practice to support a patient while awaiting transport to a remote hospital.

Antihistamines (H_1-blockers) are not useful in asthma and do not prevent histamine-induced bronchospasm in normal dosage. However, some of the newer H_1-blockers, e.g. *azelastine* and *cetirizine*, have interesting anti-inflammatory properties, including effects on kinin, LT and PG production, and may be the precursors of new anti-asthma drugs.

Many **investigational drugs** are being explored, e.g. alpha-adrenergic receptor antagonists, inhibitors of lipocortin and PGs (E series), and potassium channel activators (e.g. *cromakalim*). Intense research activity is also directed towards methods of modifying LT activity other than by the LTAs. Inhibitors of 5-lipoxygenase prevent the conversion of arachidonic acid to LTB_4 and the cysteinyl LTs (C_4, D_4 and E_4). Thus, future progress is likely to be in the more specific control of bronchial inflammation and hyper-reactivity. Interferons and inhibitors of TNFα and other cytokines have been introduced for the treatment of conditions such as rheumatoid diseases (see Chapter 12) and skin diseases (see Chapter 13), but for the present the beta$_2$-agonists and corticosteroids have a central role in asthma management.

Other allergic lung diseases

Bronchopulmonary aspergillosis

Spores of the mould *Aspergillus fumigatus* are ubiquitous and sometimes cause infections or allergy, resulting in asthmatic attacks, COPD (see below), bronchiectasis and fibrosis. Other species of *Aspergillus* are occasionally involved.

Extrinsic allergic alveolitis

Although this is a restrictive disease, not obstructive (see Table 5.4), e.g. 'farmer's lung' and mushroom worker's lung, it is convenient to include it here. A variety of environmental or occupation allergens may cause type III hypersensitivity reactions that affect the lung parenchyma (Table 5.19). Following an initial exposure to these antigens, subsequent exposure may produce a transient mild asthmatic type attack followed after 4–6 h by a 24-h episode of cough and dyspnoea with fever, chills, headache, etc. With repeated exposure, pulmonary fibrosis and a diffusion defect occur and pulmonary function tests then show marked respiratory restriction. Diagnosis is complicated by the interval between exposure and the onset of symptoms so that the connection between them is often not made.

Pulmonary eosinophilia

This term includes a number of conditions in which dyspnoea and radiologically identified

Table 5.19 Some types of extrinsic allergic alveolitis

Disease	Allergen
Farmer's lung Mushroom worker's lung Bagassosis	Spores of thermophilic actinomycetes from mouldy hay, mushroom compost and sugar cane residues
Bird fancier's lung	Avian antigens from feathers, excreta, etc. of pigeons, parrots, budgerigars, chickens
Grain handler's disease	Dust derived from the grain
Malt worker's lung	Spores of *Aspergillus* spp. in mouldy barley or malt

lung changes occur, together with a very high blood eosinophil count. Asthmatic attacks may also occur. Cases may be due to aspergillosis, drugs (e.g. sulphonamides), intestinal or other parasites and, rarely, PAN (Chapter 12).

Management. In pulmonary eosinophilia and extrinsic allergic alveolitis this involves treatment of any infection, antigen avoidance and the use of corticosteroids to minimize inflammatory lung changes.

Chronic obstructive pulmonary disease

Introduction

Chronic obstructive pulmonary disease (COPD), sometimes known as chronic obstructive lung disease (COLD) or chronic obstructive airways disease (COAD), is the collective term for a number of chronic, slowly progressive conditions, most of which are either caused by tobacco smoking or are exacerbated by it. It has supplanted the term 'chronic bronchitis'. The conditions produce widespread, persistent airways obstruction that is largely irreversible but somewhat amenable to inhaled bronchodilator and corticosteroid therapy. The conditions are the result of chronic inflammation and recurrent infection of the airways, and cause dyspnoea and abnormal blood gas levels. The underlying condition in all of these is usually **COPD** or **emphysema** (or a combination of these) but chronic asthma may also present similarly. Bronchiectasis and cystic fibrosis are less common causes.

Definitions

Members of this group of diseases may occur together. The descriptive definition of the BTS and SIGN guidelines, published in collaboration with NICE (2004), is as follows:

> 'Chronic obstructive pulmonary disease (COPD) is characterised by airflow obstruction. The airflow obstruction is usually progressive, not fully reversible and does not change markedly over several months. The disease is caused predominately by smoking.'

- Airflow obstruction is defined as a reduced FEV_1 (forced expiratory volume in 1 s), i.e. <80% predicted for a particular patient and a reduced FEV_1/FVC ratio (where FVC is forced vital capacity), such that FEV_1/FVC is less than 0.70.
- The airway obstruction is due to a combination of inflammation, mucus secretion and parenchymal damage.
- The damage is the result of chronic inflammation that differs from that seen in asthma and which is usually the result of inhaling tobacco smoke.
- Significant airflow obstruction may be present before the individual becomes aware of it.
- COPD produces symptoms, disability and impaired quality of life that may respond to pharmacological and other therapies that have limited or no impact on the airflow obstruction.
- Other factors, particularly occupational exposures, may also contribute to the development of COPD.
- COPD is now the preferred term for the conditions with airflow obstruction previously diagnosed as chronic bronchitis or emphysema, or a combination of these. There is no single diagnostic test for COPD. Making a diagnosis relies on clinical judgement based on a combination of history, physical examination and confirmation of the presence of airflow obstruction using spirometry.

The term 'bronchitis' describes inflammation of the larger airways and should now be restricted to the acute condition (see below).

COPD is usually associated with a chronic cough with the production of sputum on most days for at least 3 consecutive months of the year in at least 2 successive years. This is an epidemiological, symptomatic definition, which enables patients to be classified for statistical purposes, but a lesser degree or duration of symptoms clearly indicates the early stages of the disease.

The disability and impaired quality of life caused by airways obstruction is the principal problem for patients and occurs especially during the winter months.

Emphysema is permanent destructive enlargement of the lung parenchyma distal to the terminal bronchioles, i.e. the respiratory bronchioles, alveolar ducts and alveolar sacs. This defines a pathological lesion, not a clinical syndrome, which may occur as a separate entity but often accompanies COPD.

Acute bronchitis is occasionally caused by the inhalation of irritants but is usually due to viral infection accompanied by opportunistic bacterial infections (see Chapter 8). The outstanding symptom is cough, initially dry, but becoming productive of copious sputum. Young children may have a very severe, harsh cough with inspiratory stridor, the condition known as **croup**. Inflammation of the smaller airways (**bronchiolitis**) may also occur in infants, but this should settle in 3–4 days, though the cough may persist for 2–3 weeks. Acute respiratory distress in young children should always be taken very seriously.

A comparison of asthma and COPD is given in Table 5.20.

COPD

Epidemiology and natural history

COPD is much more common in the UK and in Eastern Europe than in most developed countries. It was known in Western Europe as the 'English disease', a consequence of being the first intensively industrialized country at a time when the health hazards of environmental pollution and the effects of occupational exposure to airborne dusts and toxins were not appreciated. The overall prevalence of COPD in the UK is about 4% in men aged about 50 years, 9% at 60 years, 12% at 80 years, but only 3% in women.

This sex difference is wholly attributable to differences in smoking habits: in fact, the difference increases with advancing age because of the cumulative effects of long-term smoking in men. However, changes in smoking habits over the past 50 years, with an increasing proportion of girls and young women smoking cigarettes, may be expected to minimize the difference. These prevalence rates are about three times that for angina pectoris.

In the 19th and early 20th centuries COPD was due to a combination of occupational and domestic air pollution, largely from the use of coal as the principal fuel, and to poor living conditions. However, there has been a switch to cigarette smoke as the prime cause of COPD since the 1920s introduction of factory-made cigarettes.

COPD is responsible for considerable morbidity and time off work, and caused about 30 000 deaths in 1999 in the UK (male:female ratio about 5:1). Almost 30% of these deaths occur before retirement, although the death rate

Table 5.20   Differentiation between asthma and chronic obstructive pulmonary disease[a]

Feature	Asthma	COPD
Symptoms under age 35 years	Common	Uncommon
Smoker or ex-smoker	Uncommon	Almost all
Chronic productive cough	Uncommon	Almost all, progressive
Breathlessness	Episodic, variable	Persistent and progressive
Night-time breathlessness and/or wheeze	Common	Uncommon
Significant diurnal or day-to-day variability of symptoms	Common	Uncommon
Reversibility with beta$_2$-agonists	>15%, except in remission	<15%

[a] These conditions may coexist.
COPD, chronic obstructive pulmonary disease (old term was 'chronic bronchitis').

is declining with reduced smoking in men, less air pollution and better treatment.

The disease is characterized by an insidious onset, starting with a 'smoker's cough' that is usually disregarded. Significant symptoms may not appear until after some 20 years or more of smoking, by which time there is appreciable irreversible lung damage. There is then a progressive decline over 10–40 years with increasing dyspnoea, exercise limitation, difficulty in expectoration and an increased frequency of alarming, acute infectious exacerbations, necessitating hospital admission. Occasionally, an acute respiratory infection is identified as the trigger for the initial onset of overt symptoms.

The prognosis can be related to the degree of exercise limitation: about 40% of patients with significantly reduced walking ability on the flat die within 5 years, usually of heart failure.

Aetiology and histopathology

The disease is multifactorial in origin, but prolonged bronchial irritation and damage is the major contributor. The prime cause is **cigarette smoking**, and almost all clinical parameters, e.g. symptoms, work lost, hospital admissions and deaths, correlate with the extent of smoking. The death rate from COPD is increased about 10-fold for each 15 cigarettes smoked daily and regularly in the past. However, the statistic usually used is pack years, i.e. (number of cigarettes smoked per day ÷ 20) × number of years smoked. **Environmental pollution** and some occupations (e.g. coal mining) potentiate the effect of smoking, and the effects of urbanization are very marked in smokers. However, the major improvement in urban pollution in the last 50 years means that there are now only very small effects in non-smokers unless it is extreme.

Climate plays a minor role, although morbidity is higher in the colder and wetter regions in the north and west of the UK, after allowing for the effects of urbanization. In Australia and New Zealand the age–mortality curve is displaced relative to that for the UK to higher age groups by about 10–15 years. This shift is due primarily to less urban pollution and differences in smoking habits. Also, the inci-

dence of severe respiratory infections is lower in the better climate.

A **low socioeconomic status** predisposes to both morbidity and mortality. The mortality in Class V (unskilled) is six times that in Class II (administrative). This is related to differences in smoking habits, hygiene, nutrition, attitudes towards achieving a healthy lifestyle and usage of healthcare facilities. Educational and cultural differences lead to a lack of awareness in the lower socioeconomic groups of the importance of symptoms, or disregard of them, the need for medical care and the benefits that modern medicine can produce. Similar considerations apply to most diseases.

There may be a slight familial tendency predisposing to bronchial mucus hypersecretion, but this is heavily outweighed by the effects of the risk factors outlined above. Respiratory infections have a very small role in causation, though they produce the severe exacerbations seen in the winter months and contribute significantly to the progressive lung damage.

The histological appearance of the lung tissues in COPD is illustrated in Figures 5.18 and 5.19.

The outstanding histopathological features in COPD leading to airways obstruction include the following:

- **Increased thickness of the bronchiolar wall** due to inflammation and hyperplasia of the mucous glands. The latter represent about two-thirds of the bulk of the increased tissue mass compared with one-third of the normal thickness (Figure 5.19).
- **Hypersecretion of mucus** from the increased number of mucous glands and from irritated goblet cells.
- Chronic insult damages the cilia, leading to impaired mucociliary clearance, and **mucus plugs** obstruct the airways partially or completely (Figure 5.18(b)).
- Numerous mucus-containing **inflammatory cells** (Figure 5.18(b)) and trapped bacteria, the latter producing the infective exacerbations.
- A modest, variable degree of **bronchoconstriction**.

In late-stage disease there is extensive destruction of the lung parenchyma (see Figure 5.20), i.e. emphysema. Fibrosis contributes to obstruc-

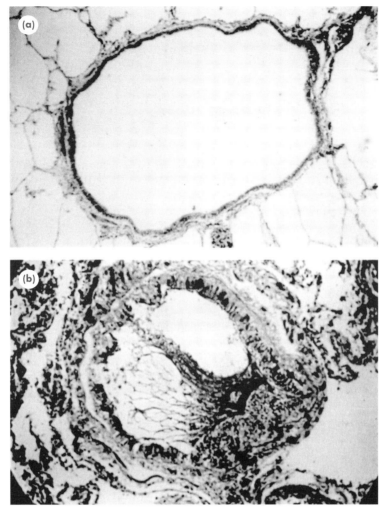

Figure 5.18   Histological appearance of the lung parenchyma in severe COPD. (a) Normal: note the thin-walled, unobstructed bronchiole surrounded by well-defined, very thin-walled alveoli. Blood vessels, lymphatics, etc. are attached to the bronchiolar wall (top right and left side). (b) COPD (chronic bronchitis), showing a thickened, inflamed mucosa, partial mucus plugging of the bronchiole, and distortion and destruction of the alveolar walls (emphysema). The mottled appearance of the tissues is largely from leucocytic (inflammatory cell) infiltration. (Reproduced with permission from Reid LM, p. 1253 in Fishman AP (1988) *Pulmonary Diseases and Disorders*, 2nd edn. New York: McGraw-Hill (Fig. 77-7 (c) and (e))).

tion, reduces lung compliance, increases the work of breathing and exacerbates dyspnoea, especially during passive expiration.

Clinical features

The **cardinal early symptoms** are as follows:

- 'Smoker's cough': initially present on winter mornings, but later throughout the year.

- Sputum: usually copious and tenacious (mucoid). It may be yellow, green or khaki-coloured (**mucopurulent**) during infective exacerbations, but clear or greyish between the infective episodes, and occasionally streaked with blood.
- Dyspnoea: as with all obstructive airways diseases expiration is the difficult phase, the spirogram being similar to that shown

(a)

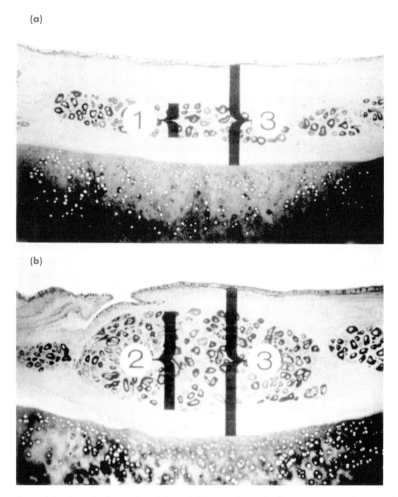

(b)

Figure 5.19 Histology of the bronchiolar wall in COPD. (a) Normal (Reid Index approximately 0.3). (b) COPD (chronic bronchitis; Reid Index approximately 0.7). Numbers in circles indicate one-third and two-thirds relationships. The Reid Index is the ratio of the thickness of the mucous gland layer to the total mucosal thickness. (Reproduced with permission from the editors of *Update*.)

in Figure 5.15(b) and (c). Wheezing may occur, especially in the morning.

• Fever and the usual signs of infection during exacerbations.

In **mild disease** cough may be the only abnormality. Patients with **moderate disease** also have excess sputum, breathlessness (with or without wheezing), and a general reduction in breath sounds on auscultation (caused by total occlusion of some airways). In **late-stage disease** there is usually breathlessness at rest or on any exertion, together with a prominent wheeze and a productive cough. The following features may also be present:

• **Cyanosis**: if the respiratory deficit is severe; frank central cyanosis is discernible when there is about 5 g/dL of deoxygenated Hb in the blood, i.e. about 30% of the total Hb, the P_aO_2 being about 6 kPa (normal = 12–13.3 kPa).

• Heart failure (**cor pulmonale**, p. 285) and peripheral oedema.

• **Plethoric complexion**: patients may have a high facial colour due to secondary poly-

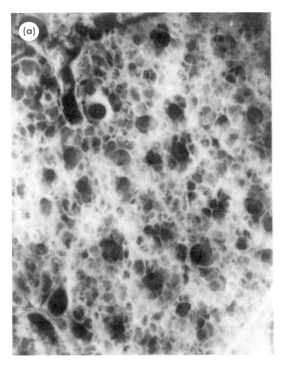
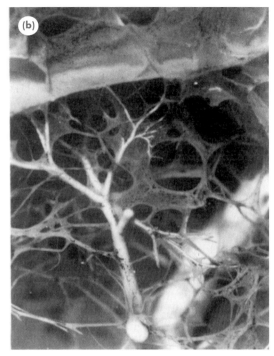

Figure 5.20   Low-power microscopic appearance of normal and emphysemic lungs. (a) Normal. (b) Emphysema showing tissue destruction and the production of enlarged air spaces, giving an increased total lung capacity. [Reproduced with permission from Heard BE (1958) *Thorax* **13**: 136.]

cythaemia (erythrocytosis, a raised red cell count), a normal physiological response to hypoxaemia, high levels of carbaminohaemoglobin (carrying CO_2) and carboxyhaemoglobin (carrying CO from incomplete tobacco combustion) that decreases the oxygen-carrying capacity of the blood. The resultant increased blood viscosity causes dilatation of the skin capillaries, which are filled with blood containing high Hb levels, thus causing the high skin colour.

• **Hyperinflation**: a consequence of air trapping.

At the extremes, two classic clinical patterns may be seen in patients. At one extreme is the type A ('pink puffer', the 'emphysemic type'), a thin, usually elderly patient with intense dyspnoea, pursed lip breathing and rapid shallow respiration, who uses the accessory muscles of respiration. The advantage of pursed lip breathing is that it creates a back-pressure in the airways and so helps to prevent them from collapse, which the inflamed, weakened airways tend to do under the increased intrathoracic pressure that occurs in forced respiration. These patients produce little sputum but have severe airways obstruction with hyperinflation and radiological and spirometric evidence of emphysema. They have good respiratory drive and maintain near-normal blood gas levels at the expense of being short of breath. Their thinness may reflect weight loss due to the energy required to maintain adequate ventilation.

At the other extreme, the type B patient ('blue bloater', the 'bronchitic' type) is obese, has a plethoric complexion and moderate dyspnoea, lapsing readily into heart failure and presenting a picture of poor respiratory drive. Type B patients adjust to their abnormal blood gases at the expense of reduced exercise tolerance, but do not experience dyspnoea at rest. There are considerable degrees of overlap between these patient groups, and their different appearances cannot be used diagnostically as most patients show elements of both types. The reasons for the occurrence of the two physical types are not clear, but may represent differences in ventilatory control.

Diagnosis

Pulmonary function tests

These show the characteristic changes outlined in Table 5.6. If peak flow testing is used, serial recordings should be made over a week to show the absence of variability. The RV may be normal or, later, be somewhat increased by air trapping and destruction of lung tissue. However, these are not the principal criteria but are aids to diagnosis and judging severity. Diagnosis is based on:

- Patient over 35 years who smokes regularly, has a chronic cough, regular sputum production, wheezing and frequent winter 'bronchitis'.
- Weight loss (usually), due to increased energy costs of respiration. Weight gain may occur later, as the result of:
  - exercise limitation (Table 5.5) and effort intolerance;
  - fluid retention, with ankle swelling, due to the oedema of right heart failure (see Chapter 4).
- Waking at night with symptoms.
- Fatigue.
- Occupational respiratory hazards.

Chest pain and haemoptysis are uncommon in COPD and suggest an alternative diagnosis, e.g. lung cancer.

Spirometry results should be used to assist diagnosis or to reconsider the diagnosis if there is an exceptionally good response to treatment, which may suggest asthma. The European Respiratory Society has published reference values (see References and further reading, p. 364), but these may lead to underdiagnosis in the elderly and are not applicable to Blacks or Asians.

Testing the reversibility of symptoms by medication is not usually part of the diagnostic procedure because it may be unhelpful (owing to poor reproducibility or inconsistency), misleading (unless the change in FEV_1 is >400 mL), and does not predict outcome. Distinction of COPD from asthma is made primarily on clinical grounds (Table 5.20).

Other useful investigations include a full blood count, to identify anaemia or polycythaemia (see Chapter 11), and a chest X-ray. The body mass index should be calculated (BMI = weight ÷ (height in metres^2).

Additional investigations that may aid management include:

- Serial domiciliary peak flow measurements.
- Alpha$_1$-antitrypsin (AAT) levels, if the condition is of early onset (<40 years), there is a minimal smoking history, or a family history of emphysema (see below).
- TLco.
- CT chest scan, e.g. to detect primary lung cancer or metastatic spread from other neoplasms.
- ECG, to assess cardiac status if there are features of cor pulmonale (see below).
- Echocardiogram, to detect pulmonary embolism.
- Pulse oximetry, to assess the need for *oxygen therapy*.
- Sputum culture, if the patient produces persistent purulent sputum, to determine appropriate antibiotic treatment.

Breathlessness

This is assessed by the ability to perform specific tasks (e.g. stair climbing, walking distance) or to manage the activities of everyday living (e.g. shopping).

Blood gases

These may be near normal until the later stages of the disease. The P_aO_2 becomes reduced gradually and this effect becomes more severe during sleep, when patients may snore heavily and show 'sleep apnoea' (i.e. brief, frequent periods of failure to breathe during sleep). Although the P_aCO_2 is usually within the normal range in the early stages, severely impaired respiratory drive may cause the P_aCO_2 to rise progressively later, when patients may be in chronic respiratory failure (p. 346).

Chest X-ray

This is usually normal, though in the later stages the heart may be enlarged and there may be evidence of emphysema and lung fibrosis.

Sputum microbiology

This is usually performed routinely in hospital. Most infections in COPD are due to *Haemophilus influenzae*, *Streptococcus pneumoniae* and viruses, so community treatment is usually initiated on a 'best guess' basis. This may compromise subsequent sputum investigation even though the patient continues to produce purulent sputum. A sputum sample should always be taken before initiating antibiotic treatment, following usual good practice.

The management of COPD will be discussed with that of emphysema.

Emphysema

When this occurs as part of the COPD syndrome it affects the alveoli closest to the respiratory bronchioles. Emphysema that is not part of COPD is uncommon and is more generalized: these patients usually show the clinical pattern of the 'pink puffer' group (p. 331).

Aetiology and pathology

The aetiology of emphysema is illustrated in Figure 5.21. The principal underlying problem is reduced AAT activity. This enzyme is a highly polymorphic glycoprotein produced by the liver

and alveolar macrophages, especially in chronic inflammation. In the lungs, the function of the enzyme is to protect the delicate alveolar tissue from autodigestion by elastase and other proteolytic enzymes that are produced to clear inhaled debris and the proteinaceous products of inflammation. Smoking produces both increased amounts of cell debris and reduced AAT levels, and may also cause lung parenchymal damage by direct toxicity.

Hereditary AAT deficiency is a rare autosomal recessive trait; it may be heterozygous or homozygous. AAT is encoded for by the *Pi* (protein inhibitor) gene on chromosome 14, of which more than 90 alleles are known. Disease is associated only with those mutations causing significant deficiency or greatly impaired function of the enzyme. The gene defects occur in between 1/2000 and 1/7000 European neonates and are the most common cause of liver disease in infancy and childhood. It is postulated that liver disease results, at least partly, from failure to clear abnormal forms of AAT. However, some further unknown genetic or environmental trigger is required because, although more than

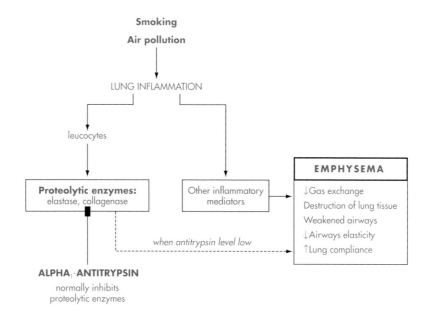

Figure 5.21 Aetiology of emphysema. The disease is characterized by proteolytic damage causing anatomical and physiological abnormalities. Normality gives normal alpha$_1$-antitrypsin levels and tissue and physiological integrity.

50% of infants with total AAT deficiency have abnormal liver function tests, only about 13% develop overt liver disease, usually by the age of 4 months. About 5% of these require liver transplantation by the age of 4 years, but the condition settles in the remainder, with a reasonable quality of life. Some 10% of the group suffer from malabsorption of vitamin K and the resultant **kernicterus** (bilirubin encephalopathy) causes permanent CNS damage if not treated early. A further 1–2% without any history of infantile jaundice present later in childhood or as adults with liver cirrhosis (see Chapter 3). Some develop emphysema as young adults. It seems likely that these various manifestations are associated with different alleles of the *Pi* gene. Symptoms are twice as common in males as in females.

The symptoms of emphysema are accelerated by environmental factors, especially smoking. Most emphysemics are smokers in whom the resultant chronic inflammation damages the alveoli rather than the airways, as in COPD. However, there is considerable overlap between emphysema and COPD.

Because lung tissue is destroyed (Figure 5.20), the TLC is increased, at the expense of an increased (unusable) RV, and the area available for gas exchange is reduced. The residual alveolar walls become thickened and fibrosed, causing a diffusion defect.

Diagnosis

Diagnosis of emphysema rests on the evidence of obstructive lung disease associated with characteristic radiographic changes, though the latter are not always present. Obstruction results from weakened, narrowed, small (2-mm diameter) airways that tend to collapse on expiration (p. 277), owing both to inflammation and atrophy of their walls and the destruction of supporting alveolar tissue. Alveolar destruction also results in loss of the elastic tissue that provides an important proportion of the expiratory force at rest. A definitive diagnosis may not be made during life and is often reached on inadequate evidence. Although any doubt can be resolved by bronchoscopic biopsy, this is rarely done because it does not influence management.

Because the damage is irreversible, treatment is usually only symptomatic.

Management of COPD

Because most patients have a combination of inflammation and AAT deficiency, their treatment is based on similar principles. There is unlikely to be a significant reversible element.

Aims

The aims of management of COPD are to:

• educate the patient about their disease and prognosis;
• prevent deterioration;
• minimize the frequency and severity of exacerbations and complications;
• give the best possible symptomatic relief;
• achieve a reasonable quality of life.

The ways in which these are achieved are discussed below, and summarized in Tables 5.21 and 5.22.

General measures

General measures in the management of COPD include the following:

• **Education** is essential to any programme of rehabilitation. In a chronic condition such as COPD, patients need to understand the relevance of the general and pharmacotherapeutic measures and appreciate what is reasonable to expect from management.
• **Stop smoking**: this may reduce the risk of further deterioration substantially, and the patient may improve somewhat. In long-standing disease, significant improvement is not a realistic objective because irreversible damage may mean that the patient's lung function does not improve, merely that the decline is slowed or arrested. However, even a small improvement in lung function can give considerable subjective benefit. *Bupropion, varenicline* and *nicotine replacement therapy (NRT)* are useful aids. Patients should be referred to a smoking cessation clinic for

Table 5.21 General approach to the management of target features in chronic obstructive pulmonary disease

Aim	Target feature	Management mode
Prevent deterioration	Bronchiolar irritation and inflammation	Stop smoking Avoid irritant and dusty environments Corticosteroids?[a]
Improve respiratory function	Poor ventilation Bronchoconstriction?	Physiotherapy Beta$_2$-agonist or antimuscarinic bronchodilators?[a] Theophylline?[a]
Symptomatic relief	Dyspnoea Excessive sputum Troublesome night cough	Oxygen Physiotherapy, inhalations Expectorants/mucolytics? Antitussives?
Treat exacerbations and complications	Infections Heart failure	Prompt antibiotics, influenza vaccination Reduce weight if obese Diuretics or vasodilators Digoxin if fibrillating Venesection
Improve quality of life	Poor mobility	Oxygen Occupational therapy Home improvements, social support

[a] These and any other potentially useful medicines (marked ?) should be tested for benefit: the patient's view is relevant. If there is no perceived benefit they should be withdrawn. COPD may coexist with asthma. The cardiovascular and diuretic actions of theophylline may be adverse or beneficial (see Chapter 4).

? = possible feature or potentially useful medication.

behavioural support, if available. The NICE guidance is that these drugs should only be prescribed via the NHS for those who have committed to a target date for smoking cessation. The initial amount prescribed should be sufficient to last only 2 weeks beyond the stop date for *NRT* or 3–4 weeks for *bupropion*, and a second prescription issued only if the patient is making a continuing effort to stop smoking. If the patient is unsuccessful, a further prescription should not normally be issued within 6 months. There is currently insufficient evidence to justify the use of *bupropion* and *NRT* together. *Varenicline* is started 2 weeks before the target stop date and continued for 10 weeks afterwards. The treatment may be repeated if necessary.

- Avoid irritant and dusty environments.
- **Weight loss and dietary advice** if obese, i.e. BMI >30 kg/m^2, to reduce the oxygen demand and the workload on the heart. Healthy eating should be encouraged and a planned exercise programme helps to improve cardiac and respiratory function. Type A patients (p. 331), in whom the respiratory effort has caused weight loss, need dietary advice and supplements to regain an ideal weight.
- **Pulmonary rehabilitation**: trained teams deliver a multidisciplinary approach to improving the use of what respiratory function remains and teach **postural drainage**. For the latter the patient lies face down and on each side in turn, and their chest wall, ribs and backs are percussed to help dislodge secretions. If secretions are very copious or tenacious, a head-down position may help.
- **Occupational therapy** (i.e. aids in the home, etc.) and **social support** (e.g. more appropriate housing and transport to day care centres) may help severely exercise-limited patients to enjoy a reasonable quality of life.
- **Influenza vaccination** annually in the autumn is recommended for all patients with chronic respiratory disease, regardless of age.

Table 5.22   Management of chronic obstructive pulmonary disease

Disease level	Symptoms and signs	Pharmacotherapy	Other considerations
Mild (FEV$_1$ 60–80%)[a]	Currently asymptomatic 'Smoker's cough'	Nil Bupropion, varenicline or nicotine replacement therapy	Stop smoking Optimize inhaler technique All treatments subject to objective ± subjective benefit as guide
	Little or no breathlessness	Beta$_2$-agonist as required **or** antimuscarinic **or** both (depends on response)	
	Infective exacerbations	Influenza + pneumonococcal immunization Antibiotics	
Moderate (FEV$_1$ 40–59%)	Exercise limitation: breathless on moderate exertion Wheeze Cough ± sputum Abnormal breath sounds	Beta$_2$-agonist as required (if responsive) **or** add, or change to, antimuscarinic bronchodilator if poor response	As above plus: Use large-volume spacer Long-acting beta$_2$-agonist only if clearly beneficial (but see p. 294)
	Infective exacerbations FEV$_1$ ≤50%[a] or two or more exacerbations/year	Antibiotics Trial of corticosteroid[b] Influenza and pneumococcal vaccination	Review medication
	Anxiety ± depression	Anxiolytic ± antidepressant (see Chapter 6)	
Severe (FEV$_1$ <40%)	Breathless at rest or any exertion	Beta$_2$-agonist + antimuscarinic Assess for home nebulizer	Oral theophylline if tolerated and other bronchodilators not beneficial
	Prominent wheeze and cough Infective exacerbations FEV$_1$ ≤50%[a] or two or more exacerbations/year	Trial of corticosteroid[b] Antibiotics Trial of corticosteroid[b] Influenza and pneumococcal vaccination	
	Cyanosis Peripheral oedema and polycythaemia	Oxygen (if beneficial) Treat for heart failure: diuretics, etc. (Chapter 3) Treat for respiratory failure: venesection?	Objective proof of benefit
	Infective exacerbations	Antibiotics	

[a] FEV$_1$, percentage of predicted value.
[b] Discontinue if there is no benefit after 4 weeks.
See text: Based on NICE Clinical Guideline 12 – COPD Guidelines 2004.

Home management

Patients with stable COPD (who are in generally good condition, have mild breathlessness and are not confused) can often be managed at home, provided they have good social support. Other factors favouring home management are S_aO_2 >90%, arterial pH >7.35 and P_aO_2 ≥7 kPa, but these will be determined in hospital.

Pharmacotherapy

A general approach to the management of COPD is given in Tables 5.21 and 5.22. The National Collaborating Centre for Chronic Diseases guidelines, published by NICE, set out the treatment of COPD according to symptoms.

Bronchodilatation

There may be an element of reversibility of airways obstruction, so bronchodilators are the cornerstone of therapy. The antimuscarinic and corticosteroid treatments used in asthma should also be given a controlled trial. The drugs should be introduced singly at first, with careful supervision to ensure that there is clinical improvement, and discontinued if ineffective. Respirometry, which is essential in asthma, is not necessary to demonstrate reversibility in COPD. Even a modest improvement in pulmonary function may give an apparently disproportionate symptomatic relief in a patient with severely compromised lung function, because a small increase in P_aO_2 greatly improves Hb saturation.

The antimuscarinic bronchodilators, *ipratropium* and *tiotropium* (p. 315), seem to be as effective as the beta$_2$-agonists and a combination of a beta$_2$-agonist and an antimuscarinic gives somewhat superior results to either used alone, but the benefit may be small.

Corticosteroid therapy and antibiotics

Inhaled corticosteroids should be prescribed to patients with an FEV$_1$ ≤50% predicted, who are having more than two exacerbations requiring treatment with antibiotics or corticosteroids in a 12-month period, to reduce exacerbation rates and slow the decline in health status. Although it has been alleged that corticosteroids are overused in COPD, a careful study of nearly 1000 patients found that inhaled *fluticasone* reduced the decline in FEV$_1$ by 32% over a 3-year trial period and the exacerbation rate by 25%. However, there is an increased incidence of bruising and oral candidiasis.

RCTs have indicated clearly that the combination of a corticosteroid plus an LABA (*fluticasone* plus *salmeterol* and *budesonide* plus *formoterol*) improve lung function and quality of life compared to the individual agents. These results were obtained in patients with moderately severe disease and are applicable to those with FEV$_1$ <50% predicted and who have frequent exacerbations, i.e. >3 in the preceding 3 years. However, the safety of such treatment in a patient group that tends to cardiac failure must be questioned (p. 294).

It is important to remember that a substantial response to treatment, especially to corticosteroids, raises the possibility that some patients diagnosed as having COPD have either chronic asthma or asthma concurrent with COPD. This should prompt reassessment, including respirometry.

Oral corticosteroids are also euphoriant in most patients, so they may feel well despite the underlying disease state, and it may be difficult to wean them from the drug. However, a proportion of patients feel anxious and/or depressed, and this may need conventional treatment (see Chapter 6).

Maintenance treatment with oral corticosteroids should be used only when they cannot be withdrawn after an exacerbation. As usual, the lowest possible dose should be used. Patients under 65 years receiving oral corticosteroids should be monitored for osteoporosis and given prophylactic treatment when indicated by X-ray densitometry, using a bisphosphonate, e.g. *alendronic acid* or *risedronate sodium*, plus *calcium and ergocalciferol tablets* if they are housebound or have a poor diet: inadequate exposure to sunlight reduces vitamin D production. Those over 65 years taking a corticosteroid long term should be prescribed prophylactic treatment routinely.

Although acute exacerbations of COPD are due to infections, the immunosuppressant action of steroids does not appear to compromise patients. However, the harmful effects of corticosteroids, i.e. bruising, oropharyngeal candidiasis and osteoporosis, must be weighed against their benefits.

Similarly, trials of prophylactic antibiotics conducted some 30 years ago showed a reduced frequency of exacerbations. However, these results are unlikely to be applicable to current practice and routine prophylactic antibiotic medication is not recommended because the benefits are outweighed by the disadvantages, notably the selection of resistant organisms (see Chapter 8).

Oxygen

Oxygen used for at least 15 h daily (**long-term oxygen therapy (LTOT)**, p. 361) improves mobility, relieves hypoxaemia and reduces mortality in those with severe hypoxaemia, i.e. P_aO_2 <8 kPa, and those who experience hypoxaemia only at night. Superior results are achieved by treatment for 20 h daily. In hospital, IPPV (p. 361) may be used to assist respiration. However, the *oxygen* concentration must always be carefully controlled because patients become unresponsive to their chronically raised carbon dioxide levels and depend on hypoxic drive to maintain ventilation (p. 360). If the P_aO_2 is raised excessively by administering *oxygen* the patient may stop breathing completely: the aim is to improve the P_aO_2 somewhat, producing a significant increase in Hb saturation (S_aO_2), without unduly increasing P_aCO_2 or exacerbating respiratory acidosis and without impairing respiratory drive. The patient's clinical condition and arterial blood gases must be monitored carefully, and the *oxygen* flow rate adjusted to give optimal oxygenation. However, such careful monitoring is not possible in a community setting, where the *oxygen* flow rate should not exceed 2–4 L/min, to give a maximum concentration of 28% *oxygen* in the inspired air with a suitable mask (p. 361) or nasal prongs. Even 24% *oxygen* may be excessive for some patients, so *oxygen* therapy should be initiated cautiously under careful supervision, preferably in hospital.

Evidence from two large trials indicates that continuous prophylactic *oxygen* used for 15 h/day in appropriately selected patients increases the untreated 5-year survival rate (30%) by at least 50%. Increasing this to 19 h/day more than doubled the survival rate without *oxygen*; use for 12 h/day did not improve survival. Thus in the late stages of the disease, if a patient has cor pulmonale or is in demonstrable respiratory failure, LTOT is indicated. *Oxygen* therapy is discussed more fully on pp. 360–364.

Treatment of complications

Heart failure.   Cor pulmonale (p. 285) should be treated (see also Chapter 4). **Venesection** (removing 500–1000 mL of blood, the old standard blood-letting treatment) may be used sometimes if polycythaemia causes such an increase in blood viscosity that cardiac function is compromised, i.e. packed cell volume (PCV) >56%.

Oxygen prevents progression of pulmonary hypertension and is the mainstay of therapy. A diuretic is indicated if there is peripheral oedema and a raised JVP. Pulmonary vasodilatation with a beta$_2$-agonist, CCB or alpha-adrenergic blocker may also be helpful.

Respiratory acidosis consequent on hypercapnia must be treated promptly (see Chapter 14).

Cough

Steam inhalations may assist expectoration by dilution of mucus, but there is no evidence that 'expectorants' can materially assist expectoration, so they are primarily placebos.

Mucolytics, e.g. *carbocisteine* or *mecysteine hydrochloride*, may reduce the frequency and duration of exacerbations, but the evidence for this is not strong, though some patients may obtain subjective relief. This issue is being addressed in a large multicentre European trial. It has been suggested that the benefits of the mucolytics are due to their antioxidant properties rather than their effects on mucus. However, mucolytics may damage the gastric mucosa, and must be used carefully if there is a history of peptic ulceration (see Chapter 3).

Short-term use of *dornase alfa* (rhDNase, phosphorylated glycosylated recombinant human deoxyribonuclease 1) to reduce sputum viscosity was not beneficial.

Cough suppressants should not normally be used because, although effective, they may cause respiratory depression. However, a few patients have a troublesome unproductive night cough and this may need to be controlled.

Prophylaxis

Pneumococcal vaccination and annual **influenza vaccination** should be offered to all patients, to reduce the frequency of exacerbations. Annual pneumococcal revaccination is not indicated because of sustained protection and the possibility of adverse reactions, but patients with splenetic dysfunction, nephrotic syndrome (see Chapter 14), or who have had their spleen removed need revaccination every 5 years.

Acute infective exacerbations

Infections may be bacterial or viral in origin (see Chapter 8) and should be treated aggressively at the first signs, especially if purulent sputum is present, but it is important to take a sputum sample for laboratory analysis before starting blind treatment because a significant proportion of bacterial strains are antibiotic-resistant.

Broad-spectrum antibiotics for empirical treatment (e.g. *amoxicillin*, *trimethoprim*, tetracyclines or a macrolide) are chosen based on **local sensitivity data**. They are those usually active against the most likely bacterial pathogens, often pneumococci, *Haemophilus influenzae* or *Moraxella catarrhalis*. *Ciprofloxacin* is present in high concentrations in bronchial secretions, but it is not clear whether this translates into additional benefit. However, it has limited activity against pneumococci and numerous side-effects (see Chapter 8) and is not usually appropriate for first-line empirical treatment.

Oral corticosteroids (e.g. 30 mg/day *prednisolone* for 1 week) may be appropriate if the patient is known to respond to them or is already being maintained on a lower steroid dose, if there is no response to a bronchodilator or if this is the first presentation of increased airflow obstruction.

Some patients whose microbial status is well established can have a reserve supply of antibiotics and corticosteroids available to start on their own initiative when they notice the first signs that usually presage deterioration in their condition. However, they should subsequently see their doctor as soon as possible. In such situations, either a bronchodilator may be added if it is not already being used, or the dose may be increased after first checking inhaler technique (see Table 5.26).

Oxygen **therapy** (p. 360) may be required if it is not already being used. **Respiratory failure** may need to be managed in hospital by IPPV or NIPPV (p. 361). **Respiratory stimulants** are used occasionally (e.g. *doxapram*, only in hospital), to tide patients over a bout of hypoventilation while other treatments are pursued.

When the patient has recovered sufficiently they should have a full medication review. If hospital treatment was required there should also be detailed consideration of social and financial circumstances when planning for discharge.

Pure emphysema uncomplicated by an appreciable element of COPD is uncommon, and patients primarily require *oxygen* because they are very breathless. *Oxygen* therapy will depend on the condition of the patient, and the 'pink puffer' type, with relatively normal blood gases, will tolerate higher *oxygen* concentrations than those with a poor respiratory drive and hypercapnia (P_aCO_2 >9 kPa). Management is otherwise as for COPD.

Natural AAT prepared from pooled plasma is available in the USA and has been given intravenously weekly, though there is little good evidence of benefit. Recombinant human AAT is in development. Inhalation of AAT is under investigation. However, the use of **AAT replacement therapy** is not supported by the evidence and is not recommended currently.

Other experimental treatments for AAT deficiency include:

- All-trans retinoic acid (see Chapter13).
- Inhalation of hyaluronidase, as a mucolytic.
- Vitamins A, C and E, to prevent oxidation of AAT, but the evidence for this is poor.
- Stem cell therapy and gene therapy are being explored, and may become feasible in the future.

Lung surgery. Rarely, the eradication of a single giant bulla (air space) in the lungs may relieve symptoms by relieving the compression of surrounding lung tissue. Patients who are still breathless, with marked restriction in the activities of daily living despite maximal pharmacotherapy and pulmonary rehabilitation, are candidates for lung volume surgery. This helps by reducing dead space (see p. 278) and so the volume of air that has to be moved in each breath. They need to meet all of the following criteria:

- FEV_1 >20% predicted.
- P_aCO_2 <7.3 kPa.
- Emphysema primarily confined to the upper lobes.
- TLco >20% predicted.

Some patients with severe COPD, who do not have significant comorbidity, may be candidates for **lung transplantation**.

However, many patients present with advanced disease that is not amenable to treatment.

Bronchiectasis

Definition and epidemiology

This is abnormal dilatation of the bronchi, their walls becoming inflamed, thickened and irreversibly damaged. It often follows pneumonia or other severe bacterial lower respiratory tract infection, which may start in childhood as a sequel to measles or whooping cough. There is impaired mucociliary clearance, and chronic local inflammation. Recurrent pyogenic infections cause massive mucus hypersecretion and airways obstruction.

Trapping of pus in the airways may also occur in **cystic fibrosis** and bronchial carcinoma and may cause similar damage. Bronchiectasis may also accompany COPD and, occasionally, asthma.

The disease is much less common in developed countries now that effective antibiotics are available, cystic fibrosis being the most common cause. Bronchiectasis persists in the Third World and in areas where natural disasters or wars disrupt social and political structures and medical services.

Clinical features

These vary greatly, depending on the severity of the disease, but the principal features include:

- chronic cough, often productive of copious purulent sputum;
- a variable degree of haemoptysis;
- breathlessness;
- febrile episodes associated with infection, sometimes pneumonia;
- anorexia and weight loss;
- night sweats;
- finger clubbing (Figure 5.7) in the later stages if there is persistent infection;
- immunodeficiency in about 10% of patients.

Investigation

Investigations of bronchiectasis include:

- chest and sinus X-rays;
- high-resolution CT chest scanning;
- sputum culture and antibiotic sensitivity testing;
- serum Igs.

Occasionally bronchoscopy, sweat sodium levels (increased in cystic fibrosis) and a test for mucociliary clearance are also required.

Management

The aims of management are to improve respiratory function and prevent deterioration by eradicating infection, if possible. Treatment includes:

- **Postural drainage** of sputum (p. 335).
- **Bronchodilators** to improve airflow.
- **Corticosteroids** (inhaled or oral), to reduce inflammation and slow disease progression.
- **Antibiotics**: selection depends on local policy and previous experience in the patient. Common practice is to use the same agents as are indicated for exacerbations of COPD or pneumonia (see Chapter 8), and *flucloxacillin* if *Staphylococcus aureus* is isolated. Other IV or inhaled antibiotics are used according to organism sensitivity. Inhaled antibiotics

may be used for prophylaxis, especially for *Pseudomonas aeruginosa*, but specific IV antipseudomonal antibiotics are required for significant exacerbations.
- **Heart/lung transplantation** in rare cases.

Cystic fibrosis

Epidemiology and pathology

This is the commonest autosomal recessive disorder, the carrier frequency being 1 in 22 in Caucasians. Characteristic symptoms occur in individuals who are homozygous for the disease allele. It affects about 1 in 2500 live births. The usual form is due to a single nucleotide deletion in the gene on the long arm of chromosome 7.

This produces a defect in the cystic fibrosis transmembrane conductance regulator (CFTR) protein, which is a crucial regulator of chloride flow across the cell membranes of exocrine glands, and there are widespread consequences. In the airways there is a decreased flow of chloride out of the epithelial cells lining the mucous glands and goblet cells. Consequent retention of chloride causes a threefold increase in sodium reabsorption into these cells. These abnormalities combine to hold water in the glandular epithelial cells, causing a greatly increased viscosity of the airways mucus. In sweat glands there is a CFTR-independent excess excretion of chloride and sodium into the sweat, which yields a concentration of >60 mmol/L and forms the basis of one of the diagnostic tests for cystic fibrosis.

Numerous other mutations occur in the cystic fibrosis gene and a precise diagnosis requires genetic analysis, but this does not affect treatment.

Clinical features

These include:

- Failure to thrive in early life. In neonates, the first sign is likely to be an abnormally viscous meconium, the green mucilage present in the ileum and colon of all newborns.

- Respiratory symptoms are the most obvious. Bouts of severe coughing are due to the very tenacious mucus. Dyspnoea and haemoptysis occur in the later stages. There is also sinusitis and nasal polyps, and spontaneous pneumothorax may occur. The end result is cor pulmonale and respiratory failure.
- Retention of mucus causes recurrent bronchopulmonary infections, often with resistant Gram-negative organisms, pneumococci and *Staphylococcus aureus*.
- Gastrointestinal effects include chronic pancreatitis, causing poor digestion and malabsorption, the latter causing steatorrhoea (see Chapter 3). In older patients, small bowel obstruction may occur and there is an increased frequency of peptic ulceration, gastrointestinal carcinoma, cholesterol gallstones and hepatic cirrhosis.
- Males are usually sterile, due to failure of the vas deferens and epididymis to develop. Females can conceive, but the normal monthly cycle fails as the disease progresses.
- In the kidney, unusually rapid excretion of antibiotics may result in inadequate plasma concentrations and treatment failure.
- Defects in other body systems include delayed puberty and skeletal growth and arthropathies. Insulin-dependent diabetes mellitus occurs in about 10% of patients.

Diagnosis

This depends on:

- A family history of cystic fibrosis: prenatal diagnosis can be done in this situation.
- High sweat sodium levels.
- Radiology, the picture resembling that of bronchiectasis.
- Finger clubbing occurs eventually.
- Absence in males of the vas deferens and epididymis.
- Genetic analysis.

Diagnosis may be difficult and children may be treated for whooping cough or asthma before a definitive diagnosis is made.

Management and pharmacotherapy

General measures include physiotherapy, i.e. postural drainage, to improve expectoration of the tenacious mucus. A nutritious high-calorie diet is needed to counter malnutrition.

Patients and their families require counselling and support. Because infection with multiple-resistant organisms is usual, and spread is person to person, they should not associate with other cystic fibrosis sufferers.

Pharmacotherapy has been revolutionized as knowledge of the disease has grown. It includes:

- Treatment as for bronchiectasis (see above), notably with antibiotics effective against *Pseudomonas aeruginosa* and *Staphylococcus aureus*. *Ciprofloxacin* is useful initially but resistance develops rapidly. *Ceftazidime* is used in hospital because it must be given by IV infusion. Nebulized *tobramycin*, etc. gives high sputum levels. Opportunistic infection with *Burkholderia cepacia* (formerly *Pseudomonas cepacia*), normally a plant pathogen, is a serious complication.
- Inhaled corticosteroids may help to reduce airways inflammation.
- Vitamins should be given and H$_2$-RAs (p. 103) are often required.
- Enteric-coated pancreatic supplements are needed, but high lipase doses in particular may cause colonic damage.
- Because some of the viscosity of the mucus is due to DNA from dead endothelial cells, inhaled *dornase alfa* (rhDNase) may reduce sputum viscosity and improve respiratory function.
- Sodium reabsorption may be reduced by *amiloride*. Chloride excretion can be increased by adenosine or uridine triphosphates (ATP, UTP).

Prognosis

The outlook has improved greatly and the average expectation of life is now over 40 years. Respiratory failure and consequent cardiac complications may lead to heart/lung transplantation.

Restrictive lung disease

In restrictive lung disease (RLD) the problem is an inability to expand the lungs normally, even though the airways are unobstructed. There are many diverse causes, some of which are given in Table 5.23.

A result of this diverse aetiology is that treatment of RLD is often symptomatic rather than specific, because by the time symptoms occur the pathological changes may be irreversible. Infections should be treated and any precipitating factors avoided as far as possible. There is clearly no effective way of treating thoracic cage deformity once it is established, although physiotherapy and surgery as soon as the problem is perceived may do much to help. Early orthopaedic surgery is highly desirable. Physiotherapy may enable patients to make the best use of their limited ventilatory function.

However, some forms of RLD (e.g. Wegener's granulomatosis, WG; see Chapter 12 and Table 12.18) are eminently treatable, so it is important to reach a definitive diagnosis. Treatment of WG usually involves corticosteroids and cytotoxic drugs.

Diseases of the pulmonary circulation

Pulmonary embolism

Aetiology, epidemiology and pathology

This important, often preventable, condition has a 10% fatality rate. Pulmonary embolism is a sequel to thrombosis in the systemic veins, especially the pelvic, abdominal and leg veins, but 10% of emboli are cardiac in origin. The latter are due to right atrial fibrillation causing right atrial thrombosis, or to right ventricular or septal infarction and resultant right ventricular thrombosis. Clot fragments break away from venous thrombi and travel through the veins, which widen progressively, then through the right ventricle and usually become trapped in the pulmonary circulation where the arteries begin

Table 5.23   Some causes of restrictive lung disease

Cause or disease	Examples, comments
Diseases causing diffuse pulmonary fibrosis	
Cryptogenic fibrosing alveolitis	Aetiology unknown. Occurs in late middle age with destruction of lung tissue
Rheumatoid and collagen-vascular diseases (see Chapter 12)	Rheumatoid arthritis, systemic sclerosis, systemic lupus erythematosus (SLE)
Iatrogenic[a]	Cytotoxic drugs: bleomycin, busulfan, cyclophosphamide Methysergide, nitrofurantoin, oxygen (>50%), sulphonamides, sulfasalazine Radiotherapy Drugs inducing SLE (see Chapter 12, Table 8.22)
Occupational	Asbestosis, pneumoconiosis (miner's lung), silicosis, siderosis (iron, iron ores: also occurs if there is chronic alveolar bleeding)
Sarcoidosis	A type IV (delayed) hypersensitivity reaction to an unidentified agent, causing granulomatous changes
Toxins	Paraquat weedkiller
Thoracic cage deformity	
Congenital	Severe kyphoscoliosis, tuberculosis
Rheumatoid	Ankylosing spondylitis
Pleural disease	
Fibrosis	Asbestos, methysergide
Effusion	Heart failure, infections (pneumonia, tuberculosis), malignancy, lymphatic disease

[a] This list of drugs is illustrative, not exhaustive. The effects may depend on dose level, accumulated dose, duration of treatment, etc. and may be reversible.

to narrow (the pulmonary arteries carry venous blood). Because the lungs receive the whole of the cardiac output, and the lungs are the first organ to receive pooled venous blood from the right heart, most emboli lodge in the lungs.

Emboli arising from the left heart lodge in the brain, causing strokes or TIAs, or in the renal arteries, leading to various degrees of renal failure. However, some renal artery occlusion may be due to *in situ* thrombosis, as is nearly all coronary artery occlusion (see Chapter 4).

The factors predisposing to venous thrombosis are dealt with in Chapter 11.

Whenever there is a risk of a **deep-vein thrombosis (DVT)**, prophylactic measures should be taken. Low-dose *heparin* is appropriate after surgery and there should be passive exercising during a period of bed rest, with early mobilization. Low-molecular weight *heparin* is preferred and may be combined with rhythmic external compression applied to the legs. Elastic stockings are also used, but are less effective. *Aspirin* taken before long-distance travel, preferably combined with elastic hosiery and avoidance of dehydration, is used widely and may help.

After embolism, the area of lung affected is ventilated but not perfused and this leads, after some hours, to failure of surfactant production and alveolar collapse. Lung tissue often does not infarct because it obtains sufficient oxygen by diffusion from the airways and the bronchial circulation.

Clinical features

The presentation will depend largely on the size and site of the emboli.

Small to medium emboli

These usually present with severe pleuritic chest pain, cough with bloody sputum and fever. Breathlessness and hyperventilation are common but may be absent. Recurrence is unlikely, but any lung damage that may have occurred is irreversible.

Massive pulmonary embolus

This produces a precipitous fall in cardiac output, the result of loss of preload to the left ventricle (see Chapter 4), so the patient will be shocked, pale and cyanosed, with marked tachypnoea and a raised JVP. Severe central chest pain occurs, due to cardiac ischaemia. There is a 30% fatality rate, sometimes immediate.

Repeated small emboli

These slowly produce progressive breathlessness and hyperventilation. Patients will become exercise-limited and may have angina pectoris (see Chapter 4) owing to widespread restriction of pulmonary perfusion and consequent severe limitation of the coronary circulation. They may also faint on exercise in the later stages, when they will also be chronically tired. Investigation will show the ECG changes associated with right ventricular hypertrophy and evidence of pulmonary hypertension. The condition is progressive.

Investigation and diagnosis

Small to medium emboli

The symptoms and signs are often non-specific, but the diagnosis should be suspected if unexplained new pulmonary symptoms or tachycardia is present. The CXR and ECG are often normal.

The extent of obstruction of the pulmonary circulation may be determined using technetium (^{99m}Tc) Macrosalb Injection [equivalents are Albumin Aggregated Injection (USP) and the Microspheres Injection (Eur. Ph.)] for **radio-isotope scanning**. The labelled particles lodge throughout the lung capillaries and so will show unperfused (non-radioactive) areas, in which the circulation is blocked by an embolus when the chest is scanned with a gamma camera. This is preferably combined with a ^{133}Xe ventilation scintigram, the two investigations (**V/Q scan**) showing unperfused but ventilated areas. However, the V/Q scan is not conclusive and must be read in conjunction with the examination and other investigations.

Medium-sized emboli are best detected by spiral CT scanning with IV contrast media, or by MRI if the CT scan is contra-indicated because the patient is allergic to X-ray contrast media. **CT angiography** (spiral CT with IV contrast agents, e.g. *diatrizoate meglumine* and *meglumine iodipamide*) or **MRI** have good specificity and sensitivity for medium-sized emboli. If **plasma D-dimer**, a breakdown product of fibrin, is not detected this positively excludes a pulmonary embolus. Raised ESR and lactate dehydrogenase (LDH) levels indicate pulmonary damage. The CXR and ECG are usually normal.

Ultrasound may be used to detect DVT in the legs, pelvic or iliac region, but is not reliable for detecting below-knee thrombosis. However, the syndrome of calf pain with swelling, redness and prominent superficial veins, and sometimes ankle swelling, is strongly suggestive. If there is doubt, venography (i.e. injecting in the foot with radiocontrast medium followed by X-radiography) is conclusive. This cannot be done if the patient is allergic to the contrast agent.

Massive pulmonary embolus

The ECG exhibits characteristic changes. Ultrasound (echocardiogram) shows an actively contracting left ventricle (an attempt to restore adequate systemic circulation) and there may be a clot in the pulmonary trunk or a main pulmonary artery. Blood gas examination shows hypoxaemia and hypercapnia. **Pulmonary angiography** will locate emboli rapidly, but the technique is hazardous and is usually undertaken as a prelude to surgery (embolectomy).

Repeated small emboli

Any of the tests described above may be done, especially CXR, ECG and V/Q scan, but may appear normal, so extensive investigations may be required.

Management

This includes:

- High-flow *oxygen*, unless the patient has COPD (p. 360).
- Analgesics, including opioids if necessary, taking care to avoid respiratory depression.
- Anticoagulants: *heparin*, to prevent further embolization, changing to *warfarin* after confirmation of the diagnosis, usually about 48 h (see Chapter 11).

For large emboli, management includes:

- Intensive care.
- Fibrinolytic therapy, e.g. *streptokinase* (by IV infusion over 24–72 h) or *alteplase* (bolus IV injection, then IV infusion over 90 min), may precede anticoagulation (Chapter 11).
- **Surgical embolectomy** (clot removal, rarely) if cardiac function is severely impaired.

For repeated small emboli, management involves:

- Anticoagulants: these are continued for 3–6 months, but lifelong treatment may be necessary if there is a chronic thromboembolic disorder.
- Antiplatelet drugs (*aspirin*, *clopidogrel* or *dipyridamole*; see Chapter 11, but note interactions with *warfarin* and other anticoagulants) may also be appropriate. The glycoprotein IIb/IIIa inhibitors *abciximab*, *eptifibatide* and *tirofiban* are used only when there is a significant risk of major cardiovascular complications.
- If the condition does not respond to anticoagulant therapy, or if anticoagulants are contra-indicated in the patient, an inferior vena cava filter can be inserted percutaneously.

Pulmonary oedema and pulmonary hypertension

Pathology, clinical features and diagnosis

Pulmonary oedema can develop precipitately, e.g. as a sequel to MI (see Chapter 4), and can be rapidly fatal. Acute pulmonary oedema is a medical emergency.

The condition is usually the result of increased pulmonary capillary pressure, due to left heart failure or mitral stenosis (see Chapter 4), which causes the accumulation of fluid in the normally minimal interstitial space of the lungs (see Figure 5.1(d)). The increased vascular pressure compresses the bronchioles and reduces lung compliance, ventilation and perfusion. These changes are more marked initially in the lung bases because of the effect of gravity. If the condition persists, or occurs acutely, fluid eventually flows into the alveoli and the terminal bronchioles, producing severe dyspnoea. Some precipitants of acute pulmonary oedema are given in Table 5.24.

If the condition is of gradual onset (**pulmonary hypertension**), the initial symptoms and signs are dyspnoea on exercise, then shortness of breath, cough, orthopnoea and paroxysmal nocturnal dyspnoea (PND; see Chapter 4, p. 195). If symptoms are untreated, or if the onset is acute, these lead to extreme dyspnoea, tachypnoea, cyanosis, and coughing up of foamy, bloody sputum. Unsurprisingly, patients are extremely anxious and fearful and sweat profusely. There is tachycardia and a raised pulmonary arterial pressure, and the X-ray shows characteristic changes. Diagnosis is based on these features.

Management

Pharmacotherapy of acute pulmonary oedema involves:

- An IV loop diuretic, which sometimes produces a dramatic improvement (see below).
- High-flow (60%), short-term *oxygen* to relieve dyspnoea.
- Opioid analgesia: *morphine* causes systemic venodilatation, reducing cardiac workload

Table 5.24   Some precipitants of acute pulmonary oedema

Pulmonary	Large embolism
Cardiogenic	Acute • arrhythmias • left ventricular failure • myocardial infarction • valvular regurgitation (aortic, mitral) • cardiac decompensation in chronic heart failure (including non-compliance with medication)
Circulatory (see Chapter 4)	Hypervolaemia • pregnancy • excessive – intravenous infusion rate – sodium intake
Renal	Renal impairment (age, etc.), renal failure (see Chapter 14)
Increased metabolic demand	Fever Excessive exercise Hyperthyroidism (see Chapter 9)

and tachypnoea, and is sedative and euphoric.
• Vasodilators to increase cardiac output.
• *Aminophylline*, given intravenously to control bronchospasm.
• Management of the underlying condition.

Diuretics have a dual action in this setting. In pulmonary oedema consequent on heart failure they reduce the blood volume and in turn the cardiac preload and cause vasodilatation, thus further reducing cardiac preload and afterload. These combined actions improve cardiac function and reduce pulmonary venous pressure. If the condition is of renal origin, diuretics also reduce the hypervolaemia consequent on activation of the renin/aldosterone mechanism. Diuretics do not act directly to clear the oedema fluid, which is cleared spontaneously when cardiac function improves and the pulmonary capillary pressure falls (see Chapter 4).

Treatment of pulmonary hypertension depends on the underlying condition, and may involve:

• Diuretics in RVF, taking care to avoid volume depletion.
• *Oxygen*. Long-term *oxygen* therapy in COPD (p. 361).

• Lowering of pulmonary artery pressure with *bosentan* (oral), sometimes nebulized *iloprost*. *Epoprostenol*, given by continuous IV infusion as an antiplatelet agent and vasodilator, is also used, especially in primary pulmonary hypertension, i.e. without discernible cause.
• *Heparin* anticoagulation initially, followed by oral *warfarin*.
• Transplantation in otherwise suitable patients who fail to respond, e.g. in those:
  – who fail to respond despite optimal medical management
  – with FEV_1 <25% predicted and no reversibility, and/or P_aO_2 >7.3 kPa
  – with raised P_aO_2 and using long oxygen therapy who continue to deteriorate
  – with no other serious chronic disease
  – who are <55–65 years, dependent on the type of operation contemplated. Older patients tolerate operations of this magnitude poorly.

Respiratory failure

Respiratory failure occurs when there is significant hypoxaemia with or without hypercapnia and may be classified into two types (Table 5.25). **Type I** respiratory failure (acute hypoxaemic respiratory failure) is the condition in which the P_aO_2 is low and the P_aCO_2 is normal or low. It occurs in pneumonia (see Chapter 8), pulmonary oedema and fibrosing alveolitis (see above). In **type II** respiratory failure (ventilatory failure) the P_aO_2 is also low and the P_aCO_2 is high.

Oxygenation of the blood is usually monitored by pulse oximetry (p. 291). Hypoxaemia is regarded as severe if the P_aO_2 is less than about 5 kPa. If sufficiently severe, hypercapnia (high blood carbon dioxide, also known as hypercarbia) causes acidosis (blood pH 7.3 or lower).

The management of type I respiratory failure involves high-flow *oxygen* (6–10 L/min), usually via a variable performance mask, and treatment of the underlying disease state. In type II failure, high-flow *oxygen* is not used because patients either require mechanical ventilation or depend on a low P_aO_2 to provide their respiratory drive, e.g. in COPD (p. 276). Mechanical ventilation is needed in opioid overdose, myasthenia gravis (see Chapter 6) and Guillain-Barré syndrome, an acute, usually demyelinating polyneuropathy causing paralysis, often following infection by cytomegalovirus or *Campylobacter jejuni*. These patients may develop severe respiratory acidosis, which must be treated vigorously (see Chapter 14).

In acute respiratory failure, extracorporeal oxygenation in an external system (for neonates and adults) or carbon dioxide removal (for adults) are controversial but are used in specialist centres.

The best **respiratory stimulant** is vigorous physiotherapy, but drugs are used very occasionally. *Doxapram* is a short-acting respiratory stimulant that is given by continuous IV infusion and should be used only under expert supervision: *oxygen* should be used with it and a beta$_2$-agonist bronchodilator added if there is significant bronchoconstriction. Active physiotherapy should also be given. *Doxapram* has numerous side-effects and regular blood gas and pH measurements should be used to guide treatment. It is contra-indicated in severe hypertension, acute severe asthma, coronary artery disease, thyrotoxicosis, epilepsy and respiratory tract obstruction. It may be used to counter the depressant effect of *oxygen* in type II failure and to treat significant respiratory depression following anaesthesia.

Table 5.25 Types of respiratory failure

Type of failure, and the metabolic abnormalities observed		Some possible causes
Type I (P_aO_2 reduced or greatly reduced <8 kPa, N = 10–13.3 kPa, S_aO_2 >90%; P_aCO_2 normal or low, <4 kPa, N = 4.8–6.1 kPa)	Acute	Cardiovascular diseases Pneumonia Pulmonary oedema
	Chronic	Fibrosing alveolitis Interstitial lung disease
Type II (P_aO_2 reduced or greatly reduced, <8 kPa; P_aCO_2 raised or greatly raised, >7 kPa; acidosis, pH <7.35)	Acute	Upper airways obstruction Severe acute asthma CNS damage COPD plus infection
	Chronic	COPD

CNS, central nervous system; COPD, chronic obstructive pulmonary disease.

Inhalation therapy

This section does not cover the inhalation of gases. *Oxygen* therapy is dealt with separately.

Advantages

The development of inhalation therapy has produced considerable benefits for patients suffering from respiratory diseases, not only asthma but also COPD, bronchiectasis and cystic fibrosis. Although simple devices had been used for many years, inhalation therapy was given a powerful impetus in 1969 with the introduction of the first selective beta$_2$-agonist bronchodilator (*salbutamol*) and the associated equipment to deliver precise doses direct to the lungs. The technique has subsequently been used successfully for the administration of:

- beta$_2$-agonists, e.g. *salbutamol* and *terbutaline*;
- corticosteroids, e.g. *beclometasone* and *budesonide*;
- anticholinergics, e.g. *ipratropium* and *tiotropium*;
- anti-allergics, e.g. *sodium cromoglicate* and *nedocromil sodium*;
- antibiotics, e.g. *bacitracin*, *aminoglycosides*, *cephalosporins*, *colistin*, penicillins and *polymyxin*, and the antifungal agent *amphotericin*.

In terminal care it is used for administering:

- mucolytics, e.g. normal and hypertonic saline, *N-acetylcysteine* and *dornase alfa*;
- opioids, e.g. *morphine*, *diamorphine* and *fentanyl*;
- local anaesthetics, e.g. *lidocaine* and *bupivacaine*.

Other applications include the administration of local anaesthetics before endotracheal intubation or bronchoscopy, water or saline for humidification of inspired air, cytotoxic agents for lung cancer chemotherapy, vaccines for immunization and DNA for gene therapy in cystic fibrosis. Inhalation is also used in one form of NRT to assist smoking cessation. It has also been proposed that many other drugs could be administered by this well-tolerated and non-invasive route, which avoids first-pass hepatic metabolism, e.g. *heparin* and *vasopressin*, and insulin is now licensed for use by inhalation in certain patients (see Chapter 9), thus avoiding the need for repeated injections. This has become possible due to the availability of virtually unlimited supplies of safe, cheap human insulin by genetic engineering.

In respiratory disease inhalation therapy is a simple, rapidly effective technique that delivers a small dose of drug directly to what is usually the desired site of action deep within the lungs. This gives a high local concentration and avoids the side-effects that occur when larger doses of drug are given systemically to achieve a similar effect. However, the inhalation route does not avoid the side-effects completely, because some is absorbed from the lungs or swallowed from impinged drug in the oropharynx (see below), but minimizes them considerably. By avoiding first-pass metabolism, the bioavailability of drugs may be enhanced. The very high pulmonary blood flow and surface area, together with the very thin alveolar walls, may also serve to enhance absorption.

Factors influencing pulmonary drug deposition

The principal factors are the particle size of the drug, the patient, the delivery system and the environment.

Particle size

The target area in the lungs depends on the site of the pathological changes, and may be the tracheobronchial region, the bronchioles or the respiratory bronchioles and alveoli. In adults, only some 8–12% of the inhaled dose reaches the distal lung, even with optimal delivery, and this may fall to below 1% in young children. The remainder is deposited in the oropharynx and is swallowed. This mechanism may also dispose of insoluble drugs deposited in the bronchi and escalated from there by mucociliary clearance.

Optimal particle size is crucial. Particles need to be about 2 µm in diameter or less to reach the bronchioles and <0.7 µm to reach the respiratory bronchioles. Below approximately 0.5 µm, particles will reach the alveolar sacs, but because this region does not possess any smooth muscle, bronchodilators will not have any effect there, although other drugs may do so, e.g. corticosteroids in extrinsic allergic alveolitis. Very small particles (<0.5 µm) may remain suspended in the alveolar gas and be exhaled (about 1% of the inhaled dose).

Larger particles (≥10 µm) are deposited in the mouth and oropharynx by inertial impaction (about 60% of the dose) and are swallowed, as are a large proportion of those in the 5- to 10-µm range. This gives rise to most of any systemic effects that occur. In the 2- to 5-µm range, particles are carried in the air stream until the velocity is slowed sufficiently by airways resistance to permit deposition in the bronchioles by gravitational sedimentation. Below approximately 2 µm, particles deposit on mucous surfaces, following diffusion, accidental contact produced by air turbulence and Brownian motion. Thus, for most purposes we need the majority of particles to be in the range of 1–5 µm, with a median aerodynamic diameter of about 3 µm.

However, recent research with respirable polymer-coated insulin particles has shown that low-density particles (<0.4 g/cm^3) >5 µm in diameter can be aerosolized more easily than the conventional higher density, smaller diameter ones. Further, the light, large particles evade pulmonary phagocytosis, giving high bioavailability and more sustained drug release (96 h versus 4 h). This technology offers exciting possibilities for controlled, systemic drug administration via the lungs of many drugs that currently are given only by injection.

Patient (physiological) factors

Although very difficult to quantify, these are among the most important considerations. Modern equipment is well designed and manufacturers take great care to produce aerosols of effective drugs having the appropriate particle size characteristics. Unfortunately, there is little control over what happens in use, especially if patients are counselled inadequately or if the

devices are used without proper ongoing supervision by knowledgeable staff. The age of the patient, their ability to coordinate breathing with drug delivery, airways geometry, inspiratory and expiratory flow rates and times, tidal volumes, breath holding and the proportions of mouth and/or nose breathing may all influence the deposition of the drug in the lungs.

We can be certain only on some points, e.g. that pulmonary deposition is reduced in proportion to the severity of the ventilatory abnormality, with poor technique and in young children. It is clearly impossible to predict the response of an individual patient to a drug delivered from a particular piece of equipment. As in most fields of therapy, there is no substitute for monitoring the actual clinical response and, if this is unsatisfactory, varying the conditions of use in a controlled way to determine whether this can be improved. If necessary, the drug and the delivery system itself may also be changed.

Drug delivery systems

There are four types available: pressurized metered dose inhalers (pMDIs), dry powder inhalers (DPIs), gas-driven nebulizers, and ultrasonic nebulizers.

Pressurized metered dose inhalers

This type of inhaler is the most widely used because it is so convenient. It consists of a metal canister filled with a suspension of a micronized drug in a propellant that is liquefied under pressure (Figure 5.22). The special metering valve gives doses that are reproducible within 5%.

The older pMDIs use CFC (chlorofluorocarbon, freon) propellants. Because of worries about the effects of CFCs on the ozone layer and the consequent environmental impact, these propellants are being replaced rapidly by hydrofluoroalkanes (HFAs). However, the latter still have some 'greenhouse' effect. The doses of propellant usually delivered are considered to be non-toxic, though they may cause small reductions in respiratory function. There do not appear to be any toxicity problems with these new inhalers.

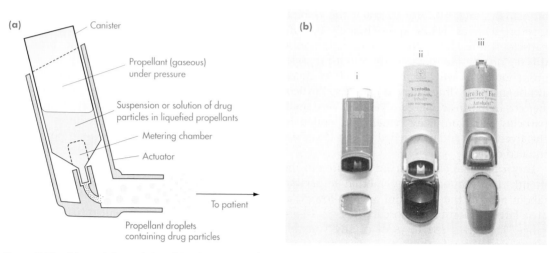

Figure 5.22 Metered dose inhalers (MDIs). (a) General arrangement. (b) Some commercial inhalers. (i) Standard MDI, (ii) and (iii) breath-actuated inhalers: the dose is released when the patient seals their lips around the mouthpiece and starts to inhale. (ii) Easi-Breathe: the unit is set by opening the mouthpiece cover. (iii) Aerobec Forte Autohaler: the unit is shown in the set position with the top lever raised.

However, in one new HFA formulation of *beclometasone* (Qvar) a change in particle size has resulted in an increase from about 25% to 60% of the dose being in the respirable range, producing significantly greater dose delivery to the small airways and acini. There is evidence that inflammation in these small airways is an important component in both acute and chronic asthma. Thus the absolute loaded dose of *beclometasone* from this device is halved compared to the older pMDIs, with a reduction of about 30% in side-effects at similar clinical effectiveness. However, the Qvar inhaler is not recommended for use in children.

There may be additional features that may worry patients when they are changed to HFA inhalers:

- An altered sound made when the dose is released.
- A change in the taste of the aerosol.
- Reduced pharyngeal impact.
- Incompatibility with their existing spacer device (see below).

Thus patients should be counselled on these points: this also provides a good opportunity to check compliance and inhaler technique (see below).

The European Commission has expressed concern about possible propellant toxicity and has urged careful supervision of patients who are changed to CFC-free inhalers. However, the propellants are regarded as being safe. Patients with 'brittle' asthma, in which there is a sudden onset of severe or life-threatening attacks, will need especially close attention.

Patients using pMDIs need careful counselling to ensure maximum benefit. Good coordination is essential for correct dose delivery and this is more difficult for the young, the elderly and the very anxious patient. It is essential to teach proper procedures and to check regularly that these are being maintained. A moderate inspiratory flow rate (about 30 L/min) gives the best lung deposition and devices are available to help train patients to inspire adequately. Pharmacists, doctors and nurses need to acquire and maintain a good technique themselves (Table 5.26) and be able to teach this to patients: one survey showed that only 28% of adult patients and 48% of hospital pharmacists had a good inhaler technique, but this situation has improved recently.

Table 5.26 Patient counselling points for the use of metered dose inhalers

Advice to the patient
- Keep the cap on the mouthpiece and keep the device clean. If necessary, remove the cartridge and wash casing with a warm, mild detergent solution; do not rinse, allow to dry thoroughly
- When using:
  - remove the cap and shake the inhaler (the drug is suspended in the propellant)
  - breathe out gently, but not fully, then immediately place the lips around the mouthpiece; start to breathe in slowly and deeply through the mouth, press down the inhaler cartridge to release the dose, and continue to breathe in steadily and deeply
  - hold the breath for about 10 s and breathe out slowly
- Good coordination to ensure release of the dose at the commencement of inhalation is essential to obtain the maximum benefit

Points for the pharmacist
- Demonstrate the correct method of use with a placebo inhaler, and ask the patient to show you how they use it. Never accept a patient's assurance that they know how to do so
- Most patients are on long-term therapy, and many develop bad habits. It is useful to ask them to demonstrate how they use their inhaler from time to time, and to reinforce correct usage. Adherence and inhaler technique should be checked with any change in medication
- Demonstration by a pharmacist, doctor or nurse is of limited value unless combined with practice and testing
- The degree of benefit can be demonstrated to the patient by determining peak expiratory flow rates before dosing and 20–30 min afterwards, if possible, thus providing strong motivation
- Patients with anything other than mild, occasional attacks will derive considerable benefit from learning about their disease and how to manage it, especially in exacerbations. They should measure peak expiratory flow rates regularly and keep a diary of the results
- If coordination is poor, a spacer device should be used

Order of inhalation of drugs
- If an attack is not too severe, it may not matter which drug is inhaled first, so compound aerosols may aid patient compliance
- If inhalation of sodium cromoglicate from a DPI causes bronchoconstriction, a beta$_2$-agonist should be used before the cromoglicate DPI
- However, in a severe attack the airways may be too constricted to permit penetration of the drug, so the patient should proceed as follows to ensure that the airways are as dilated as possible:
  - inhale one puff of bronchodilator
  - wait 5 min and inhale a second puff of bronchodilator
  - wait 5 min and inhale other products as usual
  - Unfortunately, this procedure may lead to non-compliance, owing to the waiting periods involved. If so, it is better to reduce the wait between puffs to the maximum that the patient will tolerate

If good coordination cannot be achieved, if patients dislike the sensation of the jet of cold aerosol impinging on the back of the mouth, or if it causes them to gag and involuntarily to stop inhaling momentarily, then several alternatives are available. These are the automatic (breath-actuated) inhalers, spacer devices and dry powder aerosols.

Breath-actuated inhalers
In these devices the inhaler cartridge has the same construction as in the normal pMDI, but a trigger release mechanism is set before inhaling. Release of the dose is actuated automatically when the patient seals their lips around the mouthpiece and creates a sufficient pressure differential at the start of inhalation. However,

some of these inhalers also have problems in use. Patients may dislike the sharp noise and the impact as the mechanism is activated in some inhalers. Further, a proportion of patients do not have sufficient inspiratory capacity at all times to trigger the mechanism or may not achieve a good enough seal around the mouthpiece. Recent designs have mitigated these problems. Once again, good counselling is essential for effective use.

Spacer devices

The object of these is to avoid the need for good coordination of dose release and inhalation for effective drug delivery, to maximize clinical benefit, and to minimize adverse reactions. The dose is fired into a reservoir (Figure 5.23) from which the patient then inhales, using several successive breaths if necessary. This gives comparable results to the use of a pMDI with good coordination (Figure 5.24), so patients with good inhaler technique will derive little benefit from using a spacer, apart from possibly experiencing fewer side-effects, e.g. with corticosteroid inhalers. However, another important function of the reservoir is to slow down the aerosol droplets so that there is more time for the propellant to evaporate before inhalation occurs; in this way the aerosol particles are smaller and thus more likely to penetrate the bronchiolar tree. The reduced speed of the particles also reduces oropharyngeal impaction of drug. Thus the proportion of the dose swallowed and the incidence of hoarseness and oropharyngeal thrush with the corticosteroid aerosols is reduced.

Several commercial types of spacer are available (Figure 5.23). The large-volume (750 mL) devices, e.g. Figures 5.23(a) and (b), can be used flexibly: several breaths can be taken to achieve complete inhalation of the available drug and it is possible to discharge a number of puffs into the chamber to give a higher dose. In the latter case, each puff should be inhaled separately. Research has shown that a spacer used in this way can provide an equivalent alternative to the use of a nebulizer (see below and Figure 5.24) for giving larger drug doses in severe attacks. Further, it has the considerable benefit that a patient who is not using a nebulizer can obtain a

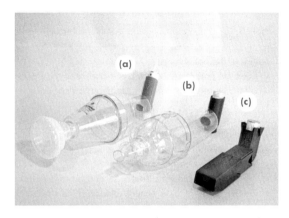

Figure 5.23 Some spacer devices. (a) Large volume (Volumatic) with paediatric mask. (b) Large volume (Nebuhaler). (c) Collapsible extended mouthpiece (Bricanyl).

larger than usual dose of inhaled drug promptly at home, before seeking medical help. However, this must be done as part of an agreed protocol and patients must not rely exclusively on this procedure in severe attacks.

Spacers increase the lung deposition from monodisperse aerosols, perhaps doubling the lung deposition from single doses (Figure 5.24), with a significant increase in clinical response. These spacers have a one-way valve through which only inspiration is possible, exhaled air and waste aerosol passing out through side vents.

However, the larger spacers are too bulky for convenient use outside the home. Many manufacturers supply smaller tube spacers with their pMDIs (see Figure 5.24(c)). Almost any tube device will have a similar, though smaller, effect to a large-volume spacer and extemporaneous devices have been used but give unpredictable results. Recently, spacers specially designed for young children have been introduced. These have a smaller volume, may be fitted with a paediatric face mask and require less inspiratory effort in use. Although spacers increase the inhaled dose, this must not be relied on to increase clinical benefit, which has to be established objectively, e.g. with improved respirometry results (not applicable in young children).

A significant proportion of the aerosol dose is deposited on the walls of the spacers, largely due to electrostatic attraction, so spacers should be

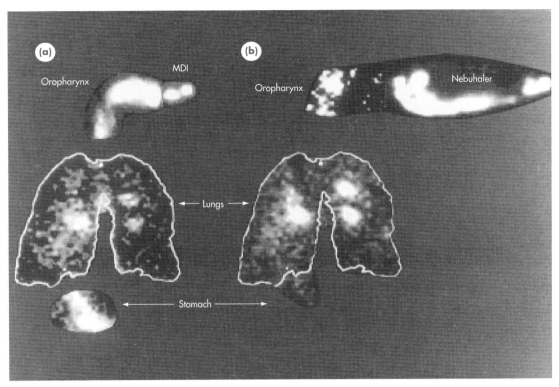

Figure 5.24 Lung deposition of particles from metered dose inhalers (MDIs) with and without a spacer device. (a) Bricanyl MDI. (b) MDI with Nebuhaler large-volume spacer. Note the absence from the stomach of ingested aerosol and its relatively low deposition in the oropharynx. (Reproduced with permission from Newman SP (1984) *Thorax* **39**: 935–41.]

washed not more than once a month with a dilute detergent solution, as an antistatic, and allowed to drain. They should not then be rinsed with water or wiped dry. More frequent washing removes the antistatic film of detergent and wiping dry increases the static charge, so there is a consequent reduction in drug delivery.

Dry powder inhalers

These devices are inherently breath-actuated and so, like breath-actuated inhalers and spacers, do not depend on good coordination for satisfactory performance. However, an adequate inspiratory airflow is still required. The dose is released into the inspired air when the patient inhales. There is no propellant, so these inhalers are more suitable for the occasional patient who is affected by the propellant or who is worried about its possible side-effects. Several types of inhaler are available (Figure 5.25), some of which use a lactose carrier for the drug, whereas others deliver pure drug. Although a number of innovative designs are in development these will have to demonstrate significant benefits in terms of clinical effectiveness or cost or both if they are to replace the Accuhaler and Turbohaler.

Some devices provide single doses from hard gelatin capsules, which have to be loaded into the device before each use. The newer ones provide a number of doses (up to 200) without recharging. They have either a dose counter or end-of-charge indicator so that the patient knows when a replacement is required. If pure, carrier-free drug is used patients are scarcely aware that a powder is being inhaled.

Like the pMDIs, the DPIs are rather inefficient devices for the delivery of drug to the lungs. Many patients distrust the very idea of inhaling a powder, and some dislike the sensation

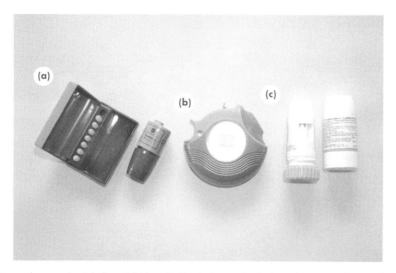

Figure 5.25   Some dry powder inhalers. (a) Ventolin Rotahaler; a single-dose device, each capsule delivers one dose. (b) Becotide Accuhaler (refillable, 60-dose) opened ready for use, showing dose counter. The mouthpiece is at 2 o'clock. A new dose is released by actuating the lever (at 10 o'clock). (c) Bricanyl Turbohaler (disposable, 100-dose) with protective cover. A new dose is released by twisting the knurled base. The small window below the mouthpiece shows a warning flag when the unit is becoming exhausted.

produced. Patients with poor respiratory function may need to inhale several times to obtain the full dose from a single actuation and coughing occurs occasionally.

High inspiration rates (approximately 60 L/min) are required to produce an adequate concentration of respirable particles to improve drug deposition within the lungs. Sustained breath holding does not seem to be necessary.

However, DPIs are simple to use and are generally more suitable for children. More importantly, the devices give a similar clinical benefit to that attainable with a pMDI. If environmental pressures against aerosol propellants are maintained, DPIs may become predominant.

Nebulizers

General principles

Nebulizers are devices for producing an aerosol from an aqueous solution of a drug. Two methods are generally used:

- **Jet nebulizers** (Figure 5.26) use a jet of compressed gas (air or oxygen) to break a fine stream of liquid into an aerosol, the smaller droplets emerging from the outlet as a fine mist.
- **Ultrasonic nebulizers** use electrically-induced ultrasonic vibrations to disperse the drug solution into an aerosol.

In the UK, nebulizers can be prescribed only via hospitals or must be purchased by patients. The following is a brief review of the topic: for more detailed information, readers are referred to the *Thorax* supplement listed in the References and further reading section (p. 364).

Indications for nebulizer therapy

Nebulizers may be preferred for a number of reasons:

- Because young children, the elderly and very infirm patients may find it difficult to use pMDIs and DPIs correctly or with sufficient benefit.
- Because some patients may require a higher dose than can be delivered by pMDIs and DPIs and may be poorly controlled on these, notably some chronic asthmatics and those with COPD and cystic fibrosis.

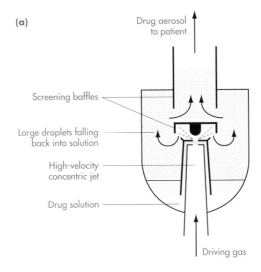

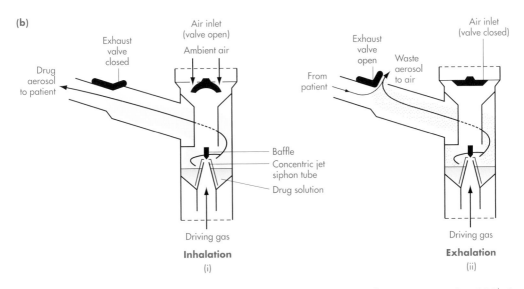

Figure 5.26   Some types of jet nebulizer. (a) A simple older type. (b) Breath-assisted, open vent type (Pari LC Plus).

- For self-medication at home, to give a larger dose of a drug when patients are inadequately controlled with a pMDI, e.g. in severe or chronic asthma, exacerbations of COPD and chronic airflow obstruction, but see above.
- In acute severe asthma, either in hospital, in the doctor's surgery, or as an alternative to parenteral medication.
- When inhalation is desirable but drugs are not produced in a convenient pMDI or DPI form.

The latter point is especially applicable in the case of:

- Antimicrobials for cystic fibrosis, bronchiectasis and HIV infection or AIDS.
- *Dornase alfa* for reducing sputum viscosity in cystic fibrosis to aid expectoration?
- In palliative care, e.g. local anaesthetics (*lidocaine* or *bupivacaine*) for relief of persistent dry cough and opioids for terminal dyspnoea.

The need for a nebulizer should be validated by proof of additional benefit (Figure 5.27). Patients must be carefully trained in the use and limitations of nebulizers because they may rely on them excessively and delay seeking effective treatment, with a consequently increased morbidity and mortality. Trials of therapy need to be continued for 3–4 weeks to assess benefit adequately and if bronchodilators are used they should normally give at least a 15% improvement over existing baseline to be considered worthwhile. However, due account should be taken of a patient's subjective perception of benefit, in addition to measurements of PEF or FEV_1.

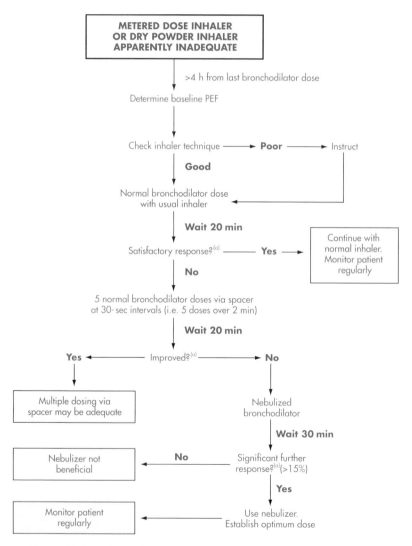

Figure 5.27   Protocol for establishing the need for nebulizer use. [a]Response or improvement is checked objectively at each stage by measuring peak expiratory flow (PEF): at least a 15% increase is required to justify a change of procedure. A trial of therapy or equipment needs 3–4 weeks to be confident of benefit or otherwise.

Types of jet nebulizer

These work on the Venturi principle. High-pressure gas (air or sometimes oxygen) is forced through a very small aperture (venturi). As the gas escapes from the venturi it expands rapidly and gains velocity as it passes across the end of a liquid feeder tube. The low pressure created sucks liquid up the feed tube and the liquid stream is broken into droplets that impinge onto a baffle. The largest droplets are trapped on the baffle and intermediate ones on the walls of the chamber. All of these drain back into the liquid reservoir. Only the smallest droplets are entrained in the gas stream and inhaled by the patient. The performance (dose delivery) depends on the precise sizes and designs of the feeder tube, venturi, baffles and chamber. The design is crucial to the droplet size produced and the presence of a baffle distinguishes the nebulizer from a simple atomizer. Two forms of modern jet nebulizer are illustrated in Figure 5.26.

Older, simple nebulizer designs that have been in use for many years are very inefficient because:

- They may produce <50% of particles in the 1- to 5-μm range.
- Some 95% of the primary droplets are trapped on internal baffles.
- About 65% remains in the chamber after nebulization and 65% of the inhaled aerosol is exhaled.

Thus only about 10% of the dose placed in a nebulizer may reach the desired sites of action in the lungs. This situation can be improved in various ways.

Open vent nebulizers (e.g. the Sidestream) have an additional vent through which the low pressure in the chamber sucks additional air. The extra gas flow entrains more respirable particles, giving shorter nebulization times and possibly reducing particle size. Further, cheaper, low-output compressors can be used. However, patients with a low inspiratory flow, e.g. young children and the elderly infirm, may inspire less drug because more is carried to waste in the increased exhaust stream.

This drug loss may be overcome by the newer **breath-assisted open vent nebulizers** that incorporate two valves (e.g. the Pari LC Plus (Figure 5.26(b)) and Ventstream). An inlet valve opens only on inspiration, admitting ambient air as with the open vent design. On expiration the inlet valve closes and an outlet valve opens, so aerosol loss is not increased by extra air flow through the inlet valve.

Aerosol loss when exhaling can also be reduced by using a holding chamber with a conventional jet nebulizer. This makes the set-up rather bulky and there is no device of this type currently available in the UK.

Some factors affecting the performance of jet nebulizers

Gas flow rate. This is the major determinant of output from a particular nebulizer, as particle size decreases markedly with increasing gas flow. The flow rate may be 6–8 L/min (high), 4–6 L/min (medium) or occasionally, <4 L/min (low), but that required to yield the desired droplet size characteristics and dose output differs appreciably with different nebulizers. The manufacturer's recommendations on air flow should be strictly observed. High flow rates are needed to nebulize viscous solutions, e.g. antibiotics and *rhDNase*. Modern jet nebulizers have output rates comparable with those from ultrasonic devices.

Domiciliary oxygen equipment cannot deliver more than 4 L/min without a special controller and is unsuitable for use with most jet nebulizers. Electrically driven air compressors are preferred unless the patient needs *oxygen* (see below). However, if patients in the community need *oxygen*, a low-flow (<4 L/min) nebulizer (e.g. Cirrus or Pari LC Plus) can be used with an oxygen cylinder. Alternatively, a flow head capable of delivering up to 8 L/min from a gas cylinder should be used with a suitable nebulizer, e.g. Permaneb (4–6 L/min); or Micromist or Ventstream (6–8 L/min). If high flow rates are used, the normal-size oxygen cylinder will have a very short life and the cost of supplying the *oxygen* will be very high. If *oxygen* is used, the patient must be capable of an adequate inhalation rate. Oxygen concentrators are unsuitable for driving nebulizers.

The inhalation rate and pattern have only a small effect on particle size, but may be very important if oxygen is used as the driving gas and in determining pulmonary drug delivery.

Driving gas.   Under hospital conditions either piped oxygen or compressed air may be used. However many patients, especially those with COPD, are intolerant of *oxygen*. At the low inhalation rates that occur with exhausted and very infirm patients, the *oxygen* concentration in the inspired air mixture may be very high (Figure 5.28), so air is the preferred driving gas for hypoxic patients with carbon dioxide retention. However, some patients tolerate *oxygen* or may need it, e.g. in an acute severe asthma attack the patient may be severely hypoxaemic and this may be aggravated by the bronchodilator, so *oxygen* is then preferred.

Diluent, volume and formulation of solution. The preferred diluent for nebulizer solutions is sterile 0.9% saline, because hypotonic solutions may cause bronchoconstriction in some patients. Solutions diluted ready for use are used in all areas of practice because there is no preservative to cause reactions and no possibility of a patient using a concentrated solution in error. However, concentrated respirator solutions are available for use with ventilators and these must be diluted with sterile 0.9% saline for use in nebulizers.

The fill volume of solution must be adjusted to suit the nebulizer being used, because some have an appreciable RV (residual volume), and to give the desired delivery rate. The delivery rate of many nebulizers falls off markedly below approximately 2 mL RV. Tapping the chamber sharply and repeatedly throughout dosing to shake solution from the walls and baffles to the bottom of the reservoir improves maximum delivery somewhat. Because of evaporation, the RV underestimates the residual mass of drug at the end of nebulization, but there is little information on this because it is influenced by numerous factors, e.g. the humidity and temperature of the driving gas. Inhalation of the more concentrated drug solution may cause respiratory irritation in some patients towards the end of a treatment session.

The fill volume also controls the time over which the dose is delivered, this being one of the advantages of nebulizer therapy because there is then adequate time (10 min) for a physiological response (e.g. bronchodilatation) to occur and so better penetration of the latter part of the dose. Patients will not usually tolerate delivery times longer than 10 min.

Solutions of lower surface tension give greater volume deliveries because they adhere less to the walls and baffles of the nebulizers. Drug solutions may be diluted with sterile 0.9% saline if a longer inhalation time is required.

Hygiene.   Nebulizers must be kept clean to avoid microbial growth and consequent infection and are best washed out after each use, or at least daily. The manufacturer's instructions must be followed closely to avoid damage to the plastic precision mouldings that are used.

Delivery of drug solution.   This is the most significant attribute of a nebulizer, and solution outputs can vary in the range 0.01–0.75 mL/min, depending on the type of nebulizer and the gas flow rate. It is impossible to predict the actual delivery of drug from a particular nebulizer to a specific patient. We can only choose the device and adjust the conditions to get the best clinical response.

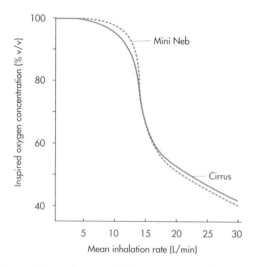

Figure 5.28   Influence of inhalation rate on the oxygen content of the inspired gas from two nebulizers (oxygen flow rate 8 L/min).

Nebulizer wear.   Some nebulizer chambers are durable, but should be replaced after about a year (e.g. Pari LC Plus, Sidestream Durable). However, most wear more rapidly and must be discarded after 3 months or if there is any sign of wear, e.g. an increasing nebulization time or a changed noise. The compressors have a very long life.

Ancillary equipment
A wide range of ancillary equipment is available from manufacturers. Either mouthpieces or face masks may be used, with similar clinical responses. Young children and exhausted or very infirm patients usually do better with face masks because they are easier to use, but it is often a matter of patient preference. Very young children are often intolerant of masks, but reasonable results are sometimes achieved by merely holding the outlet tube or mask near the child's nose and allowing normal breathing. Although this reduces dose delivery substantially, it may accustom the child to the treatment and permit subsequent use of a more effective technique.

The masks should fit the face well to avoid adverse effects on the skin or eyes. However, it is sometimes difficult to get a good fit with a mask and avoid leakage of aerosol, so mouthpieces may be preferred for use with corticosteroids, which may damage the perioral and perinasal skin, and with antimuscarinic bronchodilators, which risk causing or exacerbating glaucoma in the elderly.

There are concerns about the effects of drugs such as antibiotics on the environment and the possibility of spreading infections due to highly resistant microorganisms. For this sort of application closed systems (e.g. with exhaust filters) are used in hospitals to prevent cross-contamination. This is probably unnecessary for home use unless others in the family are at risk from respiratory infection, though nebulizers should be used in well-ventilated rooms.

Compressors must match the chosen nebulizer: many are supplied as complete outfits.

Ultrasonic nebulizers
Ultrasonic nebulization may be very fast, and output increases as the solution heats because of the associated fall in viscosity (whereas with jet nebulizers the output falls with time). The user can usually adjust the output. Some patients find the warm wet mist they produce is unpleasant, especially if a face mask is fitted, and provokes coughing. Ultrasonic nebulizers are generally quieter than jet nebulizers and do not need a compressor or gas supply.

Improvements in nebulizers
Pharmacists should be familiar with the characteristics of the nebulizers they supply, especially the gas pressures and flow rates, to be able to give good patient advice.

The British Standard for jet nebulizers (BS7711, Part 3, 1994) requires them to be marked with maximum filling levels and recommended gas flows. Manufacturers must also supply details of:

*   Intended use and any contra-indications.
*   Gas pressures, respirable outputs and RVs corresponding to the recommended, minimum and maximum flow rates.
*   Aerosol particle size distribution at the recommended flow rates.
*   Suitability for use with ventilators and anaesthetic systems.

However, BS7711 does not address many of the problems raised above.

Conclusion

Inhalation therapy has become a highly technical and sophisticated method of drug delivery that has brought tremendous advantages to sufferers from respiratory diseases. This is a research area of great interest and intense activity. Most difficult cases of asthma, in particular, can be controlled by the appropriate use of this technique, though occasionally oral medication may also be required.

Many new devices are likely to be introduced in the next few years, most of which are breath-actuated and provide more consistent dosing. For example, one new battery-powered DPI is claimed to deliver about 30% of the absolute loaded dose, i.e. some three times that from a conventional DPI. Another novel pMDI delivers a high respirable fraction at a lower velocity than current devices, similarly delivering some 30% of the absolute loaded dose. If these and similar devices perform to this level in daily clinical use they should permit significant reductions in loaded doses, and so also reduce both adverse reactions and drug costs. However, all new devices will have to demonstrate significant cost–benefit advantages.

The principal barrier to more effective control is largely a lack of appreciation of the potential benefits of inhalation therapy and inadequate understanding of the proper use of the equipment. The result is inadequate patient counselling and adherence, and sub-optimal control of the disease state. Although the situation has improved over recent years, more can, and should, be done to reduce morbidity and mortality. These comments apply to all health workers, including pharmacists.

Oxygen therapy

Aims

The aim of *oxygen* therapy is to increase the amount of oxygen carried by the blood in hypoxaemia by increasing either the Hb saturation or the amount of oxygen carried in solution in the plasma, normally 10 μmol O_2/L/kPa.

Increasing the oxygen concentration in poorly ventilated but well-perfused alveoli increases the P_aO_2 and also counteracts a reduced diffusing capacity. Patients with anaemia or heart failure may have good oxygen saturation but poor oxygen delivery to the tissues, due to low Hb levels and low cardiac output, respectively. These patients will benefit from an increase in the dissolved oxygen concentration in the plasma.

Problems

It is important to remember that *oxygen* is a drug: high concentrations of *oxygen* are toxic, especially to lung tissue and the CNS, can cause blindness in premature infants and pulmonary oedema and irritation in adults, so concentrations >60% in the inspired air are rarely used. If

high-concentration (40–60%) *oxygen* is required, it should be given continuously and patients watched for any evidence of hypoventilation (i.e. respiratory depression), which may appear rapidly or develop gradually. However, it is safe for patients with pneumonia, pulmonary thromboembolism and fibrosing alveolitis, in which carbon dioxide retention and hypoventilation are unlikely.

Patients who have had hypercapnia for some time (e.g. in COPD) rely on a low P_aO_2 to provide their respiratory drive, because the carbon dioxide and pH sensors in the respiratory centre become fatigued or down-regulated. Thus increasing the P_aO_2 artificially will inhibit this drive and may suppress respiration substantially. This aggravates the hypercapnia, and the raised carbon dioxide level finally acts as a further respiratory depressant (CO_2 narcosis). Thus those patients who most need *oxygen* are often intolerant of it. Optimal delivery of oxygen to patients with prolonged hypercapnia can only be achieved by careful blood gas monitoring and clinical supervision.

Oxygen, unless from a concentrator, is supplied as a pure gas that must be diluted with air to a suitable concentration. If the concentration exceeds 40% the gas should be humidified with a nebulizer (preferably warmed), but masks delivering 35% *oxygen* or less usually carry sufficient moisture in the entrained air.

In the UK, domiciliary oxygen equipment supplied through NHS sources will deliver up to 28% oxygen, depending on the type of mask used. If concentrations other than this are required the appropriate equipment must be purchased or provided by a hospital. This long-term low concentration *oxygen* therapy has been shown to improve survival in type B COPD patients ('blue bloaters', p. 331) with both dyspnoea and peripheral oedema (i.e. cor pulmonale) by up to 5 years. Although it does not arrest disease progression it does improve both exercise tolerance and the quality of life. In other forms of severe advanced respiratory disease it improves well-being, but does not prolong life.

In England and Wales, oxygen equipment is supplied and installed by nominated suppliers in various regions. In Scotland, oxygen cylinders and associated equipment are supplied by community pharmacists who have contracted to supply oxygen services. In this case, pharmacists who provide domiciliary oxygen must ensure that a member of the family or helper is available and properly instructed in the use of the equipment, in addition to the patient. Oxygen is a fire hazard: it must not be used while smoking or near naked flames: if patients need oxygen they should not be smoking anyway!

Methods of administration

Types of supply

In hospital, *oxygen* is piped to bedside outlets. For UK domiciliary use, either cylinders (containing 1360 L) or oxygen concentrators may be supplied; the latter provide 95% oxygen plus 5% argon at 2 L/min, dropping to 85–90% oxygen at higher flow rates. Small, lightweight, portable cylinders can be supplied by the hospital or purchased by the patient and refilled from a liquid oxygen container, giving improved mobility to suitable patients.

Oxygen cylinders are suitable only for intermittent use, giving an 11-h supply at the low setting (2 L/min) and half this at the high setting (4 L/min). When long-term *oxygen* therapy (LTOT) is required, i.e. >8 h/day or >21 cylinders per month, oxygen concentrators are used. These are small portable machines for domiciliary use that can be set to deliver 24–28% oxygen via a nasal cannula at 1–2 L/min. They are cheaper and more convenient than cylinders, but cannot meet all types of requirement. If higher flows are required, two concentrators can be linked in parallel using a Y-piece. Although the initial cost is high, this is justified when there is a need for sustained usage, i.e. 15 h or more per day over a long period.

In the USA, about half a million patients use *liquid oxygen*, which is very flexible in use. A 30- to 40-L container lasts 8–10 days at 2 L/min output. *Liquid oxygen* is available in the UK for patients requiring more than 2 h of ambulatory use, and those needing >2 L/min for >30 min. It is appropriate for patients who have exercise desaturation and in whom oxygen provides demonstrated improvement in exercise capacity and dyspnoea. It is not recommended in those with COPD if P_aO_2 >7.3 kPa and there is no exercise desaturation. Small cylinders, with or without oxygen-conserving devices, are available for patients requiring oxygen for up to 4 h.

Cylinders with normal head units, oxygen concentrators and liquid oxygen containers are unsuitable for driving nebulizers.

Tents, masks and cannulae

For hospital patients who are severely ill or debilitated, or for whom minimal attachment of equipment is desirable, an oxygen tent or 'oxygen hood' may be used, but this is uncommon. It is more usual to use masks, which cover the mouth and nose, or nasal cannulae. Fixed performance masks are preferable because the concentration delivered by variable performance masks varies with the patient's breathing pattern.

These devices are illustrated in Figure 5.29 and their characteristics are summarized in Table 5.27. Nasal cannulae have the advantage that there is no restriction on eating, drinking and talking, because the mouth is not obstructed. Further, patients in respiratory distress often do not tolerate masks. Although nasal cannulae give poor control of the oxygen concentration in the inspired air, they are generally preferred for the delivery of LTOT (see below). Endotracheal cannulae are sometimes used in hospital to achieve better control. Oxygen concentrators are designed to be used only with nasal cannulae.

Reservoir systems are available to reduce the wastage of oxygen in the expired air and can reduce the oxygen requirement by about 50%. Pulsed systems that deliver oxygen only on inspiration can reduce this to about 25%. The latter are unsuitable for use with concentrators. These arrangements are available in the UK in hospitals and for providing ambulatory oxygen (see above).

Intermittent positive pressure ventilation (IPPV)

These devices provide control of five parameters:

- Pressure of delivery of gas to the lungs.
- Duration of each pressure pulse.

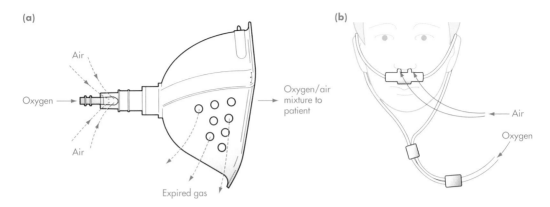

Figure 5.29   Typical oxygen mask and nasal cannula. (a) Ventimask 3 (Vickers). (b) Nasal cannula (Intersurgical).

Table 5.27   The types of oxygen masks and nasal cannulae[a], and their applications

Patient features	Type of performance[b]	Oxygen concentration delivered (% v/v)	Oxygen flow rate L/min[c]
Poor ventilatory drive, e.g. COPD	Constant	24 or 28[d]	2
Good ventilatory drive, e.g. asthma, pneumonia, pulmonary oedema	Constant Variable	31, 35, 40, 60[e] 25–60[f]	[e] [f]

[a] See Figure 5.29

[b] Constant performance masks deliver a constant oxygen concentration over a wide range of flow rates. The output of variable performance masks depends on oxygen flow rate, the breathing pattern of the patient and other factors. Nasal cannulae are the most commonly used form of variable performance device.

[c] Domiciliary oxygen equipment provided in the UK under the NHS will deliver only 2 L/min at the 'Medium' setting and 4 L/min at the 'High' setting

[d] The only type of mask that can be supplied in the UK through the NHS on prescription delivers 28% oxygen. It is unsuitable for use with oxygen concentrators with which nasal cannulae are usually preferred. If other concentrations are required the masks must be provided by a hospital or purchased.

[e] These are operable over a range of flow rates, as follows:

Oxygen concentration (% v/v)	24	28	31	35	40	60
Flow rates (L/min)	2–4	4–8	6–10	8–12	10–15	15–25

Oxygen flow rates must be sufficient to prevent inspiration of excess ambient air through the exhaust holes in the mask.

[f] See note (a); a nasal cannula operated at 2 L/min usually provides about 30% v/v of oxygen in the inspired air. These masks may be suitable for use with oxygen concentrators.

COPD, chronic obstructive pulmonary disease.

- Degree of oxygen enrichment of the air.
- Inspiratory trigger pressure.
- End-expiratory pressure.

Initially, a low trigger pressure and a long, high-pressure oxygen pulse are used, forcing gas into the lungs. This removes the work of breathing from the patient but care is needed to avoid lung damage due to excessive pressures (barotrauma). As improvement occurs, the trigger pressure is increased and the degree of assistance and oxygen enrichment reduced. A nebulizer is used to humidify the gas, so the equipment can also be used to deliver drugs.

However, if respiratory function is reasonable there is no evidence that the routine use of IPPV simply to deliver drugs is beneficial.

IPPV is instituted in hypoxaemic respiratory failure if the patient is in respiratory distress despite maximal treatment, e.g. exhaustion, inability to speak and a high respiration rate. IPPV requires endotracheal intubation, rarely tracheostomy, and also skilled initiation and supervision. A recent innovation is IPPV via a nasal mask (non-invasive IPPV, NIPPV), which is of particular value in sleep apnoea. Assisted ventilation has numerous hazards.

Guidelines for domiciliary oxygen therapy

Because of the cost of providing this service and the need to select patients and define objectives carefully, the Royal College of Physicians (RCP) has published the following guidelines:

- *Oxygen* should be given only after a careful evaluation of the needs of the patient and never as a placebo. Assessment requires measurement of blood gas tensions on two occasions at least 3 weeks apart, and not less than 4 weeks after an exacerbation of their disease, to demonstrate clinical stability.
- Patients should be supervised carefully, at least initially. A few patients may revert to an adequate P_aO_2 (>8 kPa) after several months of therapy, so *oxygen* may then be withdrawn.
- Intermittent therapy, using cylinders, is suitable for patients with:
  - Hypoxaemia of short duration, e.g. in asthma, pneumonia and pulmonary oedema.
  - Advanced irreversible respiratory disease to improve mobility and quality of life, e.g. in COPD, emphysema, pulmonary fibrosis, pulmonary thromboembolism and pulmonary hypertension.
- LTOT implies the use of *oxygen* for at least 15 h/day (including the night), so it is used for patients with chronic hypoxaemia and cor pulmonale. In these cases it is more economical to use a concentrator. The aim is to maintain the P_aO_2 at about 10 kPa without producing hypercapnia, consequent on

reducing the ventilatory drive. This can usually be achieved with a nasal cannula and a flow rate of 1.5–3 L/min. Because there are advantages for only a limited number of patients, the RCP also defines the groups likely to benefit, i.e. patients with:

- COPD (FEV_1 <1.5 L, FVC <2.0 L) associated with hypoxaemia when breathing air (P_aO_2 <7.3 kPa) and hypercapnia (P_aCO_2 >6 kPa) who have peripheral oedema.
- COPD with P_aO_2 7.3–8 kPa in the presence of secondary polycythaemia, nocturnal hypoxaemia, peripheral oedema or evidence of pulmonary hypertension.
- Interstitial lung disease with P_aO_2 <8 kPa and those with P_aO_2 >8 kPa and disabling dyspnoea.
- Cystic fibrosis when P_aO_2 <7.3 kPa or if it is in the range 7.3–8 kPa in the presence of secondary polycythaemia, nocturnal hypoxaemia, pulmonary hypertension or peripheral oedema.
- Pulmonary hypertension without parenchymal lung involvement when P_aO_2 <8 kPa.
- Neuromuscular or skeletal disorders, after specialist assessment.
- Obstructive sleep apnoea despite continuous positive airways pressure therapy, after specialist assessment.
- Pulmonary malignancy or other terminal disease with disabling dyspnoea.
- Heart failure with daytime P_aO_2 <7.3kPa on air or with nocturnal hypoxaemia.
- Paediatric respiratory disease, after specialist assessment.

Respiratory depression is seldom a problem in patients with stable respiratory failure treated with low oxygen concentrations, although it may occur during exacerbations. Patients, relatives and carers should be warned to call for medical help if drowsiness or confusion occur.

- Further criteria need to be satisfied before LTOT is prescribed:
  - Patients should be non-smokers and compliant, already on optimal medical treatment.
  - Oxygen concentrators are more economical if patients require *oxygen* for >8 h/day

or >21 cylinders/month. Exceptionally, the output from two can be combined.

- A nasal cannula is preferred but may cause nasal dermatitis and mucosal drying in sensitive individuals.

There are special arrangements for prescribing oxygen concentrators in the UK. The criteria for LTOT are liable to periodic revision and the BNF section 3.6 should be consulted for the latest information. Different criteria are used in other countries, e.g. the presence of cor pulmonale, oedema or polycythaemia (PCV >56%). *Oxygen* may be prescribed much more loosely there, possibly because of the emotive nature of the therapy, but this lacks scientific support.

Almitrine dimesilate (unlicensed in the UK) stimulates the carotid body and improves both ventilation and ventilation–perfusion mismatch. Given with *oxygen*, the drug further improves P_aO_2 levels.

References and further reading

Barnes P J, Godfrey S (1999). *Asthma (Medical Pocket Books)*, 2nd edn. London: Dunitz.

Brewis R A L (1998). *Lecture Notes on Respiratory Disease*, 5th edn. Oxford: Blackwell Science.

Brewis R A L, Corrin B, Geddes G M, Gibson G J, eds (1995). *Respiratory Medicine*, 2nd edn. London: Bailliere Tindall.

British National Formulary and *BNF for Children*. Published every March and September. British Medical Association, Royal Pharmaceutical Society of Great Britain, Royal College of Paediatrics and Child Health, and Neonatal and Paediatrics Pharmacists Group.

Devereux G (2006). ABC of chronic obstructive pulmonary disease: Definition, epidemiology and risk factors. *BMJ* 332: 1142–1144. (This is the first of 12 weekly articles by multiple authors.)

Clark T J H, Rees J (1997). *Practical Management of Asthma*, 3rd edn. London: Dunitz.

Cleghorn G J, Fortstener G G, Stringer DA, *et al.* (1986). Treatment of distal intestinal syndrome in cystic fibrosis with a balanced intestinal lavage solution. *Lancet* i: 8–11.

Cole R B, McKay D (1990). *Essentials of Respiratory Disease*, 3rd edn. Edinburgh: Churchill Livingstone.

Davies A, Moores C (2006). *The Respiratory System*. Edinburgh: Churchill Livingstone.

Engels F, Nijkamp F P (1998). Pharmacological inhibition of leukotriene actions. *Pharm World Sci* 20: 60–65.

Gross N J, Skorodin M S (1984). Anticholinergic, antimuscarinic bronchodilators. *Am Rev Respir Dis* 129: 856–870.

Insley J (1996). *A Paediatric Vade-Macum*, 13th edn. London, Arnold.

Johnson N McI (1990). *Respiratory Medicine Pocket Consultant (Pocket Consultant Series)*, 2nd edn. Oxford: Blackwell Science.

Muers M F, Corris P A, eds (1997). Nebuliser Project Group of the British Thoracic Society Standards of Care Committee. Current best practice for nebuliser treatment. *Thorax* 52 (Suppl. 2): S1–S104.

National Institute for Clinical Excellence Guideline 12. Chronic Obstructive Pulmonary Disease. *Thorax* 2004: 59 (Suppl. 1): 1–232.

Quanger P H, Tammeling G J, Cotes J E, *et al.* (1993). Lung volumes and forced ventilatory flows. Report of the Working Party on Standardisation of Lung Function Tests, European Community for Steel and Coal. Official Statement of the European Respiratory Society. *Eur Respir J* Suppl. 16: 5–40.

Rees J, Price J (1999). *ABC of Asthma*, 4th edn. London: BMJ Publishing.

Rees P J, Dudley F (1998). ABC of oxygen: provision of oxygen at home. *BMJ* 317: 935–938.

Royal College of Physicians (1999). *Domiciliary oxygen therapy services: clinical guidelines and advice for prescribers*. London: RCP.

Sugden L, Chamberlain J, eds (1997). Asthma: current topics and reviews. *J Pharm Pharmacol* 49: Suppl. 3.

The British Thoracic Society (1998). Smoking cessation guidelines and their cost-effectiveness. *Thorax* 53 (Suppl. 5): S1–S38.

The British Thoracic Society *et al.* (2003). The British Guidelines on Asthma Management: Review and Position Statement. *Thorax* 52: Suppl. 1.

West J B (1995). *Respiratory Physiology – The Essentials*, 5th edn. Baltimore: Williams & Wilkins.

West J B (1998). *Pulmonary Pathophysiology – The Essentials*, 5th edn. Baltimore: Williams & Wilkins.

Winsel S E (2006). Asthma: defining the persistent adult phenotypes. *Lancet* 368: 804–816.

Wood A J J (1986). Management of pulmonary disease in cystic fibrosis. *N Engl J Med* 335: 179–188.

6

Central nervous system

Mental illness is widespread in society but remains the object of considerable stigma and a great deal of misconception. Recurrent media scares about so-called 'maniacs' do not help the situation. Many people suffer from anxiety or depression at some stage and the lifetime prevalence of schizophrenia is about 1 in 100. In the UK, despite the admirable motives behind the campaign to depopulate the long-stay psychiatric hospitals, the Care in the Community programme appears to have overwhelmed the community organizations that have to implement it. Increasingly, people with mental health needs are seen in primary care.

Neurological disease is assuming greater importance in an ageing population, as the prevalence of conditions such as Parkinson's disease and dementia rises inexorably.

In almost all central nervous system conditions, although psychotherapy plays a vital role, drug therapy contributes substantially to making the problems manageable and relieving an enormous amount of suffering.

Physiological principles

To understand the mechanisms, symptoms and treatment of CNS disorders it is necessary to review the functions of the more important brain centres, their interconnections and the transmitters that predominate in each. Only the most simplified outline can be attempted here. An overall view is presented in this section, but further specific information appears in later sections as appropriate. More detailed accounts may be found in the References and further reading section (p. 454).

Brain functions can be considered in three broad categories:

• **Input** or perceptual, i.e. handling the mass of sensory data passed up from receptors in the sense organs.
• **Processing** that data, i.e. the cognitive function, which involves integration, association with stored data (memory, experience) and, especially in man, the addition of an emotional component.
• **Output**, i.e. the action decided by the cognitive function in response to input: this will usually be either motor (mainly voluntary muscle) or homeostatic (mainly involuntary muscle and glands); see Table 6.1 and Figure 6.1.

Brain centres and their disorder

The brain is conventionally considered in six main anatomical and functional areas:

1. Cerebrum – two hemispheres of cerebral cortex, containing the limbic system and basal ganglia.
2. Diencephalon, containing the hypothalamus and thalamus.
3. Midbrain.
4. Pons.
5. Medulla oblongata.
6. Cerebellum.

Alternatively, the brain may be subdivided into distinct regions:

• The **forebrain**, which includes areas 1 and 2.
• The **hindbrain**, which includes areas 4, 5 and 6.
• The **brainstem**, which includes the midbrain, medulla and pons.

Interconnections between these areas are manifold and complex, accounting for the richness and diversity of human activity, experience and achievement.

Cerebral cortex

The cerebral cortex is, in evolutionary terms, the youngest centre. It is the principal distinguishing feature of higher mammals. Notably developed in man, where it contains 90% of the total brain neurones, the cerebral cortex is the location of abstract thought, reasoning, judgement, creativity, the interpretation of sensory input and also memory. It functions like a computer, providing an objective, logical assessment of the environment as perceived via the senses, and then producing a plan for action depending on past experience and biological

Table 6.1 Principal anatomical centres of brain function

	Function	Centre
Input	Perception	Sensory cortex, thalamus, reticular formation
Processing	Cognitive (intellectual)	Cerebral cortex
	Emotional	Limbic system
Output	Motor	Motor cortex, cerebellum, basal ganglia
	Homeostasis	Medulla, hypothalamus, pituitary

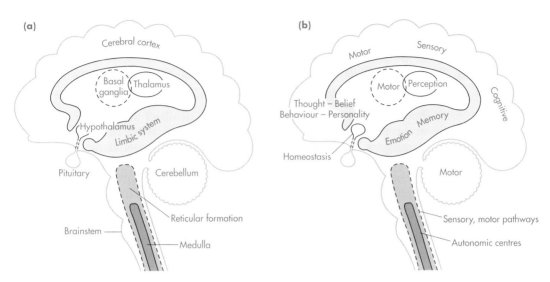

Figure 6.1 (a) Simplified schematic diagram of brain showing important anatomical areas. (b) Simplified representation of location of principal brain functions. Note: The locations of functions within the cortex are not intended to reflect specific cortical centres.

goals. Specific areas of the cortex are dedicated to subsidiary functions, such as the speech centre and the visual, auditory and motor cortexes. Anatomically, the cerebral cortex is subdivided into various lobes, i.e. the frontal, temporal, parietal and occipital.

Cortical disorders usually have a profound effect on all CNS function. They are commonly manifested as disorders of intellect, e.g. mental handicap, dementia or Alzheimer's disease, or of movement, e.g. epilepsy. Strokes are caused by obstruction of blood flow usually to discrete cortical areas. The thought disorder characteristic of schizophrenia is partly cortical, but disordered limbic or thalamic influences on the cortex are probably more important.

Most proven and putative neurotransmitters are found in the cortex. Many of the more recently discovered mediators, such as the endorphins and peptides, have yet to be definitely linked with specific CNS functions, disorders or drug actions. They may modulate the action of the traditional transmitters.

Limbic system

This interesting evolutionary development of the higher mammals provides mental activity with an emotional dimension. The limbic system is responsible for feelings rather than objective reasoning and is perceived consciously as an emotional overlay, i.e. the affect or mood, which can modify the decisions taken by the cortex. The system may mediate rage, fear, pleasure and love and, by its influence on cortical function, is responsible for beliefs as opposed to rational thought. A materialistic interpretation of one of the objectives of some Eastern philosophies, especially meditation, would be that it attempts to achieve control or even elimination of limbic influences ('the self', 'desire') on the cortex.

The contrast between limbic and cortical functions is illustrated by our response to being caught for a motoring offence. One part of us – our limbic system – is angry, fearful or ashamed (depending on our personality): at the same time, our cortex is calculating the effect on our insurance premium, the most effective way to appease the policeman, or perhaps even how to manage without a driving licence.

The limbic system has evolved from a structure in lower mammals concerned with olfaction (sense of smell), and indeed it retains this function in humans. Possibly this accounts for the emotional power that smells have on humans.

The limbic system is also involved in memory, and we are all familiar with how strongly smells can evoke even distant memories. The system is structurally complex with many component nuclei and important connections with the frontal and temporal lobes of the cortex, with the reticular system and with the hypothalamus (all of which are sometimes considered as partially within the limbic system). Dopamine is an important transmitter, as are noradrenaline (NA, norepinephrine) and 5-hydroxytryptamine (5-HT, serotonin). Gamma-aminobutyric acid (GABA) is an inhibitory transmitter here.

Normally in a stable personality there is a balance between limbic and cortical influences on behaviour: one should be neither too emotional nor too unfeeling and cold. Of course, the relative contributions in any one person, which in part defines their personality, will be determined by genetic, nurturing, social and cultural factors, providing both the diversity and the unpredictability of human behaviour. The affective dimension accounts for many of the differences between individuals, and also between man and most other animals. It is interesting to speculate on the biological advantage that the limbic system confers: possibly it is related to the social evolution of man.

Disorders of the limbic system are likely to cause inappropriate emotions, such as depression, mania or excessive anxiety. Delusions (inappropriate beliefs) may arise in the limbic system. The now discredited prefrontal lobotomy (leucotomy), an operation to sever the links between the limbic system and the cortex in severe psychiatric disorders, resulted in the patient becoming emotionally flat. A similar phenomenon is sometimes seen in patients on long-term antipsychotics.

Basal ganglia

This group of interconnected nuclei lie deep within the cerebral hemispheres and are important coordinating centres for voluntary motor activity. If the cortex decides motor strategy and the cerebellum organizes the main muscular movements, then the basal ganglia (BG) look after the fine detail, especially of posture and tone.

The BG centres include the **corpus striatum** (putamen and caudate nucleus), the **globus pallidus** and the midbrain **substantia nigra**. There are important two-way connections with higher centres (especially the motor cortex), the cerebellum and various motor nuclei of the brainstem. The BG are thus vital components in neural loops involved in the integrated control of muscular movement. They affect muscular activity indirectly by modulating motor cortex output and also directly by augmenting or suppressing motor neurones in the spinal cord via the descending extrapyramidal nerve tracts (see below). To assist them in this, the BG receive sensory information ascending from proprioceptor muscle spindles within voluntary muscle, via the reticular system (see below).

Disorders of the BG result in tremor or inappropriate muscular tone, e.g. Parkinson's disease. The three important transmitters here are acetylcholine, dopamine and GABA; the former two have opposing actions. Over 75% of brain dopamine is in the BG.

Thalamus

This important relay and preliminary processing centre for sensory data is situated in the main afferent pathway between the sense organs and the cortex. It may be involved, with other centres, in conditions where there is perceptual dysfunction, e.g. the hallucinations of schizophrenia. Dopamine is a likely transmitter in the thalamus, as are other catecholamines such as adrenaline (epinephrine) and noradrenaline (norepinephrine), and acetylcholine. The thalamus is also involved in motor activity.

Hypothalamus

Through its connections with autonomic centres in the medulla, the hypothalamus has an important influence on the output of the sympathetic and parasympathetic nervous systems. The hypothalamus itself contains centres for satiety, sleep, thermoregulation, water balance and sexual appetite. It also controls a major part of the endocrine system through its connections with the pituitary gland. Dopamine, 5-HT and noradrenaline (norepinephrine) are important transmitters in the hypothalamus. Drugs acting on dopaminergic receptors usually affect hypothalamic activity.

Brainstem

The brainstem comprises the 'lower', more primitive part of the brain (in effect the whole midbrain and hindbrain except the cerebellum). The midbrain houses visual and auditory sensory nuclei, as well as some motor centres. Throughout the brainstem is a more diffuse structure, the reticular formation.

Medulla
Many vital homeostatic centres are located here, notably the respiratory and cardiovascular centres but also controls for the GIT. These centres act via the autonomic nervous system to control many essential involuntary processes. The medulla acts partly as an executive arm of the hypothalamus, which is the brain's principal integrating centre for homeostasis.

The reticular formation
This diffuse collection of tracts and nuclei permeating the brainstem monitors and modulates much of the brain's input and output. Before describing its two components it is necessary briefly to consider spinal pathways in general.

Conventionally, neural pathways are classified according to whether they carry information to the brain or to a higher centre within it, i.e. the **ascending** or afferent pathways, or signals down from the brain to the periphery, i.e the **descending** or efferent pathways. These subserve the input and output functions identified above.

Two main pathways carry the bulk of traffic. The afferent **spinothalamic** tract brings much of the sensory information from the periphery via the thalamus to the cortex (Figure 6.2). The **corticospinal tract** (also called the **pyramidal tract** from the anatomical appearance in cross-section, where left and right tracts cross in the medulla) carries the signals to the muscles, which execute the decisions taken by the brain. The corticospinal tract is routed via the cerebellum and it receives input from the BG (Figure 6.3).

Ascending reticular formation. Some fibres leave the spinothalamic tract as it ascends through the medulla, and run via the reticular

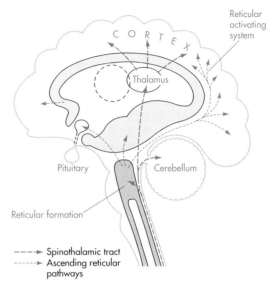

Figure 6.2   Main ascending pathways from periphery to brain.

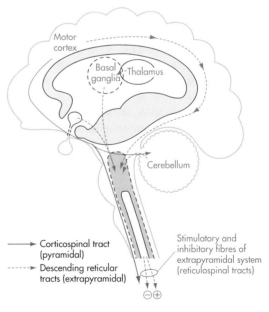

Figure 6.3   Main descending pathways from brain to muscles. Note: Only the main corticospinal efferent pathway is shown, and there are several others; the positions of pathways within the spinal cord are not intended to be anatomically accurate.

formation directly to other centres. For example, the limbic system receives information directly from the sense organs, enabling an emotional colouring to our perceptions, e.g. the fear associated with pain. Fibres to the hypothalamus allow it to act very quickly if necessary to maintain homeostasis. Output from the reticular system also bypasses the thalamus and projects directly into the cortex: this is the so-called **reticular activating system**, which is concerned with alertness and sleep.

This system may also have an important role in focusing attention because it allows unnecessary sensory 'noise' to be ignored. Clearly we are not conscious of all sensory input at all times. Just think about the messages from the various skin sensors in response to normal clothing: they are entirely ignored at the conscious level most of the time unless our attention is drawn to them. Conversely, recall how easily we are alerted, amid the noisy babble of a crowded room, the moment someone mentions our name. In a similar way the reticular formation may allow a mother to hear her baby crying in a distant room when nobody else does.

There has been speculation on the role of the ascending reticular formation in disordered perceptions, e.g. hallucinations. Although many psychotropic drugs act here, e.g. hypnotics and antipsychotics, it is difficult to link this with their clinical action.

Descending reticular formation. The descending reticular system, a vital component of overall motor function involved in the fine control and coordination, works in parallel to the corticospinal tract. The system passes signals from various brainstem reticular nuclei via reticulospinal tracts to synapses in the spinal cord with the motor neurones. These tracts run outside the main corticospinal tracts, hence the description extrapyramidal. There are both excitatory and inhibitory fibres, providing two net effects: smoothing of movement, and control of resting muscle tone that helps maintain posture.

This formation receives input from the BG (themselves connected to the motor cortex), the hypothalamus and cerebellum. The system obtains feedback on position and tone via afferents originating in the muscle spindles (proprioceptors) throughout the body. Some of these synapse in the spinal cord with the motor neurones, while others run directly to the cerebellum.

Psychiatry and neurology

It is surprisingly difficult to make an unambiguous distinction between these traditionally separate specialities. Put simply, psychiatry concerns disorders of thought, belief, perception and mood, while neurology is concerned with disorders of movement, sensation and intellect (Table 6.2). Thus psychiatrists deal with disorders of the 'mind', e.g. depression and schizophrenia, while neurologists are concerned with 'brain' disorders, e.g. parkinsonism, epilepsy and migraine. Unfortunately, some conditions exhibit both types of abnormality. For example, mood changes may occur in epilepsy, and intellectual and motor deficits may occur in schizophrenia.

Table 6.2   Distinction between psychiatry and neurology

Psychiatric disorder	Neurological disorder
Disorders of mood, thought, behaviour and perception	Disorders of movement, intellect and sensation
Primarily 'functional' in origin	Primarily 'organic'
Drugs commonly used	Drug therapy usually essential
Psychological treatment may be suitable	Surgery sometimes effective
Examples: anxiety, depression, mania, schizophrenia	Examples: epilepsy, stroke, extrapyramidal disorder, brain tumour, migraine

Looked at another way, neurological disease is generally felt to be caused by some **organic** (anatomical) lesion, whereas psychiatric disorder is **functional** – there is a problem with the way the mind functions but no identifiable structural defect. But epilepsy often has no obvious anatomical cause, and structural defects have been found in the brains of patients with schizophrenia. Changes in neurotransmitters, commonly found in CNS disorders, can be cited as evidence for either model. Moreover, there is a school of thought that regards psychiatric illness also as organic. Psychiatric disorders are generally treated by psychological means, e.g. psychotherapy and psychoanalysis, as well as with drugs, whereas surgery or drugs are usually appropriate for neurological disorders.

Although the two remain distinct medical specialities, reflecting the long intellectual tradition of mind–body dualism (see next section), increasingly the theoretical approaches to understanding the brain and its disorders are merging both disciplines. For this book, however, the traditional distinction will be observed.

Psychiatric disorder

Clinical aspects of psychiatric disorder

Definition

In considering psychiatry it is impossible to omit reference to the philosophical and sociological controversies surrounding the human mind and its malfunction. Is the dichotomy between mind (spirit, soul, etc.) and brain (a collection of neurones and chemicals, essentially a machine and therefore ultimately predictable) just a subjective artefact? Just what is meant by 'mental illness'? Behaviour, beliefs, personality types and so on vary greatly from culture to culture and in different times in history. Mental disorder might simply be regarded as behaviour that is unusual or unacceptable to most people in the society and at the time in which the 'patient' lives.

On a more practical level, a workable definition of mental illness needs to indicate when there is a need for intervention of some kind. It therefore needs to answer the question, when does a person becomes a potential patient? This is surely when they cannot cope with everyday life, or society cannot cope with them, because of their mental state. This then excludes unconventional, politically unacceptable or merely eccentric behaviour. In addition, most formal diagnostic definitions include a frequency or chronicity criterion, to distinguish the condition from reversible, temporary or secondary conditions; e.g. the symptoms must have been present for at least 6 months.

Classification

There have been countless attempts to classify mental illness and the situation changes constantly. The most widely accepted official classifications currently in use are the 10th edition of the International Classification of Disease (ICD-10) and the 4th edition of the American Diagnostic and Statistical Manual of Mental Disorders (DSM-IV). The system adopted in this chapter broadly represents a consensus of these two, with conflation or simplification where this aids understanding.

It is convenient to group psychiatric conditions into two broad types, **neurosis** and **psychosis**. As with most attempts to classify biological phenomena there is much overlap, and it must not be assumed that this classifies individual patients. Only a minority falls entirely at either end of the spectrum, showing all the classical features. Nevertheless, this distinction remains useful for differentiating the various syndromes of mental illness (Table 6.3).

Table 6.3   Classes of psychiatric disorder

	Neurosis	Psychosis
Insight	Present	Absent or reduced
Grasp of reality	Present	Absent
Hallucinations, delusions	Absent	Present
Symptoms resemble normal personality	Yes	No
Plausible external cause or precipitant	Present	Absent or incidental
Treatment options	Non-invasive possible	Invasive often necessary
Examples	Anxiety, obsession, mild depression	Schizophrenia, mania, severe depression

In general, patients with neurotic illness know they are ill and why others consider them so, and can see the effect it is having on themselves and those around them, i.e. they have insight. Although they are unable to control their symptoms, they retain a grasp of reality: they can reason and be reasoned with. They do not have **delusions**, i.e. fixed, false, irrational beliefs that they hold despite evidence to the contrary, after allowance for the context of their social or ethnic background, or **hallucinations**, i.e. false perceptions that are not perceived by anyone but them.

Thus chronically anxious patients, who are neurotic, might agree that it is foolish to worry so much, but claim that they cannot help it. There may well be something happening to them that most people would consider distressing, but their reaction seems excessive. They are likely to have been an anxious, worrying type of person even before they became ill. Such patients are often difficult to treat; they generally respond poorly to drugs, but perhaps better to psychotherapy.

People with schizophrenia, by contrast, are psychotic. They usually have very poor insight into their illness. However, it would be untrue to suppose that they do not know they are ill. They suffer miserably, partly from the vague feeling that others find them or their reported experiences strange. They often have beliefs or perceptions that others find bizarre or frankly incredible. The onset of the illness may be linked to some life event, but this may bear no direct relationship to the specific symptoms. Nor will the patient's prior personality, although they, or their relationships with others, may have seemed a trifle strange, e.g. the 'loner' child.

Ironically, the symptoms of psychosis are often easier to treat than those of neurosis, although it is unlikely that either type of disease can be fundamentally cured with current techniques.

Management

Treatment options

There are two broad categories of treatments:

- Invasive, such as drugs and electroconvulsive therapy (ECT).
- Non-invasive, including psychotherapy and conditioning methods.

These are compared in Table 6.4. The differences between these two approaches reflect the principal differences between two fundamental concepts of the causation of mental illness.

The **functional** concept assumes the problem is with the way a person thinks or feels; it is a matter of ideas and relationships. It follows

Table 6.4   Comparison of treatment options in mental illness

	Non-invasive methods	Invasive methods
Advantages	Represent a fundamental approach?	Rapid effect, cheap, relatively easy, predictable
Disadvantages	Slow effect, expensive and time-consuming, requires special skills, unpredictable, sometimes ineffective	Symptomatic relief only
Examples		
Neurosis	Anxiety management training Aversion therapy, desensitization Hypnosis, relaxation therapy Psychotherapy Counselling Group therapy, family therapy Cognitive therapy Psychoanalysis	Anxiolytics SSRIs, tricyclics MAOIs
Psychosis	Skills training Simple counselling Rehabilitation Group therapy, family therapy	Antipsychotics Lithium SSRIs, tricyclics ECT Psychosurgery

ECT, electroconvulsive therapy; MAOI, monoamine oxidise inhibitor; SSRI, selective serotonin re-uptake inhibitor.

that treatment methods should employ ideas, words, feelings and relationships; in short, psychotherapy.

Psychoanalysis is a form of psychotherapy in which the analyst explores the mental tensions or conflicts (complexes) that may underlie the psychiatric symptoms, especially anxiety. Causes are sought in experiences during infancy or childhood, or in family relationships. Psychoanalysis seeks to help the patient understand their problem on the assumption that resolution of the illness will follow. It is a lengthy, time-consuming and not always successful process. Simpler psychotherapeutic approaches often yield faster results, although some would argue that this represents a less fundamental solution.

Behaviour therapy takes a more pragmatic approach. A patient's illness behaviour is learned just like any other behaviour, i.e. it is conditioned. Being ill, and adopting the sick role, brings certain rewards, despite the suffering. Treatment should thus be aimed at modifying this behaviour, reducing its benefits as perceived by the patient.

The **materialistic** or **organic** concept of mental illness implies a distinct, and ultimately discoverable, anatomical or biochemical lesion; it is a matter of molecules. Thus drugs, physical traumas or manipulations, even including, rarely, the surgeon's knife, are seen to be appropriate.

As usual in the great schisms in science, probably the truth will ultimately be found to lie between the two extremes. Currently it seems that neuroses have a greater functional component and respond better to non-invasive methods, while psychoses are often associated with biochemical or structural defects and respond to invasive methods.

Nevertheless, either type of treatment can be appropriate and effective for either group of illnesses, depending on clinical factors. Most psychiatrists nowadays are eclectic. While non-invasive methods may be theoretically or humanely preferable, they may frequently be inadequate. For example, the first aim in treating severely depressed patients is to prevent them committing suicide, and psychotherapy is not rapid enough for this. Moreover, such patients may not have sufficient insight to allow this to be effective. Thus ECT has been found to be literally life-saving in such cases.

Diagnosis and management problems

The peculiar nature of disorders of the mind, and our incomplete knowledge of their causes, presents many problems in management (Table 6.5). Clearly, there is a difference between psychiatric diagnoses on the one hand and diagnosis of conditions such as asthma or diabetes mellitus on the other, because in the latter diseases there are agreed objective diagnostic criteria, and their pathology is relatively well understood. Further problems arise with pharmacotherapy, which are summarized in Table 6.6.

Anxiety

Definition

Anxiety is familiar to us all: the mouth dry, the heart pounding, 'butterflies in the stomach' and the sense of fear, panic or dread. It arises naturally in response to an anticipated threat of some kind and prepares us to meet that threat. The physical symptoms are part of the sympathetic nervous system's 'fright, fight or flight' response, and the

---

Table 6.5   Some problems in management of psychiatric disorders

Presentation	Often mixed, e.g. depression and restlessness
	May be masked, e.g. anxiety masked by depression
	Patient may deny illness, or compensate to mask it
Aetiology/pathology	Often unknown, so rational therapy difficult
Natural history	May be recurrent or self-limiting, so effect of treatment difficult to estimate
Diagnostic criteria	Subjective; international variation
Treatment modes	The most effective are often costly, risky or time-consuming
Compliance	Poor if patients often not fully aware of their illness

---

Table 6.6   Some problems with pharmacotherapy of psychiatric disorders

Mechanism	Mode of action of many psychotropic drugs not fully understood
Indications	Psychosis generally more responsive then neurosis
Biopharmacy/pharmacokinetics	Wide interpatient variation in drug handling
Efficacy	Often strong placebo effect
	Diagnostic uncertainties make assessment difficult
	No reliable animal models
Toxicity	Serious long-term side-effects
	Some psychiatric side-effects

subjective component (fright) is presumably a warning, rather like pain. Most are due to a rise in circulating adrenaline (epinephrine).

Anxiety then is a natural, healthy response of obvious biological value. Nowadays the kind of life-threatening dangers for which it was originally designed, like confronting wild animals, are rarely met. Instead, it has become adapted to modern life, helping us cope with less tangible stresses. These may be either **acute stress reactions**, like to public speaking, examinations or athletic competition, or more chronic **adjustment reactions**, like to unemployment or divorce. Many of us find that a certain amount of anxiety, the feeling of being properly keyed up, can improve our overall performance.

However, above a certain degree of stress and its resultant anxiety, performance levels off and then starts to decline rapidly (Figure 6.4). The point at which this happens varies from one individual to another: it is part of our personality. Some people have a low tolerance, worrying constantly and panicking easily: even quite a low stress level can impair their performance. Others, perhaps more laid-back, seem to be unmoved by normal stressors and can only work well under pressure, e.g. on the night before an examination. We also know that some people, with the so-called type A personality, are exceptionally active and seem to thrive on stress.

Normally the threat, actual or anticipated, that is generating the stress is real and would be regarded by anyone as worrying or potentially harmful. It is important to distinguish between the normal physiological response to this stress-related anxiety and the characteristics of an **anxiety disorder**. Pathological or 'clinical' anxiety, i.e. which is abnormal or counterproductive, can be thought of as occurring when:

- The threat is real but the response is out of proportion:
  - compared with the reaction of most people or
  - such that it interferes with normal functioning or everyday living.
- The threat is only imagined by the patient. It may take the form of a vague but oppressive feeling of impending doom that the patient cannot explain but which makes them anxious, worried or tense.

Thus, a pragmatic definition of anxiety disorder would be: a prolonged or exaggerated response to a real or imagined threat, which interferes with normal life.

The prevalence of anxiety disorder in the UK is estimated to be between 5% and 15% (depending on how it is defined), producing approximately 15% of GP consultations.

Pathophysiology

Figure 6.5 shows one way in which the mental and physical features of anxiety may be associated with the CNS structures discussed above. The perceived threat, if real, reaches the cortex through both the normal sensory pathways (spinal cord–thalamus–cortex) and the ascending reticular system (which runs to the limbic system).

The former path causes appropriate voluntary muscular action (e.g. flight) via the motor cortex, and the required endocrine and autonomic response (e.g. corticosteroid secretion and increased heart rate and blood pressure) via the hypothalamus and medulla. This would explain many of the symptoms associated with stress and anxiety. The limbic involvement accounts for the subjective feelings of fear or panic.

This may account for the low-tolerance type of anxiety, where the normal protective mechanisms are activated at a lower threshold than normal. But how might the anxiety caused by an imagined threat be explained? Possibly this

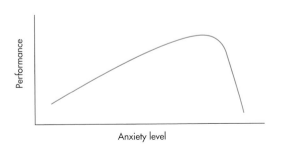

Figure 6.4 Hypothetical relationship between anxiety level and performance of tasks (arbitrary units).

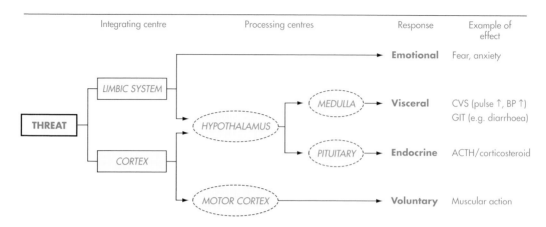

Figure 6.5 Possible pathways in the pathophysiology of anxiety. ACTH, adrenocorticotrophic hormone; BP, blood pressure; CVS, cardiovascular system; GIT, gastrointestinal tract.

originates in the limbic system, perhaps as a misinterpretation of sensory input. Impulses would then pass up to the cortex, with all the consequences of a real threat, including what are then inappropriate autonomic responses.

This might explain how chronic stress becomes associated with increased heart disease or peptic ulceration: the drive to these organ systems becomes excessive, prolonged and unnecessary. It also agrees with the finding that anxiolytic drugs act on the limbic system.

Theories of anxiety

The **psychoanalytic** or functional view of anxiety disorder is that it results from internal mental conflicts. These may arise from man's socialization, which demands the repression of primitive instincts, including the reproductive and sexual drives. This may result in inappropriate ideas or feelings in individuals who are unable to repress them effectively, and these should be susceptible to modification by psychotherapy.

The **biological** theories, on the other hand, hold that the cause is biochemical, e.g. an imbalance of amine neurotransmitters. One theory proposes that potentially anxious impulses arising in the limbic system are usually subject to inhibition via GABA-ergic and monaminergic impulses from the cortex. In anxiety there is reduced **GABA-modulin** activity, which allows

over-stimulation of the ascending reticular formation leading to excessive arousal; 5-HT receptors are also involved.

The success of drugs in controlling many of the symptoms of anxiety seems to support a biological model, but the two theories are not necessarily incompatible. Functional mental events would have to alter brain activity in order to achieve anything, and neurochemical changes would inevitably result. Thus, chemical interference would be expected to bring about a symptomatic improvement but not to affect the underlying cause. This is in accord with the apparent effect of anxiolytics in suppressing symptoms, and argues for an eclectic psychotherapeutic–pharmacotherapeutic approach to therapy.

Aetiology and classification

Both genetic and childhood developmental factors contribute to a predisposition to the illness, which usually starts in early adulthood. Environmental stressors and life events are frequently associated with its onset and persistence. In most cases the physical symptoms are similar; however, an understanding of the aetiology and also of the management is helped by classifying it according to the nature of the perceived threat and the severity and course of the illness (Tables 6.7 and 6.8).

Table 6.7   Classification[a] and features of common anxiety disorders

Class	Course	Severity[b]	Nature of threat	Features/examples
Stress-reaction (a) acute stress reaction	Acute	Usually mild	Real/plausible	Proportionate reaction to stressful life event, which will resolve itself, e.g. stage fright, examination nerves.
(b) adjustment reaction	Medium-term	Mild/severe	Real/plausible	Proportionate reaction to long-term situation, e.g. unemployment, chronic illness. Potentially reversible.
Generalized anxiety disorder (GAD)	Chronic, recurrent	Severe	Imagined, exaggerated or ill-defined	Pervasive feelings of threat or dread of ill-defined or unrealistic future events. Response disproportionate to threat; possibly related to patient's personality.
Panic disorder	Acute, recurrent	Very severe	Imagined, exaggerated or ill-defined	Sudden onset of severe disabling physical and psychiatric symptoms ('panic attack').
Post-traumatic stress disorder	Chronic	Severe	Real/plausible	Response to overwhelming events outside normal human experience, characterized by delayed chronic anxiety, avoidance behaviour and intrusive recollections (flashbacks or nightmares).
Phobia	Chronic, recurrent	Mild/severe	Imagined or exaggerated	Irrational, abnormal or excessive fear of an object or situation.
Obsessive–compulsive disorder	Chronic	Severe	Imagined or exaggerated	Irresistible bizarre thoughts or preoccupations associated with irresistible impulse to perform meaningless or ritualistic actions.
Mixed anxiety and depression	Chronic	Usually mild	Imagined, exaggerated or ill-defined	Mixture of mild anxiety and mild depression.

[a] This classification is based on the 10th edition of the *International Classification of Disease* (ICD-10) and the 4th edition of the *Diagnostic and Statistical Manual of Mental Illness* (DSM-IV).

[b] In respect of effect on patient's life or ability to cope.

Common forms of anxiety

The two international diagnostic systems (ICD-10 and DSM-IV) do not use identical classifications but largely agree on the major clinical forms.

Stress reactions arise from real external situations and are generally proportionate to them. Thus they represent a normal response to stress. Acute stress, e.g. stage fright, is usually short-term and may be relatively benign, rarely needing treatment. A key factor is that however unpleasant it is, there is a definite time when it will be over. The more chronic forms are known as **adjustment reactions**. The causes of this would be longer-term situations such as bereavement, which may also cause depression, or chronic illness or unemployment, where the anxiety arises from fear of future inability to cope. In some cases it might be expected to

Table 6.8   Other forms[a] of chronic anxiety

Class	Features/examples
Hypochondriasis	Obsession with and excessive concern for health in the absence of physical disorder.
Somatization (psychosomatic illness)	Genuine physical disorder, usually minor, brought about by mental conflicts, e.g. hyperacidity, palpitations, migraine, psychogenic pain.
Dissociative disorder (conversion disorder, hysteria)	Serious physical expression of mental conflicts as physical or psychiatric symptoms, in absence of physiological or pathological basis (e.g. blindness or paralysis).
Eating disorders	Anorexia nervosa (morbid fear of obesity, deliberate excessive weight loss, inappropriate body image). Bulimia nervosa (binge eating/vomiting; obsession with weight/shape).
Secondary anxiety	Physical illness, e.g. hyperthyroidism. Iatrogenic, e.g. caffeine, sympathomimetic, substance abuse.
Personality disorders	Enduring personal characteristics at extreme end of normal behavioural spectrum (e.g. obsessional, histrionic, schizoid, paranoid, dysthymic, cyclothymic)

[a] Based on the 10th edition of the *International Classification of Disease* (ICD-10) and the 4th edition of the *Diagnostic and Statistical Manual of Mental Illness* (DSM-IV).

resolve along with the external cause, but the sufferer may require some treatment to help manage the symptoms temporarily.

Most patients fall into the category of **generalized anxiety disorder**. There is a chronic, irrational, exaggerated but all-encompassing feeling of fear and worry. It may be unfocused or anticipate future illness, accident or poverty. Diagnosis depends on presence of symptoms for more than 6 months. It seems to be related to a person's personality, and tends to be chronic or recurrent. At its mildest it takes the form of chronic worry, but in its severest forms it can be disabling and merges into panic disorder. It may account for a third of all psychiatric consultations in general practice. It is frequently accompanied by depression.

In **panic disorder** there are sudden onsets of florid autonomic symptoms, extreme distress and often a paralysis of action or decision, usually with no discernible cause or evident stressful trigger. Patients may feel in imminent danger of death or insanity.

Post-traumatic stress disorder is a failure to adjust to or overcome a serious, life-threatening event and is characterized by recurrent sudden, panic-like symptoms associated with flashbacks.

Phobias or morbid fears are easily understood to be expressions of underlying anxiety. Examples are agoraphobia (the fear of going out, of crowds or of open spaces) and arachnophobia (fear of spiders). Recall that our definition of pathological anxiety involves the inability to cope. Thus simply being upset by spiders does not count: but if the sight or even just the anticipation of them disrupts everyday life, then there is a problem. However, the cultural and social context is also important: a fear of being eaten by a tiger might be phobic in Britain but a reasonable precaution in Bengal. Social phobia may be a form of agoraphobia. The sufferer is acutely fearful of public failure and humiliation and so avoids socializing and may cut themselves off.

Obsessional and **compulsive** states usually occur together. Obsessions are inescapable troubling thoughts: compulsions are irresistible, uncontrollable ritualistic actions. Like many neuroses they are related to the patient's personality. Obsessions are commonly seen in the rigid, inflexible person, overly concerned with neatness and order. For example, a patient obsessed by the idea of cleanliness, and perhaps their own impurity, may be compelled to wash their hands 20 or 30 times a day. **Hypochondriasis** is a particular form of obsessional disorder with a morbid fear of disease and inappropriate and inaccurate thoughts or ideas about the sufferer's own health. Such patients are constantly imagining themselves to be ill, serially consulting multiple health professionals, and self-medicating, when there is almost invariably no physical abnormality whatsoever. They may persuade doctors to carry out multiple invasive investigations but are never satisfied with the inevitable negative results. Hypochondriasis should not be confused with either **psychosomatic illness (somatization)**, when there are genuine physical symptoms, or **hysteria**, where there is little insight and the symptoms are dramatic (see below).

The commonly combined presentation of mild to moderate anxiety mixed with depression (**mild** or **mixed affective disorder**) is of particular importance to primary carers, including GPs and community pharmacists. It presents a diagnostic difficulty: is the patient depressed in reaction to prolonged anxiety, or perhaps anxious over the problems caused by their depression? The distinction in fact is not that important because as we shall see it does not influence management.

Insomnia, commonly associated with anxiety and other psychiatric illnesses, is a symptom rather than a discrete diagnosis. Nevertheless it may be a target for therapy, using hypnotics, which are largely the same range of drugs as used for anxiety.

Less common forms of chronic anxiety

A number of related neurotic syndromes with characteristic psychiatric symptoms are included in the wider definition of anxiety. They represent less common behavioural patterns with which the chronically anxious personality can present. They are summarized in Table 6.8 and a few will be briefly discussed here.

Psychosomatic illness (somatization) is not a discrete diagnosis, but frequently accompanies many psychiatric conditions including anxiety. In it there is a genuine physical dysfunction (usually autonomic) accounting for the symptoms, e.g. dyspepsia caused by gastric hypersecretion. The close relationship between the mind and the peripheral nervous system makes it easy to see how mental conflicts could alter physiological function in these cases. Indeed, psychosomatic symptoms may be the only indication that a patient is anxious: they may not complain of any mental stress, and it is the physical symptoms that are the declared reason for consultation. The clinician has to be astute enough to discern the underlying psychiatric disorder or risk merely treating the secondary symptoms.

Dissociative states usually start suddenly and dramatically, either as a neurological or neuro-muscular deficit (e.g. blindness or paralysis), or an altered state of consciousness (e.g. the amnesic patient found wandering aimlessly). However, no physical cause can be found, e.g. no problem with the eye, optic nerve or visual cortex in 'hysterical' blindness. Once again its origin seems to lie in mental conflict or instability, which is converted to a physical sign, hence the alternative term **conversion disorder**. The older term hysteria is now avoided to prevent confusion with lay concepts such as 'mass hysteria' and 'hysterical', which are quite different.

Possible causes of **secondary anxiety** must always be bone in mind when a patient first presents. Certain diseases (e.g. hyperthyroidism, phaeochromocytoma) can cause the physical symptoms of anxiety, as can certain drugs (e.g. excessive coffee consumption, alcohol or other drug abuse, adrenergic stimulants such as bronchodilators).

Clinical features

Anxiety is a neurotic disorder. The patient retains insight, is not deluded, and does not have hallucinations. They retain their grasp of reality and their illness can usually be related either to external events or their pre-illness personality. Anxiety is anticipatory (in that a future threat is perceived), whereas depression is generally retrospective.

As in all psychiatric illness the disease manifests itself as intangible features such as the patient's demeanour, body language, facial expression or phraseology: precisely measurable physical signs may be absent although there will be variable physical features. Thus great skill is needed in eliciting a psychiatric history. The presentation is highly variable but usually includes many of the following:

Psychiatric features:
- Feelings of apprehension, tension, fear, panic or terror, being 'on edge'.
- Hyper-arousal: excitability, labile mood, outbursts of hostility, insomnia.
- Circling thoughts, inability to concentrate, easily distracted, lapses of memory.

Physical (somatic) features:
- Cardiovascular: palpitations, bradycardia or tachycardia; elevated blood pressure; flushing or pallor.
- Respiratory: rapid shallow breathing (hyperventilation), or breathlessness (dyspnoea).
- Gastrointestinal: diarrhoea, dyspepsia, dysphagia, churning stomach.
- Musculoskeletal: agitation, restlessness, tremor, muscle tension.
- CNS: initial insomnia, i.e. difficulty in going to sleep.
- Metabolic: elevated blood glucose and glucocorticoids.
- Miscellaneous: excessive sweating, urge to defaecate or urinate.

This is clearly a picture of sympathetic nervous system over-activity; even the mental features resemble the central actions of adrenaline (epinephrine). However, psychiatric presentations in general may frequently be mixed, masked or disguised. An anxious patient may present as depressed (or vice versa), or the patient may complain only of the physical symptoms and deny any mental problem.

Course and prognosis

Stress-related anxiety has a generally good outlook as long as the external stressor can be eliminated or the sufferer learns to cope with it. Most other forms of primary anxiety disorder tend to follow a chronic relapsing course, with the most serious cases requiring the intermittent refuge of acute psychiatric units. An unfortunate minority of patients suffer from chronic disabling anxiety.

Management

Aims and strategy

The aims in managing anxiety are:
- to discover any immediate cause and deal with that if possible;
- to assess the severity;
- to relieve the patient's distress as soon as possible;
- to institute long-term, potentially curative treatment (in chronic anxiety).

Careful history taking and a full physical examination are important to eliminate any medical or iatrogenic causes. Family and social history are also vital. Any objective threat to the patient and its likely duration must be evaluated, as well as the patient's personality, the extent of their disability and their perceptions of the illness. It will often be necessary to address their social, economic or domestic situation.

If prompt symptomatic relief is felt essential, short-term pharmacotherapy may be indicated. However, some psychiatrists believe that this only helps patients to avoid confronting their problems and may be counter-productive in the long term. Nevertheless, drugs may enable the patient to benefit from psychotherapy because mood is stabilized, concentration improved, and the patient becomes more receptive.

Drugs obviously cannot alter the reality of unemployment, bereavement or a disastrous marriage. However, it is also vital to understand that drug therapy does nothing to alter the underlying problem in chronic anxiety. Similarly, drugs cannot cure phobias or obsessive–compulsive disorder; they merely suppress symptoms. However, the relief of temporary stress-related anxiety (e.g. stage fright or examination nerves) with appropriate drugs is simple, harmless and usually effective.

Non-drug therapy

In most cases the problem lies within the patient, so any hope of permanently overcoming the illness usually requires psychotherapy. Chronic anxiety may benefit from a combination of individual **counselling** (even a brief chat with a skilled counsellor can be very effective) and group therapy. **Cognitive behavioural therapy (CBT)** is now established as the method of choice for achieving long-term relief. It has a good evidence base and is recommended by NICE. It aims to help people understand situations that precipitate their symptoms and to devise strategies to deal with them. **Hypnosis** and **relaxation** therapies also have a place. Behavioural **conditioning** is sometimes helpful, e.g. desensitization for phobias, aversion therapy for compulsions. It has been found that, as an adjunct, providing patients with explanatory literature of an appropriate level can help significantly: this has been dubbed (rather grandly) **bibliotherapy**. **Psychoanalysis** is an option less commonly used in Europe than in North America.

Admission to a psychiatric unit may in itself sometimes be therapeutic, simply by removing the patient from a stressful domestic situation. However, some patients are regularly admitted this way. They recover partially and are returned after a few weeks or months to a life they cannot cope with, only to be re-admitted a few months later, and so on: the so-called **revolving door** phenomenon.

Psychiatric care requires a team approach, utilizing community nurses, social services, occupational therapists and clinical psychologists to improve the patient's social, domestic or economic circumstances – often a difficult task. It is also expensive compared to drug therapy and requires resources that are not always available. Thus many patients may not get optimal care.

Drug therapy

Benzodiazepines

The initial enthusiasm for the benzodiazepines as universal panaceas (based – with some justifi-cation – on their great advantages over the barbiturates) has now cooled. Although they cause little generalized CNS depression and are remarkably safe in overdose, both dependence and withdrawal symptoms are now known to be quite common. Their association with accidents and falls is also serious.

Action

The wide range of benzodiazepines available obscures the fact that there are few differences between them except in their pharmacokinetics. They all probably act at specific benzodiazepine receptors by enhancing the inhibitory activity of GABA at its receptors in many central and spinal sites, including the reticular activating system. Thus, they have a wide range of actions and that makes them very useful drugs in the right circumstances. The anxiolytic action is quite selective for the limbic system at low doses, with only a small, but not insignificant, effect on cognition and coordination; hence the rather unsatisfactory description 'minor tranquillizers' (the antipsychotic drugs being the 'major tranquillizers'). At higher doses this selectivity is lost and they act as hypnotics (sleep inducers).

Benzodiazepines have other very useful actions. They are muscle-relaxant and anticonvulsant: IV *lorazepam* is the drug of choice for status epilepticus. Parenteral use enables premedication and light general anaesthesia for minor procedures such as endoscopy, with the added benefit of short-term amnesia that covers the period of these disagreeable experiences. They are also useful adjuncts in anti-emetic regimens to cover cancer chemotherapy and are used in alcohol withdrawal therapy and for delirium tremens.

Tolerance develops during use owing to receptor down-regulation, although this should have little impact when used in the short courses currently recommended.

Pharmacokinetics

Benzodiazepines are lipophilic drugs that have good bioavailability, are widely distributed throughout the body and are avidly bound to plasma protein. They are cleared almost exclusively by the liver, the inactive glucuronide being eliminated renally. The principal difference between them is in their metabolism (Table 6.9). The shorter-acting agents (e.g. *temazepam*) are metabolized directly to an inactive form, and have half-lives of 3–15 h. The longer-acting drugs (e.g. *diazepam*) have one or more active intermediates and thus may have effective biological half-lives of up to 100 h.

One result, which is often overlooked, is that the longer-acting benzodiazepines may take several weeks to reach steady-state plasma levels. If the dose is increased too frequently during this period there will be accumulation, although the cumulative effect is to some extent offset by the development of tolerance (above). This can also occur with normal dosing in the elderly, in whom the half-lives given in Table 6.9 may be increased up to threefold. Similarly, the effects of the long-acting agents persist for similar periods after discontinuation.

Advantages

Comparison of the benzodiazepines with their predecessors, the barbiturates, explains their initial appeal to prescribers (Table 6.10). They are

Table 6.9   Comparison of some representative benzodiazepines

Half-life (h, approx.)[a]	Drug	Comment
Very short (<4)	Midazolam	Light parenteral anaesthetic
Short (4–12)	Temazepam Loprazolam Alprazolam	
Medium (12–20)	Lorazepam Oxazepam Bromazepam	
Long (>20)	Chlordiazepoxide Nitrazepam Diazepam Flurazepam	The original 'Librium' 'Mogadon' 'Valium'
Very long (>50)	Clobazam Clorazepate	Anticonvulsant Anticonvulsant

[a] Half-life likely to be much prolonged in the elderly.

Table 6.10   Advantages and disadvantages of benzodiazepines

Advantages	Disadvantages and side-effects
Effective as hypnotic/anxiolytic (symptomatic relief)	Tolerance, habituation, dependence
Specific anxiolytic effects	Subtle cognitive and psychomotor impairment
Safe in overdose	Withdrawal effects (especially short-acting agents)
Few interactions	May produce unnatural sleep pattern/sleep debt Paradoxical excitement Amnesia (may be beneficial – see text)

selective, and largely avoid drowsiness at therapeutic doses. In addition, they are extremely safe in overdose because they do not cause depression of the respiratory or other medullary centres. Death from benzodiazepine over-dosage alone is uncommon; the drugs rarely produce more than a light coma, from which the patient can be aroused.

Habituation, dependence and withdrawal phenomena were initially thought to be rare. Interactions are few. Benzodiazepines neither induce liver enzymes nor have their metabolism significantly affected by other drugs that induce or inhibit liver enzymes. They do not displace other drugs from plasma protein binding sites.

Disadvantages

The validity of many of these favourable initial impressions has been eroded. Benzodiazepines do cause unwanted CNS depression, especially a subtle impairment of motor coordination that is often unnoticed by the patient. This is thought to be implicated in a growing number of road traffic accidents. In the elderly particularly, the longer-acting agents sometimes cause paradoxical excitement, giddiness, confusion or aggression, owing to disinhibition.

Serious interactions with other CNS depressants can occur, producing potentially fatal respiratory depression. An important example is with opioids or alcohol, or both: this cocktail is commonly used in deliberate overdoses. Respiratory depression can also occur with benzodiazepines alone when used in otherwise compromised patients, such as the elderly, the very young, or those with respiratory impairment.

Flumazenil injection, a specific benzodiazepine competitive antagonist, is available to reverse overdoses rapidly.

Dependence and drug-seeking behaviour and abuse, related to down-regulation of GABA receptors, are being increasingly recognized as major problems. Withdrawal symptoms seem to be more common with the short-acting benzodiazepines, especially if they are stopped abruptly, probably because of the subsequent rapid fall in plasma level. Dependence may occur after as little as 4–6 weeks, and up to half of patients may become dependent after 3 months of continuous treatment. Currently the BNF recommends courses no longer than 4 weeks except in very exceptional circumstances.

Weaning patients off benzodiazepines is not easy, if it can be done at all. One recommended procedure is to convert the patient to *diazepam* at an equipotent daily dose (see BNF), and then reduce the dose by one-eighth of this every fortnight. Complete withdrawal can take many months.

Certain patients seem particularly prone to dependence, notably those with compliant, passive, dependent or anxious personalities, who tend to abuse prescription medication in low doses over long periods. Another group, characterised as impulsive, antisocial and more psychotic than neurotic, may abuse illicitly obtained benzodiazepines recreationally, in larger doses but with less likelihood of dependence. Pharmacists in the UK are becoming actively involved in monitoring the use of benzodiazepines and countering their misuse.

When used as hypnotics, benzodiazepines produce abnormal sleep patterns and cause a rebound sleep debt on withdrawal. There is a hangover effect from all but the shortest-acting agents.

Indications and use

The longer-acting benzodiazepines should be started cautiously with small dose increments. When stopping treatment, the dose should be reduced slowly, especially with the short-acting drugs (but see above).

A shorter-acting benzodiazepine is preferred for the elderly, for those with liver disease and for daytime use generally, even if this means more doses per day. Longer-acting drugs may be beneficial if compliance is doubtful, if the shorter-acting ones do not provide enough sleep, or if a combination of hypnotic effect and next-day sedation is desired. Doses in the elderly should start at one-quarter the usual adult dose.

The choice of agent and dose should be tailored carefully to the patient because of individual variations in clearance, response, residual effects and concurrent medication. If these precautions are observed, the value of benzodiazepines will be retained without incurring the potentially serious problems.

Other agents used in anxiety

Apart from in severe disabling acute anxiety, benzodiazepines are avoided. There are several alternatives.

Antidepressants, particularly the selective serotonin re-uptake inhibitors (SSRIs), are now the drugs of choice for many forms of chronic anxiety, primarily because of the involvement of serotonin in anxiety. Their specific antidepressant action is also helpful in mixed anxiety and depression, but effectiveness does not depend on the presence of a diagnosis of depression. Although not addictive like benzodiazepines, antidepressants do have common and distressing adverse effects (see below).

Starting dosage is lower than in primary depression (pp. 399–400) because of a risk of briefly exacerbating the anxiety, with gradual increments to the usual maxima. Owing to the slow onset of action of antidepressants (3–4 weeks), and an initial increase in anxiety symptoms, patients with acute severe problems may need initial cover with a short course of benzodiazepines. Treatment is assessed at 12 weeks and if ineffective, changed to a tricyclic antidepressant. Otherwise treatment may last up to 6 months, followed by gradual withdrawal (see p. 400).

Buspirone, a partial 5-HT agonist, is anxiolytic but not hypnotic. It is probably less liable to habituation than benzodiazepines. Its main drawback is a slow onset of activity. It must be titrated up to an effective dose and then a further 2–4 weeks are needed for full effect. This makes it unsuitable for the treatment of acute anxiety. However, it may be a suitable alternative where benzodiazepine-like activity is required beyond 1 month.

Beta-blockers are useful for pronounced adrenergic physical symptoms in some patients with stress-related anxiety such as stage fright. In addition they may indirectly reduce the associated psychiatric symptoms by sparing patients further concern about the physical symptoms. However, beta-blockers are less useful in general anxiety or panic disorder. Their principal advantages are that they can be used for long periods if necessary and have no general sedative effect.

Hypnotics

Alternatives to benzodiazepines as hypnotic drugs are the chemically distinct 'Z-drugs' (e.g. *zopiclone*, *zaleplon* and *zolpidem*), which also act on benzodiazepine receptors. They appear to offer little advantage, have similar adverse effects and are equally likely to produce dependence. Other sedative drugs sometimes used include first-generation sedative antihistamines (e.g. *promethazine*, *hydroxyzine*), chloral derivatives (e.g. *dichloralphenazone*) and antipsychotics in low doses. Barbiturates are now restricted to anaesthesia and continuing medication for epileptic patients long stabilized on *phenobarbital*. NICE recommends the short-term use of hypnotics, either benzodiazepines or Z-drugs, only after non-pharmacological methods have proved ineffective.

Drug selection

Drug therapy has only a limited role in the management of anxiety. It should usually be restricted to short periods and have specific, agreed end points, e.g. to cover an acutely distressing or disabling temporary exacerbation of the patient's circumstances. However, some chronic anxiety disorders may require up to 6 months of treatment. It must then be monitored closely to ensure that the drug is withdrawn when the specific indications resolve. For most types of anxiety the evidence of effectiveness is in the following sequence:

psychotherapy → [+? short-term benzodiazepine] → longer-term antidepressant

Psychotherapy is always preferred, but the rapid effectiveness of short-term benzodiazepines in severe acute situations allows other therapies time to start working. In particular circumstances more specific recommendations can be made (see below).

Stress-related anxiety
Short courses of anxiolytics can be very useful in acute conditions where the patient definitely needs support for a brief period before a specific stressful event. There is insufficient time for psychotherapy to produce an effect, and the dura-

tion of drug therapy is usually too short for dependence to develop, so that the benzodiazepines could be used. If the symptoms are mainly somatic (palpitations, gastrointestinal upset, tremor) beta-blockers are preferable, as they would be in situations when benzodiazepine adverse effects would be disadvantageous (e.g. musicians, actors, examination candidates). For chronic adjustment reactions, antidepressants are indicated.

Where the anxiety is secondary to an underlying medical condition (e.g. thyrotoxicosis) or drug use or misuse, obviously the aim is to diagnose and correct that.

Generalized anxiety disorder (GAD)

This category perhaps presents the greatest dangers for inappropriate drug treatment. The temptation is strong to suppress the patient's unwelcome, distressing symptoms continuously with drugs – which seem so effective – rather than uncover the true cause of the patient's problems. This is particularly so if the problems stem from an adverse social environment, such as poverty or marital distress, when the clinician may feel frustrated by their inability to tackle the underlying difficulties. However, this temptation should be resisted. Short courses of anxiolytic drugs have a place in stabilizing the patient, but the only chance of a permanent solution is to address these underlying problems. The alternative is the 'revolving door phenomenon' and anxiolytic dependence.

The idea of the 'pill for every ill' society is based mainly on the misguided drug treatment of this category of illness. The prevailing belief in the West seems to be that all distress must be avoided, all stress reactions are pathological, and life must be perpetually serene. In his *Brave New World*, Aldous Huxley prophesied and ruthlessly satirized this idealistic philosophy. Modern-day critics also claim that too frequent recourse to drugs reduces people's capacity to confront stressful situations and may mask wider sociopolitical causes. There are Valium Anonymous groups in the USA and TRANX in the UK to counter this attitude and help those who are benzodiazepine-dependent.

With growing recognition of the problems with the benzodiazepines, attention has turned to other forms of treatment. In the medium and long term, SSRIs or *venlafaxine* are far more effective than benzodiazepines and are now drugs of choice. Indeed NICE specifically advises against benzodiazepines. One notable exception is in serious organic illness and pain (Chapter 7), especially cancer, where relief of symptoms becomes the prime objective.

Psychotherapy is essential for the long term management of GAD; even so, it is not always successful.

Panic

For acute panic attacks a short course of anxiolytic therapy is often used, but this is not recommended by NICE for panic disorder. Longer-term prophylactic treatment requires antidepressants: SSRIs, the tricyclic *clomipramine*, and MAOIs are effective. However, psychotherapy (such as anxiety management or CBT) may be useful, to try to tackle the underlying problem.

Post-traumatic stress disorder; obsessive–compulsive disorder (OCD); phobias

Generally all three are treated similarly. SSRIs are the drugs of choice, usually in higher than normal dosage, followed by tricyclics then MAOIs. *Clomipramine* is licensed for the treatment of obsessive–compulsive disorders. MAOIs are effective in phobias.

Mixed anxiety and depression

Antidepressants, preferably those with a sedative action, are especially useful here, as opposed to anxiolytics.

Affective disorder: depression

Most people experience a depressed mood from time to time. Feelings of sadness are an appropriate response to a recent loss or disappointment, but they are expected to remit spontaneously sooner or later, depending on the personality of the sufferer and the cultural norms of their society.

As with all psychiatric conditions this normal response must be distinguished from an illness.

One criterion is whether it is so severe as to be socially incapacitating or whether the patient can cope. Another is whether the sufferer's culture regards the apparent cause as meriting a period of such depressed mood. Grieving for a close relative is a good example: almost all cultures recognize a period of mourning, although the acceptable duration varies greatly. In the UK, perhaps 6 months to a year is regarded as normal for a spouse. Much less would seem callous, but to dwell on it for much longer, remaining pessimistic, tearful and unable to function, would be regarded as abnormal.

On the other hand, someone who was depressed but whose life gave no apparent evidence of substantial adverse events would be regarded as suffering from a morbid, or 'clinical', depression. This distinction must be reflected in the classification of depression. It is also necessary to identify cases where there is an underlying primary medical or iatrogenic cause, to which the depression is secondary.

Note that in psychiatry the term 'affect' is an objective description of a person's transient emotional behaviour, whereas mood describes their prevailing subjective emotional state. Conventionally, affective disorder includes illnesses with abnormally high or low mood, i.e. mania and depression. Although it might seem logical to include anxiety, the complexity of anxiety disorder has always meant that it is considered as a separate major category of mental illness.

Classification and course

The difficulty in classifying depression is that it occurs in numerous forms, and different systems of classification use different criteria to distinguish between them. The range of criteria used by different classifications include:

*   Severity.
*   Presence or absence of physical (somatic or biological) features.
*   Presence or absence of psychotic features.
*   Course (duration and recurrence).
*   Presence or absence of intervening manic phases.

The first three criteria apply to a single depressive or manic episode, while the last two describe a pattern of recurrence (the course or natural history). Taken together, these represent the basis of the current ICD classification (Figure 6.6).

A depressive episode usually lasts between 3 and 12 months but a fifth of episodes last more

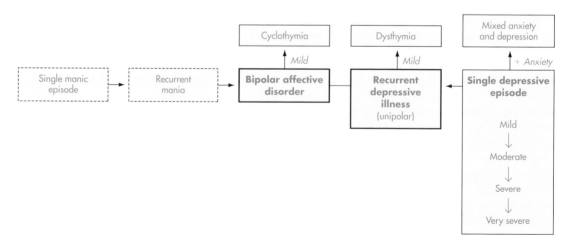

Figure 6.6   Classification of affective disorders (based on the 10th edition of the *International Classification of Disease, ICD-10*). More common conditions in bolder type.

than 2 years. A patient with the recurrent form suffers on average four episodes over their lifetime. About half of patients only ever experience a single episode, which can then be differentiated on the basis of its severity (see below). Others experience a persistent mild depression for much of their adult lives, which may be a feature of their personality. This is **dysthymia** or **chronic affective disorder**, and it may be interspersed with more severe exacerbations, when it is known as **double depression**; one-quarter of major depressive episodes occur against a background of dysthymia.

More commonly, depressive episodes, although naturally self-limiting, are prone to recurrence. A distinction is then made on the basis of whether the patient also suffers episodes of unnaturally elevated mood known as **mania**; this is **bipolar affective disorder** (pp. 405–408). A milder form, **cyclothymia**, is seen in persons subject to alternating periods of elevated or depressed mood outside what is considered as normal mood variation. Such persons are able to cope with the illness usually without resort to psychiatric support. Both cyclothymia and dysthymia are sometimes regarded as mild forms of personality disorder (see Table 6.8).

In **unipolar affective disorder** there are recurrent episodes of depression or (far more rarely) mania, with periods of remission. With unipolar **recurrent depressive illness**, which is probably the largest single category, each episode is insidious in onset, developing over the course of months, and lasting for months or even years. Many patients with apparent unipolar disease prove on closer examination to have bipolar illness, which is now regarded as more common than formerly.

In some cases there are only brief recurrent depressive episodes, although each is severe. In **seasonal affective disorder (SAD)**, depression recurs in the winter months, with either normal or hypomanic mood (p. 404) in the spring and summer. A depressive episode, particularly the milder form, may coexist with anxiety, when the description **mixed anxiety and depression** is appropriate (p. 379).

Thus affective disorder should be regarded as a continuum or spectrum of conditions rather than a collection of unique ones. At either end are episodes of either mania or depression; in between are various combinations in different degrees of severity and patterns of occurrence.

Secondary depression can be caused by some antihypertensive drugs, e.g. *methyldopa*, *clonidine*, some beta-blockers, steroids (including oral contraceptives), and many CNS depressants such as benzodiazepines, opioids and alcohol. It also occurs secondary to dementia, stroke, Parkinson's disease, hypothyroidism, other psychiatric conditions (schizophrenia, alcoholism) and many serious chronic diseases, especially those involving pain (e.g. cancer, RA).

Epidemiology

Affective disorders comprise about half of all psychiatric morbidity. Epidemiological statistics for depression are difficult to obtain because of the different definitions and the fact that most depression is encountered in primary care or is frequently unrecognized. About 20% of us develop a depressive episode at some stage in our life and in a quarter of cases it becomes chronic. The prevalence of major depression is approximately 5%. About a quarter of all depression is bipolar.

Only 1 in 20 cases is referred to secondary care, the remainder being handled by GPs, 1 in 10 of whose consultations probably involve depression. Half of these patients will only have a few minor depressive symptoms, which may well be missed, while one-quarter will have severe depression. Depression is two to three times more common in women and its prevalence increases with age.

Depression is frequently associated with other psychiatric morbidity or substance abuse, notably alcohol. Thus it must be regarded as a chronic illness, with all the implications for continuing care that this brings. Only IHD has a greater cost in disability-adjusted life-years. It increases mortality, principally from suicide.

Aetiology

As might be expected, there are both biochemical and psychological theories.

Biochemical theories

Most biochemical or organic theories of depression involve abnormalities in central monoamines or their receptors. However, the situation is still unclear and only a brief outline is given here.

The traditional model was deduced from several observations. First, depression is an adverse effect of the now obsolete antihypertensive *reserpine*, a non-specific central amine depleter. Second, the tricyclic antidepressants act by preventing amine re-uptake (following release at the nerve terminal) and hence could counteract such depletion. Thirdly, MAOIs, which enhance amine levels, are effective antidepressants. The amines believed to be most involved are serotonin (5-HT) and the catechol noradrenaline (norepinephrine); more recently, dopamine has been implicated.

Owing to its role in mood control, the limbic system is the most likely location of the abnormality. Both transmitters are found there and the levels of one or other, or both, are affected by most (but not all) antidepressants. Moreover, 5-HT is known to be involved in hypothalamic function, which could account for the sleep and appetite abnormalities of depression.

This theory has become considerably modified. The tricyclics have been found to cause amine receptor subsensitivity (down-regulation) which takes about the same time to develop as the antidepressant effect, i.e. 2–4 weeks. MAOIs and ECT have a similar action. This provides a plausible explanation of the hitherto puzzling delay in the therapeutic action of antidepressants, because amine re-uptake block occurs within hours of entry of antidepressants into the CNS. On this newer model, depressed mood is associated with an initial increase in receptor sensitivity. Amine depletion could then be explained as a compensatory fall in amine release to reduce receptor stimulation. Alternatively, depression could represent the failure of a compensatory down-regulation mechanism that normally restores emotional stability.

It is likely that these various transmitters are interlinked along the polysynaptic neural pathways involved, so that action at one type could have secondary consequences on others. We are still a long way from understanding depression at the molecular level.

Metabolic markers

The diagnostic difficulties of depression have provoked a long search for a biochemical or metabolic marker so that the degree of depression could be measured simply and reliably, like blood glucose in diabetes mellitus. The identification of such a marker might also provide an insight into aetiology.

Thyroid function was an early candidate in view of the depression associated with hypothyroidism, which must always be a differential diagnosis in assessing affective disorder. There is some correlation between depression and TSH release. There is a better, but still insufficiently consistent or specific, association between depression, raised serum cortisol and a reduced suppression of corticosteroid secretion by *dexamethasone* (the dexamethasone suppression test). However, this may be secondary to the feeding and sleep disturbances of depression. Neither measure is clinically useful.

At one time it was hoped that measuring the level of a metabolite of brain catechols, 3-methoxy-4-hydroxy-phenylethylene glycol (MHPG) would yield specific information about central amine turnover. If the depression were associated with a catecholamine depletion, then urine or CSF levels of MHPG would be low: a 5-HT deficit on the other hand would not affect the MHPG level. It is also possible, though less practicable, to measure CSF levels of 5-HT, which are frequently found to be low in depression. These measurements should then have an important bearing on drug treatment because some antidepressants selectively block noradrenaline (norepinephrine) re-uptake (e.g. *reboxetine*) while others block 5-HT re-uptake (e.g. *fluoxetine*). They might also predict when tryptophan would be a logical replacement therapy. Unfortunately this approach too has proved inconsistent, and more pragmatic considerations still determine drug selection.

Mood disorders are frequently seasonal. Depression is usually more prevalent in the spring, but in SAD it occurs each winter. Lack of sunlight is an important aetiological factor in this. Abnormalities in melatonin metabolism may be involved because melatonin secretion is suppressed by light, and in manic depressive patients (p. 403) this response is augmented. However, the relationship between melatonin and mood is unknown.

Functional theories

An alternative to this reductionist biochemical approach is the functional or psychoanalytic one, where unconscious mental conflicts are thought to be the cause of the disease (p. 373).

It is likely that a synthesis of these two approaches will eventually prevail, though at present the biochemical model probably provides a better explanation of major depression, while minor depression seems better accounted for in terms of mental conflicts and personality, or illness behaviour. A family history of depression in this respect tells us little, because the family environment is as likely as genes to influence personality development.

Genes versus environment

A family history is common in depression. Environmental factors such as social class, unemployment, domestic pressures and childhood experiences are also important. The contribution of each factor varies from patient to patient.

Although a serious loss or disappointment does not always precede major depression, an adverse or stressful event is frequently found in the patient's recent premorbid history. However, a careful history is necessary, including information from friends or relatives, to reduce the likelihood of confusing cause with effect. A depressed patient may first present with many problems in their life, any of which might plausibly have been the immediate cause of their depression. It is necessary to establish whether any did in fact predate their illness, or if they are all the consequences of depression. It may eventually become evident that there was no discernible specific trigger for the initial onset of symptoms.

Clinical features

When summarizing the various clinical features of depression it may be more helpful to adopt a pragmatic approach based primarily on severity.

Psychiatric spectrum

Traditionally, depressive episodes were divided into two broad groups depending on the presence or absence of psychotic features: this roughly correlates with severity. The milder forms resemble an exaggerated response to an adverse life event that might be expected to depress anyone to a certain extent, such as bereavement, but with which the patient is unable to cope. As such it is referred to as **minor depression**. However, the description 'minor' should not be taken to imply that, for the patient, the depression is somehow more bearable.

This was previously known as neurotic or reactive depression; the term 'reactive' being used to emphasize that the depression is a response to a life event, or that the patient still retains the ability to react emotionally to normal everyday events.

Minor depression is analogous to stress-related anxiety neurosis in that both are associated with real events and insight is preserved. However, depression is generally retrospective, whereas anxiety is anticipatory.

At the other extreme are patients with **severe** or **major depression**, where there are no obviously adverse events in the recent past. Such patients become depressed for reasons they do not understand and they have poor insight into their condition. This form is usually associated with a number of metabolic and physical (somatic) features and may or may not involve psychotic symptoms such as delusions. It is still sometimes referred to as biological or endogenous depression, and sometimes the poetic medieval (originally Greek) description melancholia is revived.

Figure 6.7 illustrates in a simplified manner how this distinction parallels some of the more important features of depressive illness. However, things are rarely as simple as this would imply and the distinctions are somewhat artificial. Biological variables within a population tend to occur as finely graded differences rather than clearly defined categories. The majority of patients appear somewhere on the continuum between the two extremes, at different points for different features, at different times in the course of their illness. Thus, a patient may have a strong family history and some delusions of guilt, but have an acute onset triggered by bereavement.

Severity

For a single depressive episode an alternative approach is to look at common presentations of the symptomatology at different degrees of severity (Figure 6.8). The core features of depression, present even in the mildest form, are:

- Depressed mood (dysphoria) with pessimism (especially regarding the likelihood of recovering) and frequent tearfulness.
- Loss of interest and capacity for enjoyment (anhedonia).
- Lethargy and fatigue.

Patients may suffer a variety of additional neurotic symptoms similar to those seen in anxiety. There are sleep and appetite disturbances and somatization (psychosomatic) problems such as constipation or dyspepsia. Anorexia is common, perhaps as an expression of general loss of interest in life's pleasures, but also possibly resulting from alterations in hypothalamic function. Patients tend to feel sorry for themselves but not guilty, i.e. 'What have I done to deserve this?' rather than 'I deserve this as punishment'.

The mood of patients with **mild to moderate depression**, although predominantly low, is labile, tending to fluctuate to some extent in reaction to the minor everyday joys and disappointments of life. They have difficulty getting off to sleep, i.e. initial insomnia or increased sleep latency, as seen in anxiety. They lose the capacity to initiate any action, and find making even quite trivial decisions difficult.

There is a marked loss of drive, vitality, ambition, libido and zest for life – a loss of appetite for more than just food. Patients have difficulty

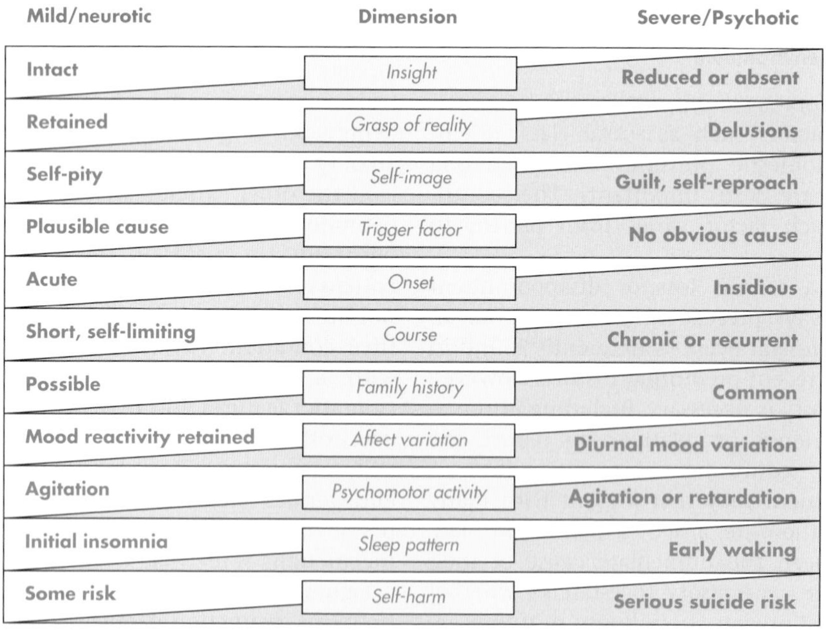

Mild/neurotic	Dimension	Severe/Psychotic
Intact	Insight	Reduced or absent
Retained	Grasp of reality	Delusions
Self-pity	Self-image	Guilt, self-reproach
Plausible cause	Trigger factor	No obvious cause
Acute	Onset	Insidious
Short, self-limiting	Course	Chronic or recurrent
Possible	Family history	Common
Mood reactivity retained	Affect variation	Diurnal mood variation
Agitation	Psychomotor activity	Agitation or retardation
Initial insomnia	Sleep pattern	Early waking
Some risk	Self-harm	Serious suicide risk

Figure 6.7   Clinical spectrum of depression. This shows the range of psychiatric and physical features (dimension) usually found in depression, and their presence, absence or quality for depressive episodes of different severity. For each feature the left-hand end represents the less serious form. An individual patient may be at different points along the spectrum for each feature. Few are wholly at one end or the other for all dimensions.

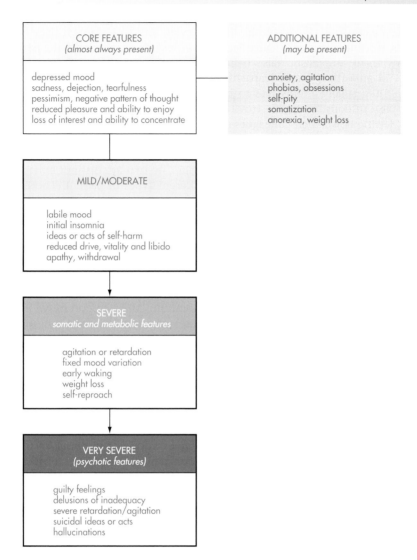

Figure 6.8   Clinical features of depressive episodes. This illustrates the general trend in episodes of depression of increasing severity. An individual patient may show a mix of features from the different stages represented here.

concentrating and suffer selective memory impairment; past mistakes in particular are forgotten, or repressed. There is a persistently negative approach to everything.

In **severe depression**, more physical (somatic) and metabolic features become evident. There may also be psychomotor impairment – either agitation, or conversely, mild retardation of thought, speech and action. Patients wake early, at 4 or 5 a.m. feeling at their worst, but things improve slightly by evening. Mood variation tends to become fixed in this pattern, whatever

the day brings. Rather than feeling sorry for themselves they somehow blame themselves for their plight: guilt, self-reproach and feelings of worthlessness are common. Because marital problems can follow the reduced libido, and impaired performance at work result from the loss of drive, the patient's low self-esteem is reinforced and justified: it becomes a self-fulfilling prophecy.

Very severe depression is accompanied by intensification of signs and symptoms, with worsening of agitation or retardation. Psychotic features also become apparent. For example, the general feeling of worthlessness and inadequacy becomes a firmly fixed, unrealistic false belief that no amount of appeals to reason can shift (i.e. a delusion). They believe themselves to be guilty, 'bad people', responsible for destroying their family and letting down their colleagues at work. These delusions may (although rarely), be reinforced with another classic psychotic sign, hallucinations (false perceptions). They may hear voices chastising them for the evil or corrupt person they believe themselves to be.

Thus it is possible to get an inkling of how people may be driven to what is, in biological terms, the highly anomalous behaviour of intentional self-harm or even self-destruction. The perpetual misery, the firm conviction that you are causing serious problems for people around you, including loved ones, and the belief that things will not improve, makes suicide an appealing, almost logical option for them.

Suicide and self-harm

There are some 5000 successful suicides a year in the UK. About 75% of these involve mental illness, mostly depression but also alcoholism, personality disorder and schizophrenia. Depressed patients are about 25 times more likely than others to attempt suicide, and 15% will eventually succeed. Prevention of suicide and attempts to change suicidal ideas are major targets in the management of depression.

In the UK, drug overdose is the usual means (up to 90% of cases) in both suicide and deliberate self-harm. Since barbiturates have become unavailable, the risk of serious consequences from drug overdose should have been reduced. However, the barbiturates have been superseded, and possibly exceeded in danger, by *paracetamol* (acetaminophen), which is freely available and hence widely believed to be safe. Yet as few as 20 paracetamol tablets can have the tragic unintended outcome of fatal liver failure. Overall, paracetamol and other analgesics are the most common choice, presumably because of ease of access (30%); sedatives are used in 15% of cases and antidepressants in 10%. Alcohol use is also involved in over half of drug overdoses. The major advantage of the SSRIs over the older

tricyclic antidepressants is their relative safety in overdose: this ameliorates the paradox that some of the most toxic medication is given to the groups of patients most likely to overdose on medication.

It is important to distinguish between **suicide**, which is intentional successful self-inflicted death, and **deliberate self-harm (DSH)**, which is deliberate self-inflicted injury (formerly parasuicide); the two are distinct entities presented by different types of patient. Those who decide to commit suicide are likely to be thorough: they will fail only through ignorance or chance, and when successful it is known as completed suicide. They plan the suicide carefully for weeks so that it almost becomes an obsession. Although ostensibly keeping it secret, they may well give covert, even unconscious hints of their intention. More importantly, if asked directly they will usually admit to suicidal thoughts. Unfortunately, the topic is usually taboo among their family so they are driven to veiled hints that, tragically, are frequently only recognized in retrospect. Suicide is more often associated with major depression than minor, and patients frequently utilize means that are more likely to succeed and less likely to permit reversal (i.e. large overdoses or jumping in front of a train).

For patients who are recovering from very severe retarded depression, a high-risk time for suicide attempts is in the early stage of recovery, when their mood remains low but their motivation and drive have started to return.

Patients with less severe depression may be driven to an ill-conceived, impulsive act of aggression directed at themselves. DSH is frequently preceded or immediately followed by a desperate phone call – the literal cry for help to complement the symbolic one. Self-harm is not usually intended to be fatal: it rarely employs irreversible measures. Often it means ingestion of a few dozen hastily assembled tablets or some clumsy slashes at the wrist. Yet if someone is so disturbed that they demonstrate their hopelessness and their need to draw attention to their plight by self-harm, they surely merit help and sympathy, however manipulative they may appear. And of course if the tablets are paracetamol the consequences might well be far more serious than intended.

The term 'attempted suicide' is now little used because it does not convey whether or not there was an intention to die.

Diagnosis

A formal diagnosis of depression is made on symptomatic grounds. There must be low mood and at least four other symptoms from among:

- pessimism;
- negative thoughts;
- weight change;
- sleep disorder;
- psychomotor agitation or retardation;
- fatigue;
- feelings of inadequacy or guilt;
- difficulty in concentrating;
- suicidal thoughts or actions.

These must have persisted for at least 2 weeks, be inconsistent with the patient's prior personality and not be secondary to another medical condition or drug therapy.

The severity of depression may be rated by applying a standard scale based on a questionnaire, such as the Hamilton Depression Rating Scale or the Beck Depression Inventory. This can also be used to assess the efficacy and progress of any treatment. However, most depressive episodes remit and antidepressant drugs are slow to act, so any observed remission may be at least partially natural, although it may be tempting to ascribe it to the therapy.

In determining treatment, the finding that the depressive episode is associated with an adverse life event, and is therefore in some way understandable or 'reactive', is no reason to avoid drugs. The key criterion is severity.

Management

Aims and modes

The aims in managing depression are, in order of priority, to:

- Prevent suicide – consider custody and compulsory treatment if suicide is a risk.

- Identify possible primary causes, such as chronic or iatrogenic illness.
- Symptomatic therapy to relieve the patient's misery.
- Investigate any adverse social, domestic or financial circumstances.
- Initiate long-term therapy to prevent relapse or recurrence.

The three main modes of treatment are physical (invasive, with drugs, ECT or custody), social and psychological therapy. The principal criteria for deciding between these for a particular patient are:

- Urgency of illness or required speed of onset of treatment.
- Effectiveness.
- Natural history and likelihood of recurrence.
- Presence of psychotic symptoms.
- Contra-indications and adverse effects.
- Cost.

A multidisciplinary team approach is preferred, involving clinicians, nurses, social workers and sometimes pharmacists. In severe depression, invasive methods are almost invariably indicated, if necessary including temporary custody and involuntary treatment to prevent patients harming themselves or making unwise decisions. Drugs and ECT are cheap and relatively rapidly effective, but in the long term, social or psychological therapies have a better chance of reducing recurrence. A distinction must be made between a depressive episode and recurrent depressive illness, for which prophylaxis must be considered. If biological or psychotic features are prominent, the illness responds better to physical therapy. In mild depression drugs are generally ineffective.

Non-drug treatment

Psychotherapy
This is the preferred treatment for mild depression and frequently all that is needed: there is little evidence that drug therapy is effective. Psychotherapy is also an important component, along with drugs, in the management of major depression after the acute stage, when patients have improved insight, although the aim of

some forms of psychotherapy is to further improve insight. At its simplest, psychotherapy may involve no more than giving the patient a sympathetic and concerned ear (see also p. 381). Preferably the patient should be involved in the treatment decision process, with discussion of the possible causes of the illness, an account of the pros and cons of the treatment options and a realistic account of possible outcomes.

Patients must be reassured that they are eventually going to get better – something that they find difficult to believe. In severe depression it is also important to try to restore the patient's self-esteem. Patients should be advised against taking important decisions while depressed.

More specific therapies include group, marital and family therapy. CBT has been used very successfully in numerous mental illnesses. In this approach, unhelpful or negative ways of thinking are countered: the patient might be encouraged, for example, to think constructively about his or her illness or to plan strategies to overcome specific symptoms. Psychoanalysis has a place in the management of neurotic depression. Psychosocial treatment involves improving the patient's social situation.

Although slow, often labour-intensive compared with drug therapy, and not always effective, psychotherapy does at least hold out hope of a recovery in that the patient becomes better able to cope and remains relatively symptom-free.

Electroconvulsive therapy

While it may seem a bizarre and unlikely procedure, and is thought inhumane by some, ECT is often rapidly effective compared with drug therapy in very severe and suicidal depression. It also helps patients who are resistant to other forms of therapy or intolerant of them, and there are surprisingly few proven harmful effects. It involves a brief electrical pulse being passed through the brain between two electrodes attached to the skull with electrode jelly (similar to that used in EEG and ECG techniques). The treatment induces electroencephalographic changes characteristic of a major tonic–clonic seizure (see p. 443). The patient is anaesthetized with a brief-acting IV anaesthetic and a muscle relaxant (e.g. *suxamethonium*) is used to prevent a physical seizure.

A course of ECT consists of treatments given about three times weekly, for 3–4 weeks. The procedure often produces a rapid elevation of mood in the severely depressed, minimizing the risk of suicide at the most vulnerable phase of depression and enabling the patient to start psychotherapy.

Psychiatry has often had recourse to what may be called trauma therapy. In less enlightened times, hydrotherapy involved drenching 'mad' patients in freezing water. Later, insulin was used to induce hypoglycaemic shock. ECT was partly an extension of this into the age of electricity. Presumably the rationale for these so-called treatments was akin to our modern predilection for kicking a recalcitrant piece of machinery, and presumably they met with the same occasional success.

The original rationale for ECT was the observation, ill-founded as it transpired, that people with epilepsy, if they developed a psychotic illness, had fewer seizures but tended to feel better after a seizure: it was therefore reasoned that more fits in psychotic patients might reduce their psychosis. Subsequent research showed that only the cranial events of a seizure are important, so that the muscular seizure may safely be suppressed.

Double-blind placebo-controlled trials, using no actual current in controls, have subsequently demonstrated convincingly that the electric shock is essential. Previously, a variety of other factors had been suggested, including the anaesthetic, the muscle relaxant, the central hypoxia, the special care and attention the patient receives (because of the slight but real risks) or even the punitive element a patient suffering from guilt might welcome. ECT appears to produce changes in brain amines and receptor sensitivity similar to those produced by antidepressant drugs.

The common adverse mental effects are headache and confusion on recovering consciousness; similar symptoms occur after a major epileptic seizure. There is some loss of recent memory, which may reduce undue anxiety about subsequent ECT procedures. These side-effects are minimized by passing the current through only the non-dominant hemisphere (unilateral ECT). Uncertainty over the possibility of long-term brain damage means that courses are kept to a maximum of about 12 treatments, although patients have had more without evident harm. ECT has none of the adverse effects or contra-indications of antidepressant drugs. It can be used safely in pregnant women, the elderly and those in whom antimuscarinic drugs are contra-indicated. There is no long-term toxicity or suicide risk. However, ECT has no place in the treatment of mild or atypical depression.

Current NICE recommendations for ECT are that it should only be used short term in severe depression where other treatments have failed, especially where suicide is a serious risk.

Other methods

In SAD, 2 h of exposure each morning to full-spectrum artificial light equivalent to bright sunlight (**phototherapy**) seems to be effective but it must be continued as long as natural sunlight is unavailable. **Transcranial magnetic stimulation** was tried experimentally with some initial success but has not yet been shown to be effective in clinical trials. It resembles ECT but requires no anaesthesia or muscle relaxant.

Drug therapy

Antidepressant drugs

The antidepressant (thymoleptic or mood-elevating) drugs can be divided into several groups, on the basis of pharmacological, clinical and adverse actions:

- Tricyclics, the original group.
- Second-generation cyclics.
- Selective re-uptake inhibitors, especially for serotonin (SSRIs).
- MAOIs.

The properties of the first two groups (referred to here generically as 'cyclics') and SSRIs are compared in Table 6.11.

Selectivity. The nomenclature of antidepressants has become somewhat confused owing to an informal classification by the principal neurotransmitter affected. The original tricyclics are non-selective. Most block both noradrenaline (norepinephrine) and 5-HT re-uptake at central synapses to varying degrees and may also restore receptor sensitivity. They also block histamine-H_1 receptors, peripheral acetylcholine (muscarinic) and alpha-adrenergic receptors to a lesser extent. Some also appear to interact weakly with dopaminergic systems. There is partial selectivity in that some (e.g. *nortriptyline*) have a greater effect on noradrenaline (norepinephrine) and others, especially *amitriptyline*, on 5-HT.

The SSRIs show high selectivity for 5-HT re-uptake. Newer agents have noradrenaline (norepinephrine) selectivity (e.g. *reboxetine*), or noradrenaline/5-HT selectivity (*venlafaxine*). *Mirtazapine* and *mianserin* appear not to affect any of the usual transmitters directly.

Certain anti-dopaminergic antipsychotic drugs also have moderate antidepressant action, particularly the thioxanthenes, e.g. *flupentixol*. However, extrapyramidal and endocrine adverse effects (pp. 419–421) limit their usefulness in depression without marked psychotic features. They are more useful in schizophrenia with associated depressive features. *Amoxapine* also blocks dopamine.

Despite this pharmacological diversity, no particular pharmacodynamic properties have been clearly shown to confer superior antidepressant efficacy. The most important clinical distinctions are the presence or absence of:

- Antimuscarinic, anti-adrenergic and antihistaminic activity (conferring adverse effects).
- Sedative action (not linked exclusively to activity on any single transmitter).
- Cardiotoxic and convulsant action, especially in overdose.

These properties, governing the adverse affect and contra-indication profile, significantly affect drug selection. Antidepressant 'selectivity' means little more than activity predominantly on one or other of the central transmitters presumed to be involved in depression.

Tricyclics and related drugs

Agents with the traditional three-ring structure, such as *amitriptyline*, are effective and cheap, and their properties well known. However, they

Table 6.11   Comparison of cyclic antidepressants with selective serotonin re-uptake inhibitors (SSRIs)

	Tricyclic and related drugs[a]	SSRI
Sedative potential	Sedative – most Less sedative – lofepramine, imipramine, reboxetine, nortriptyline	Less sedative/neutral Fluoxetine tends to be stimulant
Efficacy	Very effective in adequate dosage	Very effective in adequate dosage
Onset of activity	2–4 weeks	2–4 weeks
Side-effects CNS	Drowsiness Weight gain Activation of acute mania Extrapyramidal symptoms (rare) Hyponatraemia[b]	Stimulation – anxiety, agitation ? Suicidal ideation, esp. in young ? Weight loss 'Serotonin syndrome' Activation of acute mania Extrapyramidal symptoms (rare) Hyponatraemia[b]
Antimuscarinic	Dry mouth, blurred vision, urinary retention	
Gastrointestinal	Constipation[c]	Nausea and vomiting Diarrhoea or constipation
Cardiovascular	Tachycardia[c], hypotension	
Accident risk	Increased	? Less risk
Discontinuation	General mild GI/CNS symptoms – withdraw slowly (after 8/52)	More serious CNS symptoms inc. headache, anxiety, dizziness – withdraw slowly (after 8/52)
Overdose	Convulsions; arrhythmias, heart block	Few problems
Fatality risk (suicide)	Significant	? Less risk
Treatment	Symptomatic; not specific	Few problems
Compliance/dropout	Common problems	? Few problems (few ADRs)
Dosage	Often can be given once daily Increment dose over 1–2 weeks	Often can be given once daily Usually full dose from start
Cost	Cheap	Relatively expensive

[a] Some newer cyclic drugs have fewer adverse effects – see also Table 6.12.

[b] Dizziness, confusion, convulsions – central effect on ADH secretion.

[c] Antimuscarinic effects.

ADH, antidiuretic hormone; ADR, adverse drug reaction; CNS, central nervous system; GI, gastrointestinal; SSRI, selective serotonin re-uptake inhibitors.

have significant adverse and toxic effects (Table 6.11). Later and second-generation drugs (e.g. *lofepramine, dosulepin* (dothiepin)), some not chemically tricyclic but 'heterocyclic' (e.g. *amoxapine, mianserin, venlafaxine*), offer a number of advantages in that they have fewer adverse effects and are less toxic in overdose (Table 6.12).

Table 6.12   Comparative advantages of second and third generation cyclic antidepressants and SSRIs over amitriptyline[a]

Drug	Less sedative	Less anti-muscarinic	Less[b] cardiotoxic	Less convulsant	Less weight gain
Second and third generation cyclics					
Amoxapine	+	−	+	−	−
Dosulepin[c] (dothiepin)	−	+	+	−	−
Doxepin	−	+	−	+	−
Lofepramine	+ +	+	+ +	−	−
Maprotiline	+ +	+	−	−	−
Mianserin	−	+ +	+ +	+ +	−
Mirtazepine	−	+	+ +	+ +	−
Reboxetine	+ +	+	?	−	+ +
Trazodone	−	+	+	−	+ +
Venlafaxine	+ +	+ +	+	+ +	+ +
SSRIs					
Citalopram	+ +	+ +	+ +	+ +	−
Fluoxetine	+ +	+ +	+ +	+ +	+ +
Fluvoxamine	+	+	+ +	+ +	+ +
Paroxetine[d]	+ +	+ +	+ +	+ +	−
Sertraline	+ +	+ +	+ +	+ +	+ +

Sources: BNF; Bazire, Psychotropic Drug Directory; Taylor, Maudsley prescribing guidelines.

[a] Sources differ on the extent of the effects cited, owing to the paucity of data. The evaluations are given for qualitative comparison only.

[b] Main toxic effect is on QT interval, potentially causing arrhythmia; postural hypotension less dangerous except in elderly.

[c] As dangerous as amitriptyline in overdose.

[d] More likely to cause extrapyramidal symptoms than other SSRIs.

SSRI, selective serotonin re-uptake inhibitor; + +, significant improvement; +, moderate improvement; −, no improvement; ? uncertain.

Indications. All the traditional tricyclics and the related newer agents are very useful in moderate to severe depression, but there is no evidence that they are useful in mild depression. *Amitriptyline* and many others also have sedative as well as antidepressant action, making them particularly useful for depression mixed with anxiety or agitation. A single daily dose in the evening also aids sleep but minimizes daytime sedation. The antidepressant effect, being unrelated to plasma level, is more prolonged.

Less sedative agents (e.g. *imipramine*, *lofepramine*) may be useful where neither anxiety nor retardation are problems. This will minimize daytime sedation, which may otherwise restrict the patient's activity or occupation.

Pharmacokinetics. Generally, tricyclics are rapidly and fairly well absorbed but are subject to considerable first-pass metabolism. The extent of hepatic clearance (by demethylation and hydroxylation) varies greatly, partly accounting for wide interpatient variation in response. Among the older drugs, tertiary amine derivatives (e.g. *imipramine*) are frequently demethylated to active secondary amines (e.g. *desipramine*) with a slightly different activity profile, thus prolonging the action.

The tricyclics are quite highly protein bound. However, they have a high volume of distribution with accumulation in extravascular sites so there are no significant displacement interactions. Plasma level monitoring is not a useful guide to dose titration or efficacy, but can be used to assess compliance. The overall pharmacokinetic effect is usually a long biological half-life, which may be further prolonged in over-dosage. Although therapeutic plasma levels are achieved within 24 h, the clinical (antidepressant) effect is not seen for several weeks. Metabolism may be considerably reduced in the elderly, predisposing them to side-effects.

Side-effects. Mild to moderate antimuscarinic adverse effects, such as dry mouth, constipation, poor visual accommodation, tachycardia, etc., are common, as is drowsiness with many agents (Tables 6.11 and 6.12). Although these effects are not serious and usually remit on continued use they may be troublesome at first and contribute to poor compliance. The visual problems may result in consultation with an optician, who should be informed about the drug therapy. If not evident as drowsiness, CNS depressant effects on cognition and coordination may be difficult to distinguish from the more retarded forms of the illness. Owing to this and postural hypotension (due to peripheral alpha-adrenergic blockade), antidepressants are believed to be implicated in a large number of falls and other accidents, especially in the elderly.

Weight gain is quite common. This may be in part the resolution of depressive anorexia, but a direct effect on appetite is also seen even in non-depressives, e.g. when used for migraine prophylaxis. In patients who are susceptible to bipolar mood swings, possible (re)activation of mania is a significant risk. Indeed they may precipitate the manic episode of latent bipolar disease in what had been diagnosed as unipolar recurrent depression. A lowering of seizure threshold may destabilize patients with epilepsy or cause problems if a patient overdoses.

Hyponatraemia may occur owing to central stimulation of ADH secretion, particularly in the elderly. This causes CNS depression, including drowsiness and confusion, which may easily be attributed to other causes. Extrapyramidal symptoms occasionally occur. *Mianserin* has been implicated in bone marrow depression with leucopenia.

Toxic effects and overdose. The acute toxicity of antidepressants is important because they are often involved in suicide attempts. For tricyclics there is no specific antidote; all complications must be managed symptomatically as they arise. The main problems are:

* CNS, with seizures and confusion;
* cardiovascular, with conduction defects giving heart block; vagal inhibition giving tachyarrhythmias; and profound hypotension.

Thus such overdoses are often fatal. A principal advantage of the newer agents is a generally reduced likelihood of these complications, although *dosulepin* (dothiepin) is the most toxic of all in overdose.

Interactions. Adrenergic over-stimulation may occur when tricyclics are given with sympathomimetic drugs (e.g. as included in some OTC decongestant preparations) and MAOIs causing potentially dangerous hypertension. CNS depressants, especially alcohol, which are frequently taken in association with an overdose, produce excessive sedation or coma. The effect of anticonvulsant drugs may be diminished. Arrhythmias may occur with *digoxin* or *quinidine*.

Contra-indications and cautions. Patients with heart disease (e.g. arrhythmias, previous MI), narrow-angle glaucoma, urinary retention (e.g. prostatism) or constipation, in whom antimuscarinic effects could be harmful or dangerous, should use other drugs. Patients taking antihypertensive medication should use *mianserin*, which does not interfere with amines. Care is needed in epilepsy. The elderly are prone to over-sedation because of the long half-lives and this problem can increase until steady-state concentrations are reached. The blood count of elderly patients on *mianserin* should be monitored.

Dosage and administration. Drug treatment should be started as early as possible once major depression is diagnosed; this has beneficial effects on outcome and relapse. For optimal antidepressant effect, it is strongly recommended that tricyclics must be used in adequate doses, for example, at least 125 mg daily of *amitriptyline*, and treatment failure has been attributed largely to subtherapeutic dosing. However, one meta-analyis has suggested that lower doses may be adequate. Therapeutic levels are achieved gradually over 2 weeks by starting at half the target dose, or one-quarter of it for the elderly or children. Unacceptable adverse effects must be warned about and monitored, lest confidence in drug therapy is impaired. The inconvenience of the initial side-effects may be reduced by dividing doses unequally, e.g. two-thirds at night and one-third in the morning. If suicide is a likely or suspected risk, only small supplies should be given at any one time, although determined patients still accumulate them.

Patients must be warned that the antidepressant effect does not become apparent for several weeks, because most people expect all drugs to work very quickly. During this initial period they may only experience the adverse effects, which may be both disabling and dispiriting.

Antidepressants should not be withdrawn too quickly; otherwise there may be a discontinuation syndrome with mild mixed gastrointestinal and central effects. After 8 weeks or more of therapy, dosage should be tailed off over at least 4 weeks. These effects do not indicate dependence, which does not occur, but are probably due to receptor sensitivity changes. However, many people believe antidepressants are addictive, which reduces confidence in them and damages compliance. Exploring and correcting this misconception should be part of the initial discussion with the patient about therapeutic choice.

Newer cyclic agents

Table 6.12 shows how many of the newer tricyclic-related drugs, which have been developed to make safer antidepressants, are comparable to the class archetype *amitriptyline* for the most common adverse effects. Molecular modelling has produced a wide range of drugs with one or more improvments, greatly increasing the choice for specific circumstances. They either have fewer or less serious side-effects or less life-threatening toxic effects. However, they are no better and no faster at relieving depression.

SSRIs

Indications.   These are now the first choice in most moderate to serious depressive episodes.

The main advantages of 5-HT specificity are the absence of many of the troublesome adverse effects, toxicity and overdose problems associated with the older, less selective agents. Early hopes that they might be more effective or faster acting have not been realized, and they are used for the same purposes as the tricyclics, and generic ones are little more expensive.

Pharmacokinetics.   The SSRIs have broadly similar kinetic properties to the tricyclics, but are less likely to have active metabolites.

Side-effects.   SSRIs have a quite different profile from the tricyclics (Table 6.12). Most important is the almost complete absence of antimuscarinic, cardiotoxic and convulsant properties. Also, there may be weight loss as opposed to weight gain, and psychomotor impairment is less. However, withdrawal phenomena, hyponatraemia, activation of mania and occasional extrapyramidal symptoms still occur.

The most common problems are relatively mild gastrointestinal and central effects. However, nausea, diarrhoea or constipation may be intolerable for some. An association with gastrointestinal bleeding has recently been noted, possibly related to interference with serotonergic mechanisms in platelets. Gastro-protection (p. 777) has been recommended when SSRIs are to be taken by patients already taking NSAIDs.

Less common is CNS stimulation, presenting as anxiety, agitation, restlessness, headache or confusion. In general (i.e. apart from specific contra-indications) the SSRIs are tolerated better than tricyclic antidepressants, as measured by the dropout rate due to adverse effects; about one-third more patients cease tricyclic therapy.

Toxic effects and overdose.   Another significant advantage of this group is the absence of serious cardiotoxic or convulsant actions in overdose. Thus they are much safer than the original tricyclics, although some newer cyclic antidepressants are also safer than these (Table 6.12). It must also be remembered that SSRIs offer no greater protection from suicide by other means. Both tricyclics and SSRIs appear to increase the likelihood of suicide ideas or behaviour in the early stages of therapy. Fears that SSRIs and *venlafaxine* might be worse in this respect are probably unfounded, except in patients under 18, where their use is contra-indicated, except for *fluoxetine* in certain restricted circumstances. Patients under 30 need to be monitored closely early in treatment.

Rarely, SSRIs may cause the 'serotonin syndrome', especially when interacting with other antidepressants and especially the anti-migraine triptan 5-HT agonists. The liberation of excessive 5-HT causes CNS stimulation resulting in restlessness and hyperthermia. The syndrome is usually mild, but may prove fatal. It usually responds to discontinuation of SSRIs if they are not tolerated, but in severe cases the 5-HT blocker *cyproheptadine* can be used as an antidote.

Contra-indications, cautions, interactions. Serotonin selectivity means SSRIs can be used in many situations when tricyclics are contra-indicated. However, care is still needed in heart disease and epilepsy. They should be used with caution in patients susceptible to seizures (or undergoing ECT), cardiac disease, mania or bleeding. Suitable washout periods, usually of several weeks, must be observed when changing to other types of antidepressant (especially MAOIs) in order to avoid serious interactions. SSRIs inhibit hepatic metabolism but despite numerous theoretical interactions, few clinically significant ones occur in practice. *Sertraline* and *citalopram* may be the safest in this respect.

Dosage and administration. Most SSRIs can be given once daily. The dose–response curve rapidly plateaus above the usual effective (and tolerable) dose. Therefore full doses can often be started at once (perhaps originally fostering the impression of more rapid onset of activity). If nausea is a problem, starting on half the dose for a few days can help. However, withdrawal should still be staged over 2–4 weeks to avoid discontinuation symptoms.

Monoamine oxidase inhibitors
Indications. Frequent and hazardous dietary and drug interactions have always limited the use of MAOIs, especially in general practice. They may be of value in depression associated with atypical features characteristic of anxiety-neurosis (especially phobia or panic disorder), but they are not usually effective when used alone in severe depression. Their main role is as adjuncts or second- or third-line drugs in resistant disease. Dietary compliance is easier to ensure in hospital.

Side-effects and toxicity. The range of mild to moderate adverse effects is very wide, and the potential toxic effects of MAOIs are serious. Many central, cardiovascular and gastrointestinal autonomic disturbances occur in normal use, especially antimuscarinic and anti-adrenergic effects. Although interactions may cause hypertension, adverse effects frequently involve postural hypotension. Peripheral oedema is also common. CNS stimulation and activation of mania can occur. Overdose with MAOIs (except *tranylcypromine*) is somewhat easier to manage than with tricyclics because specific alpha-adrenergic blockers can be used, e.g. *phentolamine*.

Interactions. Normally, dietary tyramine is metabolized by MAO in the gut wall. Inhibition of MAO allows high levels of tyramine to be absorbed, causing widespread release of noradrenaline (norepinephrine) from nerve fibres, with predictable hypertensive cardiovascular consequences. Interacting prescription medication (e.g. cyclic antidepressants, CNS sedatives, opioid analgesics) can usually be avoided by professional vigilance. Greater potential problems arise with OTC preparations containing sympathomimetics (e.g. decongestants) and tyramine-containing foods (especially cheese, pickled fish and meats or meat extracts, fava beans), which is why patient counselling and warning cards are so important. *Tranylcypromine*, the most stimulant MAOI, seems to be the worst offender, especially if combined with *clomipramine*. *Phenelzine* is relatively sedating. Fatalities are still reported and MAOIs are likely to remain little used.

Because *phenelzine* causes irreversible enzyme inhibition, recovery of enzyme functions following cessation of therapy does not start for several days and may take several weeks to return to normal. Changing from an MAOI to a tricyclic requires at least a 2-week interval, but the reverse can be done safely after a week, though some SSRIs require longer.

Sometimes a tricyclic/MAOI combination is indicated, in which case a sedative tricyclic with a less stimulant MAOI (e.g. *amitriptyline* with *phenelzine*) is usually safe if managed by experienced psychiatrists. *Tranylcypromine* is the most dangerous in combination.

Other antidepressants

Moclobemide causes reversible inhibition of MAO type A (RIMA). This has two principal advantages: enzyme function is restored promptly following drug cessation, allowing quicker and safer switching to other antidepressants; and tyramine metabolism is little inhibited, so the patient is relatively free from dietary restrictions. It also has few of the autonomic adverse effects of the non-selective MAOIs and appears to be equally effective as the cyclics, particularly for retarded depression. However, it has not yet found its place in treatment protocols.

Tryptophan, a 5-HT precursor, has proved disappointing considering the strong suspicion of a 5-HT disturbance in some forms of depression. It is occasionally used as an adjuvant. *Lithium* and its use are discussed on pp. 406–408.

The herbal product St John's Wort (hypericum extract) has been shown in some trials to be as effective as other antidepressants in mild to moderate depression but is still not yet adequately standardized, nor have its active ingredients been characterized. Moreover, there is concern about interactions, especially as it is available without prescription and induces liver enzymes.

Lithium and some anticonvulsants (e.g *carbamazepine*, *lamotrigine*, *valproate*) are sometimes used as 'mood stabilizers' in bipolar disorder (see below).

Treatment strategy and drug selection

The strategy for the drug treatment of depression involves several stages (Figure 6.9). Bazire in the Psychotropic Drug Directory characterises these as the 6 Ds:

- Check the illness is not **D**rug induced.
- Select the most suitable **D**rug.
- **D**on't **D**elay treatment: start acute treatment as soon as possible.
- Titrate to full recommended **D**ose.
- Continue for the correct **D**uration, for 6 months after symptoms first respond, ensuring compliance.
- **D**iscontinue slowly.

In deciding whether or not to treat an episode of primary depression, the criteria are the severity of depression and the patient's ability to cope. Whether or not the low mood is considered an appropriate reaction to an adverse event is not important. Moreover, prompt treatment reduces the length of the episode and the likelihood of recurrence. The use of full doses for 4–6 months after symptoms have subsided or remitted is essential to prevent relapse. Unfortunately, non-compliance is common once the patient's mood has improved, especially if adverse effects are still troublesome.

Where there is a history of at least one previous depressive episode, up to 3 years' prophylactic therapy has been shown to limit recurrence. Although some would argue that the

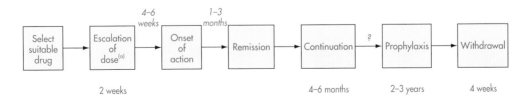

Figure 6.9 Phases in drug treatment of chronic depression. (a)Not needed with selective serotonin re-uptake inhibitor.

prophylactic dose level should be the same as that used in the acute phase, lower doses tend to be used.

Drug selection depends to some extent on a variety of specific patient or disease factors, most of which are related to tolerance or contra-indications (Table 6.13). It is conventional to distinguish different grades of depression for the purposes of treatment but there are not clear thresholds and in the vast majority of cases SSRIs are first-line when drug therapy is indicated. Other groups are used when SSRIs fail or are not tolerated, or in certain exceptional circumstances.

Mild (minor) and moderate depression

Antidepressant medication is usually unnecessary for an isolated episode of mild depression associated with an adverse life event: psychotherapy is the first choice. If drugs are needed, treatment can be stopped when the patient recovers; continuation and prophylactic therapy are not indicated. No particular types are any more effective and SSRIs are first choice. It has been claimed that MAOIs are more effective than others if there are atypical features such as anxiety, phobia, anger, hypochondria or increased appetite and sleep. However, the evidence is not strong and their dietary precau-

Table 6.13   First-line therapy in depression – special considerations

Situation/factor	Possible therapy[a]	Rationale
Mild symptoms	Consider psychotherapy	Drugs often ineffective
Mild – atypical features	MAOI	
Severe – possibly suicidal	SSRI Lofepramine, trazodone, mianserin	Less toxic in overdose
	ECT	More rapid response than drugs
Severe – psychotic	Antipsychotic[b]; ECT	Antipsychotic + antidepressant effects
Elderly, CVS disease	SSRI Lofepramine, venlafaxine	Less adverse effects, especially on CVS (arrhythmia, hypotension)
Cannot tolerate anti-muscarinic side-effects	SSRI Doxepin, mianserin	Less antimuscarinic
Cannot tolerate sedation	SSRI Lofepramine	Less sedative
Epilepsy	SSRI Trazodone	Less convulsant
Agitated, anxious, insomnia	Amitriptyline, dosulepin (dothiepin) Short-course benzodiazepine	Sedative
Recurrent bipolar	Initiate lithium therapy	See p. 406
Resistant	See Figure 6.10	

[a] Only a few examples of possible drugs are cited in each case; see text and Figure 6.10 for details.

[b] Caution needed combining antipsychotic with antidepressant and/or ECT.

CVS, cardiovascular system; ECT, electroconvulsive therapy; MAOI, monoamine oxidase inhibitor; SSRI, selective serotonin re-uptake inhibitor.

tions limit their use. Pharmacotherapy is usually indicated in moderate depression.

For patients with anxiety, initial insomnia or mixed anxiety and depression, short courses of anxiolytics or short-acting hypnotics are sometimes used. However, sedative antidepressants (e.g. *amitriptyline*) are preferable, given in the evening if needed for sleep problems.

Severe depression

Drugs are almost always necessary in severe or psychotic depression, possibly preceded by a course of ECT. SSRIs are first-line and cyclics or MAOIs are second-line. Specialist guidelines must be consulted when either switching antidepressants or combining them.

Patients suffering from psychotic symptoms, especially hallucinations, may benefit from a short course of an antipsychotic such as *haloperidol*. *Amoxapine* and thioxanthenes (e.g. *flupentixol*) have both been recommended because they have mixed antidepressant and sedative–antipsychotic actions. (In the case of the former, these effects are due to the metabolite loxapine.) However, there is little evidence to support these uses.

Where suicide is a suspected risk, the least toxic agents are essential, especially those with a lower convulsant potential, dispensed in small quantities and preferably under supervision. ECT may also be used.

Contra-indications or intolerance of adverse effects such as antimuscarinic effects or sedation can usually be circumvented by judicious drug selection (see Table 6.13). If there evidence of a recurrent pattern, *lithium* therapy may be considered. With a recurrent unipolar pattern, *lithium* may be as effective as tricyclics, but the need for plasma-level monitoring is inconvenient. However, *lithium* is the drug of choice in bipolar illness, i.e. with manic phases (p. 406).

Resistant depression

For the minority of patients who do not improve after 6–8 weeks on optimal doses of a first-line antidepressant, measuring the drug plasma level might first be considered to check for possible compliance problems or abnormal drug handling. Otherwise, changing to another antidepressant that acts in a different manner, such as from a noradrenaline (norepinephrine) to a selective serotonin re-uptake inhibitor, may help. A course of ECT could be considered. Thereafter, a wide variety of combinations are employed by psychiatrists, the only logical basis of which is that components have different modes of action (Figure 6.10).

Adding *lithium* to other antidepressants (lithium augmentation) seems particularly successful. Switching to *venlafaxine* has also been successful. *Levothyroxine* (thyroxine) augmentation is also used, presumably partly on the basis that hypothyroidism is often associated with depression. *Tryptophan* augmentation can be done on a named patient basis only.

Less common and based on even less evidence are the addition of *olanzapine* plus *fluoxetine*, *lamotrigine*, high-dose tricyclics, or a short course of steroids (e.g. *dexamethasone* 3 mg/day for 4 days). Use of these agents and combinations requires close monitoring and careful selection of agent and dose, and is too specialized to consider here.

Mania and manic-depressive disorder

Mania

Mania is a severe, usually recurrent, psychotic affective disorder that is almost the precise opposite of severe depression, although about one-tenth as common. There is an abnormally elevated mood (i.e. euphoria rather than dysphoria), unwarranted optimism, exuberance, over-confidence, inflated self-esteem, hyperactivity of thought and action, excessive libido, and little sleep. The patient has increased drive and is outgoing, but often socially tactless. The over-confidence is similar to that experienced by otherwise normal individuals during the usually pleasurable sensations of early alcoholic inebriation. In the same way, patients enjoy their episodes of mania, when they also often feel more creative, thus making compliance with treatment a problem.

A full-blown manic attack usually lasts no more than a few days, during which the patient sleeps little but appears to have boundless energy. That level of arousal, if sustained for

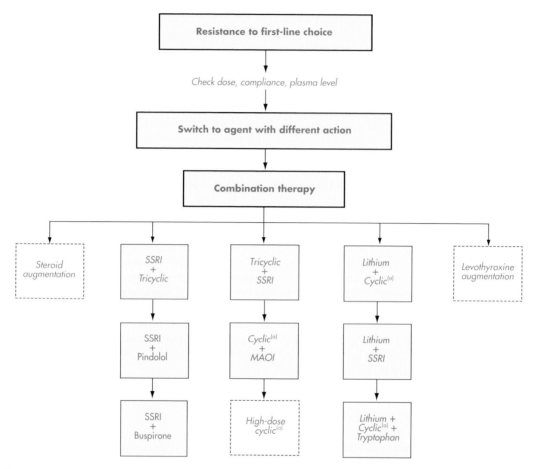

Figure 6.10 Some treatment options in resistant depression. MAOI, monoamine oxidase inhibitor; SSRI, selective serotonin re-uptake inhibitor. [a]Cyclic, tricyclic or second-generation cyclic.

longer, is potentially life-threatening. **Hypomania** is more usual, where symptoms are less florid. During a manic phase sufferers may require compulsory admission to hospital ('sectioning'; see p. 421) but others manage to function adequately in the community. At the other end of the spectrum an even milder form is seen as a (potentially advantageous) personality trait in some individuals. Such an individual retains insight, and may be thought of as simply a flamboyant character, a tireless and exuberant go-getter, a workaholic, even (colloquially) as a 'Don Juan' or a 'nymphomaniac'.

Attacks are extremely disruptive socially, domestically and financially, because overconfidence causes patients to undertake wildly ambitious commitments. Patients discover when they finally 'come down' that they are hopelessly over-committed, double-booked and in serious debt.

The accelerated mental processes produce a short attention span, flight of ideas and pressure of speech as the patient jumps rapidly from subject to subject on apparently irrational grounds, such as a rhyme or puns (the 'clang association'). The mood too may suddenly change from euphoria to irritability and aggressiveness, possibly out of frustration. The patient may thus appear quite incoherent, and the apparent thought disorder and delusions are not easily distinguished from acute schizophrenia. The differential diagnosis depends on whether mood disturbance or thought disorder predominates. An illness with elements of both is known as **schizoaffective disorder**. Clearly the lay term 'maniac' is related, but manic patients are no more criminal or violent than the general population.

Psychotic features such as lack of insight and delusions of grandeur, the counterpart of the depressive's delusions of worthlessness, are common during attacks, but the patient may seem quite normal and rational between them. Attacks rarely last more than a few weeks before the attention that patients draw to themselves means they are soon treated, although often involuntarily. Otherwise the patient would become exhausted. Mood returns to normal after a few months of therapy, or may swing into depression.

Manic-depressive disorder

Most patients experiencing mania also have episodes of severe depression, although the frequency, sequence and duration of mood swings vary enormously between patients. Depressive phases usually last longer than manic ones and are less obvious, and there are variable periods of normality between extreme swings. Mood swings can be quite abrupt, with manic phases tending to have a more rapid onset. **Rapid cycling** is when there are four or more swings per year. Fluctuations become more frequent, and more frequently depressive rather than manic, as the patient ages.

Where the symptoms are serious or psychotic, the terms **manic-depressive** or **bipolar affective disorder** are used. If manic attacks are quite frequent or predominate it is known as type I. Occasional hypomania with predominant depression is type II.

An otherwise normal person with moderately exaggerated mood swings may be described as having a cyclothymic personality; this is not a psychotic illness, and some would argue not an illness at all.

Aetiology and pathology

Major depression, mania and manic-depressive disorder may have similar aetiologies. The underlying abnormality could be in the regulation of emotional responses, both low or high, by the limbic system, and involving monoamine neurotransmitters, possibly dopamine and GABA. This hypothesis is supported by the prophylactic effectiveness of the single agent *lithium* in all three. In bipolar disease, however, cyclic antidepressants, SSRIs and MAOIs are not just ineffective but can actually be dangerous because they can trigger an exaggerated upswing from depression to mania. An electrolyte imbalance has also been proposed to account for cycling.

As with severe recurrent depression, mania is a genetically linked, chronic but generally non-progressive disease. External triggers for attacks may sometimes be found in stressful life events but equally, as with some severe episodes of depression, there may be no apparent cause. There is usually a family history and the concordance rate in twins is over 70%. The disease seems evenly spread worldwide.

Management

The aims of management are to:

• control acute manic or hypomanic attacks;
• minimize recurrence and intensity of mood swings with prophylactic therapy.

In acute severe manic attacks, initial sedation will be required. The drugs of choice are the newer atypical antipsychotics (see p. 415), particularly *olanzapine*, *risperidone* or *quetiapine* for psychotic features (e.g. loss of insight, grandiose delusions), or the mood stabilizer *valproate*. At the same time prophylactic *lithium* can be started, but it takes 7–10 days to take effect. Patients may need compulsory admission and treatment if they are a risk to themselves or others. ECT is an alternative to *lithium* in the acute phase.

If the patient is already taking *lithium* the plasma level must be checked: often patients will deliberately stop, either because of adverse effects or to induce hypomania. (This is an interesting inversion of recreational drug misuse, which more usually involves *taking* something to get high, rather than *avoiding* it.) Otherwise, *lithium* therapy is started.

If the patient demonstrates an alternating pattern (bipolar disorder) or a recurrent pattern, which is more common with mania than depression, they must be assessed for maintenance therapy. The drug of choice in the prophylaxis of recurrent mania or bipolar disorder is *lithium*. This is a potentially lifelong commitment, including mandatory regular follow-up to monitor both compliance and toxicity. As patients age, they will be more likely to start using medication for comorbidities that potentially will interact with *lithium* (e.g. diuretics, NSAIDs), so regular re-assessment is essential. *Lithium* is the only antimanic that reduces suicide risk. Theoretically, long-term antipsychotics could be used, but they are usually avoided because of adverse effects. Once a patient is stabilized, social and psychotherapeutic interventions should be introduced.

Not all patients respond to either of these traditional treatments, and a number of other approaches have become established as second-line alternatives (Table 6.14). The most promising are anticonvulsant drugs such as *carbamazepine*, *valproate* or *lamotrigine*, and *topiramate* (p. 448). These drugs may be more effective in rapid cyclers, or in those who fail to respond to *lithium*.

Additional treatment during a depressive phase of bipolar disease is problematic because of the propensity of antidepressants to activate mania. The usual antidepressant drugs are used, but with more than usual care.

Lithium

Lithium is an enigmatic drug. A monovalent cation seems an unlikely candidate for the stabilization of major affective disturbances. It closely resembles the sodium ion in charge and ionic size, and is distributed similarly in body water, which has lent support to body-water/electrolyte theories of affective disorder. However, *lithium* has also been shown to affect monoamine levels and post-receptor intracellular signalling.

Indications. For single depressive episodes *lithium* is similar to *amitriptyline* in potency and onset. However, its real value lies in the maintenance prophylaxis of recurrent unipolar or bipolar affective disorder. Here it is a safer and perhaps more effective proposition than the cyclics or SSRIs, and safer than antipsychotics or benzodiazepines, despite the need for regular plasma level monitoring.

Lithium treatment should be considered if there is evidence of recurrent episodes, either of severe depression or mania (more than one in 2–3 years). *Lithium* will reduce the frequency, duration and intensity of mood swings or abolish them. Some patients complain that it produces a flattening of normal mood (blunting of affect), and manic patients may comply poorly because they value or enjoy some aspects of their attacks of mania or hypomania. Some believe themselves to be more creative in that state.

Dosage and side-effects. *Lithium* therapy is managed by monitoring the serum level. For acute attacks, up to 1.2–1.5 mmol/L may be needed initially. For prophylaxis, the goal is to maintain a plasma level within the narrow therapeutic window (0.6–1.0 mmol/L); in many patients control is obtained below 0.8 mmol/L.

Dosage should aim for a stable plasma level throughout the day because acute adverse effects, such as nausea, polyuria, polydipsia and fine tremor, seem to be related to post-dose peak levels (Table 6.15). Thus, frequent daily doses or modified-release preparations are preferred, and

---

Table 6.14   Drug treatment options in mania and manic-depressive disorder

Acute manic phase	Maintenance treatment of bipolar disorder
First choice	
Lithium (initiate or optimize)	Lithium
Atypical antipsychotics[a]	Carbamazepine
Sodium valproate	Sodium valproate
	Atypical antipsychotic[a]
Second line	
Benzodiazepine	
Carbamazepine	

[a] e.g. olanzapine, risperidone, quetiapine.

the risk of renal damage is reduced by once-daily dosing. Change of formulation should be avoided or done gradually. Dose changes should also be gradual. Many minor adverse effects remit on prolonged use.

Plasma levels of *lithium* above 1.5 mmol/L produce warning signs of toxicity including diarrhoea and vomiting, coarsening of the tremor and CNS depression. Sustained toxic levels above 2.5 mmol/L cause hypotension, convulsions and coma, and are potentially fatal; in such circumstances dialysis may be needed to bring about sufficiently rapid reversal.

Hypothyroidism is quite a common chronic effect. The significance of long-term kidney changes remains controversial and only a minority are affected. Renal and thyroid function tests are recommended before commencing *lithium* therapy, and regularly thereafter.

Withdrawal of *lithium*, if it becomes necessary, must be gradual, staged over at least 4–12 weeks, to reduce the likelihood of rebound hypomanic symptoms or relapse.

Monitoring. Regular measurement of plasma *lithium* (12 h post-dose) is essential, at first weekly until a stable level is obtained. Subsequently the interval may be increased (up to 3–4 months) in patients who understand the precautions. Thyroid and renal functions tests (see Chapters 9 and 14) should be done at the same time. Extra measurement is indicated in suspected drug interaction or poor compliance, intercurrent illness, other circumstances that interfere with *lithium* level, or unexpected toxicity. Table 6.16 shows common circumstances that can potentiate *lithium* level and/or toxicity.

Pharmacokinetics and interactions. *Lithium* is distributed throughout body water, generally following the same pattern as sodium. It is cleared entirely by the kidney, which gives rise to many potential problems. Both fluid retention (e.g. from NSAIDs) and circumstances that promote increased renal sodium reabsorption (such as pyrexia, unaccustomed hot climate, electrolyte depletion, dehydration or diuretic

Table 6.15 Principal side-effects and toxicity of lithium, in relation to steady-state plasma level

	Minor/reversible side-effect (therapeutic range: 0.4–1 mmol/L)	Early signs of toxicity (1.5–2.5 mmol/L)	Toxicity (>2.5 mmol/L)
Gastrointestinal	Dyspepsia	Anorexia Nausea and vomiting Diarrhoea	
CVS	Benign ECG changes	Hypotension, arrhythmia	Circulatory failure
Renal	Polyuria, polydipsia Oedema	Persistent polyuria	Acute: renal damage? Chronic: renal failure??
CNS and neuromuscular	Fine tremor Incoordination Muscle weakness	Coarse tremor Muscle weakness and twitch Lethargy Dysarthria Ataxia	Convulsions Coma Permanent neurological damage Death
Other	Non-myxoedemic goitre Neutrophilia Exacerbation of psoriasis	Hypothyroidism	

CNS, central nervous system; CVS, cardiovascular system; ECG, electrocardiogram.

therapy) tend to reduce *lithium* clearance and can cause dangerously high plasma levels. Patients must be warned about this and those with renal or cardiovascular impairment need close attention. Interactions are important because of the narrow therapeutic index (Table 6.16). While most interactions increase *lithium* levels, antacids and *theophylline* can reduce them.

Clearance is increased in pregnancy. However, *lithium* may be teratogenic and use in the first trimester will depend on the relative risks of withdrawal and continuation.

Despite these potential difficulties, *lithium* is a valuable drug. It has no antimuscarinic or extrapyramidal effects, causes no amnesia, general CNS depression or psychomotor impairment, and has little effect on normal mood. Thus it has advantages over the other treatments available for depression or mania. However, in overdose it is no less toxic than conventional antidepressants or antipsychotics. All patients should be given a Lithium Treatment Card. Diligent monitoring has enabled patients to take *lithium* for decades with little ill effect.

Schizophrenia

Schizophrenia is a much misunderstood disease. It has nothing to do with a so-called 'split personality' or with Jekyll and Hyde. In schizophrenia, the split is between different components of the same personality, e.g. between mood and action, or behaviour and belief. The normally integrated aspects of a healthy personality become fragmented – literally disintegrated. A more subtle solecism is the use of 'schizophrenic' as a synonym for ambivalent.

There is a very rare, genuine split personality disorder. More properly called dissociative disorder or multiple personality, in this extraordinary condition a person alternates between two or more usually completely integrated, rational personalities. This has nothing to do with schizophrenia.

Although schizophrenia is generally what the lay public understands by madness, the popular idea (promoted by the mass media) that every 'mad axeman' has schizophrenia is wrong. Patients with schizophrenia are no more violent

Table 6.16 Circumstances enhancing lithium action or toxicity

Circumstances/concomitant drug therapy	Comment
Antipsychotics (especially haloperidol)	Accepted combination, but caution required
Cyclic antidepressants and SSRIs	Common combination. May trigger mania; enhanced toxicity (especially SSRIs)
ECT	
Increased renal **sodium** or **fluid** retention, caused by, e.g.:	Reduced lithium clearance or increased lithium reabsorption gives raised serum lithium level
• renal impairment	
• dehydration	
• unusually hot climate	
• excessive perspiration	
• pyrexia	
• vomiting, diarrhoea	
• sodium depletion	
• low-salt diet	
• NSAID	
• diuretic (especially thiazide)	
• ACEIs	

Only the main interactions are shown; see BNF (Appendix 1).
ACEI, angiotensin-converting enzyme inhibitor; NSAID, non-steroidal anti-inflammatory drug.

than the population as a whole. Violent criminals may be suffering from a 'psychopathic personality', a condition quite distinct from schizophrenia.

It must not be assumed that people with schizophrenia, being psychotic and thus out of touch with reality and lacking insight, do not suffer from their disease: they do. Moreover, there are lucid periods, possibly due to treatment, during which they have sufficient insight to remember their experiences when acutely ill. Many patients give a strong impression of perplexity and bewilderment. They are convinced of the truth of their own reality and cannot reconcile this with the reaction this causes in others.

Schizophrenia is probably the most difficult mental illness to understand because, unlike with depression or anxiety, the experience of sufferers is very remote from normal. It has been likened to that twilight world between sleep and waking, when it is difficult to distinguish between illusion and reality. Schizophrenic patients also have difficulty distinguishing between themselves and the outside world. While for most of us dreaming, thinking, saying and hearing are categorically distinct phenomena, in schizophrenia the differences are blurred. Consequently, patients may feel irrational external influences on their thoughts, or that their thoughts are available for all the world to read. This loss of the ultimate privacy – that of our thoughts – is possibly what makes schizophrenia so miserable and confusing for the sufferer.

Aetiology and pathology

Schizophrenia is a common condition: about 1% of the population are likely to have at least one episode during their life, although not all will become permanently ill. Nevertheless, schizophrenia accounts for the majority of patients in continuous psychiatric care. The condition has a uniform global prevalence. The apparent increased prevalence among lower socioeconomic groups is attributed to the 'downward social drift' of sufferers, who have difficulty maintaining jobs, eduction or relationships.

The causes of schizophrenia are unknown. Both genetic predisposition (susceptibility), early development and various environmental factors are important, as has been confirmed by studies on twins born to schizophrenic parents. Several potential genes or gene linkages have been identified. Among the biological causes suggested are autoimmune or viral encephalitis, abnormally large brain ventricles (causing reduced functional brain size), or imbalance between the right and left hemispheres. Recently, research has focused on neurodevelopmental abnormalities arising at a very early age.

Previously, postmortem studies on the brains of schizophrenic patients failed to distinguish the effects of chronic disease from those of many years of antipsychotic therapy. However, newer non-invasive imaging techniques, such as positron emission tomography (PET) and MRI, which visualize the living brain and monitor changes in its activity with far greater precision than the relatively crude electroencephalogram (EEG), reveal abnormalities in frontal, thalamic and cerebral areas. These are seen in newly diagnosed, drug-naïve patients so cannot be the result of treatment. But it is still unknown whether there are structural abnormalities in various brain centres or defective interconnections between key centres.

It could be speculated that the classical symptoms of inappropriate mood, delusions and hallucinations imply involvement of the limbic system, which is concerned with emotional responses and beliefs, and the ascending reticular system, concerned with monitoring and filtering of perceptions. On the other hand, the negative symptoms typical of chronic schizophrenia may involve lesions of frontal lobe cortical areas, and the impaired thought processes suggest cortical involvement.

The predominant biochemical abnormality seems to be functional over-activity of dopaminergic pathways between midbrain and certain cortical areas (the mesolimbic and mesocortical tracts). This is compatible with the known dopamine-blocking action of most antipsychotic drugs. Whether dopamine excess is a cause or an incidental consequence has not been established, and uncertainty remains about the relative roles of dopamine DA_1, DA_2 and DA_{3-6} receptors. GABA and 5-HT pathways are also probably involved.

Functional theories involve ideas of incomplete adjustment to society, especially to the family. The 'antipsychiatrists' suggest, on the other hand, that schizophrenia is a response to an irrational, contradictory or hostile world.

A holistic synthesis of these various theories might propose a genetic predisposition conferring susceptibility, maladaption in early life, followed by environmental triggers such as drug misuse, stress or a hostile family or social environment, ultimately leading to disease onset.

In view of the uncertainty about causes, the management of schizophrenia remains essentially symptomatic: relieve the patient's suffering, perhaps slow the progression, and help the patient to cope. As yet prevention is not possible, nor can anything be done to reverse the disease process.

Clinical features

Psychotic signs

The classification and symptomatology of schizophrenia are complex and have been endlessly debated among psychiatrists. Recently, the WHO and the American Psychiatric Association have rationalized and harmonized diagnostic criteria. Table 6.17 describes the common signs in terms of normal brain functions. All are descriptive psychiatric signs; there are no objective physical, biochemical or metabolic signs.

The defining clinical features of schizophrenia are thought disorder and delusions. A delusion is an ill-founded and irrational belief that nevertheless is implacably held, not amenable to reasoned persuasion and completely at variance with the patient's religious, social or ethnic background. Many patients have very strange ideas and make bizarre associations, sometimes inventing their own language (neologism) or using common words in an inappropriate way: "I'm in hospital because of my minarets". Some have elaborate paranoid delusions: everybody is spying on them or plotting against them, including relatives, neighbours, and governments. They may also hallucinate, hearing the voices of their tormentors talking about them,

or they see their own name in newspapers or on television (ideas of reference). No wonder they are so miserable.

Patients may believe their actions are controlled by others – often, among patients from Western countries, by means of invisible rays, magnets or electric wires. They may hear on the radio an echo of what they have just thought, or feel that they have foreign ideas inserted into their brain. One patient believed he had a telephone implanted in his head, through which his every action was dictated to him by a distant 'friend': no X-ray would have convinced him otherwise. Often their emotional responses are fatuous or inappropriate, e.g. laughing or crying at the socially incorrect time; in others mood variation is generally reduced. The combination of all these features produces the markedly unusual behaviour popularly known as 'madness'.

There is often a tragic consistency about a patient's symptom complex. Their delusions reflect their hallucinations, or their hallucinations confirm their delusions: both appear to escape the logical censorship provided by fully functional insight. However bizarre it seems, their behaviour may be consistent with their misreading of reality. Someone who believed that thoughts were constantly put into their head against their will might well believe there was a plot against them, especially if they heard voices apparently confirming this. Their reaction might well be aggressive behaviour, or shouting out loud to tell the persons whose voices they heard to go away. The novels of Franz Kafka give us some inkling of the terrors of paranoia.

Classification

Two broad syndromes are recognized (Table 6.17). Patients in the early acute stages have **type 1** (classical or florid) schizophrenia with **positive** symptoms. Loosely, these resemble disinihibited exaggerations of normal activity. **Type 2** features, usually seen in chronic schizophrenia, are predominantly **negative**, such as flat mood, apathy, social withdrawal, and lack of speech (alogia), pleasure (anhedonia) or initiative (avolition) are seen. These describe functions found in normal persons but absent in schizophrenia.

Table 6.17   Clinical features of schizophrenia[a]

Positive features (type 1)	
Cognitive	**Distorted or irrational reasoning, reduced insight**
	Loosened associations, illogical cause–effect links
	Private language
	Inattention, poor memory
	Poor problem solving and abstract thinking
Belief	Delusions
	• persecution (paranoia)
	• **external control (passivity)**
	• **thought broadcast**
	• **thought insertion**
	• grandeur
	Ideas of reference
	Delusional perceptions[b]
	Derealisation, depersonalization[c]
Perception	Hallucinations
	• **usually auditory[d]**
	• also visual
	• less common: tactile, gustatory, olfactory
Mood	Inappropriate emotional responses
Behaviour	Bizarre, irrational; occasionally aggressive, rarely violent
Negative features (type 2)	
Mood	Blunting (flattening) of affect
Behaviour	Withdrawn, antisocial, apathetic, poor self-care
	Poverty of speech, anhedonia, avolition

[a] First-rank symptoms (usually type 1) are in bold.

[b] Special personal significance attributed to everyday phenomena ('primary delusion').

[c] Feeling of distancing from external world or from self, others or own emotions.

[d] First rank if voices heard referring to patient in third person, or echoing his/her thoughts

Type 2 features may represent long-term deterioration of chronic disease, burnt-out disease or possibly consequences of long-term antipsychotic use. However, careful history taking will often reveal forerunners of these negative traits in early life, e.g. a withdrawn lonely child. At onset they are masked by the florid positive features but once the latter are under pharmacological control the former, less affected by drugs, emerge as the predominant signs of illness (Figure 6.11).

Another classification groups symptoms as either cognitive (i.e. thought disorder), positively psychotic (e.g. delusions and hallucinations) or negative (e.g. apathy, social withdrawal, lack of self-care).

Diagnosis

It is first necessary to eliminate any primary underlying cause such as iatrogenic psychosis

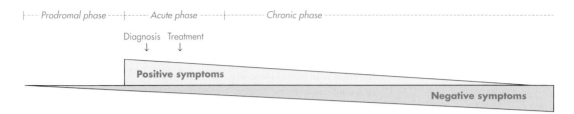

Figure 6.11   Typical course of chronic schizophrenia, showing change in type of symptoms (not to scale).

(e.g. corticosteroids), drug misuse (e.g. amphetamines), brain tumour or infection, head injury, certain rare forms of epilepsy, hyperthyroidism, etc. The symptoms must have been continuously present for at least a month, and usually with evidence of deteriorating social functioning, at work and with family and friends.

Distinguishing between borderline schizophrenia and other psychoses (mainly mania and severe depression) can sometimes be difficult. Traditionally the presence of at least two symptoms from the list given in Table 6.17, or just one 'first-rank' symptom (positive symptoms, mostly specific forms of delusion) is needed to confirm schizophrenia. Type I patients usually show several positive symptoms and the diagnosis is clear.

In chronic schizophrenia, symptoms are mainly negative and are more difficult to diagnose and to treat. Moreover they must be distinguished from iatrogenic over-sedation or extrapyramidal effects, clinical depression or 'institutionalization', i.e. the dependency and apathy that can result from long-term hospital care. The latest editions of both DSM-IV and ICD-10 include negative symptoms as primary diagnostic criteria.

In different cultures and times the symptoms take different outward forms, but the overall pattern and prevalence are consistent. Nowadays the persecutors imagined by paranoid patients are Martians or secret government spies, who control them with lasers or magnetism. In medieval Europe, and present-day pre-industrial societies, devils or evil spirits using witchcraft or curses are to blame. This is one disease for which the stress of modern industrial society cannot be held responsible.

Course and prognosis

The old medical Latin name for schizophrenia was *dementia praecox* (loosely, the madness of youth) because the most common time of onset is late adolescence or early adulthood. There may be a sudden deterioration, a form of 'nervous breakdown', which is the generic lay term for the acute onset of any psychiatric condition. However, this acute phase will usually have been preceded by a prodromal phase with gradual reduction in social, academic or work-related functioning, loss of friends, deterioration in personal hygiene or other behaviour uncharacteristic of the patient's former personality.

About a quarter of patients will suffer just a single episode, then recover and lead normal lives. Good prognostic signs are:

- The absence of a family history of schizophrenia.
- Stable premorbid personality.
- Acute onset.
- Preservation of emotional responses, initiative and coherent personality.
- Early recognition and treatment.

Conversely, a poor outlook is indicated by:

- Positive family history.
- Disturbed, eccentric, antisocial or withdrawn premorbid personality.
- Difficulty in forming relationships, from an early age.
- Disrupted domestic situation and poor social adjustment.
- Insidious onset.
- Loss of affect, initiative and drive.
- Delay in treatment.

Although most initially recover from the first episode, about three-quarters of sufferers will relapse and eventually enter a chronic phase suffering gradual decline or repeated relapses and remissions. This tends to be accompanied by the development of type 2 features. They have great difficulty forming relationships, do not marry, cannot keep jobs and drop out of education. Without treatment, follow-up and social or family support they may drift down the social scale, becoming progressively more involved in vagrancy, petty crime, illicit drug use and alcoholism. Some 10% of all patients need long-term institutional care. The same proportion commits suicide.

Between these extremes are those who, with the help of medication, adjust to their disability and manage to cope in the community, while perhaps seeming just a trifle eccentric. The importance of social and family support is emphasized by the fact that the prognosis for patients in developing countries, with their extended families and perhaps greater tolerance of eccentricity and nonconformity, is better than in the developed world. Even in the UK, many people who are obviously quite 'mad', but harmless and able to look after themselves after a fashion, are free to roam the streets.

Management

Drugs, psychotherapy and social interventions all have a place in the management of schizophrenia. Most patients are managed by a combination of family or community care with occasional hospital admission, supported by maintenance antipsychotic drug therapy. Nowadays, few schizophrenic patients need permanent institutional care.

Before the discovery of *chlorpromazine* in the early 1950s, however, things were very different. Little could be done for people with severe mental illness, if help was offered at all. There was only heavy sedation with barbiturates or, before them, bromides and straitjackets. Community care was unheard of: the idea was to keep 'maniacs' as far from 'normal' people as possible.

In the UK in the 19th century, the enlightened Victorians built asylums. Not then a pejorative term, asylum implied protection rather than imprisonment and neglect. In these enormous rambling institutions built at a safe distance outside the big cities, custodial care may have been the ethos but sedatives, locked doors, spiked walls and padded rooms were still the means (Figure 6.12).

Aims

The aims in managing schizophrenia are to:

- control acute attacks and prevent self-harm or harm to others;
- attend to social and domestic factors;
- rehabilitate the patient if possible;
- start long-term support and maintenance therapy as appropriate.

Day attendants must always have their keys attached to their person by the chain and belt provided...they are required to lock every door through which they pass.

...the patients are not to be permitted to sit or lie down on the floor or crouch in corners ...

...the patients must not be allowed to damage the shrubs and trees. Those having morbid appetites must be prevented from eating leaves, rubbish, etc.

...knives and forks must be counted and locked up in the proper box...under no circumstances must any patient be permitted to use the carving knife.

...all brooms, buckets, fire-irons, especially anything that may be used as a weapon of offence, must be kept clean, locked up, and placed in the cupboard set apart for the purpose.

Figure 6.12 Extracts from *Rules for the Guidance of the Attendants, Servants and all Persons Engaged in the Service of the Cornwall County Asylum at Bodmin*, 1900.

Social and psychotherapy

Conventional psychotherapy is of little benefit in acute schizophrenia, and psychoanalysis even less so, because patients have no insight. However, simple counselling can help many patients to adjust to a chronic illness while remaining in the community. Coping-skills training, occupational therapy and hostel or 'halfway house' accommodation may be arranged. CBT has also been found helpful. Family education and social therapy, where people in contact with the patient can be told what to expect and are encouraged to be supportive, can be very helpful in maintaining remission. Stormy home relationships and a lack of acceptance of the patient are the most common reasons for relapse, whereas a supportive home environment greatly reduces the chances of relapse.

For most types of psychotherapy a degree of insight is required, and drug therapy is usually needed to establish this. Once patients have been stabilized, such interventions can be instituted. It must be emphasized that most patients who are concordant with their medication and have a relatively stable domestic and social environment are to a greater or lesser extent lucid, have autonomy, can make decisions and should be encouraged to participate in treatment choices. Even more than a disruptive social environment, abruptly stopping medication is the greatest risk factor for relapse.

Drug therapy

When discovered in the 1950s the antipsychotic drugs, also less accurately termed neuroleptics, antischizophrenic agents or major tranquillizers, revolutionized the care of psychotic illness. For the first time many patients who would otherwise have languished in deluded misery inside custodial institutions were freed from both their mental and their physical prisons. The prototype *chlorpromazine*, perhaps surprisingly, is still used.

However, steady development since the 1950s has resulted in significant improvements in efficacy, safety and formulation. Antipsychotic drugs are now divided, although not so distinctly as some manufacturers would like it believed, into two broad classes. The 'typical' antipsychotics include original phenothiazines (e.g. *chlorpromazine*) and the butyrophenones (e.g. *haloperidol*). The 'atypical' antipsychotics include *clozapine* and *olanzapine*. These groups are distinguished mainly on the basis of their side-effect profile.

Pharmacodynamic action

The proprietary name Largactil was chosen for the original phenothiazine, *chlorpromazine*, rather prosaically because of its large number of actions. Its structural similarity to several natural neurotransmitter amines gives it antagonist activity on cholinergic, histaminic, alpha-adrenergic, serotoninergic and dopaminergic receptors. Structural alterations during subsequent development have produced a number of groups of antipsychotics with varying receptor affinities, giving a diverse range of therapeutic and adverse profiles (Tables 6.18 and 6.19).

Unfortunately, despite modern non-invasive imaging of the living brain, there is still much to learn about the relationship between receptor blockade, localization of CNS activity and antipsychotic action. One problem is that little is known of the inter-relationships and interdependencies between different receptor systems. For example, although most of the original antipsychotics are potent dopamine blockers, the newer ones preferentially target 5-HT receptors. This may be because one type of receptor is upstream or downstream of the other, with actions at either having a similar outcome. Again, the adrenergic alpha$_2$ activity shown by some agents could enhance dopaminergic transmission in the BG and thus reduce extrapyramidal adverse effects.

Typical antipsychotics

Among the typical antipsychotics, antipsychotic action correlates well with blockade of the dopamine D$_2$ receptors assumed to be in the thalamus, limbic system and cortical projections of the ascending reticular formation. However, although the onset of antipsychotic action takes weeks, receptor blockade occurs within hours of starting therapy. A similar phenomenon is seen with antidepressants, and another similarity is that measurements of changes in the metabolite of the presumed transmitter (homovanillic acid in the case of dopamine) do not correlate with clinical activity.

Dopamine blockade yields other useful actions (e.g. *prochlorperazine* used as an anti-emetic) and many adverse ones, including extrapyramidal symptoms and endocrine (hypothalamic) actions. There are at least five subtypes of dopamine receptor, and research is attempting to differentiate these in terms of their anatomical location and clinical or adverse effect.

Actions at other receptors also have either therapeutic or adverse actions (see Table 6.18). Antimuscarinic action may reduce extrapyramidal symptoms; antihistamine action is sedative, exploited therapeutically as with *promethazine*; adrenergic blockade may cause postural hypotension; and serotonin blockade has antipsychotic action.

Following the initial prolific development of the phenothiazines, other chemical structures were developed (Table 6.19). These are usually more specific for dopamine D_2 receptors, e.g. butyrophenones, which appears to accentuate the antipsychotic clinical and extrapyramidal adverse actions, but reduces autonomic adverse effects. The thioxanthene and benzamide groups are claimed to have, in addition, stimulant and antidepressant activities.

Atypical antipsychotics

The dibenzodiazepines (Table 6.19) are forerunners of the atypical antipsychotics, which have arguably greater clinical activity combined with unarguably a significant reduction in extrapyramidal adverse effects. They mark a return to broad-spectrum receptor blockade, but with a greater relative affinity for 5-HT receptors over D_2 receptors. One of the most recent, *aripiprazole*, appears to be a partial dopamine agonist, with blocking activity in the presence of high dopamine levels but mild agonist activity in the absence of dopamine. Additionally it has activity at 5-HT receptors.

The advantages of this group lie in superior activity in treatment-resistant disease, significant activity against negative symptoms, and freedom from EPS, including tardive dyskinesia (see p. 419). Generally, atypical antipsychotics are as effective on positive symptoms as the older agents and share the same autonomic adverse effects of cholinergic and adrenergic blockade. Weight gain is greater but hyperprolactinaemia

Table 6.18   Pharmacodynamic actions of antipsychotic drugs

Receptor blocked	Therapeutic effect	Side-effect
Dopamine	Antipsychotic, especially type 1 schizophrenia (D_2-receptors) Anti-emetic	Extrapyramidal symptoms ($D_{1,2}$-receptors?) Hypothalamic – ↑ prolactin (D_5-receptors?); sexual dysfunction
Acetylcholine (M_1)	Reduced extrapyramidal symptoms Sedative	Antimuscarinic, e.g. dry mouth, blurred vision, etc.
Adrenaline	? Antipsychotic (α_2-receptors)	Sympatholytic (α_1-receptors) – hypotension
Histamine (H_1)	Antihistamine Sedative	
Serotonin (5-HT_2)	Antipsychotic ? ↓ Extrapyramidal symptoms	

5-HT_2, 5-hydroxytryptamine$_2$

Table 6.19 Comparison of therapeutic and side-effects of main group of antipsychotics in relation to principal receptor-blocking affinities

Chemical group	Example	Antipsychotic		Sedative	Side-effects				
					EPS	Weight gain	Hypothalamic	Hypotensive	AntiACh
		DA_2[a]	$5\text{-}HT_2$[a]	H_1	$DA_{1,2}$	??	DA_1	α_1 Adr	ACh
Simple phenothiazine[b]	Chlorpromazine	++	++	++++	+++	++	+++	++++	++++
Piperidyl phenothiazine[b]	Thioridazine[c]	+++	++	+++	+	+++	++++	+++	++++
Piperazinyl phenothiazine[b]	Trifluoperazine	++++	+	+++	++++	++	+++	++	++
Piperazinyl thioxanthene	Flupentixol	++++	+	++	++++	+	++++	+	+++
Butyrophenone	Haloperidol	++++	+	++++	++++	+	++++	+	++
Diphenylbutylpiperidine	Pimozide	++++	–	–	+++	+	++++	++	–
Benzamide	Sulpiride	++++	+	++	++	+	++++	–	–
Dibenzodiazepine	Clozapine	++++	++++	++++	–	++++	++	++	++++
Miscellaneous atypicals[d]	(Various)	+/+++	++++	–/+++	–/+	++/+++	++	–/+++	+

Condensing inevitably entails considerable approximation, and the data are only for basic comparisons. Data compiled from various sources. Frequency/severity of effect: – none; + little; ++ moderate; +++ high; ++++ very high.

(a) There may be up to five dopamine receptor subtypes, and many 5-HT subtypes; both are simplified here.

(b) The three groups of phenothiazines are distinguished by different side chains on a common nucleus.

(c) Now little used owing to cardiotoxicity.

(d) Atypicals except the prototype, clozapine, are grouped together. See also Table 6.23.

AntiACh, antimuscarinic; DA, dopamine; α_1 Adr, alpha-1 adrenergic; H_1, histamine; ACh, acetylcholine; $5\text{-}HT_2$, 5-hydroxytryptamine$_2$; EPS, extrapyramidal symptoms.

less. Experience is not yet sufficient to be certain, but some may have a lower incidence of tardive dyskinesia and perhaps neuroleptic malignant syndrome. There may be a lower risk of suicide with *clozapine*. Nevertheless, this is not a completely homogeneous group: there are important differences in their adverse effects (Table 6.23; compare with Table 6.19).

Whether or not the atypicals really are clinically more effective than the typicals in symptom control is still debated. Initial evidence suggesting they were better than the typicals in controlling negative symptoms and resistant schizophrenia has been disputed. Re-analysis has indicated that the use of *haloperidol* as the comparator drug, and the doses used, make the results less clear-cut. The CATIE trial implied that careful selection of the right agent for a patient is more important than the class of drug used. The difference, if it does exist, is unlikely to be great. However, the unique superiority of *clozapine* in resistant schizophrenia is now firmly accepted.

Experience with *clozapine* is greatest, and it is now the benchmark. Unfortunately, because of its propensity to cause bone marrow suppression, its use necessitates patient registration on an obligatory, costly and inconvenient blood monitoring scheme. However, there are now several alternatives. Mainly because of possible orthostatic hypotension, most atypical agents need careful initiation and subsequent dose titration.

Psychotropic actions

These drugs have a wide spectrum of psychotropic actions (Table 6.20). Their ability to sedate without general impairment of consciousness (i.e. tranquillize) gives them an anxiolytic, tension-relieving effect. The antipsychotic action is a remarkable ability to banish hallucinations, diminish the power of delusions and straighten out distorted thought; this is the origin of their description as 'major tranquillizers'. Psychomotor inhibition is a specific

Table 6.20   Psychotropic properties and target symptoms of the antipsychotic drugs

Psychotropic action	Target symptom	Psychiatric condition where symptom occurs	Suitable group
Tranquillization	Anxiety Tension	Anxiety neurosis	Simple phenothiazine
Psychomotor inhibition	Hyperactivity Agitation Racing thoughts Aggression	Mania, schizophrenia	Simple phenothiazine Zuclopenthixol
Antipsychotic	Thought disorder Hallucination Delusion	Schizophrenia Schizophrenia, mania, severe depression	'Atypical'[a] Halogenated phenothiazine 'Atypical'[a], Butyrophenone 'Atypical'[a] Diphenylbutylpiperidine Benzamide
Alerting	Apathy; withdrawal; negative symptoms	Schizophrenia (type 2)	'Atypical'[a]
Mood elevation	Depressed mood	Schizophrenia; severe depression	Benzamide; thioxanthene

[a] e.g. dibenzodiazepine.

depression of overactive thought and physical activity, again not at the expense of consciousness. Some antipsychotics have a stimulant or alerting effect on withdrawn patients, and others also a mood elevating or antidepressant action. These properties are shown to a different degree by different groups and their usefulness in treating the common target symptoms of various psychiatric illnesses is indicated in Table 6.20.

Pharmacokinetics and administration

No consistent predictions about antipsychotic effectiveness in a given patient can be made either from the dose used or from plasma level measurements. Most antipsychotics have a half-life >24 h, so single daily doses are usually adequate in the maintenance phase; evening usually is the best time, especially if a sedating effect is required. There is often a first-pass effect, so parenteral doses are usually lower than oral ones. The apparent volume of distribution is high owing to the lipophilic nature and consequent accumulation in the CNS. Thus, although plasma binding is usually quite high (e.g. >95% for *chlorpromazine*), this does not present any potential interaction problems. Clearance is usually hepatic (an exception is the benzamide group), so the potential exists for hepatic drug interactions. This is also important because hepatotoxicity occasionally occurs.

Recommended maximum doses are only guides: patient response is the principal criterion. Very high doses may be given if adverse effects are absent or tolerable, provided that a clinical effect is achieved. However, persistently high doses must be avoided, especially after the acute phase has been controlled. The Royal College of Psychiatrists has issued precautions about high dose therapy (see BNF).

Side-effects

Many of the adverse effects of the antipsychotics derive from their various pharmacodynamic actions and so are, in principle, predictable. The widest spectrum of side-effects is seen with the phenothiazines (Table 6.21), but the prominence of different adverse effects varies between groups (see Table 6.19). Among the typicals, the greater the antipsychotic potency, the fewer the autonomic effects and the more likely the EPS. For the atypicals this trend has been reversed, with potent antipsychotics having greatly reduced EPS.

There are potentially serious non-specific or idiosyncratic effects. Jaundice and photosensitivity are more common than agranulocytosis. *Clozapine* is particularly liable to depress the white cell count (incidence approx. 1% of patients per year) and it is mandatory that patients are regularly monitored. As with many psychotropic drugs, seizure threshold is lowered, a problem for epileptics at normal doses and for all patients in overdose. ECG changes with prolongation of the QT interval and potential arrhythmias can occur, especially with *thioridazine* and, less commonly, the atypicals (usually in combination with other drugs). Atypical agents should not be used in the elderly with dementia because of a risk of stroke or death.

Autonomic blockade

The antimuscarinic actions and consequent precautions are similar to those of the tricyclic antidepressants (Table 6.11). Peripheral alpha-adrenergic blockade can cause cardiovascular problems, particularly postural hypotension with reflex tachycardia. Autonomic symptoms tend to remit with chronic use.

Endocrine effects

Blocking dopamine in the hypothalamus inhibits some endocrine mechanisms. Most important is the rare but potentially fatal **neuroleptic malignant syndrome**, which is probably hypothalamic in origin. The syndrome involves hyperthermia, muscle spasm, impaired consciousness and cardiovascular instability, and has a 10% mortality. Treatment is with dopaminergic agents (e.g. *bromocriptine*), muscle relaxants (e.g. benzodiazepines, *dantrolene*) and antimuscarinics (e.g. *procyclidine*), as well as cooling and rehydration.

Hyperprolactinaemia is quite common and has many consequences that are unacceptable to many patients, such as galactorrhoea, amenorrhoea, gynaecomastia, and sexual dysfunction (loss of libido and impotence).

Table 6.21   Side-effects of phenothiazines and other antipsychotics

Pharmacological effect	System	Side-effect
Dopamine blockade	Basal ganglia	Extrapyramidal symptoms (see Table 6.22)
	Hypothalamus	Hyperprolactinaemia (e.g. gynaecomastia, impotence, galactorrhoea)
		Weight gain
	Hypothalamus?	Neuroleptic malignant syndrome
Adrenergic blockade	CVS	Hypotension, especially postural; tachycardia
Cholinergic blockade	GIT	Dry mouth, constipation
	Eyes	Blurred vision, mydriasis, raised intraocular pressure
	Bladder	Urinary retention
	Heart	Tachycardia/palpitations
	CNS	Sedation, drowsiness, confusion
Membrane effects	Heart	Conduction defects; prolongation of QT interval; arrhythmias (esp. thioridazine, atypicals)
	CNS	Reduced seizure threshold, proconvulsant
Non-specific/unknown	Metabolic	Hyperglycaemia, diabetes (atypicals)
	Liver	Jaundice
	Skin	Rashes, photosensitivity (chlorpromazine)
	Eyes	Pigmented retinopathy (thioridazine)
	CNS	Impaired cognition: memory, attention, coordination
	Bone marrow	Agranulocytosis (esp. clozapine)

CNS, central nervous system; CVS, cardiovascular system; GIT, gastrointestinal tract.

Less serious, but equally likely to discourage compliance, is weight gain. The atypicals are particularly associated with this, notably *clozapine* and *olanzapine*, and they can also cause or precipitate diabetes, a condition that is anyway more common even among untreated schizophrenics. Thus regular monitoring of weight and blood glucose is essential.

Extrapyramidal syndromes (EPS)
Movement disorders, although usually harmless, are a major cause of non-compliance among schizophrenia patients. A drawback of using dopamine blockers for antipsychotic action in the limbic and reticular systems is that dopamine is also a transmitter crucial to the motor-controlling functions of the BG. (For a fuller discussion, see pp. 368–370 and pp. 427–428.) Both systems seem to involve D_2 receptors, for which most antipsychotics have a high affinity.

Thus disturbance of fine motor control has been thought almost inevitable with potent antipsychotics: the two effects seemed inextricable.

There are currently three ways around the problem:

- Intrinsic antimuscarinic activity.
- Selective affinity for dopamine receptors in the limbic system.
- Balance between 5-HT and D_2 receptor blockade

Normally, dopaminergic action in the BG is counterbalanced by cholinergic activity, whereas in the areas presumed to be disturbed in psychosis, dopamine does not appear to have a natural antagonist. Thus it is possible to counteract the adverse effects of dopamine blockade with a centrally acting antimuscarinic drug without significantly diminishing the antipsychotic action: this effect is used to treat some antipsychotic-induced EPS. Note that, by contrast, using the anti-Parkinson drug *levodopa*, although it would be effective, would also nullify the antipsychotic activity. Some standard antipsychotics with high antimuscarinic activity, especially *thioridazine*, have a lower incidence of EPS and so reduce the need for ancillary antimuscarinic drugs.

Most atypicals have a far lower incidence of EPS, perhaps because of a selective affinity for receptors in limbic and cortical areas, but not in the BG. In addition, the antipsychotic activity of most atypicals, especially *clozapine*, is more closely correlated with blockade of 5-HT$_2$ receptors, an action that has little direct effect on motor coordination but may indirectly prevent it being disturbed.

EPS can be classified into four groups (Table 6.22). Unfortunately, there are no predictors of which type will occur to which patient, or when.

Acute dystonia. Some patients react with an alarming acute muscle spasm on the first dose or within the first few days of antipsychotic therapy, especially if given in high doses or by injection. This usually occurs in the head and neck region: commonly it presents as an exaggerated and uncontrolled rolling upwards of the eyes (**oculogyric crisis**), a stiff jaw or a hyper-extended neck. Occasionally there may be a dangerous choking laryngospasm. Fortunately these reactions are easily treated by parenteral antimuscarinics (e.g. *procyclidine*) but they can severely damage the patient's confidence in the therapy.

Pseudo-parkinsonism. Early in therapy up to 50% of patients develop a motor incoordination syndrome very similar to idiopathic Parkinson's disease. (Note that Parkinson's disease involves dopamine deficit; pp. 427–428). Almost any parkinsonian symptom can occur, and though iatrogenic parkinsonism often remits spontaneously after a few months of treatment, this is of little comfort to the patient, who loses confidence and may become non-compliant.

The temptation to use oral antimuscarinic anti-Parkinson drugs prophylactically is strong. In the past they have been given routinely. However, this is now uncommon because they themselves may cause various psychotomimetic effects such as delirium; they have even been misused for such effects. In addition, their adverse antimuscarinic effects would be additive to those of antipsychotics themselves. Thus strong efforts are made to encourage the patient to tolerate the symptoms without anti-Parkinson drugs until they eventually subside.

Akathisia. Marked restlessness and anxiety seem to be the most disturbing effects for many patients. Akathisia follows a similar course to pseudo-parkinsonism but responds poorly to conventional anti-Parkinson therapy. Some patients develop a more persistent form, which resembles tardive dyskinesia. Sometimes a short course of benzodiazepines may help, and lipophilic centrally-acting beta-blockers have also been used.

Tardive dyskinesia (TD). A form of orofacial dyskinesia, TD may develop after months or years of successful therapy, or even after drugs have been withdrawn. Its bizarre symptoms involve lip-smacking, chewing and grimacing

Table 6.22	Extrapyramidal side-effects induced by antipsychotics
Class	**Common symptoms**
Acute dystonia	Neck or spine spasm Neck, jaw or larynx rigidity Oculogyric crisis
Pseudo-parkinsonism	Dyskinesia and dystonia: rigidity, tremor, bradykinesia
Akathisia	Psychomotor restlessness and agitation; inability to sit still
Tardive dyskinesia	Abnormal face, mouth or jaw movement, e.g. lipsmacking, grimacing, tongue protrusion Body writhing (choreoathetoid movements)

facial expressions. Although not directly distressing for the patient, these provoke unsympathetic or hostile reactions in onlookers because they give the patient the appearance of the popular idea of 'craziness', when paradoxically the drugs responsible for this bizarre behaviour are in fact controlling the psychotic symptoms.

The pathology of TD is different from that of other EPS and is poorly understood. It is found sometimes in schizophrenics who have never been treated, but certainly antipsychotics do increase its occurrence. The cause may be the development of dopamine receptor supersensitivity. Prevalence rates of up to 50% and annual incidences of 5% have been reported, the elderly being particularly susceptible. It has been suggested that TD is actually a symptom of severe schizophrenia rather than iatrogenic, and these patients are the most likely to be taking high doses of potent antipsychotics.

TD is unpredictable, but seems to occur more commonly after long courses and high doses of antipsychotics. Intermittent therapy, e.g. drug holidays, depot therapy, and antimuscarinic therapy seem particularly to predispose patients to TD. Perversely, reducing the antipsychotic dose temporarily intensifies symptoms, while increasing the dose may alleviate them.

Aside from a correlation with potency, generally no one drug is more likely to cause TD than another. However, *clozapine* definitely causes TD less often and indeed is a drug of choice when patients develop TD on other drugs. Other atypicals would be expected also to be favourable owing to their low EPS potential; however, the evidence for them is not as clear.

Currently the best strategy seems to be to reserve antipsychotics for serious psychosis and keep doses as low as possible. If TD occurs, it may only be mild and, with the agreement of the patient and his or her family, may be ignored, especially if the patient would be expected to relapse without antipsychotics.

Various drugs have been used, including *vitamin E, clonazepam, nifedipine, sodium valproate, reserpine* and *choline*, with little success. Currently *clozapine* and *quetiapine* are the best options. Antimuscarinic drugs should be stopped. If TD cannot be controlled, the antipsychotic must be

gradually reduced until the dyskinesia remits. If psychotic symptoms then recur, re-starting antipsychotic therapy with a different agent (especially *clozapine*) may be possible without recurrence of TD.

Drug selection

The issue of whether or not to start with an atypical is still disputed by some, but the current consensus and the recommendation by NICE is that atypicals are preferred. Their superior adverse effects profile, with consequent improvements in compliance, is now considered to outweigh by far the extra cost, both in pharmacoeconomic and patient satisfaction terms. Depending on which drug a patient is taking when treatment is being (re)considered, the progression is to start with an atypical, usually *olanzapine* or *risperidone*, then move on to *clozapine* if control is not achieved (Figure 6.13). However, if a patient is stabilized on a typical agent and is content, there is no need to change to an atypical.

Acute attack
First onset. It is now clear that prompt appropriate antipsychotic treatment at as early a stage as possible in the course of a developing schizophrenic illness is likely to produce a better outcome. Although it is not yet possible to prevent the illness progressing, therapy prolongs remission and reduces relapses and gives the patient the best chance of maintaining social functioning. To ensure the new patient is least disturbed by side-effects and thus encouraged to continue with maintenance medication, atypicals are first choice. Wherever possible, the patient should be involved in the decision about initial drug therapy.

Emergency tranquillization. An acutely psychotic patient is likely to be deluded, hallucinating, incomprehensible and quite without insight. The immediate objective is to control these features and to prevent patients harming themselves or others while their grasp of reality is impaired. In the UK, a section of the Mental Health Act allows compulsory admission to hospital for essential physical treatments in

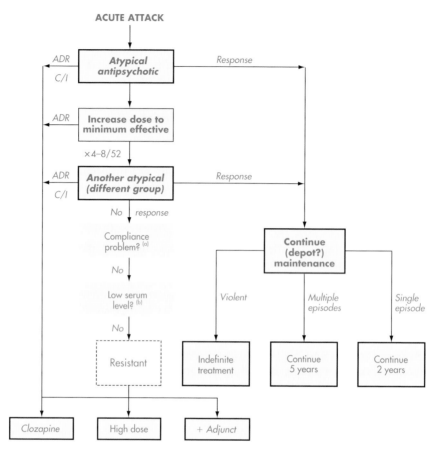

Figure 6.13   A possible algorithm for treatment of schizophrenia. [a]If *yes*, consider depot therapy; [b]if *yes*, investigate possible drug interaction or other cause of abnormal kinetics. ADR, adverse drug reaction; C/I, contra-indication.

circumstances when the patient is likely to be a danger to themselves or others; this process is known colloquially as 'sectioning'. It is proposed in the UK that compulsory treatment should be extended to community care also.

Prompt drug therapy is the only option. A sedating antipsychotic from one of the traditional or atypical groups may be given, e.g. *olanzapine* or *haloperidol*. A benzodiazepine may be added. At first, medication may have to be administered parenterally to a reluctant patient, although the onset of action is hardly quicker and there is a much higher risk of serious acute extrapyramidal complications if the dose is too high.

Drug administration during this time is carefully supervised, and the dose gradually titrated up to the minimum effective level. Tranquilliza-

tion and sedation are rapidly and reliably achieved, but control of psychotic symptoms will not be evident for up to a month or so (Figure 6.13), and full stabilization may take several months. If the patient does not respond in the first 1–2 months, some clinicians would advocate further increasing the dose; others would change to a different group for a further month. If extrapyramidal symptoms or other adverse effects are intolerable, or if there are specific contra-indications, there should be a switch from a typical to an atypical or a change of atypical. NICE recommends initiation of *clozapine* when a patient has failed after 6–8 weeks on each of two other drugs successively, including one atypical.

Treatment resistance.   This is usually defined as failure with at least two drugs, typically one typical and one atypical at optimal doses (Figure 6.13). It occurs in about one-third of patients. A true treatment-refractory state must be distinguished from poor compliance, drug interaction or possibly enhanced elimination by the patient's hepatic or renal systems.

Three strategies are currently used to manage resistance to conventional agents at maximal recommended doses. High-dose therapy can be tried, but there is limited evidence and the guidelines of the Royal College of Psychiatrists (see BNF, section 4.2) contra-indicate it for many at-risk patients, rigorous precautions must be taken and close monitoring is required. An adjunct drug can be added, such as *lithium* (especially in schizoaffective states), *carbamazepine* (especially in aggression or mood swings) or a benzodiazepine (especially if extra sedation is indicated); experience with *lithium* is greatest. Probably the treatment of choice now is to use *clozapine*. In the rare cases where *clozapine* is inadequate, NICE recommends the trial addition of *olanzapine*.

Maintenance and prophylaxis

Patients who develop chronic disease need continuation therapy, either to suppress their symptoms (maintenance) or to prevent relapses (prophylaxis). The management of such patients has undergone a number of changes in recent decades.

The first was changed social policy, which encouraged a reduction in the number of long-stay psychiatric hospital patients, many of them schizophrenic, and their return to the community. The inevitable lack of stimulation in long-stay hospitals is detrimental to recovery. Patients become institutionalized and incapable of independent existence, even if their disease eventually remits. Unfortunately, community services have not always been appropriately equipped or funded to care for this large increase in their dependent population. Only now is it realized that this discharge process has been too thorough and has become counter-productive, as the discharged patients lose contact with the care services and become homeless, vagrant or imprisoned. In a very few cases – unfortunately those that attract most public attention – they have become dangerously violent.

Second, the community care of these patients would not have been feasible without the development of long-acting depot forms of the antipsychotic drugs (see below).

Finally, recognition of the extent of TD (p. 420) provoked a further re-assessment of the role of long-term antipsychotic drugs. Fortunately this has been considerably mitigated by the advent of the atypicals, which are less likely to cause this.

Duration of drug treatment. Once the acute phase of schizophrenia has been controlled, drug dosage can be gradually reduced. At least 12–24 months' maintenance treatment is needed after a single acute attack. Some 75–85% of patients will eventually relapse following a single attack, and how best to manage these patients is still debated. A high-risk patient (i.e. who is violent, aggressive and never fully controlled) is still likely to need to be maintained on drugs indefinitely. For those who stay in remission for lengthy periods, attempts may be made to treat each acute attack aggressively, but gradually tail drugs off and stop them completely between attacks (targeted or intermittent therapy). Even so, an initial minimum 5-year maintenance period is recommended. There is a relapse rate of about 15% per month on discontinuation, which is halved by prophylaxis, so a difficult judgement has to be made, in association with the patient and their carer.

Delayed initiation of treatment or continuation therapy for less than 3–5 years predisposes to more frequent, more severe, less easily treated relapses. However, the maintenance dose might be kept low, and depot injections might allow total drug doses to be reduced further.

Depot therapy. If a patient is stabilized on antipsychotic therapy and seems to need medium- or long-term maintenance, there are a number of advantages to transferring to depot therapy:

- Lower total dose.
- Facilitation of community care.
- Regular contact with the patient by carers.
- Supervised administration prevents defaulting.
- No accumulation or abuse of unused tablets.

In most depot formulations the antipsychotic is esterified and dissolved in an oily vehicle. The deep IM dose is distributed throughout body fat during the first few days. Before exerting the clinical effect, the drug must be partitioned into the plasma from these lipid depots and then de-esterified by hydrolysis. Hence a single injection can maintain effective plasma levels for between 14 and 28 days. Depot therapy, organized either via special outpatient clinics or community psychiatric nurses, has greatly facilitated the trend to community care for chronic schizo-phrenic patients, enabling many patients who would otherwise be unable to do so to cope in the community.

There is at least one depot preparation available from each main antipsychotic group. Most reach therapeutic levels within about 1 week and steady state after two or three doses, and require 2- to 4-weekly injection. At present only one atypical preparation is available as a depot: *risperidone* absorbed into nylon globules. This has unusual release characteristics, with a lag phase of 4 weeks, during which oral therapy must be continued.

Ideally, the patient is first titrated for a main-tenance dose using the oral form of the selected antipsychotic. A test dose of the depot formula-tion is given to check for sensitivity to the vehicle. A formula may then be used to estimate the initial injected dose; e.g. one method would convert a 10-mg daily dose of *fluphenazine* into a 25-mg fortnightly dose.

A crossover phase follows, with the oral dose tapered off and the depot dose gradually increased. Subsequently, the depot dose must be titrated against effect, which is not as straight-forward as with oral therapy because of the delayed onset, prolonged action and slow reversal of effect. Moreover there is no consistent relationship between oral and depot doses needed to achieve control in a given patient. Nevertheless, the final dose is usually lower than the previous total oral dose over the injection interval, partly because of improved bioavail-ability but also possibly due to the efficiency of a constant plasma level.

There are disadvantages to this approach. Injection site problems, including pain, are common. If adverse effects occur that were not identified in the preliminary oral dose-ranging trial, the depot cannot be cleared quickly from the body. Although the lower total dose might be expected to reduce the incidence of adverse effects, including most EPS, this is not usually found; TD may be more common. These may be incidental consequences of the imposed improved compliance, or related to the stable plasma level as opposed to the constantly varying levels of oral therapy.

Equally important is the fact that there is often considerable patient resistance to this form of therapy, which is seen as controlling, punitive or detrimental to autonomy. This is likely to be particularly the case with those patients who are poorly compliant with oral therapy and there-fore one of the main target groups. Patient and family counselling and education are essential to explain the purpose and potential advantages of the technique.

Special problems

Adverse effects. The autonomic effects of the less potent drug groups (e.g. simple pheno-thiazines) may be contraindicated in certain patients, notably those with CVD, glaucoma, urinary retention, etc. Excessive sedation is unwanted in a disease associated with depression or negative features such as apathy and with-drawal. Many of these problems are found with the typical drugs but are absent or rarer in the atypicals, so a switch is indicated if they become troublesome or intolerable (see Tables 6.19 and 6.23).

The main problems that occur more commonly with the atypicals are weight gain and diabetes. For the first, either a typical drug is recommended, or *amisulpride*; for the second, either *risperidone* or *amisulpride*. In all such cases regular monitoring of weight and/or blood glucose is essential.

Compliance. Poor compliance is a perennial problem in psychotic patients. The basis is reduced insight, combined with often quite severe and frequently embarrassing adverse effects. Paranoid delusional states add to the difficulty when patients perceive carers as spies or tormentors. Apocryphal tales circulate of

Table 6.23 Relative properties of some newer atypical antipsychotics

Antipsychotic agent	Side-effects					Other comments
	EPS	Cardiac (ECG)	Sedation	Weight gain	Hypothalamic (prolactin)	
Aripiprazole	+	–	–	+	–	
Clozapine	–	+	+++	+++	–	↓ Seizure threshold, bone marrow suppression
Olanzapine	+	–	++	+++	+	EPS only in higher doses
Quetiapine	–	++	+	++	–	
Risperidone	+	+	+	+	+++	EPS only in higher doses; orthostatic hypotension
Sertindole	–	+++	–	?	–	ECG changes; monitor regularly, restricted use
Zotepine	+	++	+++	+++	+++	

The data assembled here compare some important properties of the atypical drugs, stressing differences between them. However, no thorough comparative evaluations of these differences have been done. No quantitative evaluation of relative potency or incidence of any of the properties listed is implied by this table, which should be read down each column. In most categories the atypicals generally have less potent or less frequent side-effects, apart from weight gain, than the typicals.

+++ high effect relative to others in class; ++ moderate effect; + low effect; – effect absent; ? no data.

ECG, electrocardiogram; EPS, extrapyramidal symptoms.

caches of medication found under floorboards or behind radiators when psychiatric hospitals are refurbished. In the community, once-daily dosing or depot therapy ameliorate the problem. In hospital, or in other situations allowing supervision of drug administration, nurses and carers become adept at ensuring that patients are not hiding tablets in their cheek pouch rather than swallowing them.

Concentrated oral liquid forms help because they cannot be hidden from a search of the oral cavity, but syrup-based preparations are inconvenient, messy and, in the long term, cause tooth decay and obesity. Moreover, doses are difficult to measure accurately. Newer orally dispersible formulations of *risperidone* and *olanzapine* are preferred nowadays.

In all cases counselling or other psychotherapy should also be used to encourage concordance.

Target symptoms. There is little evidence that particular antipsychotics have a preferential effect on specific target symptoms. The less potent agents are indicated where tranquillization or psychomotor inhibition is needed, e.g. in hypomania or acute panic attacks. However, antipsychotics should not be used for simple anxiety or agitation. Medium-potency agents are usually sufficient for the short-term treatment of the less intense psychotic features occasionally found in severe depression.

If there is an affective, especially depressive, component to schizophrenia then a thioxanthene may be indicated. However, fixed-dose combination preparations of tricyclic antidepressants and antipsychotics are almost never used by psychiatrists. *Zuclopenthixol* is reputed to be effective in diminishing aggressive symptoms.

Combinations. There are almost no situations where antipsychotic drugs should be combined, for no advantage is to be gained and adverse effects are likely to be inceased. Only in severely treatment-resistant cases, under specialist care, might this be attempted.

Cost. Pharmacoeconomic analysis, in comparing the conventional agents with atypicals, weighs the far greater drug costs of the latter against the resulting savings in reduced hospital admissions for relapse or inability to achieve control. Less easily quantifiable factors, such as improved quality of life and reduced drain on social services costs, are taken into account. Looked at this way, the balance between risk and benefit definitely favours using an atypical agent as soon as possible.

Neurological disorder

Parkinson's disease and the extrapyramidal syndromes

The **basal ganglia (BG)** and the **extrapyramidal pathways** play an important role in modulating and smoothing voluntary muscular movement (pp. 368 and 370; see also Figure 6.3). Disorders of movement and tone, collectively termed extrapyramidal syndromes (EPS), can result from an imbalance between excitatory and inhibitory influences in these structures. Idiopathic Parkinson's disease is the most common form; other similar conditions are often described generically as parkinsonism. Iatrogenic EPS are well-known side-effects of antipsychotic treatment (p. 419), and they can also be caused by numerous closely related neurodegenerative diseases or lesions (Table 6.24). Other causes can be circulatory, toxic or traumatic. This section will refer mainly to the idiopathic form.

Some important structures in the BG, and interconnections with other brain centres, are shown in Figure 6.14. Of the numerous stimulant and inhibitory transmitters involved, the best characterized are dopamine (mainly at D_2 receptors), acetylcholine, GABA and glutamate.

Table 6.24   Varieties of extrapyramidal syndrome and possible causes

Variety	Possible causes
Idiopathic Parkinson's disease (most common form)	Impaired dopamine metabolism owing to degeneration of nigrostriatal pathway Reactive free radical damage Neurotoxin e.g. MPTP (see text)
Other neurodegenerative disease	E.g. progressive subnuclear palsy (PSP), dementia with Lewy bodies (DLB) ('Parkinson's plus' syndromes), multisystem atrophy (MSA)
Infective	Viral encephalitis, syphilis, etc.
Iatrogenic	Antipsychotics, metoclopramide
Traumatic	Head injury, tumour
Ischaemic	Arteriosclerosis, atherosclerosis
Toxic	Heavy metals, carbon monoxide, pyridines

These complex pathways and circuits, which are still being traced, allow the brain to exercise a high degree of fine adjustment of voluntary movement; they are also responsible for the resting muscular tone required, for example, for posture. One important input comes from the substantia nigra (strictly speaking, a midbrain structure) and output from this system descends via the corticospinal tract and the extrapyramidal pathways.

Aetiology and pathology

Parkinson's disease arises from lesions of the inhibitory dopaminergic **nigrostriatal pathway** (Figure 6.14). The resulting reduction in dopaminergic inhibition allows a preponderance of unopposed cholinergic action in the nigrostriatum and increased GABA-ergic inhibitory tone downstream. These imbalances have a major destabilizing impact on the whole motor system.

Parkinson's disease is a chronic progressive neurodegenerative disease. It involves destruction of the melanin-pigmented dopaminergic cells of the substantia nigra and their axonal connections to the striatum. This results in a fall in the nigrostriatal dopamine output and a consequent increase in the activity of inhibitory GABA-ergic neurones. It is not simply a case of cellular dopamine deficiency or reduced turnover: there is a reduced number of dopamine-secreting cells. Other brain centres and transmitter systems may also be involved but most characteristic clinical signs, i.e. the motor defects, derive mainly from this lesion.

The underlying cause of idiopathic Parkinson's disease is unknown, so preventative measures cannot be taken. Neither auto-immunity nor infection is implicated. Many people developed Parkinson's disease as part of the encephalitis

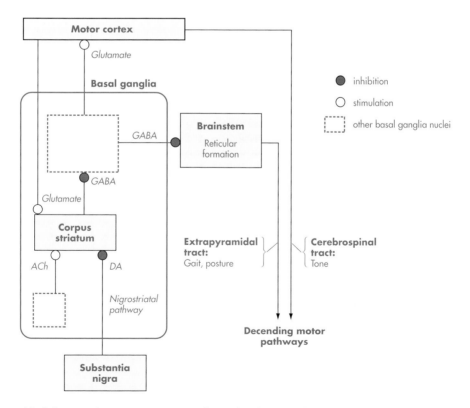

Figure 6.14 Simplified diagram showing transmitters and neural pathways within basal ganglia, and connections to other brain centres. ACh, acetylcholine; DA, dopamine; GABA, gamma-aminobutyric acid.

lethargica syndrome following an influenza epidemic in the 1920s, but although these are now dying out the prevalence of Parkinson's disease is unchanged.

There seem to be no strong genetic links, but there are suggestions of inherited susceptibility, and some studies have implicated single genes in a few patients, especially those with early-onset disease, which has been associated with mutations of the parkin gene. Within the broad classification of idiopathic Parkinson's disease there are possibly several subtly different subtypes.

Pathogenesis

The process by which nigrostriatal cells are destroyed is still not clear. A histological characteristic of affected cells is a build-up of 'Lewy bodies' (dark-staining hyaline cell inclusions). However, the specificity and direct pathological significance of such inclusions is unknown, because they also occur in some of the dementias. Theories on the pathology include accelerated ageing with increased apoptosis (programmed cell death; see Chapter 10), excessive build-up of highly destructive oxidative free radical intermediates, which are normally neutralized, and impaired energy handling.

A chance finding among drug misusers opened a fruitful line of research. A contaminant in illicitly synthesized pethidine (meperidine) produced symptomatic and histological features very similar to idiopathic Parkinson's disease. This contaminant, MPTP (methyl phenyl tetrahydropyridine), is oxidized by monoamine-oxidase-B to MPP$^+$. This toxic free radical seriously damages mitochondrial energy pathways.

This discovery provided a primate model for studying the pathology and treatment of Parkinson's disease. However, its relevance to the naturally-occurring disease in humans it still uncertain. MPTP is not common in the environment, although many herbicides and pesticides are pyridine-based and might be metabolized in a similar way. One possibility is a genetic defect in the ability to detoxify oxidative intermediates, leading to mitochondrial damage. It is unclear why only nigrostriatal cells should be affected by any of these effects.

Epidemiology

The overall prevalence of Parkinson's disease is 1–2 per 1000. Although it can affect people as young as 40, it is predominatly a disease of the elderly. The prevalence increases sharply with age and is about 3% among people aged over 65. Men and women are affected equally and there seems to be little racial or social variation. This is not what we would expect if the cause were wholly environmental or toxic. The prevalence in Europe and North America is twice that of China and Japan, which implies genetic factors, but confirmation could only come from a large-scale follow-up of migrating sufferers.

Thus the current thinking is that people may have a genetically conferred susceptibility, but whether or not they develop the disease depends on probably several environmental factors, which they may or may not meet during their life. In this, Parkinson's disease resembles many cancers.

Course

Parkinson's disease has an insidious onset, with slowly progressive non-specific signs such as vague muscle pain, stiffness, mild depression and general slowing down. A late onset may protect some patients from the worst ravages of advanced disease. Over 80% of nigrostriatal dopamine must be lost before symptoms become apparent, possibly because neurological and behavioural compensation mask symptoms before this stage. This prodromal phase may last for up to 5 years. Parkinson's disease can be considered to proceed through five phases:

1. Prodromal phase – asymptomatic.
2. Early symptomatic phase – little disability; drugs may not be needed.
3. Main treatable phase (5–7 years) – *levodopa* effective.
4. Late phase – declining *levodopa* effectiveness.
5. Terminal phase – disease extremely difficult to control.

The early symptoms can easily be mistaken for simple ageing, although when the frank clinical features emerge the condition is unmistakable.

Intellect is initially unimpaired, which may exacerbate the patient's distress. However, drug-resistant dyskinesias, cognitive degeneration, dementia and various psychiatric and other non-motor features can all occur as the disease progresses. These may be due partly to the involvement of structures other than the nigro-striatum, within or outside the BG, becoming affected by the same or related degenerative processes. It is known that brainstem areas such as the olfactory and autonomic centres and later the limbic areas can become involved.

The rate of progression of Parkinson's disease is very variable and it is difficult to determine whether treatment slows the condition in any one individual. However, progression is relent-less, with no sustained periods of remission. Untreated, the median survival is about 10 years from the onset of symptoms, and patients have three times the mortality of a matched normal population. Modern management with *levodopa* has improved the prognosis, partly by reducing the mortality and morbidity from the secondary complications of immobility. Optimal drug therapy has at least doubled the average survival time, and life expectancy now approaches normality. Death is usually from pneumonia, resulting from immobility or from aspiration due to impaired swallowing and respiratory musculature.

Clinical features

The classic signs of parkinsonism are tremor, rigidity, slowness and abnormal posture. Most may be traced to disorders of muscle tone (dystonias) or muscle movement (dyskinesias), which are usually asymmetrical. There are also signs of excess cholinergic parasympathetic activity. The clinical features are classified and described in Table 6.25.

The clinical presentation is relatively uniform and diagnosis may be straightforward, but differ-ential diagnosis between Parkinson's disease and other neurodegenerative diseases (Table 6.24) can be problematic. It is also necessary to consider possible primary causes, e.g. antipsy-chotic drug therapy, and to distinguish other conditions presenting similar features, e.g.

stroke, hypothyroidism, dementia, etc. (Table 6.24). Parkinson's disease should be excluded when investigating falls, ankle oedema (possibly the result of immobility) and reduced mobility attributed to 'ageing'. In doubtful cases imaging techniques may be helpful, including MR (magnetic resonance) and CT (computerised tomography) scanning and nuclear medicine techniques such as PET (positron emission tomography).

Clinical diagnosis is based on the following gross features:

- Flexed posture and shuffling gait.
- Expressionless face and reduced blinking.
- Distal tremor that is abolished by purposive movement.

Non-motor symptoms. A variety of non-motor problems can complicate Parkinson's disease at all stages in the disease (Table 6.25). These include psychological and psychiatric disease, autonomic dysfunction, sleep disorders and falls. They may be overlooked or mistaken for other diseases in the early stages. In the later stages they are more significant because they are generally unresponsive to dopaminergic therapy and can seriously impair quality of life and reduce life expectancy. Possibly they have become more prominent as the prognosis has improved following the introduction of *levodopa* therapy.

Their pathogenesis is still unclear. Some may be iatrogenic, originating from dopaminergic or antimuscarinic therapy; others may result from involvement of other brain centres (see above).

Management

Aims

Ideally, the aims in the management of Parkinson's disease would be to:

- reduce symptoms;
- provide general support;
- prevent further degeneration;
- induce reversal or regeneration.

At present, most success has been obtained with the relief from troublesome symptoms and

Table 6.25   Clinical features of Parkinson's disease

Motor symptoms	Example/comment
Dyskinesias	
Bradykinesia	General slowness, esp. in repetitive movements
	'Stately' walk (straight arms swinging)
	Mask-like, expressionless face (hypomimia); drooling
Hypokinesia/akinesia	Reduced voluntary movement; delays in initiating movement
	Immobility
Resting tremor	Disappears during activity and sleep
	Increases during stress
	'Pill rolling' hand movements
Other	Tiny writing (micrographia)
	Reduced blink rate
Dystonias	
Limb rigidity	Lead pipe (plastic) or cog wheel (ratchet)
Stooped posture	Stumbling, shuffling walk (festination)
Inarticulate speech (dysarthria)	
Painful cramps	

Non-motor symptoms	Example/comment
CNS	
Cognitive	Dementia
Psychiatric	Depression, anxiety, psychosis
Sleep disorder	Somnolence, insomnia
Sensory	Taste, visual and olfactory disturbance
Autonomic	
Gastrointestinal	Dysphagia, constipation
	Nausea and vomiting
	Weight loss
Urinary	Urgency, frequency, nocturia
CVS	Orthostatic hypotension
Other	Excessive sweating and salivation
Other physical signs	
Greasy seborrhoeic skin	
Falls	
Fatigue	

maintenance of the patient's independence and general health. Attempts at prevention and reversal are hampered by the lack of a clear understanding of the aetiology and pathogenesis, and so are still largely experimental.

Support
Exercise, physiotherapy, speech therapy and occupational therapy are essential to help the patient to cope with their progressive disability and maintain their independence as long as

possible. It is important to maintain muscle and tendon strength in the face of reduced mobility. Psychiatric help and medication may be needed for depression, which is common.

Symptomatic treatment: drug therapy

The primary objective of drug therapy is to enhance dopaminergic activity within the damaged areas of the BG, and this is achieved in various ways (Table 6.26). Parkinson's disease has provided an exceptionally fertile field for rational drug design and formulation to specific clinical requirements.

Residual dopaminergic activity can be mildly enhanced by inhibiting neuronal dopamine re-uptake (*amantadine*) and the excessive cholinergic tone that dopamine deficiency causes can be countered with antimuscarinics. Neither are first-line drugs but are sometimes used as adjuvants. However, antimuscarinics exacerbate the psychiatric complications of Parkinson's disease

and *levodopa* therapy, particularly in the elderly. They are helpful in tremor, but are of little use for bradykinesia and have only limited effectiveness. Thus some form of dopamine augmentation or replacement invariably becomes necessary.

Levodopa is currently the standard treatment. It is discussed in detail below. As *levodopa* inevitably becomes less effective over time, its availability can be enhanced by reducing its metabolism using a catechol-O-methyl transferase (COMT) inhibitor. Alternatively, dopamine's half-life in the brain can be increased with a monoamine oxidase B (MAO-B) inhibitor or a COMT inhibitor (Figure 6.15 and Table 6.26). Where *levodopa* is ineffective or cannot be tolerated at all (primary failure), or has become ineffective or intolerable (secondary failure), direct-acting dopaminergic agonists, e.g. *ropinirole*, can be substituted or added. These do not require central activation by dopa-decarboxylase and have a longer duration of action than *levodopa*. However, they have

---

Table 6.26   Pharmacological rationales for enhancing dopaminergic transmission in the basal ganglia

Approach	Rationale	Drug group and examples
Reduce cholinergic activity	Balance diminished dopaminergic activity	Antimuscarinic, e.g. trihexyphenidyl (benzhexol), procyclidine
Inhibit neuronal dopamine re-uptake	Maximize remaining dopaminergic activity	Amantadine
Stimulate dopamine receptors	Mimic dopamine	Dopamine agonist: • Ergot derived: cabergoline, pergolide, lisuride, bromocriptine • Non-ergot derived: ropinirole, rotigotine, pramipexole • Other: apomorphine
Supply dopamine precursor	Increase dopamine level in basal ganglia	Levodopa
Reduce peripheral destruction of precursor	Increase levodopa penetration into brain	Decarboxylase inhibitor, e.g. carbidopa, benserazide COMT-inhibitor: entacapone, tolcapone
Reduce central destruction of dopamine	Increase dopamine half-life in brain	COMT-inhibitor: tolcapone MAO-B inhibitor, e.g. selegiline. rasagiline

MAO-B, monoamine oxidase-B; COMT, catechol-O-methyl transferase.

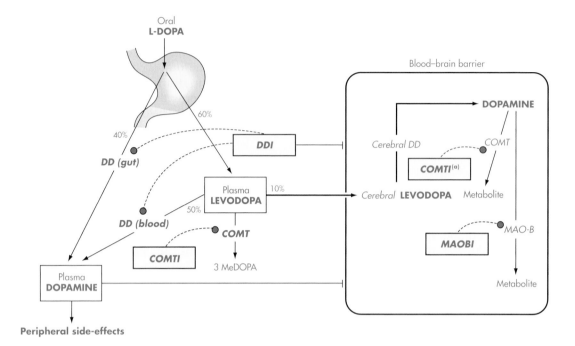

Figure 6.15 Dopamine and levodopa metabolism and pharmacological intervention. Levodopa is largely decarboxylated in the gut wall and plasma, by dopa decarboxylase. From plasma, levodopa can enter the brain but dopamine cannot. Plasma dopamine causes peripheral adverse effects. Inhibiting the metabolism of levodopa in the gut or plasma increases its availability to the brain. Dopa decarboxylase inhibitors do not cross the blood–brain barrier so do not interfere with the central action of levodopa. Percentages of levodopa metabolism refer to when in presence of dopa decarboxylase inhibitor. See text.
-----●inhibit; ⎯⎯| blocked uptake; DD(I), dopa decarboxylase (inhibitor); MAO-B (I), monoamine oxidase-B (inhibitor); COMT(I), catechol-O-methyl transferase (inhibitor). (a)Tolcapone crosses the blood–brain barrier but entacapone does not.

worse peripheral dopaminergic adverse effects, and although centrally they cause less dyskinesia, they cause more psychotic reactions.

Although drugs are the mainstay of treatment, they do not relieve all symptoms in all patients, nor do they work indefinitely. In particular, the efficacy of *levodopa* tends to decline as the disease progresses.

Retard or prevent progression
With the discovery of the possible role of free radical damage in the pathogenesis of Parkinson's disease there was hope that neuroprotection with antioxidants (e.g. vitamin E, co-enzyme Q10) or inhibitors of dopamine metabolism (i.e. MAO-B inhibitors, such as selegiline in the DATATOP trial) might prevent or retard the disease. Unfortunately, these hopes have proved unfounded.

Early observations on selegiline probably mis-attributed simple symptom control to disease retardation. On the other hand, the suggestion that selegiline might actually increase mortality has also been refuted. A more recent theory that selegiline might after all retard progression, by inhibiting apoptosis, remains unconfirmed. The final judgement on selegiline is still awaited, but MAO-B inhibitors currently retain a role in early disease and as adjuvants later.

Although the progression of the disease seems inexorable at present, modern therapy has undoubtedly improved both quality of life and survival if started promptly.

Reversal or regeneration
Rarely, highly selective surgery or deep brain stimulation to the subthalamic nucleus or globus

pallidus for treatment-resistant symptoms has been used with some benefit. This is designed to reduce or reverse the abnormal BG output. Trials of implantation of dopamine-secreting tissue into the brain have so far proved disappointing. Initially the patient's own adrenal tissue was used; more recently the transplantation of nigral tissue from aborted fetuses has been investigated.

Levodopa therapy

Rationale and development

Clearly, the ideal treatment for Parkinson's disease would be to replace the depleted dopamine in the BG. However, there is an important drug delivery problem because dopamine, being polar, is poorly absorbed orally and does not readily cross the blood–brain barrier. Further, dopamine has potent peripheral adverse effects. Thus direct delivery of dopamine to the CNS is impractical and its natural amino acid precursor *levodopa* (L-dopa, L-dihydroxy phenylalanine) is used.

Levodopa is extremely effective for all symptoms of Parkinson's disease, and especially for bradykinesia; it is up to five times more effective than antimuscarinics. Unfortunately *levodopa* is poorly tolerated, especially if given orally, when it produces severe gastrointestinal side-effects.

About 90% of Parkinson's disease patients have a good to excellent initial response to *levodopa* and failure to respond should prompt a re-evaluation of the diagnosis. However, some patients cannot tolerate *levodopa* at all, while others may have involvement of other neurotransmitter systems.

Pharmacokinetics

Levodopa is well absorbed from the GIT and, because it is the brain's natural source of neuronal *dopamine*, a proportion of the orally administered dose is transported into the brain from the plasma across the blood–brain barrier by an active uptake pump (Figure 6.15). However, owing to peripheral decarboxylation, mainly by dopa-decarboxylase (DD) in the gut wall during absorption, only about 1–3% of the administered dose actually reaches

the CNS. The free dopamine produced causes undesirable peripheral dopaminergic effects on the muscle of the gut, heart and blood vessels.

Once in the brain, *levodopa* is decarboxylated intraneuronally to dopamine. Decarboxylation is probably not confined to neurones of the nigrostriatum but also occurs in dopaminergic neurones elsewhere.

Levodopa augmentation

Dopa-decarboxlyase inhibitors

The problems of poor central *levodopa* delivery and excessive peripheral dopaminergic adverse effects are neatly ameliorated by using a peripherally acting inhibitor of dopa-decarboxylase (DDI), e.g. *carbidopa* or *benserazide*. These have been designed to be insufficiently lipophilic to cross the blood–brain barrier and so cannot interfere with the central activation of *levodopa* to dopamine. When a DDI is combined with *levodopa* (as *co-careldopa* or *co-beneldopa*) the proportion of the *levodopa* delivered to the CNS rises to 10%, the *levodopa* dose may be cut by 75% and peripheral side-effects are substantially reduced. The main problem is a predictable increase in dopaminergic adverse effects in the CNS. The DDIs themselves have few side-effects.

COMT inhibitors

Another route for the peripheral metabolism of *levodopa* is methylation by COMT (Figure 6.15). While this does not produce a metabolite with the adverse effects of dopamine, it does reduce the central availability of *levodopa*. Moreover, brain COMT is partly responsible for the clearance of dopamine. Thus further increases in *levodopa* bioavailability can be obtained by using blockers of peripheral COMT, e.g. *entacapone*, *tolcapone*. In addition, because *tolcapone* crosses the blood–brain barrier it also enhances dopamine activity in the CNS by reducing its intraneuronal catabolism. However, the use of *tolcapone* is limited by liver toxicity so it must be carefully monitored under specialist supervision.

MAO-B inhibitors

The intraneuronal catabolism of dopamine can be further reduced by inhibiting central MAO-B. MAO-B inhibitors provide a moderate improvement in cases where *levodopa* effectiveness is waning (Figure 6.15). Because they do not block MAO-A, the form of the enzyme affected by conventional antidepressant MAOIs such as *phenelzine*, they are not subject to the usual MAOI restrictions and dietary precautions.

Unfortunately, even these augmented combinations do not work indefinitely, so problems remain. First, all drug treatment is only really effective against dyskinetic symptoms. Other motor symptoms remain and indeed tend to deteriorate, especially dystonias causing gait and postural problems (Table 6.25), which are possibly mediated by defects in non-dopaminergic neuronal systems. These may be the patient's most disabling complaints despite otherwise good control. Secondly, cholinergic features may still be troublesome. Finally, there is an inexorable, imperfectly understood decline in the effectiveness of *levodopa* after a number of years of satisfactory control.

Dopamine agonists

The final option where *levodopa* is ineffective or intolerable is to use a dopamine agonist, either as an adjuvant or a substitute. There are several advantages to using a direct-acting dopamine receptor agonist. They do not require activation by DD, which is useful because concentrations of this enzyme may be reduced in late disease. Also, there may be some receptor subtype selectivity, e.g. *pergolide* (D_1 and D_2 receptors), *ropinirole* (D_2 only), although the clinical significance of this is unclear. The main disadvantage is an increase in peripheral dopaminergic side-effects because, unlike *levodopa*, they are active peripherally as soon as assimilated.

There are two main subgroups (Table 6.26). The original ones were ergot derivatives, e.g. *bromocriptine*, *pergolide*, *cabergoline* and *lisuride*, and these were widely used in Parkinson's disease. Later drugs are not derived from ergot, e.g. *ropinirole*, *pramipexole*, *rotigotine*. Unrelated to either group is *apomorphine*. The effects and adverse reactions of all are broadly similar to *levodopa*, with one important exception. All ergot derivatives (not just those used in Parkinson's disease) can cause potentially serious fibrotic reactions in the lungs, heart and peritoneum, and so drugs in this subgroup are now rarely used. If they are needed, patients must first be screened for CXR, renal function and ESR.

Dopamine agonists may be used as initial therapy, to delay the introduction of *levodopa*, or in primary or secondary *levodopa* failure.

Administration

Levodopa is routinely given with a decarboxylase inhibitor. Low doses are used to establish tolerance and then gradually increased every 2–3 days until symptoms are controlled, the limit of tolerance is reached, or a compromise between these is achieved. The precise regimen, including the best ratio of *levodopa* to inhibitor, must be carefully individualized to balance tolerance, benefit and toxicity, and must remain continually under review. A variety of different combinations of strengths and relative proportions are available. Considerable ingenuity needs to be exercised in tailoring *levodopa* drug regimens to extract maximum benefit as efficacy declines.

Divided doses are necessary to minimize gastric intolerance, caused in part by dopamine generated in the gut wall, and to prevent swings in plasma levels, which would be reflected in uneven clinical action. *Levodopa* is always taken with food; however, high-protein meals can reduce CNS penetration owing to competition for amino acid transport mechanisms at the blood–brain barrier.

Side-effects

The side-effects of *levodopa*, both peripherally and centrally, are caused exclusively by the dopamine produced after decarboxylation, which acts on dopaminergic and adrenergic receptors (Table 6.27). Elderly patients are more prone to all side-effects.

Gastrointestinal tract

Locally formed dopamine reduces gastrointestinal motility, slowing the absorption of further *levodopa*. Severe dyspepsia is minimized by taking small frequent doses with food. Nausea and vomiting are less common with the lower *levodopa* doses that decarboxylase inhibitors allow. However, if such doses remain troublesome

Table 6.27   Important side-effects of levodopa

System	Effects	Cause[a]
GIT	Dyspepsia	Local irritation
	Reduced gastric motility	Inhibition of intestinal muscle
	Nausea, vomiting	Stimulation of chemoreceptor trigger zone
CVS	Arrhythmias	Beta-adrenergic myocardial stimulation
	Hypotension	Peripheral vasodilatation
CNS	Dyskinesias and dystonias	Action in extra-striatal basal ganglia centres?
	Psychiatric symptoms	Action in limbic or thalamic centres
Endocrine	(Rare)	Action in hypothalamus

[a] All except gastrointestinal irritation and arrhythmia are due to action at dopamine receptors.

CNS, central nervous system; CVS, cardiovascular system; GIT, gastrointestinal tract.

a peripherally acting dopamine blocking anti-nauseant such as *domperidone* may be used. *Metoclopramide* and phenothiazines are unsuitable because they cross the blood–brain barrier and so would antagonize the intended central therapeutic action of dopamine, as well as causing their own extrapyramidal effects.

Cardiovascular system

Dopamine is active at both beta$_1$-adrenergic and dopaminergic receptors (it is used therapeutically as an inotrope and vasodilator; see Chapter 4). Most parkinsonian patients are in an age group that is prone to heart disease, and so care is needed in this respect. Graduated compression hosiery is helpful to minimize postural hypotension, but serious arrhythmias such as tachycardia and premature ventricular beats may require an anti-arrhythmic drug, or the cessation of dopamine treatment. Fortunately, the cardiovascular effects seem to remit on continued therapy.

CNS

Dopamine is a transmitter in other areas of the BG besides the nigrostriatal pathway, and also in centres outside the BG, and actions in these areas may be intensified by decarboxylase inhibitors. Dopamine may, ironically, produce other movement disorders, chiefly writhing (choreoathetosis) or restless legs. These tend to occur in the later stages of treatment and are difficult to distinguish from late manifestations of the disease or declining disease control. The precise picture of these complex interactions is far from clear, and strategies for countering them, discussed below, are largely empirical.

Similarly, a variety of psychiatric effects can result from an excess of dopamine in, presumably, mesolimbic and mesocortical centres. (Recall that one theory of the pathogenesis of schizophrenia attributes it to excess dopamine here; p. 409.) Psychotic features such as hallucinations and paranoia may occur, as may delirium, depression or mania. These may be exacerbated by the use of antimuscarinic drugs, e.g. antiparkinson agents and antidepressants. They may be confused with symptoms of advanced disease itself (e.g. dementia), or represent the unmasking of latent psychiatric illness, which is a relative contra-indication to *levodopa* use.

For psychosis, traditional antipsychotic dopamine blockers such as the phenothiazines clearly cannot be used. The atypical antipsychotics are preferred, especially *quetiapine* or *clozapine*, partly on the basis that the psychiatric symptoms may involve serotoninergic receptors, and partly because these drugs themselves cause few extrapyramidal problems. The 5-HT$_3$ blocker *ondansetron* has also been tried.

Care is needed when treating depression. Conventional tricyclic antidepressants with antimuscarinic effects must be avoided. There is a theoretical possibility of SSRIs worsening the parkinsonism (see above), and they also interact with *selegiline* causing hypertension. Conventional non-selective MAOIs interact with *levodopa*, causing hypertensive crisis, and with *selegiline*, causing hypotension. A sensible choice would appear to be an antidepressant with little antimuscarinic activity, such as *lofepramine*. However, in practice SSRIs are quite frequently used.

Endocrine

There is a theoretical possibility of *levodopa* mimicking dopamine's inhibition of hypothalamic-releasing hormones. However, the potential results (e.g. hypoprolactinaemia) are not seen and are likely to be less significant in the parkinsonian age group. (This effect is exploited therapeutically in the use of *bromocriptine* for hyperprolactinaemia.)

Long-term and late complications

Fortunately, no serious long-term haematological, renal or hepatic toxicity has yet been observed. However, the long-term dyskinetic and psychiatric side-effects of *levodopa* are so varied and so difficult to distinguish from late complications of the underlying disease that Parkinson's disease management has become almost a subspecialty in itself, with its own confusing taxonomy of complications. Fluctuating therapeutic responses, dyskinesias and psychiatric symptoms frequently become seriously disabling, with about half of patients experiencing problems after 5 years on *levodopa* and three-quarters after 15 years.

Numerous ingenious pharmacological, biopharmaceutical and formulation strategies have been devised to optimize delivery of dopamine to its intended site of action and to minimize adverse systemic effects. This represents a tremendous clinical pharmacological challenge.

Early experience with *levodopa* had suggested that there was a limited window for effective *levodopa* treatment in the course of the illness (phase 3, p. 428), after which these problems would arise. Thus, it was felt that *levodopa* therapy should be delayed as long as possible, conserving it for the later, more severe phases. However, many of the effects ascribed to long-term *levodopa* therapy are now considered likely to be related to disease progression, and treatment is now introduced earlier.

Difficulties in interpreting inconsistent *levodopa* activity arise because of:

- Lack of correlation between plasma and brain levels, because CNS uptake of *levodopa* depends on an active pump, the activity of which may change.
- Lack of correlation between CNS *levodopa* levels and synaptic dopamine levels, because of reliance on neuronal uptake and neuronal DD action.
- Declining ability of a reducing BG neuron population to decarboxylate *levodopa* and store dopamine, either within or outside the striatum.
- Changes in post-synaptic receptor sensitivity.
- Involvement of dopaminergic systems outside the nigrostriatal system.
- Involvement of non-dopaminergic systems.
- Normally dopamine activity in the BG varies smoothly, whereas in treatment it is pulsatile.

Management of levodopa complications

The motor problems of Parkinson's disease and *levodopa* therapy are classified in Table 6.28. It is unhelpful to attempt to specify a particular solution for each one, especially because many treatments are still experimental. Moreover, when a particular problem is not responding, other methods are tried empirically. In general, three basic approaches are employed, depending on whether problems are related to reduced *levodopa* activity, excessive *levodopa* activity, or mixed intractable fluctuations.

For reduced effectiveness (e.g. 'end of dose' and other 'off' phenomena), the aim is to increase delivery of *levodopa*, modify its time course or smooth out variations in its plasma level. Increased frequency of lower doses (without allowing plasma levels to fall below the threshold of activity), liquid formulations or enteral systems may help. The Duodopa intrajejunal system provides continuous *co-careldopa* dosing, avoiding the stomach, and the dosage rate from the portable external pump can be varied. *Rotigotine* is available as a transdermal patch. Continuous SC infusion of dopamine analogues such as *apomorphine* is cumbersome

Table 6.28   Late motor control problems of Parkinson's disease and levodopa therapy

Origin	Description	Symptoms
Levodopa-related		
Reduced effect	End of dose wearing off	Declining effectiveness before next dose, related to trough serum level
	Delayed 'on'	Increasing time before onset of activity
Increased toxicity	Peak dose dyskinesia	Writhing (choreoathetosis) or akathisia related to peak serum level
	Diphasic dyskinesia	Choreoathetosis at onset and end of 'on' period
Disease-related	'On–off'	Unpredictable acute fluctuations in symptoms, unrelated to plasma level
? Treatment resistance	'On' period freezing	Transient immobility, especially of gait, in mid-dose period
? Disease progression	'Off' period dystonia	Writhing and spasm, especially of feet in morning

'On', desired therapeutic effect; 'Off', disease-related or iatrogenic motor symptoms.

but effective. The rectal and intranasal routes are also being considered. Modified-release oral preparations are often used, but these have reduced bioavailability and so require dosage adjustment.

Dopaminergic analogues generally have a longer half-life and may be added to *levodopa*. If a regimen can be developed with the right balance between *levodopa* precursor and direct-acting agonist, it may enable an acceptable compromise between prolonged activity and increased peripheral dopaminergic problems. The addition of an MAO-B or a COMT inhibitor increases *levodopa* bioavailability. Delayed *levodopa* onset may be countered by avoiding simultaneous high-protein meals or by enteral administration.

Increased toxicity (i.e. 'on' phenomena with troublesome dyskinesias) usually necessitates a reduction in dose, although spacing out doses or using modified-release preparations may help. Reducing the dose is likely to be at the expense of increased disease symptoms and decreased mobility. Again, an acceptable balance must be agreed with the patient. Gastric toxicity can also be circumvented by the non-oral formulations.

A wide range of drugs have been tried for intractable motor problems, including atypical antipsychotics, adrenergic beta-blockers and SSRIs, but evidence is lacking. Painful dystonias may benefit from the antispastic agent *baclofen*.

'Drug holidays', once recommended, are now thought unhelpful. Because no treatment definitely retards progression of the condition, it is to be expected that even a successfully managed patient will eventually go through increasing periods of instability.

Combination products (e.g. *levodopa* + DDI + COMT inhibitor) may be helpful for patients taking multiple drug therapy at this stage.

Drug selection

Drug treatment is started when the degree of functional disability caused by the disease outweighs likely adverse effects. The NICE guidelines do not indicate a specific sequence but suggest a range of drugs from which selection must be made on the grounds of patient acceptance and tolerability, contra-indications, and concurrent morbidity or drug therapy (Figure 6.16).

The trend has been to start reliable evidence-based drugs as soon as patients find their lives appreciably affected. The principal controversy concerns the stage at which *levodopa* therapy should be introduced. The arguments in favour of early initial therapy with *levodopa* are:

- It is the most effective drug.
- It is now widely agreed that *levodopa* does not have a strictly limited window of activity – it

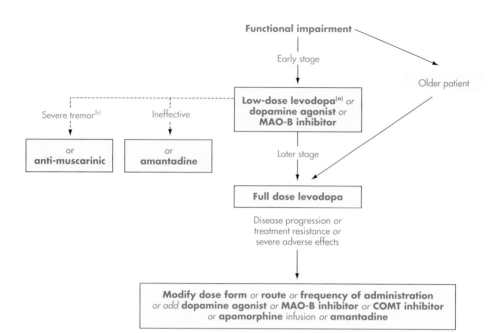

Figure 6.16 Drug selection in Parkinson's disease. [a]Levodopa always given with dopa decarboxylase inhibitor; [b] only in younger patient.

continues to benefit most patients to some degree.

- It is no longer believed that *levodopa* has long-term neurodegenerative effects that could accelerate disease progression.
- The elderly are very sensitive to the adverse effects of the possible alternatives (antimuscarinics and dopamine agonists).
- Evidence does not support the role of selegiline in disease retardation.

On the other hand, the inevitable long-term adverse effects of *levodopa*, which usually start after 5–10 years of therapy, do mean that these are experienced earlier with earlier initiation of therapy, as would be the case with younger patients. The evidence is not conclusive yet on the optimal policy in all cases.

The first choice in the early stages is between *levodopa*, in as low a dose as relieves symptoms, a dopamine agonist or an MAO-B inhibitor. Less potent and less effective drugs with a poorer evidence base could be added or substituted if control is not achieved. *Amantadine* may help, antimuscarinics can be used in young patients with severe tremor, and beta-blockers may help where there is postural tremor. Older patients should usually be started on *levodopa* as initial therapy and should avoid antimuscarinics.

Whatever treatment patients start with, all will eventually need to take *levodopa* in gradually increasing dosage and frequency (assuming they can tolerate it). However, at some stage, when long-term complications supervene or resistance develops (i.e. secondary *levodopa* failure), other strategies will be required. These fall into two groups. First, modify the dose form and route of administration, as described above. Second, use one or more of the other groups of drugs, with dopamine agonists being the first choice adjuvants (Figure 6.16).

For a few patients it seems that, eventually, no drug combination will be satisfactory and surgical options may have to be considered.

Epilepsy

The word 'epilepsy' is derived from the Greek, meaning 'to take hold of, seize'. For centuries, there has been the ancient fear that the sufferer of epilepsy has been possessed, literally taken hold of, by some malign external force. The following quotation describes many of the features of a major seizure in graphic terms.

> He begun to groan then like some terbel thing wer taking him and got inside him. He startit to fall and I easit him down I knowit he wer having a fit I seen that kynd of thing befor. I stuck the clof ... be twean his teef so he wunt bite his tung. I wer on my knees in the mud and holding him wylst he twissit and groant ... I cud feal how strong he wer tho he wernt putting out no strenth agenst me he wer sturgling with what ever wer inside him. I wunnert what wud happen it got pas him and out. It dint tho. It roalt him roun and shook him up it bent him like a bow but finely it pult back to where ever it come out of. When it gone he wunt do nothing only sleap nor I coulnt get him to walk 1 step.
> Russell Hoban, Ridley Walker
> (Reproduced with kind permission
> of the publishers)

For this reason people with epilepsy have always encountered as much prejudice as those suffering from psychiatric disorders. The lack of self-control evident during a seizure was feared, and the sufferer was therefore spurned. Yet only rarely does epilepsy directly cause psychiatric symptoms: it is predominantly a neurological condition involving disorders of movement or consciousness; moreover, patients are asymptomatic for most of the time. There may, however, be secondary psychiatric morbidity in many long-term sufferers.

Epilepsy is a chronic, paroxysmal, non-progressive disorder of intermittent disorganized electrical activity in the brain, which causes the seizure. Seizures are characterized most commonly by impairment of motor activity (convulsions), consciousness, perception or behaviour.

The term 'fit' is now avoided, as is 'epileptic' in reference to a patient, for whom the term 'person with epilepsy' (PWE) is gaining currency.

Aetiology and classification

An isolated seizure can be precipitated in anyone if their brain is suitably provoked. Transient reversible triggers include drugs (e.g. tricyclic antidepressants), cerebral infection or inflammation, intracranial hypertension, head injury, stroboscopic lights and metabolic disturbances such as glycaemic, osmotic or pH imbalance. Fever can trigger seizures, especially in children. However, an isolated attack is not considered epilepsy, which is better defined as a reduced seizure threshold with a continuing tendency to experience seizures. Because it may have a variety of causes and triggers, epilepsy is regarded as a syndrome rather than a discrete disease.

The problem may be symptomatic of a structural abnormality in the brain. In about one-third of epilepsy patients, a congenital or neurodevelopmental abnormality is found in a specific part of the brain, especially the hippocampus. Other identifiable causes include ischaemia (arteriosclerosis, stroke or perinatal hypoxia), head trauma (post-infective, perinatal, post-operative or other injury), tumour (5% overall; up to 40% of adult-onset partial epilepsy) or alcoholic brain disease. Other cases are referred to as either idiopathic (unknown cause) or cryptogenic (hidden cause).

Interestingly, even in cases where there is a clear cause (such as head injury), a family history may be found. This suggests that it is a tendency to lowered seizure thresholds that is inherited. There are strong genetic links in the generalized epilepsies, but no consistent environmental factors have been identified. The likelihood is that for many forms of epilepsy there may be a genetic predisposition that requires environmental triggers to cause active disease.

The classification of epilepsy has recently become more complex, following the system proposed by the International League Against Epilepsy (ILAE). Traditionally a patient's disease was classified simply to reflect the predominant seizure type. However, following improved investigation and diagnostic techniques, evidence has shown that outcomes are better if management takes more account of aetiology and other clinical features, and this is reflected in the new classification. Thus it is necessary first to review how individual seizures are classified, then see how this can be adapted to a more refined classification of epilepsy syndromes.

Seizure type

Partial or generalized

Many seizures clearly originate in one particular area of one side of the brain, the epileptogenic focus. The symptoms a patient displays in a **partial** seizure (focal or location-related, Table 6.29) are usually readily identified as over-activity in this area, e.g. a particular sensory experience or an abnormal muscular action, implicating an area in the sensory or motor cortex respectively. Usually, a specific anatomical lesion will be found in the area predicted from the symptom. In other words most partial seizures are secondary, and even when no lesion can be traced, one is assumed to exist. There is little evidence of genetic links, and a family history is unusual.

A **primarily generalized** seizure involves the whole of the brain, on both sides, from the outset, with symptoms involving impaired consciousness, major muscle groups, or both. This category includes the most familiar forms,

tonic–clonic ('grand mal') and **absence** ('petit mal') seizures.

Although some partial seizures may be restricted to their area of origin, in other cases they spread rapidly to many other areas on both sides of the brain. This is known as **secondary generalization**. In such cases patients may experience, before the spread, a specific sensory or other warning symptom, the **aura**. The aura is characteristic of the epileptogenic focus, and in the restricted partial form would represent the entire seizure. In some cases the partial onset is masked or unrecognized because of very rapid generalization, but an attempt should be made to identify them because it affects prognosis and treatment.

Simple or complex

This distinction among the partial epilepsies is based on whether or not consciousness is impaired during the seizure. Generalized seizures are almost invariably complex. The relationship between these different forms of seizure is illustrated schematically in Figure 6.17.

Epilepsy syndrome

The most recent classification by the ILAE at first sight seems unduly complex. The rationale is to group epilepsies taking into account their clinical features, age of onset and presumed primary causes (Table 6.30). It is then possible, on the basis of empirical trial evidence, to treat different patients in a far more targeted, if still empirical, manner than when basing selection simply on seizure type alone.

Nevertheless it still starts with the primary distinction between general and partial seizures as its chief characteristic. Next it classifies the syndrome as idiopathic, symptomatic or crypto-genic. Subsequently the syndrome is described by its various clinical factors.

Pathology

The ultimate defect in epilepsy may be a reduced threshold for neuronal membrane depolarization, for example, a reduced resting potential. Little is known of how the neuronal instability

Table 6.29	Terminology of epileptic seizures
Term	Feature
Partial	Seizure arises from specific area on one side of brain
Primarily generalized	Arises simultaneously throughout all areas of both sides of brain
Secondarily generalized	Arises from specific area on one side, but rapidly spreads to all areas
Simple	Consciousness unimpaired
Complex	Consciousness impaired
Tonic	Muscular contraction
Clonic (myoclonic)	Alternate contraction and relaxation, jerking
Atonic	Relaxation, flaccid paralysis

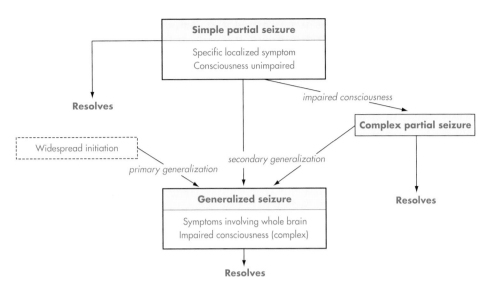

Figure 6.17   Relationship between classes of seizure.

Table 6.30   Simplified classification of epilepsy syndromes, after ILAE (International League Against Epilepsy)

Seizure	Aetiology	Example of syndrome
Generalized	Idiopathic	Generalized seizures on waking or specific triggers Childhood absence epilepsy Juvenile myoclonic epilepsy Other epilepsies characterized by generalized seizures
	Symptomatic	Epilepsies characterized by inborn errors of metabolism, cerebral malformations Early myoclonic encephalopathy
	Cryptogenic	Epilepsy with myoclonic absences
Location-related (partial)	Idiopathic	Benign epilepsy of childhood
	Symptomatic	Epilepsy with simple or complex seizures originating from specific brain areas, including those secondarily generalized
Undetermined or special		Febrile convulsions Neonatal seizures

occurs or why it should be set off by particular triggers. One possibility could be that there is an increased tendency to allow random discharges, which are normally suppressed, to spread. A neurotransmitter imbalance may be involved, such as a reduced level of an inhibitory transmitter, e.g. GABA or glutamate. Such inhibitors act physiologically by promoting chloride uptake into the neuron using the chloride ionophore membrane pump, which increases membrane potential and so stabilizes it. Recent research has focused on defective ion channels and a number of monogenic defects in these channels have been identified. However, this accounts for only a very small proportion of patients.

An amine imbalance theory is consistent with the apparent action of antiepileptic drugs (AEDs), many of which facilitate the stabilizing action of inhibitory amines. However, although several specific mechanisms have been identified for the various AEDs, it is not certain that this is how they exert their antiepileptic effect.

Epidemiology and course

About 1% of the population in the West and Asia have epilepsy, which is half the rate in Africa. There are about 250 000 patients taking AEDs in the UK. Onset is usually below the age of 30 years, with another peak in the elderly owing to cerebrovascular disease.

In general, epilepsy does not deteriorate, i.e. it is not progressive, and children especially may grow out of it. Even adult epilepsy can remit spontaneously but this can be extremely difficult to predict, and quite long seizure-free periods may, if medication is stopped, be followed by a seizure. The chances of remission are best for generalized tonic–clonic and absence seizures and poorest where these is a structural but inoperable lesion. Overall, the median period from diagnosis to being drug- and seizure-free

for at least 5 years is 20 years. However, 30% of patients continue to have seizures despite optimal therapy.

Partial and secondarily generalized epilepsies account for up to two-thirds of cases, tonic–clonic about one-third, and absence seizures, which only occur in children, about 5%. The disease usually causes no intellectual impairment, although long-term AED therapy may do so. However, repeated uncontrolled convulsions can produce brain damage owing to cerebral hypoxia, and in some cases the seizure disorder is in fact the consequence of brain damage.

Clinical features

The features of different seizures are summarized in Table 6.31. Seizures are usually very short-lived, and although usually unpredictable are sometimes triggered in a characteristic way, e.g. by flashing lights, altered mood, stress or relaxation. In all but simple partial seizures the patient is unaware of the seizure and may be unable to recall it afterwards.

If a patient presents with a fall, blackout or syncope (faint), or a transient absence, jerking, odd behavioural phenomenon or psychiatric

Table 6.31 Definitive features of common seizure types

Type	Area affected	Function affected	Clinical features of seizure
Generalized	All parts of brain affected		
Tonic–clonic[a]		Motor, consciousness	Tonic and clonic convulsions, loss of consciousness
Myoclonic[a]		Motor	Jerking of limbs
Absence		Attention, consciousness	Brief periods of reduced awareness
Partial	Specific focus, unilateral		
	Frontal lobe	Motor	Twitching, jerking (unilateral)
	Temporal lobe	Sensory	Smells, 'déjà vu', epigastric sensation, any other sensation
		Behaviour	Psychiatric
	Parietal lobe	Sensory	Tingling, etc.

[a] Other less common generalized motor seizures, usually associated with mental handicap, are purely tonic, clonic or atonic and are usually brief although equally debilitating.

symptom, this must be thoroughly investigated for a non-epileptic primary cause before epilepsy is diagnosed (see below).

Partial seizures

The effects of these highly localized seizures are mostly self-explanatory once the focus is known: or, more precisely, the features point to the focus. **Temporal lobe epilepsy** is the most common form, representing about half of all cases. This condition can be manifested in a very wide variety of neurological, and occasionally psychiatric, symptoms, including aphasia (the inability to find words), mood disorder, hallucinations and fainting. This can make differential diagnosis very difficult. There are many different types of partial seizures (see Table 6.31 and the References and further reading section), each of which usually lasts for a matter of minutes.

Tonic–clonic seizures

The classic seizure, as described in the quotation on p. 439, is the type most widely associated with epilepsy, and goes through up to five phases. In the **prodromal phase**, which is not experienced by all patients, the advent of a seizure is sensed subjectively, e.g. by a mood change.

Some patients then experience a more specific symptom, the **aura** immediately before the attack; this may be a sensory phenomenon, e.g a smell, a tingling feeling or an epigastric sensation. Auras are always the same for a given patient and suggest a primary partial seizure that subsequently becomes generalized. (There is an interesting parallel with classical migraine, which also is preceded by such auras; see Chapter 7.)

The actual convulsion then follows. In the **tonic (contractile) phase** there is a generalized contraction of many muscle groups, both somatic and visceral. Consequently, the patient loses balance and falls. The respiratory muscle spasm causes an initial brief involuntary cry, like being winded by a blow to the abdomen, followed by cyanosis.

After 30 s or so the **tonic–clonic phase** starts. This series of alternating contractions and relaxations causes the jerking that is so alarming for the onlooker, although by this time the patient is usually unconscious. There may be frothing at the mouth, incontinence and tongue biting, and this is the most dangerous phase because of the risk of self-harm. There may also be incontinence of urine or faeces. The tonic–clonic phase lasts a couple of minutes. The only first aid practicable is, if possible, to get the patient into the semi-prone (recovery) position to prevent aspiration (inhalation) of vomitus or profuse saliva. The popular idea of putting a cloth in the patient's mouth is now strongly discouraged; any potential damage would usually have been done by the time this could be arranged, and the patient might choke on it. There is also a significant chance of damage to the helper's fingers.

In the **post-ictal (after seizure) phase** there is relaxation, with flaccid paralysis and continued stupor, gradually merging into sleep. After a few hours the patient wakes with a headache, confused, and often bruised, but with no recollection of the events. A similar state follows ECT as used to treat depression.

Absence seizures ('Petit mal')

In a typical absence seizure patients will seem briefly to lose concentration. There may be an obvious stare and fluttering of the eyelids. After a few seconds they continue with what they were doing, unaware of the hiatus. In more severe forms there may be a loss of consciousness for up to 30 s, when the patient may fall; there may be muscular jerks (myoclonic seizure) but there will be no tonic–clonic convulsion. There are no prodromal signs and no post-ictal phenomena.

Such seizures usually occur in children and can easily be mistaken for 'daydreaming' or learning difficulty, or else they may be overlooked. Patients may have many attacks a day, sometimes hundreds, but the condition tends to remit as children grow up.

Status epilepticus

If a seizure does not terminate spontaneously, becoming a series of successive short fits or one long one, it is defined as **status**. This may happen with any seizure type, but most commonly with the tonic–clonic form, and it is a medical emergency. Patients may cause themselves some physical injury, but the main problem is cerebral hypoxia owing to compromised respiration.

Complications

In addition to the seizures, patients face considerable psychosocial difficulties. There is the general ignorance already referred to, as well as the associated stigma, causing difficulties with education, work, leisure and social relationships. The disease itself also imposes restrictions on such activities as driving, swimming and bathing. There may be secondary risks in infant care with an epileptic mother.

Temporal lobe epilepsy may be associated with psychiatric morbidity, including a schizophrenia-like psychosis, and depression is common. Unfortunately, most antidepressant and antipsychotic drugs lower seizure threshold and thus make treatment of these symptoms difficult. Examples of drugs with the lowest proconvulsant effects are SSRIs and *haloperidol*. The possibility of drug interactions then needs to be monitored.

Morbidity and mortality

There is an approximate doubling of the standardized mortality ratio, mostly related to refractory cases or from poor management leading to complications from seizures. There may be falls, home accidents, etc., where the link to a seizure is evident. In **sudden unexpected death in epilepsy (SUDEP)**, which affects about 0.5% of refractory cases per year, there is no obvious cause of death, which is unobserved, but is assumed to be seizure-related. There is a fivefold increased risk of suicide.

Investigation and diagnosis

The first aim when a patient presents with an unaccountable fall, blackout, etc. is to ascertain if there is any identifiable underlying cause, e.g. medical or toxic (Figure 6.18). A description of the seizure, from both the patient and especially a witness, is important. In certain circumstances a seizure may be induced artificially under controlled conditions with EEG recording, or there may be continuous ambulatory EEG recording. An ECG may also be needed to eliminate a cardiac cause.

The EEG lacks specificity and sensitivity. Some 15% of otherwise normal people will give an abnormal trace, while only 50% of patients with epilepsy will show abnormalities on random testing. An EEG is most useful in defining the seizure type, because it is possible to distinguish generalized from partial or secondarily generalized seizures. MRI has replaced radiography as the procedure for the accurate identification of cranial lesions, which it can identify in over half of chronic cases, of which 75% are partial epilepsies, 25% generalized forms. Surgery can occasionally rectify such problems, but usually it is reserved for cases where the disease is refractory to drug treatment, which is almost always tried first.

Decision to treat

Formerly it was suspected that, following only a single seizure, delaying treatment and allowing further attacks would worsen prognosis. It now seems clear that this is unlikely and further, that reduced quality of life results from premature initiation of drug therapy. This is particularly the case in children. In the UK at present the general rule is that a single attack does not automatically warrant the initiation of regular medication.

A diagnosis of epilepsy has serious legal and social implications (e.g. for driving, pregnancy, education, employment and leisure activities), and treatment involves the likelihood of adverse drug effects. Epidemiological evidence is ambiguous as to the probability of subsequent fits following a single episode, especially in childhood. Estimates of such probability range from 25% to 75%.

The circumstances of the first seizure are crucial to the decision. How likely is there to be a recurrence? Factors to consider are the cause or provoking event, if known, and whether this is persistent, e.g. was it a manifestation of a transiently reduced threshold or a unique event, such as high fever. More than two-thirds of children who have a febrile convulsion have no further problems. Is there objective evidence

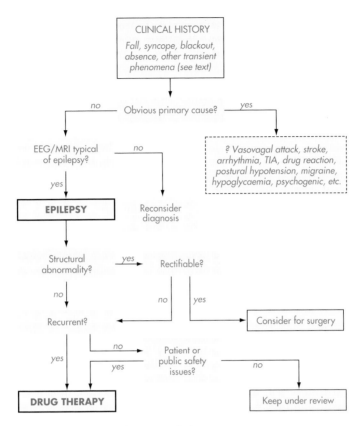

Figure 6.18 Investigation of epilepsy. EEG, electroencephalogram; MRI, magnetic resonance imaging; TIA, transient ischaemic attack.

(EEG, MRI, etc.) or neurological abnormality? Certain syndromes are more likely to recur (e.g. absences, juvenile myoclonic epilepsy).

Another factor is how serious would be the consequences of a further attack. Obviously if a patient drives a public service vehicle, for example, the risk cannot be taken. Even if treatment is delayed, avoiding driving for 1 year following a single seizure is advisable. Similar prudence might be exercised with a mother nursing an infant, who may be dropped or drowned if the mother has a seizure.

In all circumstances, decisions about starting drug treatment must involve informed discussion with the patient. Some patients who have fits no more than once every few years may prefer to risk these rather than to undergo long-term drug therapy and its associated problems.

Management

The aims of the management of epilepsy are:

- Investigate possible primary causes.
- Minimize social and psychological consequences and complications.
- Decide if active prophylaxis is necessary.
- Use drug therapy to prevent seizures or to keep seizures to minimum compatible with acceptable adverse reactions.

The over-riding consideration is to maximize the patient's quality of life by careful balancing of risks and benefits.

General measures

Careful, sensitive and thorough counselling is important, especially with children and their parents. Patients must be prevented as far as possible from being or feeling stigmatized. It must be emphasized that between attacks patients are perfectly normal, and that the disease causes no impairment of intelligence and no psychiatric disorder. It is helpful if not only the family but also a teacher, school friend or work colleague can be taught how to deal with a seizure.

Patients are encouraged to lead as normal a life as possible. There are certain legal constraints, notably on driving. In the UK the current requirement for epilepsy patients to hold a driving licence is that the patient must have had no fits at all for a year, or no daytime fits for 3 years. Patients who are well controlled and seizure-free may have normal schooling, and even swim. The number of constraints is much reduced if the patient has recognizable prodromal signs or a consistent aura.

Principles of pharmacotherapy

Drug therapy does not alter the basic lesion, whatever it is, but can be very effective in preventing seizures. The limiting factor is the adverse effects, especially as treatment is likely to be prolonged. Sometimes the doses needed for complete seizure suppression may be intolerable and it is preferable simply to aim for a reduced seizure frequency. The risks from continued seizures in the absence of treatment must be weighed against the risks of adverse effects and the potential benefits of reduced seizure frequency with treatment.

A decision tree for managing drug therapy is given in Figure 6.19. The following general principles should be observed.

Monotherapy
Monotherapy is now the accepted ideal. There are considerable benefits to avoiding polypharmacy in epilepsy in view of the many possible drug interactions. If the first drug proves inadequate or is not tolerated after optimal dose titration, another should be substituted, rather than adding another drug. Two first-line agents appropriate for the patient and their seizure type and syndrome should be tried singly before a combination is tried. Over two-thirds of patients are

satisfactorily controlled on a single drug, and those who are not are likely to prove the most difficult to control.

Formerly, insufficient care was taken to achieve the optimal plasma level with the first drug chosen, and instead of trying a second single drug, a second or even third adjunctive drug was commonly added quite early. Some older patients may still be on polypharmacy (and should remain so), but this approach probably produces more problems than it solves and is now avoided.

Dual therapy
If two first-line agents used alone fail, a further 15% of patients may be controlled on a combination of two drugs. Selection of drugs to be used in combination involves consideration of minimal overlap in adverse effects, least chance of interaction and complementary modes of action. There are few evidence-based data on the relative effectiveness of different combinations.

The remaining patients can be difficult to control, but triple therapy should be avoided if possible. Failure to achieve control with a variety of drugs as monotherapy or dual therapy at optimal plasma levels suggests the need for further investigation and perhaps a revised diagnosis. In all such cases specialist referral is mandatory.

Gradual initiation
Low drug doses are used initially and gradually increased until control is achieved or unacceptable toxic effects occur, carefully adjusting doses according to individual patient response. This requires patience: a half-life of 36 h or more (e.g. *phenytoin*) means that a new steady state will not be reached until about 7–14 days after any change in dose.

Compliance
The importance of compliance must be stressed to the patient, and this must include a clear explanation about the range and likelihood of potential adverse effects. Seizure-free patients can easily decide that they are cured and stop taking medication: this is a common cause of 'failure' of therapy. This is especially true of younger patients. Abrupt withdrawal of drugs may precipitate a seizure.

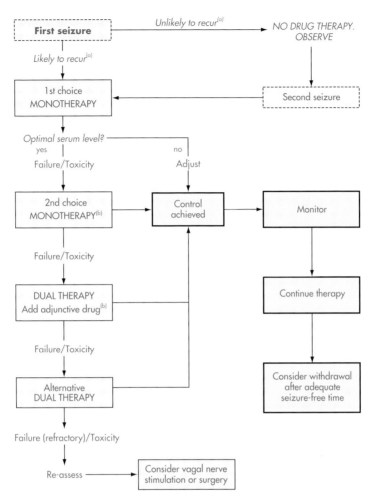

Figure 6.19 Treatment strategy for epilepsy. [a] Based on history, investigations, patient choice, etc. (see p. 444). [b] Prefer a drug with a different range of side-effects. (Adapted with permission from Beghi *et al.* (1986) Drug treatment of epilepsy: outlines, criticism and perspectives. *Drugs*; **31(3)**: 249–265.)

Switching

Particular care is needed when switching AEDs. There must be a gradual process of tapering the dose of the original while titrating up the replacement. Close monitoring is essential throughout to ensure continuity of control with minimal side-effects. Similar precautions apply when adding in an adjunctive agent.

Plasma level monitoring

It is not necessary to monitor patients' blood levels regularly. However, the non-toxic therapeutic ranges of most AEDs are known and therapeutic drug monitoring may be helpful in a number of circumstances, to check for possible abnormalities in absorption, clearance, interaction and compliance:

- During initiation, if expected response is not achieved.
- When previously stable control deteriorates.
- In pregnancy.
- In suspected toxicity.
- When doses are changed or other drugs are initiated.
- When there is renal or hepatic impairment.

Consistent formulation

Efforts should be made to ensure that patients continue taking the same manufacturer's form of AED. Unpredictable changes in bioavailability often follow changes in dose form or formulation, with loss of control or increased toxicity. Special vigilance is necessary when patients move between primary and secondary care, or between different prescribers or pharmacies, and for patients taking *phenytoin*.

Medication record

The patient should carry and maintain a complete medication record, including OTC drugs.

Antiepileptic drugs

It is possible to make some generalizations about AEDs where there are broad similarities, but the reader is referred to an official formulary for detailed information on each drug. Some of the more important features are given in Table 6.32 and discussed below.

Mode of action

Although most AEDs can be assigned a specific neuropharmacological mode of action, it is uncertain to what extent this correlates with their clinical action. Nevertheless, knowledge of the class to which a drug belongs facilitates rational combinations when these are necessary.

There are three main classes. Most AEDs interfere with voltage-dependent high-frequency sodium channels to limit the spread of the neuronal instability by inhibiting unnaturally rapid firing. This group includes the common agents used in generalized and partial seizures, such as *carbamazepine, lamotrigine, phenytoin* and perhaps *valproate*. Others facilitate the inhibitory transmitter GABA, which stabilizes neuronal membranes; this includes especially the CNS sedative agents *phenobarbital* and the benzodiazepines. *Vigabatrin* irreversibly inhibits GABA catabolism. Although *valproate* also inhibits GABA-catabolic enzymes, other actions contribute to its wide spectrum of antiepileptic activity. Some drugs active in absence seizures, especially *ethosuximide*, block voltage-dependent calcium T-receptors.

The modes of action of some of the newer AEDs have not yet been fully elucidated, e.g. *topiramate, gabapentin*. Approaches currently being explored include inhibition of excitatory transmitters such as glutamate.

Pharmacokinetics

The handling of AEDs is varied and complex. There may be great variation in plasma levels for a given dose, both between patients and even in the same patient at different times. For some drugs this may make plasma level monitoring advisable at certain times, but routinely it is usually sufficient to monitor clinically, by freedom from seizures and adverse effects.

Absorption

This may be highly formulation-dependent, especially with *phenytoin*, which makes it unwise to change brands or dosage forms. This does not preclude using generic drugs, as is sometimes erroneously believed, provided that one particular proprietary formulation is used consistently. For drugs like *phenytoin*, with a narrow therapeutic index, variation in bioavailability may permit seizure breakthrough on the one hand or excessive toxicity on the other. Similar considerations apply to potential interactions. Absorption rate and bioavailability may be reduced by food and antacids. IM *phenytoin* is very poorly absorbed, so the IV route is essential if parenteral therapy is necessary. The prodrug *fosphenytoin* causes less local irritation.

Distribution

Clearly, all AEDs are sufficiently lipophilic to enter the brain but they do so at different rates. Benzodiazepines enter quickly to act most rapidly and so are the standard treatment for status epilepticus. They have the highest volumes of distribution due to central accumulation. Most AEDs are highly plasma protein bound. Consequently, free drug levels may be sensitive to displacement owing to competition for binding by other drugs, including other AEDs. Whether or not this has clinical consequences is not easy to

Table 6.32 Antiepileptic drugs – notable features

Drug	MoA[a]	Pharmacokinetics	Main use[b] First line	Main use[b] Adjunct	Special indication	Avoid	Side-effects; other notes	Interactions
Benzodiazepine	GABA	Rapid CNS penetration/action		All forms	Myoclonus, absences		Tolerance, sedation	
Carbamazepine	Na	Potent auto-inducer; many active metabolites	Partial Tonic–clonic			Myoclonus, absences	Sedation, hyponatraemia (inappropriate ADH secretion), neutropenia	Enzyme inducer
Ethosuximide	Ca	Hepatic clearance	Absence			Partial	GI, mood changes	
Gabapentin	?	Renal clearance; no effect on liver enzymes		Partial		Myoclonus, absences	Ataxia, CNS depression	Few interactions
Lamotrigine	Na	Inducible metabolism, long half-life; low binding	Partial Generalized		Broad spectrum		Skin reactions, allergies. Numerous formulations	Metabolism induced by many AEDs; inhibited by valproate
Levetiracetam	?	Unaffected by enzyme inducers		Partial Tonic–clonic			CNS effects	
Oxcarbazepine	Na	Similar to carbamazepine but less induction	Partial Tonic–clonic					Similar to carbamazepine but fewer problems
Phenobarbital	GABA	Active metabolites, enzyme induction		Status		Absences	CNS depression Use discouraged	

continued overleaf

Table 6.32 (Continued)

Drug	MoA[a]	Pharmacokinetics	First line	Adjunct	Special indication	Avoid	Side-effects; other notes	Interactions
			Main use[b]					
Phenytoin	Na	Variable absorption, high binding, saturation kinetics, enzyme induction		Partial Tonic-clonic			Sedation, ataxia, etc. (see text); teratogenic. Narrow therapeutic index.	Many interactions
Tiagabine	GABA	Hepatic clearance, high plasma protein binding		Partial		Generalized	CNS: psychotomimetic effects, sedation, anxiety	
Topiramate	Na?	Renal clearance (partial)	Partial Tonic-clonic		Broad spectrum		Ophthalmological (monitor), CNS depression?	
Valproate	Na? GABA?	Enzyme inhibitor	Partial Generalized		Broad spectrum		Hepatotoxicity (rare), neural tube defects, menstrual changes	Potentiates some AEDs
Vigabatrin	GABA	Renal clearance		Partial	Infantile spasm	Specialist use only	Visual field defects (30%; monitor). Psychotomimetic effects	
Zonisamide	Ca	Renal clearance		Partial			Ensure adequate hydration. Avoid hyperthermia	Carbamazepine, phenytoin, antidepressants

(a) Mode or site of action class: Ca, calcium channel; GABA, enhance GABA inhibitory activity; Na, voltage-dependent Na channels.

(b) Applies to adults only; inductions in children and infants may be different; consult NICE guidance.

AED, antiepileptic drug; CNS, central nervous system; GI, gastrointestinal. Data derived from: NICE 2004; BNF 51; Duncan et al., *Lancet* 2006; **367**: 1087.

predict, partly because hepatic clearance will be increased by higher plasma levels, and a formulary should always be consulted for the latest guidance.

Clearance

Most AEDs undergo extensive hepatic metabolism but *vigabatrin, gabapentin* and *topiramate* are cleared renally. *Valproate, carbamazepine* and *phenobarbital* have active metabolites. Rates and extents of metabolism vary according to age, other disease, genetic factors and enzyme induction or inhibition by other drugs, usually in a predictable manner (see Chapter 1). A number of factors further complicate this.

Many AEDs are hepatic **enzyme inducers**, especially *carbamazepine, phenytoin* and *phenobarbital*. Some also cause auto-induction, producing subsequent difficulties in dosage adjustment; with *carbamazepine* the half-life can reduce from 50 h at the start of therapy to less than one-third of this later on. The very similar *oxcarbazepine* is far less troublesome in this regard. There is commonly a mutual interaction between AEDs, each enhancing the clearance of the other. AEDs will also enhance the clearance of other drugs by the same mechanism; *phenytoin* and others reduce the efficacy of oral contraceptives in this way, which is especially important in view of the potential teratogenic action of many AEDs. *Valproate* uniquely is an **enzyme inhibitor**, so can enhance the action of other, hepatically cleared AEDs.

The enzyme systems involved are also potentially saturable, especially with *phenytoin*. This may permit plasma levels to enter the toxic range inadvertently while treatment is initialized or the dose changed, because a dose increase similar to the previous one may produce an unexpectedly large effect (Figure 6.20). *Phenytoin* dose changes in particular must be gradual, allowing the usual five half-lives to attain steady state before alteration, and in small increments (25 mg) above about 200 mg/day.

Duration of action

Most AEDs have a sufficiently long half-life as to require only once-daily dosing. Notable exceptions are *valproate, carbamazepine* and *gabapentin*.

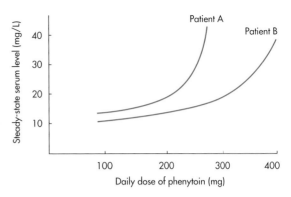

Figure 6.20 Graph illustrating effect of saturation kinetics on phenytoin steady-state plasma level. The dose/plasma level curve is linear up to 200–300 mg daily (the exact threshold varies between patients). Above that the plasma level rises disproportionately for small increments in dose because the hepatic drug metabolizing system has become saturated.

Side-effects

Consideration of the adverse effects of the AEDs is important because they may have to be given for long periods and compliance is sometimes a problem (see Table 6.32). This occurs in particular with adolescents on *phenytoin* because of the disagreeable, though not dangerous, cosmetic side-effects. In addition, as noted above, *phenytoin* causes dose-related toxic effects to occur at plasma levels that are only a little above the therapeutic range, and these are important markers of over-dosage (Figure 6.21). Other AEDs do not have such a narrow therapeutic index; for this reason *phenytoin* has fallen from favour as a first-line AED.

CNS. Most AEDs have some non-specific depressant or sedative action, but especially *phenytoin, phenobarbital* and its prodrug, *primidone*. In the long term there may be cognitive and behavioural impairment with these older drugs, especially *phenobarbital*; nystagmus and ataxia may also occur. *Vigabatrin* and *tiagabine* can cause psychiatric disturbances. *Carbamazepine* and *valproate*, and many of the newer agents, are significantly less troublesome in these respects, which is one reason why they have replaced the former three as first choices.

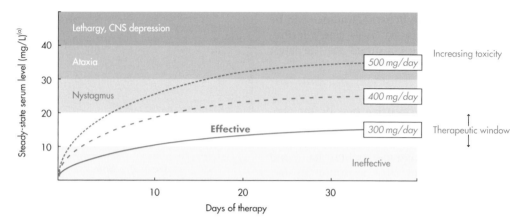

Figure 6.21   Side-effects of phenytoin in relation to plasma level. The narrow therapeutic window can be seen, and also the long time required to achieve steady state. The effect of different doses is shown for illustrative purposes only; individuals vary widely in their responses. [a] For µmol/L multiply by 4. CNS, central nervous system. (Adapted with permission from Kutt H, McDowell F (1968) *J Am Med Assoc* **203**: 969.)

Gastrointestinal tract. Many AEDs cause gastrointestinal distress (especially *valproate*), but care is needed with the use of antacids as they may impair absorption of some AEDs. Enteric-coated preparations are preferred where available. Rarely, *valproate* causes hepatic or pancreatic injury (monitoring essential).

Skin. There are serious cutaneous reactions with *phenytoin*, including acne, hirsutism (excessive hair growth), coarsened looks and gingival hyperplasia (gum overgrowth). *Valproate* can cause hair loss. *Lamotrigine* and *carbamazepine* can cause rash that is severe enough to force discontinuation.

Eyes. Both *vigabatrin* and *topiramate* require ophthalmological monitoring. The former causes visual field defects and the latter raises intraocular pressure.

Metabolic. A number of AEDs, notably *phenytoin* and *carbamazepine*, lower vitamin D and folate levels, partly because enzyme induction accelerates the catabolism of these vitamins. Osteomalacia (rickets) or megaloblastic anaemia may follow. Folate supplementation is recommended before and during pregnancy to prevent neural tube defects (see Chapter 11).

Systemic. Haemopoietic, hepatic or renal disturbances are rare. Nevertheless, blood and liver monitoring should be performed regularly. *Carbamazepine* occasionally causes hyponatraemia.

Teratogenic effects. Many AEDs present a serious dilemma in the therapy of young women. They can enhance the metabolism of oral contraceptives, possibly promoting contraceptive failure. Because most teratogenic effects occur very early in pregnancy, possibly before it is realized, any damage would already have been done. AED therapy carries a small but definite risk (about two to three times normal) of fetal abnormality; particular offenders are *valproate* and *phenytoin*. Yet both fetus and mother may suffer, the former irreversibly from anoxia, if a pregnant woman has frequent major seizures. A further difficulty in evaluating the risk–benefit is the fact that fetal abnormalities are slightly more common among female epilepsy sufferers, even if untreated with AEDs. Other potential toxic effects on the fetus include sedation, enzyme induction, and even neonatal withdrawal seizures. Neonatal bleeding may occur due to impaired vitamin K transplacental transport, and vitamin K is used immediately before delivery. In addition, the clearance of many AEDs increases during pregnancy, so plasma levels have to be monitored carefully. AEDs are secreted in small quantities in breast milk, but this does not seem to be a serious clinical problem. Whether or not AED therapy should be continued depends on the risks of withdrawal. The current view is that treatment in women should be continued, but with careful monitoring to maintain control at the lowest possible dose, preferably with a single AED. *Carbamazepine* appears to be the safest option.

Drug selection

Despite determined efforts to produce a precise classification of epilepsy and frequently quoted recommendations for different types of seizure, a systematic rationale has not emerged for linking drug to seizure type. Evidence is slim; few direct comparisons have been made and recommendations are still basically empirical. The classification by epilepsy syndrome has enabled some improved targeting and the current NICE guidelines (2004) give best choices.

Table 6.33 provides the currently agreed best choices, based on the NICE guidelines and the BNF. There seems to be no systematic distinction between choices for generalized tonic–clonic seizures and those for partial seizures, but there is between these two seizures types and for absences. Patient factors such as tolerability, adverse effects and interactions are more important criteria informing the decision on drug therapy.

Epilepsy is the sole remaining indication for *phenobarbital*, which escapes the strict legal control of barbiturates in the UK, but its use is declining.

Interest continues in the use of high-fat ketogenic diets as an adjunct in resistant childhood epilepsy. This is based loosely on the apparent antiepileptic effect of starvation, but it is not an established or widely used approach.

Benzodiazepines are the first-line drugs of choice in most forms of status epilepsy. The current recommendations for convulsive status are:

- Threatened status (i.e. premonitory stage; seizures lasting longer than 5 min, or of greatly inreasing frequency): rectal *diazepam* or buccal *midazolam*.
- Established status: IV *lorazepam*, adding IV *phenytoin* if control not achieved.
- Refractory status: referral to an intensive care unit for anaesthesia.

Table 6.33   Drug selection for epilepsy seizures

Partial (location-related)	Primary generalized – tonic–clonic	Primary generalized – absences	Myoclonic
First-line monotherapy			
Carbamazepine	Carbamazepine	Ethosuximide	Valproate
Lamotrigine	Lamotrigine	Lamotrigine	
Oxcarbazepine	Topiramate	Valproate	
Topiramate	Valproate		
Valproate			
Second line monotherapy			
Gabapentin	Oxcarbazepine	Topiramate	Lamotrigine
Phenytoin	Phenytoin		Topiramate
Adjunctive dual therapy			
Clobazam	Clobazam	Benzodiazepine	Benzodiazepine
Levetiracetam	Levetiracetam		
Tiagabine			

Adapted principally from NICE (2004).

Withdrawal of drug therapy

After a suitable seizure-free period the possibility of gradual withdrawal should be discussed with the patient. The likelihood of a lengthy remission is increased in patients with childhood onset, epilepsy of short duration, previous good control, a normal EEG, and no evidence of a primary cause, e.g. head injury, mental retardation or an adverse MRI scan.

At present it is generally agreed that the patient must have at least two seizure-free years before stopping treatment can be considered, but the more cautious would wait for up to 5 years. It also depends on patient and clinician preference (e.g. does the patient need to drive?). Withdrawal should be phased over at least 6 months, one drug at a time if on multiple therapy. Even if withdrawal is successful, the drug therapy itself cannot be considered to have brought about a cure: it is more likely that the disease has remitted spontaneously.

References and further reading

Anonymous (1995). Benzodiazepines and the newer hypnotics. *MeReC Bulletin* **15**(5): 117–120.

Bazire S (2007). *Psychotropic Drug Directory*. Salisbury: Fivepin Publishing.

Bleakley S (2006). Anxiety disorders – pharmacological management. *Hosp Pharm* **13**: 119–122.

Clarke C E, Guttman M (2002). Dopamine agonist monotherapy in Parkinson's disease. *Lancet* **366**: 1767–1769.

Davies T, Craig T K J, eds (2007). *ABC of Mental Health*, 2nd edn. London: BMJ Books.

Duncan J S, Sander J W, Sisodiya S M, Walker M C (2006). Adult epilepsy. *Lancet* **367**: 1087–1100.

Feetham C, Donoghue (2003). Antipsychotics in treatment of first episode schizophrenia. *Pharm J* **270**: 405–408.

Geddes J R, Cipriani A (2004). Selective serotonin reuptake inhibitors. *BMJ* **329**: 809–810.

Kantona C, Robertson M (1995). *Psychiatry at a Glance*. Oxford: Blackwell Science.

Khan N L, Britton T (2004). Parkinson's disease: clinical features, pathophysiology and genetics. *Hosp Pharm* **11**: 9–15.

Khan N L, Jagait P, Tugwell C (2004). Parkinson's disease: current and future aspects of drug treatment. *Hosp Pharm* **11**: 18–22.

Macmillen I, Young A H, Ferrier I N (2004). Mood (affective) disorders. *Medicine* **32**(7): 14–16.

Müeser K T, McGurk S R (2004). Schizophrenia. *Lancet* **363**: 2063–2072.

Müller-Oerlinghausen B, Berghöfer A, Bauer M (2002). Bipolar disorder. *Lancet* **359**: 241–247.

Nash J, Potokar J (2004). Anxiety disorders. *Medicine* **32**(7): 17–20.

NICE (June 2002). Schizophrenia – atypical antipsychotics: The clinical effectiveness and cost effectiveness of newer atypical antipsychotic drugs for schizophrenia (TA43). Available from http://guidance.nice.org.uk/TA43/?c=91523 (accessed 16 August 2007).

NICE (December 2002). Schizophrenia: Core interventions in the treatment and management of schizophrenia in primary and secondary care (CG1). Available from http://guidance.nice.org.uk/CG1/?c=91523 (accessed 16 August 2007).

NICE (October 2004). The epilepsies: The diagnosis and management of the epilepsies in adults and children in primary and secondary care (CG20). Available from http://guidance.nice.org.uk/CG20/?c=91523 (accessed 16 August 2007).

NICE (December 2004). Anxiety: Management of anxiety (panic disorder, with or without agoraphobia, and generalised anxiety disorder) in adults in primary, secondary and community care (CG22). Available from http://guidance.nice.org.uk/CG22/?c=91523 (accessed 16 August 2007).

NICE (December 2004). Depression: Management of depression in primary and secondary care – NICE guidance (CG23). Available from http://guidance.nice.org.uk/CG23/?c=91523 (accessed 16 August 2007).

NICE (June 2006). Parkinson's disease: Diagnosis and management in primary and secondary care (CG35). Available from http://guidance.nice.org.uk/CG35/?c=91523 (accessed 16 August 2007).

NICE (July 2006). Bipolar disorder: The management of bipolar disorder in adults, children and adolescents, in primary and secondary care (CG38). Available from http://guidance.nice.org.uk/CG38/?c=91523 (accessed 16 August 2007).

Picchioni M, Murray R M (2007). Schizophrenia: clinical review. *BMJ* **355**: 91–95.

Taylor D, Paton C, Kerwin R (2007). *The Maudsley Prescribing Guidelines*, 9th edn. London: Martin Dunitz.

Tylee A, Jones R (2005). Managing depression in primary care. *BMJ* **330**: 800–801.

7

Pain and its treatment

Pain is a common presenting symptom in primary care and an important cause of morbidity. Patients with mild to moderate pain self-medicate initially, using familiar analgesics or following pharmacist or lay advice. Those with severe pain normally present to GPs or hospitals. GP referrals to area hospital Pain Clinics are common.

The large psychological and cultural components may cause stoics to ignore a pain until the condition is difficult to salvage: doctors have dismissed the pain of their own myocardial infarction as 'indigestion'! Despite its universality and the existence of effective remedies, journal articles frequently discuss the poor management of post-operative, chronic and terminal disease pain.

This chapter discusses the characteristics and pharmacotherapy of various types of pain, to guide best practice. Morphine-like drugs are referred to here as 'opioids', although this term strictly describes only synthetic compounds, 'opiates' being of natural origin. The term 'narcotic' is not synonymous with 'opioid': it describes central nervous system depressants that relieve pain, producing narcosis (sedation and unconsciousness) in sufficiently high doses. It is widely used legally for addictive drugs of abuse.

Introduction

Although pain is a universal experience, it is difficult to define. One possible definition is:

> An unpleasant sensory and emotional experience associated with actual or potential tissue damage or described in terms of such damage. It serves biological functions, warning of external danger, e.g. excessive heat or physical trauma, and internal pathology, e.g. inflammation or blockage of a ureter by a kidney stone, enabling avoidance or treatment. It is inherently self-limiting when the provoking source is removed or cured.

This indicates that pain is not simply a physical sensation. Pain perception also depends on the patient's emotional reaction to the stimulus (see below).

Types of pain

Acute pain usually has a readily definable cause. Its biological function is protective, acting as a warning that an external threat is noxious, or signalling organ malfunction. It has a well-defined time of onset, often associated with signs of hyperactivity of the autonomic nervous system, e.g. tachycardia, hypertension and pallor, depending on the severity of the symptoms and how the patient interprets them. The best way of managing acute pain is to diagnose and treat the cause, though this is often clear, e.g. following any kind of trauma. Temporary relief with analgesics is valuable while healing and recovery proceed.

Chronic pain is usually considered to be pain that has lasted for longer than 6 months. It does not signify a danger that requires immediate avoidance and a patient may not interpret such pain as indicating serious disease. Further, adaptation by the autonomic nervous system over time may lead to the absence of objective physical signs. However, there is often progressive physical deterioration, with sleep disturbance and weight loss. In severe cases, patients undergo serious affective and behavioural changes, e.g. major depression (see Chapter 6).

Essential components in the treatment of chronic pain are the identification of any organic problem, i.e. accurate diagnosis, and the recognition and management of significant affective and environmental factors.

Pain threshold and assessment

The patient's mood, morale and the meaning of the pain for that patient affect their pain perception. Thus if a patient has chest pain and a relative or close friend has recently had an MI, the patient may interpret his or her pain as a life-threatening event. This results in the pain threshold being lowered, i.e. anxiety is algesic, resulting in less tolerance of the pain or greater awareness of it. Conversely, if another friend with a similar pain interprets it as indigestion, or it is diagnosed as such, this would not be very stressful, the pain threshold would not be lowered, and the pain may be tolerated. However, this may not be a rational response (see Chapter 3). Although it is possible to measure an individual's pain threshold, e.g. by applying a defined stimulus, usually a constant heat source at a defined distance and recording the time from application to withdrawal, this is purely a research tool, e.g. when assessing the effectiveness of a new analgesic or for comparing analgesics. However, this does not help when assessing a patient's pain. Further, attention must always be paid to factors that modulate the pain threshold (Table 7.1).

Assessment

Pain is a subjective experience, so only the individual affected knows its nature and severity: the individual patient's assessment and description are vital. Useful clues can be gained from a patient's response to a particular analgesic, e.g. if pain is described as 'severe' but relief is obtained from modest doses of *paracetamol* (acetaminophen), it is probable that there is a significant emotional component to the pain perception. Careful, empathetic exploration of this aspect may be more rewarding than the use of increasingly potent analgesics. Also, the

Table 7.1   Factors affecting the pain threshold

Threshold lowered	Threshold raised
Insomnia, fatigue	Sleep, rest
Discomfort, pain (presence or fear of recurrence)	Relief of symptoms
Anxiety, depression, sadness	Sympathy, anxiolytics, antidepressants
Fear, anger, social and mental isolation	Companionship, understanding
Boredom	Diversional activity, occupational therapy

Table 7.2   Assessment of pain[a]

The following aspects should be elucidated while taking the history:
- Site, distribution, radiation from initial site
- Severity (subjective, and score on visual analogue or other scale)
- Nature (dull, sharp, lancinating (stabbing), etc.)
- Mode of onset, duration of episodes, time course of the problem
- Aggravating and relieving factors
- Response to previous therapy, analgesics used and effective dose
- Previous history of similar pain
- Meaning of the pain to the patient, e.g. fear of malignancy
- Concurrent diseases and treatment
- Absence from occupation
- Reduction in physical activity, especially leisure
- Medicines usage
- Increased alcohol consumption

By observation of pain behaviour, i.e. signs noted by a doctor or prescriber:
- Grimacing, sighing, groaning, limping
- Guarding, i.e. touching, rubbing or holding affected area, muscular bracing of affected area or reluctance to move it
- Posture
- Reactions on examination, e.g. reflex withdrawal, apparently exaggerated response
- Use of aids/supports

[a] See also Figure 7.1.

extent to which a condition interferes with social and pleasure activities may be a better guide to severity than absence from work or school. Other clues are obtained from what a patient reports and their observable behaviour (Table 7.2).

The origin of acute pain is usually easy to diagnose, unlike that of chronic pain, which is often of obscure origin, particularly when it is due to non-malignant disease. A careful assessment should be carried out before treatment is started and patients should be re-assessed regularly. The salient features to be elucidated are given in Table 7.3.

Figure 7.1 gives some examples of pain assessment tools. The visual analogue scales are rapid and enable immediate feedback, e.g. advice on the use of medication or a decision to change

Table 7.3 The WHO 'analgesic ladder'[a]

	Type of analgesic	Preferred analgesic[b]	Possible alternatives
Step 1 Mild to moderate pain	Non-opioid	Paracetamol (acetaminophen)	Aspirin NSAIDs, e.g. diclofenac, flurbiprofen, ibuprofen, indometacin, ketoprofen, naproxen, piroxicam
	± adjuvants[c]		Amitriptyline, imipramine, diazepam, perphenazine, dexamethasone; anticonvulsants, e.g. carbamazepine, phenytoin, gabapentin, pregabalin
If pain persists, is not tolerated or increases, move to:			
Step 2 Moderate to severe pain	Weak opioid or Weak opioid + non-opioid[d]	Codeine As above	Dihydrocodeine, buprenorphine, pethidine (meperidine), possibly tramadol Any from Step 1 or Ketorolac (post-operative pain only), nefopam
	± adjuvants		Any from Step 1
If pain persists, is not tolerated or increases, move to:			
Step 3 Severe pain	Strong opioid	Morphine	Alfentanyl, buprenorphine, diamorphine (heroin)[e], fentanyl, hydromorphone, methadone, oxycodone, pethidine (meperidine)?
	+ non-opioid ± adjuvants		Any from Step 1 Any from Step 1

[a] Start at the step appropriate to the severity of the pain. If the pain is reduced by adjunctive treatment, e.g. radiotherapy, nerve ablation, surgery, the patient should be reassessed and the level of analgesia should be stepped down.

[b] If drug in one class fails after an adequate dose/time interval trial, move up the ladder: do not use another drug from the same class (see Table 7.4).

[c] See p. 479.

[d] Common combinations in the UK are paracetamol (acetaminophen) with codeine (co-codamol), or with dihydrocodeine (co-dydramol).

[e] Diamorphine is not available (illegal) in the USA and many other countries.

NSAID, non-steroidal anti-inflammatory drug.

?, not commonly used as strong opioid, but may be suitable for short-term use.

(a)

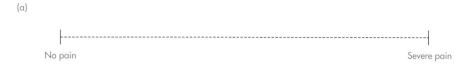

No pain   Severe pain

Place a vertical line on the dotted line to show how bad your pain is.

OR

(b)

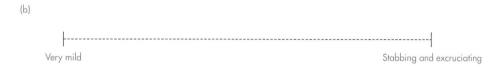

Very mild   Stabbing and excruciating

Place a vertical line on the dashed line to show how intense your pain is.

(c)

Severity		Relief	
NOW	TODAY		Over LAST WEEK
Severe	Complete		Excellent
Moderate	Good		Very good
Mild	Moderate		Good
None	Slight		Fair
	None		Poor

Place a circle round the word in each column that describes your situation

Figure 7.1   Pain assessment tools. (a) and (b) Visual analogue scales for pain level (a) and pain intensity (b); there should not be any intermediate divisions or numbering on the line: (c) Oxford Pain Chart: Categorical Scale [after Carroll and Bowsher (1993)].

medication. Patients should be given a fresh tool sheet on each occasion: if they see the previous sheet it prejudices how they respond. There are other ways, e.g. a pictorial scale of faces expressing response to different pain levels. The Short Form McGill pain questionnaire (see References and further reading, p. 511) can be completed within 5 min and is well-validated. It is important to document the results of the assessment, to provide a clear history of the progression of pain and the progress of analgesia for use by all personnel involved with a patient's care.

Pathophysiology of pain

An understanding of how the sensation of pain is generated is essential to an appreciation of how modification of these pain pathways can ameliorate the pain.

Gate theory

Various theories have tried to integrate the anatomical pain pathways and the psychological and neurological components that contribute to the perception of pain. The generally accepted model is the 'gate control theory', illustrated diagrammatically in Figure 7.2. This was first proposed by Melzack and Wall in 1965, and has since been modified as knowledge has increased. The theory proposes that neuronal impulses generated by noxious stimuli are modified in the dorsal horn of the spinal cord by a specialized mechanism ('gate'), which can tend to either inhibit or facilitate transmission of the pain impulse from peripheral organs to the brain. The gate is not an 'all-or-none' mechanism, and a balance between opposing factors determines how much of the initial nerve impulse is transmitted through it.

It has been shown recently that the SNC9A gene determines the structure of the voltage-gated sodium channels that are responsible for the transmission of signals along afferent pain fibres. Mutations in the gene may result in an inability to sense pain or excessive pain sensitivity (hyperalgesia). This discovery points the way to a new type of analgesic.

Pain receptors and fibres

Two main groups of skin receptors have been identified:

- High-threshold mechanoreceptors (HTMs), which detect local deformation, e.g. touch.
- Polymodal nociceptors, which detect a variety of types of injury (e.g. heat) and noxious (harmful) stimulation. These do not have a specialized structure and are simply bare nerve endings in the periphery.

Stretch receptors also occur in muscles, the wall of the gut and the capsules of internal organs.

Three types of nerve fibres are involved in pain transmission. The **A-beta fibres** are large, myelinated and fast-conducting (30–100 m/s). They have a low stimulation threshold and respond to light touch. The **A-delta fibres** are small, lightly myelinated and slower-conducting (5–15 m/s). They respond to pressure, heat, chemicals and cooling, and give rise to the sensation of sharp pain, producing reflex withdrawal and other prompt action. The **C fibres** are small and unmyelinated and therefore slow-conducting (0.5–2 m/s); they respond to all types of noxious stimuli and transmit more prolonged, dull pain signals. The last two of these types of fibres usually require high-intensity stimuli to trigger a response.

According to the gate control theory, A-delta and C fibres transmit pain signals to the dorsal

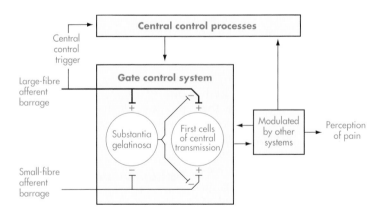

Figure 7.2   Gate control theory of the transmission of pain impulses. +, excitation; −, inhibition.

horns of the spinal cord. Impulses in these fibres can be modulated by A-beta activity that can selectively block impulses from being transmitted to the transmission cells in the **substantia gelatinosa** of the spinal cord. Such blockage prevents upward transmission to the CNS, and no pain sensation is perceived. This explains why rubbing an injured area, or applying a 'counter-irritant' such as capsaicin, which stimulates the A-beta fibres, can relieve the pain caused by an injury to that area, which stimulates the smaller C-fibres.

The gate control mechanism is believed to operate continuously, even in absence of an apparent trigger, because there is a continuous barrage of impulses from, principally, the C-fibres, whose receptors are continually active and react only slowly to stimuli. The effect is to set a threshold below which there is no effector response. Action subsequent to stimulation depends on the numbers of fibres involved, their firing rate, the proportion of large and small fibres, and the effect of central control mechanisms. The latter may over-ride the gate control, as occurs under hypnosis. When the complexities of this mechanism have been elucidated, new drugs or techniques of pain control may emerge.

Pathological pain

It has been suggested that peripheral tissue damage (e.g. from trauma, surgery or cancer) causes central sensitization, i.e. neuronal changes occur that make the spinal neurones hyper-responsive for a long period to afferent signals that would not normally trigger the gating mechanism. One consequence of this theory is that prophylactic ('pre-emptive') local, regional or opioid analgesia should be given before surgery or any predictable moderate to severe pain, to prevent central sensitization occurring. The concept also accords well with our experience of treating severe chronic pain: for effective control it is essential that the pain should not be allowed to recur (see below).

New classes of analgesics are emerging, e.g. compounds that block spinal cord receptors for excitatory amino acids such as N-methyl-D-aspartate (NMDA). One such drug is *dizocilpine*, which blocks the NMDA ion channel and resembles *ketamine*, but has a much greater potency and is more selective for the receptor. *Dizocilpine* has been shown to prevent and eliminate **central sensitization** in animals. Further, Swedish research indicates that *ketamine*, which was introduced as an IV anaesthetic, is an effective analgesic at concentrations lower than those required to produce anaesthesia, or at which central nervous side-effects (hallucinations and other transient psychotic effects) are troublesome. *Ketamine* is being used increasingly in palliative care for difficult-to-control cases and may give dramatic improvement that is maintained for several months. Other general anaesthetics are widely used for the relief of obstetric pain (p. 507).

Neurotransmitters involved in pain

Opioid receptors and endogenous opioids

The important discoveries of stereospecific opioid receptors (of which several subtypes are known) and endogenous opioids further increased our understanding of the biochemical mechanisms involved in pain transmission and perception.

Several families of endogenous opioids have been identified including the **endorphins**, **enkephalins** and **dynorphins** (p. 468). Each family is derived from a distinct precursor polypeptide and has a characteristic anatomical distribution.

Other transmitters and mediators

Physical or chemical insult can stimulate nociceptors. Inflammation, ischaemia or other pain-inducing stimuli cause the release of noxious chemicals (e.g. bradykinin, histamine and 5-HT) in injured tissues. Prostaglandins (PGs), although not directly producing pain, appear to sensitize nociceptors to various chemical and pressure stimuli. This explains why NSAIDs, which block PG synthesis, are effective analgesics in some situations.

Substance P (neurokinin-1), a polypeptide probably released by the small-diameter C-fibres, is believed to be involved in pain transmission in

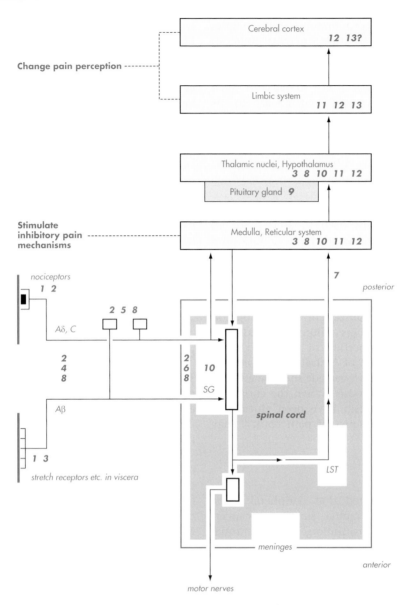

Figure 7.3 Methods of interrupting pain pathways and their possible sites of action. LST, lateral spinothalamic tract; SG, substantia gelatinosa. Aβ, Aδ, C, types of pain fibres; ?, possible effect or site. Bold numbers indicate methods or agents and their sites of action: 1, non-opioid analgesics; 2, local anaesthetics; 3, weak opioids; 4, peripheral somatic nerve block; 5, spinal somatic (extravertebral) nerve block; 6, spinal block; 7, cordotomy (usually in the cervical region); 8, electrical nerve stimulation?, acupuncture?; 9, pituitary gland ablation; 10, opioids (exogenous and endogenous); 11, psychotropic analgesic adjuncts; 12, anaesthetics (inhalation); 13, hypnosis.

the dorsal horns of the spinal cord. It is probably not the actual transmitter, but initiates a series of events leading to the recruitment of pro-inflammatory agents. The latter release media-tors, e.g. PGs, LTs, 5-HT and histamine, which stimulate the nerve endings and cause sensitiza-tion. Sensitization involves a lowering of the trigger threshold, producing **hyperalgesia**. Exci-tatory amino acid transmitters, e.g. glutamate and aspartate, may also be involved.

Pain transmission may be blocked if opioid receptors have already been occupied by endorphins at the spinal level. If successful in passing through the gating mechanisms, and several are probably involved in the total pathway, the pain impulse is transmitted via the reticular activating system of the pons and midbrain to the thalamus. From there, they are directed to the appropriate part of the cerebral cortex where the impulses are perceived as pain. The limbic system, which is anatomically close to these areas, is thought to be responsible for the emotional component of pain (see Chapter 6). Transmission of the pain impulse may be modified in the CNS by the presence of 5-HT and other chemical mediators.

It has been shown recently that pain signalling is amplified by certain ion channels in neuron membranes. There are ten isoforms of the sodium channel protein that share a common structure but have different amino acid compositions. Gene SCN9A encodes for the Na_v 1.7 sodium channel that is expressed preferentially at high levels in dorsal root ganglion and sympathetic ganglion neurons. It is deployed at the endings of nociceptive neurons close to the site of pain initiation and loss of the SNC9A gene causes inability to experience pain. This opens a new avenue for analgesia, by blocking either SNC9A transcription or translation or the Na_v 1.7 protein. Preliminary work suggests that this can be done without interfering with sympathetic nerve signalling.

The exact pathophysiology of pain is extremely complex and is still not fully understood. Figure 7.3 shows a simplified concept of the pain pathways and ways in which current treatments are thought to interrupt it.

Principles of analgesic use

The WHO recommendation on how to achieve effective analgesia is: "Dose patients by the mouth, by the clock and by the ladder." These points, and the general principles that should be employed when using analgesics, are outlined below.

Type and characteristics of pain

Because various types of treatment are available to manage pain (Figure 7.4), it is important to determine whether the pain is acute or

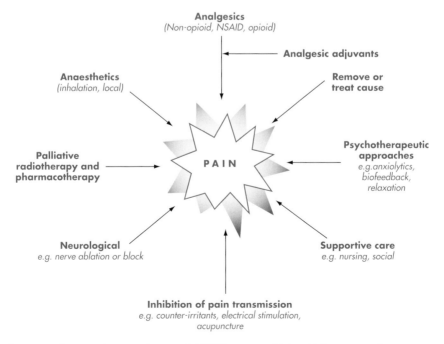

Figure 7.4 Summary of approaches to pain control. NSAID, non-steroidal anti-inflammatory drug.

chronic, to diagnose the cause, and to ascertain if any psychogenic component is present before deciding on the appropriate approach to treatment.

Acute pain generally responds well to analgesics, but chronic pain presents a far more complex problem. It often requires a multidisciplinary approach, employing several different modes of therapy. While the main emphasis in this chapter is on analgesics, alternative methods of pain control will also be discussed briefly, to place them in context.

Choice of analgesic

The type and severity of the pain will usually determine the specific drug or regimen to be used. Initiation of analgesia should be at the step appropriate to pain severity on the WHO 'analgesic ladder' (Table 7.3) and the appropriate dose and potency of analgesic is found by titrating the dose upwards, or down, until pain control is achieved at minimal dosage. Table 7.3 provides only an outline of the analgesics used, a more comprehensive listing being given in Table 7.4. The use of many of these drugs may be a matter of personal preference or convenience: it is always preferable to learn to use a few drugs well, rather than a wide range indifferently. The UK Department of Health document "Building a Safer NHS for Patients . . . ." recommends using a limited range of opioids.

Individualization of dosage

Dose requirements are affected by many variables including the severity of the pain, the patient's pain threshold, age, weight and the presence of concurrent disease. Each analgesic should be given an adequate trial by dose titration, i.e. modifying the dose until pain control is adequate or until dose-limiting side-effects occur, before switching to another drug (see, for example, Chapter 12 and the BNF, Section 10.1.1).

When using opioids in terminal disease, the only upper limit is that dose which successfully relieves the patient's pain without causing unac-

ceptable side-effects. For example, sedation is only a problem if it becomes unacceptable to the patient, but respiratory depression may be important, especially if respiratory function is already compromised, or unimportant. A recent research paper concluded that: "Properly titrated opioids have no respiratory depressant effect in adults who are awake".

The American Pain Society has recently recommended that patients and their families should be fully involved in pain assessment and management, including changes in dosage or routes of administration, and measurement of outcomes. However, it is common for patients to tolerate a lower analgesic dose when managed in a professional environment. This is due partly to better analgesic management and partly because, in the home environment, the anxiety of their families or carers that the patient should obtain complete relief leads to overdosing. Sometimes the patient seeks an excessive dose to spare their families from distress at seeing them suffer. The anxiety of families and carers is readily transmitted to patients, either overtly or inadvertently, and exacerbates the problem.

Dosage schedule

Traditionally, pain relief has been given on a 'when required' basis, so that the patient was expected to experience a return of pain before requesting more analgesic. Such an approach may sometimes be useful in acute pain, to see whether the symptoms are regressing, but is inappropriate in treating chronic pain because pain itself is a potent algesic (pain promoter): if pain is allowed to recur, a higher dose of analgesic will be required to re-establish pain control.

Thus, regular administration of analgesics is essential in chronic pain so that the patient's memory of the pain is reduced and, hopefully, gradually obliterated. This controls the psychological component and associated fear. When the patient has confidence in prescriber and treatment, the pain threshold may be raised, making it possible to reduce the analgesic dose.

The drugs, and their dose level, frequency and routes of administration, must be reviewed

Table 7.4   Some analgesics in current use

Pain severity[a]	Drug	Class[b]	PO	BC	SC	IM	IV	PR
Severe	Morphine[d]	A	✓	–	✓	✓	SL	✓
	Diamorphine (heroin)[d]	A	✓	–	✓	✓	SL	–
	Hydromorphone	A	✓	–	–	–	–	–
	Levorphanol	A	✓	–	✓	✓	✓	–
	Methadone	A	✓	–	✓	✓	–	–
	Oxycodone	A	✓	–	✓	–	SL	✓[e]
	Fentanyl[f]	A	–	✓	–	–	✓	–
	Alfentanil	A	–	–	–	–	✓	–
	Remifentanil	A	–	–	–	–	✓	–
Moderate to severe	Buprenorphine	P	–	✓	–	✓	SL	–
	Pentazocine	PAA	✓	–	✓	✓	✓	✓
	Pethidine (meperidine)	A	✓	–	✓	✓	SL	–
	Meptazinol	P	✓	–	–	✓	SL	–
	Ketorolac	N	✓	–	–	✓	✓	–
	Tramadol	A	✓	–	–	✓	SL	–
Moderate	Nefopam	N	✓	–	–	✓	–	–
	Dihydrocodeine	A	✓	–	✓	✓	–	–
Mild to moderate	Codeine	A	✓	–	–	✓	–	–
Mild	Aspirin, NSAIDs (see Chapter 12)	N	✓	–	–	–	–	✓
	Paracetamol	N	✓	–	–	–	–	–

Routes of administration[c] spans columns PO, BC, SC, IM, IV, PR.

[a] These potency groupings are only approximate. Potency is an inherent property of the drug, but the level of analgesia is usually markedly affected by the dose and route of administration, e.g. IV diamorphine (heroin) has three times the potency of oral morphine (see also Table 7.3).

[b] A, opioid agonist; P, partial opioid agonist; PAA, partial agonist–antagonist; N, non-opioid (see Table 7.5, NSAIDs, non-steroidal anti-inflammatory drugs).

[c] PO, oral; BC, buccal or sublingual; SC, subcutaneous; IM, intramuscular; IV, intravenous (SL = slow injection or infusion); PR, rectal. See below.

[d] Preferred or alternative analgesic for palliative care: diamorphine (heroin) is illegal in the USA and in many other countries.

[e] Suppositories are available by special order.

[f] Fentanyl is administered by a transdermal patch for chronic pain relief. Alfentanil and remifentanil are rapid-acting and used for induction of anaesthesia. Given intravenously, all three are short-acting adjuncts to general anaesthetics, used intra-operatively (especially remifentanil). Alfentanil is also given by SC infusion in palliative care.

The duration of action of the drugs is markedly affected by the formulation, route of administration and whether dosing is chronic or single dose. Most opioids have a single-dose duration of action of about 4–6 h, although pethidine (meperidine) is somewhat shorter-acting. Alfentanil, fentanyl and remifentanil are very short-acting.

frequently to ensure not only that analgesia is adequate but also that doses of concurrent drugs are appropriate and that side-effects are minimized and managed suitably.

Routes of administration

In selecting the most appropriate route of drug administration for a patient, factors such as 'nil-by-mouth', gastrointestinal obstruction, persistent vomiting, limited venous access or reduced muscle mass have to be taken into account.

Oral and sublingual

The **oral route** (per os, PO) is preferred if it is available although some opioids, e.g. *pethidine* (meperidine), are poorly absorbed from the gut and bioavailability can vary widely between patients. The peak effect usually occurs 30–60 min after dosing with normal oral formulations. Because peak activity occurs much later with most modified-release preparations, it is inappropriate to initiate pain control with these products. Ideally, the total daily requirement should be determined using a standard-release formulation, i.e. one with rapid release of the drug, preferably a solution. However, tablets may be used (e.g. with *morphine*) if the solution is disliked. When stable pain control has been achieved, this dose is then translated to the equivalent dose of a modified-release preparation to reduce the dose frequency.

The **sublingual route** is particularly attractive, because it provides a rapid onset of action and avoids the losses from first-pass metabolism, but may be unsuitable for very ill patients who produce little saliva. However, the Expert Working Group of the European Association for Palliative Care advises against the buccal and sublingual routes because there is no evidence for their clinical superiority over other routes and absorption may be unreliable.

Parenteral

The **intramuscular (IM) route** is commonly used post-operatively. It has the disadvantages of wide fluctuations in absorption, a 30- to 60-min lag time to peak effect, and a more rapid decline in activity than after oral administration.

In cancer patients, who are often cachectic (i.e. profoundly ill and malnourished) and have reduced muscle mass, IM administration can be painful and normal doses can give abnormally high peak concentrations. Because many cancer patients have low platelet counts, IM injection may cause severe bruising. Further, IM injection causes some muscle damage and the release of creatinine kinase, so this route must not be used within 48 h of a suspected MI (see Chapter 4) because this enzyme is used as one marker for MI. The gluteal (buttock) muscles are often used because of their large mass and it is less likely that a major blood vessel will be entered accidentally.

IM injections are preferably avoided in children because they may give rise to complications.

A bolus **intravenous (IV) dose** obviously provides the most rapid pain relief and avoids first-pass metabolism. However, rapid action also means rapid adverse reactions. This is particularly important with the opioids, which cause respiratory depression. The main determinant of the time taken to achieve a therapeutic effect with a centrally acting drug is its lipid solubility, which determines how quickly the drug leaves the plasma and is distributed into the CNS.

The IV route does not appear to confer any advantage for maintenance dosing, and opioid tolerance may occur more rapidly. However, it enables rapid titration of the analgesic dose in patients with acute, severe pain or an acute exacerbation of chronic pain. The IV infusion of analgesics after major surgery gives good post-operative pain control and has been shown to decrease the recovery period and reduce post-operative complications.

The oral route is equally effective for treating stable chronic pain, unless the patient is unable to absorb oral medications because of vomiting, dysphagia or bowel disease. In such cases, SC infusion is the preferred parenteral route.

Spinal anaesthesia is used routinely in obstetrics and increasingly for surgery on patients who are unsuitable for a general anaesthetic, post-surgically and for palliative care in a few terminally ill patients (p. 487).

The **continuous SC infusion** of opioids is used widely and achieves virtually constant blood levels (see below).

Rectal

The **rectal route** (per rectum, PR) is another alternative to oral administration in patients who are vomiting or on a 'nil-by-mouth' regimen, provided that it is not precluded by bowel disease. Several analgesics are available as suppositories (Table 7.4). This route also avoids loss of available drug by first-pass metabolism.

Rectal administration should be avoided in patients with a low platelet count due to cancer chemotherapy or to disease because it may provoke bleeding which is difficult to control.

Transdermal

This route is used currently only with *fentanyl* and *buprenorphine*. It is useful if the oral route cannot be used and continuous parenteral infusion is either unavailable or unsuitable. *Fentanyl* has a short duration of action if given orally or by parenteral bolus injection, due to rapid metabolism and tissue redistribution, whereas the transdermal patches provide prolonged dosing.

However, skin reactions may occur with the patches and the BNF advises application to dry, non-irritated, non-irradiated, non-hairy skin of the torso or upper arm, rotation of application sites when a patch is changed and avoidance of the same area for several days.

Guidelines for analgesic use

Accurate diagnosis of the cause of the pain is very important. However, there may be many underlying causes, especially in palliative care, so it may not be possible to identify a specific cause. The following guidelines are generally applicable.

- Use the oral route whenever possible.
- Only the patient knows if relief is adequate. However, treatment goals should be realistic: complete freedom from pain may be difficult to achieve. It may be helpful to set realistic stepwise goals, e.g. freedom from pain, in collaboration with the patient in the following ascending order:
  - At night.
  - At rest.
  - On movement.
- If an analgesic fails after a trial at adequate dose and frequency, move up the 'analgesic ladder' (Table 7.3): a substitute from the same class is unlikely to be more effective. If the patient is not supervised, e.g. in the community, it is worth checking that the patient is taking their analgesic(s) and any adjuvant medicines regularly and at the prescribed dose. Fear of addiction is common.

- If increased analgesia is required, the dose should be increased but the dosage interval should remain unchanged. Reducing the dosage interval below that appropriate for the drug merely makes life more difficult for the patient.
- Pain should not be allowed to recur. Drugs with a short duration of action, e.g. *pethidine* (meperidine), are unsuitable for the management of sustained severe pain.
- Opioids are not a panacea: due weight must be given to the use of adjuvants (p. 479), the management of psychosocial aspects and intercurrent disease, and the control of adverse reactions.
- Tolerance to opioids, and dependence on them, is not usually a practical problem when treating severe pain. Many patients receiving palliative care remain on a uniform dose throughout much of their illness. Opioid use should not be dictated by a short or poor prognosis, but by the needs of the patient. Physical dependence does not preclude dose reduction. If the patient's condition improves or if other treatments relieve the pain, dose reduction may be essential to avoid toxicity.
- There is some evidence that a state of hyperalgesia may occur with high IV or intrathecal doses of opioids but it is not clear to what extent this is relevant to clinical practice. The effect may be due to altered hepatic metabolism, i.e. a shift from the production of morphine-6-glucuronide (M6G), a potent analgesic, to M3G, an opioid antagonist.
- Always keep an open mind and review the treatment frequently. It may be possible to reduce the dose following a period of stable, good control. Conversely, a requirement for increasing doses is probably not due to drug tolerance or dependence but may indicate a deterioration in the underlying disease or the onset of another condition.

Analgesic drugs and techniques

Opioid analgesics

Mode of action

Opioid receptor sites

As mentioned earlier, receptor sites exist in the brain, spinal cord and elsewhere where opioids such as *morphine* bind to produce analgesia (and other pharmacological effects). The body's natural ligands for these receptors are the endorphin, enkephalin and dynorphin peptides. Receptor-binding studies have identified at least three major types of opioid receptors, designated **mu** (μ; two subtypes, μ_1, μ_2), **delta** (δ, two subtypes) and **kappa** (κ; three subtypes), each with distinct roles so that the type of pharmacological effect associated with each receptor is different. These effects are summarized in Table 7.5. About 65% of the amino acid composition of the three receptor types in animals are identical or very similar, as are most of their transmembrane regions and intracellular loops, but most of their extracellular loops differ. A further sigma (σ) receptor has been described, but its role is uncertain because opioid activity there is not antagonized by naloxone, a specific opioid antagonist.

Most of the research in this field has been carried out in rats and mice, but the evidence from them is not directly relevant to humans. A complication is that some of the receptors and their subtypes have been proposed based on drug-binding studies, but their pharmacological properties are ill defined or unknown. Because of these uncertainties and because further receptors and subtypes may exist, it is not currently possible to allocate the actions of drugs with certainty to specific subtypes in man. However, this is an active research field and drugs are likely

Table 7.5   The selectivity of opioid analgesics and their possible effects at their probable receptors[a]

Class of drug or agent	Example	Activity at receptor type		
		mu (μ)	kappa (κ)	delta (δ)
Pure opioid agonist	Morphine	Agonist	Weak agonist	?
	Pethidine (meperidine)	Agonist	Weak agonist	?
Partial opioid agonist	Buprenorphine	Partial agonist	Antagonist	?
Pure opioid antagonist	Naloxone	Antagonist	Antagonist	Antagonist
Endogenous peptide	Beta-endorphin	Agonist	?	Agonist
	Enkephalins	Agonist	?	Agonist
	Dynorphins	Weak agonist	Agonist	Weak agonist
Some effects produced by receptor activation		Supraspinal analgesia	Spinal analgesia	Analgesia
		Respiratory depression	Respiratory depression	Sedation
		Euphoria	Sedation	Hallucinations
		Miosis	Miosis	Reduced gut peristalsis
		Physical dependence		

[a] Data derived from animal experiments and may not reflect the situation in man precisely.

to emerge that act at specific receptors to achieve analgesia without the unwanted effects.

Morphine and related plant alkaloids have molecular structures similar to those of the endogenous peptides, and so activate the same receptors. *Methadone*, although chemically unrelated, can adopt a similar configuration. Naturally occurring and synthetic opioid drugs are classified according to the subtypes of receptors to which they bind, and the type of response that they thus evoke (Table 7.5). The available drugs include pure opioid agonists, partial agonists, agonists–antagonists, and pure antagonists. The affinity with which a drug binds to a receptor is important: analgesics with a high receptor affinity, e.g. *buprenorphine*, exert an analgesic action for much longer than their plasma half-life would suggest.

Opioid agonists and antagonists

Pure agonists (e.g. *morphine*) elicit a maximum response if given in sufficient concentration. However, a **partial agonist** (e.g. *buprenorphine*) can only produce a partial response irrespective of the concentration, and there may even be a decreased response if the optimum concentration is exceeded. The *morphine*-like opioids are thought to exert their agonist effects primarily at the mu receptor and to a lesser degree at the kappa receptor (Table 7.5). Partial agonists (Table 7.6) bind with the mu receptor and compete with the agonists, both naturally occurring and exogenous. If they are used in combination with

a complete agonist, they may act as competitive antagonists and the level of analgesia may be reduced, or as partial agonists, so that they show only limited activity. **Mixed agonists–antagonists**, e.g. *pentazocine*, are antagonists at the mu receptor but are still effective as analgesics through agonist effects at the kappa receptor, the agonist effect being either complete or partial.

At the other end of the spectrum are the **pure antagonists**, which are used to reverse respiratory depression post-operatively, to treat opioid poisoning (e.g. *naloxone*), and to prevent relapse in detoxified opioid addicts (e.g. *naltrexone*).

Opioid-sensitive and opioid-insensitive pain

Virtually all acute pain, with the possible exception of labour pain, falls into the opioid-sensitive category, the analgesic effect being related both to the type of agent used (weak or strong opioid) and the dose. The WHO defines **'weak opioids'** as those used to control mild to moderate pain and **'strong opioids'** are those used for moderate to severe pain.

Neuropathic pain (e.g. post-herpetic neuralgia and pain resulting from a stroke), includes **de-afferentation pain**, i.e. pain resulting from damage or interruption of afferent (sensory) nerve fibres, is partially opioid-sensitive and an adjuvant, e.g. a tricyclic antidepressant, usually *amitriptyline* or *nortriptyline*, an anticonvulsant, e.g. *gabapentin* or *pregabalin* (see Chapter 6) or nerve blocks may be required. Opioid-insensitive pains include most headaches. Pain arising from muscle spasm is best dealt with using muscle relaxants, e.g. *diazepam* and *baclofen*.

The management of post-herpetic neuralgia is discussed on p. 505.

Other types of pain may also be partially opioid-sensitive, e.g. that resulting from bone metastases is best treated with a combination of NSAIDs and opioids. NSAIDs may be adequate on their own, e.g. *diclofenac* in palliative care or as suppositories post-operatively when patients are 'nil-by-mouth', or possibly in combination with *paracetamol* (acetaminophen),. However, opioids may be needed initially or for continuing support. Some other types of cancer pain (e.g. that arising from nerve compression, raised

Table 7.6   Classification of partial agonists and mixed agonist–antagonists

Morphine-like	Nalorphine[a]-like
Buprenorphine[b]	Butorphanol[c,d]
Meptazinol[b]	Nalbuphine[b,d]
Propiram[b,d] ⎫ Investigational drug	Pentazocine[c]
Profadol[b,d] ⎭	

[a] Nalorphine is not used clinically because of side-effects.

[b] Partial agonist.

[c] Agonist–antagonist.

[d] Not licensed in the UK.

intracranial pressure and extensive tumour infiltration of tissues) may require an opioid plus an adjuvant, e.g. a potent anti-inflammatory glucocorticoid with minimal mineralocorticoid activity (*betamethasone* or *dexamethasone*). Psychogenic pain must always be addressed by identifying the underlying causes as well as by drug management, e.g. anxiolytics, antidepressants or other psychotropic agents in addition to analgesics. Analgesic adjuvants are discussed on p. 479.

Therapeutic use

Morphine

This has become the standard against which other opioid analgesics are judged and is generally the treatment of choice for chronic severe pain in advanced cancer. No other strong opioid, given orally, is consistently superior.

In addition to its central analgesic action, *morphine* causes euphoria and a sense of detachment. It also causes drowsiness for up to the first 7 days of treatment. This profile is clinically useful as it reduces the anxiety and anguish that are commonly associated with severe pain from whatever cause, e.g. MI and terminal disease. However, *morphine* should not be used primarily as a sedative. Occasional patients remain drowsy, in which case a dose reduction and a slower dose titration can be tried, and coexisting problems should be sought, e.g. the concurrent use of other sedatives. Liver impairment has little effect on the hepatic metabolism of *morphine* until it is severe, but renal damage prolongs the duration of action because 90% is renally excreted, mostly as glucuronides, and morphine-6-glucuronide (M6G) has twice the analgesic potency of *morphine*.

Morphine aggravates functional gastrointestinal pain (e.g. from colonic spasm or constipation), so it is unsuitable in patients with these problems, although the latter can be managed with stimulant laxatives.

One of the most important advances in the management of chronic pain has been the introduction of modified-release oral formulations of *morphine*, which usually give excellent control with once- or twice-daily dosing. These contain *morphine* bound to an ion exchange resin from which it is released by inward diffusion of sodium and potassium ions. Because of their slow onset of action, the appropriate dose must be established using quick-release dosage forms, e.g. solutions or normal tablets, and the first dose of a modified-release product should be given with the last dose(s) of quick-release product to cover the period until the new steady state is achieved. Adjustment of the doses of both types of product may be necessary to prevent breakthrough pain occurring. If breakthrough pain should occur in the early stages of modified-release medication, it is controlled with solution or injections (occasionally normal-release tablets) and the dosage regimen reassessed.

Suppositories are a useful alternative to injections if vomiting is a problem or if patients are unable to swallow. They are also convenient if a patient's carer cannot give injections.

The potential hazard of respiratory depression due to *morphine* may be increased because it appears to reduce the sensation of breathlessness, so the patient should be in a supervised environment when large doses are needed.

Papaveretum is a preparation of *morphine hydrochloride* (85%), *papaverine* and *codeine*, which is now rarely used in the UK. It no longer contains *noscapine*, a centrally acting cough suppressant, and the reformulated product contains a lower weight of *papaverine* but the same dose of *morphine*. This has created problems when dispensing and special care is required. *Papaveretum* has also been confused with *papaverine*, which is used to treat male impotence.

Morphine is the antitussive of choice for the treatment of the distressing cough of terminal lung cancer, with *methadone* as an alternative.

Many former traditional *morphine* mixtures, e.g. the 'Brompton Cocktail', opium tincture and camphorated opium tincture (paregoric), are no longer used in the UK because they confer no benefit over *morphine* alone.

Morphine is sometimes used for topical analgesia when local anaesthetics do not give adequate relief (unlicensed indication).

A guideline to the equi-analgesic doses of opioids is given in Table 7.7.

Table 7.7   Guide to equi-analgesic doses of some opioids[a] and their pharmacokinetic parameters

Opioid	Route of administration and dose (mg)		Pharmacokinetic parameters (h)	
	SC/IM	Oral	Half-life (h)[b]	Duration of action (h)[b]
Morphine	5–20	5–20	2	3–6
Codeine	30–60	30–60	3–4	3–6
Dextropropoxyphene	–	100	6–12	3–6
Dihydrocodeine	50	30	3.5–5	3–4
Buprenorphine	0.3–0.6	–	1–7	1–6
Diamorphine	5–10[c]	5–10[c]	0.05[c]	4–5[c]
Dipipanone	–	10	–	4–6
Fentanyl	25 µg/h[d]	–	3–12	1–3
Hydromorphone	1–2	1.3–2	2–3	3–5
Levorphanol	1–2	2	12–16	6–8
Methadone	2.5–10	2.5–10	15–60[e]	1–4[e]
Oxycodone	5	5	2–4	3–6
Oxymorphone	1–1.5	–	–	3–6
Pethidine (meperidine)	25–100	50–150	3–6	2–4
Tramadol	50–100	50–100	6	3–6

[a] Doses relative to 10 mg of morphine by SC/IM injection. Oral doses are for immediate-release products.

N.B. These are for guidance only, all patient and disease factors must be considered before prescribing or using.

[b] Approximate normal adult data.

[c] Diamorphine is hydrolysed rapidly to 6-acetylmorphine (active metabolite) and morphine.

[d] Transdermal fentanyl 25 µg/h patch is approximately equivalent to 90 mg/d oral morphine sulphate, and pro rata.

[e] Renal excretion is increased by acid conditions.

Other pure agonist drugs

Diamorphine (heroin, 3,6-diacetylmorphine)

Opinions differ over the choice between *heroin* and *morphine*. Because of its abuse potential and its disputed benefit, *diamorphine* is not available (often illegal) in most countries outside the UK.

Diamorphine itself is not an opioid agonist, but is rapidly metabolized to 6-monoacetylmorphine (6-MAM) and *morphine*, which are. Because both *diamorphine* and 6-MAM are more lipid-soluble than *morphine* they penetrate the blood–brain barrier more rapidly and so have a faster onset of action, though the final activity is due to the *morphine* produced on hydrolysis. *Diamorphine* is generally regarded as more potent than *morphine* on injection, both as a euphoriant and analgesic, and may cause less nausea and hypotension. However, the oral potencies of the two are similar because, when given orally, *heroin* is completely hydrolysed to *morphine* before absorption from the gut.

Diamorphine is unstable in solution, so *morphine* is preferred for oral solutions. However, *diamorphine* is very soluble in water and so is preferred in the UK for IM and SC administration as the injection volume is small. This may be important in very emaciated patients. Solutions are prepared from the sterile powder as required and are not stored.

Pethidine (meperidine)

This moderately potent analgesic is most commonly used peri-operatively and in obstetric analgesia. Because it is unpredictably absorbed and undergoes significant first-pass metabolism, oral bioavailability is poor and variable, with some trials showing equivalence with *paracetamol* (acetaminophen). However, some patients obtain satisfactory relief with oral *pethidine*, and saturation of metabolic pathways may increase bioavailability with chronic use (but see below). Given parenterally, it has a swift onset of action as it is highly lipophilic and crosses the blood–brain barrier readily. This property makes it useful for preoperative medication and treating acute pain. The short duration of action (1–3 h) normally makes it unsuitable for treating chronic pain, as approximately 2-hourly dosing would be required.

Further, *pethidine* is unsuitable for chronic use because its toxic metabolite *norpethidine* accumulates, causing anxiety, agitation, tremors and seizures. The latter is cleared renally and also accumulates in renal impairment. *Pethidine* probably causes more nausea, vomiting and hypotension than other opioids, and is said to have less effect on smooth muscle, so it is sometimes used for renal or biliary colic, though there is no good evidence to support this: IM or rectal *diclofenac* is usually preferred for this indication.

Although *pethidine* may produce less euphoria and sedation than *morphine*, this is disputed, and respiratory depression and postural hypotension are common at effective doses. Most of these side-effects can be corrected by using it with the antipsychotic agent *haloperidol*, which potentiates the analgesia, permitting lower doses to be used, and is anti-emetic, sedative and possibly euphoric. However, the toxicity of *haloperidol* limits the maximum dose that can be used (see Chapter 6).

Pethidine interacts with MAOIs to cause either severe hypertension or hypotension, depending on the patient and the relative doses of each, and so should not be used in patients taking hypotensive drugs or MAOI antidepressants, except under very close supervision.

Methadone

This agent is well absorbed and well tolerated by mouth and has been used with some success in pain control, particularly in the USA. However, its metabolism and excretion are complex, so the patient's physical, mental and emotional condition needs to be monitored closely. Its medicinal use in the UK is primarily for those intolerant of *morphine* and it is used widely to manage opioid dependence.

Pharmacokinetics. *Methadone* has a very long elimination half-life on multiple oral dosing (about 25 h) and is very highly bound to plasma and CNS proteins, so that accumulation can occur with chronic use. This leads to drowsiness and confusion, which may occasionally be life-threatening. The half-life is extended considerably by renal or hepatic impairment, so *methadone* must be used with special care in elderly or debilitated patients and in alcohol abusers. Steady-state blood levels are not achieved until at least 4–5 days after the initiation of therapy or a change in dose, so loading doses are sometimes used to achieve rapid control. Despite the long half-life, the duration of action is about 6–8 h initially, increasing to 6–12 h with chronic dosing, so several daily doses must be given initially. Once- or twice-daily dosing is used when steady-state blood levels have been achieved, because of the risk of accumulation and toxicity.

Although the degree of sedation and respiratory depression reflect the absolute amount of *methadone* in the body, the total body load does not influence the magnitude of analgesic response, possibly owing to different affinities for the different receptor subtypes.

Use in opioid dependence. *Methadone* is widely used in drug abuse clinics as a replacement for *heroin*, to help recreational drug users maintain a stable lifestyle. When a drug user has learned alternative strategies to *heroin* use for coping with stressful situations, the *methadone* may be withdrawn gradually. However, *methadone* may itself lead to a *morphine*-like dependence and the potential for abuse is similar to that for *morphine*. Although withdrawal symptoms are less intense than those with *morphine*, and it may relieve the physical withdrawal symptoms without giving 'highs' for the same length of time, the onset of withdrawal symptoms is slower (24–48 h) and they are more prolonged. Opioid misusers are usually given a very gradually reducing *methadone* dosage regimen, the level of which is carefully titrated to the patient's needs.

However, *buprenorphine* is now more widely used to manage opioid detoxification (withdrawal). Further, the value of *methadone* in treating opioid withdrawal has been challenged: it is not a cure and is often regarded more as a method of social control, to minimize the criminal activities often associated with drug misuse, rather than as therapy.

In these days of opioid-addicted mothers, neonatal opioid dependence should not be overlooked.

Hydromorphone

This potent analgesic, about 7.5 times as potent as *morphine*, is used in the UK when patients are intolerant of other opioids. It has a rapid onset of action but a relatively short half-life. Oral dosing is required 4-hourly, or twice daily with the modified-release preparation.

It is more widely used in the USA and Europe, probably because *diamorphine* is not available there. Like the latter it is very soluble in water and injection volumes are small, so it may be useful in syringe drivers (see below). However, the injectable preparation is not licensed in the UK.

Dipipanone

This agent is usually given orally only. Although it has been given by SC or IM injection in the past, it should not be given by the IV route because this may produce a dramatic fall in blood pressure.

The only available tablet in the UK is formulated with *cyclizine* (an antihistamine) as an anti-emetic. This makes the product unsuitable for chronic use, e.g. in palliative care.

Oxycodone

This is effective orally and is used widely in North America and elsewhere as a modified-release oral product and, combined with *aspirin* or *paracetamol* (acetaminophen), for moderately severe pain. In the UK it is available as normal-release capsules, modified-release tablets and as an injection for slow IV injection or SC use. It is sometimes used in syringe drivers for patients intolerant of other opioids, but the low concentration of the existing formulation limits the dose volume that can be given by this route.

Fentanyl and its congeners

These agents are used primarily for intra-operative analgesia. Opioids are widely used in low doses to supplement general anaesthesia with nitrous oxide–oxygen and a neuromuscular blocking agent. The muscle relaxants, e.g. *suxamethonium*, *pancuronium* and *atracurium* (there are many others), relax the diaphragm and abdominal muscles and may permit light anaesthesia to be used. In addition, they relax the vocal cords and so facilitate the passage of an endotracheal tube to assist in passing anaesthetic gases or oxygen. Patients who have received a muscle relaxant must always have assisted or controlled respiration when *fentanyl* is used.

Alfentanil, *fentanyl* and *remifentanil* have a rapid onset of action (1–2 min) and are used to reduce the induction dose of an anaesthetic, especially in poor-risk patients.

Remifentanil can be used intra-operatively as an IV infusion in adults and young children. Because it is rapidly metabolized by blood enzymes it has a very short duration of action and does not accumulate, so post-operative respiratory depression is unlikely. Because of its very short duration of action, additional analgesia is usually needed post-operatively.

Alfentanil and *fentanyl* may also be used intra-operatively as an IV infusion or as IV bolus injections. These may cause severe respiratory depression and cardiovascular side-effects, especially with *fentanyl*. Because respiratory depression may occur for the first time post-operatively, patients who have received either drug need to be observed carefully for some hours after recovery. *Sufentanil* (not licensed in the UK) is used similarly in the USA.

The side-effect of respiratory depression with *alfentanil* and *fentanyl* is used to advantage in intensive care patients on assisted respiration to manage respiration without interference from their endogenous respiratory drive. The opioid effect is reversed with *naloxone* when respiratory depression is no longer required.

Fentanyl is used widely as transdermal patches (Chapter 13), each of which lasts for 72 h, for the control of stable chronic pain when the oral route is unavailable or unsuitable. Because it takes about 12 h for the patch to produce adequate analgesia, it should be applied at an appropriate time, e.g. simultaneously with the last modified-release *morphine* dose when transferring from *morphine*. The equivalence between the *fentanyl* patches and *morphine* is that *fentanyl* 25 µg/h for 72 h is equivalent to *morphine hydrochloride* 90 mg daily.

Unfortunately, the patches are often used poorly in the community. Because of the lag time in reaching an effective concentration after a change in dose there may be too rapid titration; titration by increments that are too large; or inappropriate use in unstable pain, all of which may cause toxicity.

There is a buccal formulation, supplied with a special applicator, for breakthrough pain, but many patients find it difficult to use. An intranasal formulation is under trial for breakthrough pain when using patches, as a more convenient alternative to the buccal and IV formulations.

Fentanyl is used by SC infusion in palliative care, mainly for patients with renal failure because its metabolites are inactive.

Opioid rotation

Although oral *morphine* is the potent analgesic of choice, there is a minority of patients in whom their pain is inadequately controlled despite large doses. It is unclear why this situation occurs. Postulated mechanisms are the complex metabolism and pharmacokinetics of *morphine*, with active metabolites that may accumulate, and down-regulation of receptors or other receptor change.

These patients may benefit from a change in the route or method of administration, e.g. SC injection, patient-controlled analgesia (p. 489) or epidural anaesthesia (p. 508). Nerve blocks (Figure 7.3 and p. 487) may also be appropriate.

However, a satisfactory result may be achieved by a change of opioid, i.e. **opioid rotation** (also known as opioid switching). It is preferable to use a pure agonist, e.g. *hydromorphone*, *methadone* or *oxycodone*. Transdermal *fentanyl* or *buprenorphine* is unlikely to be useful in this context because of the pharmacokinetics of the patches. An initial dose reduction is often advocated, and is safe practice, with access to medication for breakthrough pain, taken when necessary. The dose can then be titrated according to patient response.

The reasons for benefit from rotation are not clear, but include differing metabolism, different receptor subtype responses and variable sensitivity to side-effects.

Opioid rotation is not a universal panacea, and frequent changes are undesirable. It is important to evaluate possible reasons for loss of pain control, e.g. new symptoms or intercurrent disease, and to consider alternative approaches to pain control.

Codeine and its congeners

Codeine phosphate itself is a relatively weak analgesic, but is converted to *morphine* and *norcodeine* in the liver. Although 10% of Caucasians cannot carry out this change the relevance of this to clinical practice is not known.

It is used for mild to moderate pain. It has a 'ceiling' effect, i.e. if the normal maximal dose of 60 mg fails to control the pain, further dose increases do not produce more analgesia. The side-effects of drowsiness, nausea and constipation often become intolerable at the ceiling dose. It is appropriate to co-prescribe a laxative (e.g. lactulose) in patients taking regular doses.

It is widely used as a cough suppressant and as a component of compound mild analgesics, e.g. with *aspirin* or *paracetamol* (acetaminophen). There is little evidence for the efficacy of these compound products, because the *codeine* doses are usually sub-therapeutic, i.e. <30 mg, and there is a considerable increase in side-effects. However, they are firmly entrenched in clinical practice.

Codeine formulations are best avoided in all children under 12 and should not be used in infants: the common belief that *codeine* is an effective sedative and hypnotic has resulted in fatalities.

It has the potential to cause dependence and pharmacists need to be vigilant when clients are using regular supplies of OTC products containing it.

Dihydrocodeine tartrate is possibly a more potent analgesic than *codeine* and is used for moderate to severe pain. However, both drugs are on Step 2 of the WHO ladder. Like *codeine* it is used in compound analgesic products and has similar disadvantages, including dependence. It is sometimes prescribed for dental pain.

Partial agonist and agonist–antagonist drugs

These were developed in an attempt to overcome opioid dependence problems. Although not totally devoid of abuse potential, they have less than that of *morphine* and other similar agonists.

Nalorphine was the prototype of this group but is no longer used owing to an unacceptably high incidence of psychotomimetic side-effects. Subsequently, two types of agonist–antagonist drugs have been developed that are classified according to their activity relative to *morphine* or *nalorphine* (Table 7.6).

Agents of the *nalorphine* type characteristically act only as competitive antagonists at the mu-receptor but have varying affinities and intrinsic activities at all receptor types. The mixed agonist–antagonists of the *morphine* type have a high affinity for mu-receptors, but a low intrinsic activity there.

Morphine-like opioids

Buprenorphine is a partial agonist that has a 6- to 8-h duration of action and is effective in the relief of moderate to severe pain unresponsive to non-opioid analgesics. Its potency is similar to that of *pethidine*. It is available in a sublingual formulation (but see above) and is sometimes used for premedication and peri-operative analgesia. For acute pain, the onset of analgesia of the sublingual tablets is about 30 min. However, the use of *buprenorphine* in chronic severe pain is problematic. It has a 'ceiling effect', like *pethidine* (meperidine) and *codeine*, and a low therapeutic index, like *pentazocine*, so increasing the daily dose above about 3 mg is unlikely to be beneficial. It is used to manage opioid withdrawal (see 'methadone' above). The sublingual tablets are popular among drug abusers and some health authorities have introduced a voluntary ban on prescribing these.

The transdermal patches have a lower incidence of side-effects than the sublingual formulation and are suitable for controlling moderate to severe chronic pain in palliative care and other patients. It takes about 24 h to reach a steady-state plasma level with the patches that are replaced after 72 h. Patches for replacement after 7 days are also available, the steady-state plasma level being achieved during the first application. However, the dose should be determined with the 72-h patches before switching to the 7-day formulation. Because *buprenorphine* is a partial agonist-antagonist, breakthrough pain can only be managed appropriately using the *buprenorphine* sublingual tablets: the use of other opioids gives unpredictable effects. The analgesic response should not be assessed before 24 h, but any dose adjustments should be made when the patches are changed. Due to its long terminal half-life of about 30 h, patients who suffer side-effects necessitating removal of a patch need to be monitored for a further 24–30 h. Unlike the pure opioid agonists, the effects, and side-effects, of *buprenorphine* are only partially reversed by *naloxone*.

Side-effects. Because of its high receptor affinity, large doses of other opioids may be required to displace *buprenorphine* from the receptor. This may lead, in those patients who do not obtain adequate pain relief with *buprenorphine*, to a confused situation of inadequate analgesia, despite a large opioid dose, but enhanced toxicity. If given to a patient receiving other opioids chronically, *buprenorphine* may precipitate pain and withdrawal symptoms. Thus it should be used alone. In common with most other opioids, *buprenorphine* causes dose-related respiratory depression. Because of its high receptor affinity its effect is not readily reversed by *naloxone*, making it more hazardous in overdose.

Buprenorphine is highly emetogenic in some patients but appears to be less likely than other opioids to cause constipation.

Meptazinol has about one-tenth of the analgesic potency of *morphine*. It is unusual in that it is thought to have two central mechanisms of action: a partial agonist–antagonist effect at opioid receptors, plus effects on central cholinergic receptors. It has a variable onset of action (0.25–3 h orally, 0.5 h rectally), and its duration of action is also variable (2–7 h). Thus dosing is required every 3–6 h, depending on patient response. It undergoes extensive first-pass metabolism, so blood levels after oral dosing are low and this route is better suited to the short-term relief of moderate pain, e.g. peri-operatively. For moderate to severe pain, *meptazinol* is best given by IM or slow IV injection. It is likely to cause nausea and vomiting.

Meptazinol is claimed to cause less respiratory depression than other opioids, possibly because of its cholinergic effects or its preferential action at the mu-receptor, and may be a useful analgesic to consider in patients with compromised respiratory function, but there is a divergence of opinion on this point. Some clinicians advocate the cautious use of *morphine*, despite its respiratory depressant effects, in patients with compromised lung function, believing that pain itself acts as a respiratory stimulant and reduces the risk of administering a known respiratory depressant. Further, should respiratory depression occur following *morphine* administration, this can readily be reversed by administering *naloxone*, whereas complete reversal of the effects of a mixed agonist–antagonist such as *meptazinol* cannot be achieved readily with *naloxone* and additional measures are needed, e.g. assisted respiration with *oxygen* (see Chapter 5) and possibly a respiratory stimulant.

The potential for abuse is probably less than that of *morphine* because its euphoric effects disappear with increasing dose.

Nalorphine-like opioids

Pentazocine is a moderately potent analgesic that is used infrequently nowadays in the UK as it shares the hallucinogenic potential of *nalorphine* and causes a high incidence of confusion and hallucinations. Like *buprenorphine*, *pentazocine* may precipitate a withdrawal reaction in patients who are opioid-dependent. It is unsuitable for pain associated with MI because, unlike *morphine*, it can increase the cardiac workload.

The oral efficacy of *pentazocine* is poor (slightly less potent than *codeine*) and, due to its low therapeutic index, doses cannot be increased greatly to treat severe pain without also markedly increasing the incidence and severity of side-effects. However, it is more potent when administered by any parenteral route than both *codeine* and *dihydrocodeine*.

Tramadol

This has both opioid and non-opioid modes of action, enhancing adrenergic and serotonergic actions. It is a metabolite of the antidepressant *trazodone*, so it is not surprising that it inhibits noradrenaline (norepinephrine) re-uptake and the stimulation of serotonin release at synapses. These secondary effects are responsible for the psychiatric side-effects seen in some patients, but they are also believed to facilitate the pathways that inhibit pain perception.

Tramadol is a weaker analgesic than most other opioids and appears to cause less respiratory depression. Because it causes less constipation it is often used when toileting difficulties create post-operative problems. There may also be a reduced potential for dependence, but *tramadol* should not be used if there is a history of drug dependence or convulsions. It has been used for obstetric and peri-operative pain and in MI, but is unsuitable for intra-operative analgesia during light anaesthesia.

Side-effects.   Apart from those referred to above, it may also cause occasional hypertension, anaphylaxis, hallucinations and confusion, particularly in elderly patients. Because it is not classed as a controlled drug in the UK, it is probably used more frequently than is justified.

Summary of opioid side-effects

Actions of *morphine* other than those described above are usually considered to be side-effects.

Nausea and vomiting

Morphine and its derivatives stimulate the CTZ (Chapter 3) and may cause nausea and vomiting, although this tends to be transient, wearing off a few days after initiating therapy or an increased dose. These effects may be avoided by prophylactic co-administration of an anti-emetic (see Chapter 3) over this period. Anti-emetics are also appropriate in patients who are already vomiting owing to drug use or who have a history of vomiting with opioids, and may be given initially either rectally or parenterally to bring existing vomiting under control.

Anti-emetics are not indicated in patients who are not currently nauseated and so should not be used routinely: good practice is not to prescribe a drug unless there is a positive indication. However, it is appropriate to prescribe a small quantity of an anti-emetic for use 'as required', in anticipation of possible need. Because *dipipanone* is only available combined with an anti-emetic (*cyclizine*), it is not recommended for use in palliative care.

Because the incidence of nausea and vomiting is higher in ambulatory patients, it is thought that a vestibular component is also involved. It is often helpful for the patient to lie quietly if this problem occurs.

Constipation

Opioids cause an increase in gastrointestinal sphincter tone and a decrease in propulsive peristalsis. This causes delayed gastric emptying and, almost inevitably, constipation. The regular co-administration of a stimulant laxative plus a stool softener is nearly always used in anticipation of the problem. *Dantron*, as *co-danthrusate* (*dantron* plus *docusate*) or *co-danthramer* (*dantron* plus *poloxamer '188'*), is probably the most effective agent. *Dantron* is specifically licensed in the UK only for the treatment of constipation in terminal care, but it has also been used for patients with cardiac failure or MI, to avoid cardiac stress due to bowel strain. The licence is restricted because studies in rats have indicated a potential carcinogenic risk. Products containing *dantron* may colour the urine red, and patients should be warned of this apparently alarming effect. *Dantron* may also cause a rash in the buttock area in incontinent patients, so it should

be reserved for use when other laxatives are ineffective.

The equivalent product in the USA is a combination of *casanthranol* (a natural anthracene) and *docusate* (dioctyl sodium sulphosuccinate). **Other smooth muscle effects.** *Morphine* also increases the tone in the sphincter of Oddi, which leads to increased pressure in the biliary system and occasional biliary colic. Other actions on smooth muscle include increased urethral tone, causing difficulties in micturition, and very rarely bronchoconstriction after large doses.

Respiratory depression

Morphine and other opioids can significantly depress respiration, and this is usually the cause of death from overdose. Respiratory rate, tidal volume and response to hypercapnia or hypoxaemia are all reduced. However, like many of its other side-effects, respiratory depression is not usually a limiting factor in patients who are experiencing severe pain, because pain is a potent arousal mechanism. Nevertheless, opioids must be used with great care in patients with advanced respiratory disease or otherwise depressed respiratory function. Opioid doses should be reduced if other procedures, e.g. nerve block (Figure 7.2 and p. 487) or radiotherapy, reduce pain successfully.

Effects on the eye

Stimulation of the oculomotor nerve causes constriction of the pupil, which is often a diagnostic aid in cases of *morphine* overdose and addiction. Thus, opioid analgesics are generally avoided in patients with head injury, because the opioid-induced pupillary changes, nausea and general CNS clouding may mask the signs induced by trauma and confuse the neurological examination.

Cardiovascular effects

The usual doses of opioid analgesics generally do not have major cardiovascular effects in patients with normal cardiac function. However, *morphine* may cause venous pooling and postural hypotension, through its venodilator action. The consequent reduction in cardiac preload (see Chapter 4) is an additional benefit to analgesia, and its euphoric action may help immediately following MI, to relieve severe anxiety.

Hypersensitivity

Occasionally, allergic-type reactions occur with opioid agents, and both local reactions at the site of injection and systemic allergic symptoms have been reported. If a patient is hypersensitive to *morphine*, both *codeine* and *diamorphine* (heroin) are also contra-indicated as they are structurally similar. However, *methadone* and *pethidine* (meperidine) are suitable alternatives, being chemically unrelated.

Dependence

Opioid analgesics can produce both physical and psychological dependence, although the latter appears to be a rare event when opioid analgesics are used to relieve pain. If a patient asks for increased dosages of analgesics because their pain has worsened or not been controlled, this should not be perceived automatically as drug-seeking behaviour or evidence of dependence. Physical dependence does occur, and can be managed by reducing the dose of opioid slowly when it is no longer needed for pain, rather than stopping abruptly, which causes unnecessary withdrawal symptoms.

Naloxone. Adequate doses of this antagonist will reverse completely all the actions of pure opioid agonists, so it is a complete antidote for both the actions and side-effects of *morphine*-like drugs. However, care should be taken when using *naloxone* to reverse opioid-induced respiratory depression, as patients who have been using opioid agents chronically are extremely sensitive to antagonists and too high a dose of *naloxone* can precipitate a withdrawal reaction and recurrence of severe pain. Further, it will not fully antagonize the action of partial agonist and agonist–antagonist drugs (see above).

Because the duration of action of *naloxone* is shorter than that of *morphine* and other opioids, repeated injections or IV infusion may be required. The *naloxone* dose varies widely, being dictated by the patient's condition and response. *Oxygen* and the respiratory stimulant *doxapram* (hospital use) may be needed to spare the *naloxone* dose and so maintain adequate analgesia.

Less potent analgesics

These are mainly used for the treatment of acute or chronic pain resulting from trauma, surgery and chronic systemic diseases such as arthritis. They include low-potency, centrally-acting *morphine*-like compounds ('weak opioids'), e.g. *codeine* and *dihydrocodeine*, and drugs that act on peripheral pain pathways, e.g. *aspirin*, salicylates and NSAIDs (see Chapter 12). *Paracetamol* (acetaminophen) also has central effects, but at different receptors from the opioids, and its toxicity is discussed in Chapter 3.

Weak opioids

These drugs have a ceiling to their analgesic effect, usually because of dose-limiting adverse reactions, and therefore have a limited efficacy relative to the strong opioids. Therefore combinations of these drugs with *paracetamol* (acetaminophen), provided that it is not contra-indicated (i.e. liver function is not compromised), or *aspirin* (if tolerated), may be expected to have an additive, possibly synergistic, analgesic effect. However, the BNF states that "Compound analgesics . . . . . . are commonly used, but the advantages have not been substantiated". Despite this, they are prescribed very widely. Their continuing popularity, with both patients and prescribers, may represent the triumph of experience over theoretical good practice.

Codeine is chemically related to *morphine* and is metabolized to *morphine* in the liver, so it shares its pharmacological actions. It is thought to have less abuse potential but is too constipating for long-term use.

Dihydrocodeine is mainly used for moderate pain. It has a flat dose–response curve, so there is no advantage in increasing the dose above that normally recommended: if analgesia with *dihydrocodeine* is inadequate, a change to a strong opioid is indicated.

Dextropropoxyphene (propoxyphene) resembles methadone structurally, and is less potent than *codeine*. There has been considerable controversy over its widespread use owing to serious problems if taken in overdose. In the UK, *dextropropoxyphene* has been used principally in combination with *paracetamol* (acetaminophen) as *co-proxamol*, which is unfortunately commonly used as a agent for suicide. It has been suggested that as little as 15–20 tablets of this combination can prove fatal, especially if alcohol is implicated. The main cause of death in overdose with *dextropropoxyphene* alone is respiratory depression, but in overdose with *co-proxamol* this is compounded with the hepatotoxicity of *paracetamol* (acetaminophen; see Chapter 3). Acute over-dosage with *co-proxamol* requires prompt administration of *naloxone*, to antagonize the *dextropropoxyphene*, resuscitation treatment and management of *paracetamol* overdose. If *naloxone* is not used, patients may die of cardiovascular collapse before reaching hospital.

Because of these serious toxic effects in overdose, and the fact that it is one of the most common suicide agents in the UK, *co-proxamol* is regarded as unsuitable for prescibing in the NHS and is being withdrawn from use in the UK.

Like other opioid analgesics, *dextropropoxyphene* can lead to dependence, the likelihood being about the same as with *codeine*.

Nefopam is structurally unrelated to the opioids and is sometimes useful when the pain has not responded to other analgesics. Its main advantage is that it does not cause respiratory depression, but its sympathomimetic and antimuscarinic side-effects, notably restlessness, dry mouth, urinary retention and, less often, blurred vision, tachycardia, insomnia, headache and confusion, may be troublesome. Thus, *nefopam* must be used with caution in the elderly and if there is evidence of renal or hepatic impairment, because it is extensively metabolized in the liver and largely excreted in the urine. Because of its adverse cardiovascular and CNS effects, *nefopam* is contra-indicated in MI and if the patient is liable to convulsions.

Non-steroidal anti-inflammatory drugs

NSAIDs appear to act peripherally at the pain receptor level, and so do not produce the physical dependence often associated with opioid analgesia. They are particularly useful in treating patients with chronic disease accompanied by both pain and inflammation, e.g. RA (see Chapter 12) and for the short-term treatment of mild to moderate acute pain, including musculoskeletal injuries and bone pain. Particular indications include the relief of pain accompanying dysmenorrhoea, and that associated with neoplastic bone metastases. In the latter case, combinations of an opioid with an NSAID are likely to be considerably more effective than an opioid alone.

The topical and other uses of NSAIDs are discussed in Chapter 12.

Analgesic adjuvants

These include three types of agent:

- Co-analgesics (secondary analgesics), for example an anticonvulsant, e.g. *clonazepam*, *gabapentin* or *pregabalin*, or a low-dose tricyclic antidepressant, e.g. *amitriptyline*.
- Other psychotropic agents, e.g. normal dose antidepressants, to treat the depression that frequently accompanies moderate to severe chronic pain.
- Corticosteroids, e.g. *dexamethasone*, to reduce oedema around a tumour and so prevent pressure on adjacent nerves or other tissues.

Other drugs that are used to prevent or treat the adverse effects of the primary analgesic, e.g. antiemetics or laxatives, are not discussed here.

Analgesic adjuvants tend to be used primarily in treating the chronic pain of neoplastic disease (Table 7.8). Their inclusion in a drug regimen may enhance pain relief, or it may be possible to reduce the dose of opioid, and consequently its side-effects. Other categories of drugs are also used, e.g. antispasmodics, neuroleptics and anxiolytics. The mechanisms by which these agents exert their effects are not clearly established, but are unrelated to the opioid receptor system.

First-generation antihistamines, e.g. *alimemazine*, *chlorphenamine* and *promethazine* are used primarily for their sedative properties and may also help to relieve nausea and skin irritation. However, many of these are markedly hypnotic, notably *alimemazine* and *promethazine*, and the latter has a long duration of action (about 12 h). Great care is needed when using the sedative antihistamines with other psychotropic drugs, especially opioids, because profound sedation may result. They also have marked antimuscarinic activity and may cause urinary retention, glaucoma and pyloroduodenal obstruction. Patients vary considerably in their response to antihistamines and children and the elderly are very susceptible to their side-effects.

Stabbing or shooting pains (**neuralgia**) caused by nerve inflammation or damage appear to respond particularly well to **anticonvulsant drugs**, which are thought to act by suppressing abnormal spontaneous activity in traumatized nerve fibres. *Carbamazepine* is generally the most successful agent, although side-effects can be troublesome, especially in the elderly. If *carbamazepine* is ineffective, it is worth trying *phenytoin* or another anticonvulsant before abandoning this line of treatment. Therapy should be initiated gradually, increasing the dose carefully until relief is obtained or unacceptable side-effects are encountered (see Chapter 6).

Tolerance to the side-effects of all adjuvants is improved by starting with low doses and titrating the dose slowly, especially in frail or elderly patients.

The best results with analgesic adjuvants are often obtained if they are introduced early on in the disease process, before **demyelination** (loss of the myelin sheath of nerves) has occurred. Demyelination may result from infiltration or sustained pressure by a tumour, producing nerve block, slowing of nerve conduction or nerve irritability and inflammation. It also makes nerves more liable to viral infection. The end result of these processes may be paraesthesias, partial paralysis, painful spasm, etc.

Damage to central or peripheral nerves, either as the prime cause of **neuropathic pain** (see above) or due to the secondary effects from a tumour is recognized by abnormal sensitivity in an area of autonomic, sensory or motor dysfunction.

Psychotropic drugs

Drugs from disparate therapeutic groups are used, and their modes of action in the treatment of pain is controversial. It is postulated that they block the re-uptake of certain neurotransmitters in the pain pathway, e.g. 5-HT and noradrenaline (norepinephrine), thus interfering with pain impulse transmission or its modulation. However, their pro-analgesic effect does not simply result from their psychotropic actions because they are effective at much lower doses, and act more rapidly, than in the treatment of depression (see Chapter 6). If depression needs to be treated, full antidepressant doses should be used. They may raise a pain threshold that had been lowered by the understandable anxiety and depression associated with chronic pain. Some studies have suggested that tricyclic antidepressants with an intact tertiary amine group (e.g. *amitriptyline* and *imipramine*) are the most effective. Antidepressants are thought to be most effective against the 'burning', deafferentation pain associated with sensory nerve damage, which is unresponsive to opioids.

The benefits of an antidepressant may be further increased by combination with a small dose of a neuroleptic drug, such as a butyrophenone (e.g. *haloperidol*) or a *phenothiazine* (most commonly *perphenazine*). However, these are rarely used in palliative care and such combinations should only be used by prescribers experienced in their use, because cardiac arrhythmias, postural hypotension, excessive sedation, dyskinesias (e.g. TD, p. 420), dystonias (abnormalities of muscle tone), myelosuppression and enhanced antimuscarinic side-effects may be a problem. Therefore neuroleptics are best avoided.

Anxiolytics. *Diazepam*, is especially useful because it has muscle relaxant properties in addition to its anxiolytic effect, and so is used frequently. If anxiety is not a problem and *diazepam* is too sedating, then **baclofen** is a suitable alternative for muscle spasm.

Cholecystokinin (CCK), the hormone involved in food digestion that is released by enteroendocrine cells in the gut (see Chapter 3), is also produced in the brain where it acts as a neurotransmitter involved in feelings of anxiety. It has recently been shown that CCK antagonists, e.g. *devazepide* and *proglumide*, reduce the sensation of anticipated pain. Although this points to a novel mode of analgesia, no product of this type has been marketed.

Glucocorticosteroids

These have a wide application in advanced neoplastic disease because they reduce the inflammatory swelling around tumours, and hence the pressure on nerves and in bones, thus alleviating the pain. These actions are additional to any growth-suppressant action on tumour cells, but the effect may be only temporary. Glucocorticoids also suppress the release of mediators such as histamine and kinins and are euphoric, thus raising the pain threshold. It is usual to start with a high dose to bring the symptoms under control and then reduce it as quickly as possible to the lowest effective dose, or to zero if the corticosteroid is ineffective (see also Chapters 5, 12 and 13). Slow dose reduction is not necessary if treatment has been less than 3 weeks.

Dexamethasone, and to a lesser extent *betamethasone*, lowers intracranial pressure in cerebral oedema and is especially useful for relieving the headache and associated symptoms. Low-dose corticosteroids (e.g. 2 mg *dexamethasone*) also improve mood and, possibly, appetite, but co-analgesia requires higher doses – about ten times that dose.

Anabolic steroids have been advocated to improve food utilization and increase muscle bulk and strength in patients with oesophageal, gastric and small bowel tumours who have problems with swallowing and nutrient absorption. An increase in muscle bulk would also reduce the discomfort of repeated injections. However, there is no good evidence for clinical benefit. Feeding by a nasogastric tube or percutaenous endoscopic gastrostomy (PEG), with a cannula giving direct access to the stomach to bypass swallowing problems, is preferred.

Cannabis and cannabinoids

The use of cannabis as monotherapy or as an adjunct to other analgesics is hotly debated because of its current rescheduling in the UK as a Class C Controlled Drug, to which special licensing conditions apply. Marijuana is the most widely used, or abused, psychoactive substance. It is regarded by most governments as having no therapeutic uses, although there are numerous anecdotal reports of its benefit, e.g. in relieving spasticity in multiple sclerosis. The UK Medicines and Healthcare Products Regulatory Agency (MHRA) has recently stated that it has "not objected to importing Sativex oromucosal spray for use in multiple sclerosis patients". Clearly, further research is needed, but this seems to imply that a UK licence is likely.

Only one cannabinoid, *nabilone*, is currently used in the UK, for the management of nausea and vomiting caused by cytotoxic chemotherapy uncontrolled by other drugs, and this has numerous side-effects.

The use of cannabis, especially at a young age, is a definite risk factor for the development of schizophrenia (see Chapter 6).

A major barrier to progress is that cannabis smoke contains more than 60 cannabinoids and no standardized product exists. One component, Δ-9-tetrahydrocannabinol (Δ-9-THC), seems largely to reproduce effects similar to smoking cannabis. However, it would be rash to assume that other cannabis components are not adjuncts or that they do not have potential value as co-analgesics. The precise effects of Δ-9-THC vary with the immediate environment, dose and route, and the psychological attributes of the user, similarly to alcohol.

Cannabinoid receptors are widely distributed in the brain. Why this is so, and the functions of endogenous ligands, are unknown but are of considerable interest.

Other methods of pain control

Local anaesthetics

Current agents are of two chemical types, depending on whether there is an ester or amide chain linking an aromatic lipophilic group, often a derivative of aniline or benzoic acid, to a secondary or tertiary amine residue. Table 7.8 lists those agents used most frequently.

Morphine has also been reported to be an effective local anaesthetic: low doses (1 mg in 20 mL of saline) injected into the knee joint after arthroscopy (unlicensed route) were found to be more effective than *bupivacaine* in preventing post-operative pain.

Table 7.8   Some pharmacokinetic properties of local anaesthetics

Anaesthetic	Onset of action[a]	Duration of action[b]
Ester type		
Benzocaine	T	+
Chloroprocaine	F	+
Cocaine[c]	F	++
Oxybuprocaine (benoxinate)[d]	F	+
Procaine[e]	F	+
Propoxycaine	F	++
Proxymetacaine (proparacaine)[d]	F	+
Tetracaine (amethocaine)	S	+++
Amide type		
Articaine[f]	–	–
Bupivacaine	S	+++
Cinchocaine (dibucaine)[c]	?	+++
Etidocaine	F	+++
Levobupivacaine	S	+++
Lidocaine (lignocaine)	F	++
Mepivacaine[f]	F	+++
Prilocaine	F	++
Ropivacaine	S	+++

[a] S/F, slow/fast onset; T, topical use only.

[b] +/++/+++, short/medium/long duration of effect. Formulation and the use of vasoconstrictors influences these parameters markedly. The action of prilocaine cannot be extended by vasoconstrictors.

[c] Used only in otorhinolaryngology and occasionally in ophthalmology.

[d] Relatively ineffective for topical use.

[e] Seldom used.

[f] Used in dentistry.

Mode of action

These agents depend on the ability of the lipophilic aromatic moiety of their molecules to dissolve in and attach to Na^+ channels and penetrate the lipoid nerve membrane. They prevent the large transient Na^+ flux across excitable nerve membranes by interacting directly with the intracellular components of voltage-gated sodium channels. The result is that the excitability threshold rises and nerve conduction slows and eventually fails. Although the drugs also bind to potassium channels and inhibit them at higher concentrations, this is not thought to contribute to their action.

The smaller the nerve fibre, the more sensitive it is to the action of these agents, so there is some selectivity at the concentrations used: they block transmission by small pain fibres but leave inhibitory (large) pain fibres, touch and movement relatively unimpaired.

Local anaesthetics also have important effects on calcium flux across cell membranes, so *lidocaine* (lignocaine) is the drug of choice for treating the ventricular arrhythmias that may accompany MI, heart surgery and digitalis intoxication. This effect also contributes to their systemic toxicity.

Use

Except for *procaine*, the penetration of local anaesthetic agents through ophthalmic and mucous membranes is greater than through the skin, permitting effective local anaesthesia in the eye, nostrils, throat, urethra and rectum. This property is used to facilitate the passage of endoscopes, catheters, etc. into body cavities and enables even relatively major operations (e.g. for cataract) to be carried out with minimal trauma as day-care procedures.

Local anaesthetics are not normally injected intravenously, except for the use of IV *lidocaine* (lignocaine) for treating ventricular tachycardias. However, IV regional anaesthesia (Bier's block) is used to anaesthetize a limb, intravascular spread being prevented by using a tourniquet. The use of local anaesthetics by IV infusion to produce general anaesthesia is hazardous and requires expert advice, so this route is rarely used. Regional anaesthesia can also be achieved by spinal use (see below).

Skin anaesthesia

This is difficult to achieve through intact skin, owing to poor penetration, though a *lidocaine–prilocaine* cream may be used under an occlusive dressing (to increase penetration) for 1 h before painful procedures. This is a eutectic mixture that has a low melting point and is an oil that is able to penetrate intact skin at normal temperatures. It has been used before injecting very nervous children.

A *tetracaine* gel can also be used similarly before venepuncture or venous cannulation. These must not be used on wounds, abrasions or inflamed skin because absorption may be rapid and extensive and lead to systemic side-effects.

Ophthalmic procedures

Oxybuprocaine and *tetracaine* are used extensively. Because *tetracaine* produces deeper anaesthesia, it can be used for minor surgery. *Proxymetacaine* and *lidocaine–fluorescein* eye drops are used for conventional tonometry (measuring the intraocular pressure by pressing a membrane against the cornea) as one of the procedures for diagnosing glaucoma. However, non-contact methods, e.g. firing a jet of compressed air at the cornea, are used increasingly. *Oxybuprocaine* has a similar activity to *tetracaine*, but is less irritant.

Otolaryngology

Lidocaine (lignocaine) is the preferred agent.

Nose, throat, eye and ear procedures are the only ones in which *cocaine* is still used. It is preferably avoided because of its powerful CNS stimulant action and potential for abuse. Because of its sympathomimetic effects, due to blocking of noradrenaline (norepinephrine) at synapses, *cocaine* should not normally be used with *adrenaline* (epinephrine) and similar drugs, but some surgeons believe that combination with *adrenaline* reduces *cocaine* absorption and is operatively beneficial. *Cocaine* rapidly produces effective surface analgesia that persists for at least 30 min, depending on the concentration used.

Spinal anaesthesia

Bupivacaine, *levobupivacaine* and *ropivacaine* are used to block nerve transmission at any point up to spinal cord level (see Figure 7.3), providing temporary pain relief. This topic is dealt with on p. 487. It is likely that *levobupivacaine* will replace *bupivacaine* because the L-isomer is the biologically active form and can be given at higher doses with fewer side-effects.

Prolongation and enhancement of effect

Prolongation and enhancement of local anaesthesia is usually done by combination with vasoconstrictors. Most local anaesthetics cause vasodilatation and so are often formulated with *adrenaline* (epinephrine), which produces local vasoconstriction and so prevents rapid distribution into the surrounding tissues and the circulation.

This effect prolongs the duration of action and potentiates the anaesthetic effect, owing to the increased local concentration of agent. Also, the reduced rate of systemic absorption enables drug metabolism to keep pace with administration, thus reducing the peak plasma level and so systemic toxicity. Peak plasma concentrations occur after about 10–25 min, so patients should be monitored carefully for 30 min after injection to ensure that no serious side-effects arise.

However, *adrenaline* (epinephrine) is contra-indicated if the anaesthetic is to be used in or near the fingers, toes or other appendages, because the intense vasoconstriction of their small blood vessels may result in ischaemic necrosis.

Felypressin, a synthetic derivative of the ADH *vasopressin*, may be a suitable alternative to *adrenaline* (epinephrine) and is used for dental procedures if the latter is contra-indicated in a particular patient. However, vasoconstrictors are themselves toxic and the same considerations apply as with *adrenaline*. Further, they must not

normally be used with *cocaine*, which has intrinsic vasoconstrictor and mydriatic properties. An alternative is to use a viscous vehicle, usually containing dextran 110, and this approach has been used to prolong the local action of *lidocaine* (lignocaine) for up to 10 h, though the effect is very variable.

Bupivacaine has a long duration of effect (up to 10 h), and may be useful if *adrenaline* or *felypressin* are contra-indicated. However, it has a slow onset of action (30 min), so *lidocaine* is usually used initially, followed by *bupivacaine* or *levobupivacaine*. The time of onset of action of *bupivacaine* depends on the concentration, dose and route used. It is used for peripheral nerve blocks and infiltration nerve blockade, and is the principal drug used for spinal anaesthesia in the UK (Figure 7.3). *Bupivacaine* is contra-indicated for use in IV regional anaesthesia, because of the risks of its long action, cardiovascular and central nervous toxicity, and because prolonged restriction of the blood supply would be required. Although *bupivacaine* is used widely for spinal obstetric anaesthesia, the concentration and circumstances of use in this setting require expert advice.

Side-effects of local anaesthetics

As usual, inflammation and trauma increase penetration markedly, so significant systemic absorption may then occur. On occasion, this may lead to toxicity, especially with *tetracaine* (amethocaine). This drug must never be used on mucous membranes, e.g. before bronchoscopy and cystoscopy: *lidocaine* is safer. The *lidocaine–prilocaine* cream used on the skin is irritant to the eyes and is ototoxic, and so should not be used on or near these organs.

Local anaesthetics are generally very safe, and adverse events are rare when they are used properly. However, apart from the use of the *lidocaine–prilocaine* cream and *tetracaine* gel mentioned above, they should generally be avoided for topical application to the skin because sensitization may occur. Systemic complications may also occur, usually when large doses are used to produce spinal nerve blocks. This is usually from accidental intravascular injection, which is particularly hazardous if injections contain *adrenaline* (epinephrine).

Hypersensitivity occurs occasionally: compounds of the same chemical type tend to give cross-reactions, but these do not occur between the ester and amide groups (Table 7.8).

Topical agents

Liniments and rubs have a long medical history and were once the only available treatments for localized joint and soft tissue damage. The active ingredients are mostly essential oil products, e.g. camphor, menthol, methyl salicylate, turpentine, sometimes with capsicum oleoresin or nicotinates.

More recently, several NSAIDs have been presented as gels or creams. These have the advantage that if only one or two joints are affected they can be applied to those localized areas. This avoids the need to take larger amounts of drug orally and some of the associated side-effects. Because of this, and possibly because patients are involved in the treatment, topical NSAIDs are popular. Although penetration of the drug into joints and soft tissues has been demonstrated, there is little localized effect and the therapeutic benefit is debatable.

The modes of action of most topical agents, apart from any specific NSAID activity, are alleged to be:

- Increased blood flow to the area, induced by the massage and vasodilatation.
- Counter-irritation, i.e. stimulation of C neurons inhibits local release of substance P and so attenuates the transmission of pain impulses. This mode of action has been demonstrated for capsaicin cream, which is used for the alleviation of osteoarthritis and pos-herpetic neuralgia (PHN; p. 505).

A 5% *lidocaine* (lignocaine) patch is licensed in the USA for the treatment of post-herpetic neuralgia and is occasionally imported into the UK on a named-patient basis.

Physical methods

Traction, to relieve pressure on spinal nerve roots (see Chapter 12), and manipulation and mobilization of muscles and joints are the traditional approaches of physiotherapy (PT), osteopathy (OT) and chiropractic, and are of undoubted value in some patients. PT also uses the application of heat (including short-wave diathermy), cold, ultrasound, electrical muscle stimulation and laser therapy. Ultrasound has been advocated for soft tissue injuries, PHN, facial neuritis and phantom limb pain, i.e. that apparently felt in an amputated limb.

Ice packs are widely used in the early treatment of soft tissue injuries, especially sport and similar traumas. The mnemonic 'RICE', i.e. Rest, Ice, Compression, Elevation, is used by first-aiders. Care is needed not to cause 'ice burns' by using a cloth between the skin and the cold pack.

Techniques recruiting endogenous inhibitory mechanisms

In addition to increasing the understanding of how conventional analgesics act, the gate theory has stimulated interest in alternative methods of pain relief. The emphasis has shifted from nerve destruction or blocking of pain conduction to the recruitment of the body's own inhibitory systems. This is the principle underlying the use of vibration, percussion, massage, and counter-irritation with rubefacients. The cooling produced by pain-relieving sprays may also stimulate pain trigger points (see below) or, if the cooling is sufficiently intense and prolonged, a degree of local anaesthesia may be produced. However, skin 'burns', or even frost-bite, must be avoided.

These techniques are not always successful, but they may provide acceptable pain relief to some patients with otherwise intractable conditions. Some authorities insist that these simple methods should be used first, and persevered with for several weeks, before either a maximum effect is achieved or the approach is abandoned.

Table 7.9   Modes of treatment using inhibitory pain mechanisms

Site of action	Treatment mode
Local	Acupuncture, stroking, rubbing, massage, vibration, percussion Counter-irritation, e.g. rubefacient creams containing nicotinates, salicylate esters, capsaicin etc. Reducing nerve conduction, e.g. pain-relieving sprays, ice packs Transcutaneous electrical nerve stimulation (TENS)
Central	Yoga, hypnosis, meditation, mental training (biofeedback)

Table 7.9 lists the principal alternative methods of pain control.

Neuromodulation by electrical stimulation

The most commonly used method in this category is **transcutaneous electrical nerve stimulation (TENS)**. This is normally used for the relief of chronic peripheral pain, though it has also been used to relieve acute pain, e.g. of operative incisions. Electrodes are placed over the painful area, or at the periphery of a very sensitive area, though the optimum placing needs to be found by careful trial by the patients themselves. Acupuncture sites are occasionally used (see below).

Patients wear a battery-driven pulse generator and vary the frequency, pulse width and power, normally to produce a pleasant non-painful tingling sensation. Patients usually know whether the method is going to be successful within 5–15 min. The pulse characteristics can be adjusted and the frequency of use may vary from three 1-h sessions daily upwards.

The conditions most likely to respond are postherpetic neuralgia, low back pain, phantom limb pain and post-operative scar pain. The mode of action is believed to be stimulation of the large, inhibitory A-beta nerve fibres, closing the pain gate in the dorsal horn of the spinal cord and reducing or abolishing upward transmission of the stimulus.

Invasive techniques have also been used occasionally. Electrodes connected to a miniature radio receiver have been implanted around peripheral nerves, near the posterior columns of the spinal cord, or even in the brain, and stimulated by a patient-controlled radio transmitter.

Although complications are rare, electrical neuromodulation is contra-indicated for psychoneurotic or emotionally unstable patients, and for opioid addicts. The most common problem is contact dermatitis from the electrodes.

Acupuncture

Therapeutic acupuncture, i.e. for the relief of chronic pain rather than as an operative anaesthetic, is used both by practitioners who follow the traditional Chinese system, with its over 300 sites for insertion of the needles, and some Western doctors, who may follow an empirical system. Needles are inserted to a precise depth and may be left in place for up to 30 min, or rotated, moved up and down, or electrically stimulated. Western practitioners sometimes insert the needles into sensitive trigger points, i.e. sensitive sites in muscles associated with fibromyalgia or myofascial pain that cause acute pain or muscular spasm when touched.

The mode of action is hotly disputed, but may involve interference with nerve depolarization, stimulation of inhibitory nerve fibres, release of endorphins, enkephalins or 5-HT, or hypnotic suggestion. The success of the treatment is certainly influenced profoundly by cultural and psychological factors. One estimate is that about 10% of patients are responders, a further 10% are non-responders, and the remainder experience varying degrees of benefit.

Chemical nerve blocks

Regional nerve blocks

These may be:

- **Field blocks**, i.e. SC injections at various sites around sensory nerves in the area of the procedure.
- **Peripheral blocks** involve a similar procedure, but the local anaesthetic is often injected around a nerve plexus, e.g. the **brachial plexus**, an intricate network of nerves emerging from the spinal cord at the base of the neck (between the lower cervical and uppermost thoracic vertebrae) which supply the whole arm, or the **lumbosacral plexus**, which supplies the lower back and limbs.
- **Central blocks** can be:
  - **Epidural** (extradural, peridural), outside the spinal cord between the dura mater and the inner wall of the vertebral canal.
  - **Caudal**, in the lumbar or sacral regions of the spinal cord, where it divides to form the cauda equina.
  - **Intrathecal** (subarachnoid), into the CSF between the pia mater and the arachnoid.

With intrathecal anaesthesia the level of the nerve block, and so the area and organs affected, depends on the position of the patient and the specific gravity (SG) of the anaesthetic solution. **Isobaric solutions** have the same SG as the CSF and exert their effect at the level of injection. **Hypobaric solutions** are lighter than CSF and act higher than the injection site, depending on the positioning of the patient. **Hyperbaric solutions** are heavier than CSF and flow towards the bottom of the spinal cord. They are used primarily for operations in the genital area and on the legs.

Central and other anaesthetic blocks

Local anaesthetics

These agents (see above) may be used to produce a **reversible block of afferent nerves** at any point up to spinal cord level (see Figure 7.3), including the local segment of the spinal cord. This provides temporary pain relief or anaesthesia for operations on patients in whom general anaesthesia is unsuitable, e.g. due to cardiac and respiratory problems or when central nervous sedation is undesirable. However, local anaesthetics also block other types of sensation and motor impulses, though usually to a lesser extent. The degree and extent of the anaesthetized area depends on the concentration and volume of solution injected.

Epidural (extradural) and intrathecal opioids are sometimes used for the relief of post-operative and chronic pain. Injections are usually given via a catheter located at the correct segment of the spinal cord. The effect is on the sensory, dorsal horn nerves. The release of substance P and other neurotransmitters from primary afferent nerves is inhibited by pre-synaptic opioid receptors, and effects on post-synaptic receptors reduce activity in ascending spinal tracts. However, conduction in motor and autonomic nerves is unaffected by opioids, so motor functions and blood pressure are generally not affected by the spinal use of opioids. The analgesia produced is normally insufficient for intra-operative pain so spinal opioids are used as adjuncts to general anaesthetics. Spinal *morphine* (often *diamorphine* in the UK) may provide 8–16 h of analgesia and can give months of low-dose analgesia in cancer patients without the side-effects of oral or other parenteral use. However, continuous infusions of *morphine* are safer and technically simpler and are widely used. *Alfentanil* infusions have also been used.

Such reversible nerve blocks are also used in diagnosis and to determine which nerves are involved in a particular pain process and the probable result of a **permanent nerve block**, because the production of the latter by nerve ablation with neurolytic agents can often be inaccurate and may not achieve the desired result. *Levobupivacaine* is used intrathecally for this purpose and is the agent of choice in the UK. The use of *morphine* with a low concentration of *bupivacaine* is synergistic.

Permanent nerve blocks

Once the correct site has been identified, an irreversible block produced by the injection of such agents as alcohol, phenol, chlorocresol or urethane may provide much longer-lasting relief. Unfortunately, this procedure may be too lengthy for patients who have severe intractable pain.

Alcohol produces total neurolysis, but the extent of blockage produced may be varied by using an appropriate concentration of a phenolic agent. These injections may be subarachnoid, extradural, subdural, autonomic or peripheral depending on the site of ablation that provides satisfactory relief. Surgery or heat (radiofrequency ablation) may also be used.

These are most useful in treating patients with well-defined localized pain. As expertise and knowledge increases, a wider range of destructive methods, peripheral, central or autonomic, is becoming available. Because the peripheral nerves are easily accessible, they are often chosen as sites for destruction, although nerve regeneration can occur with consequent return of the pain. Alternatively, the sensory root can be destroyed. This should theoretically result in permanent pain relief, as axonal regeneration should not occur if the nerve fibres are interrupted proximal to the sensory ganglion. Unfortunately, this is not always successful.

The procedures are potentially hazardous, and partial loss of sensation and function, thrombosis, spinal cord infarction, and even death have occurred: a skilled and experienced anaesthetist or neurosurgeon is required to conduct such procedures successfully. Because of these hazards, permanent nerve blocks are procedures of last resort.

Injection of alcohol has sometimes been used to destroy the pituitary gland, and so prevent hormone release, in patients who have widespread bilateral cancer pain, especially if the tumour is hormone-dependent. Because the alcohol spreads around the floor of the third ventricle and into its cavity, it is possible that part of the success of this technique is from direct hypothalamic injury. About 70% of patients benefit, more than half obtaining complete relief.

However, nerve blocks do not usually give complete pain relief, so adjuvant oral or parenteral opioids are usually still required, although it may be possible to use lower doses.

Neurosurgical approaches

The most common surgical procedures for pain relief are **cordotomy** (see below) and insertion of epidural, intrathecal and intraventricular catheters for opioid or local anaesthetic delivery directly to specific areas of the CNS. Subarachnoid catheter injection can sometimes be successful in cases where conventional opioid administration has failed to reach central opioid receptors.

Whereas drug therapy may not completely remove pain, an effective surgical nerve block can do so. The main problem is that it may not be possible to block the appropriate pathway without impairing other nerve pathways. It is usual to identify the nerve to be treated using low-power radiofrequency stimulation and to follow this with high-power pulses to ablate the nerve.

Cordotomy involves the interruption of the anterolateral quadrant of the spinal cord in the cervical or thoracic region. This may be done percutaneously using a diathermy probe, or sometimes by open surgery, and is most useful in treating unilateral pain below the shoulders. The method is used primarily in patients who have a limited life expectancy (about 2 years), because the development of alternative nerve pathways often allows pain to return after some time. Thus, cordotomy is used primarily in patients with advanced, irreversible disease and severe intractable pain, of whom over 80% obtain complete relief with such treatment.

Psychotherapy and hypnosis

The role of psychotherapeutic drugs has already been mentioned (see above). These behavioural approaches may be effective if there is no organic basis for the pain (i.e. it is psychogenic), if there is a minor cause but the pain is grossly aggravated by psychological factors and if anxiety and depression exacerbate pain significantly.

Meditation and **relaxation training** help patients divert their attention away from pain and facilitate their tolerance of it. **Hypnosis** sufficient to induce a light trance is a recognized form of treatment and some patients are able to self-hypnotize. It may relieve pain completely in the (highly suggestible) 20% of responders, and be a useful adjunct to other forms of treatment in many more. Hypnosis is unsuitable for patients with psychiatric illnesses who may be impossible to hypnotize or who behave in a bizarre fashion under hypnosis.

Biofeedback involves linking a patient to equipment that monitors and displays parameters such as heart rate or blood pressure (which are increased by pain) or muscle tension (which may cause pain). The patient is taught relaxation techniques and sees how this modifies their physiological responses and reduces their pain level; thus they learn to control their symptoms appropriately.

Syringe drivers and patient-controlled analgesia

Definition

This is a technique for continuous, regular or intermittent dosing with opioids, and occasionally with epidural local anaesthetics, according to the patient's perception of their own needs and pain severity. The method is used for controlling acute pain, e.g. post-operatively, following trauma and in burns patients.

The equipment usually comprises a microprocessor-driven syringe containing the drug solution, which is administered parenterally via a catheter. This may be done subcutaneously or intravenously, though the epidural route may also be used. When the patient experiences unacceptable pain, they press a button on the control unit and a predetermined dose of drug is administered.

Advantages

The advantages of PCA are:

- Patients are in control of their pain, not vice versa, and feel more secure. This alone improves the quality of analgesia obtained.
- The blood level is maintained more closely within the therapeutic range than can be achieved with injections given on demand. This should improve analgesia and minimize side-effects, but PCA has to be stopped sometimes due to severe nausea and other side-effects. Unacceptable side-effects may be due to overdosing by the patient (see below).
- Doses can readily be titrated to cope with wide variations in pain severity and patient needs.
- There is minimal delay between the perception of intolerable pain and obtaining a dose of analgesic. There is also less demand on nursing time and pharmacy provision.
- The system is very versatile and can sometimes be used in a domiciliary setting. However, some patients tend to overdose and a syringe driver delivering a SC opioid at a constant rate, which is not patient-controlled, may occasionally be used in palliative care.

Disadvantages and limitations

The following points are additional to those usually associated with opioid or local anaesthetic use:

- Highly trained staff are required to set up the equipment and supervise the patient.
- The method is only suitable for maintenance analgesia, not for dose titration. The patient's needs should be stable and established clearly, or readily estimated, and a suitable loading dose given before starting PCA.
- Some patients reject the technique.

- A patient's understanding of how to use the equipment may be limited by:
  - Extreme age.
  - Language or comprehension problems.
  - Sedation or confusion.
- Poorly controlled blood pressure may compromise perfusion of a SC injection site and the IV route has to be used.
- Changes in renal or hepatic function may cause significant variation in the plasma concentrations of drug, as for all routes of administration.

Modes of use

Two PCA arrangements are possible:

- Patient-controlled analgesia only.
- Continuous background infusion plus a patient-controlled bolus analgesic.

PCA only
This technique is best suited to acute analgesia. If excessive demand is made and the patient becomes sedated, this is a self-regulating situation, because the patient then makes less demand for analgesia until the sedation wears off.

Continuous background infusion plus PCA
This is particularly appropriate for chronic pain relief, e.g. severely burned patients, who often need opioids for long periods. It can be given as 30–50% of their predetermined hourly dose as a background infusion, the PCA function being used for breakthrough pain.

Continuous background infusion only
Strictly, this is not PCA, because there is no control by the patient. It is more useful in managing chronic pain, especially in patients who have stable analgesic needs. Further, they may be unable to manage the equipment correctly because they are confused or have little understanding of the equipment and the principles of use. It is less suitable for acute pain because of the inability to manage breakthrough pain, the risk of excessive sedation and other adverse reactions.

Technical and clinical aspects

Technical and clinical points include the following:

- The bolus dose delivered on demand in PCA must be adequate, but must not cause unacceptable side-effects.
- The time over which the dose is injected following patient triggering is adjusted according to the route used. Thus, for IM or IV injections the time may need to be lengthened to 5 min to avoid stinging or inadequate clearance from the site. Also the 'lock-out interval', i.e. the time after the end of a dose during which another bolus cannot be obtained, may need to be lengthened. Alternatively, the solution concentration may be increased so that a smaller volume is injected.
- The **lock-out interval** should be long enough to avoid adverse drug reactions. It is usually 5–8 min.
- The **maximum dose** allowed in a given period should be controlled, e.g. 30 mg *morphine* in 4 h.
- **Inadequate analgesia**. If usage is:
  - Two or less doses/hour, counsel the patient about fears of opioid use, etc. and advise more frequent use.
  - More than three bolus doses/hour, increase bolus concentration.
  - Review other possibilities, e.g. pain is not opioid-responsive or may be a new complication of the disease and/or surgery.
- **Nausea and vomiting:**
  - Use anti-emetics (see Chapter 3, p. 107), e.g. rectal *prochlorperazine* or a 5-HT$_3$ antagonist. Transdermal *hyoscine* (scopolamine) may be used occasionally in patients under 60 years if injections are undesirable. This is not suitable in the elderly because it may cause urinary retention and confusion.
  - Decrease bolus volume or increase the duration of delivery of each bolus, to give lower peak plasma concentrations.
  - Change the route, for example to IM, or possibly the opioid.
- **Urinary retention:** relieve with indwelling or intermittent catheterization.
- **Pruritus:** this is not usually a problem with

IV PCA, but may be with spinal or epidural dosing.
- Change the route or opioid.
- Use a non-sedating antihistamine.

- Use low-dose *naloxone* if the pruritis is intractable, but care is required because the analgesia may be reversed if the *naloxone* dose is too large.

Some common pain situations

The application of the principles discussed above is illustrated by discussing the management of some common pain situations.

Headache, migraine and facial pain

Epidemiology and aetiology

Headache is probably the most common of all the pain syndromes, and about 80–90% of the population have at least one headache each year. Of these, about 15% experience recurrent episodes of all kinds that interfere with their normal daily activities, and it is estimated that headaches cause an annual loss of about 70 million working days in the UK.

Peak GP consulting rates occur in the 10- to 40-year age group, the female : male ratio being about 2.5 : 1 overall. The principal causes of chronic daily headache are given in Table 7.10. There are estimated to be over 5 million migraine sufferers in the UK, though at least half have mild to moderate pain and do not consult their doctors. Pure tension-type headache is an unusual cause for a visit to a GP.

Analgesic abuse is an important cause of headache, recognition of which requires a high index of suspicion.

Table 7.10   Causes of headache by age

Occurrence	Children and teenagers	Adults	Elderly
Common	–	Tension headache Migraine	Temporal arteritis, polymyalgia rheumatica[a] Cervical spondylosis
Less common	Tension headache Migraine	Trauma Subdural and subarachnoid haemorrhage Analgesic abuse	Glaucoma Paget's disease
Uncommon	Tumours Subdural and subarachnoid haemorrhage	Glaucoma Paget's disease Cervical origin Tumours	Tension headache (first onset) Migraine (first onset) Trauma Subdural and subarachnoid haemorrhage Tumours

[a] See Chapter 12.

The main concern of pharmacists when a client requests advice is to distinguish between benign headaches and those requiring medical intervention (Table 7.11). Headache accompanied by the following features requires referral to the patient's GP.

- New pain of sudden onset, especially in those aged 60 or over.
- A marked change in the character or timing of recurrent headaches.
- Fever
- Neck stiffness.
- Impairment of cognition, motor function or vision lasting for more than 24 hours, e.g.
  - Understanding or reasoning.
  - Abnormality of gait, posture or writing.
  - Limb weakness or clumsiness.

- Eye problems, e.g. flashing lights, jagged lines, blurred vision, loss of part of the visual field (scotoma).
- Disturbance lasting <24 h is defined as a **transient ischaemic attack (TIA;** see Chapter 4) and still requires referral, especially in those already taking low-dose *aspirin.*
- Sensitivity to touch in the area of the pain (may be temporal arteritis; see Chapter 12).
- A family history of migraine.

Classification

The International Headache Society has issued modified guidelines for classifying chronic daily headache (Table 7.11). Despite this formidable

---

Table 7.11   A partial classification of chronic daily headache[a]*

Primary headache for <4 h daily
- Chronic cluster headache (patients may have >4 h headache a day, but individual attacks are usually of <4 h duration)[b]
- Chronic paroxysmal hemicrania (rare)
- Short-lasting unilateral neuralgia-like attacks with conjunctival injection and copious tear production (SUNCT)
- Headache associated with sleep

Primary headache for >4 hours daily
- Chronic migraine[b]
- Chronic tension-type headache[b]
- New daily persistent headache

Secondary headache[c]
- Head injury
- Inflammatory
  - Giant cell arteritis, polymyalgia rheumatica (see Chapter 12)
  - Sarcoidosis
  - Behçet's syndrome (see Chapter 2)
  - Non-vascular intracranial disorder, e.g. chronic CNS infection
  - Post-non-cephalic infection
- Iatrogenic, medication over-use, substances or their withdrawal
- Intracranial vascular disorders, e.g. intracranial aneurysm
- Benign intracranial hypertension

---

* This is defined as headache on 15 or more days a month due to a range of underlying mechanisms and may be complicated by, or caused by, excessive analgesic use.

[a] Based on the classification of the International Headache Society (2004) *Cephalalgia* **24** (Suppl. 1): 1–160. This includes migraine without aura.

[b] See text.

[c] This list is not exhaustive.

CNS, central nervous system.

list, most headaches are benign. Only the four most common types are discussed below, the pain patterns associated with these and other types being illustrated in Figure 7.5.

Tension-type headache

Clinical features

This common form of headache may arise from sustained muscle contraction in the cervical (neck) region or scalp, or be psychogenic in origin (e.g. caused by stress or depression). Headaches may be episodic, i.e. occurring on less than 15 days/month and having no persistent symptoms. However, they are often chronic, e.g. on more than 15 days/month for more than 6 months, present at similar times each day, every morning or evening, or on the same days each week (Table 7.12). The pain is:

- Mild to moderate.
- Typically has a bilateral 'hatband' or more generalized distribution (Figure 7.5(a)).
- Non-throbbing, no burning or pressure sensations.
- Not aggravated by head movement.

There are few abnormal signs, but the scalp and neck muscles may be tender. Bilateral pain, absence of vomiting and tendency to be chronic distinguish it from migraine (see Table 7.12), which is episodic by definition.

Management and pharmacotherapy

Treatment of this condition is often unsatisfactory because no specific pathology can be identified and it may be difficult or impossible to modify employment, social and personality trigger factors. Management and symptomatic treatment involve:

- Possible extensive investigations to eliminate serious pathology (e.g. cerebral abscess or cancer, stroke), to reassure the patient.
- Avoidance of any identifiable causes, if possible.
- Physical and psychological treatments may help, e.g. relaxation therapy, psychotherapy, hypnotherapy, ice packs or cervical manipula-

tion (provided that this has been confirmed as a safe procedure in that patient).
- **Analgesics** appropriate to severity, e.g. *paracetamol* (acetaminophen), *aspirin* (in the over-16s, if tolerated) or combinations of these with *codeine* or *dihydrocodeine*, but these may be abused. Combinations with *dextropropoxyphene* are no longer used in the UK.
- **NSAIDs**. *Diclofenac, ibuprofen* and *naproxen*, sometimes *flurbiprofen* or *tolfenamic acid* (unlicensed indication).
- **Antidepressants** (see Chapter 6) if indicated. Low-dose *amitriptyline*, 10–25 mg nightly, increasing up to 75 mg daily if required is widely used (unlicensed indication). Anxiolytics are undesirable because they may lead to habituation. Treatment is more effective if patients present soon after the onset of symptoms. Antidepressants are withdrawn gradually after about 6 months' sustained improvement.
- It has recently been shown that performing a brain scan in people who suffer chronic daily headache relieved anxiety in the short term and reduced the use of medical resources significantly, with an associated reduction in costs.

Analgesic abuse headache

This may accompany any other form of headache. Because it occurs daily it is frequently associated with tension headaches. The normal pattern is that a patient complaining of headache will manage well initially by self-medicating with simple analgesics as the need arises. There may then be a progression to regular daily simple analgesic use, seeking advice for 'something stronger', consulting their doctor and regular use of a compound analgesic (e.g. *co-codamol* or *co-dydramol* in the UK), even a potent opioid, without obtaining satisfactory relief. This adds the side-effects of the analgesic, i.e. any of the side-effects of opioids (see above), to the effects of the headache. Misuse of antimigraine drugs can cause similar problems. Opioids should not be required in tension-type headache.

The correct course of action is to stop the daily analgesic medication. This may cause rebound

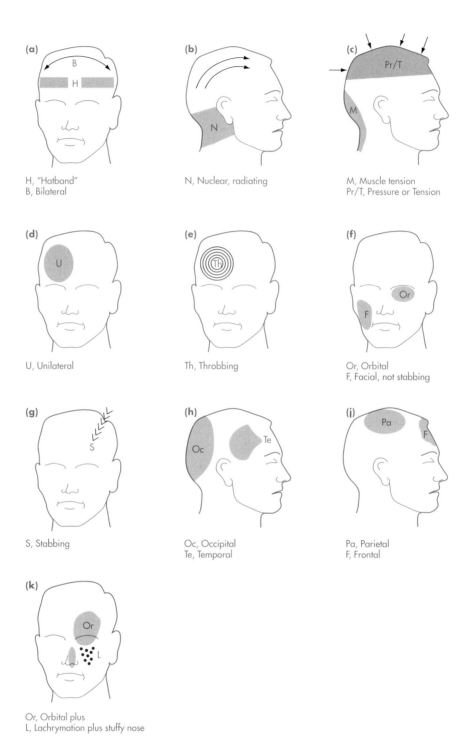

Figure 7.5 Patterns of pain in headache. (a–c) Tension headache; (d–j) migraine; (g) also neuralgia; (k) cluster headache.

exacerbation of headache for 1–2 weeks and withdrawal symptoms may need to be treated with anti-emetics and sedatives. Cognitive therapy (see Chapter 6) usually helps, but failure to improve subsequently should prompt a neurological or psychiatric investigation.

Migraine

Definitions

The International Headache Society has developed the following criteria (ICHD-II; 2004) with the intention of simplifying the diagnosis of migraine and defining those patients who are likely to respond to different treatments. The character of the headache should not be explicable by possible CNS damage. Two main types of migraine are defined:

- **Migraine without aura** (common migraine). Repeated headache attacks, lasting for 4–72 h, with the following features: recurrent moderate to severe, throbbing headache, usually unilateral but sometimes bilateral, accompanied by intolerance of light or noise, nausea, and sometimes vomiting. The pain should comply with at least **two** of:
(a) Normal physical examination.
(b) No other reasonable cause for the headache.
(c) At least two of:
    - Unilateral pain.
    - Throbbing pain.
    - Aggravation of pain with head movement.
    - Moderate to severe intensity of pain.
(d) At least one of:
    - Nausea or vomiting.
    - Photophobia and sonophobia.

Table 7.12   Features of migraine and tension-type headache

Features	Migraine	Tension-type headache
Pain	Throbbing Unilateral Worsens on head movement	Boring or pressure Bilateral No effect of head movement
Associated features	Nausea ± vomiting Photophobia + sonophobia	None or depression
Trigger factors	Too little or too much sleep Change in stress level – too much or relaxation, depression Excess external stimuli, e.g. bright or flashing lights, e.g. TV and monitor screen flicker Hunger Weather change Fatigue Menstruation Chemical • Iatrogenic, e.g. GTN, oral contraceptives • Delayed headache after alcohol • Foods, e.g. cheese, beans, onions, oranges, tea, coffee, chocolate, Chinese meals • Hormonal, e.g. menstruation, puberty, menopause • Neck pain, tooth grinding • Smoking, olfactory stimuli	Psychological stress

GTN, glyceryl trinitrate.

- **Migraine with aura** (classical migraine). Two or more headache attacks that comply with **three** of the following characteristics:
  - (e) One or more fully reversible aura symptoms indicating cerebral cortical or brainstem dysfunction.
  - (f) At least one aura symptom developing over more than 4 min, or two or more symptoms occurring in succession.
  - (g) No aura symptom should last for more than 1 h.
  - (h) Headache follows aura with a pain-free interval of less than 1 h.

'Borderline migraine' is often diagnosed when one of the criteria is not met.

The pain scale for migraine (migraine index) is a product of duration and intensity, where intensity is graded from 0 (none) to 3 (severe). The aura consists of warning of an impending attack, usually with visual symptoms, but auditory, smell and motor limb disturbances may also occur, lasting 4–60 min (see below). The headache usually follows within 60 min, or may accompany these symptoms.

Epidemiology

For epidemiological purposes, migraine patients (**migraineurs**) are defined as having had at least five attacks without aura, or two with aura.

Migraine is common worldwide, reported variously as affecting 5–25% of women and 2–20% of men. This spread is due to different definitions and trial methods. The highest incidence of migraine without aura is at 10–11 years of age in males and 14–17 years in females. That of migraine with aura is at about 5 years in males and about 12–13 years in females. There is then a slow increase in prevalence in women up to age 40 years, but the prevalence of all forms declines after the age of 45–50. Onset after age 60 of an exceptionally severe headache unlike any in a patient's previous experience is very unusual: this should raise the possibility of significant pathology, e.g. subarachnoid haemorrhage or temporal arteritis (see Chapter 12). There is a genetic predisposition in some patients, but no simple Mendelian inheritance.

Some 10% of the population are 'active migraineurs', 5% have 18 or more migraine days annually; 1% have one each day or week. The average duration of an attack is about 24 h, but may be 2–3 days in 20% of patients.

Aetiology and pathology

The aetiology has yet to be elucidated in humans. The traditional view that symptoms are simply the result of alterations in cerebral blood flow is probably incorrect. The haemodynamic changes observed during all phases of the attack cannot alone account for the symptoms. Rather, the vascular changes reflect cranial disturbance, e.g. vasodilatation of cranial or meningeal blood vessels, or oedema.

The anatomy of the cerebral circulation is complex with a high degree of redundancy, probably because:

- There is an absolute requirement for a continuous supply of glucose and oxygen.
- The brain is highly active metabolically, consuming about 20% of total blood oxygen at rest.
- Even a brief interruption of the blood supply may cause unconsciousness; 1–2 min deprivation impairs brain cell activity and 4–5 min causes permanent damage.

There is a complete circle of interconnecting arteries at the base of the brain (the circle of Willis), derived from the four main ascending arteries, two vertebral, two internal carotid. This minimizes the risk of ischaemia, e.g. due to a small clot, because the circle can be supplied by any of its ascending arteries. The cerebral veins have no valves, have very thin walls, and no muscle layer. Thus they cannot be causal in migraine but can account for the pounding nature of the headache, reflecting systolic heartbeats. There are also large venous sinuses that drain pooled venous blood from the brain and skull. Numerous anastomoses connect the arterial circle and this venous system.

There are several **pathophysiological theories** of migraine symptomatology, reflecting current uncertainties. Migraineurs probably have a genetically determined, or congenital, reduced CNS excitation threshold, i.e. they fall into an intermediate group between epilepsy and normality, but a genetic origin for this has not been demonstrated. However, mutations have been identified in genes for the voltage-gated calcium and sodium channels and for the alpha$_2$ subunit of the Na^+/K^+ pump in some types of familial migraine.

Thus the concept that vascular changes may account for the **prodrome** (see below), and that the subsequent headache is caused by vasodilatation is no longer tenable. However, opening of arteriovenous anastomoses may be expected to expose the cerebral veins to arterial pressures for which they are not designed, and this could explain the pounding nature of the headache, because the thin-walled veins would be exposed to the systolic pressure with every heartbeat. They would then expand, putting pressure on the brain, and relax during diastole. Further, it is known that stimulation of cranial nerves, especially the trigeminal, causes neurogenic plasma extravasation in the dura mater and the release of pro-inflammatory mediators.

Dilatation of the carotid arterial circulation causes stretching of arterial walls and so thickening of the meninges, producing pain.

Serotonin (5-HT), released by vascular nerves or platelets, is clearly implicated in the pathogenesis of migraine. The recent advances in treatment have been derived from the observation that injection of 5-HT can abort migraine attacks, but causes substantial side-effects. Additionally, the introduction of an NSAID that is a potent inhibitor of PG and LT B$_4$ synthesis has also focused attention on the pathogenetic role of these eicosanoids. Nitric oxide is also implicated in CNS vasodilatation.

Clinical features

Different patterns occur in individual sufferers, ranging from occasional headaches that are almost indistinguishable from tension headache to frequent disabling episodes (Figure 7.4(d–j)).

Symptoms may mimic those of TIAs (which resemble a stroke, but the patient recovers within 24 h) and are clearly associated with cerebral ischaemia. There may be dizziness or partial or complete blindness (**basilar migraine**), partial or complete hemiparesis (one-sided paralysis, **familial hemiplegic migraine**), and paralysis of the eye muscles (**ophthalmoplegic migraine**) or facial muscles. It is important to distinguish these symptoms, which arise gradually, from those of thromboembolic TIAs, which are usually of sudden onset, because both treatment and prognosis are very different for the two conditions. These atypical migraines are uncommon but are important because they are associated with ischaemia; the 5-HT$_1$ agonists, because they are potent vasoconstrictors, are contra-indicated for their treatment. These forms of migraine are now believed to be due to genetically determined abnormalities of the cerebral calcium channels and will not be discussed further here. However, the possibility is raised that this is the inherited basis of some forms of migraine.

Migraine is known to be associated with an increased risk of ischaemic stroke, and a large European study has found that this risk is increased threefold in young women with migraine. Up to 40% of strokes in this study developed from a migraine attack, and factors such as oral contraceptive use, hypertension and smoking further increased the risk.

Common migraine

This is the usual form of migraine, affecting about 75% of sufferers. The symptoms resemble those of classical migraine, but tend to comprise only headache, malaise and nausea. Occasionally, aura occurs without other symptoms. There may be considerable difficulty in distinguishing between common migraine and tension headache. Both syndromes are very common and so may be concurrent, or tension headache may exacerbate common migraine at some stage.

Migraine with aura

Triggers for attacks are listed in Table 7.12. There may be three distinct phases to an attack:

- Feelings of well-being, yawning, food rejections or cravings, etc., which may last for up to 24 h (the prodrome).
- These are followed by an aura; and
- Finally the headache and associated features occur (Table 7.13).

The aura develops over 5–20 min and lasts for 4–60 min. The aura is usually visual, including spots (**scotomas**), blurred vision, flashing lights and jagged lines. 'Pins and needles', facial tingling, speech difficulties and unusual smells may also occur, and there may be nausea.

This is followed by a severe throbbing headache that may start unilaterally and be localized, but may later become more general. Nausea increases and vomiting usually follows. Sufferers are irritable, photophobic and sonophobic and usually retreat to a dark, quiet bedroom. The attack lasts from hours to days and often terminates with sleep, often followed by a longish, variable pain-free period. Because attacks are associated with smooth muscle inhibition there is often urinary retention followed by a delayed diuresis towards the end of an attack.

Investigation

A typical history and a normal neurological examination are usually conclusive. The presence of atypical features should prompt further examination to exclude meningitis, subarachnoid haemorrhage, TIAs, partial epilepsy, stroke, a brain tumour or other serious pathology. Patients are normal between attacks.

The possible involvement of all of the factors listed in Table 7.12 should be assessed, possibly with a patient diary.

Management

Apart from the mildest form of common migraine, this requires pharmacotherapy, but some general measures are important, as follows:

- Effective identification and treatment of any associated diseases.
- Counselling:
  - For identification and avoidance of possible trigger factors (Table 7.12), especially changing or stopping a combined oral contraceptive in young women.
  - Strong reassurance that the condition is benign, because many patients think that they have a brain tumour or are going 'mad'.
  - The importance of prompt treatment at the first sign of an impending attack.
  - Rest, usually in a quiet, darkened room.

The principles of treatment of are outlined in Table 7.13.

Table 7.13   A stepped approach to migraine management[a]

Step	Clinical features	Pharmacotherapy[a]
Step 1 (mild migraine)	Occasional mild symptoms Minimal interference with lifestyle	Simple analgesics, compound analgesics or NSAID Anti-emetic if required
Step 2 (moderate migraine)	Moderate to severe throbbing headaches, one attack a month or less Significant nausea ± vomiting Interferes with lifestyle, e.g. attacks last 2–3 days, quiet rest essential	Compound analgesics Anti-emetic Tolfenamic acid or 5-HT$_1$ agonist (second-line drugs if these are ineffective[a])
Step 3 (severe and/or frequent migraine)	More than one severe attack a month Severe nausea ± vomiting Significant interference with lifestyle, e.g. frequent time off work, often unable to carry out tasks of normal living	Treat acute attacks as Step 2 Prophylactic pharmacotherapy[a]

[a] See text.

5-HT$_1$, 5-hydroxytryptamine$_1$ receptors.

Acute attacks

General considerations

Gastric stasis and generally poor gut peristalsis develops during an attack, so drug absorption from the gut may be compromized with all drugs in migraine, especially with conventional tablets and capsules. Absorption is improved by using effervescent oral formulations and by using an anti-emetic and prokinetic drug, e.g. *metoclopramide* or *domperidone*, 30 min before an analgesic if possible, or simultaneously. Routes of administration that avoid first-pass metabolism, e.g. buccal dosage forms (sublingual tablets and oral aerosols), nasal sprays and injections, are pharmacokinetically preferable, because many of the drugs used undergo extensive first-pass metabolism. Suppositories are useful if the patient is nauseated and vomiting. Patient dislike of suppositories and repeated injections may be outweighed by the rapidity and extent of benefit derived from a product.

It may take experimentation over a few attacks to establish the optimum drug, dosage and route of administration. Patients do not always require the same treatment: mild attacks may respond to simple analgesics, while severe ones in the same patient may require specific treatment. The relative responses to different drugs may be different in different attacks, but the response to specific treatment seems to be more consistent than that to simple analgesics.

Opioid analgesics should be avoided, because they are ineffective, exacerbate nausea and vomiting and, if taken regularly for attacks, may cause analgesic overuse headache.

Drugs should not be used during the aura, which is unresponsive to treatment and may not always be followed by headache. However, if it is known that headache always supervenes, simple analgesics should be taken before the headache is established.

Specific anti-migraine drugs, the 5-HT$_1$ agonists (triptans), should be reserved for established headache, on grounds of toxicity, in patients who find simple analgesics and anti-emetics ineffective. Although all triptans are effective, the response varies between patients, as do the incidence and severity of side-effects.

Headache recurrence following response to treatment limits the benefits of treatment significantly, not least because patients may regard it as treatment failure. Recurrence occurs in about 35% of responders, for unknown reasons.

The 'therapeutic gain' (TG) is the response rate to treatment minus the response to placebo or comparator, and is used below. However, trial results are difficult to compare due to different end-points, time of measurement of the response, use of 'escape medication' and comparison in only one attack or over several attacks.

There are two approaches to management: the traditional **stepped-care model** (ladder), i.e. simple analgesic to compound analgesic to a triptan (see below) or *ergotamine*, or to decide on the appropriate treatment for a particular patient depending on their symptoms, the **stratified-care model**. The latter is gaining ground with the introduction of the triptans, which are effective and less toxic than *ergotamine*.

Simple and compound analgesics

These have been discussed above and in Chapter 12. Adequate doses should be used, i.e. *aspirin* 600–900 mg every 4–6 h, provided that it is tolerated and not contra-indicated, or *paracetamol* (acetaminophen) 1000 mg every 4–6 h (to a maximum of 4 g daily). Effervescent *aspirin* is preferred and is sometimes as effective as *sumatriptan*.

Non-steroidal anti-inflammatory drugs

Tolfenamic acid is an NSAID that is specifically licensed for the treatment of acute migraine attacks. It has the general properties and side-effects of NSAIDs and may also cause dysuria (mostly in men), tremor, euphoria and fatigue, but it seems to be well tolerated. *Tolfenamic acid* is reported to be as effective as the 5-HT$_1$ agonists and is formulated as a tablet that disintegrates rapidly and has good bioavailability. Other NSAIDs that are licensed for migraine treatment are *ibuprofen* (1.2–1.8 g daily in divided doses), *diclofenac*, *flurbiprofen* and *naproxen*, at equivalent dosage. *Flurbiprofen* and *diclofenac* are also available as suppositories, which are useful if the patient is vomiting.

Serotonin agonists (5-HT$_1$ agonists, 'triptans')

All of these are effective in relieving migraine headaches, but they are not suitable for prophylaxis. Unlike simple analgesics and NSAIDs, there is evidence that they are most effective when used at the first signs of the headache and not during the aura.

The $5\text{-HT}_{1B/1D}$-receptor agonists licensed in the UK are *sumatriptan* and the newer *almotriptan*, *eletriptan*, *frovatriptan*, *naratriptan*, *rizatriptan* and *zolmitriptan*. These drugs act highly selectively on specific subsets of 5-HT_1 receptors, 5-HT_{1D} and, to a lesser extent, 5-HT_{1B}. They have a much lower affinity for other 5-HT_1 receptors and are inactive at 5-HT_2, 5-HT_3, adrenergic, dopaminergic, muscarinic and benzodiazepine receptors.

The role of 5-HT_{1D} and 5-HT_{1B} receptors is uncertain. They are believed to be pre-synaptic 'autoreceptors' that control the release of neurotransmitters at the nerve terminal.

Because of their vasoconstrictor action, 5-HT_1 agonists are likely to aggravate any condition caused by arterial blockage, spasm or inflammation and are contra-indicated in such situations, e.g. IHD, previous MI, atypical angina, uncontrolled or severe hypertension and intermittent claudication (see Chapter 4), temporal arteritis and Raynaud's disease (see Chapter 12).

Non-responders. *Zolmitriptan* is the only antimigraine drug that can be repeated for the same attack by those who fail to respond to a first dose; this should be not less than 2 h after the first dose. For all other triptans non-responders should not repeat the dose. This also minimizes the risk of analgesic-induced headache. Non-responders will not gain any benefit from a second dose of the same or any other triptan, because this will increase or prolong vasoconstriction and the risk of ischaemia and thromboembolic stroke, without relieving the migraine. Further, the maximum dose of all triptans that may be used within 24 h is limited.

However, the same drug, given by a different route or in a higher dose, may be successful in another attack. Non-responders are more likely to benefit from a change to a different drug class. If a small dose has proved to be inadequate, a larger dose may help in a subsequent attack.

Partial responders. If an attack responds to a first dose only one repeat dose of a triptan should be used for the same attack if there is inadequate relief or in those in whom the headache remits and recurs. The precise details vary with the drug and dosage form: the BNF and patient information leaflets should be consulted.

Although more expensive than previous treatments, the cost–benefit ratio for triptans is probably no worse than for older drugs. There is less time off work and a better quality of life.

Sumatriptan is poorly absorbed from the tablets (14% bioavailability), taking 2 h to reach a peak plasma concentration which is 75% of that obtained by SC injection. The latter is the preferred mode of use, which avoids first-pass metabolism. An autoinjector device has been produced (peak plasma concentration at 12 min, 97% bioavailability; TG in 51% of patients initially, 71% at 1 h).

The oral route is not suitable if there is nausea and vomiting, and it clearly gives slower relief than the injection. However, some patients who do not wish to inject find it adequately effective (TG 33%, 58% of patients, 100-mg dose). Alternatively, a nasal spray is available for those not wishing to inject or who are vomiting and gives rapid absorption, but the peak plasma concentration (at 1–1.5 h) is only about 20% of that from the injection, partly due to pre-systemic metabolism. Some patients find the nasal spray inconvenient and irritant: it is also expensive. The terminal elimination half-life is about 2 h.

Sumatriptan may also help in the management of cluster headache (see below).

Side-effects include drowsiness, a transient increase or reduction in blood pressure, bradycardia or tachycardia and, occasionally, fits. However, these side-effects are usually mild and fairly brief. Caution is required in renal impairment and, following reports of chest pain and coronary vasoconstriction, they are contraindicated in patients with ischaemic syndromes (see above).

Interactions. Because of the similar modes of action, *sumatriptan* must not be used with *ergotamine*: nor within 24 h of stopping *ergotamine*, which must not be used within 6 h of taking *sumatriptan*. Use with MAOIs, SSRIs and *lithium* increases the risk of CNS toxicity, and use of *sumatriptan* with these must be avoided.

Second-generation triptans have better bioavailability, greater potency at active receptor sites and longer half-lives than *sumatriptan*. Because they are more lipophilic, CNS penetration is also improved and they reduce neuroexcitability, especially in the trigeminal ganglion.

Naratriptan is similarly effective to *sumatriptan*, and is available as tablets. Used at the lower dose (2.5 mg) it may have fewer side-effects than *sumatriptan* and has similar interactions, but the TG is also lower. At the higher dose (5 mg) it resembles *sumatriptan*. Because it has a longer duration of action it may be useful in patients who regularly suffer from relapses.

Zolmitriptan is another recent introduction in tablet form, designed to be a potent 5-HT$_1$ partial agonist and more lipophilic than *sumatriptan*, giving better CNS penetration. It has a slightly higher TG than *sumatriptan* but a higher incidence of adverse reactions. It is also available as orodispersible tablets and as a nasal spray. It is not clear whether the orodispersible tablets are superior to normal ones and are clearly unsuitable if they cause a dry mouth.

Rizatriptan is available as tablets and 'melt' wafers that are dissolved on the tongue and swallowed. It is consistently effective and well tolerated, and is cost-effective. *Rizatriptan* metabolism is reduced by *propranolol*. Patients taking *propranolol* must not take *rizatriptan* within 2 h of a dose of *propranolol* and should take only the minimum dose of *rizatriptan*.

Frovatriptan has the longest half-life of the 5-HT$_1$ agonists and may be particularly useful in menstrual migraine. It is somewhat less effective, and cheaper, than other triptans.

Possible side-effects with all these agents include drowsiness and transient hypertension; dry mouth, unpleasant sensations in any part of the body, and muscle pain and weakness may also occur. Absolute contra-indications for this entire group are given above.

Arrhythmias due to accessory cardiac conduction pathways are an additional contra-indication for *zolmitriptan*. It is also contra-indicated in those who have had a TIA or a stroke.

There is inadequate information on their use in the elderly.

Second-line drugs

These include *ergotamine* and *isometheptene mucate*. Low cost has ensured the continued use of *ergotamine*, despite its complex actions and long list of side-effects. The BNF states that both of these are "less suitable for prescribing", and their use is declining.

Ergotamine tartrate is the oldest antimigraine drug, with ergot preparations having been in use for at least 2000 years. The isolation and pharmacological characterization of the ergot alkaloids in the mid-20th century (pure *ergotamine* was isolated by Stoll in 1920) was a major event in the development of modern pharmacology. It is an amino acid alkaloid derived from the lysergic acid nucleus. Preparations contain about 40% of the relatively inactive ergotaminine, due to spontaneous epimerization. Because of its long history, well-conducted controlled trials have not been carried out, so there is no objective evidence for its level of benefit. Actions of ergotamine include:

- At 5-HT$_1$ and 5-HT$_2$ receptors:
  - Partial agonist in many blood vessels (it is a powerful vasoconstrictor).
  - Mixed agonist/antagonist actions in the CNS.
  - A non-selective 5-HT antagonist in many smooth muscles.
- At alpha-adrenergic receptors:
  - Partial agonist/antagonist in blood vessels and smooth muscles, promoting uterine contraction and vasoconstriction.
  - Antagonist in the central and peripheral nervous systems.
- At dopaminergic D$_2$ receptors:
  - Powerful stimulation of the CTZ, especially with injections, causes nausea and vomiting.

While the vasoconstrictive effects of *ergotamine* contribute to its benefit in migraine, these non-selective, wide-ranging actions mean that it also has a formidable array of side-effects. These, and the risk of habituation, which limits its use to not more than twice per month, have contributed to its increasingly rare use. It is less effective than *sumatriptan* and probably also less so than *naproxen*.

Ergotamine is available as compound tablets with *cyclizine*, as an anti-emetic, and with caffeine, allegedly to promote absorption. The benefit from caffeine is debatable and it may even cause analgesic headache (see above). Oral bioavailability is poor, about 1–3%, with extensive first-pass metabolism and large inter-individual variations in absorption. The use of a buccal aerosol or sublingual tablets may provide improved absorption, but the aerosol has a very nauseating taste. Suppositories give about a 20-fold increase in peak plasma concentration, and this is probably the preferred route. Pharmacokinetic data are rather imprecise due to assay difficulties (peak plasma concentrations are only about 10–500 pg/mL).

Because *ergotamine* binds irreversibly to receptors it has a longer duration of action than the triptans. This may be beneficial in patients with lengthy attacks or those in whom headache recurs frequently after triptans. However, there are restrictions on dose frequency because of its strong peripheral vasoconstricting action, i.e. not more than four tablets in 24 h, not to be repeated within 4 days, and not more than eight tablets/week.

Patients have lost fingers because of failure by GPs and pharmacists to adhere to these dosage restrictions, or to recognize inappropriate prescribed dosage.

Although injections of *ergotamine* have been used, they usually contain a mixture of ergot alkaloids. They therefore have numerous side-effects and, in addition, are highly emetogenic (20% of patients) and are often poorly tolerated. The side-effects, contra-indications, etc. of *ergotamine* are given in Table 7.14.

Dihydroergotamine preparations have been withdrawn in the UK but the nasal spray is widely used in North America and continental Europe.

Isometheptene, an indirect sympathomimetic agent, is marketed in the UK combined with *paracetamol* (acetaminophen). It may cause circulatory disturbances, dizziness, rashes and, rarely, blood dyscrasias. Its numerous side-effects, cautions, contra-indications and interactions are considered to outweigh its clinical usefulness.

Prophylactic pharmacotherapy

This may not be necessary if attacks are infrequent or of mild to moderate severity and if this situation is well tolerated by the patient and is well controlled by acute drug usage. However, opinion differs as to when prophylaxis should be considered. In the UK, it is often recommended if there is more than two moderate to severe attacks a month, if they suffer increasing headache frequency or significant disability despite suitable treatment and if they cannot take appropriate migraine treatment. In the USA the borderline is drawn at three or more attacks per month. Much

Table 7.14 Ergotamine: some side-effects, cautions and contraindications

Side-effects[a]	Gastrointestinal: nausea, vomiting, abdominal pain, diarrhoea, peritoneal fibrosis (excessive use)
	Cardiovascular: chest pain, angina pectoris, myocardial infarction (rare)
	Respiratory: pleural fibrosis (excessive use)
	Muscle cramps
	Habituation and ergotamine-induced headache may occur
	Peripheral vasospasm
Cautions	Elderly
	Not for prophylaxis
	Peripheral vasospasm: numb or tingling fingers or toes (stop treatment; risk of gangrene)
Contraindications	Peripheral vascular disease, Raynaud's syndrome
	Coronary heart disease
	Sepsis
	Severe/uncontrolled hypertension
	Pregnancy, breastfeeding

[a] This list is not exhaustive (see text).

depends on what level of pain and disruption to their lives, balanced against side-effects, patients are able to tolerate.

The drugs used comprise:

*   Beta-blockers: *propranolol, metoprolol* (possibly *atenolol, nadolol, timolol*).
*   5-HT antagonists: *pizotifen* (pizotyline), *methysergide*.
*   Tricyclic antidepressants: e.g. *amitriptyline* (whether the patient shows depressive symptoms or not; unlicensed indication).
*   *Sodium valproate* and CCBs (unlicensed indication).

The modes of action of these drugs in migraine are unclear, especially because the effects of other beta-blockers and anticonvulsants are similar to those of placebo.

The use of *methysergide* for resistant cases is restricted to hospital consultants in the UK, because of its toxicity, especially retroperitoneal fibrosis.

All of these drugs are, at most, 50% effective in only about half of the patients, but one can usually be found useful by trial and error. Further, it is difficult to be sure of the true benefit because there is a large placebo effect, up to about 40%. Each of the drugs needs to be tried for at least 2–3 months before it is discarded as ineffective. If the patient responds, treatment should continue, with 6-monthly medication reviews: complete remission is common.

It has also been suggested that trials of high-dose riboflavin or NSAIDs might be worthwhile. If NSAIDs are used (this is an unlicensed indication), the drug selected would have to be relatively free of side-effects (e.g. *ibuprofen*) because long-term use is involved. As usual, there needs to be a balance between benefit and harms.

Beta-blockers, usually *propranolol*, are usually regarded as the drugs of choice for migraine prophylaxis. Their utility is limited by their side-effects (see Chapter 4) and, in the past, by their interaction with *ergotamine*, because both drugs cause peripheral vasoconstriction. This interaction is less of a problem if one of the newer 5-HT$_1$ agonists is being used to treat attacks.

Pizotifen (pizotyline) is probably the second choice, but good evidence of benefit is lacking. This also has antihistaminic properties and causes marked drowsiness initially, so the minimum dose should be taken at night and increased gradually, as tolerance is achieved, to the minimum dose that gives satisfactory control. Increased appetite and weight gain often make it unacceptable, especially to women. Its weak antimuscarinic properties may cause urinary retention and closed angle glaucoma, so it may not be suitable in middle-aged to elderly patients. Another 5-HT$_1$ agonist/antihistamine, *cyproheptadine*, is sometimes used in refractory cases.

Clonidine has been used but is regarded as unsuitable in the UK because it may cause or aggravate severe depression, with an increased risk of suicide. Migraine sufferers may often be depressed due to the condition

The highly desirable introduction of more effective prophylactic drugs presumably awaits a better understanding of migraine pathophysiology.

Cluster headache (migrainous neuralgia)

This name derives from the fact that episodes tend to occur in clusters of attacks, lasting several weeks, interspersed by remissions of months to years. Despite its synonym, it is unrelated to migraine, though many of the same drugs are used.

Clinical features

There are abrupt episodes of excruciating, unilateral pain ('suicide headache') which affect the eye, temple or forehead and increase over about 30 min and may last for several hours. The affected eye waters copiously and there is often flushing of the same side of the face (Figure 7.5(k)), though this may vary. Attack frequency is between eight per day and one on alternate days, usually once or twice a day for a few weeks or months, often at night and at predictable times. The prodromal signs of classical migraine and the aura do not occur, and the attacks do not usually cause vomiting.

Sufferers are mostly men aged 30–50 (male : female ratio, 10 : 1), but remission tends to occur by the age of 60. There is no persistent major deficit. The cause is unknown, but alcohol may provoke attacks, especially during a cluster. The fact that high-dose *oxygen* may abort an attack points to the possibility of oxygen starvation in part of the CNS.

Pharmacotherapy

Sumatriptan, by SC injection, is the only drug licensed for cluster headache. It may be taken in anticipation of an imminent attack (unlicensed indication), because the timing is usually consistent once a cluster has started. High-flow (100%) *oxygen* often provides relief within minutes.

Pizotifen and *verapamil* (also *methysergide*, hospital-only; see above) are used for prophylaxis throughout a cluster. Regular oral *lithium* (see Chapter 6) may help chronic sufferers.

Trigeminal neuralgia

Definition

This is a neuropathy of the fifth cranial (trigeminal) nerve that causes episodes of agonising, lancinating (stabbing or 'electric shock') pain, usually on one side of the face. Each episode lasts for a few seconds.

Clinical features

The trigeminal (Vth cranial) nerve is mostly sensory and has three branches:

- **Ophthalmic**; carrying sensory fibres from the anterior half of the scalp, forehead, the eye and surrounding structures, the nasal cavity and side of the nose.
- **Maxillary**; contains fibres serving the lower eyelid, nose, palate, upper teeth and lip, and parts of the pharynx.
- **Mandibular**; serving the anterior tongue (not taste), lower teeth and jaw, cheek and side of the head in front of the ear.

Trigeminal neuralgia is usually of unknown cause, but it can also occur in multiple sclerosis and due to a fifth nerve tumour. It may also be a form of post-herpetic neuralgia, when it usually affects the ophthalmic branch. Other neuropathies can affect the trigeminal nerve, but these are usually chronic and distinct from trigeminal neuralgia.

The severe spasms of pain usually affect the mandibular division and may spread upwards to involve the other branches. The characteristics and localized distribution of the pain are diagnostic: no neurological abnormality can be detected.

Spasms may occur several times a day, usually in response to trivial triggers, e.g. cold wind, touching, shaving or washing the face, chewing or tooth brushing. Episodes remit spontaneously for anything from months to years, but always recur. Middle-aged and elderly patients are mostly affected.

Management

Most patients respond to pharmacotherapy with *carbamazepine*, taken at the commencement of an attack. This usually reduces the severity, duration and frequency of attacks and is not beneficial in other forms of headache.

Carbamazepine is a rather toxic antiepileptic drug with a long list of side-effects and interactions, being a liver enzyme inducer (see Chapter 3). Consequently, it is usual to start with a low dose in a first attack and build up slowly (fortnightly) until symptoms are controlled. This is especially necessary if dizziness occurs. Like *phenytoin* and some other anticonvulsants, *carbamazepine* has a narrow therapeutic window, so plasma-level monitoring should be instituted if high doses are used.

Phenytoin may be effective in those not responding to *carbamazepine*. If the side-effects of high-dose *carbamazepine* are not tolerated, a combination with *phenytoin* is sometimes used, the doses of each being reduced appropriately. However, these interact (both are liver enzyme inducers) and such combinations are rarely justified (see Chapter 6).

The dose and build-up in subsequent attacks depend on the patient's reaction and tolerance to the drugs.

Tricyclic antidepressants are more useful in post-herpetic facial neuralgia and in non-specific facial and jaw pain associated with depression (see below).

Surgery or nerve ablation with alcohol injections may be required in those not responding to pharmacotherapy.

Post-herpetic neuralgia

Definition

This is a chronic pain syndrome in the **dermatome** (the skin area served by a single sensory nerve) affected by **herpes zoster**, an acute skin infection (**shingles**) due to reactivation of **varicella-zoster provirus** (VZV, see Chapter 8).

Clinical features

VZV causes chickenpox, a common acute skin infection. Most patients (90%) are children under the age of 10. Infections in older people are generally severe and occasionally fatal, and are usually associated with immunosuppression, e.g. drug treatment (transplant, autoimmune and cancer patients), radiotherapy, some neoplastic diseases (especially lymphomas), and AIDS, or waning immunity in old age.

During recovery from chickenpox the virus tracks up sensory nerve axons to the local dorsal root ganglia and becomes incorporated in the nuclear DNA there as a provirus. This location is protected from immunological defence mechanisms, so the provirus persists until it is reactivated by a reduction in host immunity. The virus then tracks back down the nerve axon to cause a skin infection in the dermatome innervated by that sensory nerve. This pattern may be repeated. There are usually three distinct phases:

- **Prodromal**, with malaise, unilateral nerve pain or paraesthesia lasting 3–5 days (range 1–14 days), the skin being very sensitive to touch, and sometimes mild fever.
- **Active**, vesicles appear over 3–5 days and crust over during several days to 3 weeks, accompanied by nerve and skin pain which seems excessive relative to the skin involvement.
- **Chronic post-herpetic neuralgia (PHN)** lasting months to years.

Occasionally, the nerve may be affected without any skin eruption. The affected area is unilateral, sharply demarcated at the mid-line front and back, and may involve a few adjacent dermatomes. The principal sites are the thorax (50% of cases), head and neck (20%) and lumbosacral area (15%). Involvement of the eye or ear requires specialist advice.

Management and pharmacotherapy

Shingles

Mild cases
Only simple or compound analgesics and soothing and drying lotions (see Chapter 13) are required.

Moderate to severe cases
These require prompt treatment, especially if the patient is immunocompromised:

- Early antiviral treatment, to minimize the risk of PHN and complications, e.g. eye or ear involvement. However, diagnosis may be difficult because the prodromal symptoms may mimic migraine, heart disease or acute abdominal problems. The antivirals (see also Chapter 8) used include:
  - *Aciclovir* orally, or by IV infusion in the immunocompromised, plus topical application to the eye or ear if these are affected. Alternatives are *famciclovir* and *valaciclovir*, oral prodrugs of *penciclovir* and *aciclovir* respectively, with superior bioavailability.
  - *Foscarnet*, occasionally *amantadine*, for resistant strains of VZV (unlicensed indications in the UK).
- Antibacterials for bacterial opportunistic infections of the rash (see Chapter 8).
- Pain control with:
  - Analgesics, including opioids (see below) if needed, though most have not been assessed. Side-effects may become unacceptable before effective analgesia is achieved.
  - Local anaesthetics (p. 482), especially topical *lidocaine*, or nerve block (p. 487) if pain is severe.

- A sedative tricyclic antidepressant, e.g. *amitriptyline* or *trimipramine*, at night, as an analgesic adjunct, hypnotic and antidepressant.
- Anticonvulsants, i.e. *gabapentin* or *pregabalin*, reduce the pain.
- There is conflicting evidence for the benefit of *capsaicin*, and this may cause skin reactions (see below).
- TENS (see p. 486).
- Soothing soaks to the affected skin.

Chronic post-herpetic neuralgia

Severe pain in the prodromal or early active phases indicates the likelihood of severe PHN, so early aggressive antiviral treatment is indicated. Prolonged PHN requires any of the analgesic treatments listed above (depression is a feature of moderate to severe PHN). There is no evidence for most opioid analgesics in PHN, but *tramadol* and oral *oxycodone* are effective and the risk of dependence must be weighed against the possible benefit for this condition, which is not life-threatening although very debilitating.

Capsaicin cream, a counter-irritant, is also used **after the rash has healed**. This is very irritant and must not be applied until the lesions have healed completely. It should be applied not less than three, nor more than four times daily. If applied less frequently the transient burning sensation may be more severe and prolonged; the skin needs to become habituated. More frequent application also causes skin irritation. Application sites must not be occluded and the hands must be washed thoroughly immediately after application. The area around the eyes must be avoided.

Corticosteroids are contra-indicated in the acute phase because they may promote widespread viral dissemination across the skin. They may help when the rash has healed and a short trial course of *prednisolone* is worthwhile. Intrathecal *methylprednisolone* is also helpful, but its safety has not been established.

Non-drug measures (e.g. TENS, p. 486) may help to minimize the dose of analgesic and the risk of opioid dependence.

Prophylaxis

A varicella vaccine is available. Use of the vaccine in non-immune individuals, especially those at risk of varicella infection, may prevent an attack of shingles in later life.

Shingles is not contagious, because the syndrome develops only after a previous chickenpox infection and reactivation of dormant provirus. However, chickenpox may occur in a non-immune patient due to contact with a case of shingles.

Some special pain situations

Certain categories of patient present particular problems in pain control. This can be from the type of pain itself or may relate to the constraints that their disease state may impose on any choice of therapy.

Opioids and other sedatives in surgery

Premedication

The objectives of pre-anaesthetic medication are to:

- Relieve anxiety without excessive drowsiness, so that the patient remains cooperative and the various preparative procedures can proceed smoothly.
- Give an amnesic effect and so avoid unpleasant memories.
- Relieve any preoperative pain.
- Minimize:
  - the dose of the general anaesthetic, usually inhalational.
  - the undesirable effects of anaesthesia, e.g. vomiting, headache, coughing and excessive secretions.
  - post-operative stress.

Several agents may be required to achieve these ends.

Surgery is often preceded by organic or traumatic pain, and itself obviously causes moderate to severe pain. Even mild preoperative pain interferes with the smooth induction of general anaesthesia and increases the amount of anaesthetic required.

Oral benzodiazepines are widely used. They are sedative, anxiolytic and amnesic, but have no analgesic effect. Short-acting ones are preferred, e.g. *lorazepam, midazolam* or *temazepam,* but *diazepam,* which is long-acting, is also used in adults.

Diazepam is used to provide mild sedation, but it is unsuitable for children because its effects in them are unreliable and it may cause paradoxical excitation. *Alimemazine,* a sedative antihistamine, may be used in children, but this may cause post-operative restlessness. It is unsuitable for use in elderly patients because of its antimuscarinic effects, e.g. urinary retention and blurred vision.

Opioids are no longer widely used for premedication. The choice of opioid is determined by their duration of action and the incidence of side-effects. *Morphine,* and sometimes *pethidine* in obstetrics, are used occasionally, but their side-effects are particularly undesirable in surgical patients, e.g. prolonged recovery time, nausea and vomiting, constipation and urinary retention, bradycardia causing hypotension, respiratory depression (especially in those patients with an asthmatic tendency or frank asthma) and spasm of the bile duct and ureters. However, premedication with an opioid may minimize the occurrence of agitation during recovery. They are more usually used at induction and to reduce the dose of a general anaesthetic required by about 15%. They also enhance analgesia during general anaesthesia. Drugs with a rapid onset and short duration of action are now preferred because any side-effects resolve rapidly. *Alfentanil* and *fentanyl* can be administered by IV injection or infusion. *Remifentanil* is given by IV infusion only. They are also used as analgesics to prevent the pain due to procedures, e.g. dressing changes. Their side-effect of respiratory depression is beneficial in ventilated patients, to prevent spontaneous respiration interfering with the ventilation provided by the equipment.

Patients with severe adrenal suppression due to corticosteroid use may have a dramatic fall in blood pressure due to operative stress, so a high-dose glucocorticoid with mineralocorticoid properties, e.g. *hydrocortisone* and especially *fludrocortisone,* may be used in anticipation of intra-operative shock.

Antimuscarinic drugs, e.g. *hyoscine (scopolamine) hydrobromide,* are now rarely used for premedication, whether alone or in combination with an opioid. They reduce the excessive bronchial and salivary secretions that occur with some inhaled anaesthetics, due to airway intubation. *Hyoscine* produces some sedation and amnesia and reduces vomiting, but may cause undesirable bradycardia and CNS side-effects, e.g. excitement, hallucinations and drowsiness, especially in the elderly.

However, modern anaesthetic techniques and the increasing use of day-case surgery largely avoid the need for traditional premedication routines.

Induction agents

Propofol provides rapid recovery without hangover and causes little undesirable muscle activity. It is an oil at room temperature: 1% injections are given intravenously, but 2% injections are emulsions and are given by IV infusion. *Propofol* is also used as a sedative for short surgical and diagnostic procedures, but there is a significant incidence of bradycardia, allergic reactions and convulsions.

Obstetric pain

The use of analgesics to control the pain of labour presents several problems and poses risks to both mother and fetus. The ideal agent should meet the following criteria:

- Provide adequate pain relief.
- Interfere minimally with the course and duration of labour.
- Have little effect on fetal vital signs during labour and after birth.

Pethidine (meperidine) is the most common obstetric analgesic as it is short-acting and generally meets these criteria. However, problems still occur, notably respiratory depression in the neonate, the incidence of which can be reduced by giving the drug early in the course of labour and using the IM route, the IV route being associated with more neonatal respiratory depression.

Common alternative forms of analgesia include the epidural administration of local anaesthetics, and the inhalation of sub-anaesthetic doses of 50% nitrous oxide in oxygen.

Palliative treatment of cancer pain

Great advances have been made in this field, and most patients can be maintained virtually free of pain by application of the principles of the WHO 'analgesic ladder' (Table 7.3). It is essential to appreciate that pain is not an invariable accompaniment to cancer, and about one-third of cancer patients remain pain-free. A clear understanding of the common pain syndromes associated with neoplasms and their pathophysiological mechanisms, the psychological state of the patient, and the indications and limitations of the available therapeutic approaches, is vital to effective management. Short-acting drugs, e.g. *pethidine* (meperidine), are unsuitable because they require frequent dosing, without additional benefit.

Several different types of pain may be associated with cancer (see Table 7.15), and these often co-exist: some 80% of patients who are experiencing pain have two or more types and about 20% four or more types. The pain may be due to the disease itself or to the debility it causes, and to coexisting disease or treatment, and so a combination of therapeutic approaches is often required. Thus a multidisciplinary approach, including specialist 'Macmillan' pharmacists, has been adopted increasingly to form pain teams, which take a holistic approach to the patient's needs. The clinical aspects of cancer and its overall management are discussed in detail in Chapter 10.

Types of pain

Because pain can have many causes, some of which are not directly related to neoplastic activity, especially careful assessment and diagnosis of the pain is essential in cancer patients. Regular reassessment is required to take account of disease progression and the occurrence of unrelated intercurrent disease. Depending on its aetiology, the pain in terminal disease may only

---

Table 7.15   Some types of pain in cancer patients

Pain caused directly by the tumour
Tumour infiltration of viscera, nerves and bone
Nerve compression
Raised intracranial pressure (headaches)

Pain caused by complications of therapy
After surgery, e.g. phantom limb pain, neuropathic pain, adhesions
After chemotherapy, e.g. peripheral neuropathy caused by vinca alkaloids
After radiotherapy, e.g. fibrosis, myelopathy
Mucositis
Gastrointestinal distress, constipation
Post-herpetic neuralgia (as a consequence of immunosuppressive treatments)

Incidental pain, i.e. not caused by the tumour
Pre-existing chronic pain, e.g. arthritis
Bedsores
Headache
Gastrointestinal pain, e.g. due to opioid treatment causing constipation

be partially responsive to opioid analgesics, so a combination of analgesics with different pharmacological actions is often necessary. Adjunctive agents, radiotherapy or surgical approaches may be appropriate in special circumstances.

Tumour infiltration of tissues

Visceral organs

Tumour invasion of the stomach, biliary tract, intestine, uterus or bladder causes intense contraction of the local smooth muscle with increased pressure and local ischaemia. Visceral pain is characteristically increasing in intensity, diffuse, unlocalized and continuous. Opioid drugs are the most effective in these circumstances, but treatment must be started on the appropriate step of the WHO 'analgesic ladder' and must be given in adequate doses. A simple analgesic, usually *paracetamol* (acetaminophen), added to the opioid is often helpful. A regular laxative, combining both a stimulant and a stool softener (see Chapter 3), is also needed to prevent constipation that would otherwise add to the pain and complicate the picture.

Nerves

Infiltration or compression of local nerves by a tumour may cause a variety of symptoms according to the site of involvement. These include hyperaesthesia (increased sensitivity), dysaesthesia (painful sensation), neuralgia (paroxysmal nerve pain), allodynia (pain elicitated by light touch). Motor disturbances and sensory loss may also occur. The tumour may cause persistent mechanical stimulation of high-threshold nociceptors, i.e. those not readily stimulated, and partial damage to axons and nerve membranes, resulting in increased sensitivity to sympathetic stimulation and pressure. Nerve pain may respond to standard opioid analgesics, at least partially, but unacceptable side-effects often occur before adequate analgesia is achieved, so a combined approach is often required. Analgesic adjuvants, nerve blocks or neurosurgical procedures (see above) may be more successful, but the last two of these may not always be achievable (see above), or desirable in very frail patients, and may add their own problems.

Bones

Bone pain is common in cancer and may be due either to a primary tumour (e.g. multiple myeloma) or to metastases (e.g. from breast, lung or prostate cancer). Bone tumours stimulate local pain receptors directly and induce the production of PGs that may cause osteolysis (solution of the mineral component of bone), sensitize free nerve endings and augment pain perception. Inhibitors of PG release, e.g. NSAIDs (see Chapter 12), are thus the logical choice to treat bone pain. Although NSAIDs exert their main analgesic action at peripheral sites, there is also a central component. It is worth maximizing the dosage of individual agents and changing drugs if side-effects are excessive or the response is poor, because individuals vary considerably, both in their response to different NSAIDs and in the occurrence of side-effects. Bisphosphonates, e.g. *alendronic acid, disodium pamidronate, ibandronic acid, sodium clodronate* and *zoledronic acid*, can also help by inhibiting osteolysis. *Strontium ranelate* both inhibits osteolysis and stimulates mineralization and may also be helpful (unlicensed indication). However, cytotoxic chemotherapy or single-dose local palliative radiotherapy, if appropriate (see Chapter 10), may have a dramatic, if temporary, analgesic effect.

Opioids are generally not very effective in relieving bone pain and can sometimes be reduced in dose or withdrawn totally after the introduction of an NSAID, though many patients use the combined therapy.

Morphine in palliative care

Optimal use follows the guidelines given on pp. 470 and 490. Oral *morphine* is the first-line opioid in palliative care. Initially, the oral dose of plain tablets or liquid is given 4-hourly, with rescue medication as required. Doubling the bedtime dose usually enables the patient to sleep throughout the night. With a 4-h duration of action, *morphine* takes about 24 h to reach steady state, so patients need re-evaluation daily. Once stabilized, the change is made to modified-release tablets (not to be crushed), usually formulated for 12-hourly dosing. If pain increases, the dose should be increased but the dose interval retained.

If oral dosing is not possible or not tolerated, rectal (dose equals oral dose) or SC routes (potency relative to oral is 2, as a bolus or continuous infusion) can be used. The choice may depend on the availability of the desired dosage form (see Table 7.4) and its suitability, e.g. the IM route gives more pain with *morphine* and should not be used. The IV route is uncommon in palliative care because pharmacological tolerance develops, leading to escalating doses.

A change to *diamorphine* (heroin) or *hydromorphone* (in North America or elsewhere that heroin is not licensed) may be needed if high doses are required, because *morphine* is not very soluble and only small volumes can be injected by the SC route. Also, if the SC route is unsuitable due to generalized oedema, coagulation problems, poor peripheral circulation or local adverse drug reactions, the IV route may be used (potencies relative to oral *morphine*: *diamorphine* (heroin), about 3; *hydromorphone*, about 15).

About 20% of patients fail to respond to these measures. These will need spinal opioids, with local anaesthetics and other adjuncts (see above).

Patients with liver failure

These patients often present a therapeutic dilemma because most of the commonly used analgesics are contra-indicated. In particular, the effect of liver failure on the pharmacokinetics and pharmacodynamics of the analgesic has to be considered (see Chapters 2 and 3). Most opioids are significantly metabolized by the liver and will accumulate in liver disease if dosing intervals are not adjusted. Further, the oral bioavailability of opioids may be increased owing to reduced first-pass metabolism.

Patients with liver failure are particularly sensitive to the effects of opioids, as to other sedatives, because they are metabolized hepatically and relatively small doses can precipitate encephalopathy (see Chapter 3). Those with cirrhosis are liable to develop oesophageal varices (see Chapter 3), and NSAIDs should be used cautiously as the gastrointestinal irritation caused may precipitate catastrophic bleeding. Chronic administration of large doses of hepatotoxic drugs, e.g. *paracetamol* (acetaminophen),

can further exacerbate the liver failure. Fortunately, the severity of liver failure usually encountered in cancer patients does not require large dosage changes.

In practice, an estimate of the dosage interval required to prevent accumulation occurring is obtained by giving a cautious dose of opioid, the subsequent dose being withheld until the pain reappears. It is particularly important in this situation to use drugs in which the analgesic half-life is similar to the plasma half-life, e.g. *morphine* (plus its active metabolite, morphine-6-glucuronide), because the risk of accumulation is then minimized, as the loss of analgesic effect should correlate with drug clearance.

Patients with renal failure

Choosing an appropriate analgesic in this group of patients does not usually present a problem (but see Chapter 14). Some analgesics however (e.g. the NSAIDs) can cause nephropathy, so taking a medication history is important, to determine whether the renal failure may initially have been due to analgesic over-dosage or misuse. NSAIDs may also be contra-indicated because they may exacerbate fluid retention and precipitate decompensation in developing heart failure (see Chapter 4).

Opioid analgesics may present a significant problem in renal failure. *Morphine* and its glucuronide metabolites accumulate, requiring an increased dosing interval or dose reduction.

Fentanyl is said to be safer in renal impairment and can be given intravenously. If injections are not tolerated, then transdermal patches can be used. However, it takes about 24 h after application of the first patch to reach an adequate *fentanyl* plasma concentration. Further, the long half-life of *fentanyl* (about 17 h) creates problems if the drug accumulates, and replacement with an alternative must be started at a low dose concurrently with the removal of a patch, and increased gradually thereafter. *Alfentanil* is being used increasingly in palliative care for patients in renal failure.

Pethidine (meperidine) should be avoided because the toxic metabolite norpethidine accumulates in renal failure and can lead to seizures.

References and further reading

Carroll D, Bowsher D (1993). *Pain Management and Nursing Care*. Oxford, Butterworth-Heinemann.

Cox J J, Reimann F, Nicholas A K, *et al.* (2006). An *SCN9A* channelopathy causes congenital inability to experience pain. *Nature* 444: 894–898.

Goadsby P J (2006). Recent advances in the diagnosis and management of migraine. *BMJ* 332: 25–29.

Headache Classification Committee of the International Headache Society (2004). The international classification of headache disorders (second edition). *Cephalalgia* 24 (Suppl. 1); 1–160.

Hawthorn J, Redmond K (1998). *Pain: Causes and Management*. Oxford: Blackwell Science.

Lance J W, Goadsby P J (2005). *Mechanism and Management of Headache*, 7th edn. New York: Elsevier.

McQuay H J, Moore A (1998). *An Evidence-based Resource for Pain Relief*. Oxford: Oxford University Press.

McMahon S, Koltzenburgh M (2005). *Wall & Melzack's Textbook of Pain*, 5th edn. Edinburgh: Elsevier.

Melzack R (1987). The short form McGill pain questionnaire. *Pain* 30: 191–197.

Melzack R, Wall P D (1996). *The Challenge of Pain*. Harmondsworth: Penguin.

National Institute for Health and Clinical Excellence (2004). Improving Supportive and Palliative Care for Patients with Cancer.

North West Medicines Information Service, Pharmacy Practice Unit (2005). Systematic review of opioids for non malignant neuropathic pain. *Medicine Digest* Number 415, p. 1 (available from http://www.mmnetwork.nhs.uk/downloads/news/Med%20Digest%20415.pdf).

Quigley C (2005). The role of opioids in cancer pain. *BMJ* 331: 825–829.

Regnard C F B, Tempest S (1998). *A Guide to Symptom Relief in Advanced Disease*, 4th edn. Hale, Cheshire: Hochland & Hochland.

Scottish Intercollegiate Guidelines Network (SIGN) (2000) Guideline 44.
This is about to be updated.

Stannard C, Booth S (2004). *Pain*, 2nd edn. Churchill's Pocket Books, Edinburgh: Churchill Livingstone.

de Stoutz N D, Bruera E, Suarez-Almazor M (1995). Opioid rotation for toxicity reduction in terminal cancer patients. *J Pain Symptom Manage* 10: 378–384.

Sykes N, Fallon M T, Patt R B (2003). *Clinical Pain Management: Cancer Pain*. London, Arnold.

Twycross R G, Wilcock A (2001). *Symptom Management in Advanced Cancer*, 3rd edn. Edinburgh: Churchill Livingstone.

Twycross R G, Wilcock A, Charlesworth S, Dickman A (2002). *PCF2: Palliative Care Formulary*. Abingdon, UK: Radcliffe Publishing.

Waddell G, Bircher M, Finlayson D, Main C J (1984). Symptoms and signs: physical disease or illness behaviour? *BMJ* 289; 739–741.

Wellchew E (1995). *Patient Controlled Analgesia*. London: BMA Publishing Group.

Internet references

http://www.i-h-s.org (the International Headache Society).

http://www.prodigy.nhs.uk/guidance (National Library for Health: Clinical Knowledge Summaries – gives very comprehensive and clear information on palliative care, migraine, headache, shingles, post-herpetic neuralgia and trigeminal neuralgia).

http://www.painassociation.com and http://www.cancerbackup.org.uk are both sources of good practical advice from patient support groups on coping with chronic pain.

8

Infections and antimicrobial therapy

At some point in their life, everybody is likely to suffer an infection that will require treatment with antimicrobial agents. However, such an infection is unlikely to prove serious unless there is some underlying chronic condition, a complication, or a highly resistant pathogen is implicated. Only 65 years ago death from acute infection was common and antimicrobial chemotherapy was still in its infancy.

Antimicrobial chemotherapy began with the introduction of the sulphonamides in the 1930s, and this was followed by penicillin in the 1940s. The original benzylpenicillin had an enormous impact on the early therapeutics of infection, but now has only limited applications. This illustrates the important principle that the therapeutics of infectious disease must be developed continually in order to remain effective. Compare this situation with that of diabetes, in which the major therapy (insulin) was introduced in the 1920s and remains largely unchanged up to the present. The disease itself has neither changed nor 'adapted' to the treatment. By contrast, the staphylococcal organism against which benzylpenicillin was originally so dramatically effective is now almost universally resistant to antimicrobials.

It must be emphasized that recommended antimicrobials and doses change from time to time and depend on the location of patients. Current local guidance must be consulted before making any therapeutic recommendations.

Introduction

The constantly changing pattern of microbial sensitivity has been a prime factor contributing to the proliferation of antimicrobial agents. Most of this chapter addresses the treatment of bacterial infections but similar principles apply to the treatment of fungal and viral infections. We use the term **antimicrobials** when describing chemotherapeutic agents generally, and **antibacterial**, **antifungal** and **antiviral** for those used specifically to treat corresponding infections. The term 'antibiotic' was originally applied only to those agents derived from living organisms, usually fungal or bacterial. However, many antimicrobials are now manufactured synthetically or semi-synthetically, e.g. chloramphenicol and the more recent penicillins, so 'antibiotic' is now synonymous with 'antimicrobial'. Similarly, the unqualified term 'chemotherapy' is now usually applied to the treatment of neoplastic disease, discussed in Chapter 10.

Although there is a very wide range of antibacterials available, patients may commonly be prescribed agents from among the penicillin, cephalosporin, macrolide, tetracycline or quinolone groups. However, in some situations (e.g. a lower urinary-tract bacterial infection) the most likely pathogen is known to be *Escherichia coli*, an organism against which only some of these agents are effective. The prescriber then has to choose the most appropriate antimicrobial for treating that infection in their particular patient, guided by advice from the pathologist or the results of laboratory tests.

This chapter first describes the various groups of antimicrobial agents, and then discusses the principles of selection by considering the various steps in the decision-making process that should be taken when diagnosing and treating an infected patient. The final part of the chapter will consider the application of these principles in the treatment of some important infections. Although the treatment of HIV/AIDS is a speciality, the principles of its treatment are discussed, together with some AIDS-related infections. The chapter also discusses antibiotic-associated colitis.

Before considering individual agents, we review a simple classification system for microorganisms and define the concepts of minimum inhibitory and microbicidal concentrations.

Classification of microorganisms

Table 8.1 presents some aspects of bacterial classification. Bacteria may be described as **Gram-positive** or **Gram-negative**, depending on whether the bacterial cell wall retains the Gram stain used for microscopy, and by their shape, i.e. bacillus (rod), coccus (spherical) or spiral. **Aerobic** organisms only grow in the presence of oxygen and **anaerobic** species require the absence of oxygen for growth. **Facultative** organisms are able to grow with or without oxygen, reflecting a more adaptable metabolism.

Thus *Escherichia coli* is described as a facultatively anaerobic, Gram-negative rod. Refinements of classification include whether a stain cannot be removed by acid, i.e. they are acid-fast, e.g. *Mycobacterium* spp. If an organism is found in the human GIT, the name used often indicates this, e.g. the species *Enterococcus faecalis*. Some of these descriptions may help predict likely sensitivities to antibacterials. In general, it is more difficult for antibacterials to penetrate the cell wall of Gram-negative bacteria than Gram-positive ones.

Antibacterials that are predominantly effective against a restricted range of either Gram-positive or (less commonly) Gram-negative bacteria are said to possess a **narrow spectrum of activity**, whereas those that are effective against several types of organism are termed **broad-spectrum**. Anaerobes may be either Gram-positive, e.g. the clostridia, or Gram-negative, e.g. *Bacteroides* spp., and usually require special groups of agents. The antimicrobials used to treat other classes of microorganism, such as viruses, fungi or protozoa, are largely narrow-spectrum agents, though some newer antifungal agents, e.g. *caspofungin* and *voriconazole*, are active against a range of fungi. Antiviral agents usually have a fairly

Table 8.1   Some ways of classifying bacteria

Classification method	Criterion	Classes	Examples
Gram stain	Retention of stain by cell wall	Gram-positive	*Staphylococcus aureus*
			Clostridium tetani
		Gram-negative	*Acinetobacter baumannii*
			Escherichia coli
			Neisseria meningitidis
			Pseudomonas aeruginosa
Metabolism	Oxygen requirements	Aerobe	*Streptococcus pneumoniae*
		Anaerobe	*Bacteroides fragilis*
			Clostridium tetani
		Facultative anaerobe	*Staphylococcus aureus*
			Haemophilus influenzae
Morphology	Shape	Rod	*Escherichia coli*
		Coccus	*Staphylococcus aureus*
			Neisseria meningitidis
		Spiral	*Treponema pallidum*
Source	Resident in the GIT	Enterobacteria	*Escherichia coli*
			Enterococcus faecalis
Structure	Cell wall	Most bacteria: wall in Gram-positives differs from that in Gram-negatives	
	No cell wall	Mycoplasmas	*Mycoplasma pneumoniae*

GIT, gastrointestinal tract.

restricted spectrum, e.g. *aciclovir* is effective only against herpes viruses.

Table 8.2 gives an approximate guide to the sensitivity of some bacterial pathogens to the antimicrobials in common use.

Minimum inhibitory and microbicidal (bactericidal) concentrations

For an antimicrobial agent to be effective in treating a particular infection it must be able to inhibit the growth of the causative organism or to kill it. The **minimum inhibitory concentration (MIC)** is the minimum concentration of an antimicrobial that is capable of inhibiting the growth of an organism and the **minimum bactericidal concentration (MBC)** is the lowest concentration that will kill it. Because of statistical uncertainties in counting very low numbers of survivors, it is common to deter-

mine the concentration of an antimicrobial agent that kills 50% of a population, i.e. the MBC_{50}. If the MIC or MBC for an organism is higher than the concentration of an antimicrobial that can reasonably be achieved clinically, that organism is described as being resistant. Thus, an antimicrobial agent will possess a spectrum of activity, those organisms inhibited at low MIC being termed sensitive and those inhibited only at a clinically unattainable MIC being resistant.

However, the distinction between MIC and MBC is often clinically irrelevant, because inhibition may be perfectly satisfactory if immune mechanisms (Chapter 2) are able to eliminate the inhibited organisms. Table 8.2 gives the approximate sensitivities of a range of Gram-positive and Gram-negative pathogens to the common antibacterial agents. However, many factors other than intrinsic sensitivity or resistance are involved, e.g. acquisition of resistance

Table 8.2   The antibacterial spectra of some antimicrobial agents[a]

Antimicrobial agent	Staph. aureus	Staph. aureus coag. −ve	Strep. pyogenes	Strep. pneumoniae	Enterococcus faecalis[b]	N. meningitidis	N. gonorrhoea	H. influenzae	Moraxella catarrhalis	Escherichia coli	Klebsiella spp.	Enterobacter spp.	Proteus spp.	Salmonella spp.	Ps. aeruginosa	Bacterioides fragilis	Clostridium perfringens	Clostridium difficile
Gram reaction	+	+	+	+	+	−	−	−	−	−	−	−	−	−	−	−	+	+
Benzylpenicillin[c]	G	G	S	V	G	V	V	R	R	R	R	R	R	R	R	G	S	R
Flucloxacillin[d]	V	G	S	V	R	V	V	R	R	R	R	R	R	R	R	R	V	R
Co-amoxiclav	V	G	S	V	V	V	V	S	S	V	V	G	G	V	R	V	V	R
Azlocillin/piperacillin	G	G	S	V	V	S	V	V	V	G	V	G	G	G	V	G	S	R
Piperacillin + tazobactam	V	G	S	V	V	S	S	S	S	V	V	V	V	V	V	V	V	R
Cefradine[e]	V	G	S	V	V	V	V	G	V	G	V	G	G	G	R	R	V	R
Cefuroxime	V	G	S	V	V	V	V	G	V	G	V	G	G	G	R	R	R	R
Cefixime	R	G	S	V	R	S	S	S	S	S	V	V	V	V	R	R	S	R
Cefotaxime[f]	V	G	S	V	R	S	S	S	S	S	V	V	V	V	R	R	S	R
Ceftazidime	V	G	S	V	R	V	V	V	V	S	V	V	V	V	V	V	V	R
Chloramphenicol	V	G	V	V	V	V	V	S	S	V	V	V	V	V	R	V	R	R
Ciprofloxacin/ofloxacin	V	V	V	V	V	S	S	S	S	S	S	V	V	S	V	V	R	R
Clindamycin	S	V	S	V	R	R	R	R	R	R	R	R	R	V	R	S	S	R
Erythromycin[g]	V	G	V	V	G	V	V	V	V	R	R	R	R	R	R	R	V	R
Gentamicin	V	G	R	R	V	V	V	S	V	V	V	V	V	V	V	V	R	R
Imipenem + cilastatin	V	G	S	V	V	G	S	−	−	−	−	−	−	−	−	−	−	−
Metronidazole/tinidazole	R	R	R	R	R	R	R	R	R	R	R	R	R	R	R	S	S	V
Nitrofurantoin	R	R	R	R	R	V	V	G	V	V	V	G	G	V	R	R	R	R
Rifampicin	V	V	V	V	V	V	V	V	S	V	V	V	V	V	R	R	S	R
Sodium fusidate	V	G	S	V	V	S	S	R	R	R	R	R	R	R	R	R	V	R
Tetracyclines	V	G	V	G	V	V	V	V	S	V	V	G	G	V	G	G	G	R
Trimethoprim[h]	S	S	S	S	S	R	R	S	−	V	V	−	V	−	R	R	−	−
Vancomycin/teichoplanin	S	S	S	S	V	R	R	R	R	R	R	R	R	R	R	R	S	S

[a] This table is an approximate guide only and cannot be used as a basis for prescribing. Increases in resistance usually occur with time. Up-to-date local sensitivity data should always be consulted.

[b] *Enter. faecium* is generally more resistant to antimicrobials; amoxicillin + gentamicin is usually effective.

[c] Includes phenoxymethylpenicillin.

[d] Includes meticillin (discontinued in the UK).

[e] Includes cefaclor and cefalexin.

[f] Includes cefpirome and ceftriaxone.

[g] Includes azithromycin and clarithromycin.

[h] Includes co-trimoxazole (trimethoprim + sulfamethoxazole), which has only limited applications in the UK.

G, globally-acquired resistance (more than 10% of strains) or drug is unsuitable; R, intrinsically resistant; S, sensitive, acquired resistance is rare; V, strains vary in resistance.

Modified from Ledingham JGG, Warrell DA, eds (2000). *Concise Oxford Textbook of Medicine*. Oxford University Press, with permission.

factors and the emergence of new mutants. Further, if a sufficiently high, non-toxic dose of, for example, a penicillin is used, many organisms that are normally considered to be resistant will be inhibited. With some diseases, e.g. bacterial endocarditis, it is essential to use bactericidal agents, to penetrate the vegetations in which the organisms are protected (p. 564), so that the organisms are killed, not merely inhibited, in order to prevent relapse. In such cases the MBC is more relevant.

Classification and properties of antimicrobials

Antimicrobials may be classified by their chemical structure, mode of action or spectrum of activity.

Chemical structure

For many purposes, the classification of an antimicrobial by its chemical structure (Figure 8.1) may be the most convenient because the group, having similar basic structures, will cause similar adverse reactions, e.g. allergic reactions with penicillins or ototoxicity and nephrotoxicity with aminoglycosides. This type of classification depends on the chemical nucleus of the original (parent) drug. Different side chains are attached to this basic nucleus to form the various members of the group, which often possess properties different from those of the parent compound. Such derivatives may have an extended spectrum of activity, the ability to overcome normally resistant organisms, improved bioavailability, resistance to acid inactivation in the stomach or fewer adverse effects.

Mode of action

The modes of action of antimicrobials (Table 8.3) are of little practical therapeutic relevance, though it may determine the spectrum of activity. However, there is one aspect in which

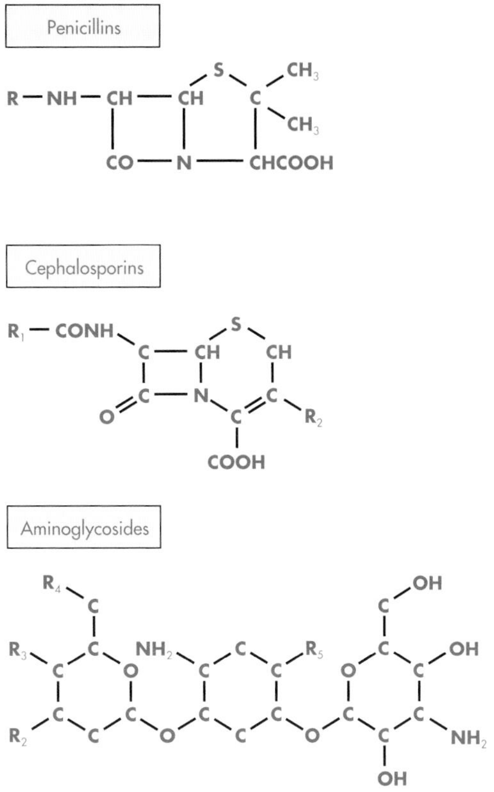

Figure 8.1   Structures of some important antimicrobials, showing the parent nuclei. $R-R_5$, various side chains.

the distinction between **bacteriostatic** agents and **bactericidal** ones may be important. Thus tetracyclines, sulphonamides and low doses of *erythromycin* are bacteriostatic agents. The penicillins and most other antibacterials are bactericidal and it is this group that must be used if it is necessary to eliminate organisms completely to avoid persistent problems, e.g. in bacterial endocarditis (p. 564). This distinction may sometimes be a concentration effect (see above). Furthermore, host defence mechanisms play an important part in eliminating the effects of an infection (e.g. pus), even with bactericidal agents.

The ability to use antimicrobials effectively to cure human disease relies on **selective toxicity**, i.e. structural or metabolic differences between the microbial and host (human) cells. Because penicillins specifically inhibit a step in the

Table 8.3   Modes of action of some antimicrobial agents

Mechanism	Examples
Antibacterials	
Inhibition of wall synthesis	Penicillins, cephalosporins, macrolides, vancomycin
Interference with protein synthesis	Aminoglycosides, chloramphenicol, tetracyclines
Interference with DNA replication	Quinolones
Inhibition of folate synthesis	Sulphonamides, trimethoprim
Antifungals	
Alteration of cell membrane permeability	Amphotericin, nystatin
Antivirals	
Incorporation into nucleic acid chain to give inactive nucleic acid	Aciclovir, cidofovir, ganciclovir, foscarnet, inosine pranobex
Reverse transcriptase inhibitors	
Nucleoside/nucleotide	Abacavir, lamivudine, tenofovir disoproxil, zidovudine
Non-nucleoside	Efavirenz, nevirapine
Protease inhibitors	Indinavir, ritonavir, saquinavir
Prevention of adhesion to host cell	Enfuvirtide
Interacts with influenza virus neuraminidase, preventing of penetration into host cell and new virion release	Oseltamivir, zanamivir

formation of bacterial cell walls, which are not present in mammalian cells, they are virtually non-toxic to animals. The aminoglycosides (e.g. *gentamicin*) interfere with bacterial ribosomal activity and, fortunately, bacterial ribosomes differ from human ones sufficiently to enable relatively selective action. However, these antimicrobials may still be toxic to man, due to their action as allergens in low concentration or causing other toxicities when present in sufficiently high concentration.

Activity spectrum

The problem faced by prescribers is to decide which of many antimicrobials will be the most effective against the organism responsible. In the absence of sensitivity testing and identification this decision must be based on a knowledge of the spectrums of activity of available antimicrobials (Table 8.2) and local knowledge of the most likely infective agent in a particular

patient: this is **empirical treatment**, sometimes described as treating 'blind' or on a 'best guess' basis (see p. 538). Monotherapy with the single most effective narrow-spectrum agent is the usual aim.

Penicillins

Chemical structure

The penicillins possess a **beta-lactam** group as part of the parent nucleus (6-amino-penicillanic acid; Figure 8.1). The cephalosporins, monobactams and carbapenems are also beta-lactam antibacterials, although the parent nuclei differ somewhat in each case. The substitution of different side chains on the parent nucleus has produced compounds with an extended spectrum of activity, the ability to overcome the resistance of some bacteria to the parent compound and improved bioavailability.

Spectrum of activity

The original *benzylpenicillin* (penicillin G) was active only against Gram-positive organisms (e.g. *Staphylococcus aureus*) and Gram-negative cocci (e.g. *Neisseria meningitidis* and *N. gonorrhoea*). Despite resistance problems, this drug remains the most effective agent for the treatment of streptococcal infection in the UK and streptococcal resistance is rarely a problem, except for *Enterococcus faecalis*. *Benzylpenicillin* also remains the first-line treatment for both *Neisseria meningitidis* (the meningococcus) and *N. gonorrhoea* (the gonococcus), both Gram-negative species, although acquired resistance is limiting its use as a sole agent for the latter. All other Gram-negative organisms are inherently resistant.

Beta-lactamase-resistant penicillins

Staphylococcus aureus, one of the most important wound pathogens, was initially satisfactorily treated with *benzylpenicillin*. However, 90% of *Staph. aureus* isolates now produce the enzyme **beta-lactamase** (penicillinase), which splits the beta-lactam nucleus and renders the antimicrobial ineffective. Indeed, most beta-lactam antibacterials may be inactivated by staphylococcal beta-lactamase. Penicillins have been developed that are beta-lactamase resistant; notably *methicillin* and *flucloxacillin*. *Methicillin* is not used clinically now, but resistance to it is used as a marker for **methicillin-resistant Staph. aureus** (MRSA; see below). *Flucloxacillin* is now the most widely prescribed penicillin in *Staph. aureus* infections, because it is resistant to penicillinase and has superior oral bioavailability. However, as a result of gaining beta-lactamase stability, the spectrum of this group is narrowed. Even though *flucloxacillin* retains activity against streptococci, its MIC against these organisms is greater than that of *benzylpenicillin*.

Flucloxacillin is therefore restricted to the treatment of suspected or confirmed *Staph. aureus* infections, all of which are assumed to be resistant to *benzylpenicillin*. If more than this single species is suspected in a particular infection, another antibacterial must be added. Alternatively, a beta-lactamase inhibitor, e.g. *clavulanic acid* or *tazobactam*, may be used with a broad-spectrum penicillin, e.g. *amoxicillin* plus *clavulanic acid* (as *co-amoxiclav* in the UK) and *piperacillin* plus *tazobactam* (marketed as Tazocin).

Broad-spectrum penicillins

Ampicillin was the first broad-spectrum penicillin developed and extended the Gram-negative range of penicillins to include *Haemophilus* and *Escherichia coli* species. However, a common observation is that as the spectrum of activity of an antimicrobial is extended into the Gram-negative range, its usefulness against Gram-positive organisms diminishes. Unfortunately, many strains of Gram-negative organisms are now resistant to *ampicillin*, its activity against many other Gram-negative organisms is unimpressive and it is completely ineffective against *Pseudomonas* spp. *Amoxicillin*, a prodrug of *ampicillin*, has better bioavailability (see below), but a similar activity spectrum, and is widely used.

Carbenicillin was the first antipseudomonal penicillin, but this has now been superseded by the ureidopenicillins, e.g. *piperacillin* and *ticarcillin*, which are available only for IV use. There is little to choose between these. Although the ureidopenicillins are also active against Gram-positive organisms, the older penicillins are usually used against these infections because they are often effective at lower concentrations, are cheaper, and may be administered orally.

As well as being used for the empirical treatment of septicaemia, the ureidopenicillins are also used prophylactically in certain surgical procedures or in immunocompromised patients. However, they are beta-lactamase susceptible and so are available only as co-formulations with beta-lactamase inhibitors, e.g. *tazobactam* or *clavulanic acid*. *Ticarcillin* and *piperacillin* are available only in combination with *clavulanic acid* and *tazobactam*, respectively.

The data in Table 8.2 may be taken to imply that most infections could be adequately treated with a ureidopenicillin, and that there could be little reason to prescribe any other type of penicillin. However, drug penetration to the site of infection, cost, ease of administration, resistance of certain strains, toxicity and other factors may affect antimicrobial choice in addition to activity spectrum (Figure 8.2).

Bioavailability and formulation

A particular problem of *benzylpenicillin* is that it can only be administered parenterally because it is inactivated by gastric acid. The substitution of a phenoxymethyl group for benzyl, giving *phenoxymethylpenicillin* (penicillin V), confers improved acid stability and absorption, but it is less active. Oral bioavailability is improved still further by synthesizing a derivative, e.g. *amoxicillin*, a prodrug of *ampicillin*. It is acid-stable, well absorbed orally and absorption is not affected by the presence of food, making for simpler dosing, the blood levels achieved orally being similar to those following IM injection of ampicillin. It is used widely in clinical practice and is the preferred aminopenicillin, except for the treatment of shigellosis (p. 569). However, it is penicillinase-sensitive and so is often used in combination with the penicillinase inhibitor, *clavulanic acid*.

It is sometimes advantageous to administer a single high dose of penicillin intramuscularly, using the depot product *procaine benzylpenicillin* (unlicensed, available through the named patient mechanism in the UK), but this is only slowly absorbed and is now used only to treat syphilis, to avoid the need for repeated injections of *benzylpenicillin* and the consequent likelihood of patients dropping out from treatment. For other purposes, alternative antimicrobials are now available.

Because *benzylpenicillin* is a polar compound, it is distributed widely in the tissues in body water. However, it does not pass the blood–brain barrier in significant amounts unless very high doses are used, the patient has renal failure or the meninges are inflamed (see meningitis, p. 548). It is excreted rapidly in the urine, mostly as the unchanged compound, and the effect of severe renal failure may be dramatic, e.g. the elimination half-life of *amox-*

icillin is increased from 0.9–2.3 h to 5–20 h, and for *benzylpenicillin* the normal $t_{1/2}$ of 0.5 h is increased to 10 h.

Side-effects

The penicillins have a very wide therapeutic index, i.e. blood levels far higher than those required for treatment need to be attained before dose-related side-effects occur.

A disadvantage that broad-spectrum penicillins share with many other broad-spectrum oral antibacterials is the tendency to cause diarrhoea, owing to the suppression of sensitive species in the gut flora. Consequently, resistant species become dominant, because they no longer have to compete for nutrients with the very large numbers of sensitive organisms. This effect is particularly true of the less well-absorbed, broad-spectrum antimicrobials (e.g. *ampicillin*), whereas the closely-related, well-absorbed *amoxicillin* tends to cause far less diarrhoea.

The main problem associated with penicillins is a **hypersensitivity reaction**. This results from their action as haptens (see Chapter 2), and hypersensitivity developed to one member of the group may preclude the use of all other related compounds. The further a compound is from the basic penicillin structure, the less the chances of a cross-reaction. An individual who is hypersensitive to a penicillin has about a 10% chance of reacting similarly to a cephalosporin or carbapenem (Figure 8.1), but the chances of developing a cross-reaction to a monobactam (e.g. *aztreonam*) are reduced. However, there are reports that patients with an allergy to *ceftazidime* react also to the monobactam *aztreonam*, probably due to a common side-chain moiety.

The hypersensitivity reactions experienced are very variable. The most serious form is **acute anaphylaxis** (see Chapter 2), but a delayed pruritic rash is much more common. Other reactions include urticarial rash (Chapter 13), fever and organ damage. Although a patient presenting with a mild reaction need not necessarily develop a life-threatening reaction on subsequent treatment, penicillins are not prescribed if there is any previous history of allergy to them or the patient claims to be 'allergic'. A careful history of such allergy should be taken, as patients may confuse true allergy with non-allergic side-effects such as diarrhoea, although relying on patients' recall and understanding of an incident is very unreliable. However, if hypersensitivity is a possibility it is safer to choose a different class of antibacterial completely, such as a macrolide (e.g. *erythromycin*), rather than risk a major hypersensitive reaction.

We have noted that penetration into the CNS is normally poor. However, very high doses may produce a concentration sufficient to cause a rare encephalopathy, which may be fatal. This hazard is clearly greater in a patient with renal failure or severe renal impairment. Because of this potential side-effect, penicillins should not normally be given intrathecally.

From a therapeutic standpoint, an important advantage of the structural classification of antimicrobials is to be able to predict and avoid the hypersensitivities or other adverse reactions associated with a particular group.

There is concern over the occurrence of cholestatic jaundice associated with the use of *flucloxacillin*. This reaction is rare, reversible and more likely in older patients, but may occur up to several weeks after treatment has ceased. The UK's CSM advises that:

- *Flucloxacillin* should not be used if there is a patient history of hepatic damage associated with it.
- *Flucloxacillin* should be used with caution in patients with a history of hepatic impairment.
- Careful enquiry should be made about hypersensitivity reactions to beta-lactam antibacterials.

Amoxicillin also carries a risk of cholestatic jaundice and this is about six times greater if it is combined with *clavulanic acid* (as *co-amoxiclav* in the UK), because *clavulanic acid* reduces the renal clearance of *amoxicillin* and so higher concentrations are produced.

Another problem with high doses of penicillins is the increased load of potassium or sodium, according to which salt is used, and should be avoided in patients with renal impairment, e.g. the elderly who are likely to be taking diuretics. The interaction with potassium-sparing diuretics is particularly hazardous. A further group of patients particularly susceptible to electrolyte disturbances is those with **myasthenia gravis**, an autoimmune condition in which antibodies are developed against the acetylcholine receptor protein. Antigen–antibody complexes are deposited in neuromuscular junctions, causing destruction of synaptic acetylcholine receptors, resulting in weakness and fatigability of the respiratory, ocular, eyelid and proximal limb muscles. Large increases in electrolyte concentration may precipitate a crisis requiring respiratory support.

Therapeutic role of penicillins

Benzylpenicillin and *flucloxacillin* are generally used for **cellulitis**, an infection of the loose SC tissue, and in combination with *gentamicin* for **endocarditis** (p. 564).

Amoxicillin is used for simple, i.e. uncomplicated, urinary-tract infection (p. 576) and community-acquired pneumonia. It is also used prophylactically for dental procedures in patients who have had rheumatic fever (see Chapters 4 and 12), because these patients are at risk of endocarditis from organisms liberated into the blood from the mouth.

Phenoxymethylpenicillin or *amoxicillin*, being orally active, are used for prophylaxis post-splenectomy because these patients are at high risk of infections by encapsulated bacteria, e.g. *Strep. pneumoniae*, *Haemophilus* spp. and *Neisseria* spp.

Newer broad-spectrum agents, e.g. *piperacillin* and *ticarcillin*, are used with beta-lactamase inhibitors for the initial empirical therapy of serious hospital-acquired chest and abdominal infections, in which a wide range of organisms are usually implicated.

Cephalosporins

Chemical structure and mode of action

This is the antimicrobial group most closely related structurally to the penicillins, because they all possess a beta-lactam ring (Figure 8.1). As with the penicillins, substitutions on the parent nucleus, 7-amino-cephalosporinic acid, produce agents with differing pharmacokinetic profiles, spectrums of activity and adverse effects. Cephalosporins are conventionally classified in terms of 'generations', three to date, each new generation producing members with improved Gram-negative activity.

Spectrum of activity

Orally active cephalosporins

The **'first-generation'** cephalosporins, *cefadroxil*, *cefalexin* and *cefradine*, and the **'second-generation'**, *cefaclor* is orally active and have a similar spectrum of activity to *ampicillin* (Table 8.2), but these have been largely supplanted by the newer agents. *Cefuroxime axetil* is another second-generation drug that is available in an oral formulation, but is absorbed poorly. It has the same antibacterial spectrum and indications as *cefaclor*, but is less susceptible than earlier cephalosporins to inactivation by beta-lactamases.

As a further complication to this somewhat awkward classification system, there are now **'third-generation'** oral cephalosporins, e.g. *cefixime*, which have improved Gram-negative activity compared with 'second-generation' agents. However, unlike the 'third-generation' parenteral agents they are ineffective against pseudomonads. They have long durations of action and can be given once or twice daily.

Cefixime is long-acting and can be given once or twice daily.

Although cephalosporins are more stable to staphylococcal beta-lactamase than *benzylpenicillin*, they are not completely unaffected by the enzyme, so *flucloxacillin* is a more rational choice for treating staphylococcal infection. Gram-negative organisms also inactivate many of the first- and second-generation cephalosporins by the production of beta-lactamases. Thus, the first-generation cephalosporins, especially *cefradine*, have limited use.

Parenteral cephalosporins

Cefpirome has greater activity against pseudomonads and the greatest beta-lactamase stability of the third-generation cephalosporins. It is licensed in the UK for treating lower respiratory tract, urinary-tract and skin infections, bacteraemia and septicaemia, especially in infections in neutropenic patients (see Chapter 2).

The parenteral third-generation agents, *cefotaxime*, *cefpirome*, *cefpodoxime*, *ceftazidime* and *ceftriaxone* are more active than second-generation cephalosporins against some Gram-negative bacteria, including pseudomonads. However, as often happens, they are less active against Gram-positive organisms, notably *Staph. aureus*. Their broad spectrum of activity may encourage superinfection by fungi and resistant bacteria.

The main application of *ceftriaxone* is in the management of severe infections, e.g. bacterial meningitis (see p. 548), septicaemia and bacterial endocarditis (see p. 564). Its long half-life allows for convenient once-daily dosing and use in Outpatient Antimicrobial Therapy (OPAT) schemes in which patients are discharged from hospital and either attend daily clinics to receive IV antimicrobials, or have them administered at home. This is a recent innovation in the UK. Typical patient groups include those requiring 6 weeks' IV therapy for MRSA osteomyelitis and those needing prolonged therapy for deep-tissue or implant-associated infections.

Therapeutic role

This is much debated, because the spectrum of action of cephalosporins can be covered by various penicillins and other cheaper antibacterials. The use of IV cephalosporins as first-line agents is often determined by the local antimicrobial policy, where recommendations for antimicrobial prescribing in a particular area are made by the local hospital microbiology department. Thus a hospital might employ *ceftazidime* as first-line therapy for severe *Pseudomonas* infection, often in combination with an aminoglycoside, in preference to an aminoglycoside–ureidopenicillin combination.

This is because of the risk of *Clostridium difficile*-associated diarrhoea (antibiotic-associated colitis, AAC; p. 570) with *ceftazidime*, its propensity to select for extended-spectrum beta-lactamase (ESBL) producers, and because of a preference to avoid aminoglycosides, owing to their potential toxicity (p. 524). Additionally, many hospitals now find it necessary to include carbapenems in their treatment protocols because of the increased prevalence of ESBL producers.

The first- and second-generation oral cephalosporins remain useful for urinary-tract infections unresponsive to other antibacterials, especially in pregnancy, and for respiratory tract, middle ear, paranasal and frontal sinus, skin and soft tissue infections. However, antimicrobials are not recommended for the first-line treatment of **otitis media**, because many of these infections are viral and clear without antimicrobial intervention. An antimicrobial is indicated if the infection does not settle in 3 days or if there are complications. The agents usually used to treat infected **otitis externa** are those not used sytemically, e.g. *neomycin* and *clioquinol*, but these should not be used for more than about 7 days because prolonged treatment may cause local sensitivity reactions and predispose to resistant fungal infections.

First-line uses of agents such as *cefuroxime* may include acute pancreatitis, prophylaxis before surgery (e.g. appendectomy), treatment of severe community-acquired pneumonia requiring hospital admission, and pyrexia of unknown origin (PUO; p. 539). *Cefradine* and *cefalexin* are more suitable for dental use, largely for their activity against the *Streptococcus viridans* group. However, if resistant bacteria are known to be present, prophylaxis and therapy must be guided by the results of laboratory tests, as usual. Other possible applications for first-line use include exacerbations of COPD (see Chapter 5) if *H. influenzae* is suspected, and PUO. However, a carbapenem is often preferred in acute pancreatitis.

Ceftriaxone is used for the late symptoms of Lyme disease, caused by a tick-borne spirochaete *Borrelia burgdorferi*, which is widespread in rural wooded areas of Europe and North America. Although the initial symptoms are mild (arthralgia, skin rash, fever, etc.) this is an increasingly important disease, because some weeks to months later patients often develop arthritis and severe, persistent cardiovascular and neurological problems. *Ceftriaxone* is also used in some types of endocarditis (p. 564), the empirical treatment of meningitis (p. 551) and brain abscesses, and in OPAT schemes (see above).

Cefadroxil and the oral prodrug of *cefuroxime*, *cefuroxime axetil*, have poor oral bioavailability, but are useful in the treatment of *H. influenzae* chest infections that are resistant to *ampicillin*. However, it is doubtful whether they should be used as first-line agents in the community on grounds of cost and the danger of development of cephalosporin resistance.

Side-effects

Although the very early cephalosporins, *cefalotin* and *cefaloridine*, caused significant renal damage, this does not occur with later members of the group.

Hypersensitivity reactions similar to those with the penicillins are encountered and cross-reactions may occur.

Diarrhoea, and sometimes AAC (p. 570) can occur, together with nausea and vomiting and malaise. Blood disorders, e.g. haemolytic anaemia and leucopenia, may also arise. The indiscriminate use of third-generation cephalosporins is thought to promote the spread of ESBL-producing organisms (see above).

Aminoglycosides

Chemical structure and mode of action

Streptomycin, first isolated from the fungus *Streptomyces griseus* in 1944, revolutionized the treatment of TB. However, this has been supplanted by newer antimicrobials (p. 574).

The class name describes the chemical structure of this group; they are glycosidally linked aminosugars.

The most widely used are *gentamicin*, *tobramycin* and *amikacin*, which are members of the kanamycin group, although *kanamycin* itself is no longer used in the UK. Despite the availability of numerous derivatives, the properties of the kanamycin group vary little. The other aminoglycosides have few clinical applications.

The aminoglycosides act by interfering with bacterial protein synthesis via actions on bacterial messenger and transfer RNAs (mRNA, tRNA). Miscoding causes incorrect amino acid insertion into peptide chains, causing loss of the protein activity and suppressing cell growth, eventually causing cell death.

Spectrum of activity

Gentamicin is the aminoglycoside of choice in the UK. The other clinically useful members of the kanamycin group (*tobramycin, amikacin* and *netilmicin*) have very similar activity against a wide variety of Gram-negative bacteria (Table 8.2), particularly pseudomonads, and there is little to choose between them. *Amikacin* is claimed to have greater stability to inactivating enzymes produced by *Pseudomonas* spp. and is active against some Gram-negative species with acquired *gentamicin* resistance. All aminoglycosides are active against *Proteus* spp., but anaerobic bacteria are resistant. *Gentamicin* is useful for treating staphylococcal infections but has only moderate activity against streptococci. It is synergistic with penicillin against these organisms, e.g. *Enterococcus faecalis*, possibly by increasing cell permeability to penicillin. *Gentamicin* is the basis of treatment for most types of endocarditis (p. 564).

Other aminoglycosides have more specific uses. *Spectinomycin* is highly effective against gonococci but is inactive against other organisms, so it is only used for the treatment of penicillin-resistant gonorrhoea. *Streptomycin* is rarely used in the UK because of problems with toxicity and resistance and because it can only be administered intramuscularly. However, it is used occasionally as a second/third-line agent for resistant TB (p. 574) and for some cases of enterococcal endocarditis. It is also used as an adjunct to *doxycycline* for **brucellosis**, a rather unpleasant localized (two-thirds of patients) or systemic (one-third) infection that may persist for a year. It is usually contracted by drinking unpasteurized cows' or goats' milk and is rare in the UK because it has been eliminated almost completely from cattle there.

Gentamicin is used as single low-dose prophylaxis before changing urinary catheters, when an infection has been confirmed, and in larger doses as part of the therapy of severe Gram-negative infections.

Amikacin is sometimes used in place of *gentamicin* when resistance to the latter has been demonstrated, and as a second-line agent for treating multi-drug-resistant TB (MDR-TB).

Tobramycin is used as a nebulized formulation in the management of cystic fibrosis.

Neomycin is too toxic for parenteral use. Given orally, it retains its antibacterial activity in the gut lumen and has been used to reduce the gut flora before gastrointestinal surgery. Although it is often used as an antiseptic in topical corticosteroid preparations, e.g. in some skin creams and eye drops, it is liable to cause skin and conjunctival sensitization.

Pharmacokinetics

The aminoglycosides are highly polar, not significantly absorbed orally, and are largely excreted unchanged via the kidney. Good renal function is an important factor in their safe use. They are usually administered parenterally unless intended for topical use (e.g. in eye drops), and are generally well distributed in the tissues after parenteral administration, but penetrate the CSF poorly unless the meninges are inflamed.

Toxicity

The aminoglycosides are among the most toxic antimicrobials. **Nephrotoxicity** is a rare, but serious, problem if used in patients with previous renal impairment, but **ototoxicity** is more common and may cause hearing impairment or even deafness. These effects are related to plasma levels, although it has been suggested that some ototoxicity may occur even with careful control of *gentamicin* dosage if this is given for longer courses than usual. Courses are preferably no longer than 7 days. Other rare side-effects include hypersensitivity reactions and neuromuscular blockade. For the latter reason they must be avoided in **myasthenia gravis** (see above).

When aminoglycosides are used, especially in high doses for serious infections, initial and maintenance doses are calculated from the patient's weight and serum creatinine level or determined using a nomogram, to ensure appropriate blood levels and adequate renal clearance. Adjustments are then made, based on the results of therapeutic drug monitoring to determine plasma peak and trough levels. As toxicity appears to be associated with sustained trough levels rather than the peak level attained immediately post-dose, once-daily dosing of an aminoglycoside is now the treatment mode of choice in most situations.

The activity of these drugs is concentration-dependent and they exhibit a long post-dose antimicrobial action, retarding regrowth of organisms despite the absence of significant drug levels, because regrowth requires extensive anabolic synthesis. Therefore a single daily dose of *gentamicin* would be expected to produce blood levels adequate to treat *Pseudomonas* infections and accumulation is avoided, allowing trough levels to fall below the 2 mg/L known to be associated with both ototoxicity and nephrotoxicity. In practice, the target trough level is <1 mg/L and regular plasma level drug monitoring is still prudent. Once-daily dosing is unsuitable in endocarditis, where regular smaller doses are required to produce maximal synergy with penicillin therapy.

Other antibacterial agents

The penicillins, cephalosporins and aminoglycosides are the most widely used groups of antibacterials, and provide the first-line agents for the treatment of many infections. The groups discussed next are older agents whose use is diminishing (e.g. sulphonamides), recent introductions whose full potential has yet to be realized (e.g. new beta-lactams), or groups represented by only a few related agents in clinical use (e.g. the macrolides).

Newer beta-lactam antimicrobials

Two relatively new classes, the carbapenems and monobactams, have widened the choice.

Imipenem is a very broad-spectrum carbapenem that is active against most Gram-negative organisms, including *Pseudomonas*, and has useful activity against a range of Gram-positive bacteria and anaerobes. Metabolism of *imipenem* by renal dihydropeptidases tended to shorten the half-life of the antimicrobial considerably, but this problem has been overcome by co-administration with *cilastatin*, an alpha-dihydropeptidase inhibitor that prevents inactivation in the kidney. However, this combination has been largely superseded by *meropenem*, which has a similar spectrum of activity, and does not require the co-administration of *cilastatin*, because it is not metabolized similarly. Further, *imipenem* has significant potential to cause convulsions if overdosed with respect to renal function. *Meropenem* has less seizure potential and so lessens this risk in renal failure.

Ertapenem is a new carbapenem that has the advantage of once-daily administration, but does not cover *Pseudomonas* infections. This limits its utility as an empirical agent, but may be advantageous in the hospital setting due to the potential reduction of selection for carbapenem-resistant pseudomonads.

Faropenem, which is active orally, is not available in the UK, but is used in Japan and the USA for the treatment of upper respiratory tract infections.

Aztreonam is the only monobactam in general use in the UK. It is active only against aerobic Gram-negative organisms, notably *Ps. aeruginosa*, and must be given parenterally. Its clinical utility is limited by its narrow spectrum of activity, but it is used in drug trials as a comparator agent.

Macrolides

The most important member of this group is *erythromycin*. Other macrolides, such as *clindamycin* and *lincomycin*, are now less used in the UK owing to their associated incidence of AAC (pp. 570 and Chapter 3). *Clarithromycin* and *azithromycin* are recent additions with superior bioavailability to *erythromycin*, and reduced potential to cause nausea and vomiting, the chief adverse effects of the latter.

Erythromycin is bacteriostatic at the serum levels achieved with usual oral doses, but the higher levels achieved with IV use are bactericidal. It interferes with bacterial protein synthesis by inhibiting the transfer of amino acids from tRNA to growing peptide chains. *Erythromycin* is particularly effective against Gram-positive organisms (Table 8.2) and is a very useful alternative for patients who are hypersensitive to penicillins, or believed to be so, but resistance is now common. It has limited application in the treatment of Gram-negative infections because cell wall penetration is poor, although some *Haemophilus* strains are sensitive. Activity is particularly good against bacteria that do not have a cell wall, e.g. mycoplasmas, and it is the agent of choice for treating *Legionella* pneumonia, but high doses must be used, e.g. 4 g/day. Gastrointestinal upset is reported to be less of a problem with low doses, e.g. 1 g/day, and with *clarithromycin* and *azithromycin*.

Clarithromycin, is more active than *erythromycin* and is given twice daily, or once daily as an extended-release formulation, although the latter is not suitable for use in renal impairment. A further important advantage of both *clarithromycin* and *azithromycin* is enhanced activity against *Haemophilus* spp. A major distinction between these two agents is that while *azithromycin* has superior tissue penetration it achieves poorer sustained blood levels than *clarithromycin*, so the latter is preferred to treat septicaemia. Due to its long tissue half-life *clarithromycin* can be given only once daily for tissue infections and so is preferred for conditions such as impetigo and carbuncles.

The main indications for *azithromycin* are to treat Lyme disease (p. 523), as a convenient single-dose therapy for treating *Chlamydia trachomatis*, the commonest cause of blindness worldwide, and for the prophylaxis of endocarditis (unlicensed application, see p. 564 and Chapter 4) in children. Chlamydias are the most common cause of sexually transmitted infection and these are inreasing, especially in women, and *Chl. trachomatis* is present in about 40% of these.

Telithromycin, a ketolide derivative of *erythromycin*, has a similar activity spectrum and is especially useful for treating sinusitis, community-acquired pneumonia, exacerbations of COPD (see Chapter 5), and pharyngitis and tonsillitis caused by resistant streptococci. However, it has been reported recently to cause an increased rate of hepatic side-effects, including cholestatic jaundice, so it should not be used in patients with hepatic or renal impairment. It may also prolong the QT interval (see Chapter 4) and is contra-indicated if there is a personal or family history of QT prolongation.

Chloramphenicol

This synthetic, bacteriostatic agent has a very broad spectrum of activity. The mode of action is by inhibition of bacterial protein synthesis, competing with mRNA for bacterial ribosomal binding. It also inhibits peptidyl transferase, thus preventing the addition of amino acids to growing peptide chains.

Major drawbacks to its use include bone marrow toxicity and the development of resistance. Being among the cheapest of broad-spectrum agents, *chloramphenicol* has been used extensively and often inappropriately in the Third World for treating many types of infection. Consequently, this very useful agent has become virtually ineffective in the treatment of various serious endemic infections, e.g. typhoid fever, in some countries.

The incidence of aplastic anaemia associated with *chloramphenicol* has led to the general recommendation that it should only be used systemically for life-threatening infections resistant to other agents. Plasma level monitoring is required for neonates, who metabolize and excrete it poorly, so it is best avoided in this patient group. Monitoring is also desirable for children under 4, in the elderly and in patients with hepatic impairment. Peak concentration, 1 h after IV use, should not exceed 25 mg/L and trough concentrations determined immediately pre-dose should not exceed 15 mg/L.

Owing to the development of many safer broad-spectrum antibacterials, the only principal systemic indication for *chloramphenicol* is the treatment of meningitis caused by *H. influenzae*, when cephalosporins cannot be used owing to severe drug allergies. In this case, the risks of brain damage or death from the infection outweigh the risks from the drug.

Chloramphenicol still has valuable topical use in the treatment of eye infections, e.g. severe conjunctivitis, because it penetrates well into optic tissues. There have been occasional reports of aplastic anaemia, possibly associated with the small doses used in eye preparations, and this has led some physicians to advise against its use for bacterial conjunctivitis. However, there is little direct evidence of a causal relationship and the incidence of such reactions seems no greater than that observed for aplastic anaemia in the general population, so the eye drops are now available OTC from pharmacies without prescription. Although ear drops, formulated in propylene glycol, are available there is a high incidence of sensitivity reactions to the vehicle and are regarded as less suitable for general prescribing. Moreover, the OTC prescribing of ear drops for the treatment of moderate to severe ear pain, usually due to otitis media, is highly undesirable (p. 531) because of lack of efficacy, the risk of hearing loss, or even meningitis, and the risk of missing a diagnosis of meningitis. Instead, ear drops of *ciprofloxacin* and *ofloxacin* are available on a named-patient basis for treating chronic otitis media associated with perforation of the ear drum (unlicensed indication) and avoid the use of the potentially ototoxic aminoglycosides or polymyxins.

Tetracyclines

Like *chloramphenicol*, and introduced at the same time, the tetracyclines are broad-spectrum bacteriostatic agents that inhibit bacterial protein synthesis. Their Gram-negative activity is unimpressive because many organisms, including *Pseudomonas* and *Proteus* spp., are intrinsically resistant, and resistance has emerged with *Haemophilus*. Even in Gram-positive infections, acquired resistance has led to reduced usage.

The group contains a number of closely related compounds, all of which have a very similar spectrum of activity but different pharmacokinetic profiles. *Oxytetracycline* has largely replaced *tetracycline* for oral use owing to its superior bioavailability.

The long half-life of *doxycycline* allows once-daily dosage and *minocycline*, another long-acting agent, requires twice-daily dosing. The latter has an extended spectrum, being active against *N. meningitidis*, but it causes dizziness and vertigo and has been superseded by *rifampicin* (see below) for prophylaxis in meningitis contacts.

Their low toxicity has made this group a popular choice for the treatment of chest infections in the community. Interestingly, it has been claimed by some that the fall in popularity of the tetracyclines, due to resistance, has produced a decline in certain resistant strains of bacteria.

These agents are used principally for gonorrheal and chlamydial infections, which often occur together in sexually transmitted disease and for treatment of other chlamydial infections, e.g. trachoma, urethritis, salpingitis (infection of the Fallopian tubes, possibly causing infertility in women) and psittacosis. Tetracyclines (and *rifampicin*) are also used to treat brucellosis, an infection contracted from infected cows, sheep and goats (p. 524), and Lyme disease (p. 523).

Tetracyclines are still widely used for the treatment of acne, when they are given orally at low dosage for courses lasting many months, and are also applied topically. Topical application is also used for infections of the skin or eyes.

Doxycycline and *minocycline* are the only tetracyclines that can be administered safely in renal impairment. However, caution is required in patients with hepatic impairment. *Doxycycline* is also used for malaria prophylaxis in high-risk areas.

Because they cause irreversible staining of teeth in children and possibly dental hypoplasia (by complexing with calcium in developing teeth and bone), they are contra-indicated in pregnancy and in children under 12 years of age. These drugs are chelating agents, reacting with salts of calcium in supplements and milk, aluminium and magnesium in antacids, and iron and zinc. This results in decreased absorption if taken with food, so they should be taken on an empty stomach.

Sulphonamides and trimethoprim

Sulphonamides were the earliest synthetic antibacterials to be used, but have been largely replaced by more effective agents. They are bacteriostatic, being competitive inhibitors of *p*-aminobenzoic acid uptake in bacterial folate synthesis (see Figure 11.4). Because humans cannot synthesize folate and require it to be supplied preformed in their diet, sulphonamides are not toxic to humans by this mechanism.

Determining true MICs for sulphonamides is difficult because their action is markedly affected by *p*-aminobenzoic acid in the culture media used. Because many previously susceptible strains are now resistant it is difficult to be sure of their true spectrum of activity.

Sulphonamides have been used in the treatment of a variety of infections, and both Gram-negative and Gram-positive organisms may be sensitive, so the theoretical spectrum is quite broad. Their slow onset of action, high incidence of side-effects (e.g. renal and hepatic damage, hypersensitivity and blood dyscrasias) and pattern of resistance have greatly limited their use. Until recently, the only widely used member of the group was *sulfamethoxazole*, usually in combination with another folate synthesis inhibitor *trimethoprim* (as *co-trimoxazole* in the UK; Table 8.2). Synergism occurs between these two agents that act at different points in the folate synthetic pathway, but in clinical practice *trimethoprim* alone is equally effective in most situations.

Recent fears over the incidence of bone marrow suppression have further limited the indications for *co-trimoxazole*. The most important remaining indication is the prevention and treatment of *Pneumocystis jiroveci* (formerly *Pn. carinii*) pneumonia in HIV-positive patients and in those who are immunosuppressed, e.g. following organ transplantation. The UK CSM advises that *co-trimoxazole* should now be considered only for treating acute exacerbations of COPD (see Chapter 5) and sensitive urinary-tract infections (p. 576), and then only when there are good reasons to prefer it. It should also be used for treating the protozoal infection, toxoplasmosis, which is acquired from cats, and nocardiosis.

Nocardia is branching bacterium, and infections are acquired by walking barefoot on infected soil, producing a local lesion known as a mycetoma, or by inhalation. The pulmonary disease is seen in immunocompromised individuals, causing fever, cough and haemoptysis. If immunosuppression is severe, this becomes a widespread systemic infection.

Nitroimidazoles

The principal agent in this group is *metronidazole*, originally employed successfully in the treatment of trichomoniasis, and now a widely used antiprotozoal agent, e.g. for amoebiasis and giardiasis (see Chapter 3). It is also effective and used frequently in the treatment and prophylaxis of anaerobic bacterial infections, caused by either *Bacteroides fragilis* or clostridia, especially following gut surgery or similar 'dirty' surgery. *Metronidazole* is also used to treat mouth infections, e.g. acute ulcerative gingivitis, a gum infection caused by spirochaetes or other mouth commensals if oral hygiene is poor. Further common uses are the eradication of *H. pylori* from the stomach (see Chapter 3) and the treatment of rosacea (see Chapter 13).

Resistance to *metronidazole* is uncommon. Its use is limited by gastrointestinal disturbance and the occurrence of a 'disulfiram-like' reaction in patients drinking alcohol, a consequence of the inhibition of acetaldehyde hydrogenase. The resultant accumulation of acetaldehyde causes flushing, orthostatic hypotension, causing faints, central nervous effects, e.g. dizziness, headache and epileptiform seizures, and peripheral neuropathy.

Disulfiram is used as an adjunct to psychotherapy in the treatment of alcohol dependence, but is of doubtful value because heavy drinkers usually prefer to give up the disulfiram. Further, the reaction is triggered by contact with the very small amounts of alcohol used in some medicines, even that used in some mouthwashes.

The newer compound *tinidazole* is used similarly to *metronidazole*. Its longer duration of action means that it can be given less frequently.

Quinolones

The prototype of the class, *nalidixic acid*, has the disadvantage of low activity, poor tissue concentration and the rapid development of acquired resistance, and so is now rarely used.

The more recently introduced fluoroquinolones have wider therapeutic applications. *Ciprofloxacin*, the first to enter clinical use, is active against Gram-negative and, to a lesser extent, Gram-positive organisms (Table 8.2). Important exceptions include the anaerobic species *Bacteroides fragilis* and *Cl. difficile*, some pseudomonads, *Ent. faecalis* and *Strep. pneumoniae*. Its main indication is therefore in the treatment of aerobic Gram-negative infections. Its principal advantage over other antimicrobials is that it is the only orally active antipseudomonal agent.

Ciprofloxacin is used with other antimicrobials as a first-line treatment for pulmonary or gastrointestinal anthrax, but definitive treatment depends on laboratory data.

The newer 'third-generation' quinolones, *levofloxacin* and *ofloxacin*, which is a racemic mixture of the S-isomer *levofloxacin* and the R-isomer, have increased activity against Gram-positive organisms, e.g. *Strep. pneumoniae*, and may be administered once daily.

Norfloxacin is given twice daily, but is licensed only for urinary-tract infections and prostatitis.

Quinolones act by interfering with bacterial DNA gyrase, responsible for the supercoiling of DNA. The resultant aberrant DNA cannot fit the bacterial cytoplasmic space, resulting in rapid cell death. This mode of action has the advantage of preventing plasmid formation and therefore plasmid-mediated resistance, although resistance can still develop by chromosomal mutation.

Levofloxacin, *moxifloxacin* and *ofloxacin* are recent additions to this group, with the important advantage of greater activity against Gram-

positive pathogens. However, *ciprofloxacin*, *levofloxacin* and *ofloxacin* are not active against MRSA and are contra-indicated if this organism is suspected.

Moxifloxacin is used as a second-line agent for treating community-acquired pneumonia and sinusitis, and as a reserve agent for acute exacerbations of COPD (see Chapter 5), if all other treatments have failed or are contra-indicated: because this group comprises an older population the risk of side-effects is increased. It has some activity against anaerobes.

Side-effects

Almost any body system may be involved. All quinolones are liable to cause a range of gastrointestinal disorders, but AAC (p. 570) is rare. CNS effects include headache, dizziness and sleep disturbance. Although convulsions are uncommon, quinolones should not be used in patients with epilepsy (see Chapter 6) or those who have a reduced seizure threshold. Taking NSAIDs at the same time may increase the seizure risk. The risk of neurological impairment is increased by alcohol and this is one group of antimicrobials for which the appropriate response to the question "Can I drink with this?" is a firm "No".

Pruritis and rashes may occur (see Chapter 13), but the latter are rarely serious. Patients should avoid excessive exposure to sunlight and if photosensitization occurs the drug should be discontinued: this also applies if psychiatric, neurological or hypersensitivity reactions occur, including severe rash.

The occasional occurrence of tendon damage and rupture within 48 h of use has led the UK CSM to issue specific advice. Previous tendon inflammation with any of this group is an absolute contra-indication to quinolone treatment. The risk of tendon damage is increased by the concomitant use of corticosteroids and elderly patients are more prone to tendonitis. If tendonitis is suspected the drug must be discontinued immediately.

They should be used with caution in pregnancy, during breastfeeding and in young children or adolescents, because of possible damage to weight-bearing joints.

Moxifloxacin is not suitable for use in hepatic impairment or with other drugs that prolong the QT interval or if there is a history of IHD, electrolyte disturbances or heart failure with a reduced left ventricular injection fraction (see Chapter 4).

Levofloxacin appears to be less likely to cause problem side-effects than other quinolones.

Rifamycins

The chief member of this group, *rifampicin*, will be considered in greater detail in the treatment of TB in combination with other antibacterials (p. 574). It is also active against *M. leprae* (causing leprosy), staphylococci, various mycoplasmas, meningococci and *Legionella pneumophila*, although its wider application has been limited by fears of *M. tuberculosis* resistance. However, it is used prophylactically in close contacts of meningococcal meningitis and, in combination with other drugs, e.g. *fusidic acid*, for the treatment of serious infections due to *rifamycin*-sensitive MRSA. It is also used to treat brucellosis, but this disease is rare in the UK because it has been virtually eliminated from cattle.

Rifabutin has similar properties. It is also used for the treatment of non-tubercular disease due to other mycobacteria and for the prophylaxis of *M. avium-intracellulare* complex in immunocompromised subjects, e.g. in HIV/AIDS and post-transplant patients.

The rifamycins have numerous side-effects, e.g. gastrointestinal symptoms, including AAC (p. 570), headache, drowsiness, influenza-like symptoms, shortness of breath, thrombophlebitis, collapse and shock, haemolytic anaemia (see Chapter 11), acute renal failure (see Chapter 14), jaundice, oedema, thrombocytopenic purpura (see Chapter 11) and exfoliative dermatitis. They are hepatotoxic, so liver function tests should be done before commencing treatment and regularly during treatment, especially in the first 2 months (see TB; p. 574). Jaundice is a contra-indication to the use of rifamycins.

They induce liver enzymes, with potentially serious consequences (Chapter 3). The effectiveness of many drugs will be reduced when *rifamycin* treatment commences and will return to normal when treatment ceases, but will be enhanced if doses have been increased recently. The plasma levels of essential drugs, e.g., corticosteroids, *phenytoin*, sulphonylureas (in type 2 diabetes mellitus), and oral contraceptives, should be monitored. Other end-points, e.g. clotting function with anticoagulants, should also be determined.

Vancomycin and teicoplanin

These glycopeptides, which inhibit cell wall synthesis, have a bactericidal action against aerobic and anaerobic Gram-positive bacteria. They are ineffective in Gram-negative infections.

Vancomycin is not significantly absorbed from the gut, but is given orally every 6 h for up to 10 days to treat AAC with *Cl. difficile* overgrowth. It is given by IV infusion for the treatment of endocarditis (see Chapter 4 and p. 564) caused by Gram-positive cocci, though there are persistent reports of resistant enterococci (e.g. *Ent. faecalis* and *Strep. viridans*). It has been particularly useful systemically as a treatment for MRSA infection and has been used for treating peritonitis in peritoneal dialysis patients (see Chapter 14). For this latter purpose, it has been added to the dialysis fluid, but this is an unlicensed route. Because of its long half-life it can be given 12-hourly.

Because resistance has been reported it should be reserved for treating serious, resistant infections and used under laboratory guidance.

Although relatively expensive and somewhat nephrotoxic there is often little alternative when treating MRSA (but see below).

Teicoplanin is similar to *vancomycin* and is also indicated for the treatment of MRSA, with similar precautions. Advantages are its long half-life, allowing once-daily dosing, and that it can be given by IM injection, though this is painful.

Linezolid

This is the first of a new class of antimicrobials, the **oxazolidinones**, which inhibit protein synthesis by preventing the association of mRNAs with ribosomes. It is effective against MRSA and other Gram-positive bacteria, including **vancomycin-resistant enterococci (VRE)**, but is ineffective against Gram-negative species.

The chief problems with this agent are reversible myelosuppression and neurotoxicity. It has excellent tissue penetration, but resistance can develop readily, especially if doses below those recommended are used and if treatment is prolonged.

Thus this is another reserve antimicrobial for treating infections resistant to other drugs or if other agents are not tolerated.

Sodium fusidate

This is the only antibacterial of steroid structure in clinical use. It is a narrow-spectrum agent, the only indication being the treatment of staphylococcal infection. It is used in conjunction with either *penicillin* or *erythromycin* because resistance is likely to occur if used alone.

It is used in staphylococcal endocarditis (p. 564) and because it is concentrated in bone, combinations with *sodium fusidate* are often used in osteomyelitis, a difficult-to-treat, usually staphylococcal, bone infection.

Sodium fusidate is also used topically for staphylococcal skin infections and the ocular preparation has gained in popularity for the treatment of conjunctivitis, as an alternative to *chloramphenicol* with its potential adverse effects on bone marrow.

It is cleared hepatically and renally, so clearance may be delayed in hepatic and gallbladder disease and biliary obstruction. Renal impairment may be accompanied by jaundice. Because of these associations, hepatic monitoring should be used if treatment is prolonged.

Peptide antimicrobials: polymyxins

Only two members of this group of decapeptide antimicrobials are used currently, *polymyxin B* and the related compound *colistin* (polymyxin E). They act by binding to Gram-negative cell membranes, altering their permeability.

Being highly polar, they are not absorbed orally. Reports from 30–40 years ago recorded serious neurotoxicity and nephrotoxicity when given parenterally. Thus they have been used only topically until recently, e.g. in the eradication of nasal carriage of MRSA prior to surgery, and in eye drops. They are active against many Gram-negative organisms, including *Ps. aeruginosa* and *colistin* is sometimes used orally, usually with *nystatin*, for reducing the normal gut flora in immunosuppressed patients. However, resistant Gram-negative species occur, e.g. strains of *Ps. aeruginosa*, so they are not recommended for treating gastrointestinal infections. *Colistin* is also used as a nebulized inhalation to treat *Ps. aeruginosa* lung colonization in cystic fibrosis.

Multidrug-resistant Gram-negative organisms, e.g. *Acinetobacter baumannii*, *K. pneumoniae* and *Ps. aeruginosa*, are increasingly causing problems in the intensive care units of large hospitals. Some strains are now sensitive only to *colistin* and *polymyxin B*, thus forcing the use of agents that had previously been abandoned owing to their toxicity. Accordingly, the utility and toxicity of these agents are being reappraised for use against multidrug-resistant Gram-negative organisms (see References and further reading).

They are not used in ear drops because of the risk of serious ototoxicity. Members of this group have been used topically, often in combination, to treat infected wounds and in eye drops, and are included in some OTC topical products. However, the use of any topical antimicrobial for wounds is to be discouraged owing to problems with acquired resistance, healing and skin sensitization: it would be a seriously retrograde outcome if the potential value of the polymyxins as rescue drugs in serious Gram-negative infections were to be lost as a consequence of their trivial use.

Streptogramin antimicrobials

There are only two members of this group, *quinupristin* and *dalfopristin*, which are always used together in a fixed combination. Their sole applications are in the treatment of serious Gram-positive infections that are resistant to other antimicrobials and in patients in whom other treatments cannot be used. They are not active against *Ent. faecalis* and should be used with other antimicrobials for mixed infections involving Gram-negative bacteria.

Newer antibacterial agents

Tigecycline is now licensed in the UK for treating complex bacterial skin infections, e.g. impetigo and erysipelas, and complex skin and soft tissue infections (cSSTIs), e.g. cellulitis and intra-abdominal infections (peritonitis). It is a very broad-spectrum agent, active against Gram-positive organisms, including MRSA and VRE, and most Gram-negatives, but excluding *Proteus* and *Pseudomonas* species.

Daptomycin is licensed in the USA, also for treating cSSTIs, but is active only against Gram-positive organisms, including MRSA and VRE. It has a novel mechanism of action, involving Ca^{2+}-mediated membrane disruption. It is rapidly bactericidal *in vitro* and can be given once daily.

Oritavancin and *dalbovancin* are extended half-life glycopeptides, designed to permit dosing once weekly. They are not yet licensed in the UK.

Antifungal agents

Fungal infections require quite separate agents from those effective against bacteria. Included here are agents active against true filamentous fungi, e.g. *Aspergillus* spp., and those used for treating yeast infections, e.g. *Candida albicans*.

Candida infections, e.g. oropharyngeal and vaginal **thrush**, are common and troublesome, and two principal groups of agents are used in their treatment: the polyene antimicrobials and the imidazoles.

Another common fungal infection in humans is **tinea**, caused by the filamentous fungi known collectively as dermatophytes. Tinea may affect various areas of the body surface, causing the skin infections known as ringworm and athlete's foot. Fungal infections of the skin and, especially, nails are usually difficult to eradicate, so therapy is often prolonged.

More serious systemic fungal infections, e.g. pulmonary aspergillosis, or those caused by *Cryptococcus* and *Pneumocystis* spp. are usually opportunistic infections in immunocompromised patients, in whom they may be life-threatening. Cryptococcosis is treated with prolonged IV infusion of *amphotericin* plus *fluconazole* (see below) and is followed by *fluconazole* PO for 8 weeks. *Pneumocystis* pneumonia requires parenteral therapy with high-dose *co-trimoxazole*. IV *pentamidine isetionate* is used in patients with severe disease who cannot tolerate *co-trimoxazole*, but this may cause severe hypotension during the infusion or immediately afterwards. Mild to moderate infections in patients who cannot tolerate *co-trimoxazole* can be treated PO with *atovaquone*, or the antileprotic agent *dapsone* plus *trimethoprim* (unlicensed indication). A combination of *clindamycin* and the antimalarial *primaquine* is also used (unlicensed indication), but is rather toxic.

A 21-day course of a corticosteroid is used in HIV-positive patients with moderate to severe disease, started at the same time as the anti-pneumocystis medication. The latter should be continued for several days after the corticosteroid is withdrawn and continued until all infection has been cleared. Some patients will need long-term prophylaxis.

Because *Pneumocystis* infection is so common in HIV/AIDS patients, antimicrobial prophylaxis with oral *co-trimoxazole* or inhaled *pentamidine isetionate* is used widely. However, inhaled *pentamidine* does not protect against extra-pulmonary disease. *Dapsone* can also be used. *Atovaquone* is used occasionally, but this is an unlicensed indication.

Imidazoles

Clotrimazole, miconazole and *niridazole* are all used topically in the treatment of vaginal thrush. *Miconazole* gel is a useful alternative to *nystatin* for the treatment of oropharyngeal thrush. The newer imidazoles are well absorbed. The first of the orally active agents was *ketoconazole*, but this is associated with severe, even fatal, hepatotoxicity if administered at high doses or in long courses so it should be reserved for serious systemic infections.

Newer, less toxic agents, e.g. *fluconazole*, are available and are useful for the treatment of candidiasis. However, resistant candidiasis, e.g. caused by *Candida glabrata* and *C. krusei*, is a recurring problem in sexually transmitted disease clinics. *Fluconazole* is used parenterally for these and other invasive fungal infections, but resistance is common.

Parenteral *voriconazole* may be used for fluconazole-resistant and life-threatening fungal infections. However, it is rather toxic and has very many side-effects, including blurred vision, photophobia and altered visual perception, which affects 30% of patients, but usually disappears with continued treatment. The IV formulation is unsuitable for patients with a creatinine clearance <30 mL/min, owing to the accumulation of a carrier molecule (sulphobutylether beta cyclodextrin sodium). Careful monitoring is essential, e.g. hepatic, renal, respiratory and cardiac function both before and during treatment and, similarly, blood counts and serum electrolytes. The drug has many interactions, notably with anti-HIV and immunosuppressant agents. *Voriconazole* is active against *Candida* and *Aspergillus* species and is often the agent of choice for confirmed pulmonary aspergillosis. Because it is available in an oral formulation it can be used to switch patients from IV administration, thus permitting the discharge from hospital of patients being treated for serious fungal infection once the initial hazard is passed.

Itraconazole has a similar activity spectrum to *voriconazole* and is available as oral and IV infusion formulations. The oral liquid form has a much higher bioavailability than the capsules. However, even when the oral liquid is used for the prophylaxis of fungal infection in neutropenic patients (see Chapter 2), serum levels should be monitored to ensure adequate protection. Parenteral *itraconazole* is less toxic than *voriconazole*, but may cause rare, life-threatening hepatotoxicity. Patients should therefore be warned to report immediately any fatigue, anorexia, nausea, abdominal pain, or dark urine, due to cholestasis (see Chapter 3).

Polyenes

Examples of these are *amphotericin* and *nystatin*, which damage the fungal cell membrane to cause cytoplasmic leakage. They are not absorbed orally and may be administered as lozenges or mouthwashes for treating oropharyngeal thrush. For vaginal thrush, *nystatin* is administered as a pessary, but has largely been replaced by the imidazoles.

Amphotericin is administered parenterally for serious systemic fungal or yeast infections, but may cause severe renal damage, even at low doses, and also severe neurological side-effects, including deafness and convulsions. Skin rashes may necessitate stopping treatment. Anaphylaxis (see Chapter 2) is fortunately rare, but the CSM recommends giving a test dose before any IV use, the patient being supervised for 30 min afterwards.

Liposomal formulations are somewhat more effective and less toxic than the original sodium deoxycholate complex for IV use. However, nephrotoxicity may still be a problem. They are very expensive compared to the sodium deoxycholate complex.

Other antifungals

Fungal infections of the scalp and nails respond well to oral *griseofulvin*, which accumulates in those tissues, although this may need to be administered continuously for up to 6 months, possibly 12 months for infection of the toenails. Shorter courses of treatment and better cure rates are achieved by using more modern agents such as *terbinafine*, but they have greater toxicity. Tinea pedis (athlete's foot) may respond to topical antifungals such as *tolnaftate* or an undecanoate, but is now often treated with topical imidazoles.

Ketoconazole is used as a shampoo to control dandruff, which is associated with the yeast *Pityrosporum ovale*, which also occurs in a hyphal form, known as *Malassezia furfur*.

In the treatment of systemic candidiasis, *amphotericin* may be used in combination with *flucytosine*, an antimetabolite of *cytosine* that has no action on the true filamentous fungi.

Flucytosine may cause serious blood and hepatic disorders, so careful monitoring is required.

Caspofungin is the first of a new class of anti-fungal agents, the **echinocandins**, which interfere with fungal cell wall synthesis through their action against 1,3-beta-D-glycan synthase. These agents appear to be less toxic than *amphotericin* and may be used to treat invasive candidiasis and aspergillosis. *Caspofungin* is also used for the empiric treatment of suspected fungal infections in neutropenic patients. However, it may cause hepatic damage and blood dyscrasias.

Antiviral agents

The search for useful antiviral drugs has intensified since the emergence of HIV/AIDS. Because the life cycles of viruses are intimately associated with those of their host cells, it is difficult to find agents that selectively inhibit virus replication without damaging human cells. However, there are certain events in the synthesis of viral DNA and RNA that differ from those of the host, and these have been exploited with the nucleoside group of antivirals. These act either by inhibiting DNA or RNA polymerases or by incorporation into nucleic acid to form 'nonsense' nucleotide sequences.

Influenza and HIV/AIDS are dealt with on pp. 553–554 and 557, respectively.

Herpesvirus infections

These DNA viruses have the ability to migrate up sensory nerve axons and integrate with nerve cell nuclei in the regional nerve ganglia as proviruses. Their persistence in the nerve cells is due to the production of a microRNA from the only viral gene that is active during herpesvirus latency. This promotes the degradation of host cell messenger RNAs that code for molecules involved in apoptosis and thus keeps the nerve cell alive.

Although the primary infection may be minor, a subsequent trigger event, such as high sun exposure, major physical stress or immunosuppression, may activate the provirus, which then tracks back down the nerve axon to produce skin lesions. Reactivation may occur from the trigeminal ganglion in most people who have had **herpes labialis** ('cold sore'), sometimes causing painful neuralgia as the provirus is activated. **Chickenpox** is similar, but reactivation of the **varicella-zoster virus** causes shingles (see Chapter 7).

One of the first nucleoside antivirals, *idoxuridine*, is now rarely used and has been supplanted by *aciclovir* and its congeners. Table 8.4 lists the antiviral drugs currently in use in the UK, including their applications, except those used to treat AIDS.

Human **cytomegalovirus (CMV)** infection is a complication in severely immunosuppressed patients, including those with AIDS, and has been successfully treated with *ganciclovir*, a nucleoside analogue.

These antiviral treatments are similar in concept to the use of the purine and pyrimidine antimetabolites used in cancer chemotherapy (see Chapter 10).

Interferons are the body's own natural antiviral agents (see Chapter 2), and recombinant genetic engineering techniques have now produced them in commercially useful quantities. In addition to their antiviral properties, some interferons have cytomodulating and cytotoxic effects. **Interferons alpha** and **beta** can be produced by most cells in response to a variety of stimuli, e.g. viruses, dsRNA, ILs 1 and 2, and TNFα. **Interferon gamma** is produced only by T cells and natural killer cells (see Chapter 2). Those used in medicine are non-glycosylated proteins with a molecular weight about 19.5 kDa.

The interferons have several modes of action, e.g.:

* Block mRNA synthesis.
* Activation of enzymes that:
  – Degrade viral RNA.
  – Inhibit mRNA translation.
  – Block tRNA function.
* Block protein glycosylation that confers final protein functionality.
* Block:
  – Viral protein maturation.
  – Release of mature virions from host cell.

Interferon gamma-1b is licensed to reduce the frequency of infections in chronic granuloma-

Table 8.4   Applications of some antiviral drugs

Infections	Drugs and dosage forms										
	Aciclovir				Valaciclovir	Penciclovir	Famciclovir	Ganciclovir	Valganciclovir	Cidofovir	Foscarnet sodium
	Oral[a]	Cream	Ointment	IVi[b]	Oral	Cream	Oral	IVi	Oral	IVi	IVi
Herpes (HSV1) infection[b]											
– lips	S	✓	EO	–	S[d]	✓[g]	–	–	–	–	–
– immunocompromised[b]	✓	–	–	✓	–	–	–	✓[i]	–	–	✓[k]
– in neonates and infants <6 months old	✓	–	–	✓	–	–	–	–	–	–	–
– herpetic stomatitis	✓[a]	–	–	–	✓[e]	–	✓[e]	–	–	–	–
– eyes	–	–	EO	–	–	–	–	ED	–	–	–
Genital herpes (HSV2)	✓	✓	–	✓	✓[e]	–	✓h	–	–	–	–
Varicella-zoster virus (VZV)	✓[c]	–	✓[d]	–	✓	–	✓	–	–	–	–
Cytomegalovirus (CMV)	–	–	–	–	✓[f]	–	–	✓[i]	✓[i]	✓[i]	✓[k]

[a] Tablets or capsules. Oral suspension can be used as a mouthwash and then swallowed.

[b] IVi, intravenous infusion, used for all severe or disseminated disease. Adequate hydration should be maintained, especially with high doses.

[c] Also used for attenuation of chickenpox if immunoglobulin is contraindicated (unlicensed use).

[d] Use with eye ointment if there is eye involvement.

[e] For treatment and suppression of recurrent infections of skin and mucous membranes.

[f] Prevention of CMV disease in renal transplant patients.

[g] Should not be used in the mouth.

[h] For treatment and suppression of recurrent genital infections. Virus is transmitted in semen. Strict contraception is essential in both sexes during treatment and for 90 days afterwards. Contraindicated in pregnancy and breastfeeding, severe anaemia, and low neutrophil and platelet counts. Specialist advice is required for the treatment of chickenpox in pregnancy.

[i] For life-threatening and sight-threatening CMV infections in immunocompromised patients only.

[j] For CMV retinitis in AIDS patients and prevention of CMV infection in solid-organ transplant patients.

[k] For CMV retinitis in AIDS patients for whom other drugs are inappropriate.

[l] For CMV retinitis in AIDS patients and for mucocutaneous HSV in immunocompromised patients unresponsive to aciclovir.

Note: This listing is not exhaustive. The BNF and manufacturer's literature should be consulted for further details or in cases of doubt.

S, in severe disease and prevention of recurrence; ED, eye drops; EO, eye ointment.

tous disease, in which the intracellular bactericidal mechanisms of neutrophils and monocytes are impaired (see Chapter 2).

Interferon alfa (IFN alfa) is used to treat chronic hepatitis B (only 50% response; see Chapter 3) and for chronic hepatitis C, preferably as a combination of *peginterferon-alfa* with *ribavirin*. Early use in acute hepatitis C may reduce the risk of chronic infection. *IFN alfa* is also used as an antineoplastc agent in some lymphomas and solid tumours.

Interferon beta-1b is used in relapsing, remitting multiple sclerosis and possibly for secondary progressive multiple sclerosis.

Despite their biological origin as antiviral agents, the interferons have numerous side-effects, but are proving useful in the management of viral hepatitis B and C.

Therapeutic decisions in antimicrobial therapy

Simply possessing a knowledge of the organism involved and spectrum of activity of various antimicrobials is usually insufficient to treat suspected infections effectively. The full therapeutic decision-making process is summarized in the flow diagram (Figure 8.2).

General clinical features of infection

The first decision to be made is whether the symptoms are in fact caused by microbial infection.

Local infection

Any tissue injury, including infection of mucous membranes (e.g. sore throat) or the skin surface (e.g. impetigo), causes inflammation (Chapter 2). However, localized inflammation can have origins other than infection, e.g. contact dermatitis may often be restricted to a particular area of skin. Non-infective inflammation can be complicated by the presence of a secondary (opportunistic) infection invading the damaged issue and increasing the inflammation. Pus formation usually indicates the presence of a localized bacterial infection and is most commonly associated with staphylococcal infections. However, provided that the infection does not penetrate the dermis or traverse mucous membranes and is not caused by MRSA, patients are unlikely to suffer much harm if they are otherwise healthy.

Systemic infection

Physicians need to be particularly vigilant for the signs of progressive or systemic infection. An initially localized infection may invade deeper tissues, sometimes progressing to become more generalized and even life-threatening. When bacteria penetrate the dermis or SC layers, resulting in **cellulitis**, there is widespread inflammation. The pathogen, usually a streptococcus, may then enter the blood directly or via the lymphatic system. The subsequent systemic spread via the blood can be very rapid and severe **septicaemia** may cause septic shock (Chapter 2), e.g. in meningococcal and streptococcal infections and listeriosis. In the absence of effective antimicrobial therapy, hypothermia and life-threatening hypotension may ensue. In hospital patients, most cases of septicaemia are associated with breaches of skin and mucosal integrity, e.g. by catheters and other implanted devices and traumatic or surgical wounds. Similar, though less dramatic, long-term complications such as **endocarditis**, **rheumatic fever** and **glomerulonephritis** (see Chapters 4, 12 and 14) may follow a streptococcal sore throat.

The early signs of a systemic infection tend to be non-specific: lethargy, tiredness, chills and muscular and joint aches are common. The cardinal sign of systemic infection is **fever** (pyrexia; raised body temperature). However, this does not always indicate the presence of living organisms in the bloodstream because **endotoxins** (pyrogens) derived from Gram-negative bacteria, and WBCs that have ingested them, may be responsible. The biological advantage to the host of an increase in body temperature in response to infection is obscure. Possibly a slight rise in temperature may be less favourable to the growth of the invading organism, or it may stimulate host defence mechanisms more than it does microbial activity.

Many non-microbial systemic inflammatory diseases, e.g. RA (Chapter 12), may also cause fever. Body temperature can also be raised by tumour growth, as a presenting, non-specific symptom, and following severe trauma. Medicines may also be implicated, as 'drug fever' can give rise to influenza-like symptoms, e.g. *rifampicin*, penicillins, *phenytoin* and *carbamazepine*. All these possibilities must be considered before infection is diagnosed and antimicrobials are prescribed.

Some signs of systemic infection can be determined from blood samples. The ESR and CRP (Chapter 2) will be raised, but this will also occur with any systemic inflammatory process. The neutrophil count has a greater diagnostic value, and may be extremely high in bacterial infection. However, there may be neutropenia in

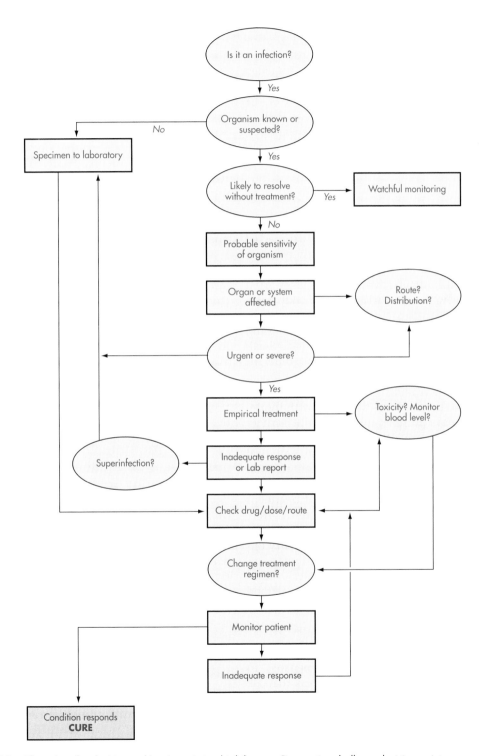

Figure 8.2   Flow chart for decision-making in antimicrobial therapy. Box, action; balloon, decision point.

severe bacterial infection, e.g. typhoid fever, and in viral infection. In addition, the occurrence of WBCs in normally sterile body fluids, e.g. urine or CSF, may indicate the presence of pathogens.

Finally, if a particular organ becomes inflamed it may eventually malfunction. Almost any organ can become infected, from parts of the GIT (e.g. the appendix) to vital organs such as the heart, kidney, brain or liver. In severe cases, and in the absence of effective treatment, organ failure may lead to death.

Laboratory culture and sensitivity testing

In hospital, the identity of any suspected infecting organism and its sensitivity to a representative range of antimicrobials, are usually determined routinely. Swabs will be taken from infected wounds, and a wide range of body fluids is sampled. Samples are then inspected microscopically and cultured in appropriate media and the organism is provisionally identified. Small filter paper discs impregnated with different antimicrobials are placed on an agar plate inoculated with the organism, and its sensitivities are determined by observing areas of growth inhibition. Wherever possible, culturing and sensitivity testing are performed before antibacterial treatment is initiated. Sampling before empirical treatment (see below) is started is the minimum requirement, because the presence of antibacterials in the sample, or the effect of treatment on the organism, may inhibit the test culture sufficiently to give negative or inconclusive results. Sometimes, the laboratory will carry out detailed identification and typing, to direct treatment and to support epidemiological monitoring, e.g. to trace the origin of a food poisoning outbreak or MRSA infection.

Limitations of culturing and sensitivity testing

Not all sites of infection are amenable to culturing and sensitivity testing. Areas that are heavily colonized with commensals, such as the skin, GIT and the superficial genitourinary tract, often yield unhelpful, false-positive results because a large variety of organisms will invariably be cultured, including organisms that may be potentially pathogenic but are unrelated to the current infection. *E. coli* is a ubiquitous enteric commensal, but only certain toxigenic or enteropathogenic strains are responsible for gastrointestinal upsets.

Similarly, identification of *Staph. epidermidis* in a wound swab does not necessarily mean that antibacterial therapy should be given. It is only when the patient's immunity is compromised, or a particularly heavy infection leads to cellulitis or septicaemia, that treatment is required. In some gastrointestinal and genitourinary infections, the use of antibacterials, especially broad-spectrum ones, can permit over-growth and infection by resistant but normally non-pathogenic organisms.

Because all laboratory culture media and methods are artificial, they cannot provide the ideal conditions appropriate for fastidious or damaged microorganisms and may give false-negative results. Thus failure to grow pathogens should not be taken as evidence of their absence in samples. Other techniques may be required if a patient's condition clearly points to infection, e.g. serology for the detection of *Chlamydia* and spirochaetes. Staining and microscopic examination of sputum for acid-fast bacilli is an example of this in diagnosing TB, and permits the commencement of treatment long before culture can give positive evidence.

New techniques of DNA multiplication by the polymerase chain reaction are now available for microbial identification and, being automated, can give rapid results. This is being done already for TB and should also be capable of predicting antimicrobial sensitivity, but the process is still relatively expensive and so is not used routinely. However, these techniques are bound to grow in popularity as the genomes of pathogens are determined, because they are sensitive and specific, can be automated and are applicable even after antimicrobials have been used.

Treating in the absence of sensitivity tests (empirical treatment)

Culturing and sensitivity testing can take days (e.g. in meningitis) or even weeks (e.g. in TB, p. 574), and treatment may have to be started on an empirical ('blind', 'best guess') basis. This is usually based on knowledge of the epidemiology of the disease, the site of infection, and local experience. Table 8.5 lists some organisms most commonly associated with different infections. However, organisms other than those described may be responsible: for example, *E. coli* causes 95% of urinary-tract infections, but other Gram-negative organisms, such as *Klebsiella aerogenes*, *Ps. aeruginosa* or *Proteus* spp. have been implicated, especially in hospital-acquired (nosocomial) infections. After deciding on the most likely organism, local knowledge of the spectrum of activity will determine the choice of antimicrobial, although strain resistance may confound even the most astute choice. These empirical decisions are later modified when the results of laboratory tests become available.

Pyrexia (fever) of unknown origin (PUO, FUO)

This may be defined as a temperature $>38°C$ persisting for 2–3 weeks without a clear diag-nosis being made, despite a range of carefully targeted examinations being done.

Provided that possible non-infectious causes have been excluded, a more detailed history needs to be taken. This will include information on travel, occupation, animal contact, leisure activities (especially water sports), recreational drug use, tattooing or body piercing, blood trans-fusions, sexual activity and medication usage. A wider range of blood tests, examination of biopsy material (including washings or scrap-ings) and additional imaging may be needed. There needs to be a systematic examination of all body systems.

While these investigations are proceeding only general supportive measures should be taken, i.e. no antimicrobial agents or corticosteroids, etc. that might obscure the signs of infection should be used unless the condition compromises patient safety. Blood tests, etc. may need to be repeated regularly.

Despite all this, no definitive diagnosis can be made in a small proportion of patients. Such patients may feel unwell for several months, until

Table 8.5 Some common infections and their probable pathogens

Infection	Likely organism[a]	Suitable antimicrobial[b]
Ear, nose and oropharynx		
Sore throat	Two-thirds of cases are viral	None
Tonsillitis	*Streptococcus pyogenes*	Penicillin V
Otitis media (in infants)	*Haemophilus influenzae*	Amoxicillin or a cephalosporin
Respiratory tract		
COPD (exacerbations)	*Haemophilus influenzae*	Amoxicillin or trimethoprim
Pneumonia (uncomplicated)	*Streptococcus pneumoniae*	Amoxicillin or erythromycin
Urogenital		
Cystitis	*Escherichia coli*	Trimethoprim or nitrofurantoin
Vaginitis	*Candida*	Clotrimazole (topical)
	Trichomonas	Metronidazole
Skin		
Cellulitis	*Streptococcus pyogenes* and/or *Staphylococcus aureus*	Phenoxymethylpenicillin plus flucloxacillin Co-amoxiclav

[a] Other organisms may be responsible.

[b] Antibacterials other than those indicated may be suitable. Local pathologist advice is essential for unusual or resistant infections.

the condition finally resolves, often without specific treatment.

Antimicrobial resistance

The high incidence of bacterial resistance makes culture and sensitivity testing essential, especially in hospital. There is a lesser problem in the community because severe infections are less frequent and the true scale of the problem is unknown. Knowledge of local patterns of resistance is therefore important, especially when treating empirically.

Mechanisms of resistance

An organism may protect itself from antimicrobial attack in a number of ways (Table 8.6), enzyme degradation of the antimicrobial being the most important. Extracellular beta-lactamases tend to be produced by Gram-positive organisms, whereas intracellular lactamases may be found in the periplasmic space of Gram-negative organisms. Prevention of access to the target due to decreased penetration is more likely to be found in Gram-negative organisms and binding of antimicrobials in the periplasmic space is a particular problem for beta-lactam antimicrobials. A further mechanism is efflux resistance, in which an antimicrobial is actively expelled from the bacteria.

Resistance develops primarily by selection from a small population of genetically resistant strains in the general infective pool under the selective pressure imposed by the antibacterial, so the 'fittest' (i.e. resistant) organisms survive. Mutation during treatment, with a genetic change conferring resistance, is rare except with some highly mutable pathogens, e.g. influenza A virus (p. 554).

Plasmid transfer, whereby one or multiple resistance genes are transferred together from one bacterium to another, plays a key role in spreading resistance rapidly throughout a microbial population. This may even occur between unrelated species. Less commonly, DNA can be transferred by two further mechanisms: **transduction** by bacteriophages and **transformation** by uptake of soluble DNA.

Patterns and causes of resistance

The development of resistance by previously sensitive organisms has been a problem ever since the introduction of the sulphonamides in the 1930s. A number of factors are involved in this phenomenon, with the resistance of organisms responsible for **nosocomial** (hospital-acquired) infections playing a central role.

The emergence of resistance in the community and hospitals are closely inter-related. Recent problems with resistance in the community by organisms such as streptococci and staphylococci may have contributed to the level of resistance of these bacteria in nosocomial infections, or vice versa. Also, the use of antimicrobials in animal feeds is believed to have contributed to the prevalence of antimicrobial resistance, and the prohibition of using clinically useful antimicrobials in animal husbandry is usual in developed countries.

Of particular concern in the UK is the emergence of penicillin-resistant pneumococci in community-acquired pneumonia. In this case, it

Table 8.6   Mechanisms of microbial resistance

Process	Examples
Enzymic degradation	Beta-lactamase
	Extended spectrum beta-lactamases
	Aminoglycoside inactivators
	Various specific enzymes
Modification of target enzymes	Non-binding of trimethoprim to dihydrofolate reductase
Prevention of access to target	Resistance of some strains of *Staphylococcus aureus* to
(efflux pumps)	tetracycline

has been suggested that the problem can largely be overcome by administering higher than usual doses.

Although 80% of antimicrobials are prescribed in the community, hospitals and nursing and residential homes are regarded as the major reservoir of resistant organisms. The reasons behind this are not fully understood, although the broadest-spectrum agents are used most heavily in these settings, with their populationss of at-risk patients. Both appropriate and inappropriate antimicrobial use can drive the emergence of resistance, so reduction of inappropriate use is a priority.

The spread of resistance within hospitals and, increasingly, residential care units is of prime concern and may be associated with a lack of adequate isolation facilities. Simple infection control procedures, e.g. hand washing, scrupulous ward cleaning, mask wearing and the sterilization of uniforms, should be rigorously enforced. Barrier nursing can be used either to protect a vulnerable patient from ward infection or to protect patients on a ward from an infected patient. In the 1990s doctors in Holland reduced the incidence of MRSA infections by a rigorous 'search and destroy' process that involved identification of MRSA carriers on admission and their isolation in single rooms. However, this would now be much more difficult in the UK, because of greater pressure on beds and the higher incidence of MRSA infection.

Immunocompromised patients, e.g. those with febrile neutropenia following cytotoxic chemotherapy or high doses of steroids, the frail and elderly, cancer patients and AIDS sufferers, will often require intensive empirical cover with very broad-spectrum agents. Additionally, sub-therapeutic antibacterial concentrations can occur in the immediate patient environment due to the indiscriminate use of topical antimicrobials and sub-therapeutic dosing.

Resistant organisms cause particular problems in intensive therapy units, where antimicrobial use is high, with many staff in direct patient contact, and where patients have impaired resistance to infection.

Patterns of resistance vary on the national and the international scale. For instance, the incidence of beta-lactamase-producing *H. influenzae* is far lower in the UK (about 6%) than in the USA (>30%). High-level penicillin resistance is prevalent in about 10% of *Strep. pneumoniae* isolates in the USA, and lower level resistance in a further 40%. This compares with figures of between 10 and 40% and up to 70% respectively in mainland Europe. In the UK, high-level penicillin resistance is found currently in less than 5% of pneumococci. Local changes in the resistance of *E. coli* to *trimethoprim* and *ampicillin* have been observed within the UK.

Patients receiving multiple or prolonged courses of treatment are more likely to experience a resistant infection subsequently. Resistance can also develop within an individual either quite rapidly or some time after commencing treatment, usually by transfer of resistance factors between conjugating bacteria. Microbial resistance in an individual patient is a particular problem in intensive care and burns units where staphylococcal, coliform, pseudomonad and *Haemophilus* infections are often implicated. As well as resistant organisms occurring in an individual they can be transferred between patients, unwittingly, by health workers.

Resistance usually starts to be reported quite soon after the introduction of a new antibacterial into clinical use. Thus resistance to *ciprofloxacin* was observed only a year after its introduction, and even the newest antimicrobials (e.g. *linezolid*) have been the subject of clinical reports of resistance.

Certain organisms tend to cause more problems than others. *Ps. aeruginosa* has a particularly high tendency to develop resistance, and there have been reports of isolates that are resistant to both *ciprofloxacin* and the ureidopenicillins. Another group of Gram-negative organisms causing concern is *Klebsiella* spp., particularly because of their propensity to carry genes coding for extended spectrum beta-lactamases (ESBLs). The latter can hydrolyse most penicillins and cephalosporins, may be mediated by plasmid or chromosomal genes and are selected for by the use of the third-generation cephalosporins and *clavulanate*. Such resistant organisms are causing increasing concern because of their greater frequency of occurrence in urinary-tract infections in the community. These infections require hospital treatment, because only parenteral anti-microbials are effective, e.g. carbapenems and *aminoglycosides*.

After a period during which staphylococcal resistance appeared to stabilize, *Staph. aureus* has re-emerged in the form of MRSA, posing a major problem. Once these occur in a hospital ward the most stringent infection control measures are required. Community-onset MRSA (C-MRSA), where a patient presents with MRSA infection without traditional risk factors being present (e.g. prior hospital in-patient treatment), is increasingly present in the USA and a number of cases have been reported in the UK. There have been 11 cases of nosocomial infection recently (end 2006) by a virulent, highly toxigenic strain of MRSA that produces Panton-Valentine leucocidin (PVL), infections which may be fatal within 24 h of symptoms occurring. Disturbing features of PVL + MRSA infection are:

• The speed of attack, placing a premium on rapid diagnosis and correct empirical treatment.
• It will infect young, previously healthy individuals, unlike most other strains of MRSA that affect immunosuppressed and debilitated people.
• PVL+ MRSA is present in the community and there have been five deaths from community-acquired infection in the UK over a 2-year period. Despite their pathogenicity, these strains tend to differ from those acquired in hospital because they are still susceptible to many antibacterials.

However, most MRSA strains are not 'super-bugs': many strains are weak pathogens, but cause problems because they infect patients who are already seriously ill or are exposed to surgical wound infections from major procedures. Further, despite media attention, there is not a current epidemic of MRSA in the UK, and TB is a far greater international problem (see below).

Overcoming resistance

Methods of counteracting the problem are either to find new antimicrobials to which resistant organisms are sensitive, or to use compounds capable of neutralizing any enzymes produced by the bacteria that inactivate antimicrobial agents, e.g. *clavulanic acid* and *tazobactam* for penicillinases.

However, it is less costly to prevent resistance occurring in the first place, by controlling the way in which these agents are used – particularly in the hospital – through the introduction of **antimicrobial policies**. Because breakdown of infection control in one hospital unit inevitably affects the whole, there needs to be a multidisciplinary infection control team (IFT) under the direction of a senior staff member, with adequate laboratory and secretarial support and direct access to the chief executive. The latter carries overall responsibility for the performance of infection control procedures in the hospital. There is a UK Nosocomial Infection National Surveillance Scheme to assist hospitals and ensure quality.

Part of infection control measures involves periodical change of the antimicrobials in common use for particular organisms or procedures, preventing inappropriate prescribing and ensuring the prescribing of full courses at adequate doses. Full courses are particularly important to individuals, as they will prevent either the re-emergence of an infection with potentially resistant organisms, which might follow incomplete kill, or superinfection with another pathogen. A further method is to use combinations of antimicrobials. This is an essential element in the treatment of TB and endocarditis (pp. 574 and 564), where it is essential to kill the organism involved, but there are few other applications.

Infection control is integral to clinical governance and is part of the responsibilities of all staff members, including cleaners, maintenance engineers, caterers, pharmacists, nurses, doctors and managers.

Combination therapy

Apart from attempting to circumvent resistance, there are a few other instances when combinations of antimicrobials might be indicated. These include:

- To achieve synergy, e.g. the concurrent use of an aminoglycoside and a ureidopenicillin in the treatment of pseudomonad infection.
- In life-threatening infections (e.g. septicaemia), where urgent empirical treatment is essential, a combination may be used until sensitivity testing has been performed.
- When the immune system is compromised, as in the chemotherapy of leukaemia, where very broad prophylactic cover is required using a combination of both antibacterial and antifungal agents. This also applies in the early stages of bone marrow transplantation, until the implanted tissue has acquired adequate function. Similarly, in HIV/AIDS, the immune system is severely compromised because of the destruction of CD4+ Tн cells and combinations of antiretroviral drugs are always used (p. 558 Table 8.11).

The problems of TB treatment are dealt with below (p. 574).

Penetration to the site of infection

Even if the pathogen is sensitive to an antimicrobial agent, the drug must reach the site of infection in order to be effective. Factors that impair the achievement of adequate local antibacterial concentrations include:

- Perfusion problems.
- Internal barriers.
- Route of elimination.

Perfusion problems

Any systemically administered drug must be transported in the blood to the desired site of action before it can have an effect. Thus, well-perfused tissues will be the most accessible to systemic antimicrobials. The alveoli of the lung are particularly well perfused, because they receive the whole of the cardiac output. Thus, if they become infected (pneumonia, p. 559) appropriate antibacterial therapy is almost invariably successful if the patient is otherwise healthy. Conversely, an infection within the poorly perfused pleural cavity (e.g. in

pleural **empyema**), may require longer courses of treatment and higher doses.

The treatment of **wound infections** can be made particularly difficult when the peripheral circulation is impaired. This is important in diabetics (see Chapter 9), in whom atherosclerotic arterial damage and microangiopathy slow wound healing and impair the penetration of antimicrobials. The elderly also tend to have a poor peripheral circulation, predisposing to pressure sores and venous ulcers and such lesions are very difficult to treat should they become infected (see Chapter 2).

Connective tissue infection is similarly problematical, e.g. staphylococcal bone infections (**osteomyelitis**) can be very difficult to treat if the organism becomes sequestered in bone following orthopaedic surgery or a compound fracture. A combination of antibacterials is then needed, e.g. *sodium fusidate* plus *flucloxacillin* and/or *gentamicin*.

Internal barriers

In several circumstances infections may occur in body sites that are not easily accessible to antimicrobials. In others, the infection itself will create a barrier to penetration.

If large amounts of infected sputum are produced in pulmonary infections, as in bronchiectasis and cystic fibrosis, the mucus protects the organisms and prevents ready access by antimicrobials, necessitating frequent high-dose treatment. Although it has been claimed that *amoxicillin* is better than *ampicillin* in treating chest infections owing to a superior penetration into sputum, the difference is probably of minor clinical significance, provided that adequate blood levels of *ampicillin* are attained. Similarly, when the infection results in the formation of large quantities of pus, as in a staphylococcal boil or abscess, the bacterial coagulase enzyme causes a fibrin clot to be formed around the lesion that inhibits penetration of the antibacterial. Surgical drainage must then precede antimicrobial therapy. A cyst, which is not surrounded by a fibrin clot, is more amenable to antibacterial treatment.

Penetration of the CNS by antimicrobials is also extremely variable due to the blood–brain barrier that usually prevents the penetration of hydrophilic molecules. Fortunately, IV *benzyl-penicillin*, cephalosporins and other antimicrobials attain therapeutic concentrations in the CSF and cure bacterial meningitis (p. 548) because meningeal inflammation opens the tight cell junctions of the blood vessels' endothelium that form the barrier and so permits antimicrobial penetration.

Route of elimination

This is of particular importance when dealing with urinary-tract infections (p. 576). *Nitrofurantoin* is excreted unchanged in the urine in concentrations that exceed the MIC for likely urinary pathogens, even though the plasma concentration is inadequate to treat a systemic infection. This is fortunate because adequate antimicrobial plasma levels would cause unacceptable side-effects. In contrast, penicillins achieve both adequate urine and plasma levels.

With biliary tract infections it is essential that a sufficient amount of the unchanged antimicrobial is eliminated by biliary excretion to obtain therapeutic levels. This occurs with penicillins and cephalosporins, which consequently may be effective in the treatment of infective cholecystitis.

Indications for antimicrobial therapy

Before antimicrobials are prescribed it is important to consider whether this is the most appropriate therapy: there may be very positive indications for their use or they may be of limited value. Thus, most **viral infections**, especially of the respiratory system, do not respond to currently available antiviral therapies. The major exceptions to this are the herpesvirus and cytomegalovirus infections that can be cured with *aciclovir* and *ganciclovir*, respectively (see above), and HIV/AIDS, which can be treated, but not cured.

Even if the organism is sensitive, treatment may still not be worthwhile if the infection is **self-limiting**, e.g. herpes labialis, mild streptococcal throat infection or mild staphylococcal skin infection. In an otherwise healthy individual such infections will be overcome by host defences within 5 days. Salmonellosis of the GIT (p. 567) does not respond well to antimicrobial treatment and some agents may actually prolong the carrier state, i.e. the time during which the organism will be found in the stools.

In summary, injudicious use of antimicrobials increases the risk of resistance developing, and may also cause serious toxicity.

Severe and systemic infection

Many systemic infections require prompt empirical treatment owing to the danger of spread to vital organs or the development of septicaemia and, in extreme cases, septicaemic shock. Clinical judgement of severity is important and the physician needs to consider several factors:

• Degree of pyrexia and other signs associated with fever, e.g. fits in young children, rigors and malaise.
• Likely time course of the infection.
• Patient's immune status.

The choice of an empirical agent is determined by what is known of the probable aetiology of the infection. However, this must be kept under review, e.g. *Vibrio valnificans*, a warm-water species usually found in the waters around Mexico has now been detected in the Baltic sea, a result of global warming. This could become a novel cause of serious wound infections and cellulitis in Europe.

Impaired resistance to infection is associated with a number of diseases. Major inherited disorders of the immune system (e.g. hypogammaglobulinaemia, impaired phagocyte activity and deficiency of complement components) predispose to infection, but most are rare. A more common problem occurs in leukaemia, where the WBCs, although produced in large numbers, are ineffectual in combating infections. Also, the use of cytotoxic agents for treating neoplasms often causes myelosuppression and so compromises the immune system. Leukaemic patients are thus particularly prone to infection by a variety of organisms, some of which are opportunistic. Even commensals normally resident in the gut may cause opportunistic infections under these conditions, and any infection occurring in these patients must be treated aggressively.

Immunosuppressive therapy is given to prevent rejection following an organ transplant, so antimicrobial therapy and barrier nursing are employed prophylactically until the danger of early organ rejection has passed. Immunosuppression to treat autoimmune diseases also renders patients more susceptible to infections.

Immunodeficiency associated with disease is now a worldwide problem owing to HIV/AIDS infections, in which destruction of CD4+ TH cells (see Chapter 2) exposes the patient to a variety of unusual infections. One of the most common and serious of these is pneumocystis pneumonia, which is treated with high-dose *co-trimoxazole*. Nebulized *pentamidine* may be administered prophylactically for this. TB is common in HIV patients and about 50% of these are believed to be infected with TB in southern Africa. HIV patients are also unable to deal immunologically with human herpesvirus (HHV) infections and these cause neoplasms and serious infections, e.g. HHV6, a common commensal, may cause severe pneumonia and HHV8 is associated with Kaposi's sarcoma.

Elderly debilitated patients are also at risk, and prompt treatment may be indicated for even a mild infection in such cases. This occasionally raises ethical problems, because the prognosis may be extremely poor owing to other medical conditions, and treating such an infection may prolong a life of greatly reduced quality.

Prophylaxis

Antimicrobial prophylaxis is contentious. Inappropriate prophylaxis may not only lead to increased populations of resistant organisms but also adds significantly to drug costs. However, prophylaxis against infection may sometimes be appropriate.

In some surgical procedures prophylaxis is essential, particularly in 'dirty' surgery involving the GIT or lower abdomen, when the antimicrobials used must protect against opportunistic infection by gastrointestinal commensals. A combination of a cephalosporin, to cover coliforms, and *metronidazole* for anaerobic bacteria, is usual. The aim is to prevent such organisms from causing a systemic infection if they should reach the patient's bloodstream and to prevent sepsis along suture lines. The practice of oral pre-surgical gut 'sterilization' using *neomycin*, or a non-absorbed sulphonamide, is now rarely used: antimicrobials are preferably given intravenously just before surgery and for one or two doses afterwards, although there is evidence that single-dose prophylaxis prior to surgery is usually adequate. Antimicrobials are similarly used after major orthopaedic surgery, e.g. total hip replacement. A further example is in dental surgery, where those with a history of heart valve disease or endocarditis (p. 564) may require prophylaxis before any procedures are carried out, however minor.

Prophylaxis may sometimes be required over longer periods. Those with sickle-cell anaemia (Chapter 11) can suffer an extremely painful, and sometimes fatal, sickling crisis, which predisposes to infection with *Salmonella* (osteomyelitis) and *Strep. pneumoniae* (pneumonia or meningitis). Because streptococci are so common, continuous low-dose *penicillin* prophylaxis is often prescribed. Splenectomy greatly increases the risk of infection by encapsulated organisms, e.g. *Haemophilus* and *Neisseria* spp. and *Strep. pneumoniae*, and long-term *penicillin* prophylaxis is prescribed. Vaccinations are also given.

Cystic fibrosis patients may also require continuous, lifelong prophylaxis in order to prevent the chest infections that are a major feature of this disease. *Ps. aeruginosa* is commonly implicated and frequent courses of parenteral or inhaled aminoglycosides are often prescribed.

Finally, prophylaxis is often indicated when there has been contact with certain virulent infections, e.g. meningococcal meningitis (p. 548). Close contacts require only short courses of *rifampicin* or *ciprofloxacin* (unlicensed applications) in such cases.

Side-effects

Hypersensitivity is a major contra-indication to using a particular antimicrobial. This is well recognized with the penicillins, but can occur with any agent. Close questioning is necessary to ascertain the status of claimed hypersensitivity reactions because patients sometimes confuse these reactions with minor adverse effects such as gastric disturbance, reporting that they are 'allergic' to a particular antimicrobial. Taken at face value this may preclude the use of an otherwise useful drug because prescribers will always avoid the possibility of a major allergic reaction, however unlikely it seems to be from the history. If no suitable alternative is available, and the treatment is essential, or when an antimicrobial is given intravenously for the first time, it is common practice to prepare for the possibility of an anaphylactic reaction by having injections of *adrenaline*, *hydrocortisone* and an antihistamine readily available. *Penicillin* desensitization, whereby the patient is exposed to gradually increasing concentrations of *penicillin*, is rarely employed as it is a perilous procedure, potentially causing anaphylaxis, and it is usually possible to choose an alternative antibacterial.

Some serious adverse effects, such as the nephrotoxicity and ototoxicity associated with aminoglycoside therapy, are dose-related (see above), as is encephalopathy with excessive doses of penicillins. Other adverse effects may be more difficult to predict and may not resolve on discontinuation of treatment, e.g. the bone marrow toxicity associated with *chloramphenicol*. Table 8.7 summarizes some of the most common adverse reactions to antimicrobials. Apart from these there are various rare idiosyncratic and unpredictable reactions, such as the lupus syndrome with *isoniazid* and blood dyscrasias with cephalosporins. Gastrointestinal adverse effects are discussed in Chapter 3.

Interactions

Consideration should also be given to potential interactions between antimicrobials and other drugs, although these are uncommon. The use of *gentamicin* and a loop diuretic has been reported to increase the incidence of ototoxicity. Similarly, the combination of a cephalosporin and a loop diuretic may increase nephrotoxicity, although this is a problem only with the early, first-generation cephalosporins, e.g. *cefradine*.

There is a theoretical interaction between bactericidal and bacteriostatic agents because bactericidal agents depend on microbial reproduction or active metabolism for their effect, so activity may be reduced by agents that inhibit cell division. However, such combinations are rarely necessary. When they are used together, e.g. in the treatment of an atypical chest infection with *amoxicillin* and *erythromycin*, the

---

Table 8.7 Some adverse effects of antimicrobials

System affected	Severe effect	Mild effect
Gut	Clindamycin	Most broad-spectrum agents
Renal	Aminoglycosides	
	Amphotericin	
	Some sulphonamides and cephalosporins	
Liver	Rifampicin	
	Ketoconazole	
	Co-amoxiclav	
Hearing loss	Aminoglycosides	
Bone marrow	Chloramphenicol	
Hypersensitivity	Penicillins[a] and cephalosporins	Penicillins
	Sulphonamides	Sulphonamides

[a] Especially ampicillin (rashes).

combination does not seem to present any problems.

The potential of certain antimicrobials to affect the activity of liver enzymes is well recognized. The rifamycins are hepatic **enzyme inducers** (Chapter 3), which results in low concentrations of many drugs. This may be very important if adequate blood levels are critical for the activity of essential drugs, and patients taking oral contraceptives, anticonvulsants, oral hypoglycaemic agents or *theophylline* should be warned that they will be less effective. Failure of contraception has been reported after women had taken short courses of *rifampicin* for prophylaxis against meningococcal infection.

The converse, **enzyme inhibition**, has been reported with *erythromycin* and *quinolone* antimicrobials. This causes increased blood levels of, e.g. *theophylline*, causing convulsions, and *warfarin*, causing bleeding. These effects make it difficult to maintain proper control of plasma levels of affected drugs, because the levels will rise or fall during therapy with an enzyme inhibitor or inducer, and then change again when that treatment ceases (see also Chapters 2 and 3; Table 3.34).

Dose and frequency

These parameters are often determined on the usual age and weight basis, and with due regard to renal and liver function. Precise dose calibration is not particularly important with the beta-lactams, because they have a wide therapeutic range. However, they have a concentration-dependent killing profile, so blood levels of these should be maintained above the MIC for most of the interval between doses. However, close monitoring is essential for more toxic agents, e.g. *gentamicin*. Antimicrobials such as the aminoglycosides and quinolones exhibit a concentration-independent microbicidal profile, so it is necessary to exceed the MIC for only a short time to kill the organism.

The aminoglycosides are eliminated via the kidneys, and *gentamicin* clearance correlates well with glomerular filtration rate, as estimated from the plasma creatinine level. However, with longer courses of *gentamicin* treatment it is necessary to monitor plasma levels directly because the volume of distribution can vary markedly between individuals. Also the toxic effects, especially ototoxicity, are more likely if trough levels are too high. Once-daily administration may be appropriate (see p. 524, *gentamicin*).

Antimicrobials eliminated by hepatic metabolism can accumulate in liver failure, but this is difficult to predict or calculate. It is probably best to avoid giving antimicrobials such as *erythromycin* and *rifampicin* if liver dysfunction is suspected. If these are essential, plasma level monitoring should be used, at least initially, until the extent of the liver problem is defined.

The frequency of administration is important, not least because of the level of non-compliance associated with this group of drugs. Patients tend to stop in the middle of a course if the regimen proves too irksome or if they feel better, as they often do after 24–48 h of antimicrobial therapy. Therefore, the fewer doses that are taken each day the greater the likely compliance.

The half-lives of the penicillins and many cephalosporins are only a few hours. Ideally, doses should be timed to the half-life of the drug, but this would be impractical in most cases of penicillin therapy. Therefore, with these less toxic antimicrobials, doses are chosen that achieve plasma levels several times greater than the MIC. In this way the frequency of administration can then be reduced, as the plasma level will still exceed the MIC before each subsequent dose. Antimicrobials that can be given just once a day, such as *ofloxacin* and *cefixime*, may offer advantages for patient compliance.

Duration of therapy

A balance must be achieved between eliminating pathogens completely, to limit the emergence of resistant organisms, and giving too long a course, with which the patient may not comply, and with the increased risk of adverse effects and resistance.

The usual recommended course for most antimicrobials is 5–10 days, but this is not evidence-based in most cases and there are numerous exceptions to this empirical generalization. Thus uncomplicated lower urinary-tract infections in women are usually adequately treated with 3-day courses, but common practice is to treat upper respiratory tract infections, in the absence of any chronic lung disease, with a 5–7-day course. *Chlamydia* infection can be treated with a single dose of *azithromycin*. Other treatments may require weeks (e.g. endocarditis) or months (e.g. TB) of antimicrobial treatment.

Failure of therapy

Even after the most diligent choice of antimicrobial, therapy may still fail. Table 8.8 summarizes the possible reasons for such failure and reflects the main points made in this section regarding appropriate therapeutic choice.

Some important infections

Meningitis

Aetiology

The term meningitis strictly refers to inflammation of the meninges, the triple membrane covering the CNS, which is not necessarily due to infection. It may also be caused by invasion of neoplastic cells in association with cytotoxic chemotherapy (see Chapter 10), of blood after a subarachnoid haemorrhage, or rarely by drugs. This non-infective inflammation is more correctly called meningism, the term meningitis being reserved for infective causes.

The causative microorganisms vary with age, between countries and regionally within countries. This brief account is confined to UK experience.

Table 8.8 Possible reasons for the failure of antimicrobial therapy[a]

1. Diagnosis	No infection; viral infection
	Non-responsive condition
2. Drug	Non-sensitive organism
3. Dose	Age, causing renal/hepatic dysfunction affecting metabolism or excretion
4. Route	Drug destruction in the gut
	No absorption from site
	Site inaccessible to drug, e.g. abscesses
5. Absorption	Nausea, food, compliance
6. Distribution	In CSF. pus, urine, bile, fat etc.
7. Duration	Early apparent resolution causing non-compliance
	Impatience
	Need for long duration of treatment to eliminate pathogens completely
8. Disease	Underlying serious disease, e.g. tumour, COPD, immunodeficiency
9. Drug interaction	Immunosuppressives, e.g. steroids, cytotoxics
10. Drug resistance	Selection of resistant strain from original population
	Supra-infection
	Mixed infection from start

[a] Failure may arise because of wrong decision in factors 1–7 or failure to appreciate factors 8–10.
COPD, chronic obstructive pulmonary disease. CSF, cerebrospinal fluid.

In the first 3 months of life the common bacteria causing community-acquired meningitis are group B streptococci, *E. coli* strain K1 and *Listeria monocytogenes*. *Neisseria meningitidis*, *Strep. pneumoniae* and *H. influenzae* are less common. However, the last three of these are the most common species in older children up to 14 years, with most cases being due to *Neisseria meningitidis* serogroups B and C. *H. influenzae* is becoming rare in the UK due to effective immunization with Hib vaccine.

Table 8.9 summarizes the probable pathogens, which can usually be deduced from the age of the patient and any predisposing factors, e.g. skull fracture, ear disease and occupational or recreational history. Of the organisms listed, *N. meningitidis* is the most likely in an adult. *Listeria* meningitis is occasionally found in both neonates and the elderly. A completely different group of Gram-negative bacteria is usually implicated in neonatal meningitis.

About 75% of teenage and adult cases of bacterial meningitis are infected with *Neisseria meningitidis* and *Strep. pneumoniae*. In the remainder, *L. monocytogenes*, *E. coli* K1 and *H. influenzae* and similar Gram-negative bacteria predominate: *Staph. aureus* may also be involved. Secondary infection, e.g. following a fracture of the skull, may allow skin surface organisms to reach the meninges and staphylococci and streptococci are then the usual pathogens but occasionally *Pseudomonas* may cause problems, because of its antimicrobial resistance.

However, viral meningitis is the most common type in the UK, but it is usually mild and self-limiting. A number of viruses may be involved (Table 8.9). Unlike bacterial meningitis, which causes most of the severe cases, there may be only minimal changes in the appearance and cellular components of the CSF, so it is sometimes erroneously termed 'aseptic meningitis'. However, this merely means that there is no growth on laboratory media, which are designed to cultivate non-fastidious bacteria and fungi. Viral meningitis will not be discussed further here.

Other rarer forms of meningitis usually occur in immunocompromised patients, caused by fungi, mycobacteria and protozoa.

Table 8.9   Aetiology and treatment of meningitis in the UK

Age group	Likely organisms	Initial therapy
Adult and children	*Neisseria meningitidis* *Streptococcus pneumoniae*	Cefotaxime
Elderly	*Neisseria meningitidis* *Streptococcus pneumoniae* *Listeria monocytogenes* Aerobic Gram-negative bacilli	Cefotaxime or ceftriaxone plus amoxicillin
Neonate	Group B streptococci *Escherichia coli* Other Gram-negative bacilli *Listeria monocytogenes*	Cefotaxime plus amoxicillin or amoxicillin plus aminoglycoside
Viruses: infections are normally mild and do not usually need treatment	Herpes simplex Human immunodeficiency virus Enteroviruses Epstein-Barr virus (normally causes glandular fever) Mumps	See Table 8.4 See Table 8.11 Supportive. No specific treatment available
Fungi	A fungal aetiology is rare in the UK	Fluconazole Voriconazole if organism is resistant to fluconazole or if infection is life-threatening

Epidemiology

Although nasal carriage of *N. meningitidis* is common, being present in about 5% of adults, the annual incidence of meningococcal meningitis in the UK is only about 10 per 100 000. Occasional local epidemics are caused by the group B serotype.

The most vulnerable groups are infants up to 1 year and elderly residents in institutions and nursing homes. Neonates are infected via the birth canal but environmental organisms cause most infections later in the first year, after which the incidence falls sharply with age up to about 14 years, alongside the maturation of the immune system, and then declines slowly due to the acquisition of minor infections with likely pathogens, specific immunity and nasal carriage of the meningococcus (see Chapter 2). Above the age of 70 the incidence increases due to impaired health and infections, notably pneumonia, urinary-tract infections and otitis media, and immunosuppression, either for treating autoimmune diseases or as a side-effect of the management of other diseases.

Although the overall incidence of primary meningitis is fortunately low, local epidemics are favoured by crowding, e.g. in army units, boarding schools, residential homes and prisons, due to the ease of transmission from an index case. **Secondary meningitis** usually occurs following spread in the blood of non-CNS infection (e.g. urinary-tract infections, otitis media and pneumonia), or accidental or surgical trauma to the head, neck or spinal cord.

Pathology and clinical features

The outermost layer of the meninges, the dura mater, is in intimate contact with the skull and vertebral column. The innermost pia mater is in contact with the brain and spinal cord. Sandwiched between these is the arachnoid. Between the arachnoid and pia mater is the subarachnoid space that contains CSF. This has little intrinsic immunological activity, containing only small numbers of leucocytes. Consequently, if even a few organisms reach the CSF they proliferate very rapidly.

Bacterial infection causes leucocyte recruitment, the pia and arachnoid becoming engorged with polymorphs (see Chapter 2).

Acute bacterial meningitis

Primary bacterial meningitis is usually a sequel to sore throat or an ear or respiratory tract infection, which is followed abruptly by only mild generalized malaise and possibly drowsiness, so diagnosis in the early stages is difficult, especially in infants. Rapid diagnosis is essential because the disease can progress very quickly, particularly in fulminating (explosive) meningococcal infection, and a brief delay may result in the death of young children or permanent brain damage. Later, a high fever together with symptoms indicating CNS involvement (headache, photophobia, neck stiffness and other neurological signs, e.g. Kernig's sign (inability to extend the leg when sitting or when the thigh is flexed against the abdomen)), will confirm the diagnosis. However, these classical diagnostic neurological features are seen in only 50% of cases.

N. meningitidis from the nasopharynx, which may be transported via the bloodstream to the CSF, produces meningeal inflammation. As with any acute inflammation, WBCs and protein then pass from the bloodstream into the CSF and examination of this by lumbar puncture produces a turbid sample instead of being clear, with a low glucose level in bacterial meningitis. Most of the damage to the CNS is not actually due to the microorganism, but to the host inflammatory response, allowing vascular leakage and a raised intracranial pressure. Endotoxins (i.e. lipopolysaccharides from bacterial cell walls and engulfed bacteria in leucocytes) also play a role, causing fever. The increased cerebral pressure from inflammatory exudation is responsible for most of the neurological signs.

Meningococcal infection is often accompanied by the appearance of a haemorrhagic (purpuric) skin rash within the first 18 h, which can be distinguished from an inflammatory rash because it does not blanch under pressure with a drinking glass or a clear plastic ruler. The combination of the rash with fever and headache is pathognomonic of meningococcal meningitis. However, diagnosis cannot wait for classical signs because of the rapid progress of the disease, particularly in fulminating meningococcal infection. In this case, there are severe systemic complications, e.g. shock, disseminated intravascular coagulation (see Chapter 2) and renal failure. Death may occur within 24–36 h of the onset of symptoms. Most mortality is due to meningococcal septicaemia rather than direct CNS damage.

The complications of meningococcal sepsis are believed to result from endotoxin production (see Chapter 2). Patients may occasionally deteriorate rapidly on initial treatment with antimicrobials owing to a release of endotoxins from killed bacteria. If prompt appropriate treatment is given, healthy adults will suffer no permanent CNS damage. In children, however, serious neurological sequelae such as blindness and mental retardation may occur in up to 30% cases, despite antibacterial therapy.

Chronic microbial meningitis develops slowly and is usually caused by *M. tuberculosis* or *Cryptococcus neoformans* (a yeast), the latter especially in AIDS patients.

Diagnosis

Apart from the clinical signs described above, a lumbar puncture is performed before initiating therapy, if possible and advisable, and the CSF examined by direct Gram staining, culturing, sensitivity testing and immunoelectrophoresis for antigens. Both *N. meningitidis* and *Strep. pneumoniae* are diplococci, but the former is Gram-negative and the latter Gram-positive. Prior treatment usually results in negative CSF findings but diagnosis is still possible through serological tests for bacterial antigens in the CSF.

Lumbar puncture may be contra-indicated if there is clinical suspicion of raised intracranial pressure, e.g. papilloedema with headache and vomiting. It is often avoided in meningococcal meningitis.

It may be difficult to distinguish the headache of meningitis from that of migraine and subarachnoid haemorrhage. Differentiation is important because of the imperative of the different treatments of these two conditions. A first attack of migraine is very unusual over the age of 50.

Bacterial DNA testing, using the polymerase chain reaction, offers improved speed and accuracy of diagnosis in doubtful cases, but should not delay immediate empirical antibiotics.

Pharmacotherapy

Because the CSF has a low intrinsic immunological activity, some time will elapse after the invasion of the organism before an effective immunological response can be mounted, and this can result in an overwhelming infection. Therefore, it is important to achieve high CSF concentrations of antimicrobials promptly. A limiting factor in the choice of antibacterials is their ability to cross the blood–brain barrier sufficiently to achieve adequate CSF levels. Some antibacterials (e.g. *chloramphenicol*, antitubercular drugs and *amphotericin*) readily enter the CSF whereas others (e.g. cephalosporins and penicillins) will provide high CSF levels only if the meninges are inflamed, as they are in meningitis. The more polar antibacterials (e.g. aminoglycosides and sodium fusidate) always achieve poor CSF concentrations and must be administered intrathecally if they are needed. This procedure requires careful aseptic technique, is technically difficult to perform on neonates and should only be used with specialist advice.

Immediate empirical treatment

If there is a delay of more than 1 h before a lumbar puncture can be performed, then IV **empirical antibacterial therapy** is usually administered immediately because of the potentially serious consequences of delay. Because of this and the severity of the condition there are no RCTs to guide best treatment.

If meningitis is suspected, GPs are now recommended to administer an initial high dose of *benzylpenicillin* (e.g. 1.2 g in adults, preferably by slow IV injection), after obtaining a blood sample. Urgent transfer to hospital is mandatory. Alternatively, and if there is a history of penicillin allergy, *cefotaxime* (2 g in adults) or *cefuroxime* (1.5 g in adults) should be used. *Cefotaxime* is likely to be effective against meningococci, streptococci and *H. influenzae*. *Chloramphenicol* may be substituted if there is allergy to both penicillins and cephalosporins (see below). These recommendations may be varied according to local policy.

Steroid therapy is contentious, but may improve survival in bacterial meningitis by reducing cerebral oedema. *Dexamethasone phosphate*, e.g. 0.15 mg/kg four times daily in adults, should be given by IM or slow IV injection before or with the first antimicrobial dose. The benefit of this is unknown in meningococcal disease, but reduces the overall risks of severe hearing loss in children and all-risk mortality in adults. However, *dexamethasone* is contraindicated in immunocompromised patients, if there is septic shock or if meningitis occurs after surgery.

Acute infection

The initial treatment in hospital will depend to some extent upon the age of the patient and the results of direct CSF examination (Table 8.9). The third-generation, broad-spectrum cephalosporins (e.g. *cefotaxime* and *ceftriaxone*) are widely used. Their spectrum of activity offers a superior alternative to the *benzylpenicillin* regimen used previously. They are active against *N. meningitidis*, streptococci and the Gram-negative organisms that may be responsible. If *L. monocytogenes* is suspected, e.g. in the young and elderly, *amoxicillin* plus *gentamicin* are used for 10–14 days. If penicillin-resistant strains of pneumococci are suspected or proven, *vancomycin* or *rifampicin* is added to *ceftriaxone*. *Dexamethasone* may be helpful, but reduces penetration of *vancomycin* into the CSF.

Cefotaxime is used if *H. influenzae* is implicated, but *chloramphenicol* is indicated if the patient is hypersensitive to penicillins and cephalosporins, or if the organism is resistant to *cefotaxime*. This is one of the few indications for *chloramphenicol*, because the severity of the disease outweighs the risk of *chloramphenicol*-induced agranulocytosis. *Rifampicin* is given for 4 days before hospital discharge in cases of proven *H. influenzae* type b (Hib) infection, though this is increasingly uncommon.

Treatment of neonatal meningitis is more problematic than that of other age groups owing to the variety of possible pathogens, and initial therapy is often a matter of local policy. The combination of *amoxicillin* and a third-generation cephalosporin is effective against a wide range of Gram-negative organisms and provides adequate cover against streptococci. If Lancefield group B streptococci are implicated, IV *benzylpenicillin* plus *gentamicin* are used.

Once the results from lumbar puncture have been obtained, therapy can be continued for the specific organism.

Following a head injury, the risk of secondary meningitis may require different antimicrobial treatment. Thus, a high-dose regimen of *flucloxacillin* and *ampicillin* would be required to cover staphylococci and streptococci. Occasionally, an anaerobic organism may be implicated and *metronidazole*, which crosses readily into the CSF, is used.

Chronic disease is treated as usual for the identified organisms.

Prophylaxis

Meningococci are highly transmissible, so prophylaxis is advised for close family contacts or for those living in closed communities such as residential care homes, boarding schools and prisons. *Rifampicin* is the drug of choice, owing to an increased incidence of sulphonamide resistance. *Ciprofloxacin* or *ceftriaxone* are off-label alternatives.

Vaccines have been developed against the A, C, W135 and Y meningococcal polysaccharide serotypes of meningococci and this 4-valent vaccine is recommended as routine prophylaxis for travellers to endemic areas, i.e. most of Africa. Saudi Arabia requires proof of vaccination for all Muslims making the Hajj and Umrah pilgrimages to Mecca. Guidelines for the public health management of meningococcal disease in the UK have been published (see References and further reading).

Meningococcal Group C Conjugate Vaccine and Haemophilus Type b Conjugate Vaccine (Hib vaccine) are included in the immunization schedule for the first year of life and give satisfactory protection against the relevant organisms. In 2006 it was announced that a 7-valent pneumococcal vaccine is to be provided for all infants in the UK.

There is currently no vaccine against meningococcal group B organisms.

Summary

The treatment of meningitis illustrates the following general points:

- Vaccination against the commonest types of bacteria that may cause meningitis is preferable to the antimicrobial treatment of infection.
- This type of infection is a medical emergency. Prompt empirical treatment with an appropriate antimicrobial is essential, based on patient age.
- Risks of the infection may outweigh the potential adverse effects of treatment if *chloramphenicol* is required to treat severe disease. The risk–benefit balance is always a consideration in treatment selection.
- Samples for culturing and sensitivity testing should be obtained before initiating therapy but treatment must not await the results. Immediate microscopical examination of Gram-stained CSF may provide valuable clues to appropriate therapy.
- Factors other than the site of infection may indicate the most likely organism involved. In meningitis age is the most important determinant.
- Adjunctive treatment with *dexamethasone* is often given to reduce elevated intracranial pressure due to meningeal inflammation, but may interfere with antimicrobial penetration into the CSF. The evidence of benefit for this intervention is inconclusive.

Influenza

Viral structure and physiology

This mostly respiratory disease is caused by an enveloped, roughly spherical RNA virus, about 125 nm in diameter (Figure 8.3). Each virion

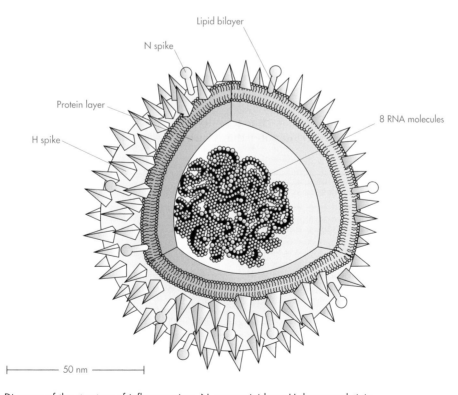

Figure 8.3   Diagram of the structure of influenza virus. N, neuraminidase; H, haemagglutinin.

consists of eight RNA molecules of different lengths, surrounded by an inner protein shell and an outer lipid bilayer. There are three major types of the virus that are defined by the proteins of their inner shells. Type A strains are genetically labile and are responsible for all the major epidemics and pandemics. Type B is also genetically labile and causes occasional milder, more localized epidemics. Type C is genetically stable and is rarely implicated in outbreaks.

The surface carries two different types of protein projections, comprising about 500 **haemagglutinin** (H) 'spikes', which are responsible for the recognition of the target respiratory cells and attachment to them (incidentally causing the agglutination (clumping) of RBCs), and about 100 **neuraminidase** (N) spikes, which are concerned with the release of newly-formed mature virions from infected cells. There are 16 types of haemagglutinin, of which H1–H3 are found in human virions, H1–H12 in domesticated poultry and H13–H16 in wild birds. Of the nine types of neuraminidase only N1, N2 and N8 occur in human strains and all are found in domesticated poultry and in pigs. Thus most human outbreaks originate from poultry.

Small changes in these spikes are described as **antigenic drift** and are probably due to single amino acid changes. This may mean that host resistance is partial, because some immunity has been acquired by previous contact with the parent strain. Major changes in the spikes (**antigenic shift**) denote the emergence of new virulent, potentially epidemic or pandemic strains characterized by the precise physicochemical structure of each of these spikes, e.g. the H3N2 strain of 'Hong Kong' virus responsible for the 1968 pandemic.

Because humans in South-East Asia often live in close contact with domestic poultry and pigs it is possible for an avian strain to infect pigs that are also carrying specific swine strains. There can then be reassortment of RNA strands between the two strains of virus, with the potential for the creation of a novel strain that can infect humans. The likelihood of this is increased because the avian virus has already made the jump to mammals. Further, infected bird carcases are often fed to other domestic animals, and cats develop a syndrome that resembles human influenza closely. It is therefore not surprising that all modern epidemics arise in South-East Asia and are spread from there by infected wild fowl and human carriage. The ease of transcontinental air travel greatly facilitates the latter, so that epidemics can now spread very rapidly to cause a global pandemic.

Thus there are potentially about 150 strains or serovars (serological variants). Those associated with epidemics that occurred in the 20th century are given in Table 8.10.

At the time of writing, the virulent H5N1 strain of avian virus is causing great anxiety because of its novel surface structure, its ability to cause severe human respiratory infections with a 30–50% fatality rate and its ready spread

Table 8.10 Strains of type A influenza virus responsible for major epidemics and pandemics 1900–2006

Period	Trivial designation	Serovar	Comments
1901–1917 and 1968 onwards	Hong Kong	H3N2	Characterized by serology of recovered elderly patients.
1918–1928	Virulent 'swine', 'Spanish'	HswN1	Severe pandemic. Precise H antigen is unknown, but is related to strains in pigs.
1929–1946	–	H0N1	First isolate to be identified serologically. H0 may be a minor variant of H1
1947–1956 and 1977 onwards	–	H1N1	–
1957–1967	Asian	H2N2	Pandemic
1968 onwards	Hong Kong	H3N2	Severe pandemic
1997 onwards	Avian	H5N1	Potentially pandemic

by migratory birds. Although it appeared in Hong Kong as long ago as 1997, with 18 human cases and 6 deaths, the fact that there was no major epidemic, even in that crowded city, leads to cautious optimism that it has only a limited ability for bird-to-human spread, even less chance of human-to-human spread and presents only a low risk of a pandemic. All of the humans involved in outbreaks in South-East Asia have been infected by very close contact with domestic poultry, in which the disease spreads throughout all their tissues. However, a new virulent human serovar may emerge at any time.

The H1, H3, H4, H7 and the N1, N2 and N7 strains are also of particular concern, because all of these have been able to jump the species barrier into mammals, especially pigs, horses and seals. These phenotypes are therefore potentially capable of transmission into humans.

Clinical features

There are two basic forms of presentation of the infection, conjunctival and respiratory. The former is associated with H7 strains, which are of low pathogenicity.

H5N1 infection in birds spreads rapidly to all their organs, causing death within about 48 h. In humans, the infection has an incubation period of up to 7 days, followed by high fever, cough and shortness of breath and over 80% of patients have a severe illness with a brief or longer period of respiratory failure and signs of multi-organ failure, e.g. abnormal liver function tests and lymphopenia. A small number of H5N1 cases have presented with early fever and gastro-intestinal disturbance, including diarrhoea, but obvious respiratory symptoms developed late and caused acute respiratory distress. A high index of suspicion is needed for these early symptoms to be recognized as influenza.

Virus shedding in influenza A infection peaks at about 7 days after symptom onset and may continue for up to 10 days. Neutralizing anti-bodies are detectable about 10–14 days after infection, so these cannot be used for early specific diagnosis, which can be done reliably only by genomic identification using the reverse transcriptase polymerase chain reaction on lower respiratory tract samples.

Recovery from the infection may be followed by a prolonged post-viral syndrome, causing debility and depression.

Pharmacotherapy and prophylaxis

Oseltamivir may be used for the treatment of influenza A and B in adults and children over 1 year, but only if given within 48 h of the onset of symptoms. It is recommended primarily for use in at-risk patients, e.g. those who are immuno-suppressed, the elderly, or people who live in residential homes where influenza is current. In otherwise healthy individuals the drug shortens the duration of symptoms by 1–1.5 days.

Oseltamivir is also licensed for the prophylaxis of influenza in at-risk adults and adolescents over 13 years, if given within 48 h of exposure during epidemics. The timing of treatment is critical: if used outside the window of opportunity the benefit is lost. In epidemics, prophylaxis may need to be continued for up to 6 weeks.

Further, it has recently been shown in Vietnam that resistance of the H5N1 strain to *oseltamivir* can arise during treatment in about 1% of cases, and this is more common in children. However, the infected population was small and the resistant strain was not trans-mitted between humans, so this observation needs further investigation. If this is replicated in a larger cohort the implications are far-reaching, e.g. stockpiling of *oseltamivir* may prove to be a waste of resources and raises expec-tations of beneficial treatment that may not be achievable. Further, it may be necessary to use higher doses or to institute combined treatment with other antiviral agents.

If *oseltamivir* cannot be used because of intol-erable side-effects, *zanamivir* is licensed for use in adults and adolescents aged >12 years, and is less toxic. *Zanamivir* is available only as a dry powder inhalation for twice-daily use. However, it may cause bronchospasm, respiratory impairment, angioedema (see Chapter 2), urticaria or other rashes, so a short-acting bronchodilator should be available immediately (e.g. *salbutamol* or *terbutaline sulphate*), and patients should be monitored carefully, at least initially. If patients are already taking other agents by inhalation, *zanamivir* should be inhaled last and care is needed in patients with asthma or other respiratory diseases. This may limit its usefulness in those patients who might need it most.

Both of these agents inhibit viral neuraminidase and so prevent the release of new virions from infected cells.

The anti-Parkinson drug *amantadine* is no longer recommended by NICE, although it is licensed for the prophylaxis and treatment of influenza A infections, the most common type. It has been supplanted by the drugs mentioned above.

Nebulized *ribavirin* has been shown to be effective against influenza A and B in adults (unlicensed indication) and may be appropriate in those with severe infection. However, it may cause respiratory deterioration, bacterial pneumonia, pneumothorax, non-specific anaemia and haemolysis, so its use needs to be confined to hospitals with full facilities for respiratory support and fluid and electrolyte management. Pregnant women and those planning conception should not be exposed to the aerosol, because of teratogenic risk.

Vaccination

Pharmacotherapy of influenza is no substitute for annual autumnal vaccination. Both H and N molecules are highly antigenic, especially the haemagglutinins. Influenza vaccines are prepared using a WHO-recommended strain grown in hens' eggs, with added *neomycin* and *polymyxin B* antimicrobials, and possibly thiomersal antiseptic to suppress bacterial contamination during processing. They contain either purified virus inactivated with formaldehyde (Split Virion vaccine) or purified H+N particles inactivated with propiolactone (Surface Antigen vaccine). Neither is capable of causing influenza, but must not be given to individuals who are sensitive to egg protein or the antimicrobials used in manufacture. Although the vaccines are effective, the problem is to identify the strain(s) current in humans and to produce adequate stocks of vaccine. This takes about 7 months at present, though faster production methods using tissue culture fermentation are being explored. Tissue culture has the additional advantages of a much cleaner microbiological process than egg culture and a reduced need for antimicrobial and

antiseptic cover. Because all outbreaks start in the Far East, this may give the UK sufficient time to develop and produce stocks of vaccine, but whether these would be adequate for large-scale immunization depends on the rate of spread of the virus.

There is also the ethical problem that all influenza vaccine production is done in Australia, the UK and the USA, and no policy has been proposed to deal with the needs of the developing world. This is not an entirely altruistic question, because the existence of very large unprotected populations promotes the spread and long-term carriage of the virus. India has a large and efficient pharmaceutical industry with good UK industry connections and it seems logical that vaccine manufacture should be established there.

The UK Biological Products Research Laboratory has a novel approach to the need to accelerate vaccine production. They have used genetic manipulation to create a bank of a virulent strains of the H5N1 serovar in the expectation that at least one of these will match the characteristics of the next virulent pandemic strain when it arrives, as it surely will. This will save at least 2 months of lead time for vaccine production.

The experimental vaccines produced to date require the addition of an immunological adjuvant and two doses are needed to produce an adequate antibody response. One British company has already tested a vaccine (GSK, mid-2006) that has given a satisfactory response using one-quarter of the dose of the normal influenza vaccine, thus enabling the vaccine to be available to a much larger population.

Annual immunization is currently recommended for:

- All people aged over 65 years.
- Residents and staff in residential or nursing homes for the elderly or other long-stay facilities.
- Healthcare workers and those caring for people whose welfare would be compromised if the carer falls ill.
- Individuals aged over 6 months with any of the following chronic conditions:
  - Asthma or any chronic respiratory disease.
  - Heart, liver and renal disease.

- Diabetes mellitus.
- Immunosuppression, including prolonged corticosteroid treatment and asplenia or splenic dysfunction.
- HIV infection, regardless of immune status.

Epidemic spread of H5N1 influenza in 2005/06 was aborted in Indonesia by rigorous public health measures, i.e. large-scale culling of domestic poultry and banning the sale of poultry in open markets.

Summary

In the absence of effective specific treatment the management of influenza illustrates:

- The importance of rigorous public health measures to prevent disease dissemination.
- The value of large-scale immunization of at-risk groups to protect individuals and the general population.
- The importance of rapid characterization of epidemic strains to permit early manufacture of effective vaccines.
- The value of good medical records to identify those at risk.
- The importance of prompt diagnosis to enable the most effective use of drugs to abort influenza and opportunistic bacterial infections.

HIV/AIDS

This is a specialist field (see References and further reading), but the general principles of treatment are discussed here.

The virus

The human immunodeficiency virus (HIV) is a two-stranded RNA virus enclosed in an envelope composed of the usual bilamellar lipopolysaccharide layer with surface globular proteins that are concerned with attachment to host cells. A molecule of **reverse transcriptase** is attached to each RNA molecule and, after penetration into CD4+ T-lymphocytes (TH [helper] cells; see Chapter 2), the enzyme synthesizes a complementary DNA molecule on the viral RNA template. This process is the reverse of the process of transcription in human cells (DNA → RNA), hence the generic name 'retrovirus'. The viral DNA is converted into double-stranded form by host enzymes and incorporated into the host cell genome as a provirus and may remain in this protected environment for many years.

Some later event, e.g. immunosuppression, triggers activation of proviral DNA, which then directs the synthesis of virus intermediates, e.g. viral proteases that break down host cell components and synthesize viral core and envelope proteins, viral RNA and reverse transcriptase, and the viral components are assembled into new virions. Only the viral complementary DNA is active in infected cells, because the reverse transcriptase also breaks down host RNA and so prevents new host protein synthesis. The new virions that are released invade other CD4+ immune cells, e.g. macrophages, APCs, some monocytes and B cells. The infected cells are not usually killed but their functioning is impaired profoundly, eventually causing severe immunosuppression. Infected individuals die of infections and neoplasms against which they cannot mount an effective immune response.

Antiretroviral therapy aims to reduce the plasma viral load (virions plus viral RNA), and keep it low for as long as possible, and to prolong life of a good quality: there is no current cure. Although there have been many attempts to produce a vaccine, the virus mutates readily to change the characteristics of its envelope. Combination therapy with antiretroviral drugs from two or more classes, i.e. highly active antiretroviral therapy (HAART), is the most effective current treatment for the management of HIV-positive individuals.

Treatment benefit, i.e. survival, has to be balanced against drug toxicity, because the drugs used are very toxic, particularly to the liver. Any infections that occur need their usual, but aggressive, treatment in the absence of the patient's ability to mount an immune response.

A recent report indicates that some drugs in HAART do not penetrate all areas of the body, e.g. the brain, where the virus selectively attacks the motor, language and cognitive centres, and testicles. If these findings are replicated, it is clear that we need new lipophilic drugs that penetrate the CNS or an effective vaccine for at-risk subjects if we are to deal adequately with HIV/AIDS.

Antiretroviral pharmacotherapy

Four classes of drugs are available (Table 8.11):

• **Nucleoside reverse transcriptase inhibitors**, which interfere with synthesis of proviral DNA and the functioning of viral RNA.
• **Non-nucleoside reverse transcriptase inhibitors**, which bind irreversibly to the enzyme.
• **Protease inhibitors**, which prevent viral damage to host cells.
• **Fusion inhibitor**. Only one of these is available currently. This prevents the fusion of virions with the host cell envelope, and so the release of mature virions from infected cells and their penetration into uninfected cells.

Drug regimens

Treatment should be initiated by specialists before there is irrevocable damage to the immune system. The factors involved in a decision to treat are:

• CD4+ lymphocyte count.
• Plasma viral load.
• Clinical condition of the patient.

HAART (Table 8.11) consists of:

• Two nucleoside reverse transcriptase inhibitors **plus**
• A non-nucleoside reverse transcriptase inhibitor or a protease inhibitor, which is often administered with a small dose of *ritonavir* (another protease inhibitor) to increase blood levels of the former.
• *Enfuvirtide* is used as third-line therapy, if there is an inadequate response to any of the other agents, or when the patient is unable to tolerate a drug.

Ensuring adequate doses will minimize the possibility of drug resistance and the patient is monitored carefully for drug toxicity and interactions with any other drugs. Drug interactions are likely because most of these agents are metabolized in the liver, protease inhibitors and non-nucleoside reverse transcriptase inhibitors via the cytochrome P450 system.

Side-effects such as hepatitis, pancreatitis, anaemia and glucose intolerance can be monitored by haematology tests. Discontinuation or treatment for them is instituted before they become a major problem. Antimicrobial and general support is given as required, for as long as required, but the severe immunodeficiency caused by the underlying disease commonly predisposes to unusual infections and tumours. Kaposi's sarcoma causes widespread lesions of

Table 8.11   Antiviral drugs used for the treatment of HIV/AIDS[a]

Reverse transcriptase inhibitors		Protease inhibitors	Inhibitor of fusion of virus with host cell
Nucleoside/nucleotide	Non-nucleoside		
Abacavir	Efavirenz	Amprenavir	Enfuvirtide
Didanosine	Nevirapine	Atazanavir	
Emtricitabine		Fosemprenavir	
Lamivudine		Indinavir	
Stavudine		Lopinavir with	
Tenofovir disoproxil		ritonavir[b]	
Zalcitabine		Nelfinavir	
Zidovudine		Ritonavir	
		Saquinavir	
		Tipranavir	

[a] See text for combinations of these used in HAART (highly active antiretroviral therapy). A number of ready-formulated products are available to reduce the number of different medications to be taken regularly and so improve adherence

[b] Low doses of ritonavir increase the effectiveness of some protease inhibitors. It is used in combination with a nucleoside reverse transcriptase inhibitor.

the skin, mouth, bowel and lungs. Non-Hodgkin's lymphoma of the brain also occurs. Unusual infections include *Pneumocystis jiroveci*, which is treated with IV *co-trimoxazole*, inhaled *pentamidine isetionate* or other drugs (p. 560). The latter is a very toxic agent that requires special care in handling. Infections by *Cryptococcus neoformans* require treatment with *amphotericin*, with or without *flucytocine*. Prophylactic antimicrobials are often necessary.

Clinical deterioration requires a change of the drugs used, but a stage will come when the effects of drug toxicity outweigh the benefits of treatment. Treatment benefit, i.e. survival, has to be balanced against drug toxicity, because the drugs used are very toxic, particularly to the liver. Any infections that occur need usual, but aggressive, treatment.

Pneumonia

Definitions and epidemiology

The absolute mortality from pneumonia in the UK is greater than for any other common type of infection, despite the availability of effective treatments and the continuing sensitivity of the organisms to antimicrobials. This largely reflects the types of patient most susceptible – the elderly and the very young.

In the UK, pneumonia accounts for about 50 000 hospital admissions per year, the majority being elderly. The mortality rate is 16–40%. Pneumonia also causes greater problems in chronically ill, frail patients and those with otherwise impaired immunity, e.g. patients with lymphomas or AIDS and those taking immunosuppressants, in whom it is a common secondary opportunistic complication.

The term pneumonia indicates inflammation of the lung alveoli and associated airways (see Chapter 5), accompanied by exudation into the alveoli that produces consolidation (hardening and non-compliance) of the lung parenchyma.

Pneumonia is usually a result of infection, often following aspiration of bacteria from the upper respiratory tract into the lower airways and alveoli. However, it may be caused by any physical, chemical or allergic irritant, e.g. **lipoid pneumonia** (pneumonitis) caused by accidental aspiration of liquid paraffin from laxatives or nose drops. **Aspiration pneumonitis** is a consequence of the inhalation of gastric contents during sleep, especially sleep induced by hypnotics, but sometimes following reflux oesophagitis with an oesophageal stricture (see Chapter 3). There is a high mortality due to the destructive effect of gastric acid and pepsin on the delicate lung parenchyma, and the inevitable associated infection.

The term 'chest infection' is often used to indicate pneumonia, but it is important to distinguish pneumonia from other causes of respiratory distress, because it is a serious disease and it may not be necessary to treat uncomplicated lower respiratory tract infections with an antimicrobial, e.g. most viral pneumonia.

Although pneumonia has been classified by its old anatomical terms, **bronchopneumonia** (widespread and involving the airways and alveoli) and **lobar pneumonia** (localized to one or more lobes), these terms are of little clinical relevance. The usual classification is into community- or hospital-acquired and opportunistic pneumonia (Table 8.12).

This is another example of a disease which, like meningitis, may be life-threatening, and which, because of its associated severity and mortality, must be treated immediately on an empirical basis before the results from sensitivity testing are known.

Aetiology

In community-acquired infection the most likely organism is *Strep. pneumoniae*, causing pneumococcal pneumonia. If bacteraemia develops as a complication, there is a 25% mortality rate. Influenza A is an occasional cause of viral pneumonia and although this will not respond to antibacterial therapy, complication with opportunistic bacterial infections, especially *Staph. aureus*, is serious and requires prompt antimicrobial treatment.

Community-acquired infection due to *Mycoplasma pneumoniae* and *Legionella pneumophila*, for example, also occur. The former is probably the second most common cause of pneumonia, with epidemics occurring in

Table 8.12   Classification and aetiology of pneumonia

Class	Aetiological agents	Approximate percentage of cases
Community-acquired	Streptococcus pneumoniae	60–75
	Mycoplasma pneumoniae	5–18
	Legionella pneumophila	2–5
	Viral	2–8
	Haemophilus influenzae	4–5
	Staphylococcus aureus	1–5
Hospital-acquired	Gram-negative organisms, e.g. Klebsiella, Pseudomonas, Proteus spp.	50–60
	Gram-positive organisms	10–20
Opportunistic[a]	Pneumocystis jiroveci	50
	Aspergillus fumigatus	–
	Candida	Common

[a] In immunocompromised or immunosuppressed patients, e.g. AIDs.

4-yearly cycles. *Legionella* infection is now recognized as originating overwhelmingly from water-cooled air-conditioning systems. Both of these used to be described as 'atypical' pneumonias, but the term has been dropped because there is considerable overlap in symptoms between pneumonia caused by all of the organisms. These are all examples of **primary infections** where the initial infecting organism alone is responsible for the illness.

Common examples of **secondary (opportunistic) pneumonias** are those that occur as complications of COPD (see Chapter 5). *H. influenzae* may be aspirated from the upper respiratory tract in COPD patients, although pneumococci may also be implicated. Aspiration pneumonitis following the inhalation of stomach contents or vomit can be associated with staphylococcal, streptococcal and, rarely, anaerobic organisms. Staphylococcal pneumonia is often associated with an underlying viral infection, e.g. influenza, and carries a very high mortality.

A different range of organisms is likely to be responsible for **hospital-acquired pneumonia**. MRSA is often carried as a nasal commensal and is an organism of low virulence that can cause a severe pneumonia, and wound infections, which are very difficult to treat when it is imported into the hospital environment where it infects patients with poor resistance and many avenues for infection, e.g. catheters, IV lines and surgical wounds. Artificial ventilation of patients is associated with a high mortality in intensive care units because the patient's defences are breached by the equipment. Multiply-resistant MRSA and Gram-negative organisms are more prevalent in the hospital environment, and the risk of infection by these organisms is increased greatly by the immobility and sedation of seriously ill patients.

Yet another group of organisms is encountered in immunocompromised patients. Cytotoxic chemotherapy renders patients susceptible to pneumonias caused by *Klebsiella pneumoniae* or, particularly seriously, fungi such *Aspergillus*. AIDS patients often contract pneumonias that previously were rarely seen. *Pneumocystis jiroveci* (see above) is one such organism, which carries a high mortality and was previously seen only in some patients with abdominal cancer. Other types of pneumonias contracted by AIDS patients include those caused by *Mycoplasma pneumoniae*, *Actinomyces israeli* and cytomegalovirus.

Clinical features

The symptoms and signs vary with the pathogen involved and the prior immune status of the patient. There is often a prior upper respiratory tract infection, followed usually by an abrupt onset of a chill and then high fever (38–40°C). A dry cough, high shallow respiration rate and pleuritic pain on coughing develop over a few days. Sputum production, sometimes haemoptysis (coughing of blood or blood-streaked sputum), acute dyspnoea and hypotension with a blood pressure <60 mmHg develop later, if inadequately treated. Herpes labialis often occurs (see below).

Diagnosis

Diagnosis is based primarily on the symptoms and clinical signs outlined above, but some of these may not be present. In particular, elderly patients may not have fever and present with confusion. *L. pneumophila* infection is often associated with a non-productive cough and in 60% of *Mycoplasma* infections there are minimal respiratory signs.

In severe infections with an at-risk patient, or in hospital-acquired infection, appropriate investigations must be carried out immediately, e.g. CXR, sputum for microscopy, culture and antimicrobial sensitivity testing, and blood for a full blood count and microbiology. If sputum is not produced readily it can be induced by giving nebulized hypertonic saline.

In doubtful cases fibre-optic bronchoscopy may be required to obtain specimens of secretions and bronchoalveolar lavage specimens.

If the pneumonia is community-acquired and the patient is seriously ill, particularly if immunosuppressed, has HIV/AIDS, is over 65 years or has other predisposing factors (e.g. smoking, excessive alcohol consumption or pre-existing lung disease), urgent admission to hospital is required. Pneumonia in previously well patients with influenza or chickenpox carries the possibility of serious *Staph. aureus* infection.

In such patients, and those with hospital-acquired infection, empirical treatment must be commenced immediately. This must be aggressive if there is any indication of serious systemic disease, e.g. septicaemia, confusion, a high respiratory rate or a fall in blood pressure suggestive of septic shock (see Chapter 2).

Management

General measures
Patients with fever and pleuritic pain require analgesics, but opioids must not be used because they may depress respiration.

Patients should be well hydrated, possibly intravenously, and well nourished. *Oxygen* by assisted ventilation is often required.

Pharmacotherapy
Prompt treatment is essential. Unfortunately there are few adequately powered controlled trials comparing antimicrobial regimens to guide treatment. Trials that have been done indicate the probable equivalence of all proposed treatments. In the UK, some guidelines for treatment of community-acquired pneumonia are included in the BNF (Section 5.1, Table 1).

In uncomplicated infection, high-dose *amoxicillin*, or *benzylpenicillin* in previously healthy patients, given for 7 days, is felt to be sufficient to deal with the pneumococci responsible for most mild to moderate cases. *Erythromycin* is used if there is a history of penicillin allergy and is also used with the penicillin if atypical pathogens are suspected. *Flucloxacillin* is added if staphylococci are possibly involved.

In more severe cases hospital admission is usual, and treatment with *cefuroxime* or *cefotaxime* plus *erythromycin* is used, *flucloxacillin* being added if staphylococci are suspected. If pneumonia is a sequel to influenza or measles, *flucloxacillin* is added because *Staph. aureus* infection is more likely.

Because high-level penicillin resistance in pneumococci is uncommon in the UK, and less than 20% of *H. influenzae* are resistant, empirical treatment of mild to moderate pneumonia with antimicrobials other than *amoxicillin* remains controversial. In areas where penicillin resistance is a greater problem, a macrolide or *tetracycline* are often given as first-line therapy.

For severe infection of unknown aetiology, quinolones (e.g. *levofloxacin* or *moxifloxacin*) have recently been added to the armoury and these are likely to be used increasingly as the level of penicillin resistance increases. *Cefuroxime* or *cefotaxime* plus *erythromycin* or *clarithromycin* are also used. *Flucloxacillin* is added if staphylococcal infection is suspected. *Erythromycin* is used if an 'atypical' pathogen is possible and *rifampicin* is added if *Legionella* is likely. A tetracycline is used for infection suspected to be caused by *Chlamydia* or *Mycoplasma*.

This regimen is occasionally varied in those who have co-morbidity (e.g. COPD, diabetes or renal/hepatic failure), to cover the possibility of encountering resistant organisms. In such cases *co-amoxiclav* (*amoxicillin* plus *clavulanic acid*) or *clarithromycin* are sometimes used, due to the possibility of beta-lactamase-producing *H. influenzae*.

For seriously ill patients who cannot be managed at home, IV antimicrobial therapy should be instituted as soon as possible in hospital. The suggested regimen is to use a second-generation cephalosporin, e.g. *cefuroxime*, which would provide good cover against *H. influenzae*, combined with *erythromycin*, *azithromycin* or *clarithromycin* in atypical infection. If a pneumococcal infection is confirmed, *benzylpenicillin* should be used, but there are increasing reports of resistance. If the patient responds, oral therapy may be substituted after a few days.

Treatment is longer than normal, 7–10 days being usual. In severe infections, e.g. suspected or proven infection with *Staph. aureus*, *L. pneumophila*, Gram-negative enteric bacteria, *Chlamydia* or *Mycoplasma*, 14–21 days' treatment is required.

For **hospital-acquired (nosocomial) pneumonia**, treatment using agents effective against Gram-negative organisms is indicated, the choice being dependent on the prevailing antimicrobial policy. A third-generation cephalosporin, e.g. *cefotaxime* or *ceftazidime*, or a ureidopenicillin, may be used, with the addition of an aminoglycoside in severe illness. *Vancomycin* is often added empirically if the patient is carrying MRSA.

Hospitals often have a protocol in place to cover the progression from first-line empirical cover, through second- and third-line agents. For example, if the first-line treatment with a cephalosporin fails, a quinolone may be used and if that fails in turn or septicaemia supervenes, cover may be broadened to include *piperacillin* with *tazobactam*, a beta-lactamase inhibitor. The combination of the last two agents is available commercially.

Other antibacterials are occasionally indicated for certain atypical infections e.g. *co-trimoxazole* for *Pn. jiroveci*.

Prophylaxis

Two types of pneumococcal vaccine are available and are provided in the UK via the NHS. The 23-valent pneumococcal polysaccharide vaccine (unconjugated) contains purified polysaccharides from the 23 most common capsular types of *Strep. pneumoniae*. It is used to immunize all those over 5 years who are at special risk, i.e. those who:

- are aged over 65 years;
- are asplenic or who have splenic dysfunction, including those with homozygous sickle-cell anaemia (see Chapter 11), and those with coeliac syndrome (see Chapter 3) that may lead to splenic dysfunction;
- have a chronic respiratory disease, including asthma, requiring frequent or regular treatment with an inhaled or oral corticosteroid (see Chapter 5);
- have diabetes mellitus or chronic cardiac, renal or hepatic disease;
- are immunodeficient due to HIV infection (see p. 557), prolonged systemic corticosteroid treatment, or immunosuppressive treatment, e.g. following organ transplantation (see Chapter 14) or neoplastic disease (see Chapter 10);
- have a permanent implant for certain types of deafness (cochlear) or to shunt CSF from a distal site to the brain (CSF shunt), e.g. in spina bifida, due to a developmental failure of the vertebral canal to close, or a peritoneovenous shunt in hepatic failure (see Chapter 3) with ascites (fluid in the peritoneal cavity).

A single dose of the 23-valent vaccine is given, preferably 2 weeks before initiating planned treatment, for example:

- Chemotherapy, because of the risk of neutropenia and immunosuppression.

- Surgery for splenectomy, because asplenic patients are at special risk from infection by capsulated bacteria.
- Implantation of a device, if possible.

The 7-valent pneumococcal polysaccharide conjugated vaccine is prepared from capsular polysaccharide-diphtheria toxoid complexes adsorbed onto aluminium phosphate, to increase antigenicity. Two doses at least 1 month apart are given to at-risk children under 5 years, plus a booster dose after their first birthday, i.e. to infants 2 to <6 months, starting at 2 months of age and unimmunized infants 6–11 months. Unimmunized children 1–5 years should receive two doses 2 months apart.

All children who have received this 7-valent conjugated vaccine should be given a single booster dose of the 23-valent unconjugated vaccine after their second birthday, at least 2 months after the final dose of the conjugated vaccine.

Revaccination of immunized individuals is not generally recommended, because of the risk of severe adverse reactions. However, those at special risk, e.g. asplenic patients, those with splenic dysfunction and with nephrotic syndrome (see Chapter 14), should receive regular revaccination at 5-year intervals.

Summary

The treatment of pneumonia can be summarized as follows:

- Empirical treatment of likely organisms dictates the initial antimicrobial therapy.
- The environment in which the infection was contracted, i.e. hospital or community, and the age and immune status of the patient indicate the most likely pathogen.
- Results of laboratory tests determine the definitive treatment.
- Implantation of a device increases susceptibility to infection.
- Prophylaxis by active immunization is given to young children and others at risk of pneumococcal infection.

Infective endocarditis (IE)

This is an infection of the endocardium, especially the heart valves, usually caused by bacteria, but sometimes by fungi. It is a serious disease that requires prompt, prolonged antimicrobial treatment.

Aetiology and pathology

Two factors interact to enable infection to be established: microorganisms must gain access to the blood and the endocardium must permit their attachment and growth.

The underlying predisposition may be due to a prosthetic heart valve, or to previous heart valve damage, e.g. prior rheumatic fever, mitral valve prolapse or congenital heart disease (see Chapter 4). All of these cause local turbulent blood flow and consequent small intracardiac thrombi, often on the heart valves which provide sites for the attachment of bacteria. Most microorganisms cannot attach to healthy endocardium. Thrombi with adherent or embedded microbial growths are known as vegetations. Antimicrobials penetrate poorly into these, hence the need for prolonged bactericidal treatment.

Diabetic patients are also an at-risk group, as are hospital patients with an indwelling venous cannula, IV drug abusers and those with poor dental hygiene.

The organisms usually involved include oral alpha-haemolytic streptococci ('*Strep. viridans*'; about 30–50% of cases), *Enterococcus faecalis* (about 20%) and *Staph. aureus* (about 30%, especially if hospital-acquired; 50% of those with prosthetic valves). MRSA is reported increasingly, but a large range of occasional organisms has been implicated.

Clinical features

The symptoms and signs may be very non-specific, but fever and a new heart murmur are the most common signs (90% of cases). The patient may present with malaise, night sweats, fatigue, weight loss, muscle and joint pain and haematuria. The left side of the heart is usually more involved than the right.

The disease often follows a prolonged, moderate course, hence the term 'subacute bacterial endocarditis' (SBE), but this term is falling into disuse because not all the infections are bacterial. In subacute disease, heart failure, finger clubbing (see Chapter 5), a haemorrhagic (petechial) rash and 'splinter haemorrhages' of the nail bed often develop. Strokes and MI are a result of embolization from vegetations, and occur in about 20% of cases.

However, *Staph. aureus* infections often cause severe, acute disease and MRSA is increasingly common. Infected aneurysms may occur.

Investigation

The following tests are very useful:

- Blood for culturing, serology, antimicrobial sensitivity tests, and ESR or CRP. If cultures are negative (about 25% of cases), at least two further sets of samples are taken. A negative result does not exclude a diagnosis of IE if appropriate clinical signs are present. Serology may provide evidence of infection when cultures are negative.
- Echocardiography will show vegetations and blood regurgitation across abnormal heart valves and may identify those patients needing urgent surgery. Trans-oesophageal echocardiography is sensitive for small lesions and is 90% specific.
- Serial ECGs may show evidence of developing conduction defects, due to valve ring involvement, or MI. Embolization from vegetations is responsible for many deaths.
- CXR.
- Urine, for proteinuria and haematuria, which occur in about 70% of patients as a result of renal infarction.

Pharmacotherapy

Treatment with bactericidal antimicrobials is desirable to prevent relapse, if they are suitable for the patient.

Initial empirical treatment is with *benzylpenicillin* plus *gentamicin*. *Flucloxacillin* is substituted for *benzylpenicillin* if symptoms are more severe, in anticipation of staphylococcal infection.

Vancomycin plus *rifampicin* are substituted for the penicillin if the patient is allergic to penicillins, if there is an artificial heart valve, or if MRSA is suspected. If *flucloxacillin* is being used, *rifampicin* is added for at least 2 weeks.

If fully sensitive streptococci are confirmed, *benzylpenicillin*, or *vancomycin* if the patient is allergic to penicillin, alone for 4 weeks is satisfactory. Alternatively, *benzylpenicillin* or *vancomycin*, plus *gentamicin* for 2 weeks are used if the organism is highly penicillin-resistant. If the organisms are more resistant, if *Enterococcus faecalis* is suspected or proven, or if there are complications, *gentamicin* plus either *amoxicillin* or *vancomycin* is used. If the organisms are gentamicin-resistant, *streptomycin* is substituted, one of its very few indications nowadays.

There is a group of difficult-to-treat bacteria, known collectively as 'HACEK' organisms, i.e. *Haemophilus*, *Actinobacillus*, *Cardiobacterium*, *Eikenella* and *Kingella* species, for which *amoxicillin* (or *ceftriaxone* if amoxicillin-resistant) plus low-dose *gentamicin* is used. The combination is used for 2 weeks, the *gentamicin* is stopped and treatment with either *amoxicillin* or *ceftriaxone* is continued for a further 2 weeks. If the patient has a prosthetic heart valve, treatment is prolonged to a total of 6 weeks.

Summary

The treatment of IE illustrates:

- The need for prompt treatment to prevent serious cardiac damage and stroke.
- The necessity for prolonged treatment with bactericidal antimicrobials to ensure the elimination of the infectious agent from protected sites in the vegetations.
- The role of prosthetic devices, heart valves in this case, acting as a focus for infection.

Rheumatic fever

Rheumatic fever (RhF) has been described as a disease that licks the joints but grips the heart, i.e. the joint problems are minor and the delayed cardiac consequences are the major problem.

This syndrome follows infection with group A streptococci. It is probably an autoimmune disease, triggered by a cross-reaction between streptococcal antigen(s) and the laminin in the basement membrane of human heart valves. There is a less important reaction against cardiac myosin.

Epidemiology

Acute rheumatic fever (ARhF) is a disease of poor living conditions, including malnutrition, overcrowding and lack of hygiene. Consequently it is now uncommon in Western, developed countries, having started to decline in the late 19th century, a process that was accelerated by the introduction of antimicrobials.

However, it remains a major public health problem in the Third World and the WHO estimates that about 5×10^5 people acquire the condition annually. Children and adolescents aged 5–15 years are most at risk and high incidences (between 80 and 500 per 100 000 children) have been recorded in the indigenous populations of Australia and New Zealand. It is rare in adults over 30 years of age. Attacks may recur in adolescents and young adults, but become increasingly less frequent in adults and are rare over the age of 40–45.

Pathogenesis

Infections by many strains of group A beta-haemolytic streptococci are the trigger event and outbreaks of ARhF follow those of streptococcal pharyngitis, so-called 'strep sore throat', but not all patients notice this. However, it is known that ARhF may follow other streptococcal infections, e.g. impetigo. There is no specific test for causative strains, nor is it possible to identify those who will subsequently develop **chronic rheumatic fever (CRhF)**. Familial clustering is a reflection of shared poor living conditions.

The cardiac complications involve all tissues, i.e. endocardium, myocardium, valves (especially the mitral valve) and pericardium.

Clinical features

The initial presenting symptom is the sudden onset of a fleeting palindromic arthropathy of the larger joints (see Chapter 12). There may also be non-specific symptoms, e.g. abdominal pain, fever with apparently excessive tachycardia, epistaxis, raised ESR and CRP, etc. that are not of diagnostic value. The anaemia of chronic disease (see Chapter 11) is common.

Arthritic symptoms
The migratory polyarthritis affects the large joints, initially of the legs, each joint being affected for about a week. Joint involvements tend to overlap. However, a monoarthritis is common in endemic regions.

Cardiac involvement
Symptoms may be difficult to detect in mild disease. Auscultation may give the signs of a pericardial rub, due to inflammation, valve murmurs, due to regurgitation initially but valve stenosis later. There is usually some pericardial pain. The ECG commonly shows a sinus tachycardia faster than that expected from the fever, but with a paradoxical, prolonged PR interval – the PR interval is expected to be shorter than normal in tachycardia. Heart failure may be life-threatening.

Central nervous system involvement
Chorea (i.e. neurogenic, rapid, involuntary, jerking limb movements that disappear during sleep) may be the sole manifestation, and develops later. Other CNS involvement may be associated with muscular weakness. Very labile moods, with restlessness, crying bouts and anger or other inappropriate behaviour often occur.

Skin symptoms and signs
SC firm, painless, uninflamed rheumatoid nodules (see Chapter 12) appear over the tendons or bony surfaces after several weeks. Erythema marginatum occurs in about 10% of patients. It is a usually fleeting, pinkish rash, lasting a few hours that extends centrifugally, reminiscent of urticaria or ringworm (see Chapter 13).

Diagnosis

The WHO criteria are as follows:

- Chorea and indolent (persistent) carditis do not require evidence of prior group A streptococcal infection.
- **First episode**
  - Major criteria: carditis, arthritis, chorea, erythema marginatum, SC nodules.
  - Minor criteria: arthralgia (joint pain without inflammation), fever, raised ESR or CRP levels, prolonged PR interval on ECG.
  - Evidence of prior group A streptococcal infection, i.e. a positive throat culture or rapid antigen test for group A streptococcus or a raised or rising streptococcal antibody titre.
- Diagnosis requires: two major criteria or one major and two minor criteria
- **Recurrent episode**

  In a patient without established rheumatic heart disease as first episode, or in a patient with established rheumatic heart disease, requires two or more minor criteria, plus evidence of prior group A streptococcal infection (by serology).
- **Differential diagnoses** include:
  - Reactive arthritis (see Chapter 12). Post-streptococcal reactive arthritis is difficult to distinguish from ARhF and is best treated as the latter.
  - Joint infection: septic arthritis, viral arthropathy.
  - Infective endocarditis (see above).
  - Lyme disease (pp. 523, 526).
  - Sickle-cell anaemia (see Chapter 11).
  - Neoplastic disease: leukaemia or lymphoma

Unfortunately the criteria were established for epidemiological and not for diagnostic purposes. In many parts of the world where ARhF is common, the prompt availability of laboratory tests, ECG and echocardiography is limited, so diagnosis must be based on clinical judgement. This enables treatment to be initiated promptly and so helps to avoid the possibility of serious sequelae.

Treatment

The aims are to:

- give symptomatic relief;
- minimize inflammation and so serious heart damage;
- eliminate carriage of streptococci in the nasopharynx.

These are accomplished by:

- Rest (bed or chair).
- *Phenoxymethylpenicillin* for 10 days or *erythromycin* if penicillin-sensitive.
- Anti-inflammatories when the diagnosis is clear, e.g. *aspirin* 100 mg/kg/day in children (risk of Reye's syndrome in those under 16), up to 8 g/day in adults or *prednisolone* 2 mg/kg/day, for about 14 days, and then reduced gradually (20%/week) according to clinical improvement or levels of ESR or CRP. Cover *prednisolone* withdrawal with *aspirin* if necessary. There is no permanent joint damage after the arthropathy.
- Treat heart failure if present (see Chapter 4).
- Valve replacement, if available, if there is regurgitation or significant stenosis.

Prophylaxis with twice-daily *phenoxymethylpenicillin* is maintained until 5 years after the last attack or age 20–21, whichever is the longer. Patients who have had a valve replacement require *warfarin* (see Chapter 11).

Inadequate treatment or prophylaxis may lead to death 20–30 years after the initial attack.

Gastroenteritis and acute diarrhoea

The human bowel, being in contact with the external environment, contains a range of non-pathogenic commensals, but some of these are potentially pathogenic if they gain access to another site. These organisms live in a state of balanced competition with each other for food. However, problems arise when this balance, or that between them and their host, is upset (e.g. by broad-spectrum antimicrobial treatment) or an unusual organism is involved. The predominant potentially pathogenic bacteria include anaerobes (e.g. *Bacteroides fragilis* or *Cl. difficile*), and there are also coliforms (e.g. *E. coli* and *Klebsiella* spp., *Ent. faecalis* and *Proteus* spp.). Fungi (e.g. *Candida* spp.), viruses and protozoa (e.g. *Entamoeba histolytica* and *Giardia intestinalis* (formerly *G. lamblia*)) may also be involved.

The term **gastroenteritis** describes any non-specific inflammation of the stomach and bowel, but is often applied to any bowel infection resulting in diarrhoea. The causative organisms tend to be different for adults and infants. Other species are responsible for specific infections, e.g. cholera, dysentery and typhoid. This section deals only with acute, non-specific infective diarrhoeas; non-infective chronic diarrhoeas and those of other origins are covered in Chapter 3.

Antimicrobials are used for gut infections only if symptoms are severe and prolonged, if a specific pathogen is confirmed, or in immuno-suppressed and elderly subjects. Antimicrobial treatments are discussed below.

Treatment with antidiarrhoeals, i.e. *loperamide*, *diphenoxylate* or opioids, should be avoided if at all possible, as this will tend to retain inflammatory exudate in the bowel and prolong symptoms.

Acute diarrhoea in children (infantile gastroenteritis)

This is rarely fatal in otherwise healthy children, but with malnourishment and poor housing there is a high risk of mortality. Viruses (especially rotaviruses) are usually responsible. An important feature of infantile gastroenteritis is the depression of gastrointestinal luminal disaccharidase levels, resulting in an osmotic diarrhoea (see Chapter 3). Oral rehydration therapy is the mainstay of treatment, as the young are particularly vulnerable to dehydration. Antimicrobial therapy is likely to be useless and may prolong symptoms by causing further disturbance of the gastrointestinal flora.

Bacterial gastroenteritis in infants is often caused by self-infection from their own bowel with enteropathogenic strains of *E. coli*. These either produce an exotoxin that increases gastrointestinal fluid secretion, resulting in the production of a watery diarrhoea, or cause damage to the mucosa that results in a bloody diarrhoea. *E. coli* infections are usually self-limiting and require only simple oral rehydration therapy, which provides sodium, potassium and chloride, usually with glucose to provide energy and assist electrolyte absorption (see BNF, Section 9.2.1). However, certain uncommon strains, e.g. enterohaemorrhagic *E. coli* O157:H7 (EHEC), can cause a more severe or even fatal outcome. This has occurred in food poisoning outbreaks in several countries, where this strain caused a high incidence of complications, even including renal failure. Enterotoxigenic *E. coli* (ETEC) is the most common cause of travellers' diarrhoea (see below).

The organisms are transmitted via the faecal-oral route. *Campylobacter jejuni* is a worldwide commensal in many farm animals and dogs and may be ingested from animal faeces, often through children playing in contaminated soil or with pets. *Camp. jejuni* causes severe abdominal pain and antimicrobials may be required.

Antimicrobial treatments are similar to those used in adults.

Acute adult diarrhoea

Acute infective gastroenteritis is usually attributed to 'food poisoning' or 'travellers' diarrhoea' in the lay mind. However, toxins are involved only occasionally, the symptoms usually being caused by microbial overgrowth. Table 8.13 shows that a variety of organisms may be responsible, but antimicrobial therapy is rarely indicated. In other cases, e.g. dysentery, typhoid fever or giardiasis, the organism responds to specific antimicrobial therapy.

Salmonella infections
Infection by *Salmonella enteritidis* and *S. typhimurium*, but not *S. typhi* or *S. paratyphi*, are

Table 8.13 Diarrhoea in adults

Common name	Likely organisms
Food poisoning, traveller's diarrhoea	Salmonella enteritidis or S. typhimurium (NOT S. typhi or S. paratyphi)
	Clostridium welchii
	Yersinia enterocolitica
	Escherichia coli
	Campylobacter jejuni
	Staphylcoccus aureus
	Brucella spp.
	Bacillus cereus
Bacterial dysentery	Shigella spp.
Amoebic dysentery	Entamoeba histolytica
Giardiasis	Giardia intestinalis
Cholera	Vibrio cholerae
Typhoid and paratyphoid	Salmonella typhi, S. paratyphi
Antibiotic-associated	Non-specific, but especially Clostridium difficile

still an important cause of food poisoning, but *Campylobacter* infections are now the major cause of diarrhoea in developed countries. *S. enteritidis* and *S. typhimurium* strains are sometimes named after the location in which they were first isolated, e.g. *S. enteritidis* serotype Dublin, a common cattle commensal. Lack of basic hygiene after toileting, e.g. hand washing, including nail scrubbing, is the usual cause of human-to-human spread or self-infection. Symptoms usually last for a few days, rarely a week, and range from a watery stool to a severe diarrhoea with abdominal pains, vomiting, fever, blood and pus. The latter symptoms are caused by invasion of the bowel wall, usually by *Campylobacter* or virulent strains of *E. coli*, and may lead to systemic disease.

Even for severe attacks healthy adults usually require only oral rehydration. Indeed, antibacterials may increase the duration of symptoms, by further disturbance of the bowel flora, and prolong intestinal carriage. However, if there is severe sepsis, symptoms lasting more than 3 days, or if the patient has some underlying problem, e.g. is frail and elderly or immunocompromised, antimicrobials may be indicated.

Oral rehydration therapy (see above) is still required as a first-line treatment. *Ciprofloxacin* is usually the first choice if antimicrobial treatment is required, but resistance is an increasing problem. *Erythromycin* or *co-trimoxazole* are

alternatives, but the latter may cause serious side-effects.

Severe disease causing dehydration is an indication for hospital admission, where patients should be isolated and barrier-nursed. Children under 2 years are rarely given antimicrobials, but should be supervised by a Paediatric Consultant.

Travellers' diarrhoea

This may be caused by a variety of organisms, depending on local conditions, although ETEC is usually responsible. If the symptoms are severe (e.g. nausea, vomiting and bloody stools), prolonged, or if signs of septicaemia are present, *ciprofloxacin* may lessen the severity and reduce duration of symptoms from about 5 days to 24 h. The once popular prophylactic use of sulphonamides is undesirable as the risk of infection is reduced by only 50% and adverse effects are common.

Typhoid fever

Clinical features

In contrast to food-borne salmonellosis, *Salmonella typhi* infections require antimicrobial treatment. A similar but milder disease is caused by *S. paratyphi*. Infection is usually spread by sewage-contaminated water. Man is the only natural host for the organisms, so personal hygiene is very important.

Typhoid fever is not always associated with diarrhoea. Patients may have constipation in the early stages, and the systemic complications are more important than local gut symptoms. This is because the organism can penetrate the gastro-intestinal mucosa and proliferate within the local reticuloendothelial cells before spreading throughout the body. After about 3 weeks, the gut wall is damaged and penetrated by sufficient bacteria to cause the initial symptoms of dehydration, fever and confusion. The most serious complications are gastrointestinal haemorrhage and perforation.

Following recovery, some 5–10% of patients become convalescent carriers and continue to excrete typhoid bacteria, and 1–4% become chronic carriers, who continue to excrete organisms for many years. Gallbladder carriage is usual in the West and is associated with gallstone formation (see Chapter 3).

In the Third World up to 30% of patients die and a further 10% relapse after apparent recovery. This contrasts with 1–2% deaths in developed countries.

Treatment

Ciprofloxacin is the antibacterial of choice. Broad-spectrum antibacterials (*ampicillin*, sulphonamides and *chloramphenicol*) are active against some strains of *S. typhi*, but resistance is a major problem. Indiscriminate use in some Third World countries has led to the loss of previously effective antimicrobials, e.g. *chloramphenicol*. Thus treatment must be guided by early diagnosis, sensitivity testing and local knowledge.

IM immunization with capsular polysaccharide antigen of *S. typhi* must be renewed every 3 years to maintain immunity. A live, attenuated, oral vaccine is available (Ty21a) and gives superior immunity.

Cholera

The insidious onset of typhoid fever contrasts markedly with infection by *Vibrio cholerae*. The current strain has been the El Tor biotype, named for the Red Sea port from which it was first identified. This organism does not invade the gut wall and the tissues, but produces a toxin

that acts rapidly on the bowel to induce an intense, watery diarrhoea, resulting in dehydration. Over the years cholera has tended to become less virulent than the 'classic cholera' encountered earlier in the last century, when diarrhoea and death from dehydration could follow quite rapidly. In otherwise healthy people the course is often mild. Cholera is very rare in Western travellers to endemic areas and may even pass as a bout of simple travellers' diarrhoea. However, present-day cholera, which tends to cause epidemics when sanitary conditions are very poor, does cause many fatalities amongst the young, elderly or malnourished in developing countries.

A new pathogenic strain, *V. cholerae* O139, has been identified and may cause future epidemics.

Oral rehydration can be life-saving, but IV fluids are needed in very ill patients. The disease is otherwise self-limiting.

Antimicrobial therapy plays only a small part in the management of cholera. Antibacterials such as the tetracyclines will reduce fluid loss to some extent, but availability is limited in countries where cholera is endemic, and resistance is a problem.

Because the organism does not invade the tissues, immunity following natural infection is poor.

Prophylaxis with current vaccines give poor immunity and a new killed whole cell vaccine is available and an attenuated live vaccine is being investigated.

Chemoprophylaxis with *tetracycline* is effective but is not a substitute for scrupulous personal and food hygiene.

Dysentery

Bacterial dysentery

Classical **bacillary dysentery (shigellosis)** is caused by *Shigella* spp., which are found only in the bowel of man and the higher primates. Similar symptoms may be caused by *Campylobacter*, *Yersinia* or enteroinvasive *E. coli* (EIEC). The disease is associated with overcrowding, poor sanitation and hygiene and is usually seen in the UK in kindergartens, nursery schools and residential homes.

Shigella sonnei and *Sh. flexneri* are the commonest species in the UK and usually cause a mild to moderate diarrhoeal disease, often indistinguishable from gastroenteritis.

Sh. shigae causes severe, bloody diarrhoea, with dehydration and prostration and a high mortality if untreated. The stools contain inflammatory exudate, WBCs, blood and mucus. Arthritis and renal damage may also occur. Fluid replacement is essential, using oral rehydration salts, or IV fluids if dehydration is sufficiently severe.

In terms of antimicrobial treatment, *ciprofloxacin* is again the treatment of choice, but there have been reports of resistance to this, so sensitivity testing is an essential guide to therapy in severe disease.

Protozoal dysentery

Amoebic dysentery is caused by *Entamoeba histolytica* and has similar symptoms to shigellosis but systemic effects are uncommon. Only a small proportion of those carrying amoebic cysts develop invasive disease. Part of the reason for this is that the cysts are those of a non-pathogenic species, *Ent. dispar*, which cannot be differentiated from *Ent. histolytica* microscopically. Identification is by serology using fluorescent antibody. It is not known why the asymptomatic carrier state is so common and the epidemiology of amoebic dysentery remains uncertain.

Transmission is mostly by the faecal–oral route, but person-to-person transmission can occur by vaginal and anal intercourse and cunnilingus. The condition tends to be longer-lasting than shigellosis and may be mild or severe. Severe infection may be indistinguishable from severe UC (see Chapter 3) and may require colonic biopsy. Important complications of severe infection are toxic megacolon and intestinal perforation. Invasion of the liver to cause abscesses may occur (mostly in men), without prior gastrointestinal symptoms, and infection may break through into the peritoneal, pleural and pericardial cavities, with life-threatening consequences.

The treatment of choice for invasive disease is *metronidazole* in high doses for 5–10 days or *tinidazole* for 2–6 days. This should be followed

by *diloxanide furoate* or *paromomycin* to eradicate cysts from the gut lumen. The latter can also be used to eliminate the asymptomatic carrier state.

Giardia intestinalis (formerly *G. lamblia*) causes diarrhoea of long duration, sometimes months if untreated, referred to as **giardiasis**. There is no blood in the stools, but owing to malabsorption a frothy foul-smelling diarrhoea with copious wind (steatorrhoea) may result. *G. intestinalis* is common in the water supplies in the Third World and in areas affected by war and economic deprivation. Diagnosis is by the clinical symptoms and signs and a history of travel to an endemic area, faecal microscopy and more specifically by enzyme-linked immunoassay.

Initial treatment is with a nitroimidazole, i.e. *metronidazole* for 3–5 days or single-dose *tinidazole*. *Albendazole* and *mepacrine* are second line drugs in the event of treatment failure.

Other protozoal infections have become important with the rise of HIV/AIDS, e.g. those due to *Cryptosporidium cayetanensis, Isospora belli, Dientamoeba fragilis* and the microsporidium *Encephalitozoon intestinalis*. *Cryptosporidium* may cause life-threatening diarrhoea with high mortality in HIV/AIDS patients not on HAART (Table 8.11).

Treatment is with *co-trimoxazole* for *Cryptosporidium* and *Isospora* infections and *albendazole* for *Encephalitozoon*.

Dientamoeba is co-transmitted with the pinworm *Enterobius vermicularis*, so treatment needs to cover both organisms, i.e. *metronidazole* or *tinidazole* for *Dientamoeba*, and *mebendazole*, in patients aged over 2 years, for *Enterobius*.

Antibiotic-associated colitis

The use of oral broad-spectrum antibacterials, particularly if poorly absorbed, can lead to overgrowth of resistant organisms in the gut lumen. This may cause a mild diarrhoea that resolves on discontinuation of treatment. In some cases the disturbance is drug-specific, e.g. *erythromycin* causes a decrease in drug transit time and *tetracyclines* can inactivate lipases. The latter action prevents fat absorption, which then passes into the colon to produce steatorrhoea.

AAC is more serious and is the result of overgrowth with *Clostridium difficile*. This organism releases an exotoxin that causes a local inflammation and formation of a membrane of necrotic tissue over the bowel wall, which in about 20% of cases leads to a form of chronic diarrhoea, sometimes called **pseudomembranous colitis**. This is an intense, potentially fatal diarrhoea that requires oral treatment with *vancomycin* or *metronidazole* and is currently a serious problem in the UK.

Summary of acute diarrhoea treatment

- Most cases of diarrhoea will not require antimicrobial treatment. Exceptions to this are when:
  - Systemic effects are present.
  - The patient is either very young or elderly.
  - The patient has some other debilitating condition.
- Oral or IV rehydration are the most important treatments for the management of severe or persistent diarrhoea.
- Antimicrobial therapy may benefit patients suffering from infection caused by certain specific organisms, particularly when there are systemic complications. Conversely, the indiscriminate use of antimicrobials may exacerbate symptoms. Although the 4-quinolones are the treatment of choice for most bacterial infections, if indicated by the clinical condition of the patient, *metronidazole* is used to treat anaerobic bacterial infections, e.g. by *Bacteroides* and *Clostridium* spp., giardiasis and amoebic dysentery.

Tuberculosis

Epidemiology

During the 19th and early 20th centuries, tuberculosis (TB) was the cause of 50% of all deaths and morbidity and was described as "The Captain of the Armies of Death". The old term for the disease, consumption, describes the extreme wasting of the tissues of those with untreated disease. Today it is far less common in the UK, affecting 5–10 per 100 000 of the native population, though it is much more prevalent among some immigrant groups. Although the fall over the last century in the incidence of TB in the West can be linked to general improvements in nutrition, hygiene and general living standards, immunization and antimicrobial chemotherapy have played an important part since the 1950s, so that death from TB is now rare in the West.

Recently, however, TB has again become a serious worldwide health issue. The WHO has declared the disease to be a global emergency. It estimates that TB is now responsible globally for 4 million deaths annually, and rising. TB is the major cause of death from infectious illness among those over 5 years of age in developing countries. Much of the problem is related to the emergence of HIV/AIDS, which renders affected individuals highly susceptible. Approximately 10% of cases, rising to 30–50% in some sub-Saharan African countries, are related to HIV infection. In Third World countries overall, TB is responsible for some 25% of avoidable deaths. India and China have 1.8 and 1.3 million cases, respectively, but these figures are likely to be considerable underestimates. The financial, logistical and manpower burdens of TB and its treatment are a significant constraint on economic development.

Aetiology

Pulmonary TB is caused by *Mycobacterium tuberculosis* transmitted via airborne droplets coughed or sneezed by infected individuals. Rarely, **bovine TB**, transmitted via cow's milk, causes TB of the GIT. Mycobacteria are unusual in that they possess an outer waxy coat, which makes them particularly resistant to drying, the host's defence mechanisms and to most antimicrobials. The bacterium becomes a focus for chronic inflammation, and granuloma (**tubercle**) formation (see Chapter 2) is a particular feature.

Pathogenesis

The progression of TB is summarized in Figure 8.4. Following primary infection, usually in the lungs, neutrophils are attracted to the site of infection and replaced by macrophages after about a week. These cells engulf and attempt to digest the organisms, which however may

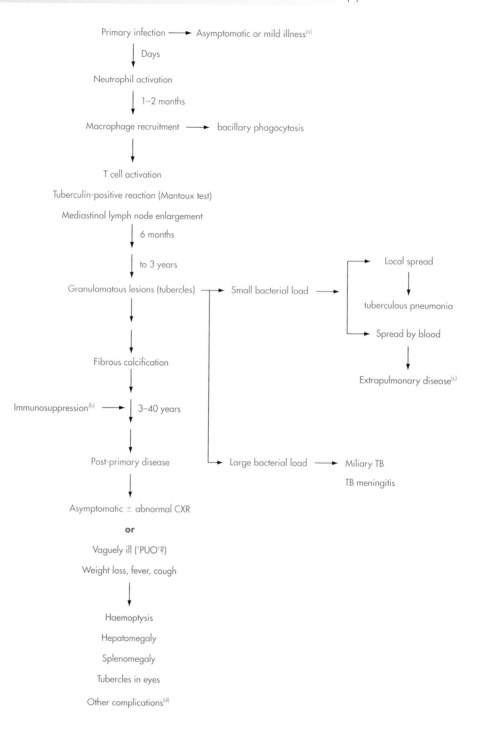

Figure 8.4   Pathogenesis of tuberculosis. [a]Only a small proportion of those infected show signs and frank symptoms, which are usually non-specific, i.e. poor appetite, cough ± slight wheeze, occasionally a small transient pleural effusion and a rash over the lower legs (erythema nodosum). [b]May be due to ageing, drugs, concurrence of some neoplastic diseases (especially lymphomas; see Chapter 10), chronic diseases, e.g. severe diabetes mellitus,

remain unharmed and viable owing to their waxy coat. T cells are also activated and their lymphokines attract and maintain the population of macrophages around the focus of infection. Two groups of T helper cells are known to be involved in this immune response; the TH_1 and TH_2 cells are distinguished by their CD antigens and the different cytokines that they release (see Chapter 2). It is believed that TH_1 activity is responsible for macrophage activation, but that the action of TH_2, or a mixed TH_1/TH_2 activity, renders cells highly susceptible to killing by TNF. This activity of the immune system and its proinflammatory cytokines is responsible for much of the lung damage associated with TB. This process eventually leads either to the formation of tubercles, which may heal completely leaving a small, often calcified, scar, or to spread via the lymphatics into the lymph nodes, where the bacteria form a more widespread 'primary complex'. In immunosuppressed patients or the elderly, mycobacteria occasionally spread via the bloodstream to various tissues, e.g. the spleen, liver, kidneys and eyes, a condition known as **miliary TB**. Bacteria may also reach the CNS, causing **tuberculous meningitis**, or become sequestered in bones (usually the spine) where they become centres for granulomatous lesions and cause deformity.

At about 1–2 months after infection, individuals become sensitized to mycobacterial proteins, displaying a local type IV hypersensitivity reaction that causes further tissue damage. This is the basis of the Mantoux test for immunity to TB. At this stage all the characteristic clinical features of TB are apparent (see below).

The major complications usually occur on reactivation of the disease (**post-primary TB**), as a result of reduced immunity or another concurrent infection. Post-primary infection of the lung produces the typical symptoms of pulmonary TB, the primary infection often having been mild or asymptomatic. Re-infection

is another uncommon cause for post-primary infection.

High-dose corticosteroid and other immunosuppressive treatments and diabetes mellitus can trigger post-primary TB, so many clinicians give prophylactic *isoniazid* (see below) before initiating such therapy in patients with evidence of previous TB infection.

Although it is estimated that about 30% of people worldwide are carriers of *M. tuberculosis*, only about 10% of these develop symptoms, because of containment by carriers' immune response or differences in the pathogenicity of different strains. A major TB school outbreak in Leicester, England, in 2001 was caused by the CH strain and affected over 250 pupils. This strain is more pathogenic than usual, causing symptoms in about 25% of those infected. It has recently been discovered that, surprisingly, this increased virulence is probably due to a single gene deletion that, although the CH strain grows less well in culture, makes it less immunogenic. Thus the CH-infected patient does not mount a normal inmmune response.

In this connection, it is known that a heat shock protein of *M. tuberculosis* (Hsp70) modulates the patient's immune response by stimulating the CCR5 receptors of dendritic, antigen-presenting cells to group together with T cells, thus activating more T cells and increasing the immune response. Hsp70 is now being evaluated as a new agent for the treatment of TB and, incidentally, for enhancing the immune response to cancer cells. Other possible agents for stimulating the CCR5 receptors of dendritic cells are also being investigated.

Clinical features

In most subjects, primary infections are asymptomatic or mild, i.e. a vague malaise, sometimes with cough and wheezing. Symptoms normally disappear as the tissues heal, but viable mycobacteria persist for years in the tubercles. Although

---

HIV/AIDS. [c]Extrapulmonary disease may affect the lymph nodes, bones and joints, gastrointestinal tract and kidneys. [d]Other complications include pleural effusion; emphysema (pus in the pleural cavity); laryngeal and more distant spread; *Aspergillus* lung infection; haemoptysis (see Chapter 5); may be fatal. CXR, chest X-ray; PUO, pyrexia of unknown origin (see p. 534); TB, tuberculosis.

patients become tuberculin-positive, i.e. hypersensitive to mycobacterial protein, the immunity may not be complete, leading to more severe lung problems. If the bacterial load is heavy, miliary disease, tubercular pneumonia, and tubercular meningitis may occur within the first year. If the bacterial load is light, the lymph nodes, bones and joints, the gut and kidneys may become infected within 5 years.

In young children the disease progresses rapidly and early diagnosis is essential to avoid mortality.

Advancing age, with declining immunocompetence, chronic disease and immunosuppression may allow reactivation of the mycobacteria in granulomas years later, to cause post-primary infection. The classic respiratory symptoms of a post-primary infection include the slow development of tiredness, weight loss, fever and a cough productive of mucoid or purulent sputum, which may be bloodstained. There may also be chest wall pain, dyspnoea and wheeze, and a history of recurrent colds. Finger clubbing (see Chapter 5) occurs in advanced disease. The CXR is abnormal but is not necessarily diagnostic, so bacteriological evidence is needed.

Without adequate therapy, lung damage will lead to progressive disability and a slow, lingering death.

Diagnosis

This depends on the following:

- Symptoms and signs.
- CXR, and CT scan if the X-ray is equivocal.
- Sputum microbiology. Lung washings or biopsy specimens of suspected lung lesions, lymph nodes and pleura may be necessary in doubtful cases.
  - Microscopy for acid-fast rods.
  - Culture and sensitivity testing
- DNA testing, if speed is required or if microbiology is negative in a patient with suggestive symptoms.

The Mantoux test cannot usually be used in the UK to diagnose active TB, because of widespread BCG vaccination (see below).

Prophylaxis

Immunization

In the UK, **Bacillus Calmette-Guérin (BCG)**, a live attenuated vaccine against TB, has been offered to all tuberculin-negative children aged 10–13 years, reducing the risk of overt TB by up to 75%. However, the low incidence of TB in some areas has caused this to be stopped. In deprived areas, and where there is a high immigrant population, immunization is being offered to children at birth, reducing new infections considerably. In other countries efficacy may be much higher (e.g. in Scandinavia) or much lower (e.g. in the tropics), and a more effective vaccine is being investigated. In addition, immunity may be lost in later life, but the efficacy of BCG in older adults has been less well studied.

TB is spread from person to person, so **contact tracing** of all newly diagnosed patients is essential to reduce the risk of disease spread. All those in the same house, and sometimes people in the same school or workplace, are screened for TB. If they are unwell, rigorous investigation for TB is required. If they are well, a CXR and tuberculin test are done. If the CXR is negative in adults no further action is required, even if they are tuberculin-positive (see above).

If the tuberculin test is negative in children and young adults, the test should be repeated after 6–8 weeks and if it is still negative BCG vaccination should be given. However, if it has become positive, and if BCG vaccine has not been given, this indicates active infection and treatment should be started immediately.

All medical and paramedical hospital staff should be immunized with BCG if they are tuberculin-negative. BCG immunization is not given to tuberculin-positive subjects because this is likely to provoke a severe hypersensitivity reaction.

Chemoprophylaxis

People at high risk who are in contact with the public in areas with high levels of TB, e.g. teachers and catering staff, are often given *isoniazid* for 6 months, which reduces the infection risk but there is a risk of hepatotoxicity. This is also required for patients who are taking immunosuppressive agents, including high-dose corticosteroids, and are starting renal dialysis. Some consultants routinely give *isoniazid* before starting prolonged or high-dose corticosteroid treatment.

HIV infection is immunosuppressive by definition and patients cannot respond to BCG vaccination, so all are given *isoniazid*. There is a risk of peripheral neuropathy in this situation, but *pyridoxine* may help prevent this. An *isoniazid*-resistant strain of BCG vaccine must be used if a patient is to be given *isoniazid* later.

Liver function tests should be done before starting *isoniazid* treatment and regularly thereafter during therapy.

Pharmacotherapy

The purpose of chemotherapy is to eradicate the organism completely, but there are major problems associated with this. It can take 6–8 weeks to culture the slow-growing *Mycobacterium*, and a further 4–6 weeks for sensitivity testing. This means that therapy must be started empirically. However, newer DNA probe techniques are being developed that reduce this to about 48 h and should lead to earlier, more effective treatment.

M. tuberculosis is resistant to many common antibacterials owing to poor penetration of the agents. Moreover, because resistance is so widespread, treatment failure is inevitable if a single agent is used. During active disease, the growing bacteria must be dealt with quickly, but there will also be dormant or semi-dormant bacteria that require protracted therapy for elimination.

Antitubercular drugs are rather toxic, and must be used long term: both of these factors tend to reduce compliance. In addition, compliance is often poor because patients tend to feel much better soon after initiating chemotherapy: they become non-infective after 2 weeks. Poor compliance results in an incomplete kill of the organisms and, almost inevitably, future relapse with drug-resistant disease.

There has been much interest in finding ways of improving compliance. Uniquely this has become very much a public health issue, where it has been shown that good compliance with a regimen actually reduces the rate of TB notification. A useful strategy might be to monitor urine levels of the various agents. A directly observed therapy, short course scheme (DOTS) has also been used successfully. In this, patients are invited to attend clinics three times each week, the dosages being adjusted accordingly to allow for the increased interval between them. This is one situation in which combination products are preferred to aid compliance, unless that is not possible due to drug toxicity.

Figure 8.5 summarizes the current recommendations made by the WHO for the treatment of pulmonary TB.

It is assumed that the organism will be drug-resistant, so a combination of *isoniazid*, *rifampicin*, *pyrazinamide* and *ethambutol* is given for the first 2 months. *Isoniazid* and *rifampicin* are then usually given for another 4 months, if laboratory results indicate that these two agents are effective. It is important to continue with all four agents until efficacy is confirmed by laboratory tests. *Rifampicin* and *isoniazid* are somewhat faster-acting than *ethambutol* or *pyrazinamide*. All drugs are administered as a single daily dose, 30 min before breakfast and often as combined preparations (*rifampicin/isoniazid* or *rifampicin/isoniazid/pyrazinamide*) in order to improve compliance.

Rifampicin, *isoniazid* and *pyrazinamide* can all cause liver damage, so liver function must be monitored throughout treatment. *Ethambutol* at high doses has been associated with retinal damage and should be discontinued if visual disturbance occurs. *Isoniazid*-induced peripheral neuropathy can be avoided by giving *pyridoxine*.

Rifampicin can turn urine or tears an orange-red colour and patients must be warned of this to avoid undue alarm and unnecessary visits to the doctor. It may also cause staining of contact lenses.

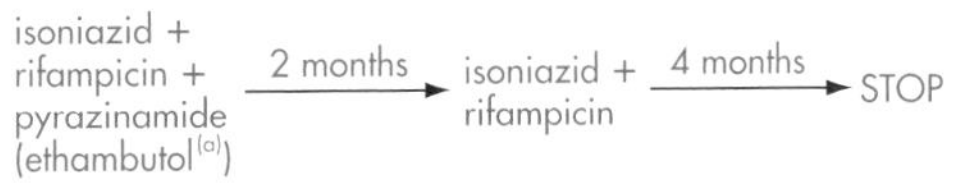

isoniazid + rifampicin + pyrazinamide (ethambutol[a]) — 2 months → isoniazid + rifampicin — 4 months → STOP

Figure 8.5 Standard treatment of tuberculosis. [a]Add if isoniazid resistance is likely.

If sputum samples are still positive by acid-fast staining and microscopy or by culture in months 5–6, or relapse occurs, an 8–9-month treatment regimen incorporating second-line agents is necessary (see below).

Multiple resistance

The emergence of multiple drug-resistant strains of TB (MDRTB) is of great concern. In the UK, resistance to *isoniazid* alone occurs in about 3% of isolates, and dual resistance to *isoniazid* and *rifampicin* in about 0.6%. Overall, the prevalence of MDRTB is about 0.8% of cases in the UK and about 3.4% in India but these figures mask large differences in the absolute number of cases, i.e. about 55 cases annually in England and Wales and about 63 000 in India. Resistance may be primary, where a person has been infected by a resistant strain, or strains, or secondary where a resistant strain has emerged owing to incomplete treatment.

If *isoniazid* resistance has been confirmed, treatment should continue with *rifampicin* and *ethambutol* for a year. If *rifampicin* resistance is confirmed, treatment with *isoniazid* and *ethambutol* should be continued for 18 months. In both cases *pyrazinamide* is added for the first 2 months of treatment.

If a patient's strain is known to be resistant to *isoniazid* at the outset, *streptomycin* or *amikacin* may be substituted for *isoniazid* in initial treatment, but this involves IM or IV injections and serum level monitoring to ensure an appropriate peak level 1 h after injection and trough (pre-dose) concentration. If there is renal impairment or the patient is aged over 50 years, the trough concentration needs to be reduced considerably. *Streptomycin*, unlicensed in the UK, is used only rarely, and is available only through the named-patient mechanism.

The high costs of patient monitoring of liver function, and possibly aminoglycoside blood levels, clearly causes problems of supplying the facilities and trained personnel in Third World countries.

Strains of TB resistant to the usual combination of first-line drugs are rare in the UK, except in immigrants, but are increasingly common in some other countries. In such cases, second-line drugs such as *capreomycin*, *cycloserine* (neurotoxic) and *ethionamide* are added to the drug cocktail. Encouraging results have also been obtained with 4-quinolones, e.g. *ciprofloxacin*. *Amikacin* and *clarithromycin* have been used rarely (unlicensed indications).

In the UK, people with drug-resistant disease are treated as in-patients in specialized units, where second-line drugs are commonly used. At least five drugs, including *amikacin*, are used until cultures are negative, followed by a minimum of three drugs for up to 9 months. The cost of such treatment is considerable (about £60 000 per patient).

Summary

The treatment of TB illustrates the following:

- Need for multiple agents to overcome drug resistance.
- Importance to patients and contacts of completing courses of treatment even though they feel well soon after treatment commences.
- Problems of poor compliance associated with prolonged courses of treatment with agents that have serious or unpleasant side-effects.
- Benefit of closely supervised treatment to ensure compliance.

Urinary-tract infection

Symptoms and diagnosis

Infection of the lower urinary tract (see Chapter 14, Figure 14.1) occurs either in the bladder (**cystitis**) or the urethra (**urethritis**) and is estimated to affect 15% of women each year and occur in up to 50% of women at some time in their lives. Their very short urethra predisposes to ascending infection with perineal bacteria.

The symptoms of frequency, haematuria, suprapubic pain and dysuria (i.e. painful micturition), though not life-threatening, may be extremely uncomfortable and have a 50% probability of cystitis. The urine may appear turbid due to the presence of bacteria and pus, and may have an unpleasant fishy smell due to the production of microbial metabolites. Recurrence (2%) and reinfection (8%) are common.

The condition is uncommon in men because their longer urethra acts as a barrier to ascending infection from the penis. Consequently, urinary-tract infections in men are regarded more seriously.

Despite apparently minor symptoms, urinary-tract infections may involve the kidney (**pyelonephritis**), even causing renal failure, and pathogens may then gain access to the circulation and cause septicaemia.

Diagnosis may be difficult if symptoms are present but bacteria cannot be seen microscopically in the urine nor cultured. This is known as **abacterial cystitis**, which can occur in up to 50% of cases. Conversely, because bacteria are often isolated from the urine in the absence of any overt symptoms (**covert bacteriuria**), the diagnostic criterion for significant bacteriuria is normally taken to be more than 100 coliforms/mL plus ≥ 10 leucocytes/mm^3 (in a microscope counting chamber) or $\geq 100\,000$/mL of any pathogens. The coliform count alone is insufficient. More vigorous treatment may be indicated for certain groups of patients, particularly in the presence of recurrent or ascending infections: this includes pregnant women, children, patients with learning difficulties and all men. The elderly may also be prone to complications, which may present as confusion in the absence of the usual signs of infection. Undiagnosed urinary-tract infections in infants and young children may have serious renal consequences in later life.

The full spectrum of urinary-tract infections, including pyelonephritis, is discussed in Chapter 14. Here, we will discuss only the treatment of cystitis.

Aetiology

The majority (90%) of acute uncomplicated cases of cystitis are due to self-infection with *E. coli* from the anus that colonize the perineal area. Other Gram-negatives, e.g. *Proteus* and *Klebsiella* may be implicated, particularly if infections are chronic. Infections due to staphylococci are the second most common in the community but are less usual in hospital.

Pseudomonas infection is usually associated with an anatomical abnormality of the urinary tract.

Organisms other than *E. coli* are also more likely in hospital-acquired infections, especially in catheterized patients. In cases that fail to respond to usual treatment, organisms such as *Chlamydia* or *Candida* should be considered.

Investigation

A urine specimen that is minimally contaminated by commensals from the genitalia is necessary for culturing and sensitivity tests. This is obtained through a 'clean-catch midstream urine' (MSU) sample, usually collected into a sterile sample jar at home by the patient: the genital area is first washed with mild soap and dried, and the first and final parts of urine are rejected. The sample is collected first thing in the morning when the bacterial count is likely to be highest due to undisturbed overnight growth. However, an uncontaminated sample is difficult to collect in some circumstances, e.g. young children and the elderly, and a more reliable method is via a catheter, although this may itself introduce infection into the bladder. Rarely, suprapubic bladder aspiration with a syringe may be required when it is difficult to collect a sample, e.g. from a young infant.

Apart from culturing, which may take some time, other changes in the urine can indicate the presence of microorganisms. Reagent strips can be used to detect the presence of nitrite produced as a result of bacterial metabolism. The pH of the urine may be low in the presence of *E. coli* or high if due to *Proteus* spp. or other urease-positive, ammonia-producing, species.

Further investigations for potential complications are indicated in all cases of male or childhood urinary-tract infection, in women with recurrent or persistent symptoms and when sterile urine has not been achieved after standard therapy (see Chapter 14).

Management

Aims

The immediate aim of treatment, from the patient's view, is the rapid relief of uncomfortable symptoms. This is best achieved by the eradication of the responsible organism using a short course of an appropriate antibacterial agent. The prevention of recurrent and chronic infections and of subsequent renal damage is a further aim that may require longer courses of treatment.

Choice of antibacterial

Samples for laboratory investigation must be taken before treatment is commenced. As *E. coli* is the most likely organism, the initial antibacterial choice is relatively simple. The final decision will depend on local, known patterns of resistance. *Trimethoprim* may be appropriate for blind treatment and achieves high urine concentrations. Strains of bacteria resistant to *trimethoprim* are becoming increasingly common in hospitals and, to a lesser extent, in the community, and a first-generation cephalosporin, e.g. *cefalexin*, is a useful alternative.

Nitrofurantoin is also suitable, although its use is limited by toxicity and good renal function is required. *Proteus* spp. are also resistant. The 4-quinolones are active against a wide range of organisms including pseudomonads, but should be reserved for infection of proven sensitivity that are resistant to other agents, or for treatment failures. The quinolone *norfloxacin* is restricted to treating urinary-tract infections because it achieves sub-therapeutic blood levels, but a high urine concentration.

The last dose of the day of any agent should be taken just before going to bed in order to achieve high urine concentrations when bacterial count is likely to be maximal. Symptoms should begin to clear within 48 h, and a 3-day course is usually sufficient for uncomplicated cystitis in women; 5-days' treatment is necessary in men.

Frequent urinary-tract infections may require prophylactic use of antibacterials. In children, low-dose *trimethoprim* can be used, given last thing at night for many months. In adults, prophylaxis with low-dose *nitrofurantoin* is an alternative and rarely causes problems.

Other treatment modes include alkalinization of the urine with potassium or sodium citrate or sodium bicarbonate may provide some symptomatic relief if the urine is very acid (pH <4), and will inhibit growth of *E. coli*. However, the use of potassium or sodium citrate may be hazardous in

elderly patients and others with impaired renal function, owing to the cardiovascular effects of accumulated sodium or potassium. Moreover, *Proteus* spp. thrive in a high pH, but not under acid conditions, so acidification of the urine with ammonium chloride is then appropriate. Thus, simple pH testing with indicator paper should guide this type of treatment.

Advice should always be given to increase fluid intake and to ensure regular voiding in order to obtain maximum washout of organisms from the bladder. Also, women should be advised to wipe from front to back after toileting, though the value of this has been questioned. 'Pushing' fluids, e.g. 200 mL three times an hour for several hours, may wash out the bacteria and abort an infection without the need for antimicrobial treatments, provided that it is started promptly when symptoms occur. It is also important to void completely in order to leave the minimum of infected urine in the bladder.

Summary of urinary-tract infections

Treatment of urinary-tract infections illustrate the following general principles:

- *E. coli* is responsible for the majority of acute urinary-tract infections, so initial empirical therapy can be chosen with a high degree of confidence.
- Local patterns of resistance will indicate which of a number of possible antimicrobial agents should be used.
- The antimicrobial must be present in high concentrations in the urine. Only those agents that are rapidly excreted unchanged in adequate concentration in the urine are suitable for the treatment of urinary-tract infections.

References and further reading

Anon (1995). Drug-resistant tuberculosis. *Drug Ther Bull* 33: 28–29.
Anon (1997). The management of urinary tract infections in women. *Drug Ther Bull* 35: 65–69.
Anon (2004). Drugs for parasitic infections. *Med Lett Drugs Ther* 46: 1–12 (available from www.medletter.com/freedocs/parasitic.pdf).

Bartlett J G (2002). Antimicrobial-associated diarrhoea. *N Engl J Med* 346: 334–339.

British Thoracic Society (2004 update). Guidelines for the management of community-acquired pneumonia in adults (available from http://www.brit-thoracic.org.uk/bts_guidelines_pneumonia_html).

Bryan C S, ed. (2002). *Infectious Diseases in Primary Care*. Philadelphia, PA: W B Saunders.

Carapetis J, McDonald M, Wilson M J (2005). Acute rheumatic fever. *Lancet* 66: 155–168.

Commerford P J, Mayosi B M (2006). Acute rheumatic fever. *Medicine* 34(6): 239–243.

Falagas M E, Kasiakou S K (2005). Colistin: the revival of polymyxins for the management of multidrug-resistant Gram-negative bacterial infections. *Clin Infect Dis* 40: 1333–1341.

Falagas M E, Michalopoulos A (2006). Polymyxins: old antimicrobials are back. *Lancet* 367: 633–634.

Finch R G, Woodhead M A (1998). Practical considerations and guidelines for the management of community-acquired pneumonia in adults. *Drugs* 55: 31–45.

Gemmell C G, Edwards D I, Fraise A P, *et al.* (2006). Guidelines for the treatment and prophylaxis of methicillin-resistant *Staphylococcus aureus* (MRSA) infections in the UK. *J Antimicrob Chemother* 57: 589–608.

Greenwood D, Finch R D, Davey P, Wilcox M (2007). Antimicrobial and Chemotherapy, 5th edn. Oxford: Oxford University Press.

Griffin G E, Harrison T S eds (2001). Infections *Medicine* 29 (Parts 1–3); 1–129.

Hawker J, Begg N, Blair I, *et al.* (2001). *Communicable Diseases Control Handbook*. Oxford: Blackwell Science.

Heyderman R S (2003). Early management of suspected bacterial meningitis and meningococcal septicaemia – second edition. *J Infect* 50; 373–374.

Macfarlane J T, Brody D (2004). Update of the BTS guidelines for the management of community acquired pneumonia in adults: What's new? *Thorax* 59; 364–366.

Ormerod L P (2005). Multi-drug resistant tuberculosis (MDR-TB): Epidemiology, prevention and treatment. *Br Med Bull* 73–74: 17–24.

Scott G M, Kyi MS eds (2001). *Handbook of Essential Antibiotics*. Amsterdam, The Netherlands: Harwood Academic Publishers.

Shanson D C (1999). *Microbiology in Clinical Practice*, 3rd edn. Oxford: Butterworth-Heinemann.

The British Thoracic Society (1993). Guidelines for the management of community-acquired pneumonia in adults admitted to hospital. *Br J Hosp Med* 49: 346–350.

The Writing Committee of the World Health Organization (WHO) Consultation of Human Influenza. (2005). Avian influenza (H5N1) infection in humans. *N Engl J Med* 353: 1374–1385.

Tunkel A R, Scheld W M (1995). Acute bacterial meningitis. *Lancet* 346: 1675–1679.

9

Endocrine system

Endocrine control of physiological functions represents broadly targeted, slow acting but fundamental means of homeostatic control, as opposed to the rapidly reacting nervous system. In endocrine disease there is usually either an excess or a lack of a systemic hormonal mediator, but the cause may be at one of a number of stages in the endocrine pathway. Thyroid disease and diabetes mellitus represent contrasting extremes of endocrine disease and its management. Diabetes is one of the most serious and probably the most common of multisystem diseases. Optimal control of diabetes requires day-to-day monitoring, and small variations in medication dose or patient activity can destabilize the condition. Therapy requires regular review and possible modification. Furthermore, long-term complications of diabetes cause considerable morbidity and mortality.

Thyroid disease is a disorder of thyroid hormone production that has, compared to diabetes, equally profound overall effects on metabolic and physiological function. However, it causes few acute problems and has far fewer chronic complications. Moreover, management is much easier, requiring less intensive monitoring and few dose changes. Furthermore, control is rarely disturbed by short-term variations in patient behaviour.

Diabetes mellitus

Diabetes mellitus is primarily a disorder of carbohydrate metabolism yet the metabolic problems in properly treated diabetes are not usually troublesome and are relatively easy to control. It is the long-term complications of diabetes that are the main causes of morbidity and mortality. People with diabetes suffer far more from cardiovascular and renal disease than other people, and diabetes is the principal cause of acquired blindness in the West. Most people with diabetes do not die from metabolic crises such as ketoacidosis but from stroke, MI or chronic renal failure.

Diabetes is associated with obesity and lack of exercise, and the steady increase in prevalence in the West is being reproduced in large parts of the developing world as they adopt that life-style. Diabetes is in danger of becoming almost pandemic. Particularly worrying is the rise in the incidence of diabetes of both types in ever younger patients. This threatens to put an intolerable strain on health services, particularly in developing countries.

Physiological principles of glucose and insulin metabolism

Insulin action

Insulin is the body's principal **anabolic** hormone. It expands energy stores during times of adequate nutrition against times of food shortage. Opposing this action are several **catabolic** 'counter-regulatory' or 'stress' hormones that mobilize glucose for use when increased energy expenditure is necessary. The most important of these are adrenaline (epinephrine), corticosteroids, glucagon, growth hormone and growth factors. These two opposing systems work in harmony to maintain glucose homeostasis. Insulin also enhances amino acid utilization and protein synthesis, the latter action being shared with growth hormone.

Insulin action has three main components (Figure 9.1):

- **Rapid**: in certain tissues (e.g. muscle), insulin facilitates the active transport of glucose and amino acids across cell membranes, enhancing uptake from the blood.
- **Intermediate**: within all cells, insulin promotes the action of enzymes that convert glucose, fatty acids and amino acids into more complex, more stable storage forms.
- **Long-term**: because of increased protein synthesis, growth is promoted.

One important consequence is the prompt (though not complete) clearance of glucose from the blood after meals. Glucose would otherwise be lost in the urine because of the kidney's limited capacity for reabsorbing glucose filtered at the glomerulus.

Glucose transport

Glucose uptake into cells across the cell membrane is dependent on the concentration gradient between the extracellular medium (e.g. blood plasma, gastrointestinal contents) and the cell interior. However, because glucose is such an important metabolite, there exist a number of membrane transport pumps or facilitators in certain tissues. There are special insulin-

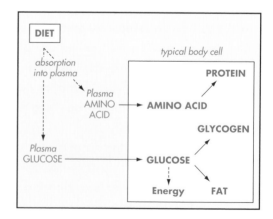

Figure 9.1 Simplified scheme showing the anabolic actions of insulin. Insulin aids the uptake of metabolites into body cells and enhances the action of enzymes that utilize them as precursors to synthesize more complex molecules. Note: not all actions shown occur in all body cells.

independent sodium-dependent transporters (SGLT) for uptake from the GIT into intestinal cells and a variety of insulin-dependent and insulin-independent glucose transporters (GLUT) for most other tissues or organs (Table 9.1).

In muscle and adipose tissue the transporter depends on an insulin-requiring active pump for glucose uptake, so insulin deficiency deprives them of glucose. Other cells, particularly in the liver, brain, kidney and GIT, do not absolutely require insulin for glucose uptake, but diffusion is nevertheless facilitated by it. In the liver, enhanced phosphorylation of glucose drives intracellular concentrations down, encouraging uptake. Insulin lack does not deprive tissues such as these of glucose; on the contrary, the hyperglycaemia associated with diabetes can produce intracellular glucose overload, and this may be responsible for some diabetic complications (p. 593). This is particularly relevant to tissues such as nerves, which are freely permeable to glucose.

Insulin also facilitates the uptake of amino acids into liver and muscle, and of potassium into most cells. This latter effect is exploited therapeutically for the rapid reduction of hyperkalaemia (see Chapter 14).

Metabolic effects

By facilitating certain enzymes and inhibiting others, insulin has wide-ranging effects on intermediary metabolism in most tissues (Table 9.2; Figure 9.1). The synthesis of the energy stores (glycogen in liver and skeletal muscle, fat in liver and adipose tissue) is facilitated, and their break-

down is inhibited. Tissue growth and cell division are also promoted by enhanced nucleic acid (DNA, RNA) synthesis, amino acid assimilation and protein synthesis.

Overall effect

Only a general appreciation of how insulin and the catabolic hormones control everyday metabolic variations is given here (see also References and further reading).

Anabolic actions of insulin

Following a meal, glucose is absorbed from the GIT into the blood and rapidly transported into the cells, to be converted into forms suitable for storage and later use.

In the liver some glucose is converted into glycogen and stored but most is converted into lipid (free fatty acid, FFA [or non-esterified fatty acid, NEFA], and triglyceride). Lipid is released into the blood as very-low-density lipoprotein (VLDL), to be taken up and stored in adipose tissue. However, the release of glucose into the blood is inhibited. Hepatic regulation of glucose output is an important mechanism for limiting the uptake of glucose into tissues where transport is independent of insulin.

In adipose tissue, fat breakdown is inhibited and glucose uptake promoted. The glucose provides glycerol for esterification with FFAs, and the resulting fat is stored. Adipose tissue also takes up the fat-containing chylomicrons obtained by digestion (see Chapter 3). In muscle, fat metabolism is inhibited and glycogen is

Table 9.1   Insulin requirement and transporters for glucose uptake into different tissues

Tissues not requiring insulin	Transporter	Tissues requiring insulin	Transporter
Gastrointestinal – uptake	SGLT	Adipose	
Gastrointestinal – release to blood	GLUT2	Muscle – skeletal, cardiac, smooth	GLUT4
Liver	GLUT7	Other tissues	
Nerves, brain	GLUT1,3		
Kidney tubules	GLUT2, SGLT		
Eye – retinal vessels, lens	SGLT		
Leucocytes	GLUT		
Blood vessel endothelium	GLUT		
Pancreatic beta cells	GLUT2		

SGLT, sodium-dependent glucose transporter; GLUT, glucose transporter.

Table 9.2   Metabolic effects of insulin

Metabolite	Process	Liver	Tissue Muscle	Adipose
Carbohydrate				
Increased	• Glycogen synthesis (glycogenesis)	✓	✓	↔
	• Glucose oxidation (glycolysis)	✓	✓	✓
Decreased	• Glycogen breakdown (glycogenolysis)	✓	✓	↔
	• Glucose synthesis (gluconeogenesis)	✓	↔	↔
Lipid				
Increased	• Fat synthesis (lipogenesis)	✓	↔	✓
	• Utilization of dietary fat	✓	↔	✓
Decreased	• Fat breakdown (lipolysis)	↔	↔	✓
	• Fatty acid oxidation (ketogenesis)	✓	✓	✓
Protein				
Increased	• Protein synthesis	✓	✓	✓
Decreased	• Protein breakdown (proteolysis)	✓	✓	↔
Nucleic acid				
Increased	• DNA and RNA synthesis	↔	✓	↔
	• Cell growth and division	↔	✓	↔

✓, insulin has important effect (increase or decrease) on process in this tissue; ↔, no effect.

synthesized, which increases glucose availability for immediate energy needs. Amino acid uptake is promoted so that growth can be continued.

Catabolic actions of counter-regulatory hormones

During stresses such as 'fight or flight', infection or any major trauma, catabolic hormones reverse these processes. Blood glucose is rapidly raised to supply energy for the muscles and if this is insufficient fats can also be mobilized. Peripheral oxidation of FFAs produces large amounts of energy, but in the liver excess acetyl-CoA is produced. This is condensed to produce high-energy ketoacids such as acetoacetate, which many tissues can utilize in small amounts. In insulin insufficiency these 'ketone bodies' may accumulate in the plasma, causing ketoacidosis.

Insulin deficiency

The consequences of insulin deficiency, and thus many of the clinical features of diabetes, can be deduced from these considerations (Figure 9.2).

It will be explained below that obese type 2 patients may not at first have an absolute deficiency of insulin; rather, there is a degree of insulin resistance. This may be described as a relative lack because the result is the same; moreover, eventually their insulin levels do fall. There are important differences between the physiological effects of partial (or relative) deficiency and total insulin deficiency.

Partial deficiency (type 2)

Even small amounts of insulin will prevent severe metabolic disruption, especially accelerated fat metabolism, i.e. ketosis. Thus, although fasting blood glucose levels may be raised, the main problems only arise after meals; these arise from impaired glucose transport and cellular uptake resulting in impaired clearance from the blood. Adipose and muscle tissue cannot take up glucose efficiently, causing it to remain in the blood, and glucose deficiency in muscle may cause weakness. Becuse other tissues cannot compensate sufficiently to assimilate the entire postprandial glucose load, the blood

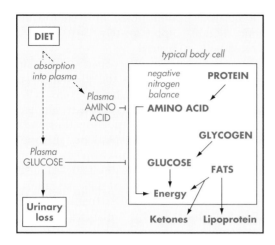

Figure 9.2 Metabolic consequences of insulin lack. Cellular uptake of glucose is prevented so that after exhausting their glycogen supplies, cells need to use fats and even protein for their energy needs. Compare with Figure 9.1. Note: not all actions occur in all body cells.

glucose level rises causing **hyperglycaemia** (>11 mmol/L).

When the blood glucose level increases so that the concentration in the glomerular filtrate exceeds the renal threshold (see Chapter 14, p. 876), glucose is lost in the urine (**glycosuria**). Urinary glucose acts as an osmotic diuretic carrying with it large volumes of water (**polyuria** and **urinary frequency**), resulting in excessive thirst and fluid intake (**polydipsia**). Because of reduced fat uptake by adipose tissue, plasma lipid levels rise, especially triglycerides (**dyslipidaemia**). LDL is relatively unaffected but HDL is reduced, increasing atherogenic risk (Chapter 4). Protein synthesis may be reduced but patients are often still relatively obese. However, they usually do lose weight in the weeks before first diagnosis, in part due to dehydration.

Total deficiency (type 1)

With no insulin at all there is severe hyperglycaemia at most times. This may raise the blood osmotic pressure sufficiently to cause neurological complications including coma; this is discussed on pp. 594–596. Cellular metabolism is profoundly disturbed. No glucose is available for energy metabolism, and the first result is a depletion of liver and muscle glycogen stores.

Subsequently fat is mobilized, mainly from adipose tissue, so that plasma triglyceride and FFA levels rise, as does lipoprotein. These supply energy needs for a little longer while the patient loses yet more weight. The brain cells switch to metabolizing the hepatically produced keto-acids. Fat stores are not replenished, and eventually may be exhausted. Finally, protein must be broken down into amino acids, which can be converted to glucose in the liver (**gluconeogenesis**), at the expense of lean muscle mass. Other than in uncontrolled diabetes, this process normally occurs only in times of prolonged starvation; it is a desperate remedy that is akin to burning the house down to keep warm. Further, without insulin, any glucose so produced cannot be utilized effectively anyway. This situation is inevitably fatal within months.

Thus many of the clinical problems in type 2 diabetes are a direct consequence of hyperglycaemia, while in type 1 diabetes there is also disrupted intracellular metabolism. In addition, chronic complications occur in both types, related to both hyperglycaemia and dyslipidaemia. These are discussed below.

Insulin physiology

Insulin (molecular weight about 5800 Da) is composed of 51 amino acids in two chains of 21 (A chain) and 30 (B chain) amino acids connected by two disulphide bridges. It is synthesized in the pancreatic islet beta-cells. Other cells in the islets are the alpha-cells (producing glucagon) and the delta-cells (producing somatostatin). Islet cells altogether comprise less than 3% of the pancreatic mass. Insulin is stored in granules in combination with **C-peptide** as proinsulin (molecular weight 9000 Da), which is split before release into the portal vein. Insulin has a plasma half-life of only about 5 min. Approximately 50% of insulin is extracted by the liver, which is its main site of action, and after utilization it is subsequently degraded. Eventually, kidney peptidase also metabolizes some insulin. C-peptide is less rapidly cleared and is thus a useful index of beta-cell function. The main control of insulin level is plasma glucose: a rise stimulates both the release and the synthesis of insulin. Amino acids and possibly fats also promote insulin release (Figure 9.3).

A wide variety of other neuronal, endocrine, pharmacological and local influences on insulin release have been identified (Figure 9.3), but their physiological or pathological significance is not established. Adrenergic beta-receptors mediate release, so beta-blockers can theoretically inhibit this, though stimulation of inhibitory adrenergic alpha-receptors, magnified during the hyperglycaemic stress response, usually predominates.

Interestingly, glucose is a more powerful stimulant orally than parenterally, and various gut hormones have been implicated in this. Glucagon also promotes insulin release, possibly to facilitate cellular uptake of the glucose that it causes to be released into the plasma.

Pattern of secretion

It is important to note also that there is a continuous basal level of insulin secretion throughout the 24 h, independent of food intake, which contributes to the regulation of metabolism and promotes glucose uptake into cells. This amounts to about 1 unit/h. Following a meal there is an additional bolus secreted, which is biphasic. Within 1 min of blood glucose levels rising, preformed insulin is released from granules in beta-cells into the blood. This release is stimulated by certain antidiabetic agents (insulin secretagogues) and is the first component to be compromised in early diabetes. Should hyperglycaemia persist, further insulin synthesis is stimulated and there

is a delayed second phase of secretion after about 45 min. Appoximately 5–10 units are secreted with each meal.

Thus the plasma insulin concentration curve normally closely parallels the plasma glucose concentration curve throughout the day, reflecting every small change in nutrient supply or demand (Figure 9.4). Considering these subtle and sometimes rapid adaptations, it can be appreciated how far current therapeutic methods fall short of mimicking the physiological ideal.

In non-diabetics, the total daily secretion of insulin is probably rather less than the average daily requirement in type 1 diabetes of 50 units of exogenous insulin, mainly because of losses at the injection site.

Amylin

The 37-amino acid peptide amylin is co-secreted with insulin from beta-cells. It appears to contribute to glucose regulation by a local (paracrine) action on islet cells, which moderates intestinal glucose uptake, thereby reducing the load presented to the pancreas, or by suppressing glucagon secretion. In diabetes, amylin deficiency parallels that of insulin and it is believed that patients whose postprandial hyperglycaemia is not adequately controlled by conventional therapy may benefit from amylin agonists, although none is yet in clinical use.

Insulin receptors

These are present on the cell surfaces of all insulin-sensitive tissues and are normally down-

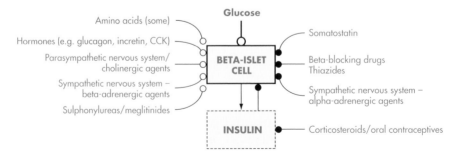

Figure 9.3 Factors affecting the release or action of insulin. CCK, cholecystokinin. ──────● inhibition/antagonism; ──────○ stimulation/potentiation.

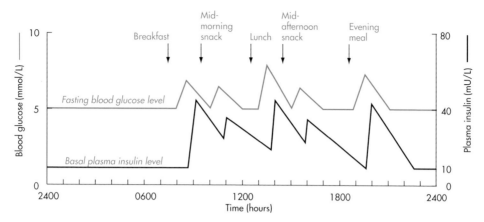

Figure 9.4 Schematic representation of normal diurnal variations in blood glucose and plasma insulin levels. As the blood glucose level rapidly rises after a meal, it is closely followed by an increase in insulin level to limit the rise. The insulin returns towards the basal level as blood glucose reaches the normal fasting level once more. Note how the two substances follow almost parallel curves, the insulin a little later than the glucose. The small but positive constant basal insulin level emphasizes that insulin has functions other than just dealing with dietary glucose. Note: this diagram does not differentiate the two phases of insulin release.

regulated by insulin, especially if it is present at continuously high levels, e.g. the hyperinsulinaemia of over-eating, obesity or obesity-related type 2 diabetes. This may account for the reduced insulin sensitivity (insulin resistance) found in some patients and the beneficial effect of weight reduction, especially of abdominal fat, on glucose tolerance: there is a vicious cycle whereby hyperglycaemia and reduced insulin action reinforce one another. Long-term insulin treatment also often gradually reduces the insulin requirement, perhaps owing to reduced glucose levels. However, there is still much to be learned about the interactions between insulin, insulin receptors and carbohydrate metabolism.

Epidemiology and classification

The hallmark of diabetes is hyperglycaemia, owing to abnormalities of insulin secretion or action. There are two primary forms of diabetes and a variety of minor secondary ones. In type 1 diabetes there is usually gross destruction of the insulin-secreting pancreatic beta-cells. In type 2 diabetes insulin is secreted but is either inadequate or insufficiently effective to meet metabolic needs.

The current WHO definition of diabetes is based on standardized measurements of plasma glucose concentrations. It defines three classes, diabetes, impaired glucose tolerance and impaired fasting blood glucose (Table 9.3). Patients in the second category are borderline and about half will progress to frank diabetes eventually (up to 5% per year). However, they need not be treated immediately, depending on age and the presence of other risk factors: older patients or those with no cardiovascular risk factors may just be monitored. More recently the category of impaired fasting glucose has been introduced in an attempt to identify at an even earlier stage those with latent or 'pre-diabetes' who should be monitored. It is a less reliable predictor but has the advantge that it does not require a glucose tolerance test (see below).

Often, a single random plasma glucose of >11.1 mmol/L (blood glucose 10 mmol/L) is sufficient for diagnosis in a patient with classic symptoms, although this should be confirmed with a fasting plasma glucose >7 mmol/L.

Table 9.3   WHO definitions of diabetes mellitus (based on plasma glucose levels, as measured in laboratory)

Class	Plasma glucose (mmol/L)		
	Fasting		**OGTT at 2 h**
Diabetes mellitus	>7	and/or	>11.1
Impaired glucose tolerance (IGT)	<7	and	7.8–11.1
Impaired fasting glucose (IFG)	6.1–7		
Normal fasting glucose	<6.1	and	<7.8

If whole blood is used (as obtained by finger prick) all figures would be approx. 10% lower (e.g. 6.1 and 10 mmol/L for diabetes mellitus).

The apparently non-uniform thresholds derive from conversion from old mg/100 mL units, as still used in North America.

OGTT, oral glucose tolerance test.

Laboratories may report plasma glucose levels, as specified by the American Diabetic Association diagnostic criteria, whereas finger prick tests measure blood levels; nevertheless, it is customary always to refer to blood glucose in discussing diabetes. In borderline cases the **oral glucose tolerance test (OGTT)** can be performed: the patient's blood glucose is measured before and at 2 h after a standardized 75-g glucose load, given orally following an overnight fast.

Epidemiology

Diabetes is known to affect more than 2% of the UK population, and probably as many again are likely to have impaired glucose tolerance or even frank diabetes if screened. The prevalence varies considerably between populations. For example, Europeans are prone to type 1, especially in northern Europe, whereas the incidence in Japan is less than 10% of that in Finland.

Type 2 seems to be related partly to the affluence of a population, possibly through the prevalence of obesity, inactivity or both, which are major risk factors. However, genetic factors are also important. In some ethnic groups the prevalence is very high, e.g. in some Pacific Islanders and the North American Pima Indians it reaches 50%. Among South Asian immigrants to the UK it is five times that in the host population, suggesting a possible genetic susceptibility to changed environmental factors, e.g. a diet richer in fats and sugar.

Classification

Primary diabetes – type 1 and type 2

In the vast majority of cases there is direct damage to the pancreatic islet cells. Different attempts to classify diabetes comprehensively have been confounded by the use of criteria that are not mutually exclusive (e.g. age at onset, patient build or need for insulin). For example, some older ('maturity onset' or type 2) patients eventually require insulin, some older patients need it from the start ('latent autoimmune diabetes in the adult', LADA) and a few younger patients may not ('maturity onset diabetes of the young', MODY). Whether the patient needs insulin may be the most practical distinction, but does not correspond consistently with other important parameters.

A classification based on the pathogenesis of the pancreatic damage is now accepted as the most meaningful. This distinguishes two broad types (Table 9.4), which correspond roughly with insulin dependency. The key criterion is the mode of pancreatic damage, but many other distinctions follow from this classification, including natural history, family history and patient type. These will be discussed in the following sections.

Secondary diabetes

A minority of cases with identifiable primary causes (e.g. severe pancreatitis, steroid-induced diabetes) do not fit readily into either of the conventional categories. They may or may not require insulin for treatment (p. 591).

Table 9.4   Comparison of the main types of primary diabetes mellitus

	Type 1	Type 2
Endogenous insulin	Absent	Present
Insulin deficiency	Absolute	Relative or partial
		Insulin receptor defect?
Insulin resistance	Usually absent	May be present
Pancreatic islet damage	Severe (destruction)	Slight/moderate
Immunology	Auto-immune; islet cell antibodies	No antibodies demonstrated
Usual age of onset	<30 years	>40 years
Build of patient	Thin	Obese (usually)
Therapeutic class	Insulin-dependent (IDDM)	Non-insulin-dependent (NIDDM; but may require insulin)
Genetics	Weak family history; HLA-linked	Strong family history
Ketoacidosis prone?	Yes	No

Aetiology and pathogenesis

Primary diabetes

Despite having similar clinical pictures and complications, types 1 and 2 primary diabetes have very different causes (Table 9.5).

Type 1 diabetes

In type 1 diabetes the islet beta-cells are almost completely destroyed by an autoimmune process. Antibodies against all islet cells, and beta-cells specifically, are found in 80% of patients. However, interestingly, it is not these anti-islet antibodies that mediate cell destruction but T-cells; the islets are invaded by inflammatory cells causing insulitis. Insulin autoantibodies may also be found but their significance is uncertain. As is usual with autoimmune disease, there is rarely a strong family history: siblings or children of people with type 1 diabetes have about a 5% chance of developing the disease. However, there is a correlation with the patient's HLA tissue type (see Chapter 2) and in a minority of patients an association with other autoimmune diseases, especially of endocrine tissues (e.g. thyroiditis, pernicious anaemia).

Table 9.5   Aetiology and pathology of primary diabetes

	Type 1	Type 2
Risk factors	HLA antigens (DR3, DR4)	Family history
		Over-eating; lack of exercise
		Toxin? Amyloid?
		Ethnic group
Trigger factors	Viral infection	Obesity
	Metabolic stress/excessive demand	Metabolic stress/excessive demand
	Environmental toxin?	
Pathogenesis	Rapid autoimmune destruction of islet cells	Gradual islet cell degeneration / depletion
		Peripheral insulin receptor defect?

Overt diabetes may follow many years of subclinical pancreatic damage, and when it occurs there is usually less than 10% of functional islet cell mass remaining. Clinical onset is usually abrupt, over a few weeks, and often associated with, or precipitated by, a metabolic stress such as an infection, which acutely increases insulin demand beyond capacity. This might account for the winter seasonal peak in incidence and also the brief temporary remission that frequently follows, as the infection remits and the marginal insulin levels once again just compensate. Subsequently, full-blown disease irreversibly takes hold. As with other autoimmune diseases, viral infection may be causing the expression of a normally suppressed HLA receptor, which subsequently activates lymphocytes (see Chapter 2). Other environmental triggers such as toxins or certain foods (including milk protein) may also be involved.

Autoantibodies may be found in some patients up to 15 years before the onset of acute disease. This could eventually provide a means of early identification of prediabetes, so that they may be treated prophylactically, possibly by immunotherapy. However, such markers are also often found in close relatives who never develop the disease, and the chance of the identical twin of a diabetic patient subsequently developing diabetes is less than 50%. The introduction of the category of 'impaired fasting glucose' was another attempt at early identification of potential sufferers.

Thus it seems that in type 1 diabetes there is a genetically determined HLA-dependent susceptibility that requires an environmental trigger for full expression. Following contact with this trigger, which may never be encountered, swift deterioration and complete insulin dependence are inevitable. There is still considerable ignorance of the relative contributions of genes and environment and of specific environmental factors.

Type 2 diabetes

These patients have one or more of the following fundamental abnormalities, and in established disease all three commonly coexist:

- Absolute insulin deficiency, i.e. reduced insulin secretion.
- Relative insulin deficiency: not enough insulin is secreted for metabolic increased needs (e.g. in obesity).
- Insulin resistance and hyperinsulinaemia: a peripheral insulin utilization defect.

In most cases type 2 diabetes is associated with obesity (particularly abdominal obesity) on first presentation, and in a quarter of all people with diabetes simple weight reduction reverses the hyperglycaemia. This is commonly associated with peripheral insulin resistance owing to receptor-binding or post-receptor defects. Obesity and reduced exercise also contribute to insulin resistance and are modifiable risk factors for type 2 diabetes. The resultant hyperglycaemia induces insulin hypersecretion, hyperinsulinaemia and insulin receptor down-regulation, i.e. further insulin resistance. Hyperglycaemia itself is known to damage beta-cells owing to the direct toxic effect of excessive intracellular glucose metabolism, which produces an excess of oxidative by-products; these cannot be destroyed by natural scavengers such as catalase and superoxide dismutase. The vicious cycle eventually depletes ('exhausts') the beta-cells, intrinsic insulin levels fall and some patients may eventually come to require exogenous insulin therapy. Thus, type 2 diabetes is usually a progressive disease, although the late onset usually means that some patients die before requiring insulin.

There is still debate as to the primary defect of type 2 diabetes. It has also been proposed that the amyloid deposits (insoluble protein) long known to be found in the pancreas of type 2 patients are related to abnormalities in amylin secretion (p. 586) and contribute to the pancreatic defect.

There is an association between abdominal obesity, hyperinsulinaemia, insulin resistance, hyperlipidaemia, type 2 diabetes and hypertension, and this combination of risk factors is termed **metabolic syndrome**. However, despite much research, as yet it is not known which of these factors (if any) is the prime cause, or if there is another underlying reason.

Genetics

The genetic component in type 2 diabetes is much greater than in type 1. A family history is very common, often involving several relatives. Identical twins almost always both develop the disease, and offspring with both parents having diabetes have a 50% chance of developing the disease. The 'thrifty gene' hypothesis proposes that the ability to store fat efficiently – and hence develop obesity – conferred a survival advantage in more primitive societies where famine was a regular phenomenon, hence its persistence in the genome. This may explain why some pre-industrial groups (e.g. Pacific Islanders) readily develop diabetes when exposed to the industrialized lifestyle.

Secondary diabetes

Most diabetes results from primary defects of the pancreatic islet cells. However, there are occasionally other causes of ineffective insulin action, impaired glucose tolerance and hyperglycaemia (Table 9.6).

Natural history

Onset

About 80–90% of diabetic patients have type 2 diabetes, which tends to occur late in life, hence the obsolete description 'maturity onset'. Onset is usually insidious and gradual, patients tolerating mild polyuric symptoms perhaps for many years.

The other 10–20% have type 1 diabetes and require insulin at the outset. Almost invariably they become ill at an early age: the peak onset of type 1 is around puberty, starting most commonly in the winter months. Although the disease may be present subclinically for some considerable time (months, or possibly years), clinical onset is invariably abrupt.

Presentation

Type 2 diabetes is usually first diagnosed following one of three common presentations (Table 9.7):

Table 9.6   Some causes of secondary diabetes

General mechanism	Aetiology	Example
Hepatic glucose metabolism defect	Liver failure	Viral hepatitis, drugs
Pancreatic destruction	Cirrhosis	Alcoholism
	Pancreatitis	
Anti-insulin hormones	Corticosteroids	Cushing's disease
		Steroid therapy
		Pregnancy ('gestational diabetes')
		Major trauma/stress
	Growth hormone	Acromegaly
	Adrenaline (epinephrine), etc.	Phaeochromocytoma
	Glucagon	Glucagonoma
	Thyroid hormones	Hyperthyroidism
		Major trauma/stress
		Adrenergic drugs
Hyperglycaemic/anti-insulin drugs		Thiazide diuretics, diazoxide
		Oral contraceptives
Insulin antibodies	Autoimmune disease	
Abnormal insulin receptors	Congenital lipodystrophy	

- About half of patients first complain of increasing polyuria and/or polydipsia.
- In about a third it is a chance finding of glycosuria or hyperglycaemia at a routine medical examination.
- In less than 20% of cases the patient complains of symptoms subsequently found to result from a complication secondary to diabetes.

Type 2 patients may be asymptomatic or may have been only mildly symptomatic for several years. Commonly, they ignore these symptoms or attribute them to ageing, and only present when classical symptoms such as polyuria, thirst, tiredness or recent weight loss (even though the patient may still be relatively obese) become unacceptable. In many other cases their diabetes is only detected when they undergo a medical examination, e.g. for insurance purposes or a new job. Alternatively, the complaint may be of an infective complication not obviously linked to diabetes, at least not in the patient's mind, such as recurrent candida infections or boils, a non-healing foot lesion or a persistent urinary-tract infection. Rarely, as the complications proceed insidiously even during this early period, the primary reason for consultation may result from vascular disease, nephropathy, neuropathy, retinopathy or impotence. In some cases IHD, even MI, is the first presentation.

A common manifestation of the complications is the 'diabetic foot'. The patient presents with a possibly gangrenous foot lesion, probably following a recent injury and subsequent infection.

Only very rarely will a type 2 patient first present with metabolically decompensated disease (ketoacidosis). These patients will probably have had impaired glucose tolerance for some time and then have undergone some major stress such as MI or serious infection. Another possible trigger factor could be starting a drug that impairs glucose tolerance, e.g. a thiazide diuretic or an atypical antipsychotic. Such stresses may also uncover latent disease in a less dramatic manner.

Unfortunately, a severe acute presentation is far more common at the onset of type 1 disease. This is usually associated with some metabolic stress (e.g. infection), and presents with rapid weight loss, weakness, extreme thirst, severe polyuria, urinary frequency and multiple nocturia. Some may even go on to acute metabolic decompensation (ketoacidosis) and even coma, being practically moribund on hospital admission. Following recovery with insulin therapy there may follow some months of apparent remission with a reduced or absent insulin requirement, the so-called 'honeymoon period', but these patients then deteriorate rapidly. Before the isolation and therapeutic use of insulin in the 1920s they inevitably died shortly thereafter.

Progression

Insulin secretion in type 2 diabetes declines relatively slowly, but up to one-third of patients may eventually need exogenous insulin, i.e. they are 'insulin-requiring' as opposed to insulin-dependent.

In most type 1 diabetes, pancreatic beta-cell destruction is already almost complete at diagnosis, and routine insulin requirements do not generally increase. However, in both types the multisystem complications progress throughout life at rates that vary considerably between patients and will very likely be the eventual cause of death. People with diabetes have a reduced life expectancy, although the prognosis has greatly improved with advances in treatment. Younger patients have mortality rates of up to five times that of the general population, while for older ones it is about twice normal. The precise prognosis for any given patient will depend on many factors, but particularly the overall consistency of control of blood glucose.

Table 9.7   Different presentations of type 2 diabetes

Typical diabetic symptoms (see text)	55%[a]
Chance finding	30%
Complication – infective	15%
– other	2%

[a] Approximate figures; after Watkins (2003) (See References and further reading).

Clinical features

Symptoms

The symptoms of diabetes as summarized in Table 9.8 are best understood in relation to their pathogenesis.

Symptoms due to hyperglycaemia

The classic symptoms, which give diabetes mellitus its name ('sweet fountain'), are easily explained by the osmotic effect of the elevated blood glucose levels that occur when glucose is denied entry to cells. They are more pronounced when the blood glucose level rises rapidly, e.g. in decompensation or acute onset. The osmotic effect of chronic hyperglycaemia will to some extent be compensated by compensatory hyponatraemia and an increased intracellular osmolarity (see Chapter 14).

When the blood glucose level exceeds the renal threshold (about 10 mmol/L), glucose appears in the urine in large quantities. The traditional method of distinguishing diabetes mellitus from diabetes insipidus – almost the only two idiopathic causes of chronic polyuria – was simply to taste the urine: in the former case it is sweet, and in the latter literally insipid (tasteless). Glycosuria predisposes to urinary-tract infection, partly because of the favourable growth medium presented to perineal organisms and partly because diabetic patients are generally more susceptible to infection (see below).

Diabetic urine dries to leave a white glucose deposit, a clue that sometimes leads to diagnosis: there may be underwear stains or white specks on the shoes of elderly males (from careless micturition). Severe plasma hyperosmolarity may reduce the intraocular pressure, causing eyeball and lens deformity, and glucose may alter lens refraction: both lead to blurred vision. This is sometimes a prodromal sign of hyperglycaemic crisis in type 1 diabetes.

Impaired metabolism and complications

The metabolic consequences of insulin lack were discussed in detail above. The pathophysiology of hyperglycaemia and ketoacidosis is now considered.

Complications

Most complications of diabetes are due to either acute metabolic disturbances or chronic tissue damage.

Acute complications

The most common acute complications are disturbances in glycaemic control. Optimal management of diabetes aims for a delicate balance, preventing excessive glucose levels but not forcing glucose levels too low. A variety of circumstances can drive the glucose level outside

---

Table 9.8   Clinical features of diabetes

Direct consequences of high blood glucose levels
Polyuria, frequency, nocturia, polydipsia (osmotic diuresis)
Visual disturbance (osmotic changes to intra-ocular pressure)
Urethritis, pruritis vulvae, balanitis (urogenital infection)
Metabolic consequences of impaired glucose utilization
Lethargy, weakness, weight loss (intracellular glucose deficit)
Ketoacidosis (increased fat metabolism)
Long-term complications of hyperglycaemia and hyperlipidaemia
Vascular disease, heart disease, renal disease, neuropathy, eye disease, infections, arthropathy

these narrow limits, and if treatment is not adjusted accordingly, the result is either excess or insufficient glucose in the blood (Table 9.9).

Hyperglycaemia/ketoacidosis

Causes, pathogenesis and symptoms

Hyperglycaemia in treated diabetes usually arises because normal medication is somehow omitted or becomes insufficient to meet an increased insulin requirement. Drugs that raise blood glucose levels can also interfere with control. When diabetic control is lost, blood glucose rises and the symptoms develop gradually over a number of hours. Above a blood glucose level of approximately 15–20 mmol/L, both hyperosmolar and metabolic problems develop (Figure 9.5; Table 9.10).

Blood glucose levels can exceed 50 mmol/L and this high osmotic load (which is also in the extracellular fluid) cannot be matched within those cells from which glucose is excluded owing to the absence of insulin. Thus, water is drawn from the intracellular compartment and this causes tissue dehydration. This particularly affects the brain where the resultant reduced intracranial pressure leads to CNS depression. The skin is also dehydrated, and loses its elasticity; this reduced skin turgor can be detected by pinching a fold of skin and noting its delay in

Table 9.9   Causes of acute disturbances in diabetic control

Hypoglycaemia	Hyperglycaemia/ketoacidosis
Excess (mis-measured?) dose	Missed antidiabetic dose
Potentiation of oral hypoglycaemic (drug interaction)	Hyperglycaemic drugs, e.g. thiazides, steroids
Missed meal; dieting	Excess dietary intake
Unexpected physical activity	Metabolic stress, e.g. infection, surgery, pregnancy
Excessively tight blood glucose control	
Alcohol	

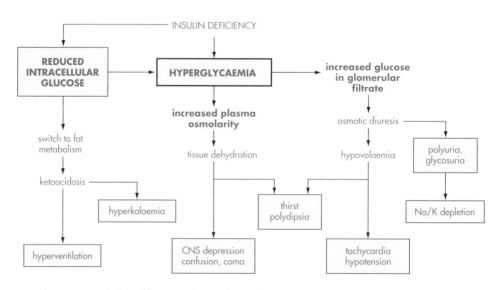

Figure 9.5   Pathogenesis and clinical features of acute hyperglycaemia and ketoacidosis.

Table 9.10   Clinical features of hyperglycaemia and ketoacidosis

Glycosuria, ketonuria
Polyuria, nocturia
Thirst, polydipsia

Hypotension
Rapid (bounding) pulse and respiration

Dry mouth, reduced skin turgor
Visual disturbance

Hyperkalaemia, acidosis, ketonaemia
Sweet smell of ketones on breath

Weakness, drowsiness, eventually coma

springing back, but this is less conclusive in the elderly, in whom skin elasticity is already reduced.

In the kidney the high load of glucose in the glomerular filtrate, not all of which can be reabsorbed, produces an osmotic diuresis. This results in a reduction in circulating fluid volume, leading to hypotension and reflex tachycardia. The high urine volumes also cause a loss of electrolytes, especially sodium and potassium. However, the plasma potassium level may be paradoxically high because acidosis inhibits the Na/K pump throughout the body, preventing intracellular potassium uptake (see below and Chapter 14, p. 891). Osmoreceptors and baroreceptors detect the electrolyte and fluid losses, causing thirst, but as CNS depression and confusion develop the patient often cannot respond by drinking.

In the absence of glucose, many cells start to metabolize fat instead. Adipose tissue releases fatty acids, and the liver converts some of these to acid ketones that can be readily utilized as an alternative energy source by many tissues. The resulting metabolic acidosis (diabetic ketoacidosis) is misinterpreted by the respiratory centre as carbon dioxide retention, resulting in an increased respiratory drive and hyperventilation. Acidosis impairs oxygen dissociation from Hb, exacerbating the gasping (overbreathing, 'air hunger'), and also causes peripheral vasodilatation, exacerbating the hypotension. Both respiratory rate and blood oxygen level fall as coma supervenes. Ketoacidosis is more likely to develop in type 1 patients, although fortunately it is uncommon.

People with type 2 diabetes usually secrete sufficient insulin to prevent them developing ketoacidosis (except during severe stress), but they may still suffer hyperosmolar non-ketotic hyperglycaemic states. This may result in coma and is associated with a higher mortality than ketoacidosis.

Management

Diabetic ketoacidosis is a medical emergency with about a 15% mortality rate. Close monitoring and very careful attention to the patient's fluid and electrolyte balance and blood biochemistry are essential (Table 9.11). Immediate attention is life-saving, but the patient may take several days to stabilize.

IV soluble insulin is essential. An initial bolus of about 6 units is followed by continuous infusion (6 units/h). Fluid replacement needs are estimated from measurements of the CVP and plasma sodium level. Hyponatraemia ('appropriate hyponatraemia', glucose having

Table 9.11   Principles of the management of ketoacidosis

Problem	Treatment
Underlying cause	Discover and treat
Hyperglycaemia and hyperosmolarity	Insulin (soluble): small bolus plus continuous infusion
Dehydration	IV infusion: saline/dextran/plasma
Acidosis	Bicarbonate?
Hyperkalaemia/potassium deficiency	Careful potassium repletion, after correction of acidosis
Hypoxaemia	Oxygen, up to 60% initially

osmotically displaced sodium in the plasma) and/or sodium depletion require 0.9% saline administration. However, if the dehydration has caused hypernatraemia, especially in the non-ketotic patient, hypotonic saline (e.g. 0.45%) may be indicated. Severe hypotension or shock require plasma replacement (see Chapter 14 p. 903). Potassium replacement is difficult to manage because the initial hyperkalaemia masks a total body potassium deficit. However, once insulin is started and potassium moves intracellularly, closely monitored IV potassium replacement is required. Acidosis will often resolve spontaneously with conservative therapy as ketone production falls and existing ketones are metabolized. Many clinicians would not use bicarbonate unless blood pH was below 7.00 for fear of overcompensating.

Hypoglycaemia

Causes

In all forms of diabetes, hypoglycaemia (blood glucose <3 mmol/L) is much more common than symptomatic hyperglycaemia, and it develops very rapidly, sometimes within minutes. Usually, either an excessive insulin dose is accidentally injected (many patients have eyesight problems) or else the normal dose of insulin or antidiabetic agent is not matched by an adequate dietary intake (Table 9.9). Insulin-induced hypoglycaemia is usually associated with injections of short-acting insulin. Deliberate overdosing is not unknown.

Hypoglycaemia induced by sulphonylurea antidiabetic drugs is rarer but more prolonged, more severe and more difficult to treat than insulin-induced hypoglycaemia. The elderly are especially prone, partly because the drugs are cleared more slowly and partly because of impaired homeostasis. Drug interactions that might potentiate oral antidiabetic drugs are considered on p. 615. Alcohol not only causes hypoglycaemia by inhibiting hepatic gluconeogenesis but also impairs the patients' perception of it, reducing their ability to respond.

Pathogenesis and symptoms

Hypoglycaemic symptoms fall into two main groups (Table 9.12). At glucose levels below about 4 mmol/L insulin release is inhibited and the counter-regulatory hormones such as glucagon and adrenaline are released in an effort to raise blood glucose. At a glucose level below 3.5 mmol/L the body responds by activating the sympathetic nervous system and adrenal medulla (the 'fight or flight' response). The consequent **sympathetic/adrenal** symptoms (Table 9.12) should provide the patient with a preliminary warning (but see below).

As the glucose level falls below about 2.5 mmol/L, neurological signs develop owing to the deficiency of glucose in the brain. These **neuroglycopenic** features may be noticed more by others than by patients themselves, although many patients do report an awareness of subjective prodromes. Sometimes the signs are subtle changes in mood or visual disturbances, but eventually there is almost always erratic behaviour resembling drunkenness. This has sometimes led to police arrest and delayed treatment, occasionally with fatal results. Frequent hypoglycaemic attacks may have a cumulative deleterious effect on higher brain function (cognition), especially in the elderly. All people with diabetes should carry, in addition to a readily available sugar source such as dextrose tablets, a card or

---

Table 9.12   Clinical features of hypoglycaemia

Adrenergic (autonomic) – enhanced sympathetic activity

- tremor, sweating
- shivering, palpitations
- anxiety, pallor

Neuroglycopenic – reduced CNS glucose delivery

- drowsiness, disorientation, confusion
- apparent drunkenness; aggression, inappropriate behaviour
- convulsions, coma, brain damage; death

Other effects – multiple or indirect pathogenesis

- hunger, salivation, weakness, blurred vision

bracelet stating that they have diabetes and should be given sugar if found acting strangely.

A patient's ability to recognize 'hypos' (their **hypoglycaemic awareness**) should be checked regularly because it tends to diminish. Long-term diabetes patients become less sensitive to the warning signs and thus more vulnerable. This may result partly from autonomic neuropathy and partly from reduced counter-regulatory hormone response. It is also possible that frequent attacks may reduce the patient's ability to recognize them. Awareness is pro-gressively reduced by frequent hypogly-caemic episodes but may be at least partially restored by minimizing or eliminating episodes through relaxing control slightly, more careful monitoring and patient education.

Most of the adrenergic symptoms are medi-ated by beta-receptors, and so may be antago-nized by concurrent beta-blocker therapy. Although this rarely presents a serious problem, such drugs should be avoided in people with diabetes if they already experience hypogly-caemic unawareness. Otherwise, there is no contra-indication but a cardioselective beta-blocker is preferred. Theoretically, beta-blockers might help by preventing beta-mediated insulin release (Figure 9.3), but this is swamped by the symptom-masking effect.

Management
Although both hypoglycaemia and hypergly-caemia can result in coma, there is rarely any problem distinguishing them, especially as rapid blood glucose test stick methods are readily available. A test dose of glucose would clinch matters because hypoglycaemia will be very rapidly reversed, whereas glucose would have no significant effect, either helpful or harmful, in hyperglycaemia. In contrast, insulin given blindly would severely exacerbate hypogly-caemia and should never be given where there is doubt.

The conscious patient must take glucose tablets, or sugar, chocolate, sweet tea, etc. Semi-conscious or comatose patients require IV glucose 20% or IM glucagon (1 mg). The response is usually satisfyingly prompt, occur-ring within minutes. Glucagon injection can usually be managed easily by patients' relatives, who should be fully informed on how to recognize and deal with hypoglycaemic episodes. Unless patients or their relatives are taught to recognize the early signs, the patient may become comatose before being able to correct it.

Persistent hypoglycaemic attacks require reassessment of therapy. Dietary modification may be required (e.g. increased carbohydrate), although this might compromise weight reduc-tion efforts. Modern intensive insulin therapy regimens aimed at producing 'tight' glycaemic control have increased the likelihood of hypoglycaemia, and a judgement of risk and benefit has to be made when such regimens are considered (p. 626).

Unstable diabetes

A small proportion of people with type 1 diabetes prove exceptionally difficult to control, experiencing frequent episodes of hypogly-caemia, hyperglycaemia or both. They are vari-ously termed **brittle**, **unstable** or **labile**. It is unlikely that this condition is inherent to their disease, and specific causes are always sought. Poor compliance through error, ignorance or disability, e.g. visual problems measuring insulin doses, unrecognized intercurrent illness and drug interaction must first be eliminated. In older patients with recurrent hypoglycaemia the possibility of reduced hypoglycaemic awareness must be investigated.

Recurrent hyperglycaemia/ketoacidosis is more common in young patients and may sometimes be associated with psychological or psychopathological factors such as teenage rebel-lion or illness denial, self-destructive impulses or other emotional instability. A particular subgroup has been identified of slightly obese females aged 15–25 years who may be covertly manipulating their therapy adversely. Supervised IV therapy in some of these patients seems to resolve the problem temporarily.

Chronic complications

In many patients, even before diagnosis, widespread damage occurs in the kidney, nerves, eyes or vascular tree (Figure 9.6). These long-term complications are to different degrees common to both types of diabetes, and their prevention or treatment are the real challenges for diabetes management and research.

Pathogenesis

It is important to determine whether or not these chronic problems are a direct consequence of hyperglycaemia. If so, then optimal control to achieve normoglycaemia would be expected to minimize them. Evidence has accumulated that this is broadly true for the so-called microvascular complications (mainly kidney, eye, nerves). The fact that similar complications arise in most types of diabetes, despite their different aetiolo-

gies, supports the hyperglycaemia hypothesis. The extensive Diabetes Control and Complications Trial (DCCT; 1992) confirmed that better control is associated with less severe complications in type 1 diabetes. The UK Prospective Diabetes Study (UKPDS; 1998) supported the same hypothesis in type 2 patients.

Other hypotheses have been proposed. It could be that an as yet unidentified primary lesion in diabetes is responsible independently for both the hyperglycaemia and the complications. If so, correcting one would not necessarily improve the other. Some complications could be secondary to the abnormal pattern or amount of insulin secretion, which is not completely rectified by conventional treatment. For example, the hyperinsulinaemia seen in many type 2 patients may contribute to blood vessel disease (macrovascular complications) or hypertension. Alternatively, the abnormally high levels of counter-regulatory hormones

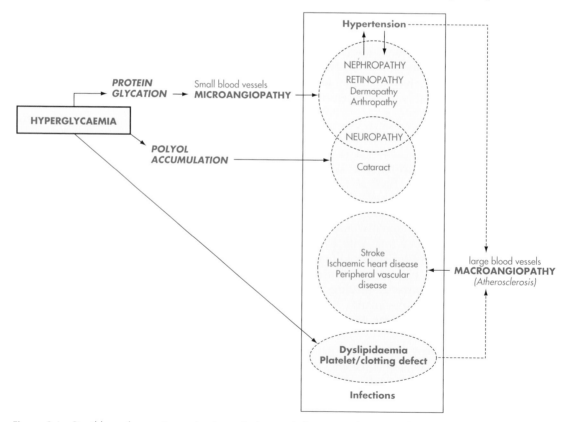

Figure 9.6 Possible pathogenetic mechanisms of chronic diabetic complications. The central box lists the clinical features. Also shown is possible interlinking of pathogenetic mechanisms.

usually found in diabetes may be deleterious. The involvement of growth hormone and insulin-like growth factor in angiopathy has also been investigated but no clear pattern detected. Finally, there seems to be a genetic variation in the susceptibility to different complications, regardless of the degree of glycaemic control.

Thus there is unlikely to be a simple answer, but the general strategy of normalizing blood glucose is well established as the best we currently have for minimizing complications.

Three general mechanisms are proposed for the pathological basis of the complications: **protein glycation** (glycosylation), abnormal **polyol** metabolism and accelerated **atheromatous** arterial changes.

Glycation

Normally, almost all body protein is to some extent glycated, i.e. glucose molecules from body fluids are covalently bound to free amine groups on protein side chains. The degree of glycation is directly proportional to the average blood glucose level. An accessible marker for this is Hb glycation, particularly the HbA1c fraction. Other proteins, and also lipids and nucleoprotein, throughout the body are similarly affected. In excess, one result is the formation of abnormal crosslinks between different regions of protein chains. Protein configuration is thus changed, disrupting secondary and tertiary structure and hence function. Basement membrane proteins seem particularly susceptible to glycation, the result being thickening and increased permeability (i.e. reduced selective barrier function). As basement membranes are present in most tissues, and especially in blood vessels, this could account for the widespread, multisystem distribution of diabetic complications. Chronic hyperglycaemia also results in oxidative stress through increases in mitochondrial superoxide formation, producing **advanced glycation end-products (AGPs)** that can cause a variety of damaging effects.

Basement membrane damage in capillaries and smaller arterioles can cause **microangiopathy** and subsequent ischaemia in almost any organ. **Retinopathy** is undoubtedly caused in part by this mechanism. **Neuropathy** may

result from a combination of this and direct glycation of the sheaths of small nerve axons, e.g. sensory nerves. Similarly, glycation of the glomerular basement membrane probably causes the characteristic glomerular sclerosis of diabetic **nephropathy**, although renal arterial disease probably also contributes. Glycation of tendon sheaths and joint capsules may be responsible for the joint problems, particularly the stiffness in hands and feet, that some patients suffer; glycation of collagen in skin sometimes gives it a thickened, waxy appearance. The myocardium may also be affected, as may immune cells such as macrophages and leucocytes.

Polyol metabolism

Some tissues do not require insulin for glucose transport into their cells (Table 9.1), relying instead simply on diffusion down a concentration gradient. Thus, while other tissues are glucose-depleted in diabetes, these will accumulate excess glucose in the presence of hyperglycaemia. Being surplus to energy needs, some of the excess glucose is reduced to polyols such as sorbitol by the enzyme aldose reductase via an otherwise little used pathway (Figure 9.7).

The resulting polyols are not readily eliminated from the cells, possibly because they are more polar than glucose and of greater molecular weight. Furthermore, low dehydrogenase activity, particularly in the eye lens and nerve sheaths, means that they are not metabolized efficiently. The resultant accumulation of osmotically active molecules draws water into the cells, causing them to expand, severely disrupting their function and possibly killing them. Retinal blood vessels, the eye lens and the glomeruli may be damaged in this way, contributing to retinopathy, cataract and nephropathy, respectively. It has long been known that an analogous intracellular accumulation of galactitol in the lens is linked to the high prevalence of cataracts in the inherited metabolic disorder galactosaemia.

A further abnormality may also contribute. Myoinositol, an important intermediate in energy handling, may (although also a polyol) instead of accumulating become deficient. By a poorly understood series of steps this deficiency may impair nerve conduction (Figure 9.7).

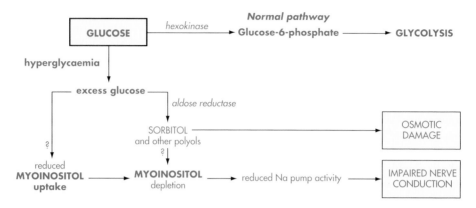

Figure 9.7   Polyol pathway and effects of polyol accumulation.

Macroangiopathy

Almost all people with diabetes suffer from increased obstructive vascular disease owing to a greatly increased predisposition to atherosclerosis. Several factors contribute to this. Because of their more active lipid metabolism, people with diabetes have raised plasma levels of triglycerides and lowered HDL, producing an unfavourable, atherogenic lipoprotein ratio (see Chapter 4, Figure 4.28). Furthermore, many type 2 patients are initially hyperinsulinaemic and insulin may itself be a growth factor for atheroma. Platelet aggregating ability is also usually raised, and hypertension is common. Thus major risk factors for atherosclerosis are intensified and cerebrovascular disease, stroke, IHD and peripheral vascular disease are common. Macroangiopathy also contributes to kidney disease.

Other mechanisms

As illustrated in Figure 9.6, other complications of diabetes occur, the pathogenesis of which remain obscure. Moreover, different complications may be inter-related or coexistent. Neuropathy may result partly from direct neuronal damage and partly from impaired blood supply to the nerve sheaths. Microangiopathy may result partly from glycation, partly from polyol accumulation and partly from hyperinsulinaemia. Once nephropathy is established, it promotes hypertension and vascular disease.

Diabetes and hypertension. There is an association between diabetes (especially type 2) and hypertension, as part of the metabolic syndrome. The precise cause and effect relationships have not yet been elucidated. Many hypertensives have insulin resistance, hyperinsulinaemia and impaired glucose tolerance, and insulin may have several hypertensive actions including promoting renal sodium retention, increasing sympathetic vasoconstrictor activity and directly increasing vascular reactivity, via an effect on sodium handling. In some cases hypertension may be secondary to diabetic kidney disease, although the converse may also be true (see Chapter 4, p. 213). Alternatively, it may be that a third, as yet unknown, independent factor first causes insulin resistance, which then leads to both type 2 diabetes and hypertension. Hyperinsulinaemia could then be a common link in the vascular complications of both diabetes and hypertension.

The UKPDS (1998) found that rigorous control of blood pressure in diabetes reduced complications. However, prolonged therapy with two common antihypertensive agents, thiazide diuretics and beta-blockers, while effectively lowering blood pressure, can also lead to glucose intolerance or even overt diabetes. For this reason beta-blockers are not recommended as first-line treatment for hypertension in diabetes, and extra care is needed with both.

Clinical consequences

Almost any system in the body may be affected by diabetic complications, which is why diabetes is regarded as a multisystem disease (Table 9.13).

Eyes.   Diabetes is the most common cause of acquired blindness in developed countries. After 30 years of diabetes, about 50% of patients have some degree of retinopathy, and up to 10% become blind. The blindness is due to small-vessel damage in the retina, with dilatation, haemorrhage, infarction and ultimately excessive proliferation of new vessels that project into the vitreous humour (neovascularization). Retinopathy is frequently associated with nephropathy. People with diabetes also have an increased incidence of glaucoma and cataract.

Nervous system.   Diabetic neuropathy may affect any part of the peripheral nervous system, but most commonly starts with the peripheral sensory nerves, causing tingling and numbness (paraesthesias), loss of vibration sense or the sense of balance and limb position. It may interfere with the ability of blind people with diabetes in reading Braille. Autonomic neuropathy is potentially devastating because it can seriously disturb cardiovascular, gastrointestinal or genitourinary function, causing numerous symptoms; postural hypotension and impotence are common. Voluntary motor nerves are less commonly affected.

Renal.   Diabetic nephropathy is the cause of death in about 25% of type 1 diabetes. Predominantly a form of sclerosis of the glomerular basement membrane, it develops very slowly and so most commonly occurs in type 1 patients, up to 40% of whom may be affected. The increased glomerular filtration rate ('hyperfiltration') in early diabetes, which is due to hypertension and to the osmotic loading of hyperglycaemia, may overload renal capillaries. Nephropathy is heralded by microalbuminuria, with increasing proteinuria frequently progressing to end-stage renal failure, associated with worsening hypertension. Diabetic nephropathy is one of the most common causes of chronic renal failure, with people with diabetes comprising about 15% of the caseload of UK renal replacement therapy units. Renal decline is hastened by inadequate or tardy treatment of associated hypertension.

Cardiovascular.   About half of diabetic deaths are from the consequences of macroangiopathy. People with diabetes have a twofold greater risk of stroke and a fivefold greater risk of MI compared with matched non-diabetic subjects. Peripheral vascular disease is also common, with a 50-fold higher risk of peripheral gangrene. Some patients undergo progressively extensive amputation; usually the lower limbs (especially the feet; see below) are affected, but fingers are also at risk.

Hypertension is often associated with diabetes. Up to 50% of type 1 patients have it, and it is probably secondary to nephropathy. About a

---

Table 9.13   Clinical consequences of diabetic complications

System	Clinical features
Eyes	Retinopathy, glaucoma, cataract; blindness
Nerves	Sensory, autonomic and motor defects
Renal	Glomerulosclerosis; chronic renal failure
Cardiovascular	Ischaemic heart disease (angina, MI), peripheral vascular disease, stroke; cardiomyopathy; congestive heart failure
Locomotor	Slow-healing peripheral lesions; 'the diabetic foot'; amputations; joint stiffness
Immune	Increased susceptibility to infection

MI, myocardial infarction.

fifth of type 2 patients are hypertensive; the aetiology is uncertain but related to the metabolic syndrome, with obesity and hyperinsulinaemia contributing.

A rare complication is diffuse cardiac fibrosis (cardiomyopathy), which may lead to heart failure.

Locomotor. The 'diabetic foot' is a common problem. In normal people minor foot injuries, such as a blister or a lesion from ill-fitting footware, usually heal before being noticed. In people with diabetes, however, these often develop into non-healing painless ulcers that become infected and irreversible damage sometimes occurs before medical attention is sought. In some cases this results in osteomyelitis or gangrene, both of which can lead to amputation. This results from a combination of poor peripheral sensation (neuropathy, so that the wound is not felt), poor peripheral circulation (angiopathy, so that healing is impaired) and reduced resistance to infection. All people with diabetes should see a chiropodist regularly. Correctly fitting footwear is essential. No pharmacist should attempt to treat any foot problem in a diabetic, or sell them 'corn plasters' or similar products. Any foot problem, however minor, should be referred to their chiropodist or doctor urgently.

Diabetes can also cause soft tissue damage resulting in limited joint mobility (stiffness), and a characteristic arthropathy, usually in the feet, where angiopathy and sensory neuropathy also contribute (Charcot joints; see Chapter 12).

Systemic. People with diabetes are very prone to infections owing to an impaired immune response caused by defects in immune and inflammatory cells. Recurrent bladder infection is common, which can ascend to cause pyelonephritis: urinary retention and stasis due to autonomic neuropathy exacerbate this. Skin infections are also frequent, and contribute to foot problems.

Management of complications

General strategy
The overall approach to preventing diabetic complications, minimizing them or delaying their onset combines control of blood glucose, risk factor reduction and regular monitoring.

Optimal glycaemic control. Although the aetiology and pathogenesis of the complications are still uncertain and likely to be multiple, the main clinical approach has been to aim for scrupulous control of blood glucose levels, keeping them within the normal range, in an attempt to mimic physiological normality. This is based on the assumption that complications are due to hyperglycaemia. This seems to be particularly likely for the microvascular, possibly polyol-related, complications in nerves, eyes and kidney. Evidence derives from clinical trials, including those using the more 'physiological' treatments such as continuous SC insulin infusion (p. 624) or other methods of achieving 'tight' glycaemic control. This means keeping fasting blood glucose levels below 7 mmol/L and not exceeding 11 mmol/L after meals, and may necessitate conversion to insulin therapy in poorly controlled type 2 patients.

Good control has been shown to reduce the incidence of complications. The most convincing evidence in type 1 diabetes was the DCCT trial, which reported significant slowing of deterioration in retinopathy, microalbuminuria and, to a lesser extent, neuropathy. The UKPDS trial found broadly similar benefits in type 2 patients and also strongly demonstrated the synergistic role of hypertension in exacerbating complications and the importance of achieving normotension as well as normoglycaemia. Unfortunately, this study failed to identify clearly the treatment mode that offered the best protection, although this had been one of its aims.

An unwanted side-effect of tight control is that by keeping the average blood glucose low the incidence of hypoglycaemia is increased, especially among elderly and unstable diabetics. In the DCCT trial there was a threefold increase in the incidence of hypoglycaemia when under tight control. This means that in some circumstances a compromise is necessary because of the acute and the long-term complications of frequent hypoglycaemic attacks. Thus, older patients in whom the diabetes onset occurred quite late, i.e. type 2, are usually allowed to run higher average levels. The long delay in onset of complications will mean that life expectancy may be little reduced, whereas quality of life would be markedly reduced by frequent hypoglycaemia.

For the macrovascular complications (cardiovascular, cerebrovascular and peripheral atherosclerosis) this approach is less successful, perhaps because insulin and related endocrine abnormalities and hypertension may contribute directly, independently of glycaemia. It is still unknown whether the generally higher insulin levels associated with tight control regimens can actually exacerbate some macrovascular problems.

Minimize risk factors. It is important to control any additional risk factors that could exacerbate organ damage, especially via atherosclerosis. These include smoking, hypertension, obesity, hyperlipidaemia and hyperuricaemia.

Monitoring. This essential component in minimizing complications is discussed below (see also Table 9.22).

Reduce polyol accumulation. According to the polyol hypothesis for certain of the complications, it should be possible to impede this process by interfering with the metabolism of polyols. Unfortunately, aldose reductase inhibitors (e.g. sorbinil), although they do minimize sorbitol accumulation and prevent myoinositol depletion, have not proven clinically successful in reversing or even retarding neuropathy, cataract, nephropathy or retinopathy. Dietary myoinositol supplementation has also been unsuccessful.

Specific complications

Nephropathy. There are currently four methods that have been shown to slow the rate of deterioration in renal function:

- Careful glycaemic control.
- Control of hypertension.
- Use of ACEIs or ARAs.
- Moderate protein restriction (in more advanced nephropathy).

It is essential that people with diabetes are monitored annually for the onset of hypertension and microalbuminuria. In treating hypertension, ACEIs (and ARAs) seem to have an additional direct beneficial effect in diabetes, dilating intrarenal (efferent glomerular) vessels and thus minimizing glomerular hypertension. ACEIs are increasingly used early unless contra-indicated e.g. by bilateral renal artery stenosis, which is always a possibility in someone with diabetes. ACEIs are indicated when there is hypertension with proteinuria or microalbuminuria; in type 1 diabetes their use is recommended if there is microalbuminuria, even with normotensive patients. However, at present there is no evidence that ACEIs benefit normotensive diabetes with no evidence of nephropathy. Other antihypertensives may not offer similar extra benefits but another antihypertensive should be used if ACEIs are contra-indicated or inadequate at reducing pressure.

Once established, renal failure is managed as usual (see Chapter 14), although haemodialysis is more difficult because of vascular and thrombotic complications. Continuous ambulatory peritoneal dialysis is particularly suitable in diabetes because insulin may be administered intraperitoneally (thus directly entering the portal circulation, which is more physiological). However, there may be a problem with the glucose, which is usually added to dialysis fluid to promote water removal. People with diabetes are nowadays unlikely to be given low priority for renal transplantation, as they tended to be in the past, and this is sometimes combined with pancreatic transplantation (p. 605). There are however some problems: the poor general health of these patients and multiple organ damage increase the operative risk, and there is an increased likelihood of post-transplant infection owing to the immunosuppression required. Nevertheless, graft survival is only about 10–15% poorer than the average for renal transplants.

Macroangiopathy. The usual dietary constraints on saturated fat and cholesterol are important. Monounsaturated fats, especialy olive oil, are recommended. The HPS study supported the use of statins for all people with diabetes of either type at cardiovascular risk, whatever their lipid level, and this is now accepted. The CARDS study extended the recommendation in type 2 diabetes to those patients with even normal or low lipids, regardless of CVS risk. However, such routine use is not yet officially recommended. In the PROactive trial type 2 patients with pre-existing macrovascular disease used pioglitazone in addition to their usual treatment. A small but significant reduction in all-cause mortality, MI and stroke was achieved but at the expense of weight gain and an increase in heart failure.

Other conventional atheroma risk factors such as smoking and hypertension must also be scrupulously addressed (see Chapter 4).

Neuropathy and neuropathic pain.   Little can be done for diffuse neuropathy, but neuropathic pain can be partially relieved and fortunately severe attacks, although prolonged, tend to remit. Drug therapy may be of help in the sometimes excruciating pain. Conventional analgesic or anti-inflammatory drugs are generally ineffective. A variety of other drugs have been tried and the first-generation tricyclic antidepressants (e.g. *amitriptyline*) are standard first-line therapy. Second-line agents include anticonvulsants such as *carbamazepine*, *gabapentin* or *topiramate* (see also Chapter 6).

Retinopathy.   Retinal disease is conventionally treated by laser photocoagulation.

Management

Aims and strategy

Preventative methods for diabetes are as yet poorly developed. More progress has been made with potentially curative surgery. However, at present the vast majority of people with diabetes require long-term management of established disease.

The cardinal aim of management in diabetes is to keep blood glucose levels within the normal range; this should produce patterns of glucose and insulin levels in the blood similar to those that follow normal changes in diet and activity (see Figure 9.4). Blood glucose levels should remain below the maxima in the WHO defini-

tion for impaired glucose tolerance (Table 9.1). Ideally, this would require a continuous basal level of insulin to maintain metabolism, supplemented by rapid pulses following meals and a reduced level during exercise.

Optimal management should attain three important interlinked aims:

• Prevent symptoms.
• Maintain biochemical stability.
• Prevent long-term complications.

At present, this ideal is not achievable. Even if pancreatic transplantation were to be perfected, insulin receptor defects might still remain. Current therapy is limited to artificially manipulating diet and insulin (endogenous or exogenous) in order to mimic normal patterns as closely as is practicable.

The older directive, paternalistic medical model for such manipulation is no longer acceptable, clinics preferring to negotiate a 'therapeutic contract' with the patient. The aim is to agree a desired level of control – optimal, prophylactic or perhaps merely symptomatic – based on the severity of the disease and the patient's age, understanding, likely compliance and normal way of life.

Sometimes it is inadvisable to strive too zealously to approach the ideal. For the elderly, where long-term complications are of less concern, keeping symptoms at a tolerable level without excessive disruptions to normal life patterns may be adequate. For this, the target need only be to achieve random blood glucose levels below 12 mmol/L. In some patients the incidence of hypoglycaemic attacks is unacceptably high if control is too tight. The advent of the insulin pen has enabled the flexibility to achieve these differing aims.

Prevention

Because type 1 disease involves immune destruction of the pancreas, immunotherapy has been attempted experimentally, as early as possible after initial diagnosis or even in the pre-symptomatic stage in at-risk individuals, e.g. where there is a strong family history or impaired glucose tolerance. In animal models anti-T cell antibodies, bone marrow transplantation, thymectomy, *azathioprine* and *ciclosporin* have been tried. In the Diabetes Prevention Trial-1 early introduction of insulin therapy, to 'spare' the beta cells and perhaps to reduce their expression of autoantigens, was unsuccessful. Another trial using *nicotinamide* to inhibit macrophages has also failed to reduce progression.

However, considerable pancreatic damage has usually occurred by the time symptoms are noticed. Only about 10% of functional islet cells then remain, so no great improvement can be expected. Research is now concentrating on discovering reliable early prognostic markers, such as islet cell antibodies. Patients at risk could then be identified by screening.

No specific aetiological agents have been identified for type 2 diabetes, but risk factors are well known. These correspond with many of the well-established cardiovascular risk factors associated with the lifestyle of industrialized countries, i.e. diets high in sugar and fats and low in fibre and slowly absorbable complex carbohydrates, lack of exercise and obesity. Weight loss in particular has been shown to delay development of the disease in high-risk individuals and achieve remission in severely overweight people with diabetes. In the Diabetes Prevention Programme both intensive lifestyle intervention and *metformin* significantly reduced the risk of developing diabetes in people with impaired glucose tolerance. Another trial showed benefit with *acarbose*. In the Finnish Diabetes Prevention Study dietary modification and exercise was similarly beneficial. More recently the DREAM trial with *rosglitazone* over 3 years showed significant reduction in progression from impaired glucose tolerance/impaired fasting glycaemia to overt type 2 diabetes.

Cure: organ replacement

Pancreatic transplants are now a realistic option. Dual renal plus pancreatic transplantation is especially considered for people with diabetes with advanced nephropathy, because such patients are going to have to undergo immunosuppression anyway. One-year patient survival exceeds 90% and 5-year graft survival exceeds 50%. Transplantation substantially increases the quality of life, although of course is still limited by the risks of surgery and the penalty of lifelong immunosuppression (Chapter 14).

The implantation of donated **beta-islet cells** is still experimental but looks promising. Stem cells may offer even more fundamental a solution for the future. A number of **artificial pancreas** devices have been devised, although none is yet available for routine use (p. 624).

Therapeutic strategy

Using conventional methods, the only way for a diabetic to enjoy relatively normal eating and activity (i.e. unpredictable, unplanned and uncontrolled) would be to have frequent, precisely calculated injections of soluble insulin (or appropriate doses of a rapidly acting oral hypoglycaemic [insulin secretagogue] drug). The dose would be based on blood glucose measurement or guided by experience and recent diet and activity level: thus insulin is supplied on demand in a manner emulating normal physiology (see Figure 9.4). With the introduction of insulin pens, such an 'insulin demand-driven' strategy is becoming practicable, although dosage adjustment is still imprecise. The artificial pancreas, if perfected, may prove a better option.

'Insulin supply drive'

The alternative (and original) approach, still used for many older patients, is to turn physiology on its head and to accept a model driven by insulin supply. Instead of matching insulin supply to instantaneous changes in demand, demand in the form of diet and activity is adjusted and controlled to conform to available insulin (whether endogenous or administered exogenously). Because both drugs and insulin must be given prospectively this is in effect 'feeding the insulin', as opposed to the normal situation where insulin follows feeding. Meals and activity must be regular and of predictable composition: explicit adjustments in drug or insulin dose must be made to allow for deviations (Figure 9.8).

This places considerable constraints on patients, particularly children. Education and counselling are extremely important and Diabetes UK performs a valuable role here.

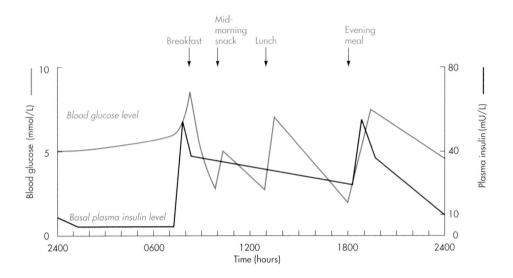

Figure 9.8 Matching food intake to available insulin – schematic representation. In the insulin supply-driven model, insulin levels are maintained artificially either by direct injection or by augmentation using oral hypoglycaemic agents. To prevent hypoglycaemia, sufficient glucose must be provided by the diet at regular intervals. Note what would be the effect of missing the mid-afternoon snack: blood glucose would start to fall dangerously low just before the evening meal. Unusual activity, by causing increased glucose demand, would complicate this picture.

People with type 1 diabetes are inevitably reasonable compliers in the strictest sense, in that the severe metabolic upset precipitated by drug defaulting is a powerful motivator. Nevertheless, excellent compliance with diet, and the very tight control of blood glucose demanded for avoidance of long-term complications, is less common, especially in type 2.

Treatment modes

Dietary management is the bedrock of treatment. All people with diabetes, irrespective of other treatments, require some control of their eating and exercise patterns, both in terms of total calorific intake, types of nutrients and eating schedule. Indeed, about half of patients will need no more than this, especially those who lose weight. A further 25% will need to augment their natural insulin with drugs. The remainder will need insulin.

The initial choice is usually related to how the patient first presents (Figure 9.9). Younger patients, who are frequently non-obese, usually present unambiguously with type 1 insulin-dependent diabetes, although a variable insulin-independent ('honeymoon') period may occur following diagnosis.

Older patients, who are often obese, will almost always be type 2 and must be tried first on diet alone. Should this fail, drug therapy will be added. All drugs used in diabetes are classed in the BNF as **antidiabetic**, and this term will be used generically here (although NICE refers to these drugs as 'glucose-lowering drugs'). The older term 'oral hypoglycaemic' is obsolescent, owing to the development of classes of drugs that do not directly lower blood glucose. Those that do, i.e. sulphonylureas and meglitinides, are more accurately described as insulin **secretagogues**.

Type 2 patients are usually to some extent overweight on presentation, and a biguanide is the first choice. Otherwise a sulphonylurea is selected. Sometimes a synergistic combination of the two types will be required. For those for whom these measures are ineffective a glitazone may be added. For some patients even this is

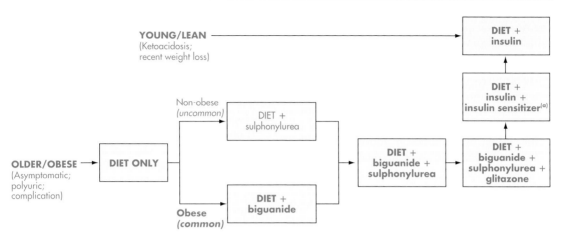

Figure 9.9   Treatment strategy for diabetes related to presenting symptoms. Meglitinides may be substituted for sulphonylureas. A glitazone or glucosidase inhibitor can be added or substituted at any stage to attempt to improve control before moving to next stage (but avoid meglitinide + sulphonylurea). See text. [a]Insulin sensitizer = metformin or glitazone.

unsatisfactory and, especially if ketoacidosis occurs, insulin treatment is needed, as it will be eventually in those whose disease progresses faster. Type 2 patients may also need insulin temporarily during periods of increased requirement such as major infection, surgery or pregnancy. Combining antidiabetic drugs with insulin therapy is being used increasingly (see below).

At any point in this sequence, an adjunctive drug that reduces intestinal glucose absorption or reduces insulin resistance may be added.

Initiation of treatment

On first diagnosis, all patients will be fully examined and investigated to establish baseline measures for monitoring development and progression of any complications. This will include ophthalmological, renal, cardiovascular, neurological, lipid and foot assessment.

Some patients will need to be treated first in hospital, especially type 1 patients first presenting with ketoacidosis. Blood glucose levels will be measured 3-hourly during this period, to establish the diet and possibly the drug or insulin dosage necessary to achieve the agreed level of control. After discharge some will continue to attend as outpatients. Others will be managed by general practice clinics, which often

include specialist diabetic nurse practitioners. However, regular diabetic clinic visits are desirable if they have developed complications or management becomes difficult. Some type 1 and most type 2 patients without acute complications may be treated by their GP from the outset.

Diet

Most type 2 patients must first be encouraged to try to control their disease on diet alone, and no patient taking antidiabetic drugs or insulin should believe that these obviate the necessity to control their diet. Recommendations about diet have evolved in several important ways. Fats are now discouraged, while complex carbohydrate and fibre are encouraged, and the overall approach is now far less restrictive. The recommended diabetic diet, save in a few respects, now closely resembles the normal healthy diet that everyone should eat: regular meals low in fats, simple sugars and sodium and high in complex carbohydrate (starch) and fibre.

Formerly, inflexible, unrealistic or impractical prescriptions and restrictions (diet sheets, 'exchanges') took little or no account of the psychological importance of individual dietary habits, dietary preferences and ethnic variations.

The result was poor compliance complicated by guilt and anxiety. The modern approach recognizes that:

- Dietary records or recall are an imprecise basis for future modification.
- Nutrient uptake varies even from precisely regulated and measured portions, owing to the interactions between foodstuffs, variations in temperature, physical form and degree of chewing, etc.
- Compromise is needed to devise a regimen with which the patient can be concordant.

Thus a perfect diabetic diet is difficult to achieve in practice, and although the pursuit of it is worthwhile, this could be counter-productive in some patients. Rather, efforts are made to ensure that patients understand, in their own fashion, what the aims are. Counselling and education are then used to maximize motivation. Advice from a dietician with experience in modifying diabetic diets to suit individual lifestyles can help achieve good compliance.

Four aspects of diet need to be considered (Figure 9.10):

- Total energy intake.
- Constituents.
- Timing.
- Variation.

Energy intake

All patients need to adjust their calorific intake to achieve and maintain the desired bodyweight for their size, aiming for a body mass index of about 22 kg/m^2. For most people with type 2 diabetes, who are frequently obese, this implies a weight-reducing diet. Reliable tables are now available to predict the required energy intake according to age, gender, activity level and lifestyle.

Constituents

Macronutrients
The unselective restriction on carbohydrate that used to characterize diabetic diets is now considered misconceived. Carbohydrate is not harmful if taken mainly as slowly absorbed complex polysaccharides, e.g. starch. Such carbohydrates allow people with type 2 diabetes to make best use of their limited endogenous insulin secretory capacity by not raising postprandial blood glucose too rapidly. Foods can be classified

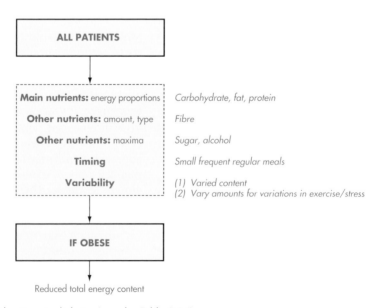

Figure 9.10   Dietary considerations in diabetes (see also Table 9.14).

according to their **glycaemic index**, which represents the ratio of the total glucose absorption they produce compared with that from a standard test meal of wholemeal bread and cottage cheese. The lower the index the better, and representative values are rice 80%, potatoes 77%, pasta 60% and lentils 45%. Foods acceptable to various ethnic minorities, such as chappatis, kidney beans, chickpeas, etc. are also now encouraged where appropriate.

The relatively high fat content of early diabetic diets, which was needed in a carbohydrate-reduced diet to provide calories more cheaply than with protein, is now seen to be dangerously atherogenic. A reduced fat intake, low in saturated fats and comprising about one-third polyunsaturated and one-third monounsaturated fat (e.g. nuts, fish, olive oil) is now encouraged. Cholesterol itself is usually reduced inherently along with saturated fats. There are no particular constraints on protein except for patients with suspected nephropathy, when restriction is indicated.

Other nutrients

A small amount of simple sugar (sucrose) is now considered acceptable, if the calorific content is accounted for. This is usually consumed as a constituent, e.g. of baked products. Artificial non-nutritive sweeteners are still preferred and patients must be advised to monitor their intake of 'hidden' sugar in processed foods. So-called 'diabetic foods' often contain sorbitol or fructose and, while they may not raise blood glucose as much as sucrose, have a high energy content and cause diarrhoea in excess. They are also expensive, offer nothing that a well-balanced diabetic diet cannot offer, and are not recommended by Diabetes UK.

Alcohol is not prohibited if its high calorific content is accounted for and its hypoglycaemic effect is appreciated, i.e. it should be taken with some carbohydrate. Recent evidence of its protective effect against heart disease suggests that once again similar recommendations should apply to the diabetic population as to the population as a whole. There should be little added salt, to minimize rises in blood pressure.

Fibre is extremely important. Although fibre is primarily carbohydrate, the terminology is somewhat inconsistent; however, the distinctions are relevant (Figure 9.11). Starch, in staple foods like bread, potatoes and rice, is the main digestible carbohydrate energy source. Older classifications grouped all other indigestible matter together as 'dietary fibre', but there are important and distinct components. The non-starch polysaccharides (NSP) are now known to be particularly important in diabetes. They provide no energy but further delay absorption of glucose from starch digestion (see above), and by forming intestinal bulk promote a feeling of satiety that may reduce appetite and therefore help weight control.

The (semi)soluble or viscous fibres and gums found in fruit, vegetables and pulses (Figure 9.11) produce in addition a modest reduction in blood cholesterol, possibly by binding bile salts and thereby preventing their enterohepatic recirculation. The insoluble NSP fibres, as in bran and unmilled cereals and grains, have little effect on cholesterol, but contribute to stool bulk along with other fibrous residues, e.g. lignin. Although undigested in the ileum, some of this material is hydrolysed by colonic flora to release absorbable and metabolizable carboxylic acids.

Proportions

The recommended proportions of macronutrient energy intake are approximately 60:30:10 (carbohydrate:fat:protein; Table 9.14); traditional diabetic diets used to be nearer 25:65:10. Within the fats, only a third should be saturated fats. How the patient implements this has also changed. Clinics no longer issue rigid menus, kitchen scales and detailed tables of what can be exchanged for what. More generalized recommendations with much wider variability are found to be more successful.

One such approach simply visualizes a meal plate divided into segments (Figure 9.12). About two-thirds contains polysaccharide: equal parts staple carbohydrate sources such as rice, pasta or potatoes starch and fibre such as fruit or vegetables. The remainder is mostly composed of fats and protein sources such as meat, fish and dairy products. A small amount of sugar is allowed. The patient is advised to construct each meal in these proportions. This roughly conforms to the recommended proportions, allowing for some

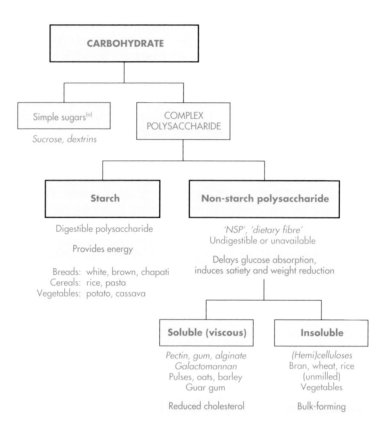

Figure 9.11   Different forms of dietary carbohydrate, including fibre; with functions and examples of foodstuffs. [a]Avoid as far as possible.

fat and protein being included along with the carbohydrate.

Timing

Small, regular, frequent meals are important. This means similar calorific intake at all main meals and regular snacks in between. For type 2 patients this minimizes the load put on the pancreas at any one time. For both types it helps to keep blood glucose levels within closer limits, minimizing the risk of hypoglycaemia between drug or insulin doses and the risk of postprandial hyperglycaemia. There is some evidence that this too is a pattern that might benefit the general population. Nibbling or 'grazing' appears to produce lower average plasma lipid and blood glucose levels and less obesity compared with a similar calorific intake obtained from intermittent, larger meals.

Variation

People with diabetes need to understand that these constraints do not prevent them having a varied, appetizing and nutritious diet. They should also understand how to augment their diet to match any unplanned or unusual exercise or stress so as to avoid hypoglycaemia. Temporary changes in a patient's metabolic requirements (as in serious illness) or oral absorptive capacity (e.g. gastroenteritis) require appropriate adjustment, which may involve temporary insulin therapy in a type 2 patient, and regular blood glucose monitoring is then essential.

Type 1 patients using the 'insulin pen' will generally be even more flexible (see below). In mildly diabetic elderly patients the diet will also be far less rigid, for reasons already discussed. On the other hand, the diets of growing children need constant reassessment. The availability of

Table 9.14   Nutrients in diets recommended for diabetic and general population[a]

	Nutrition Subcommittee of the Diabetes Care Advisory Committee of Diabetes UK [b]	National recommendations for optimal UK diet[c]
Carbohydrate	50–60%	50–60%
Total fat	30–35% [saturated fat 10%]	30–35%
Protein	1 g/kg body weight	10%
Simple sugars	≤10%	60 g
Cholesterol[d]	Not specified	Not specified
Soluble fibre[e]	Not specified	18 g
Alcohol	2 units (female)	2 units (female)
	3 units (male)	3 units (male)

[a] Percentages are rounded and given as maximum proportion of total energy intake. Amounts are per day.

[b] Diabetes UK, *Diabetic Medicine* 2003; **20**: 786–807.

[c] Based on reports from National Advisory Committee on Nutrition Education (NACNE, UK DoH) and Committee on Medical Aspects Of Food Policy (COMA, UK DoH).

[d] Cholesterol intake usually automatically reduced sufficiently if saturated fat intake less than 10%.

[e] 15 g soluble fibre equivalent to 18 g non-starch polysaccharides (NSP) or 30 g total dietary fibre.

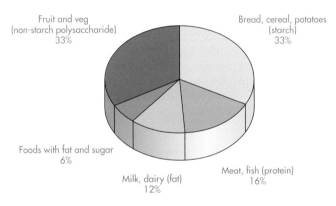

Figure 9.12   The 'plate model' of meal planning recommended by Diabetes UK. Each meal should be constructed roughly of the types of foods and in the proportions shown, visualizing them as making up the complete plate of food. (Adapted from www.diabetes.org.uk/eatwell/food_diabetes/index.html).

nutrients and the habits and constraints of different ethnic groups also need to be taken into account. Dieticians are an essential part of the diabetic team.

Diet as sole management may fail in up to two-thirds of type 2 patients. Primary failure is usually due to poor compliance, poor motivation or inadequate counselling. Secondary failure usually results from disease progression, with falling insulin production. The next stage is to introduce oral antidiabetic drugs.

Oral antidiabetic drugs

Aim and role

Oral antidiabetic drugs (OADs) are used as the next step for type 2 patients in whom diet has failed to control their condition adequately. The majority may then be controlled by a combination of diet and oral drugs for a number of years, but some type 2 patients may eventually require insulin treatment.

There are four main therapeutic targets for OADs (Table 9.15). Doubts over the safety of some of these drugs have now been resolved. The results of the University Group Diabetes Programme (UGDP) trial in the 1970s, which suggested significant toxicity in the sulphonylureas, are now discredited. *Phenformin*, an early biguanide, caused numerous deaths from lactic acidosis and was withdrawn. Newer biguanides are much safer: only *metformin* is currently available in the UK; elsewhere *buformin* is used.

Novel incretin analogues are undergoing trials. Incretin is a newly discovered peptide hormone, secreted in the small intestines following food intake, which enhances insulin secretion and suppresses glucagon, slows gastric emptying and reduces food intake. It was isolated from a lizard that eats only four times a year. *Exenatide* has been shown to lower glycated Hb levels and weight. Sitagliptin inhibits incretin inactivation.

All OAD strategies depend on endogenous insulin secretion and are therefore effective only in patients with type 2 disease who retain appreciable beta-cell function. Ketosis-prone patients, patients with brittle disease or those whose fasting blood glucose exceeds 15–20 mmol/L, almost invariably need exogenous insulin, in both type 1 and type 2 patients.

Action

These drugs have different, albeit complementary and sometimes overlapping, actions on the underlying abnormalities in type 2 diabetes, so combination therapy is indicated if monotherapy fails.

Alpha-glucosidase inhibitors (*acarbose*) inhibit the final stage of the digestion of starch within the intestine by blocking the enzyme disaccharidase. This reduces the rate of glucose absorption and thus the postprandial glucose load presented to the islet cells. Thus, a pancreas with a limited insulin secretory rate might be better able to handle this load with less hyperglycaemia. It can be regarded as anti-hyperglycaemic rather than a hypoglycaemic agent. It has a relatively small effect on glycaemia and is used only as an adjunct to other therapy, but may be added at any stage to improve control.

Sulphonylureas enhance the release of preformed insulin in response to circulating glucose, partly by increasing beta-cell sensitivity to blood glucose. This mimics the acute phase of the normal response to hyperglycaemia. However, sulphonylureas do not directly stimulate subsequent insulin synthesis. Inhibition of

Table 9.15 Oral antidiabetic drugs

Therapeutic target	Site of action	Group	Examples
Reduce or retard glucose uptake	Intestine	Alpha-glucosidase inhibitors	Acarbose
Enhance insulin secretion[a]	Pancreas	Sulphonylureas	Tolbutamide, glibenclamide, glipizide, glimepiride, gliquidone
		Meglitinides	Repaglinide, nateglinide
Enhance insulin action	Peripheral receptors	Biguanides	Metformin, buformin[b]
Reduce gluconeogenesis	Liver		
Reduce insulin resistance	Peripheral receptors (esp. adipose tissue)	Thiazolidinediones (Glitazones)	Rosiglitazone, pioglitazone

[a] Insulin secretagogues.

[b] Buformin not licensed in UK.

glucagon has also been suggested. Pharmacodynamically, they differ only in relative potency but there are important pharmacokinetic differences between them. Sulphonylureas can be combined with most other OADs except the meglitinides. Although some doubt was cast over the safety of the long-established combination with *metformin* by the UKPDS, this has not been confirmed and the combination is still widely used.

Meglitinides (prandial glucose regulators) also stimulate insulin release but not at the sulphonylurea receptor. They are claimed to do so more specifically in response to the blood glucose level and thus to mealtime glucose load, making them more glucose-sensitive. They have two main advantages over sulphonylureas. A more rapid onset means they can be given 15 min or less before a meal, giving patients more flexibility and control; and their shorter duration of action reduces the likelihood of postprandial hyperinsulinaemia and between-meals hypoglycaemia. In addition, if a meal is missed they can easily be omitted. *Nateglinide* has a prompter and shorter action than *repaglinide*. Currently *nateglinide* is only licensed for use with *metformin*, whereas *repaglinide* can be substituted for sulphonylureas at any stage. The combination of a meglitinide with a sulphonylurea is irrational.

Biguanides do not stimulate or mimic insulin but are insulin sensitizers. They have two main actions: they increase peripheral glucose uptake and utilization and they inhibit hepatic gluconeogenesis and release of glucose from the liver into the blood. The underlying effect is probably via a general inhibitory action on membrane transport. Intracellularly, this would prevent glucose entering mitochondria, thus promoting anaerobic glycolysis in the cytosol. Because this is less efficient than aerobic glycolysis, cellular glucose uptake and utilization are increased. This may also account for a tendency to cause lactic acidosis. In the intestine, reduced membrane transport may be useful in slowing and reducing glucose absorption. There may also be intestinal lactate production. They may also have an anti-obesity action. Only *metformin* is licensed in the UK.

Biguanides can be combined with most other OADs.

Glitazones (thiazolidinediones: *rosiglitazone* and *pioglitazone*) are also insulin sensitizers. They activate a nuclear transcription regulator for an insulin-responsive gene (peroxisome proliferators-activated receptor-gamma, PPARγ), which has numerous complex effects on lipid and glucose metabolism. An important component is to promote triglyceride uptake and peripheral adipose growth. The effect of this is to reduce triglyceride availability, increase glucose utilization, reduce insulin resistance and thus reduce insulin levels. They also shift fat from visceral, muscle and hepatic sites to peripheral adipose tissue, which although resulting in an increase in weight, produces a more favourable cardiovascular risk. This is partly because they alter blood lipids favourably, lowering triglyceride and raising HDL levels.

The PROactive study suggested this group may reduce complications, both macrovascular (by reducing insulin and lipid levels) and microvascular (by reducing hyperglycaemia) complications, but this has not yet been confirmed. The prototype, *troglitazone*, was withdrawn soon after release owing to liver toxicity but *rosiglitazone* and *pioglitazone* are safe and effective either alone or in combination if other OADs fail to achieve control, although their precise role has not yet been determined. Currently NICE recommends that they should not be added as second-line drugs to either *metformin* or a sulphonylurea, except when these latter two drugs cannot be used in combination owing to contra-indications or intolerance.

Biopharmacy and pharmacokinetics

Sulphonylureas are generally well absorbed although potential bioavailability differences mean that patients should avoid changing formulation or brand. Most sulphonylureas are more than 90% protein-bound (except *tolazamide*, 75%), and so are liable to competitive displacement interactions.

There are important differences in clearance, half-life and duration of action, which determine frequency of administration, precautions and contra-indications. Clearance is usually hepatic with subsequent excretion of inactive or less active metabolites (Table 9.16; Figure 9.13), usually renally. The older *chlorpropamide* is partially cleared renally and also has active metabolite, which accounts for its long half-life. Those with inactive metabolites (e.g. *tolbutamide*) generally have the shortest half-lives. Some sulphonylureas have metabolites that are chiefly excreted in the bile, which makes them more reliant on hepatic function.

The duration of action, or biological half-life, is related to the plasma half-life but is often longer, owing partly to the activity of metabolites. *Chlorpropamide* has too long a duration of action and frequently produces between-meals hypoglycaemia; it has little if any role now and is contra-indicated in the elderly. The other popular first-generation sulphonylurea, *tolbutamide*, fell from favour because its action was felt to be too short, requiring frequent dosing. However, for this reason it may be useful in the elderly, to minimize hypoglycaemia. Most newer second-generation drugs avoid these problems, but there are wide interpatient variations in the handling of all sulphonylureas and dose regimens must be individualized. *Glibenclamide* is a special case because it is concentrated within beta-cells so its biological half-life is considerably longer than its plasma half-life. For this reason, it too is avoided in the elderly.

Biguanides differ substantially from the sulphonylureas, being poorly absorbed, little protein-bound and cleared predominantly by renal excretion (with about 30% cleared by hepatic metabolism). *Metformin* has a short half-life and may require thrice daily dosing at higher doses. However, modified-release preparations are available for dosages up to 1 g twice daily; higher doses need standard-release therapy. *Buformin* is longer-acting.

Renal clearance of biguanides may exceed glomerular filtration rate, implying some tubular

Table 9.16 Relative duration of action of sulphonylureas

Relative duration of action[a]	Very short	Short	Medium	Long	Very long
Daily dose frequency	2–3	2–3	1(–2)	1	1
Examples	Gliquidone	Tolbutamide	Glimepride, glipizide, gliclazide	Glibenclamide	Chlorpropamide[b]

[a] Approximate descriptive indication of relative durations: precise time will vary from patient to patient.

[b] No longer recommended.

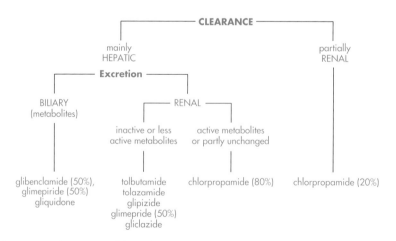

Figure 9.13 Clearance and excretion of the sulphonylureas.

secretion. Thus minor renal impairment, un-noticed because of a normal serum creatinine level, might still permit significant accumulation, and renal function monitoring is essential with their use.

Meglitinides are rapidly absorbed, reaching a peak within 1 h and have a very short half-life, being cleared and eliminated hepatically. This means they may be useful in controlling blood glucose in close association with meals.

Glitazones (thiazolidinediones) are rapidly absorbed and hepatically metabolized. Although the half-life is less than 24 h, and once or twice daily dosing is adequate, full effect takes at least a week, owing to the slow speed of fat redistribution.

Alpha-glucosidase inhibitors are not absorbed, acting slowly within the gut.

Adverse reactions

Sulphonylureas are well tolerated and free from serious long-term adverse effects. The principal problem is hypoglycaemia, which may be protracted and even fatal. A related drawback is the tendency to produce or maintain obesity. Both effects can be linked to increased insulin levels, which also are giving concern over a possible exacerbation of macrovascular complications, insulin being a possible growth factor in arterial walls.

Hypoglycaemia may be caused by an overdose, an interaction, a missed meal or unexpected activity and occurs more commonly with the longer-acting drugs (*glibenclamide* and *chlorpropamide*), especially in the elderly, who must avoid them. (The possible compliance advantage is far outweighed by the likelihood that a meal will be forgotten while plasma drug levels are still significant.) With the newer, shorter-acting drugs any hypoglycaemia that does occur is brief and more easily rectified.

Chlorpropamide can occasionally cause a mild disulfiram-like flush with alcohol (due to acetaldehyde dehydrogenase inhibition), and occasionally hyponatraemia and a syndrome of inappropriate secretion of ADH. These effects, as well as minor idiosyncratic reactions, are uncommon with second-generation sulphonylureas.

Meglitinides do not present such risks of hypo-glycaemia and weight gain as the sulphonyl-ureas. No serious class effects have become apparent so far.

Biguanides (with the exception of *phenformin*) cause minor adverse effects, being somewhat less well tolerated than sulphonylureas. The nausea, diarrhoea, muscle discomfort and occasional malabsorption experienced may be due to the membrane effects inherent in their mode of action. Malabsorption of vitamin B_{12} can occur. Biguanides are best taken with food, the dose being increased gradually to improve tolerance. Iatrogenic lactic acidosis, which has a high mortality, occurs rarely with *metformin* and the risk can be further reduced by careful monitoring of renal and hepatic function and ensuring that it is avoided in patients with renal impairment and hypoxic/hypoxaemic conditions such as cardiopulmonary insufficiency. Because biguanides do not release insulin, they cannot cause hypoglycaemia and they do not cause weight gain.

Alpha-glucosidase inhibitors frequently cause uncomfortable and sometimes unaccept-able or intolerable gastrointestinal problems owing to the increased carbohydrate load deliv-ered to the large bowel. Subsequent bacterial fermentation causes distension, pain, flatulence and diarrhoea.

Glitazones can cause a number of problems. Fluid retention results in oedema, and heart failure in up to 3% of patients: this is potentiated in combination with insulin. There may also be a mild dilutional anaemia. Hypoglycaemia is rare but weight gain is common. In view of the hepatotoxicity of the withdrawn troglitazone, monitoring of hepatic function and avoidance in hepatic impairment is needed, but they are safe in renal impairment if allowance is made for the fluid retention.

Interactions

Interactions with OADs are potentially serious because the patient's delicate biochemical balance is maintained by a specific dose. Potenti-ation can rapidly cause hypoglycaemia, whereas antagonism could lead, more slowly, to a loss of glycaemic control and a return of polyuric symptoms. Pharmacokinetic interference with absorption, binding or clearance occurs almost exclusively with the sulphonylureas, when the temporary introduction of an interacting drug can alter the free OAD plasma level, with potentially dangerous consequences. A number of drugs cause a pharmacodynamic interaction by a direct effect on glucose tolerance (Table 9.17). Fortunately, clinically significant problems are relatively rare, and certainly far fewer than the theoretical possibilities. Moreover, different drugs, especially among the sulphonylureas, have different tendencies to show a given interaction.

Pharmacokinetic potentiation
Drugs that increase gastric pH may enhance absorption of sulphonylureas. Highly plasma protein-bound drugs can theoretically displace sulphonylureas. However, following redistribution and alterations in clearance there may be little overall change in free drug levels. Moreover, the newer sulphonylureas bind to different plasma protein sites and are less prone to this effect. The hepatic clearance of sulphonylureas can be reduced by severe liver disease and by enzyme-inhibiting drugs and enhanced by enzyme inducers; similar considerations apply to

Table 9.17 Important interactions and precautions with antidiabetic therapy

Potentiation → hypoglycaemia	Antagonism → hyperglycaemia
Interference with antidiabetic therapy generally[a]	
Beta-blockers – mask/may cause hypoglycaemia	(Beta-blockers, calcium-channel blockers)[b]
ACEIs – increase glucose uptake	Corticosteroids
Alcohol – potentiates hypoglycaemia	Thiazide (and loop) diuretics
Fibrates	(Antipsychotics)
MAOIs	
Interactions with sulphonylureas[c][d]	
Absorption	
(Antacids, H$_2$-RAs)	
Binding displacement	
Salicylates (high doses)	
Hepatic clearance	
Sulphonamides ⎫	Chloramphenicol ⎫
Warfarin ⎬ enzyme inhibition	Rifampicin ⎬ enzyme induction
Antifungals: imidazoles ⎭	Anticonvulsants ⎭
Liver failure	Excess alcohol
Renal clearance	
NSAIDs	
Sulfinpyrazone	
Renal impairment	
Interactions with biguanides	
Renal/hepatic impairment	
Alcohol (potentiates lactic acidosis)	

[a] Problems possible with either oral or insulin therapy.

[b] Entries in parentheses are known to be rare or minor.

[c] There are wide variations in the significance of specific interactions with individual oral antidiabetic drugs, and not all possible interactions are indicated. This table is merely to show possible effects and mechanisms. A detailed text is recommended to ascertain clinical significance of an interaction.

[d] Meglitinides have similar pharmacokinetic properties to the sulphonylureas.

ACEIs, angiotensin-converting enzyme inhibitors; H$_2$-RAs, H$_2$-receptor antagonists; MAOI, monoamine oxidase inhibitor; NSAIDs, non-steroidal anti-inflammatory drugs.

the meglitinides. The glitazones have not been reported to cause any hepatic enzyme interactions. The renal clearance of unchanged drug or active metabolites of any of these drugs can be reduced by renal impairment and by certain drugs that cause fluid retention (e.g. NSAIDs).

Pharmacodynamic potentiation

Alcohol is directly hypoglycaemic in fasting conditions, and it may also potentiate biguanide-induced lactic acidosis. Both MOAIs and beta-blockers tend to cause hypoglycaemia; the former may inhibit glucagon secretion and the latter inhibit hepatic glycogenolysis. Beta-blockers can 'mask' the effects of hypoglycaemia as perceived by the patient. Beta-blocker interactions are seen mainly with non-cardioselective agents if at all, but aside from those with *propranolol* they are rare and usually insignificant. ACEIs enhance glucose uptake and utilization by cells, although the effect may diminish with continued therapy and is of uncertain significance.

Antagonism

Drugs that induce liver enzymes can increase the clearance of hepatically metabolized sulphonylureas. Various drugs tend to raise blood glucose, either directly or via the suppression of insulin release. Paradoxically, given the masking effect referred to above, beta-blockers can block insulin release.

As a consequence of the inhibited disaccharide digestion, oral treatment of hypoglycaemia in patients taking glucosidase inhibitors should preferably be with glucose/dextrose rather than sucrose preparations.

Contra-indications and cautions

The main precautions may be summarized thus:

- People with diabetes need to take particular care when changing dose, brand or type of antidiabetic medication.
- Medication records should be monitored to identify the introduction of potentially interacting drugs.
- The elderly are particularly prone to hypoglycaemia with the longer-acting OADs;

these patients may be forgetful about meals, less able to recognize hypoglycaemia, and less tolerant of it homeostatically and neurologically.

- Alcohol use must be carefully controlled: although initially it may cause hyperglycaemia (owing to its caloric content), it enhances hypoglycaemia and may impair the ability to respond to it.
- Alcohol also dangerously enhances the possibility of lactic acidosis with biguanides and it causes unwelcome flushing with sulphonylureas, particularly *chlorpropamide*.
- Some clinicians manage all patients with significant renal impairment (common in people with diabetes) or hepatic impairment (less common) with insulin.

Selection

Combinations

Most type 2 patients are overweight and a biguanide is the preferred first choice. It is also satisfactory for others but a sulphonylurea might be started in the non-obese. Patients who fail to achieve blood glucose control on either regimen use a biguanide in combination with a sulphonylurea. Meglitinides, with their faster, shorter action may be substituted for the sulphonylurea at any stage if the patient prefers it, especially if they are tending to suffer hypoglycaemia or weight gain. A glitazone can be added as a third agent when dual therapy fails, especially if the patient has persistent postprandial or between-meals hyperglycaemia, both of which imply insulin resistance. However, if *metformin* plus a sulphonylurea combined fail to control the patient, it is likely that they have very little beta-cell capacity left and the introduction of insulin should be considered rather than adding a third drug (see below).

Acarbose could be added at any of these stages to improve control but has a limited benefit and is often poorly tolerated. *Sitagliptin* and *exenatide* (p. 612) are available as third-line agents.

Constraints

In addition to these pharmacodynamic considerations, the choice of any OAD must take account of:

- duration of action;
- mode of clearance;
- age;
- renal and hepatic function;
- tolerance of adverse effects;
- patient preference for number of daily doses.

The elderly must avoid the longer-acting drugs, while other patients may have particular reasons for preferring more or less frequent dosing. By analogy with insulin regimens, a combination of a single daily dose of a long-acting drug, combined with regular top-up doses of a short-acting one, has been recommended, but is little used. In general there is little to choose between the sulphonylureas, but patients with renal impairment might do better with *gliquidone* (Figure 9.13).

Some patients cannot be controlled on maximal tolerated doses of combined OADs. This may occur after many years of therapy as the beta-cell function inexorably declines (i.e. secondary failure), occurring in up to one-third of type 2 patients within 5 years of diagnosis. Alternatively some patients present late, when there has already been considerable degeneration (primary failure). In either case the situation signifies that there remains insufficient residual beta-cell function, and exogenous insulin supplement becomes mandatory.

At that stage small doses of insulin may be added to OAD therapy to provide a basal level. This may delay the onset of full insulin therapy, and may be preferred by patients anxious about full insulin dependence. When type 2 patients eventually need to be controlled with insulin they do not of course become type 1, and they may more accurately be referred to as having **insulin-requiring type 2 diabetes**. Insulin-augmented OAD therapy will be considered below after insulin has been discussed (see p. 627).

Insulin

About two-thirds of people with diabetes are treated with insulin, about half of whom are truly insulin-dependent type 1 and others are type 2 in secondary failure of OAD therapy.

Patients using insulin require much finer control of all aspects of management, including diet, activity and dose measurement, than other people with diabetes. There is less margin for error because patients rely totally on the injected dose. In contrast to type 2 patients, they lack the small basal insulin secretion that, although insufficient to prevent hyperglycaemia, keeps the type 2 patient free from metabolic complications like weight loss and ketosis.

Aims and constraints

In theory, it should be possible to attain glycaemic control with insulin that closely mimics the natural physiological variations in response to food intake, exercise and metabolic requirement. However, until recently it was not possible even to approach that.

Recall that natural insulin secretion from the pancreas into the portal vein is finely and continuously tuned to variations in blood glucose level (p. 586; see Figure 9.3): this is very different from the usual exogenous insulin therapy. An approximation might be attained with a continuous basal injection plus regular IV boluses of a rapidly acting insulin preparation to coincide with meals and, ideally, continuously titrated against the blood glucose level. This would resemble the natural pattern except for the portal delivery to the liver. However, such a regimen is impractical for most patients.

Absorption from the usual SC injection sites, whether as depot injections or by continuous delivery, can vary in any one patient from time to time and from site to site, particularly with the otherwise more convenient longer-acting preparations. Moreover, whereas exercise inhibits normal insulin secretion, it tends to speed absorption from an injection site by promoting peripheral circulation; thus when less insulin is required, more is delivered exogenously. It is also likely that SC injections administered by some patients are effectively IM now that perpendicular injection is recommended, changing absorption characteristics. Alternatively, some patients retard absorption by injecting into fat, which is less painful. Furthermore, the clearance of most forms of injected insulin is generally slower than endogenous insulin, the half-life of soluble insulin after SC injection being about 1 h.

Until recently the most common compromise was to give a mixture of a fast-acting and a moderately long-acting preparation before breakfast (e.g. *soluble* plus *lente*), perhaps with a booster dose of soluble in the evening. With appropriate 'feeding the insulin' throughout the day (p. 605) acceptable control can be achieved. However, it results in relative hyperinsulinaemia, a tendency to hypoglycaemia during the day and after midnight (especially if a meal or snack is missed or there is unanticipated exertion), and hyperglycaemia before breakfast (Figure 9.8).

Three recent advances have brought treatment closer to the ideal for many patients. Ultra-short-acting analogues such as *lispro* allow closer matching to meals; long-acting analogues such as *glargine* provide more consistent basal levels; and 'insulin pen' systems permit easier and more accurate injection.

Insulin types

Developments in insulin technology have produced a range of chemically pure, immunologically neutral preparations of standard strength (100 units/mL in the UK and North America) with a wide range of pharmacokinetic parameters.

Pharmacokinetic differences

Formulations of insulin can be divided into four broad groups depending on their duration of action; their times of onset and periods of peak activity also vary considerably (Table 9.18). The fastest action is provided by solutions of insulin. In solution, insulin molecules normally associate non-covalently into hexamers, which are progressively dissociated by dilution in body fluids to the active monomer. This process, which delays onset and prolongs duration, can be accelerated by small rearrangements of molecular structure that affect association characteristics but not pharmacodynamic activity. Increased duration may also be provided by forming stable suspensions of carefully controlled particle size that gradually dissolve in a uniform manner. Alternatively, solubility char-

acteristics can be manipulated. Other chemical manipulation produces ultra-long-acting (basal) formulations. A number of premixed formulations provide combinations of these properties.

Ultra-short (rapid) action. By substituting different amino acids at key positions, insulin analogues have been produced that exist in monomeric form with little tendency to associate but retain full activity at insulin receptors. In *insulin lispro* lysine and proline are placed at positions B28 and B29 near the end of the B chain; *insulin aspart* has aspartic acid at B28. These agents have an onset of less than 15 min, reach a higher peak within about half the time of conventional soluble insulin (1 h as opposed to 1.5–2.5 h) and a duration of action little greater than 5 h (as opposed to 6–10 h). Thus, they can be injected less than 15 min before a planned meal, or even just after one has been started; the optimal time will need to be determined for each patient. The advantages include:

- Less imposed delay between injection and food intake (especially breakfast), and/or reduction of postprandial hyperglycaemia if delay not observed.
- Convenient pre-meal bolus doses, as part of basal-bolus regimen (below).
- Easier adjustment for unexpected food intake or missed meal.
- Reduction of between-meals hypoglycaemia, caused in some patients by excessive duration of action on regular short-acting preparations.
- Less reliance on foods with a low glycaemic index.

However, there is no advantage in using these intravenously instead of soluble insulin in emergencies or as part of a 'sliding scale' regimen (see below). Patients who switch need careful re-education about the relative timing of injection and food intake.

Short action. Clear solutions of soluble (neutral) insulin act less rapidly than ultra-short analogues and are cleared within 6–10 h. They are useful:

- when IV use is required, e.g. for ketoacidosis;
- when titrating a newly diagnosed patient's requirement;

Table 9.18 Approximate pharmacokinetic parameters of insulin preparations[a]

Insulin preparation		Duration of activity (h)[b] 1 2 3 4 5 6 7 8 10 12 14 16 18 20 22 24 36	Retarding agent
Ultra-short	Lispro/aspart		
Short	Neutral/soluble 1[c] Neutral/soluble 2		
Intermediate/ prolonged	IZS amorphous		Zinc
	Biphasic isophane 1[c] Biphasic isophane 2 Biphasic isophane 3		Protamine
	Isophane (NPH)		Protamine
	IZS mixed		Zinc
	IZS crystalline		Zinc
	Protamine zinc suspension		Protamine + zinc
Basal	Insulin glargine/detemir		

(a) Data given are only approximate comparative indications. Activity in patients varies with manufacturer, dose, site and technique of injection, etc. (see Table 9.20).

(b) ▢ Duration of biological activity

▢ Peak activity

(c) Numbers indicate representative different preparations available in UK.

IZS, insulin zinc suspension; NPH, neutral protamine Hagedorn; Biphasic, generic name for range of mixtures of short- and medium-acting preparations.

- in a continuous SC infusion system;
- for the temporary insulin therapy of type 2 patients during pregnancy, surgery or severe illness.

Soluble insulin is being replaced by ultra-short-acting preparations when a booster dose is needed rapidly, or when frequent injections are needed for patients with brittle diabetes.

Soluble insulin to cover a particular meal should be injected 15–30 min, or occasionally 45 min, beforehand. When newly diagnosed type 1 patients are being assessed they are usually put on an **insulin sliding scale** regimen, with 4-hourly soluble insulin doses adjusted according to the current blood glucose level.

Intermediate and prolonged action. Many patients still receive part of their daily insulin dose as a depot injection. This is intended to provide a continuous basal level of insulin for metabolic activity, with little effect on postprandial glucose disposal. The particular regimen is dictated partly by life pattern and patient preference, but ultimately by trial and error. Depot preparations are formulated by complexing insulin with either zinc or protamine, a non-allergenic fish protein. This produces a fine suspension that is assimilated at a rate that is dependent on particle size and injection site perfusion. Being a suspension, it cannot be given intravenously. Available products span a wide spectrum of times of onset, peak activity and duration, allowing flexibility in tailoring regimens (Table 9.18).

The *insulin zinc suspension* (IZS) range contains an insulin–zinc complex in either crystalline or amorphous form, the latter being more readily absorbed. *Insulin zinc suspension mixed* is 30% crystalline and 70% amorphous, and *insulin zinc suspension crystalline* is 100% crystalline, with proportionate increases in duration of activity. (Insulin zinc suspension amorphous, which is no longer available, was purely amorphous and combined prompt onset with quite prolonged, but rather variable, action). *Isophane insulin* containing protamine as the retarding agent also has an intermediate activity.

Protamine zinc insulin and *insulin zinc suspension crystalline* are the longest-acting prepara-

tions available. If an excessive dose of this type is injected, the hypoglycaemic effect is correspondingly prolonged and glucose or glucagon injection may be needed to reverse it. Because the variability in response between different preparations increases with the duration of action (even in the same patient), these very long-acting forms are little used unless patients of long standing are stabilized on them.

A variety of premixed *biphasic* preparations (compatible combinations, usually of soluble and isophane forms) are available to provide further flexibility. Some patients mix specific combinations immediately before injection.

Basal. A more physiological approach to insulin provision has recently evolved. The **basal-bolus regimen** is designed to provide a continuous backgound level of insulin supplemented by bolus doses at mealtimes. Existing prolonged action formulations, while lasting 24 h or more, did not provide the required consistency of release: they all tended to give a peak at 6–12 h (Table 9.18). Two different strategies have been devised to solve this problem. In *insulin glargine*, amino acid substitutions have changed the isoelectric point of the molecule from below pH 7 to neutral. As a result it is soluble when administered in a slightly acid solution but precipitates out as microcrystals at body pH after injection. Subsequent dissolution and absorption from the depot provides a predictable, consistently sustained action with an essentially flat activity profile for up to 24 h (Table 9.18). In *insulin detemir*, attaching a C14 fatty acid chain to the insulin molecule substantially increases reversible binding to albumin in body tissue, with a similar result.

Purity and antigenicity

There are two significant factors here: chemical, and therefore immunological, similarity to human insulin; and contamination with extraneous antigenic material. Originally, all insulin was extracted from ox or pig pancreases supplied by slaughterhouses. (Approval for insulin treatment from these sources has been obtained from most major religions, but strict vegans may present a problem.) Beef insulin differs from the human insulin polypeptide sequence by three amino acids, and porcine by just one. These differences affect antigenicity but not hypogly-caemic potency. As may be expected, porcine is the better tolerated, but neither causes great problems.

Contaminants derived from the extraction process (e.g. pro-insulin), insulin breakdown products and other unrelated proteins, can stim-ulate the production of insulin antibodies, and allergic reactions used to be quite common. Consequently, chromatographic purification is now used giving highly purified or mono-component animal insulins that cause far fewer problems.

Human insulin is made either semi-synthetically, by chemically modifying the single variant amino acid in purified porcine insulin (emp, enzyme-modified porcine), or biosynthetically (crb, chain recombinant-DNA bacterial; prb, proinsulin recombinant-DNA bacterial; pyr, precursor yeast recombinant). Biosynthesis is becoming the preferred process and human insulin now costs less than animal forms.

Unfortunately, the expectation that human insulin would be vastly superior has not been realized. Anti-insulin antibodies are not signifi-cantly less common with human insulin than with the highly purified porcine form, and allergic phenomena still occur, probably due to breakdown products occurring during manufac-ture, storage, etc. Nevertheless, almost all new patients are started on human insulin, and use of animal-derived insulin is now rare.

Human insulin is slightly more hydrophilic than animal forms. Thus, although it has an identical biological action to pork insulin when given intravenously, it is assimilated more rapidly from SC sites and acts more quickly in otherwise identical formulations. It is also cleared more rapidly, possibly by binding more avidly to those hepatic and renal enzymes that destroy it. These differences are slight and only relevant to patients transferring from one form to the other.

Adverse reactions

The chief adverse effects of insulin are hypogly-caemia, injection site problems, immunological

phenomena and resistance. These may be partially inter-related.

Hypoglycaemia
This is the most common complication of insulin therapy and potentially the most harmful; the clinical aspects were discussed on pp. 596–598. Insulin can cause hypoglycaemia either through an excessive (e.g. mis-measured) dose or through an unexpectedly reduced insulin requirement (most commonly, a missed meal).

Human insulin has been associated with an apparent increase in the incidence of hypogly-caemic attacks, including some deaths. This was initially attributed to a reduced hypoglycaemic awareness, i.e. hypoglycaemia is not more common but is permitted to progress more frequently. The autonomic warning symptoms of hypoglycaemia (see Table 9.12) seemed to be experienced less intensely or at a later stage when using human insulin, perhaps owing to autonomic (sympathetic) neuropathy.

There is no pharmacodynamic rationale for this phenomenon and it has been suggested that it is only incidentally related to human insulin use. The change to human insulin came at a time when the need for tighter control became apparent and aids to this, e.g. injector pens and home blood glucose monitoring, were devel-oped. Improved control produces lower mean glucose levels and therefore an increased risk of hypoglycaemia. Thus it is not now regarded as a serious problem of human insulin, although it is stressed that great care is necessary in transfer-ring a patient to human insulin. Close moni-toring is essential and the daily dose may need to be reduced, particularly when changing from beef insulin or for patients with a higher than average daily insulin requirement.

Injection site lipodystrophy
Some patients develop unsightly lumps (**lipo-hypertrophy**) or hollows (**lipoatrophy**) at frequently used injection sites if they fail to rotate the sites regularly. These are not due to scar tissue but are caused by local disturbances of lipid metabolism. Lipoatrophy seems to be an immunological phenomenon; immune complex deposition may possibly stimulate lipolysis in SC

adipose tissue. It responds to changing to a purer form of insulin, initially injected around the depression. Lipohypertrophy is more common with the newer insulins and may result from enhanced local lipogenesis, a known insulin action. It is reversed when the site is no longer used. Although patients may prefer to inject at these easily penetrated, relatively painless sites, such an approach results in delayed and erratic absorption.

Insulin antibodies and insulin resistance

Insulin antibodies (insulin-binding globulins) occur in up to 50% of insulin-treated patients. It might be expected that they would speed the clearance of insulin by forming immune complexes that would be eliminated in the usual way by the monocyte–macrophage system. However, on the contrary, insulin antibodies delay assimilation and prolong the action and so are potentially beneficial. They are otherwise usually harmless, although they may sometimes be responsible for insulin resistance (see below).

Insulin allergy ranges from minor local irritation to, very rarely, full-blown anaphylaxis. The less serious reactions commonly remit on prolonged use and are minimized by using the highly purified modern insulin formulations as first choice. The size of the insulin molecule is borderline for antigenicity. Hyposensitization has been used to treat insulin allergy, by injecting extremely dilute insulin solutions at progressively higher concentrations to induce tolerance. Very occasionally, local steroid injections need to be given with the insulin.

The term insulin resistance tends to be used in an ambiguous manner (Table 9.19). In pathogenetic terms, it refers to one of the common underlying problems of type 2 diabetes, namely reduced receptor sensitivity. As an adverse effect of insulin treatment, it refers to the requirement in some insulin-dependent diabetes for doses of insulin far above the physiological norm.

In the latter sense, insulin resistance occurs only rarely and may be defined as an insulin requirement >1.5 units/kg/day (about 100 units daily in an average patient). There are many possible causes; probably the most common is simply obesity, but poor injection technique may be an unsuspected problem. Insulin resistance is less common now with the use of the monocomponent and human formulations. Treatment involves eliminating any obvious cause and then gradually switching to highly purified or human insulin. As a final resort, systemic steroids, which are themselves diabetogenic, may be needed.

Administration

Delivery systems

Pen injectors. Multidose insulin reservoir injector pens are now the most popular delivery system. Each pen has a replaceable cartridge

---

Table 9.19   Possible causes of insulin resistance

Metabolic	Obesity
	Increased catabolic hormones
	Interacting diabetogenic drugs (e.g. steroids)
Immunological	Anti-insulin antibodies
	Anti-insulin-receptor antibodies
Pharmacokinetic or biopharmaceutic	Poor injection technique
	Increased insulinase activity
	Reduced assimilation from injection site
	• local enzymic degradation
	• scar tissue
	• lipohypertrophy
Genetic	Receptor defect

loaded with up to 300 units (3 mL), representing up to 1 week's supply for some patients. There are various forms of metered-dose injectors. One automatically delivers a 2-unit dose for each depression of a trigger, i.e. 2 units per 'click', a situation that is particularly beneficial to visually impaired people with diabetes; another form permits full doses to be preset visually on a digital scale, which may be palpable or audible. Most have a maximum deliverable single dose to minimize the risk of overdose. Each type of pen should only be used with the appropriate cartridge. The main advantages are correct dose measurement, and hence less error, and the facilitation of multiple daily dosing as part of a basal-bolus regimen.

Standard syringe.   The use of disposable plastic syringes with fixed needles is no longer the norm in the UK. If stored in a fridge, these syringes may be re-used for up to 1 week, without significant contamination of the vial contents (which contain a bacteriostat) and no increase in skin reactions. Patients change the syringe when the needle is blunted or the barrel graduations become unclear. Injection through clothing, long practised by some people with diabetes, has also been reported to not cause significant problems. Patients must use a safe method of contaminated waste and 'sharps' disposal.

Artificial pancreas.   The ideal replacement pancreas has not yet been constructed. One experimental approach involves a feedback-controlled, blood-glucose driven 'closed loop' system. A sensor in an IV catheter monitors blood glucose continuously and the results are fed to a microprocessor that calculates the instantaneous insulin requirement. This drives a portable pump, strapped to or implanted in the patient, delivering the appropriate dose. The main problem is in designing a suitably sensitive indwelling blood glucose sensor. In another experimental system, an implanted insulin reservoir enclosed in a glucose-sensitive gel membrane permits insulin diffusion in proportion to external glucose concentration. The reservoir is replenished percutaneously.

Continuous SC insulin infusion is a more practicable but still relatively expensive 'open loop' option, without the automatic dosage control. An external reservoir/pump strapped to the body delivers a continuous basal level of insulin via an indwelling catheter, with meal-time boosts being activated manually. Modifications include an implanted pump, contolled by radio, and the use of an intraperitoneal catheter, which has the theoretical advantage of more closely mimicking the natural insulin secretion. Clearly this method would only suit patients who are able to manage the technology and understand the relationship between blood glucose, diet, activity and insulin dose. However, current prototypes are as yet too bulky, expensive and demanding of patients' motivation for general use.

Other forms.   Simple oral administration of insulin is impossible owing to intragastric enzymic destruction. Systems are being developed that avoid this but do not require the complications of injection. One approach is to incorporate insulin into liposomes that would be taken orally. The lipid coat would act as an enteric coating and the liposomes would be absorbed unchanged from the gut, as are chylomicrons. Percutaneous **jet injection** has also been tried. **Intranasal administration** is being explored, using a liposomal or polymer vehicle. People with diabetes with advanced nephropathy on peritoneal dialysis find it convenient to add insulin to their **dialysis fluid**.

A *metered dose inhaler* (inhaled human insulin, Exubera) for pulmonary absorption is now available in the UK. It seems to offer an activity profile similar to injection with the rapidly acting insulin analogues but may be more acceptable to some patients in combination with a single basal insulin dose by injection. Concerns remain over cost and possible lung damage, especially in smokers, who should not use it. Moreover, bioequivalence is an issue for patients switching to inhaler, not least because the dose is expressed in milligrams, 1 mg being equivalent to 3 units.

Storage
Insulin should always be kept cool, but is stable at room temperatures for up to 28 days. Formulations incorporating polyethylene-

polypropylene glycol, specially developed for prolonged reservoir use, are stable for even longer. Thus, insulin may safely be used in pens and continuous SC infusion, etc. and while travelling. Pharmacy stocks and patients' reserve supplies are refrigerated (but not frozen). Before withdrawing a dose, the vial should be warmed to body temperature and gently mixed by inversion or rotation (but not shaken).

Mixing

If a combination of two preparations of different durations is required, specially formulated proprietary mixtures should be used whenever possible, and extemporaneous mixing avoided. The *insulin zinc suspension* formulations are intended to be stable after intermixing but others are not, and mixtures of these must be injected within 5 min. One problem is the adsorption of the soluble form onto the retardant from the longer-acting one, which may seriously interfere with the expected rapid action of the former. The order of mixing is important: the soluble form is drawn up first, then the depot form. This avoids contamination of the whole vial of soluble insulin with zinc or protamine.

Injection

Now shorter needles have become available, deep SC injection perpendicular to the skin is universally recommended. Most patients cope well, but instruction and counselling when treatment is started are clearly important, especially with children. Diabetes UK and a number of interested manufacturers produce helpful literature on this and all other aspects of diabetes care.

Equally important is the need to rotate the site of injection regularly so that any one site is only used once in 10–20 injections. Seven general areas are recommended by Diabetes UK (upper arms, thighs, buttocks, abdomen), but within these areas the precise injection site used on one occasion can be avoided on the next; they provide a template to assist such variation. This minimizes skin reactions, especially lipohypertrophy. Patients can also use the slower assimilation sites, e.g. thighs, for the overnight dose. Sites usually covered by clothing are preferred. Factors that may alter absorption from the injection site, possibly upsetting control, are summarized in Table 9.20.

Dosage regimens

An initial dose titration period on first starting insulin will indicate the total daily dose required, but decisions on how this is to be distributed throughout the day require discussion with the patient. With fewer, medium-acting injections overall control is poorer and

Table 9.20   Factors affecting insulin absorption from injection site

Factor	Example	Effect on absorption	
		Slower/reduced	Faster/increased
Pharmaceutical	Incorrect mixing of delayed and rapid forms (especially if injection delayed)	+	
	Depth of injection	+	+
Local inactivation	Proteolytic enzymes	+	
	Insulin antibodies	+	
Local perfusion	Regional differences (abdomen > arm > thigh)	+	+
	Exercise (in limb sites); massage		+
	Skin temperature	+	+
	Angiopathy	+	
	Scar tissue	+	
	Lipohypertrophy	+	

there is the added risk of hypoglycaemia, with the threat of coma if a meal is missed. However, when multiple injections are linked with close blood glucose monitoring, aimed at achieving lower glucose levels (so-called 'tight glycaemic control') there is the risk of more frequent episodes of hypoglycaemia. On the other hand, use of multiple short-acting regimens can lead to hyperglycaemia between injections and poorer control. For each patient a balance must be struck that imposes no more restriction on their life than they are prepared to tolerate, which as closely as possible meets their treatment objectives. Achieving this is not easy. Factors to consider are:

- the patient's pattern of glycaemia (e.g. nocturnal hypoglycaemia, morning hyperglycaemia);
- age;
- severity of complications;
- occupation, social habits and routine;
- compliance;
- physical disabilities;
- comprehension of disease, prescribed regimen and associated equipment;
- patient preference;
- ethnic and religious constraints.

The blood glucose targets are usually:

- never below 4 mmol/L;
- fasting (preprandial) 4–7 mmol/L;
- postprandial and bedtime <9 mmol/L.

Specialized units can organize test periods of 24-h blood glucose monitoring via temporary indwelling sensors to plot the patient's pattern of glycaemia. However, the interpretation of these data is complex and it is an uncommon technique. Somewhat easier is for the patient to perform a short period of self-monitoring and recording, the results of which can be discussed with their diabetologist.

There are also more general considerations, especially when first starting insulin. Many people have a distaste for injections or fear them, and the psychological stress of accepting reliance on injections for life can be substantial. This is more of an issue with type 2 patients as they approach secondary failure on OADs, which is considered below.

The choice ranges from multiple daily injections of short-acting insulin closely co-ordinated with eating and activity pattern, to a convenient but very unphysiological single daily dose of a longer-acting preparation (Table 9.21).

Whatever the regimen, the total daily dose required is usually 0.5–1.0 unit/kg (about 50 units). This is usually divided as ⅔ during the day and ⅓ at night for minimum frequency regimens and 50/50 for basal-bolus regimens.

Minimum dose frequency regimen

Because of the potential compliance benefits of fewer daily injections, this method used to be favoured. However it is no longer preferred because it imposes inflexibility on activity patterns and mealtimes, and risks both poor control and episodes of hypoglycaemia. The regimen usually consists of morning and evening doses of a combination of short- and medium-acting preparations, the relative doses being determined by trial and error.

There are numerous possible variations. For example, the morning dose could be a mix of about one-third soluble and two-thirds intermediate-acting forms, which covers breakfast and provides a sustained level throughout the day. This may be repeated in the evening, or later in those patients who get serious pre-breakfast hyperglycaemia. Alternatively there may simply be a booster dose of soluble before the evening meal. If one of the commercially available premixed combinations can be used it is certainly convenient, especially with a pen. More flexibility is provided by individually determined combinations, but a pen cannot then be used.

Some patients can be controlled satisfactorily with just a single dose of a long-acting form. This includes type 2 patients with significant residual endogenous insulin production in whom OADs have failed, and some elderly patients requiring only symptomatic relief and for whom the threat of long-term complications is less critical.

Multiple injections

These are now preferred for all patients who can manage to self-inject frequent doses of short-acting insulin throughout the day, before each food intake. In addition, an evening dose of

Table 9.21   Examples of insulin regimens

Regimen	Before breakfast	Before lunch	Before evening meal	Bedtime	Examples of patient groups suited to the regimen
1a	Long[a] ± short	–	–	–	Insulin-requiring type 2 (with metformin)
1b	–	–	–	Intermediate	Some elderly patients
2	Intermediate + short	–	Intermediate + short	–	Some type 1
3	Intermediate + short	–	Short	Intermediate	Some type 1
4	Short	Short	Short	Intermediate	Well-motivated type 1 Unstable Morning hyperglycaemia and/or nocturnal hypoglycaemia
5 (Basal-bolus)	Ultra-short-acting analogue[b]	Ultra-short	Ultra-short	Long-acting analogue[c]	Well-motivated type 1 Many newly diagnosed type 1

[a] Duration of action.
[b] E.g. Insulin aspart or lispro.
[c] E.g. Insulin glargine or detemir.

long-acting insulin is given for basal needs. The most recent variation of this basal-bolus regimen utilizes ultra-short-acting and long-acting analogues, e.g. Table 9.21, regimen 5.

A multiple injection regimen is especially useful for brittle patients requiring close control, or for temporary transfer of patients to insulin, e.g. type 2 patients during pregnancy or with serious infections. However, many clinics are starting most new patients on such a regimen, for which injector pens are ideal. Existing patients are also being converted. Many patients can, with experience, finely judge the dose required according to their food intake and exercise. Others, more committed, will measure their blood glucose level immediately before the next scheduled dose and adjust the insulin dose accordingly.

The improved, more physiological control provided by this type of regimen reduces the development or progression of complications; in some trials they have even remitted. Such regimens can also, if used properly, minimize the risk of hypoglycaemia between meals and of overnight hyperglycaemia.

Insulin for type 2 patients
Most type 2 patients will eventually need insulin as their beta-cell capacity become exhausted (secondary failure). Owing to the insulin resistance common in type 2, their insulin requirement when they become completely insulin dependent will often exceed that of a type 1 patient. However, it may be preferable not to wait until insulin is absolutely necessary to initiate treatment. It may be psychologically preferable to start patients on a combination of oral agents and small insulin doses. They will invariably note an improvement in their well-being and can adjust to insulin injections before becoming completely reliant on them. The combination can also be helpful in difficult to control type 2 patients with high insulin resistance, or those with persistent morning hyperglycaemia. Another situation where the combination is useful is with patients who are already using insulin but are showing resistance: adding *metformin* may reduce their insuin requirement.

The most logical combination is insulin plus an insulin sensitizer. *Metformin* is the usual choice. Combining insulin with a secretagogue such as a sulphonylurea or a meglitinide is irrational. One regimen is to add a small dose of about 15 units of medium-acting insulin each evening. When switching to this regimen, OAD doses are reduced.

Summary

Diabetes therapy must be individualized following regular close consultation between patients and their clinicians. To a certain extent the optimal result is found by trial and error, but this must be supported by diligent monitoring of blood glucose and reporting of all hypoglycaemic episodes and other disturbances of control.

Monitoring

People with diabetes require self-monitoring of their biochemical control, and regular assessment by a clinician of the development or progress of long-term complications. The former has recently been much simplified and improved. Type 1 patients need much closer monitoring than type 2.

Biochemical control

While even moderate control relieves symptoms and prevents serious biochemical abnormalities, tight control is believed to be essential if complications are to be minimized. In general, diligent monitoring is more important for type 1 diabetes, but all patients should record all test results.

Glucose

Urine glucose

This has been the traditional way of assessing control. A few elderly patients still use the colour reaction based on Benedict's test for reducing substances. It is imprecise, non-specific and cumbersome, even with the ingeniously formulated Clinitest reagent tablets.

Urine glucose estimations can never provide precise information about current blood glucose levels, particularly low, potentially hypoglycaemic ones. Urinary concentrations will vary according to urine volume independently of blood glucose. Furthermore, aglycosuria does not necessarily guarantee normoglycaemia, owing to differences in renal threshold between patients and in the same patient at different times.

Nevertheless, urine testing remains useful as a simple initial screen and for type 2 patients not prone to hypoglycaemia when tight control is not essential, e.g. the elderly and patients averse to repeated skin puncturing. A few patients may be monitored adequately by regular urinalysis and occasional blood glucose measurements, once the relationship between the two has been established.

Urinary glucose measurement also has the advantage that timing is less important than with blood testing because urine concentration reflects control over the previous several hours. Thus, newer glucose oxidase-based urine dipsticks have been developed that are more specific for glucose and far more convenient because they can simply be passed through the urine stream.

Blood glucose

There are three main uses for blood glucose monitoring: to detect hyperglycaemia or incipient hyoglycaemia; to monitor closely in times of changing glucose/insulin need (e.g. intercurrent illness); and to determine a new patient's diurnal glucose profile so as to construct an appropriate insulin regimen.

Most patients, especially with type 1 disease, measure their blood glucose directly using a drop of blood from a finger prick on a glucose oxidase stick. This provides an immediate measure of glycaemia that is reasonably accurate and reliable, not overly prone to error from poor technique, and easy to read. Sticks for unaided visual reading are being replaced by ones to be inserted into automated meters that display the result digitally and may give audible warnings. Some meters can store the most recent results, for reporting at clinics.

Various spring-operated skin puncture devices may be used to help obtain the blood drop easily and safely, and percutaneous techniques of measurement are being developed.

A few type 1 patients regularly test four times daily, including at the lowest points, before meals and in the morning, and at the high point after meals. This is necessary only in the more erratic, brittle patients, in intensive multiple-dose regimens in younger patients, or when previously well-controlled patients start to experience problems. Others, once stabilized, will test randomly a few times weekly and some may perhaps use urine dipsticks daily. The main guideline is to identify a patient's risk times (e.g. between-meal hypoglycaemia or postprandial hyperglycaemia) and subject those to special scrutiny.

Once type 2 patients have become stabilized, weekly or even monthly fasting blood glucose measurement is usually sufficient.

Dose modification falls into two basic strategies. Well-motivated patients on the basal-bolus regimen who are suitably trained by the diabetic team will be able to modify their *next* insulin dose, based on the results of their preprandial glucose level and the glycaemic content of their next meal. This is termed 'dosage adjustment for normal eating (DAFNE)'.

For patients who prefer regular dosing, frequent changes following this apparently logical DAFNE strategy is both inconvenient and inappropriate. More systematic is to note pre-meal blood glucose over several days. If it is consistently unsatisfactory, they must alter the *previous* scheduled dose on future days, because the current pre-meal level is a reflection of the previous dose.

Glycated (glycosylated) haemoglobin

The abnormal, quantitative glycation of systemic protein as a consequence of excess blood glucose (p. 599) applies also to blood proteins, including Hb and albumin, as well as to plasma fructosamine. Because these substances remain in the blood for long periods (120 days for Hb, 7–14 days for the others), their glycation gives a long-term, integrated picture of blood glucose levels over those periods. This can be measured at diabetic clinics and is useful in tracing any problems with control that might not be revealed by patients' tendency to be extra meticulous on the few days before each clinic visit.

Care must be taken to ensure adequate time between successive measurements, especially after a treatment change. This allows the level to restabilize, bearing in mind the normal 120-day red cell lifespan. A reading taken too soon will give a falsely high reading because the glycosylated red cells originally measured will not have died. One the other hand, when there is a reduced red cell number or increased cell turnover, e.g. in haemolysis or blood loss, a falsely low reading may be given.

The glycated Hb level gives the best index of the control needed to minimize complications and is now regarded as the 'gold standard'. Non-diabetics have about 5% of glycated Hb (HbA_{1c}) and the target level for optimal diabetes control is currently <7.5%, or <6.5% in patients at increased arterial risk, e.g with hypertension.

Ketones

Regular ketonuria monitoring is unnecessary for type 2 and most type 1 patients, but is essential in brittle ketosis-prone people with diabetes, and in all patients during periods of metabolic stress such as infection, surgery or pregnancy. Great accuracy is not required and urine dipsticks are adequate because any ketonuria at all in the presence of glycosuria indicates a dangerous loss of control. Combined glucose/ketone sticks are preferred, especially as heavy ketonuria may interfere with some standard glucose sticks.

Clinical monitoring

In addition to biochemical monitoring, regular medical examination is important in the long-term care of people with diabetes. This will identify as early as possible the development of any of the many possible systemic complications. Table 9.22 lists the factors that need to be monitored at intervals that will vary from patient to patient.

Table 9.22   Regular assessment in diabetic clinic

System	Test or examination
Biochemical	Glycated haemoglobin
	Blood lipids, body weight
Feet	Chiropody; pulses
Eye	Fundoscopy, acuity, cataract
Renal	Proteinuria, creatinine (clearance)
Neurological	Detailed sensory, motor and autonomic neurological examination
Cardiovascular	Blood pressure, ECG, peripheral perfusion (pulses, etc.)
	Symptoms of ischaemia

Thyroid disease

Thyroxine is a simple catechol-based hormone but it has multiple crucial subcellular actions essential to life. It is involved with oxygen utilization within all cells, and thyroid abnormalities have profound effects on most organ systems in the body. Thyroid disease is one of the most common endocrine disorders, yet fortunately it is relatively straightforward to treat and to monitor. This is partly because the thyroid axis is largely independent of other endocrine systems and partly because the long half-life of thyroid hormone means that dosing is not as critical as for insulin replacement. Thus frequent variations in thyroid hormone levels do not normally occur and the acute disturbances of control seen with abnormal insulin and glucose levels are rare. Furthermore, long-term complications are few and uncommon.

Physiological principles

Synthesis

Thyroid hormone is synthesized from the aromatic amino acid tyrosine (closely related to phenylalanine and catecholamine) in the thyroid gland, which sits across the trachea in the front of the neck. Iodine is an essential ingredient, and the conversion from dietary inorganic iodide to iodinated thyroid hormone is termed the organification of iodine. Ionic iodide in the blood is taken up by the thyroid gland by an active **sodium/iodide symporter** (Figure 9.14) then, catalysed by **thyroid peroxidase**, oxidized to give I_2, which is then bound to the aromatic ring of the tyrosine residues.

Mono- and di-iodotyrosine are covalently attached to thyroglobulin within the colloid-filled thyroid follicles, dimerized with another tyrosine ring, then further iodinated to either **tri-iodothyronine** (T_3) or **thyroid hormone** (T_4). T_3 is five times more potent than T_4, but 75% of thyroid hormone is synthesized and transported as T_4. This is largely converted in target tissues to T_3. Several weeks' supply is stored in the gland in the bound form, but it is released into the blood as free hormone.

In this chapter the term **thyroid hormone(s)** will be used when referring to the natural physiological hormone. Thyroxine (T_4) when used as a drug is officially termed *levothyroxine*, and tri-iodothyronine (T_3) when used as a drug as *liothyronine*.

Control and release

Control of thyroid function is an example of a classic endocrine negative feedback loop, which enables fine control of many body systems according to need. A relatively simple peripherally active hormone (**thyroid hormone**) is

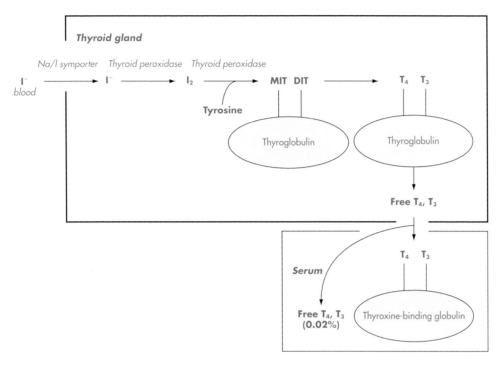

Figure 9.14   Thyroxine synthesis. I, iodine; MIT, mono-iodotyrosine; DIT, di-iodotyrosine; T_3 tri-iodothyronine; T_4, thyroxine; Na/I symporter, see text.

released from an endocrine gland that is its site of synthesis, stimulated by a peptide trophic hormone (**thyroid-stimulating hormone**, thyrotropin, TSH) from the pituitary and also under CNS influence via a releasing hormone (**thyrotropin-releasing hormone**, TRH) from the hypothalamus (Figure 9.15). Both the synthesis and the release of trophic and releasing hormones are inhibited by the active hormone.

TSH is a 221-amino acid glycoprotein with receptors on the thyroid that mediate both the synthesis and the release of thyroid hormones. It is the main physiological control on thyroid function, an important clinical indicator of thyroid malfunction and a component in the aetiology of some thyroid diseases. Hypothalamic control via the tripeptide TRH is less important because low thyroid hormone levels can stimulate TSH release directly, but it enables the CNS to exert an influence on thyroid function; it is particularly concerned with temperature control. Disease of this arm of the thyroid axis is rare.

Distribution and metabolism

Approximately 80 µg of thyroid hormones are released daily, peaking overnight when TSH levels are highest. It has a biological half-life of about 7 days, being cleared by de-iodination in the liver and kidneys. It is carried in the blood almost entirely bound, mostly to **thyroid-binding globulin**; only 0.02% is carried as free T_3 and free T_4 (FT_3, FT_4). However, only the free hormones are biologically active.

Actions of thyroid hormone

Thyroid hormone enters target cells and after conversion to T_3 interacts with nuclear receptors to influence the expression of genes coding for proteins invoved in energy metabolim, oxygen consumption and general tissue growth; thus it has far-reaching effects on metabolism, growth and development (Table 9.23). In some ways the action resembles that of catecholamines (e.g

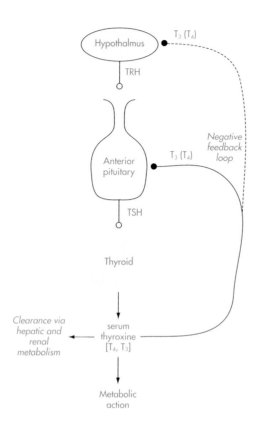

Figure 9.15 Control and release of thyroxine (hypothalamic-pituitary-thyroid axis). ●——— inhibit; ○——— stimulate; T_3, tri-iodothyronine; T_4, thyroxine TSH, thyroid-stimulating hormone; TRH, thyrotropin-releasing hormone.

adrenaline), to which it bears a structural resemblance, but the effect is far more prolonged and more fundamental, whereas the catecholamines have a very brief action.

Metabolism and growth. Thyroid hormone has a generally catabolic effect, stimulating metabolism and increasing oxygen consumption, basal metabolic rate and body temperature. However, in children there are anabolic effects leading to protein synthesis and growth. Carbohydrate absorption is increased and plasma lipid levels fall.

Cardiovascular and renal. There are inotropic and chronotropic effects mediated via up-regulation of numerous systems, including beta-receptors. In addition the calorigenesis promotes peripheral vasodilatation and secondary fluid retention to maintain cardiac output and blood pressure.

CNS. The action on the CNS is known mostly through the consequences of thyroid malfunction, considered below. There are important effects on mentation and CNS development. However, little is known of the precise mechanisms.

Investigation

The three key parameters of thyroid function are serum levels of FT_3, FT_4 and TSH. Older tests measured protein-bound iodine and total thyroid hormone, but now the precise radio-immunoassay of free hormones and TSH gives a far better correlation with physiological and

Table 9.23   Actions of thyroid hormone

System	Effect
Metabolism	
Calorigenesis	↑ oxygen consumption and oxygen dissociation
	↑ basal metabolic rate, ↑ temperature
Lipid	↓ total cholesterol (↑ hepatic LDL receptors)
Carbohydrate	↑ absorption from GIT
Cardiovascular	Inotropic: beta-receptors up-regulated
	↑ heart rate, ↑ cardiac output
	Peripheral vasodilatation
Renal	Fluid retention
Neurological	Essential for nervous system development
	(No calorigenic effect in brain)
Growth	Essential for normal growth, including bone

clinical status. It is possible to measure the binding proteins, and several factors can change binding, but the feedback control is sensitive and precise, so FT_4 levels tend to be very stable. It is not usually necessary to measure TRH. The measurement of FT_4, FT_3 and TSH together is know as a **thyroid function test (TFT)**. It has become clear that TSH levels are the most important index of thyroid status, and management now stresses normal TSH levels.

In the initial investigation of thyroid disease an autoantibody screen should be done for antithyroid antibodies, and also for anti-intrinsic factor and anti-gastric parietal cell antibodies, because there is an association with other autoimmune diseases including pernicious anaemia. Liver function, lipid profile, blood glucose and full blood count are also necessary.

The possibility of primary hypothalamic or pituitary disease should always be borne in mind when thyroid dysfunction is detected, particularly hypothyroidism. In this case both thyroid hormone and TSH levels will be low.

Thyroid disease

Normal thyroid function is described as **euthyroidism**. **Hypothyroidism** (underactivity) and **hyperthyroidism** (overactivity) are about equally common and together constitute the most prevalent endocrine abnormalities. Usually the cause is idiopathic, often involving autoimmuity, although iatrogenic causes occur. Detection and diagnosis are usually straightforward, and management of hypothyroidism is also simple. Hyperthyroidism is more complex to manage and may develop complications.

There are several potentially confusing aspects to thyroid disease. Firstly, certain aetiological factors, such as autoantibodies, amiodarone and iodine, are common to both hypo- and hyperthyroidism; similarly, an enlarged thyroid gland (goitre) can occur in both. The action of iodine/iodide can seem paradoxical, causing either stimulation or inhibition in different circumstances. Long-term hyperthyroidism can eventually evolve into hypothyroidism, and some forms of hypothyroidism can have a hyperthyroid phase.

Hypothyroidism

Aetiology and epidemiology

Hypothyroidism is far more common in women than in men (prevalence 1.5% vs 0.1%) and more common in the elderly, although it can affect the very young and is then far more serious. It is usually due to intrinsic thyroid gland disease although rarely it may occur secondary to hypothalamic or pituitary disease, or to drugs (Table 9.24).

Simple **atrophy** is the commonest cause, mainly affecting elderly women. There may be an autoimmune component as it is sometimes associated with other autoimmune disease, but no antibodies are found. Autoimmune destruction is the main cause of **Hashimoto's thyroiditis**, which can affect the middle-aged and elderly. Also common is hypothyroidism secondary to the treatment of hyperthyroidism (see below).

In the developed world dietary **iodine deficiency** is now almost unknown, partly owing to iodination of salt, but it is far more common in developing countries. Congenital hypothyroidism secondary to maternal iodine deficiency affects the developing nervous system of the fetus to produce **cretinism**.

The term **myxoedema** is sometimes used as a synonym for hypothyroidism but more precisely describes one characteristic dermatological sign.

Pathology

Low levels of thyroid hormone compromise many crucial metabolic processes, as can be inferred from Table 9.23. There is a general slowing of basal metabolic rate, a fall in temperature, and slowing of physical and mental processes. More detail is given on p. 635.

Investigation and diagnosis

The standard thyroid function test is definitive. When thyroid hormone levels fall there is almost invariably a compensatory rise in TSH. However, a small rise in TSH may precede both clinical signs and a fall in thyroid hormone level by many months; this is known as **subclinical hypothyroidism** (see below).

In rare hypothalamic-pituitary causes the combination of low FT_4 and low TSH levels is diagnostic.

Screening for autoantibodies to thyroid peroxidase or thyroglobulin is not necessary for diagnosis but can indicate a possible cause, and can act as an alert for possible autoimmune complications in Hashimoto's thyroiditis. Occasionally there may be anti-TSH receptor antibodies with a blocking effect, although such antibodies are usually stimulant, causing hyperthyroidism (Graves' disease, see p. 637).

Hypothyroidism is often diagnosed following vague generalized complaints of tiredness and lack of energy. However, these common symptoms can of course have many other causes, which sometimes makes diagnosis of mild

---

Table 9.24   Causes of hypothyroidism

Aetiology	Example
Common (90% of cases in developed countries)	
Atrophy (idiopathic)	Commonest form; no goitre
Autoimmune destruction	Hashimoto's thyroiditis
Iatrogenic	Secondary to treatment of hyperthyroidism (antithyroid drugs, surgery, radiotherapy)
Less common	
Dietary	Iodine deficiency where natural level low; goitre present
Congenital	Cause of cretinism (1/4000 in UK)
Iatrogenic	Lithium, amiodarone
Secondary	Hypothalamic or pituitary disease

disease problematic. Thyroid disease should always be borne in mind as a differential diagnosis of depression in the elderly.

Clinical features

Most of the features of hypothyroidism can be understood from a knowledge of the physiological action of thyroid hormone (Table 9.25). The overall clinical impression is of slowness and dullnes of intellect combined with an unprepossessing appearance. Therefore a history from a relative might be helpful, to identify recent or specific changes, which may be less apparent to the patient because onset is usually insidious. The two most common erroneous diagnoses in mild disease would be simple ageing, owing to the slowness, stiffness and general aches and pains, or depression.

The most characteristic symptoms are the general physical and mental sluggishness,

Table 9.25   Principal clinical features of hypothyroidism

	Common feature	Less common
Systemic/metabolic	Tiredness Weight gain Cold intolerance Goitre Hyperlipidaemia	Hypothermia, cold periphery

Haematological		Anaemia – iron deficiency
		          – pernicious/macrocytic
		          – normochromic normocytic

Cardiovascular	Bradycardia	Pericardial/pleural effusion Hypertension Heart failure
Dermatological	Dry, thick skin	Dry, thin hair; alopecia Myxoedema (non-pitting oedema) Periorbital oedema Vitiligo
Musculoskeletal	Delayed relaxing reflexes Slow movement Myalgia, arthralgia, stiffness	Peripheral myopathy Carpal tunnel syndrome Ataxia (unsteadiness) Deafness Hoarseness
Neuropsychiatric	Depression Slow thought Poor memory	Dementia Psychosis
Gastrointestinal	Constipation	Anorexia
Reproductive	Menorrhagia/oligomenorrhoea	Infertility Delayed puberty
Developmental		Growth retardation Mental retardation; cretinism

lethargy, intolerance of cold, weight gain and coarsening of the skin. The voice is hoarse and hair is dry, brittle and falling. There may be a characteristic swollen thyroid, visible in the neck as a **goitre**.

The classic dermatological feature is **myxoedema**, which is an accumulation of mucopolysaccharide in the dermis that causes widespread skin thickening and puffiness. This form of oedema is non-pitting because it is not caused by excess fluid accumulation (contrast with the pitting oedema of heart failure; see Chapter 4, p. 184).

The heart rate is slowed and this may cause heart failure. The periphery is cold.

Thought processes and memory are impaired and mild depression is common. There is usually weight gain and constipation, despite anorexia.

Biochemically, in addition to abnormal thyroid functions tests (low FT_3 and FT_4, raised TSH), there is usually hyperlipidaemia and possibly abnormal liver enzymes. Haematology (see Chapter 11) may show a mixed picture of iron deficiency (hypochromic, microcytic anaemia), folate and/or B_{12} deficiency (macrocytic anaemia) or simply a normochromic, normocytic pattern.

Subclinical hypothyroidism

In some patients there are few if any symptoms and FT_4/FT_3 levels are within normal limits but TSH is elevated; this might be identified as a chance finding. The pathogenesis is probably an early stage of thyroid insufficiency being compensated by slightly elevated TSH level, initally keeping thyroid hormone levels adequate. Eventually the slowly progressive nature of idiopathic hypothyroidism will lead to frank insufficiency that does not respond to increasing levels of TSH: thyroid hormone levels then fall and symptoms develop. Regular monitoring is all that is required during the asymptomatic phase.

Complications

If thyroid hormone levels are corrected there is no reduction in life expectancy and there are no long-term problems.

Heart failure or 'myxoedemic' coma can be precipitated by severe metabolic stress, such as trauma, infection or hypothermia, which may acutely increase thyroid hormone requirement. Psychosis can also occur ('myxoedemic madness'). If the fetus is exposed to inadequate thyroid hormone *in utero*, irreversible neurological damage leads to cretinism. Hypothyroidism in children results in retardation of mental and physical development that is partially reversible on thyroid hormone treatment. Newborn are routinely screened.

Management

The management of hypothyroidism is relatively straightforward, simply requiring oral thyroxine for life. The general aim is to restore T_4, T_3 and TSH levels to within the normal ranges. TSH should not be suppressed too much in an attempt to maintain T_4/T_3 at high–normal levels: this represents overtreatment and can lead to long-term cardiovascular complications. Thus a mid-range TSH level is usually regarded as the primary objective, ensuring of course that T_4/T_3 are also within range. However, low-end TSH levels are regarded by some as preferable.

Levothyroxine

This is the synthetic replacement drug used for maintenance therapy, which is identical to natural thyroxine (T_4). (This has completely replaced the original dried thyroid gland, a natural product derived from animal sources, with all the quality control risks these entail.) *Levothyroxine* is well absorbed on an empty stomach, but absorption is delayed and possibly reduced by food. Dosing is not nearly as critical for *levothyroxine* in hypothyroidism as it is for insulin in diabetes, because *levothyroxine* has a half-life of about 7 days and a gentle dose–response curve. Moreover, day-to-day requirements do not change even with intercurrent illness, nor do they tend to alter over the long term. Owing to the natural diurnal variation of TSH secretion, which peaks overnight, a single dose is usually taken each morning before breakfast.

Levothyroxine is initialized at 50 µg daily and increased by 50 µg daily every 2–4 weeks depending on response. Clinical improvement is usually evident within the first month of therapy. Thyroid function testing is required 6 weeks after each dose change. Most patients are stabilized on 100–200 µg daily; subsequently only annual TFTs will be needed.

More care is needed when initializing treatment in the elderly or those with known IHD, using a lower starting dose, e.g. 25 µg on alternate days, and smaller increments, because the cardiac over-stimulation could precipitate ischaemic symptoms or even an MI. Sometimes *liothyronine* (T$_3$) is used for its shorter half-life, permitting a more rapid correction of overdosing. Regular ECGs are advisable and beta-blocker cover may be needed to limit the heart rate.

Side-effects

The adverse effects of excess *levothyroxine* (thyrotoxicosis) are exactly what would be predicted from the physiological action of excess thyroxine and are described below (p. 640). With overdosage, as with untreated hyperthyroidism, there is the possibility of osteopenia or osteoporosis in women, which should be monitored.

Cautions and interactions

The dose may require increasing in pregnancy. Hepatic enzyme inducers (e.g. *rifampicin, phenytoin*) increase clearance. Some drugs reduce absorption, so *levothyroxine* should be taken at a different time from *sucralfate, aluminium hydroxide* and iron salts (Table 9.26). Other factors that affect the control of hypothyroidism are also shown in this table.

Liothyronine

Liothyronine (tri-iodothyronine, T$_3$) has a swifter onset and shorter half-life than *levothyroxine* and it is about five times more potent. It is mainly used for emergency treatment of severely hypothyroid states such as coma, or for initiating treatment in those with CVD. It is available in injectable and oral forms.

Hyperthyroidism

For several reasons, hyperthyroidism is not simply the opposite of hypothyroidism. The causes are more diverse, there are more potential complications and there are more treatment options with worse side-effects. Note that the term **thyrotoxicosis** is used to describe the syndrome resulting from excess thyroid hormone levels, but **hyperthyroidism** refers specifically to when the syndrome is due to excessive secretion from the thyroid gland.

Aetiology and epidemiology

Hyperthyroidism is about 10 times more common in women, in whom the point prevalence is about 1%. However, the lifetime incidence in women is over 2%, some forms being acute or reversible.

Graves' disease, caused by IgG autoantibodies that stimulate the TSH receptor, is the commonest form, representing some 75% of all cases (Table 9.27). It typically follows a fluctuating but progressive course, eventually leading to hypothyroidism, either naturally or as a result ot treatment.

Autonomous growth of multiple, hypersecreting 'toxic' nodules in the thryoid gland is the second most common form and this is more often seen in elderly females, but isolated 'toxic' adenomas (benign tumours) can also occur. These are usually associated with goitre. Occasionally

Table 9.26 Cautions and interactions of levothyroxine therapy

(a) Factors affecting thyroid function or levothyroxine treatment	Increased thyroid hormone action or thyroid function	Reduced thyroid hormone action or thyroid function
Interfere with thyroid hormone action	–	Enzyme inducers (e.g. rifampicin) ↓ absorption (e.g. aluminium hydroxide, iron, etc.) ↓ TSH secretion (corticosteroids, dopamine)
Interfere with thyroid status	Amiodarone (inhibit peroxidase) Lithium (unknown effect)	Amiodarone (excess iodine) Lithium (blocks iodine uptake and thyroid hormone release) Iodide/iodine excess, e.g. older 'expectorants' Iodine deficiency Monovalent anions e.g. pertechnetate (TcO_4^-), perchlorate (ClO_4^-), thiocyanate (SCN^-): compete for iodine uptake. Pregnancy (↑ thyroid hormone requirement)

(b) Drugs affected by levothyroxine treatment	Drugs with action enhanced	Drugs with action diminished
Drug interaction	Sympathomimetic (mimic action) Warfarin (potentially ↑ action – monitor)	Propranolol, digoxin (↓ serum level) Insulin/oral hypoglycaemic (↓ glucose tolerance)

Table 9.27   Causes of hyperthyroidism

Aetiology	Examples
Most common (75%)	
Autoimmune stimulation	Graves' disease (stimulatory anti-TSH receptor antibody)
Less common	
Multinodal goitre	
Adenoma	
Thyroiditis	Post partum, viral, autoimmune
Iatrogenic	Amiodarone, excessive levothyroxine dose
Dietary	Excess iodine
Rare	
Secondary	Pituitary – excessive TSH secretion
	Other endocrine abnormalities

general thyroid inflammation (**thyroiditis**) occurs following radiation, childbirth or viral illness; there may be an underlying auto-immune aetiology to this. It usually remits without recurrence. **Thyroid cancer** is one of the most common radiation-induced tumours, via ingestion of radioiodine (^{131}I), e.g. after radiological accidents such as at Chernobyl.

Amiodarone, which has a high iodine content, frequently causes mild hyperthyroidism, possibly leading to thyrotoxicosis on prolonged therapy. It can also cause hypothyroidism (Table 9.24). Very rarely hyperthyroidism can be secondary to pituitary hyperactivity (Table 9.27).

Pathology

High levels of thyroid hormone cause a general acceleration of metabolic processes with increased metabolic rate and energy utilization, hyperthermia and increased cardiovascular activity (see below). There is a compensatory fall in TSH, often to undetectable levels.

Investigation and diagnosis

Owing to the several possible aetiologies, more extensive investigation is required than for hypothyroidism. Typical clinical features will invariably be borne out by a TFT, which will usually show raised FT_4 and FT_3 and barely detectable TSH.

Further investigation will depend upon the degree of suspicion of different aetiologies, but could include:

- Autoantibody scan; thyroid peroxidase and thyroglobulin antibodies are usually found, but there is a 10–20% false-negative rate because they may also occur in unaffected individuals. TSH-stimulating receptor antibodies are difficult to assay and are not routinely sought.
- Imaging is best done with radiolabelled sodium pertechnetate (^{99m}Tc), which is preferentially taken up into the thyroid by the symporter but not organified. This will show the overall size of the organ, with concentration in any nodules, showing their number and size. It is a prerequisite if ablation therapy is planned. Ultrasound is less invasive. MRI or CT scanning is used if ophthalmopathy (see below) is suspected.
- Biopsy: if a tumour is suspected.

Clinical features

The clinical features of hyperthyroidism (Table 9.28) should be contrasted with those of hypothyroidism (Table 9.25): the picture is strikingly different. The range of features varies slightly according to aetiology but is broadly consistent. Typically the patient is thin, nervous, agitated, hyperactive, hot, thirsty and sweaty.

Examination will show a raised heart rate, possibly even atrial fibrillation; in severe cases there may be signs of heart failure. The neck will usually be swollen and auscultation of the goitre will reveal bruits (the sound of rapid, excessive blood flow). There are also usually diarrhoea and anxiety.

In Graves' disease the common complication of ophthalmopathy (see below) will cause bulging eyes and an unblinking stare, known as **exophthalmos** – the classic sign of thyrotoxicosis. Another characteristic Graves' feature is **pretibial myxoedema**, where the deposition of fibrous material causes painless dermal nodules on the shin.

Course

Graves' disease may follow a relapsing and remitting course, with remissions facilitated by therapy. However, remissions become decreasingly likely following each successive relapse. Paradoxically, the end-stage for some patients may be autoimmume hypothyroidism. There is an increased risk of osteoporosis and heart disease in untreated disease.

Table 9.28   Principal clinical features of hyperthyroidism

	Common feature	Less common
Systemic/metabolic	Fatigue, weakness Hyperactivity, restlessness Weight loss Heat intolerance, sweating Polydipsia Goitre	Hyperthermia, warm periphery Polyuria Bruit over gland (excess perfusion)
Cardiovascular	Tachycardia, atrial fibrillation Palpitations	Heart failure (high output) Hypertension
Musculoskeletal	Hyper-reflexia Tremor	Myopathy Lid retraction, lid lag
Neuropsychiatric	Irritability, anxiety, dysphoria Insomnia	Depression Psychosis
Gastrointestinal	Increased appetite	Diarrhoea
Reproductive		Oligomenorrhoea Loss of libido
Dermatological		Pruritis Pretibial myxoedema[a]
Ophthalmopathy[a]	Grittiness Periorbital, conjunctival oedema Scleral injection ('red eye') Proptosis (exophthalmos)	Diplopia Impaired acuity
Family history	Autoimmune disease e.g. Graves' disease, pernicious anaemia, vitiligo, type 1 diabetes mellitus	

(a) Only in Graves' disease.

Complications

Ophthalmopathy (thyroid eye disease)

A characteristic eye disease affects about half of Graves' disease patients. It is potentially serious and for unkown reasons it is associated with smoking. The cause is autoimmune inflammation of the oculomotor muscles, with fibrous overgrowth. This pushes the eyes forward and impairs eye movement. The overexposed corneas can become dry and painful, and there may be diplopia (double vision). In the most severe form (<10% cases) the retro-orbital swelling can compress the optic nerve and threaten sight.

It can be detected by examination of eye movement and testing for double vision at the extremes of lateral eye rotation, but MRI scanning is needed for precise assessment. Its severity is not related to thyroid hormone levels nor is it relieved if euthyroidism is achieved by medical or surgical means, probably because it is due to antithyroid antibodies rather than excessive thyroid hormone itself. For most patients it is an unsightly inconvenience rather than a threat to sight.

Thyroid crisis ('storm')

This rare condition, which occurs when there are very high levels of thyroid hormone, is potentially fatal. There is excessive cardiovascular stimulation, high fever and extreme agitation. It can be triggered in hyperthyroid patients by extra metabolic stress, such as infection, by mental stress, or by radioiodine therapy.

Autoimmune disorder

Other autoimmune diseases including pernicious anaemia, myasthenia gravis, type 1 diabetes and vitiligo are more common among Graves' disease sufferers.

Management

The aims of management are symptom control and reduction of thyroid hormone output. For the latter, three modes are available:

- Pharmacological suppression.
- Radio-isotopic thyroid gland reduction/ablation.
- Surgical thyroid gland reduction/ablation.

Beta-blockers are used for symptom control while other therapy is initialized. This is effective because many of the effects of thyroid hormone are sympathomimetic and resemble those of adrenaline (epinephrine), including cardiac stimulation, tremor and anxiety (Table 9.23). *Propranolol* is preferred, probably because it is non-selective and crosses the blood–brain barrier, helping the anxiety. Agents with intrinsic sympathomimetic activity (e.g. *pindolol*; see Chapter 4) should not be used.

Patients may use different modes at different stages in their illness. Typical paths are shown in Figure 9.16. After initial stabilization with antithyroid drugs patients may go into remission after a year or so and drugs may be withdrawn. However, relapse is common and remission is then less likely. Thyroid gland reduction aims at a graded reduction in thyroid mass, hoping to leave enough remaining to produce normal amounts of thyroid hormone. However, judging this is difficult and it is always preferable to err on the side of greater destruction, obviating the need for further invasive therapy at a later date. Consequently, eventual iatrogenic hypothyroidism is common. Alternatively, a full ablation may be decided on at the outset, removing doubt and easing management by starting the patient on thyroxine replacement immediately. Thus the choice of options depends on the cause, severity, patient age and patient preference.

Pharmacotherapy

Antithyroid drugs are usually first-line treatment. They block thyroid peroxidase rapidly, but symptom control takes 2–4 weeks owing to stores of thyroid hormone and its long half-life. The most common agents are the thionamides. *Carbimazole* is preferred in the UK but *propylthiouracil* is used in the USA. The latter also blocks T_4–T_3 conversion but this may not be clinically significant. Most antithyroid drugs also have immunosuppressant activity, reducing TSH-receptor antibodies, which may account for the

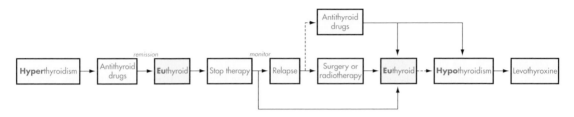

Figure 9.16   Treatment pathways for hyperthyroidism.

sustained remission seen in about half of patients after withdrawal of drug therapy It may also be related to the most serious side-effect, agranulocytosis.

A high initial dose (e.g. 40–60 mg *carbimazole*, depending on initial TFTs) is tapered after 4–6 weeks, with advice to the patient to be alert for overtreatment (sluggishness, constipation, slow pulse, etc). Repeated T_3/T_4 level estimations guide dose reduction at 4- to 8-week intervals. TSH takes longer to rise than thyroid hormone levels do to fall. A maintenance dose of 5–10 mg daily is continued for 18 months, after which a trial withdrawal can be attempted. About half of patients remain in remission and are monitored annually. Some eventually relapse; others develop autoimmune hypothyroidism. Those who relapse have less chance of a further remission and either long-term pharmacotherapy or an alternative mode of therapy is then indicated.

Block and replace

An alternative strategy is to continue antithyroid drugs at a high dose for the same period of 2 years, effectively producing a chemical ablation. Standard replacement doses of *levothyroxine* are given, eventually withdrawing all drugs if euthyroidism is achieved. This strategy is simpler, requiring less monitoring and titration, and it allows for a more sustained immunosuppressant action from higher doses of antithyroid drug. However, there is little evidence that it is more effective, and there is an increased risk of side-effects.

Side-effects include minor dermatological problems, avoided by changing to another antithyroid agent, and other minor non-specific drug side-effects. Most important, however, is bone marrow suppression and agranulocytosis,

which can affect 0.1% of patients. This is usually rapid in onset, occurring during the first 3 months of treatment, so not easily detected from blood counts. All patients must be warned to watch for swollen glands, throat infections and bruising. If these occur they should stop their drug and consult their GP urgently. The problem is reversed on withdrawal but antimicrobial cover (for neutropenia) and *filgastrim* (to stimulate leucocyte recovery) may initially be required. A change of drug may subsequently be tried: the effect may not recur.

Iodide/iodine have an antithyroid effect and are sometimes used as an adjuvant in thyroid storm or before thryoidectomy, to reduce gland size, but they are no longer first-line therapy.

Radiotherapy

Selective thyroid reduction using sodium radioiodide (^{131}I) exploits the concentration of iodide in the thyroid, which minimizes exposure of other organs and allows a low total body dose. In the USA it it often the first line treatment for those over 50, owing to the potential cardiovascular risks of hyperthyroidism. In Europe it is preferred to surgery for medical failure to control hyperthyroidism or following relapse. Although the aim is to spare enough gland to permit normal thyroid hormone output, there is a 10–20% chance of hypothyroidism in the first year following treatment and subsequently up to a 5% annual incidence. Sodium radioiodide is taken as an oral solution. Little special contact avoidance is necessary afterwards, except for avoiding public transport and sustained close contact with children for about 4 weeks. It is contra-indicated in pregnancy.

Complications

The effect takes several months to develop, during which thyroid hormone levels may rise temporarily, and antithyroid drug or beta-blocker cover may be needed. Ophthalmopathy is a relative contraindication because it may be exacerbated. There is a small increase in the risk ot thyroid cancer.

Thyroidectomy

Surgery has a similar aim to radiotherapy, i.e. subtotal thyroid gland reduction, but has the same imprecision and is more invasive. It is particularly indicated if there is a large goitre. It is important that patients are rendered euthyroid before surgery, to avoid thyroid storm. Some are given oral iodine (Lugol's iodine) or potassium iodide for a few weeks before surgery, to inhibit thyroid hormone synthesis and reduce gland vascularity. As with radioiodine, many patients eventually become hypothyroid. Potential surgical complications include laryngeal or parathyroid damage.

Ophthalmopathy

Milder cases need symptomatic treatment, including artificial tears and eye protection. If sight is threatened, high-dose corticosteroids, surgery or radiation therapy may be indcated.

Thyroid storm

Urgent antithyroid therapy with thionamides and iodine are required to reduce thyroid hormone output. Symptomatic cover with beta-blockers, corticosteroids and possibly IV fluids will usually be necessary. The precipitating cause must be discovered and treated.

References and further reading

Alberti K G M M, Defronzo R A, Zimmet P, eds (1997). *International Textbook of Diabetes Mellitus*, 2nd edn. Chichester: John Wiley.

Bloomgarten Z T (2004). Diabetes complications. *Diabetes Care* **27**: 1504–1512.

Davies M, Srinivasan B (2005). Glycaemic management of type 2 diabetes. *Medicine* **34**(2): 69–75.

Devendra D, Liu E, Eisenbarth G S (2004). Type 1 diabetes: recent developments. *BMJ* **328**: 750–754.

Diabetes Control and Complications Trial Research Group (1993). The effect of intensive treatment of diabetes on the development and progression of long-term complications in insulin dependent diabetes mellitus. *N Engl J Med* **329**: 977–986.

Dinneen S F (2006). Management of type 1 diabetes. *Medicine* **34**(2): 63–7.

Franklyn J A (2005). Hypothyroidism. *Medicine* **33**(11): 27–29.

Marshall S M, Flyvbjerg A. Prevention and detection of vascular complications of diabetes. *BMJ* **333**: 475–480.

Nathan D M (1998). Some answers, more controversy, from UKPDS. *Lancet* **352**: 832–833.

NICE (September 2002). Type 2 diabetes – blood glucose: Management of type 2 diabetes – Managing blood glucose levels (Clinical Guideline). Available from http://guidance.nice.org.uk/CGG/?c=91523 (accessed 16 August 2007).

NICE (July 2004). Type 1 diabetes: Diagnosis and management of type 1 diabetes in children, young people and adults (CG15). Available from http://guidance.nice.org.uk/CG15/?c=91523 (accessed 16 August 2007).

Nutrition Subcommittee of Diabetes UK (2003). The implementation of nutritional advice for people with diabetes. *Diabetic Med* **20**: 786–807.

Phillips P (2002). Insulins in 2002. *Aust Prescr* **25**: 29–31.

Shepphard C S (2005). Goitre and thyroid cancer. *Medicine* **33**(11): 35–37.

Stumvoll M, Goldstein B J, van Haeften T W (2005). Type 2 diabetes: principles of pathogenesis and therapy. *Lancet* **365**: 1333–1346.

Watkins P J (2003). *ABC of Diabetes*, 5th edn. London: BMJ Publishing Group.

Weetman A P (2005). Thyrotoxicosis. *Medicine* **33**(11): 30–34.

Internet resources

http://www.diabetes.org.uk (website of Diabetes UK, the charity for people with diabetes).

10

Neoplastic disease

Cancer is a common condition and causes much suffering. It has a high morbidity and a very high mortality, being the second most common cause of death in the developed world. This is mainly because of the tendency to spread to secondary sites and initiate new tumours. Tumours affect health and threaten survival in part simply because of their bulk, but also for more indirect reasons.

Because the causation of cancer is complex and still incompletely understood, the prevention of most cancers is currently not feasible. Moreover, the natural history of cancer means that it is not usually detected until a late stage, when treatment is difficult and, with some exceptions, currently offers limited hope of success. However, this situation is improving rapidly as insight into the control of cell division is developed and targeted biological treatments are discovered. Cancer therapy currently stands at a watershed and for perhaps the first time it is not overly optimistic to expect significant advances in the near future.

Classification and epidemiology of cancer

Terminology

Cancer is the general term for a group of disorders caused by the abnormal and unrestricted growth of cells. The term derives from the crab-like histological appearance of an invasive tumour, which seems to extend claws or tentacles into surrounding tissue. Each primary tumour derives from a single aberrant cell following mutation.

The term **neoplasm** ('new growth') describes this tendency to excessive, uncontrolled growth. It is synonymous with the less technical 'tumour' (swelling). **Benign tumours** enlarge but do not invade surrounding tissue. They are generally much less dangerous than **malignant tumours**, which do invade local tissues and also spread to distant sites (**metastasis**). However, the term 'benign' can be misleading because a large growth, even if not disseminated, can nevertheless be fatal by interfering locally with a vital organ or function, e.g. tumours in the brain or endocrine glands, or those obstructing a major blood vessel.

The nomenclature of cancer is complex and inconsistent (Table 10.1). It attempts to classify three characteristics, all of which have a bearing on prognosis and treatment:

• The tissue of origin (in the histological sense).
• The organ of origin.
• Whether it is benign or malignant.

Table 10.1   Classification and nomenclature of neoplasms, with common examples

Tissue and organ of origin	Examples	
	Benign	Malignant
Haematopoietic	Polycythaemia	–
Lymphoreticular		
Granulocytes	–	Myelocytic leukaemias
Lymphocytes	–	Lymphocytic leukaemias
Lymphoid tissue	–	Lymphomas, e.g. Hodgkin's lymphoma
Plasma cells	–	Myelomas
Connective tissue/mesenchyme		
Bone	Osteoma	Osteosarcoma
Fatty tissue	Lipoma	Liposarcoma
Mesothelium	Mesothelioma	Malignant mesothelioma
Epithelial tissue		
Glandular	Adenoma (e.g. thyroid adenoma)	Adenocarcinoma, e.g. adenocarcinoma of breast or lung
Squamous	Squamous papilloma	Squamous cell carcinoma
Melanocytes	Moles	Malignant melanoma
Nervous tissue		
Meninges	Meningioma	Meningiosarcoma
Embryonic, germinal	Teratoma	Testicular teratoma Choriocarcinoma Nephroblastoma

Usually, but not universally, malignant tumours end in '-carcinoma', '-sarcoma' or '-aemia', while benign tumours usually end simply in '-oma'. For historic reasons there are a number of exceptions, e.g. melanoma and lymphoma are malignant (and so are usually explicitly so described), while neither anaemia nor granuloma is a tumour at all.

The suffix -oma simply denotes a tumour, e.g. osteoma (bone tumour), adenoma (gland tumour). Malignant tumours are predominantly **carcinomas** (epithelial origin, e.g. adenocarcinoma), **sarcomas** (connective tissue, e.g. osteosarcoma) or **leukaemias** (haematological). Most malignant human tumours are carcinomas, partly because epithelia have the greatest exposure to potentially carcinogenic environmental agents and partly because they usually have a high cell turnover, with an attendant greater likelihood of neoplastic mutation.

Epidemiology

Prognosis in cancer is usually quantified in terms of **median survival**, i.e. the time after which 50% of patients might be expected to have survived; or as the **5-year survival**, which is the proportion of patients expected to be alive after 5 years. Figure 10.1 shows the survival for the most common tumours. Recent improvements in treatment have meant that overall, a third of males and almost a half of females have a better than 50% survival at 5 years, while only about one-fifth of all patients have a poorer than 10% 5-year survival. There is still a poor prognosis for some forms of cancer, notably of the lung and GIT, despite modern treatment. However, the prospects for breast cancer continue to improve, 5-year survival having risen from 50% to over 80% between 1950 and the present. Ironically, the higher survival rates are often for the less common tumours such as testicular and skin cancer.

Cancer causes about a quarter of all deaths in developed countries, only slightly less than CVD. The incidence started to increase early in the 20th century owing partly to increasing longevity and reduction in deaths from other serious illnesses, which gives tumours more time to develop, and partly to improved diagnosis. One in three people will develop cancer at some time. Part of the increase is also undoubtedly due to environmental features of industrialized

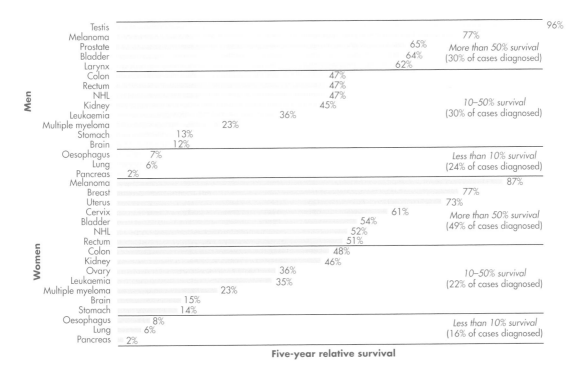

Figure 10.1 Survival rates for common tumours (England and Wales). Five-year relative survival, adults diagnosed 1996–99. Source: Cancer Research UK News & Resources website (2007), CancerStats. http://info. cancerresearchuk.org/cancerstats/ (accessed 13 August 2007). NHL, non-Hodgkins lymphoma.

life, such as atmospheric pollution, smoking and diet.

There are wide variations in the incidence and prevalence of cancer for different anatomical sites, sexes, ages, and racial, ethnic and geographical groups. These give tantalising but largely unresolved glimpses into the aetiology of different tumours.

Site and sex

In developed countries lung cancer is the single most common tumour in men but the incidence is falling slowly. The most common tumour in UK women is now not breast cancer but lung cancer (Figure 10.2), due both to improved breast cancer treatment and to increased smoking among young women, particularly in Scotland. For both sexes, gastrointestinal tumours, especially of the stomach and colon, are the second largest group, followed by skin cancer.

Age

Cancer incidence generally increases with age. For certain tumours in the very aged the prevalence can be very high, e.g. >50% for prostatic carcinoma in males over 80 years (although much remains asymptomatic), but less for breast cancer in females. However, some tumours are more common in childhood, such as leukaemia and tumours of the CNS.

The increase with age may be related to at least two factors. Firstly, the longer one lives the greater the chance of unfavourable carcinogenic events such as mutation or environmental toxin exposure, the effects of which may be cumulative. Secondly, with age there is a reduced efficiency of the immune system, which may normally be protective.

Occupation

The first cancers where a definite cause was demonstrated were those associated with exposure to certain industrial chemicals. These included scrotal cancer among chimney sweeps, bladder cancer among azo-dye workers, and bone cancer among watch workers painting luminous dials with radium paints and licking

(a)

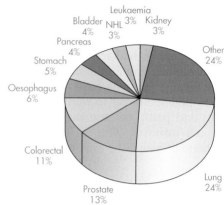

Male

All malignant neoplasms – 80 220

(b)

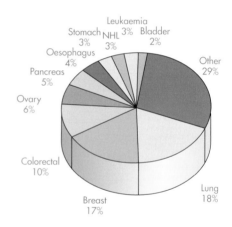

Female

All malignant neoplasms – 74 327

Figure 10.2 Relative and absolute mortality for commonest cancers (males and females), UK 2003. Source: Cancer Research UK News & Resources website (2007), CancerStats. http://info.cancerresearchuk.org/cancerstats/ (accessed 13 August 2007). NHL, non-Hodgkins lymphoma.

the brush. The inhalation of asbestos dust has been linked to an unusual form of lung cancer (mesothelioma) and its incidence is growing. Although such instances currently represent only a small proportion of all tumours, they are important because they are preventable.

Geographic and ethnic variation

Different nationalities have strikingly different incidences for certain tumours. Stomach cancer is far more common in Japan and Chile than in the USA or Israel, while the incidence of colon cancer is particularly low in Asia and Africa. Jewish women, nuns and virgins have a low incidence of cervical cancer. Skin cancer is common in Australia. Prostate cancer is highest among Africans, lowest among East and South Asians. On the other hand, the prevalence of leukaemia is remarkably constant between nations.

Although genetic factors may explain some of these variations, environmental associations are often found to be more important. Thus, immigrants sometimes eventually assume the incidence rate of the host population, depending on the extent of cultural assimilation: Japanese immigrants to the USA have a reduced incidence of stomach cancer, possibly owing to reduced intake of raw fish. Conversely, colon and prostate cancer are far higher among Japanese immigrants to the USA than among native Japanese. Furthermore, it has been established that cervical cancer is strongly associated with the infection with human papilloma virus (HPV).

Trends

Changes in incidence and mortality over time reflect a combination of changes in longevity, detection rates, treatment success and exposure to environmental risk factors. For the more common cancers, mortality is gradually falling (Figure 10.3), e.g. breast cancer in women and gastrointestinal cancers in men and women. Prostate cancer mortality in men is rising owing mainly to greater longevity. For tumours such as stomach cancer, small reductions in incidence are significant and produce large reductions in mortality, because survival is poor. The incidence of testicular cancer has risen but successful treatment has produced significant falls in mortality.

Although overall cancer rates are generally lower in the developing world, incidence is increasing in most countries. This is probably because of greater longevity and improved screening.

Aetiology

Any theory of the causation of cancer must account for both genetic and environmental

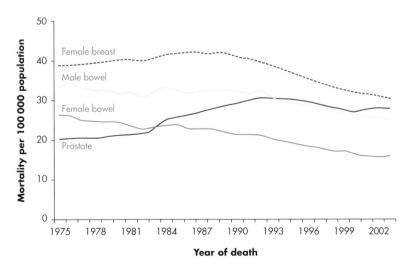

Figure 10.3 Trends in common male and female cancer deaths (Europe). Source: Cancer Research UK News & Resources website (2007), CancerStats. http://info.cancerresearchuk.org/cancerstats/ (accessed 13 August 2007).

factors. It is unlikely that a single cause accounts for all cancers. Almost certainly, cancers form a heterogeneous group of diseases with multifactorial causes. Individuals may have an inherited predisposition, but this may never be expressed unless an appropriate combination of environmental triggers is met. There are also several steps between initiation and clinical disease, and arrest at any of these will prevent the tumour from developing.

There are two distinct aspects to genetic considerations of cancer. First, the aetiological: to what extent is cancer, or predisposition to cancer, inherited? This is discussed here. Second, the pathological: to what extent, and by what mechanism, are changes in the genetic code of tumour cells responsible for their neoplastic characteristics? Only occasionally, when there are mutations in germ cells, i.e. spermatozoa or ova, do these aspects coincide.

The current consensus is that, although DNA changes are involved in all cancers, hereditary factors contribute only about 20% to the overall causation, while environmental factors contribute 80%. Most known associations between environmental factors and cancer have been discovered empirically: the evidence is epidemiological rather than biochemical. How some of these factors might be encompassed within a unified concept of the pathological mechanism is discussed on pp. 657–668.

The process of causing cancer is called **carcinogenesis**, and material factors such as toxins, radiation, etc. that contribute are called **carcinogens**. The terms 'oncogenesis' and 'oncogenic', although sometimes used in this context, are best avoided because of a potential confusion with the newer concept of the 'oncogene', which derives from recent discoveries about the involvement of certain genes in cell proliferation (p. 656).

Genetic factors

From the viewpoint of natural selection, it is unlikely that genes simply coding for a disease with such a high mortality would survive in the gene pool. Moreover, most cancer patients do not usually present with a strongly positive family history. However, there is some evidence for genetic links in certain cancers:

- Some chromosomal abnormalities are associated with malignancy, e.g. Down's syndrome (trisomy 21) with leukaemia.
- Certain rare tumours do run in families, e.g. nephroblastoma.
- There is an association between certain histocompatibility antigens (see Chapter 2) and some malignancies, e.g. HLA-B8 and Hodgkin's lymphoma.
- Certain hereditary tumours are associated with known mutations, e.g. retinoblastoma.

There is a tendency for some common tumours (e.g. breast, ovary and colon) to cluster in family groups. A breast cancer patient's sisters or daughters have double the risk of suffering the same disease; this risk is trebled if there are two first-degree relatives with the disease. There is a known association between familial breast and ovarian cancer and mutations of certain genes whose products are crucial to DNA repair mechanisms (the BRCA genes). Unfortunately, this has not so far produced a reliable screening method.

With familial tumours it is important to try to differentiate between a shared genetic predisposition and shared environmental factors. In general, and fortunately for the prospects for prevention, evidence indicates that whatever the importance of genetic predisposition, for common tumours one or more environmental triggers seem to be essential for a cancer to develop in most people.

Environmental factors

Despite the tremendous efforts to identify specific carcinogenic factors, considerable doubt remains about the extent of their contribution. This may reflect a multifactorial causation. A summary of the most likely candidates and their estimated relative contribution to all cancers is given in Table 10.2. The possible contributions of immunological factors, trauma (e.g. local irritation) and psychosocial factors are unknown. Strong circumstantial evidence for the importance of environmental factors comes from the observation that the most common tumours

Table 10.2 Environmental factors in cancer aetiology: estimates of contribution of various factors to total tumour burden

Factor	Contribution[a]
Chemicals	
• smoking	35
• diet[b]	30
• occupation	3
• alcohol	3
• medicines	1
• hormones	7
Infection (e.g. *Helicobacter*)	10
Radiation	5

[a] Current best estimate of the percentage contribution to the world cancer burden.

[b] High end of the estimated range, and still controversial.

Smoking is by far the largest single contributor, although a wide variety of industrial carcinogens have also been positively identified. The link between smoking and lung cancer is one of the best examples of how epidemiological methods can elucidate the cause of a cancer. Recent trends in UK lung cancer deaths (Figure 10.4) can be correlated with evidence of a reduction in the prevalence of smoking among males from a maximum in 1950 of 65% in men and 40% in women. Nowadays less than 25% of the UK population smoke, although the fall has been greater among men, and there is a rising trend among young women. As a result the lung cancer trend for women has been rising while there has been a significant fall in men (Figure 10.4). Furthermore, while smoking is currently on the decline in most developed countries, an even more worrying trend is for a dramatic increase in developing ones. This is presumably because legislative and social changes lag behind economic advances (which afford greater access to manufactured cigarettes), aided perhaps by a switch in the focus of a tobacco industry under increasing legislative pressures in the developed countries.

The statistical effort needed to confirm the link between smoking and lung cancer was enormous. Despite the fact that probably 90% of lung cancers (bronchial carcinomas) are

in developed countries (lung, breast, gut and prostate) are rare in many developing countries.

Chemicals

Chemicals seem to be the chief culprits. Most chemical carcinogens are mutagens, i.e. they damage the genes, producing mutations. This provided one of the first clues to the underlying pathological basis of cancer.

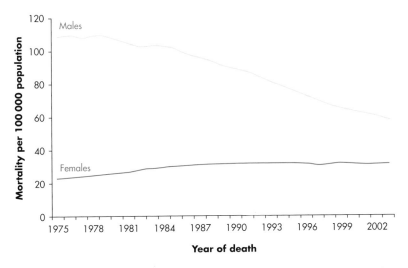

Figure 10.4 Trends in lung cancer deaths (UK). Source: Cancer Research UK News & Resources website (2007), Cancer-Stats. http://info.cancerresearchuk.org/cancerstats/ (accessed 13 August 2007).

smoking-related, only one in six heavy smokers is likely to develop the disease. Other common tumours such as breast cancer defy such analysis; links between breast cancer and the intake of fat and alcohol have been claimed but not proven. The carcinogenicity of the oestrogens in oral contraceptives and hormone replacement therapy is still debated. How much more difficult then to trace the causation of less common cancers with more subtle or less biologically plausible aetiologies, especially because allowance must always be made for the long lag time between cancer induction and clinical presentation.

Dietary factors are increasingly seen to be important, although the specific carcinogenic constituents remain largely unknown. Excess fats, red meat, food additives, nitrates and numerous other factors have been implicated, as has the insufficiency of fibre or antioxidants, but strong evidence of a causal link is lacking. Evidence implicating alcohol is growing; for example, it may act synergistically with smoking in oropharyngeal tumours. It has been estimated that dietary factors account for three-quarters of gut, breast and prostate tumours.

Drugs may cause cancer in a number of ways. The main offenders are the cytotoxics, which are both mutagenic and immunosuppressant (see p. 689). Hormones, especially the sex hormones (e.g. oestrogens), may encourage tumours in hormone-dependent tissues. The possible relationships between sex organ tumours and factors such as endogenous hormonal activity, breast-feeding, the age of onset of sexual activity, male circumcision, etc. are under investigation.

Other factors

Infection. A number of viruses have been causatively linked to certain tumours. Examples are cervical cancer and human papilloma virus (HPV), Burkitt's lymphoma and Epstein–Barr virus, hepatatis B and hepatitis C infection and liver cancer, and HIV infection and Kaposi's sarcoma.

Radiation. There are well-demonstrated links between cancer and both ionizing and ultraviolet radiation, which are known to produce genetic damage. Radiation from the nuclear industry,

nuclear weapons (early testing and actual use), high levels of environmental radon gas in certain geographical areas, and medical equipment (diagnostic and therapeutic), have all produced cancer. The possible carcinogenic effects of microwaves from mobile phones, and electromagnetic radiation from overhead power cables, are currently debated. Fair-skinned people in very sunny regions, e.g. Australia, California, have a significantly increased incidence of skin cancer. Like smoking, this is a cause that is understood, quantifiable and avoidable.

Immunological. One important potential factor in carcinogenesis is a loss of the body's ability to identify and eliminate cells that have become neoplastic. Normally the immune system is continually checking for the presence of abnormal, non-self cells ('immunosurveillance'). Neoplastic cells transformed by genetic mutation often have altered cell surface receptors, and if they are sufficiently different as to become antigenic, they are promptly detected and destroyed by the immune system. If the immune system is compromised owing to e.g. immunodeficiency disorder, immunosuppressant therapy, stress or age, or alternatively if the surface changes are minor, then tumour cells are more likely to escape this control.

Trauma. Sometimes chronic irritation seems to initiate tumours, although usually there is an associated infection. This may account for the correlation between oral cancers and ill-fitting dentures and between vaginal cancer and early intercourse or poor genital hygiene. Similarly, chronic inflammation in poorly controlled UC may be responsible for an increased incidence of colon cancer. The explanation may lie in the faster rate of tissue proliferation found in the repair phase of chronic inflammation (Chapter 2), which increases the likelihood of a neoplastic mutation.

Psychosocial. Psychological factors probably do not play a significant part in carcinogenesis, although it has been claimed that people who repress emotions rather than express them are more likely to develop cancer. Nevertheless, major stress often does precede the onset of a tumour, as with many other diseases, particularly autoimmune disease, possibly due to a consequent dysfunction of the immune system.

Pathobiology

So far, factors involved in the genesis of a neoplasm have been discussed, but not the mechanism. The nature of many carcinogens suggests that the first step is a mutation: a small chemical change in the genetic code. Advances in molecular biology are promising eventually to lead to an understanding of how this change transforms a normal cell into a neoplastic one.

In this section, the normal control of cell growth and proliferation is reviewed, and how this might go wrong is examined. The process of single cell division and the consequences for the whole tissue of normal and abnormal division are then examined in detail. Finally, the possibilities for therapeutic intervention in the process are discussed.

Normal cell proliferation

Two important parameters of normal cellular growth are division rate and differentiation of function.

Stem cells and differentiation

Each nucleated cell in an organism has within its DNA the theoretical potential to produce all the gene products capable of performing the function of any cell in the whole organism. (Exceptions include mature RBCs and platelets, because they have lost their nucleus.) In mammals, this **totipotency** is suppressed, and effectively lost, early in the embryonic stage. Precursor **pluripotent stem cells** remain; these are less flexible and by **differentiation** are eventually **committed** to one particular cell type and function (Figure 10.5). The process continues through several stages during which the stem cell becomes progressively less generalized and more committed. A final division gives a mature functional **end cell** that performs a specific physio-

logical role (e.g. neutrophil, epidermal cell) but is no longer capable of division.

Capacity for division

During the growth phase of an organism, cell proliferation clearly exceeds cell death, but subsequently cell numbers remain relatively stable throughout mature life. However, tissues retain the ability to proliferate in response to either physiological demands or losses (e.g. bone marrow, gut lining) or pathological ones (e.g. injury). Thus, in most tissues there is a reservoir of stem cells, which remain dormant until their division is needed to provide either replacement stem cells or more functional differentiated (end) cells. In the bone marrow, the most vigorously dividing body tissue, there are multipotent marrow stem cells that differentiate into more specific stem cell lines, e.g. erythroblasts for erythrocytes, myeloblasts for granulocytes, etc. (Chapter 11).

The rate of growth of a tissue as a whole depends not just on the rate of division of the dividing stem cells within it (i.e. mitotic activity or turnover rate) but also on the proportion of cells that are dividing. Different tissues have different proportions of stem cells: the gut epithelium, the bone marrow and the basal layer of the dermis have the highest proportions. In tissues that are renewed less frequently there is a lower proportion, but the number can increase in the appropriate circumstances. For example, although the liver normally has low cell losses, if part is removed surgically the remainder will regenerate rapidly. On the other hand, nerve and skeletal muscle cells are almost never replaced (in adults), so presumably few stem cells remain in these tissues.

Ideally, the death of one functional end cell should result in one stem cell dividing to produce another stem cell and a replacement functional one (see Figure 10.6). Alternatively, if the stem cell population is depleted, the remaining stem cells must divide to replace the loss by producing two new stem cells after each mitosis.

Cancer involves uncontrolled division and impaired differentiation, and because stem cells are both incompletely differentiated and still capable of division, neoplasms generally derive from stem cells. These considerations have

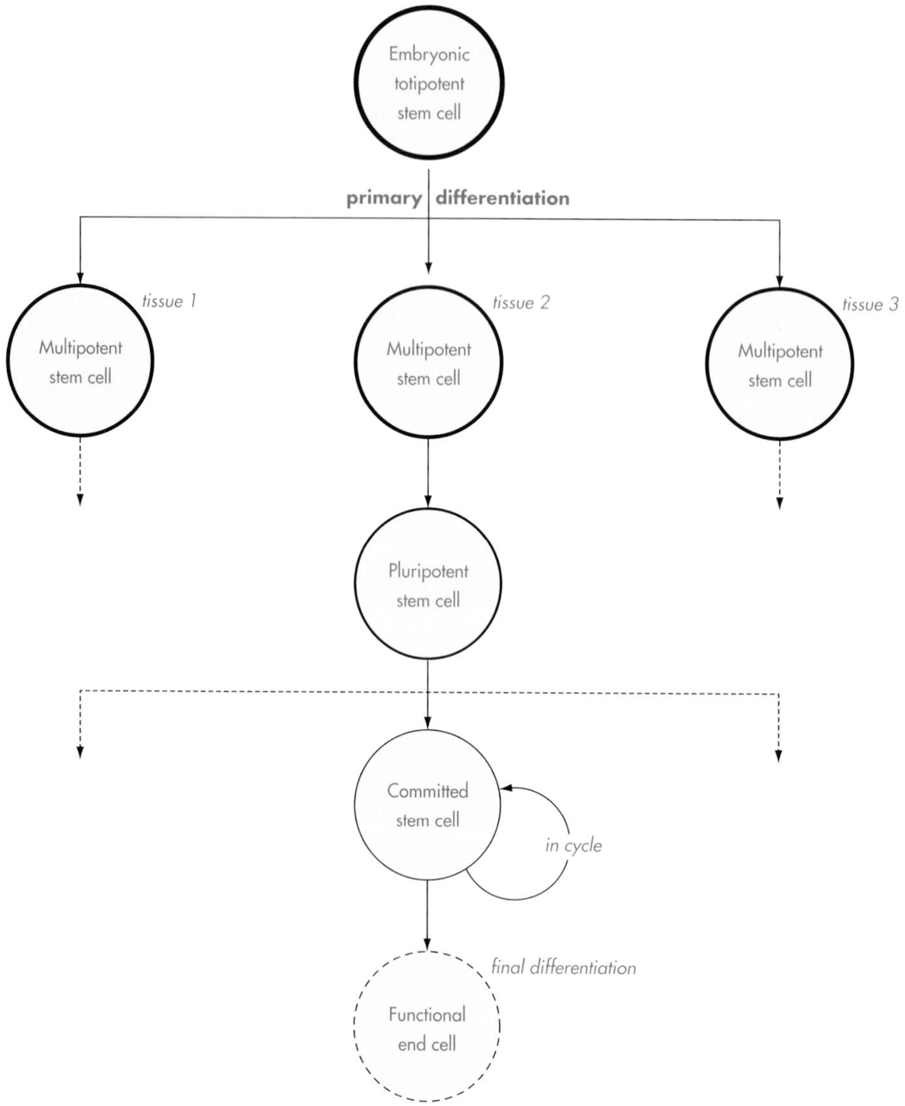

Figure 10.5   Stem cells and differentiation.

important consequences for the treatment of cancer: stem cells are the main target of chemotherapy (pp. 677–687).

Control of growth and differentiation

Stem cells need a signal to tell them when to divide and to stop, and the daughter cells need to know whether or not to differentiate. This is accommodated by their responding to a complex network of **cytokines** with growth stimulant or growth inhibitory properties (Chapter 2). Cytokines are generally polypeptides of about 50–100 amino acids (molecular mass 15–30 kD). Some cytokines may pass directly from cell to cell, producing negative feedback that inhibits growth in response to increasing population density in the tissue, so-called contact inhibition. Others diffuse through a tissue, establishing a concentration in direct proportion to the number of secreting cells. Some cells release **autocrines** that act on receptors on their own surfaces.

Numerous growth factors specific for particular cell types are known, e.g. platelet-derived growth factor (PDGF), epidermal growth factor (EGF), epoetin, thymopoietin, granulocyte colony stimulating factor (G-CSF). Some tumours also secrete their own transforming growth factors (TGF), which closely resemble EGF. Generally these are growth stimulants (mitogenic) and they may be secreted in excess in some cancers. Other factors are growth inhibitors and are presumed deficient in cancer. There are also more general, systemic endocrine stimulants such as somatotropin (growth hormone) and the adrenocorticoids. The sex hormones have a similar but more specific role.

The process is well illustrated by the normal reaction to skin injury. The mitotic activity of basal layer stem cells is strongly stimulated and that tissue temporarily becomes **hyperplastic** (see below); it may even overshoot somewhat, causing bulky scars (keloids). Quite soon after the lesion is healed, however, cell turnover returns to normal (see also Chapter 2). Another well-known physiological example is the increase in epoetin secretion in response to sustained low blood oxygen levels, stimulating RBC production.

Biochemical basis of control of growth and differentiation

The signals for the production of such growth factors, and for transducing their stimuli from the cell surface receptors where they bind to the nucleus where the signal is converted into mitotic activity, has been the subject of intense and productive research in the last decade, resulting in novel approaches to the targeted pharmacological control of cell division. The intracellular mitogenic factors needed to promote cell division are at the end of a complex signalling chain of kinase enzymes whose production is reduced during quiescent, i.e. non-dividing, phases, by repression of the genes controlling their synthesis. Normal cell division is then seen as the expression, by de-repression, of mitogenic genes (oncogenes). Repression and de-repression are well-known processes in the

control of cellular metabolism. This is covered in detail below (see p. 659).

Unusual growth patterns

Cell growth is usually well controlled and organized to meet the needs of the body. There are a number of ways the system can become deranged; however not all result in cancer.

Hyperplasia.   This is a form of increased proliferative activity, usually a response to injury. It must be clearly distinguished from neoplasia in that it is:

- still under control and ceases when the task is accomplished;
- purposeful: the cells produced are fully developed specific functional cells;
- restricted to the affected tissue.

Hypertrophy involves an increase in cell size, but not cell numbers. An example would be muscle hypertrophy in response to chronic high loading, e.g. myocardial ventricular hypertrophy following untreated hypertension.

Metaplasia.   Pluripotent stem cells retain the ability to change their differentiation slightly in response either to normal needs, such as the loss of related tissue, or to irritant damage. For example, gut epithelial cells can change function and become either glandular or absorptive to compensate for losses after gut surgery. Like hyperplasia, metaplasia is usually protective and controlled. However, exceptionally, it may presage neoplastic change. In Barrett's oesophagus, chronic gastric reflux produces metaplastic columnar epithelium that may be pre-neoplastic, and smoking produces some bronchial metaplasia, columnar cells becoming squamous.

Dysplasia describes an occasional moderate abnormality of differentiation producing a variety of unusual cells (pleomorphism) rather than a uniform cell population. Dysplasia often accompanies hyperplasia, e.g. during inflammation or repair, and as such is transient and insignificant. However, it sometimes represents a pre-neoplastic condition, especially where there is no evident cause for the hyperplasia. Thus, biopsy samples are examined for evidence of dysplasia when investigating possible cancers, e.g. cervical smears, gastroscopy specimens.

Abnormal proliferation and differentiation

Insensitivity to local growth control mechanisms, permitting an unnecessary and even self-destructive overgrowth, has long been recognized as a characteristic feature of neoplastic tissue. Often de-differentiation also occurs, i.e. reversion to a more primitive cell type that does not perform the normal function of the tissue involved.

Oncogenes

This breakdown in control may involve abnormal secretion of growth factors, an abnormality in growth factor receptors, or abnormal signalling beween the cell surface receptors and nuclear receptors coding for growth or differentiation. It is now known that the genes coding for mitogenic proteins or their receptors can become expressed inappropriately (amplified). This is partly based on findings linking the rare human tumour viruses to the far more numerous non-viral tumours. Although viruses seem to be uncommon causes of human cancer, genes resembling tumour virus RNA (i.e. with a similar nucleotide sequence) have been found in all human cells; they are known as cellular oncogenes.

This remarkable discovery implies that viruses can cause cancer by mimicking genes that already exist in the host genome. Some viruses may have evolved in this way, a survival advantage having been conferred by the acquisition of a gene that promoted clonal expansion, providing a greater potential for further viral replication. Alternatively, the viruses may have formerly been part of the human genome but have evolved to become semi-independent.

How do oncogenes cause cancer and how are they related to other factors, such as chemical or viral carcinogens? One possible model is as follows. In normal cells:

* Human oncogenes are normally present but repressed.

* When activated by the need for proliferation, they code for growth factors, or growth factor receptors, or other mitogenic promoters.
* These factors are essential for a cell's entry into the cell cycle and movement through it as a prelude to cell division (pp. 657–661).
* Expression of oncogenes is strictly controlled and turned off when no further growth is required.
* 'Anti-oncogenes' (tumour suppressor genes) may be expressed to control excessive cell growth.

However, neoplastic transformation may result in abnormal proliferation by one or more of the following mechanisms:

* A carcinogen causes the inappropriate expression of a human oncogene, often by mutation of a controlling gene, e.g. a repressor or de-repressor gene.
* Viral oncogenes mimic activated human oncogenes.
* An anti-oncogene (or tumour suppressor gene) malfunctions through mutation, permitting neoplastic transformation.

Details of the various stages in the control of cell division are discussed below.

Role of mutation

It is now clear that neoplastic change originates from a chance genetic mutation in a single cell; this would explain the carcinogenic action of mutagens. Any permanent alteration in the DNA structure of a single cell is passed on to all daughter cells, and a tumour is a clone of that first single abnormal cell. However, the majority of random mutations are so disruptive as to be lethal, preventing proliferation. Moreover, cells have a sophisticated capacity for the self-repair of damaged DNA, or for self-destrucion if repair is impossible. Thus, few mutations actually persist to cause cancers.

It is also likely that several mutations are necessary for complete transformation; this could explain the long lag times between exposure and disease. Mutations are usually somatic, i.e. not in germ line tissue, but if an initial mutation did occur in a spermatozoon or an ovum, this could be passed on to offspring as a predisposition to the tumour, which would need a further somatic mutation for full expression. Furthermore, owing to the rate of proliferation and the genetic instability characteristic of neoplasia, as a tumour grows it probably becomes polyclonal, which may partially explain multiple drug resistance.

The original mutation is usually caused by chemicals or radiation. Other possible causes are random mutations from faulty cell division accumulating in old age, or the introduction of foreign, viral DNA or RNA. The overall process of **neoplastic transformation** occurs in several stages. One of the environmental carcinogens identified in Table 10.2 may alone cause the appropriate mutation, but usually a sequence of initiator and promoter factors are required.

Summary

The ultimate cause of cancer is probably that the normal mechanisms that control cell division and differentiation are activated or suppressed inappropriately. There is a failure in the processes by which these mechanisms are usually inhibited from functioning during times when they are not needed.

Thus, cancer may eventually prove to be precisely what it has always intuitively seemed to be – a disorder of the controls on cell proliferation. The precise mechanisms are difficult to elucidate but great strides are being made in discovering precisely how differentiation itself is controlled and how this control is lost.

These concepts are gradually coming to be applied to the cure of cancer. The present strategies for treating cancer are based on a growing knowledge of the growth characteristics of individual neoplastic cells and the neoplasm as a whole. They are still directed primarily towards killing every existing neoplastic cell with minimum damage to normal host cells. Traditional methods using cytotoxic drugs are insufficiently discriminating and thus crude, unsatisfactory and often unsuccessful. The new understanding of cell division mechanisms and control is leading to a more fundamental targeted approach, involving intervention in the expression or de-repression of oncogenes or intracellular signalling.

Cytokinetics

In order to control cancer, it must either be prevented from developing or else differences must be found between neoplastic and normal cells that can be exploited therapeutically. Because of current uncertainty over the aetiology, few tumours can be prevented from starting. The notable exception is smoking-related lung cancer. Moreover, tumours do not have unique biochemical or metabolic processes crucial to their persistence and that can be targeted pharmacologically, as is done successfully when antibiotics are used against microorganisms. Cell division and differentiation in neoplastic cells use essentially the same processes as do normal cells.

The differences between normal and neoplastic cells that we can exploit are quantitative rather than qualitative: the extent of expression and signalling of growth-promoting factors, the rate of growth, the degree of differentiation, and the rate of cell death. Thus, in order to understand how a tumour might be treated, it is necessary to study how it grows, i.e. its **cytokinetics**. In the following sections the stages in the life cycle of normally dividing individual cells and the controls on these are first described. This analysis is then applied to whole cell populations; at this level other factors then need to be considered, notably the ability of tumour cells to migrate and to develop their own blood supply. This leads to a description of natural history of a tumour.

The cell cycle

Phases

The original studies of cell division concentrated on the stages of mitosis that can be distinguished microscopically, i.e. prophase, metaphase, anaphase and telophase. More relevant for cancer is what happens between one mitosis and the next. This is the interphase, common to all dividing cells, and it can be further subdivided into several phases in which there are different types of metabolic activity (Table 10.3). The whole process from one mitosis to the next is known as the cell cycle, and cells that are regularly dividing are termed 'in cycle'.

On this model, the four traditional stages of mitosis are known collectively as the **M phase** (Figure 10.6). If further division is not immediately required, the cell enters the G_0 phase. Alternatively, if it is to divide again there is a subsequent period of intense protein and RNA synthesis, the G_1 **phase** (for historic reasons, from 'gap-1'). During this phase the new daughter cells are synthesizing the materials

necessary for physical enlargement. This is followed by the **S phase** and a further gap phase, the G_2 **phase**.

Sequences of signals control a cell's entry into and passage through each of these phases, initially determined by the expression of oncogenes and ultimately mediated through the activity of **cyclin** proteins. The cyclins are activated upstream by protein kinases, the **cyclin-dependent protein kinases (cdk)** (Figure 10.7). Protein kinases catalyse the activation or deactivation of proteins by phosphorylation, often in association with nucleotide intermediates such as guanosine triphosphate (GTP). Because this area of cell biology is relatively new, a glossary of

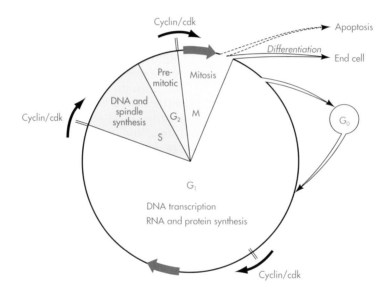

Figure 10.6   Cell cycle in stem cell.

Table 10.3   Phases of the cell cycle

Phase	Approx. duration (h)[a]	Principal mitotic activity
M	1	
G_0	?[b]	None (resting phase)
G_1	480	RNA (transcription) and protein (translation)
S	16	DNA (replication), spindle protein
G_2	8	Nucleoprotein

[a] Times for skin basal layer cells are given, to show the relative times in different stages; other tissues may have different patterns.
[b] Time in G_0 is extremely variable (see text).

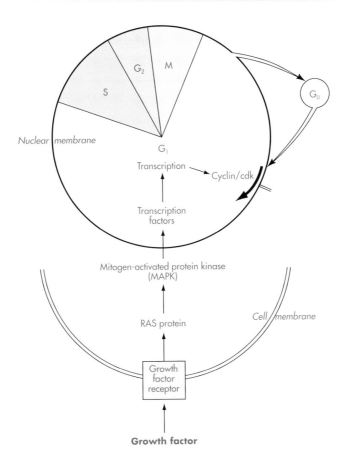

Figure 10.7   Control of cell cycle. Stimulation of growth factor receptor, showing signal transduction to the nucleus and subsequent release from the G_0–G_1 restriction point. cdk, cyclin-dependant kinase; M, mitotic phase; G_1, first gap phase; S, synthesis phase; G_2, second gap phase. ‖ Restriction- or check-point.

some of the relevant terminology is given in Table 10.4.

Within the cycle there are specific **check-points** or **restriction points** at which it can be arrested or aborted, if for example a fault has developed in DNA replication. This may allow DNA repair before onward progression, or it may trigger death of the cell. The main checkpoints occur to control re-entry to the cycle from the G_0 phase, and movement from the G_1 to S and from G_2 to M phases (Figure 10.6).

This signalling is shown in simplified form in Figure 10.7, illustrating the signal pathway from stimulation of a cell membrane-bound growth factor receptor to a cell's release from the G_0–G_1 restriction point. Thus proliferation and differentiation are tightly controlled, and it is a break-

down of these controls that is the hallmark of cancer. Elements of these pathways have provided fruitful areas for the development of therapies targeted more specifically at neoplastic cells, in which the pathways are more highly activated.

The G_1 phase has the most variable duration. The time between one M-phase and the next is known as the **intermitotic** or **cell cycle time**. In the example given in Table 10.3 of normal human skin basal layer cells this is about 20 days. For the hyperplastic (but not neoplastic) basal cells in psoriasis it is about one-tenth of this, owing mainly to a shorter G_1 phase. For some bone marrow and gastrointestinal epithelial cells the cell cycle time may be <10 h; for liver cells it averages weeks.

Table 10.4   Some common terms in molecular biology relevant to cell cycle, cell signalling and oncogenesis

Term	Definition	Function
AP-1	Protein transcription factor	Binds to DNA → expression
Cadhedrin	Cell surface adhesion molecule (CAM)	Cohesion of mass of cells
cdk	Cyclin-dependent kinase	Binds to cyclin
c-fos, c-jun	Cellular oncogene (c-onc) (v-onc = viral oncogene)	Code for transcription factors (API) affecting growth
cpki	Cyclin-dependent protein kinase inhibitor	Inhibits division
cyclin	Protein in cell cycle, coded by cyclin genes	Control cell cycle progression
EGF-R	Epidermal growth factor receptor	Tyrosine kinase receptor
HER1,2	Human epidermal growth factor	Tyrosine kinase receptor
jun	Part of AP1 gene family (above)	Binds to DNA → expression
MAPK	Mitogen-activated protein kinase	Signal transducer
p53	Cellular anti-oncogene	Transcription factor: inhibits division by inducing p21, which is a cpki
pk	Protein kinase	Mediates activation or deactivation of protein by phosphorylation
pki	Protein kinase inhibitor	
Protease	Proteolytic enzyme secreted by tumour cell	Facilitate invasion and destruction of local connective tissue
Protein kinase	Signal transducer (membrane, cytoplasm, nuclear)	Activate/deactivate signalling proteins by phosphorylation; work with nucleotides
Proteosome	Intracellular complex of proteolytic enzymes	Scavenging and destroying damaged proteins or protein fragments that have been tagged by ubiquitin
RAS	Protein family involved in signal transduction	
ras, raf	Oncogenes	Code for RAS protein
tka	Tyrosine kinase inhibitor	
VEGF	Vascular epidermal growth factor	Growth of new blood vessels (angiogenesis)

M phase

There are three possible outcomes to the M phase (Table 10.5). Normally it will result in one daughter cell becoming a committed end cell and the other remaining a stem cell. This stem cell may then continue in cycle to another mitosis if it is suitably stimulated because the tissue requires further proliferation. However, if the mitosis has been in some way faulty the daughter cell may embark on a programmed sequence of changes resulting in cell death, termed **apoptosis** (see below).

Dividing cells are not immortal. Each mitosis reduces the chromosomal length by a fixed number of base pairs, lost from an otherwise redundant series known collectively as the

Table 10.5 Possible outcomes to the M/G_0/G_1 phases

1. Cycle continues:
   - no restriction; cell proceeds to the S phase

2. Cell temporarily leaves cycle:
   - mitotic cycle is arrested at restriction point: G_0 phase entered

3. Cycle resumes:
   - cell recruited back into cycle and proceeds to the S phase

4. Cell permanently leaves cycle:
   - daughter cell may undergo apoptosis owing to a defective mitosis
   - cell may differentiate, maturing into a functional cell, after which there will be no further division

telomere, found at the end of each chromosome. This acts as a mitotic counter and ensures senescence: after a predetermined number of divisions the cell will usually cease replicating and enter growth arrest. Certain stem cells can increase their replicative life by repairing telomeres with **telomerase**. Neoplastic cells can exploit this method indefinitely, rendering them effectively immortal, and some cytotoxic drugs target telomerase in order to counter this.

G_0 phase
Cells in the G_0 phase cease all mitotic activity, although of course they continue normal metabolism. It is also likely that DNA repair mechanisms, if needed, are active during this phase. Thus, resting cells form a reservoir of quiescent stem cells, but they may be recruited back into cycle by an appropriate mitogenic stimulus.

Tissues that are capable of proliferation or regeneration but only need to do so intermittently (e.g. the liver) have a high proportion of their stem cells in this phase. The same may be true of certain tumours such as the leukaemias during periods of remission, which thereby retain the ability eventually to resume the malignant process. Because cells in G_0 are not dividing, they are usually insensitive to the cytotoxic drugs. Thus resistance to chemotherapy may sometimes occur because there are a high proportion of G_0 cells in the tumour.

G_1 phase
Different cycle times between cell populations or cell types are usually the result of differences in the G_1 phase. However, the G_1 phase in tumour cells is not invariably shorter than that of normal cells from the same tissue; often it is longer. It is a popular misconception that neoplasia is simply a more rapid cell division: there is no consistent relationship between cell cycle time and malignancy (see also p. 663).

From the G_1 phase the cell may enter the G_0 phase or proceed to the next mitosis. However, it can only progress if it passes a restriction point. This requires an appropriate signal, and it is such a signal that gives the cell control over progression through the cycle and hence the rate of division (Figure 10.7).

Other phases
During the short S phase the cell is synthesizing new DNA and related histones in preparation for the next mitosis. There follows a shorter G_2 phase when essential mitotic components such as chromosomal protein are synthesized.

Apoptosis and the p53 gene
Natural cell death is now known to be an organized process rather than merely a wasting away or decline in metabolic functions; it is sometimes called **cell suicide**. Following signals responsible for regulating the cell population, characteristic changes occur that prepare a cell for death and eventual phagocytosis. This seems to be a normal and necessary component of the same general control mechanisms that govern the viability of a cell or tissue population considered above. Apoptosis includes controlled cleavage of DNA and expression of cell surface receptors that facilitate macrophage activity.

So far apoptosis has not been effectively exploited in therapy, but clearly it is a potential target. Selectively triggering it in neoplastic cells would represent a cytotoxic effect that is highly selective for tumour rather than normal tissue.

The *p53* gene is an important controller of the cell cycle. Its gene product is a protein that modulates the expression of other genes directly responsible for a variety of aspects of the cycle. In particular, *p53* can halt progress at phase boundaries, e.g. G_1–S. The trigger for such activity seems to be DNA damage: *p53* can allow time for DNA repair mechanisms, thus preventing a potentially harmful mutation becoming permanently encoded. It can also trigger apoptosis if a mutation does persist. Thus, *p53* has been dubbed 'the guardian of the genome' and also an anti-oncogene.

Neoplastic cells seem to evade these controls and so are effectively immortal. At least half of all tumours have been found to have defects in *p53*, implying that if this protection is lost, neoplastic transformation can persist. Furthermore, *p53*-deficient tumours tend to be the more aggressive and more treatment-resistant, perhaps because apoptosis cannot be triggered even after some degree of damage.

Therapeutic intervention

Conventional cytotoxic drugs and radiation act by interfering at the nucleoprotein level in one or more of the active phases of the cell cycle, but are generally ineffective in the G_0 phase. The numerous biochemical events that occur in the cycle offer a variety of possible pharmacological interventions, e.g. alkylation of nucleic acid or inhibition of protein synthesis, but because the same events occur in all normal dividing cells, these may also be damaged.

It is important to know in which phase a drug acts so that logical combinations can be chosen; the resultant synergistic effect is well established. It would also be helpful to know when the tumour cells are in particular phases, or the proportions in each phase, but this is rarely practicable. The theoretically attractive strategy of synchronizing all cells to the same phase is sometimes attempted, with only limited success.

By contrast, newer 'biological' treatments target the cell signalling pathways. This offers the possibility of greater selectivity because in many cases these are inappropriately activated in cancer cells. Targets include the growth factor receptor, e.g. *trastuzumab*, and the protein kinases, e.g. *imatinib* (see p. 697).

Cell compartments

The population of cells in any tissue, normal or neoplastic, can be divided into a number of different groups or cell compartments (Table 10.6). Some cells will be capable of division, i.e. stem cells, and these may be actively cycling or resting. Most cells will be functional and non-dividing. There will also be some dead cells awaiting scavenging by the reticuloendothelial system. The relative sizes of these compartments will vary between tissues. Moreover, there are usually considerable differences in the relative compartment sizes between normal tissue and the neoplastic tissue derived from it, and these are potentially more significant therapeutically than possible differences in intermitotic times (Figure 10.8 and below).

Measures of tissue growth

Growth rate

What then affects the rate at which a tumour, or any tissue, grows? In normal adult tissue the growth rate is zero, because generally new cell production rate precisely equals cell loss: we have seen that complex feedback mechanisms ensure that this is so. Only in children, or in injured tissues, does growth exceed losses (p. 653). The tissue growth rate depends directly on the proportion of cells in the tissue that are dividing (the **growth fraction**, representing cycling stem cells) and inversely on the intermitotic time. The cell loss rate (**cell loss fraction**) is

Table 10.6 Cell compartments

Cell type	Compartment	Features
Stem cells	Resting	In G_0
	Cycling	Undifferentiated; intense metabolic activity (in G_1, S, G_2 or M phases)
Differentiated ('end cells')	Functional	Main component in normal tissue
	Dead	Variable proportion (usually small, owing to effective scavenging)

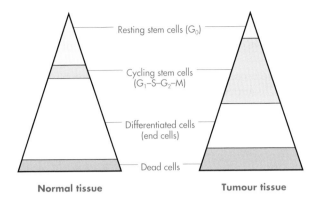

Figure 10.8   Relative sizes of cell compartments in normal and neoplastic tissue.

dependent on several factors (see below), but is most simply considered as the proportion of dividing cells that do not survive.

The growth rate of a tissue, especially a solid tumour, is usually expressed as the time taken for it to double in size, i.e. number of cells or mass. Thus a higher growth rate means a shorter doubling time. The relationship between doubling time and the factors discussed above can be represented empirically as:

$$\text{Doubling time} = \frac{\text{Intermitotic time}}{\text{Growth fraction} - \text{cell loss fraction}}$$

A tumour is by definition a lesion in which cell production exceeds cell loss. If the tumour consisted entirely of cycling stem cells and all daughter cells survived (and none differentiated), the doubling time would be equal to the intermitotic time and growth would be exponential, i.e. follow first-order kinetics. In this respect, the growth would resemble bacterial growth in optimal conditions, and some young solid tumours do approach this condition. However, generally not all cells in a tumour are cycling stem cells and a proportion of cells die after division (Figure 10.8).

In neoplastic tissues the growth fraction is often high. It can be up to 0.9 (90%) in young tumours as more cells leave G_0 and enter the cycle and there is far less differentiation than normal, i.e. both daughter cells remain as stem cells. However, the increased number of mitoses in a tumour produces more faulty divisions,

resulting in non-viable cells, apoptosis and cell death. Furthermore, a rapidly growing solid tumour often outstrips its ability to grow new blood vessels (angiogenesis), so that relatively hypoxic, even necrotic, regions with a high cell loss develop, especially in the centre of the tumour. A further proportion of tumour cells may be destroyed by the immune system. Thus, the cell loss fraction may also sometimes approach 0.9 (90%).

Growth in tumours

It is clear from the above discussion why the intermitotic time of individual cells in neoplasms need not be short. Usually, the main cytokinetic difference between normal and neoplastic tissue is the proportion of dividing cells rather than the rate of division. Moreover, the doubling time may not be high in a tumour even compared with normal tissue, owing perhaps to a high cell loss fraction. Many primary tumours are slow growing, particularly at first. For example, the doubling time in normal leucopoiesis (white cell production) is 2 days, with a growth fraction of about 50%: in acute leukaemia the corresponding figures are 2–10 days and <30%. In solid tumours, malignancy derives predominantly from local invasiveness and metastasis rather than simple growth.

As a tumour grows, its need for nutrients increases, and thus for blood vessels to transport them. To facilitate this process the tumour may produce vascular growth factors that promote angiogenesis (see below), or other factors that switch off signals that normally inhibit angiogenesis. This offers further possibilities for therapeutic intervention.

The 'population pressure' produced by these various factors, e.g. increased competition for oxygen and nutrients, may be part of the reason for metastasis: some cells in effect seek a better environment. Angiogenesis is also important here.

Chemosensitivity
Because cytotoxic drugs only act on cycling cells the chemosensitivity of tumours is often closely related to the growth fraction and doubling time (Table 10.7).

Differentiation

Along with their lack of sensitivity to normal feedback inhibition, neoplastic cells usually display abnormal differentiation. Neoplastic cells may revert to a more primitive form that has little functional capacity beyond replication, i.e. more like a stem cell. There are three main ways in which differentiation may be abnormal.

Excessive normal function. This is particularly noticeable with tumours of hormone-secreting cells, e.g. ovarian carcinomas producing high oestrogen levels, or when an adrenal adenocarcinoma produces Cushing's syndrome. Here,

aspects of normal cellular function persist, at least at first. It may be due to an increased number of secreting cells, but insensitivity to feedback inhibition is also very important. Tumour growth may sometimes be detected and monitored by the abnormal levels of these hormones, or by their effects. Mature tumours however tend to lose this exaggerated normal function and regress.

Abnormal differentiation. The disorganization of genetic expression (abnormal repression or de-repression) may cause the cell to behave like a completely different functional type, i.e. a different phenotype. An example is the secretion of large amounts of ADH by some bronchial carcinomas. Such abnormal secretions sometimes offer an easy method of detection and objective monitoring.

De-differentiation. The most common pattern is for the neoplastic cell to exhibit no particular function whatsoever: it simply divides. Although often grossly abnormal microscopically, the tumour usually makes its presence felt clinically only by pressure of numbers. By this time it is often too late for curative treatment. Some neoplastic cells demonstrate their phenotypic regression by secreting substances that are more usually associated with the embryonic development stage, e.g. **alpha-fetoprotein (AFP)** and **carcinoembryonic antigen (CEA)**, which may

Table 10.7   Cytokinetic parameters[a] of some human tumours

Histological type	Doubling time (days)	Growth fraction (%)	Cell loss fraction (%)	Relative chemosensitivity[b]
Embryonal	25	90	90	++
Lymphoma	30	90	90	++
Sarcoma	40	10	70	–
Squamous cell carcinoma	60	25	90	+
Adenocarcinoma	80	5	70	+ or –

[a] Approximate values only.
[b] Sensitivity to cytotoxic chemotherapy: ++, very sensitive; +, sensitive; – resistant.

be measured for diagnostic or monitoring purposes.

The natural history of a tumour

Growth curve

Let us assume that a tumour starts as a single cell and continues to divide at a constant rate. Its growth can be traced by plotting its mass or cell number against time (equivalent to the number of doublings; Figure 10.9). After a slow start, possibly during the various initiation and promotion stages, growth becomes exponential (the vertical scale in Figure 10.9 is logarithmic), but the rate falls as the tumour size increases. This decrease is related to a reducing growth fraction and an increased cell loss fraction, and there may also be an increased intermitotic time. In solid tumours these factors, which often make the tumour less sensitive to therapy, result partially from relatively poor vascularization.

A vital clinical point is illustrated. The tumour mass will not reach 100 mg until after approximately 30 doublings have produced about 10^8 cells: how long this takes will depend on the doubling time. At this stage, being so small, it will usually be unnoticed by the patient. There will be no obvious or palpable ('feelable') lump, and it is unlikely to be causing symptoms, except possibly for certain hormone-secreting tumours. A mass of 100 mg is the smallest lesion that can be detected on X-ray, although more recent scanning techniques, e.g. ultrasound, CT, MRI and positron emission tomography (PET) have reduced this threshold. Nevertheless, even mass screening, were it feasible, would miss many significant, slightly smaller tumours. Yet by the 100-mg stage many tumour types will have already have metastasized.

The tumour size would have to increase a further 10-fold before becoming palpable, if it were near the body surface; even then distinct symptoms might not be noticed. Yet there are now 10^9 cells, almost certainly there has been some invasion of local healthy tissue, and some metastases are likely. The task of complete eradication is now daunting, as every one of these cells must be removed or killed, with acceptable, or at the very least, survivable damage to the healthy host tissues.

Most tumours are diagnosed in the window between 1 g and 100 g, when symptoms become troublesome. This growth pattern explains why many tumours seem to start so suddenly and

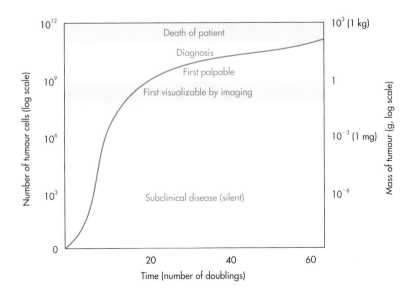

Figure 10.9   Hypothetical growth of solid tumour.

progress so rapidly. If they are not diagnosed at this stage, or treatment is ineffective, death will usually occur as the tumour burden approaches 1 kg. It can thus be seen why early detection is so important if cancer is to be treated successfully, and why successful cancer therapy is generally so difficult to achieve.

Local invasion

As a tumour grows, its bulk (a 'space-occupying lesion') puts pressure on local structures such as nerves, blood vessels, the gut lumen, etc. with predictable symptomatic consequences. Benign tumours tend to be self-contained and have definite margins, so this is their main adverse effect. Conversely, malignant tumours, partly because of their insensitivity to the presence of other cells and also because of a lower adhesiveness to their basement membrane, are far more invasive. They expand in a very disorganized way, their margin is indistinct and they cause considerable disruption to their environment.

This process is aided by the secretion of proteases (proteolytic enzymes such as matrix metalloproteinase) from tumour cells, which facilitate their passage through basement membranes and into the extracellular matrix of local connective tissue. Eventually, measurement of the activity of these enzymes might offer an estimate of prognosis, e.g. high levels may predict further growth, metastasis or relapse, and thus provide a basis for deciding if further therapy is warranted.

Metastasis

Migration of neoplastic cells away from the primary tumour to distant sites is the key stage in malignancy. Most morbidity and almost all mortality from cancer is associated with metastatic deposits. This process probably starts very early in the natural history of a tumour, and perhaps has already begun in some 50% of all cases at diagnosis. At first there may be multiple, completely undetectable **micrometastases**. These may remain dormant for variable periods before suddenly starting to grow, usually signalling a relapse. Angiogenesis is crucial to this resurgence in growth.

The mechanisms of metastasis are becoming better understood. Probably, single cells are always detaching themselves and being carried away in the blood or lymph, or are shed into a local body cavity, e.g. from abdominal epithelial tumours. Most such cells are destroyed immunologically. Inevitably, however, some will find a new site to colonize and start a new neoplastic clone; well-perfused areas like lung, liver and bone marrow are common sites.

There are two important stages: escape from the primary cell mass by a loss of adhesion, as with invasion; and arrest at a distant site. The most important **cell adhesion molecules (CAMs)** are cell surface-transmembrane molecules known as **cadhedrins**. Possibly reduced activity of these, owing to gene down-regulation, allows some cells to escape. Migrating cells then become trapped by other adhesion receptors called **integrins**, which are normally involved in localizing cells involved in defence mechanisms, e.g. leucocytes.

The rate and pattern of metastasis is partly determined by the site of the primary and its route of local invasion. For example, local lymph nodes – part of whose function it is to trap such debris – are frequent metastatic sites for many types of tumour, e.g. the axillary nodes in breast cancer. The liver is frequently involved in gastrointestinal tumours, which shed cells into the portal circulation.

Even if the pattern cannot be explained by such considerations, it is usually empirically consistent and predictable, e.g. breast cancer commonly causes bone and liver secondary tumours. Knowledge of these patterns is clearly important in treatment and prognosis. The extent of metastasis is part of the basis of 'staging' (p. 672).

Metastases usually grow considerably faster than their parent primary tumour, partly because they are smaller and thus better perfused. In patients who have been exposed to previous chemotherapy they also tend to be more chemoresistant, i.e. survivors have been selected; this is one reason why disseminated disease is more difficult to treat.

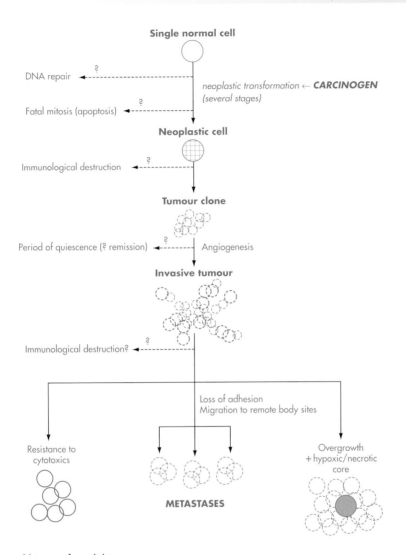

Figure 10.10   Natural history of a solid tumour.

Angiogenesis

Otherwise known as **neovascularization**, this process is vital for normal tissue expansion. As a tissue grows it requires extension of its vascular supply, and tumours, especially metastases, can hijack the process to maintain their own growth. Angiogenesis can be triggered by hypoxia or by oncogenic proteins increasing the expression of growth factor receptors on the vascular endothelium, signalling the requirement for proliferation. One such is **vascular endothelial growth factor (VEGF)** and inhibitors of this are already in clinical use.

Resistance

The longer a tumour grows, the more likely it is to develop resistance to chemotherapeutic agents. As more cell divisions occur, the chances are greater of a mutation favourable to resistance (p. 684). Another factor in resistance is the degree of vascularity.

Summary

Figure 10.10 illustrates in a diagrammatic form some important stages in the growth of a tumour.

Differences between normal and neoplastic tissues

The differences between normal and neoplastic cells and tissues can now be summarized (Table 10.8). Although some of the characteristics, especially the cytokinetics, of a given tumour may be little different from normal, taken together they render a neoplasm unmistakable. Each of these differences is a potentially target for therapeutic exploitation. They emphasize that the simplistic view of cancer as no more than 'abnormally rapidly dividing cells' is inadequate.

To illustrate this point, consider why the proliferative skin disorder psoriasis (Chapter 13) is not a neoplastic disorder. Certainly, the cycle time of the basal cells in a psoriatic lesion is much reduced compared with normal; possibly there is also a greater cell loss fraction. Clearly growth and proliferation in a hyperplastic tissue is not under full control, because it is obviously inappropriate for normal epidermal development. However, the psoriatic growth is not totally unrestrained. There remains some local inhibition because there is no invasion of the dermis. Moreover, there are no metastases, no primitive basal cell colonies in lymph nodes or bone marrow: in fact, no de-differentiated cells at all. The hyperactive basal cells do more or less what their more sedate cousins, normal basal cells, do: they become prickle cells, which move upwards through the epidermis, become keratinized, and are shed. In other words, they are normally differentiated.

Clinical features

Mechanisms of host damage

Cancer rarely kills because of a functional failure of the primary organ affected. In the case of breast cancer this is obvious, but patients with

Table 10.8 Some differences between neoplastic and normal cells or tissues

Characteristic	Normal	Neoplastic
Contact inhibition	Present	Absent or diminished
Adhesion to neighbours	Present	Diminished
Growth promotion	Controlled	Excessive, autonomous
Growth inhibition	Sensitive	Insensitive, evaded
Doubling time	Average for tissue	Low, average or high
Growth fraction	Average for tissue	Average or high
Apoptosis	Normal	Evaded
Cell loss fraction	Average for tissue	Average or high
Differentiation	Typical of tissue	De-differentiation (atypical or excess activity)
Invasion of local tissues	Absent	Usual
Spread to distant tissues	Absent	Common
Immune recognition	Normal	Reduced, evaded
Angiogenesis	Not usually activated	Activated

lung cancer do not usually die of respiratory failure and those with stomach cancer do not die from malabsorption and starvation. Certainly, malfunction of the affected organ can often cause specific symptoms (Table 10.9). However, the clinical consequences of most tumours are generally indirect, being related either to their bulk or to the invasion of local or distant tissues. There is also a diverse group of remote, obscure or secondary effects collectively termed **paraneoplastic phenomena**, some of which may be caused by toxins or other abnormal metabolites released by the tumour, e.g. TNF.

Symptoms and presentation

The range of possible symptoms from a tumour is almost unlimited. Because of variations in tumour type, size and location, cancer can mimic almost any other disease on first presentation. The classic story of a 'lump' is not the most common and, even so, lumps may be neither malignant nor even neoplastic. Pain is also an unusual first symptom. Most commonly there is a period of feeling vaguely unwell which is often associated with anorexia and recent significant weight loss.

Table 10.9   Mechanisms of host damage by tumours

Altered organ function	Example
Excessive normal	↑ Gastrin (in Zollinger–Ellison syndrome)
Diminished	Haemopoietic tumours such as leukaemia
Atypical	ADH-secreting lung tumours
Abnormal or toxic metabolites	Tumour necrosis factor
Space-occupying lesion	
Pressure on local structures	• nerves → pain • blood vessels → ischaemia, haemorrhage • gastrointestinal → obstruction • brain → neurological symptoms (central and peripheral)
Local invasion	• inflammation • ulceration • effusion (e.g. pleural, abdominal)
Metastasis: disruption at distant sites	• bone → pain, fractures, hypercalcaemia • liver → hepatic failure
Paraneoplastic phenomena	
Cachexia: debility, anorexia, wasting	
Depressed immune response	
Anaemia, fever	
Electrolyte imbalance	Hypokalaemia, hypercalcaemia
Metabolic disturbance	Hypoglycaemia
Psychological effects	

Table 10.10 lists common symptoms that may be caused by cancer. If several of these coexist, or they are persistent and unexplained by other circumstances or diseases, then the possibility of cancer must be fully investigated. The presence of known risk factors, such as age, immunodeficiency, environmental exposure, family history, sex or occupation will increase the suspicion. Many symptoms are related to the site of the primary neoplasm, but certain tumours – especially haematopoietic, bone marrow and some endocrine tumours – can cause less obvious effects. For example, different marrow neoplasms may cause aplastic anaemia, thrombocytopenia, leucopenia, etc. leading to tiredness, bleeding or infections.

Specific problems in cancer

Cachexia

The profound debility and wasting typical of advanced cancer probably has a number of causes. Various toxins, metabolites and electrolyte abnormalities, notably hypercalcaemia, contribute. These may act through anorexia, exacerbated by malabsorption and the patient's depressed mood. Very large tumours may compete with the host for nutrients. There may also be an abnormality in the regulation of metabolic rate and thermogenesis. A non-specific, hypoplastic, iron-resistant anaemia is also a common feature of many serious chronic diseases (Chapter 11). Cachexia may eventually become the predominant feature and often appears to be the main cause of death.

Psychological factors

These are significant as they undoubtedly affect the patient's response to the illness and the rigours of therapy, particularly chemotherapy. Depression is common and requires appropriate treatment. Some suffer so severely from the nausea and vomiting of chemotherapy that they decide not to continue with it, and face the consequences, although this is unusual nowadays with the advent of more effective anti-emetic treatments (see Chapter 3).

Psychological factors may significantly affect the course and severity of the disease and thus have a bearing on management. Some of the

---

Table 10.10 Warning signs of cancer. The list of signs and symptoms Cancer Research UK recommends people look out for, which might suggest cancer. If persistent and unresponsive to normal treatment, medical advice should be sought

---

A new or **unusual lump** or **swelling** anywhere on your body

A **sore** that will not heal, anywhere on your body or in your mouth

A change in the shape, size or colour of a **mole**

Blood in your urine or bowel motions

A **cough**, croaky voice or difficulty swallowing that lasts longer than **4 weeks**

A change to looser or more frequent **bowel motions** lasting longer than **4–6 weeks**

Difficulty passing urine

Unexplained **weight loss**

Bleeding from the vagina after the menopause or between periods

Unexplained pain or ache that lasts longer than **4 weeks**

Source: http://info.cancerresearchuk.org/healthyliving/signsandsymptoms (accessed March 06)

successes of 'natural' healing methods may be explained in this way. There is evidence that personality can have an effect on outcome, bearing out the common empirical observation that a positive outlook and 'will to live' may promote longer remissions or even full recovery.

One interesting study compared the psychological profiles and outcomes of therapy in a group of women who all had breast cancer at a similar stage and received similar treatment. Those who responded to the original diagnosis by aggressively 'fighting' the tumour had the better survival, while those who were overwhelmed and surrendered did worst. Perhaps surprisingly, those who reacted with 'stoic acceptance' did almost as badly as the overwhelmed group, while 'denial' was almost as favourable as aggression. The conclusions of this study have been challenged. It has also been pointed out that to imply to patients that a positive fighting spirit is essential for recovery may be counterproductive in some patients, who suffer feelings of inadequacy and failure if they do not improve.

All such considerations must be subsumed by the global assessment of patients' quality of life with or without treatment.

Pain

This is far less consistent a feature of cancer than is commonly imagined. Most patients with solid tumours experience pain at some time, but many have either little pain or pain only for short periods. Although pain remains the most feared symptom, modern methods of pain control (see Chapter 7), with their emphasis on active prophylaxis, mean that no patient need suffer unduly, and about one-third of cancer patients never experience pain. The origin of cancer pain is usually direct pressure on nerve endings, or the result of the compression against bones causing entrapment neuropathies. Compression within bones from metastases is often one of the most intractable forms. There may also be direct stimulation of nerve endings by toxins or abnormal metabolites. Hypercalcaemia is a common feature of many tumours, and this may also cause or exacerbate pain; optimal treatment currently utilizes bisphosphonates and rehydration.

Death

The causes of death from cancer are poorly understood. The immediate terminal event may be heart failure, respiratory failure or 'multiorgan failure' but this does not really explain the process. Failure of the organ primarily affected by the tumour is rarely responsible. Often, death seems to be the end result of prolonged cachexia, which makes the patient more susceptible to a variety of secondary illnesses, especially overwhelming infection. Immunosuppression is a feature of many cancers.

Investigation and diagnosis

The diagnosis of malignancy is ultimately histological. However, the whole panoply of modern investigative techniques are exploited. The aims of investigation may include:

- screening;
- locating a suspected lesion;
- obtaining a biopsy and characterizing it;
- 'staging' the illness;
- monitoring the patient's progress.

Screening

Although early detection is highly desirable if the tumour is to be treated effectively, most cancers will have already grown to about 75% of their fatal size before symptoms become apparent. Thus, it might then seem that extensive mass screening should be implemented. However, cost-effectiveness and the potential problems of the anxiety and unnecessary treatment resulting from false-positives have limited the trend.

Nevertheless, screening techniques are becoming increasingly reliable and are starting to make a substantial impact. For certain tumours they are now regarded as highly beneficial in identifying disease at an early stage. Programmes currently operating successfully include breast screening by mammography and Papanicolaou cervical histology smears. In Japan, gastroscopy is helping to detect gastric carcinomas earlier. Colon cancer screening (detecting faecal occult blood) has been implemented in the UK in 2006, and prostatic cancer screening for older men (detecting prostate-specific antigen, PSA) is undergoing trials. Intensive screening of high-risk groups such as those with a cancer family history is also being evaluated.

One of the limitations of some programmes is their failure to reach the most at-risk groups. However, there is no doubt that overall these programmes have saved many lives, prevented much suffering and obviated much treatment. Perhaps a fuller understanding of the aetiology of various tumours is required before prevention becomes more generally feasible. Even so, the experience with smoking and lung cancer unfortunately suggests that even positive proof of causation is no guarantee that the public, industry or governments will react appropriately.

Imaging

Some form of imaging is almost always carried out, depending on the suspected location of the lesion. Techniques used include radiology, ultrasound, CT, MRI, radioisotope scanning, thermography and fibre-optic endoscopy. The increasing sensitivity of modern techniques permits the identification and location of ever smaller lesions, but at present the visualization of micrometastases is not feasible.

Characterization

Biopsy and histological examination are essential to the diagnosis of cancer. Access to biopsy specimens increasingly uses minimally invasive methods such as fibre-optic endoscopy, possibly linked to keyhole laparascopic surgical techniques, e.g. for the gastrointestinal, urinary, genital and respiratory tracts, whereas in the past exploratory major surgery was required, e.g. laparotomy. The histological appearance of the cells will indicate the tumour type, tissue of origin (e.g. epithelial or germ cell), degree of differentiation and extent of dysplasia. From this the seriousness of the condition can be estimated, how advanced it is, its propensity for metastasis, and its likely response to different forms of therapy.

Tumour markers

The presence and extent of the tumour may sometimes be indicated indirectly by the plasma levels of certain specific markers that they produce. Embryonic and fetal substances (e.g. AFP, chorionic gonadotrophin) can be measured by radioimmunoassay. An elevated level of normal hormones from endocrine tumours, such as thyroxine from thyroid or, indirectly, pituitary tumours, or ectopic hormones, e.g. ADH from lung cancer, can readily be quantified.

Staging and monitoring

Staging, which is an attempt to quantify the severity of a tumour, is essential following diagnosis. Although detail varies from tumour to tumour, in general the following qualitative system can be applied to most tumours:

- Stage 1. Tumour confined to original site, with no local invasion (in situ).
- Stage 2. Local invasion.
- Stage 3. Spread to local lymph nodes.
- Stage 4. Metastasis in distant sites.

A more rigorous method, which allows progress or response to therapy to be quantified, is the so-called 'Tumour/Node/Metastasis' or TNM system, where the size of the primary tumour, the extent of local lymph node involvement and the presence of metastases are determined.

The stage of a tumour has implications for the choice of therapy, for prognosis and for monitoring. For example, the involvement of tissue outside the original mammary lump in breast cancer indicates the extent of surgery required. The 5-year relative survival for Stage 1 cervical cancer (i.e. relative to comparable women without cancer) is 80%, while for Stage 4 it is less than 10%.

Prognosis

Despite sophisticated investigative techniques, empirical and epidemiological means are still important in estimating prognosis. Clinical experience has shown that most primary tumours have a characteristic natural history. Their rate of growth, the degree, rate and pattern of metastatic spread, and their sensitivity to certain types of therapy and even to specific drugs, can often be predicted on this basis.

From these data, and depending on the stage that a patient's tumour has reached, estimates of the prognosis can be made in the form of median survival figures, i.e. 50% of patients at that particular stage usually survive 6 months, 5 years, etc. This is the origin of the frequently heard but misguided assertions such as 'the doctors gave him only 6 months to live' – these claims often prefacing enthusiastic but naïve accounts of 'miracle cures'.

Management: aims and strategy

The three priorities in dealing with cancer are, in order of importance:

- Prevention.
- Early detection.
- Total eradication.

In most cases these are as yet largely unrealized ideals. Our incomplete knowledge of the causes of most cancers, coupled with inadequate screening, usually rule out the first two priorities. Smoking and lung cancer is potentially a major exception. For breast cancer, various preventative techniques including reduced-fat diets (to minimize oestrogen production) and prophylactic *tamoxifen* (an anti-oestrogen) have been advocated, but evidence is lacking. Screening was discussed above (p. 671).

Modern management is ensuring the third priority is increasingly achieved. Once diagnosed, the ideal treatment would remove or kill every neoplastic cell, because in theory even a single remaining cell could generate a new neoplastic clone. However, current methods of therapy still do not in the majority of cases permit this without unacceptable, even fatal, damage to the patient. On the other hand, when a tumour mass is reduced below a certain size the patient's immune system, by analogy with microbial infections, may mop up the remainder; thus complete eradication by therapy may not in fact be

required. However, it must also be remembered that the immune system in cancer sufferers might well have been compromised by the chemotherapy or the disease itself, and neoplastic cells may escape immune recognition.

Aims

When therapy is contemplated there must be a careful and realistic identification of the therapeutic goals. These may be considered in a hierarchy (Table 10.11). The success of treatment is usually measured in terms of timed survival, i.e. the proportion of patients still alive after a given period. A greater than 75% survival rate at 5 years is now achievable for several cancers.

Realistic assessment
The most appropriate level in this hierarchy for a given patient will depend on the nature of the tumour, the stage of the disease, and clinical experience. The risks of untreated disease (the prognosis) and the potential benefits of treatment (the likelihood of a response) must be balanced objectively against the predictable risks of treatment, e.g. adverse drug effects. This evaluation must be made in consultation with the patient and his or her family.

The term 'cure' is relative: it can never be certain that all metastatic cells have been eliminated. As yet, it can be claimed for only a small number of cancers that a large proportion of patients survive

Table 10.11   Hierarchy of aims in cancer management

1. Prevention	
2. Cure	Eradication of tumour and metastases
3. Remission/mitigation ('response')	Significant reduction in tumour load Increased survival
4. Symptomatic/palliation	Treatment of secondary complications Relief of symptoms
5. Terminal care	Improve quality of life Optimize symptom control

to an extent comparable with disease-free individuals of similar ages. These include testicular teratoma, chorionic carcinoma, some childhood leukaemias, and Hodgkin's lymphoma. A significant proportion of breast, colorectal and some lung cancers can also be cured.

For most treatment regimens in the majority of malignancies, induction of remission, i.e. a response, is the most realistic goal. The aim is to reduce significantly the number of neoplastic cells and hence the bulk of the tumour. In this way patient survival may be improved and symptoms usually reduced. In some tumours, particularly if far advanced at presentation, even this cannot be expected. The aim then is simply palliative, i.e. to deal with any secondary effects that may be causing the patient pain, distress or other serious symptoms. For example, partial surgical excision may reduce pressure on local nerves or blood vessels, or relieve gastrointestinal obstruction.

Terminal care and quality of life

Finally, if treatment fails, strenuous efforts are still made to ensure that the patient's remaining life is as comfortable as possible, with optimal symptom control, optimal nutrition, counselling, attention to psychosocial and spiritual needs, etc. Increasing importance is being attached to the quality of the patient's life with or without therapy. For some patients with advanced disease, even heroic treatment, necessitating mutilating surgery or serious adverse drug effects, may produce only a moderate improvement in survival. In the past there might have been unrelieved therapeutic efforts of increasing harm until the patient's death was often secondary to the adverse effects of the therapy, such as overwhelming infection or haemorrhage. However, cancer teams are now more realistic and accord the patient a peaceful, dignified and pain-free end: much depends on the attitudes and wishes of the patient and, perhaps, their family.

Modes of therapy

The method of treatment will largely be determined by a realistic assessment of the therapeutic goal. The usual modes are:

- Surgery (excision of primary tumour).
- Radiotherapy.
- Pharmacotherapy (cytotoxic chemotherapy, endocrine therapy, biological therapy, immunotherapy, gene therapy).

If neoplasms were always benign, simple surgical removal would suffice. Unfortunately, malignant neoplasms invade the tissues surrounding them, making it difficult to determine accurately how much tissue to remove. Furthermore, complete surgical removal of widespread metastatic deposits ('secondaries') is not practicable; besides, many are microscopic and cannot be identified by present techniques. Thus, surgery alone is rarely adequate and some additional form of 'mopping up' of potential secondaries is usually necessary. This is termed **adjuvant therapy**.

The type of adjuvant therapy used depends partly on the likely distribution of presumed secondaries. Local invasion and lymph node spread can be treated by radiotherapy. For disseminated disease, drugs are more suitable because of their potential to reach most tissues in the body. Indeed, for most tumours this is the main role of drug therapy, although in some cases it is the chosen primary therapy. It may also be used before surgery to debulk (reduce in size) the tumour, limiting the extent of surgery required and its potential disfigurement. This is termed **neoadjuvant chemotherapy**.

Three other factors govern the choice of treatment. The first is the evidence base and derived guidelines. The second, especially where guidelines do not exist, is clinical experience: some tumours are known to be particularly radioresistant; others are chemoresistant, etc. The third involves practical considerations (Table 10.12).

Surgery

Surgery is usually the most appropriate treatment for solid tumours in sites where it would neither threaten a vital function nor be too mutilating, and where reconstruction is possible. However, surgery may inadvertently facilitate metastatic spread, displacing tumour cells and liberating them into the local circulation or lymph. Where

---

Table 10.12   Factors governing the choice of treatment in cancer

Surgery	Well-defined solid tumour
	Non-vital region, e.g. mastectomy
	Non-mutilating result, e.g. unsuitable for some head and neck tumours
	Resection/reconstruction possible, e.g. gut
Radiotherapy	Diffuse but localized tumour, e.g. lymphoma
	Vital organ/region, e.g. head and neck, CNS
	Adjuvant therapy, e.g. post-mastectomy
	Palliation
Pharmacotherapy	Firm evidence base
	Adjuvant therapy following surgery or radiotherapy
	Neo-adjuvant therapy prior to surgery or radiotherapy
	Combination with radiotherapy (chemoradiation)
	Widely disseminated/metastasized (Stage 4)
	Diffuse tumour, e.g. leukaemia
	Some primary tumours, e.g. Hodgkin's lymphoma
	Palliation

---

lymphatic dissemination is known to occur as part of the natural history of the tumour, local lymph nodes, which may have trapped potential metastasizing cells, are also excised; breast cancer is a prime example. Such **radical surgery** is becoming less common nowadays with the advent of the 'multimodal' approach (below). In some cases it is not appropriate at all.

Radiotherapy

Radiotherapy is suitable as primary therapy in some local tumours when surgery is inappropriate. Other common applications include adjuvant therapy for diffuse local spread, e.g. after mastectomy or lumpectomy for breast cancer, and de-bulking palliative treatment for inoperable tumours. Radiotherapy may be administered externally as high-energy ionizing radiation, or systemically by radioisotope administration, e.g. oral radioiodine [^{131}I] for thyroid tumour, or implantation, e.g. intrauterine radiocaesium [^{137}Cs] needles for cervical cancer.

Radiotherapy is often seriously damaging to normal tissue, and strategies have been devised to minimize collateral damage, some of which are analogous to ways of reducing drug toxicity discussed below. These include fractionating the dose and highly specific targeting, which has become much easier with improvements in imaging.

Pharmacotherapy

The ideal antineoplastic drug would have completely selective toxicity for neoplastic cells, just as antimicrobial agents are toxic to microbial but not human cells. Unfortunately, save for one minor exception (the utilization of *crisantaspase* by some leukaemic cells; see below), human neoplastic cells do not differ in any qualitative biochemical way from normal cells.

Thus other, usually quantitative, differences between normal and neoplastic tissue have to be exploited. These occur in several broad areas:

- Neoplastic tissues have different growth parameters, which are amenable to **cytotoxic** intervention.
- The growth of some neoplasms is sensitive to natural **hormones** and other **growth factors**.
- Cell signal transduction pathways are activated to a different (greater or lesser) degree in neoplastic cells; these processes can be selectively modified by **biological** agents including cytokines.

- Genomic expression may be inappropriate in neoplastic cells, making them targets for **gene** therapy and **biological** agents that interfere with gene expression.
- Neoplastic cells may express a different immunological phenotype, making them a target for **immunological** agents.

At present, owing to rapid developments in novel targeted agents, the terminology of anti-neoplastic agents is in flux and needs refinement. It is usual to distinguish the traditional relatively unselective cytotoxic agents, which act on nucleoprotein within the nucleus, from newer biological agents that act primarily on cell signalling and cytokines within the cytoplasm or on the cell surface. The former kill cells, hence the name **cytotoxic**; the latter tend to be **cytostatic**, inhibiting further growth but not necessarily killing the cell. The parallel with antimicrobial therapy, with its bactericidal and bacteriostatic agents, is again an instructive analogy. Consequently biological agents tend to have fewer severe side-effects on normal cells. However, many do affect both neoplastic cells and healthy bone marrow cells and some retain conventional cytotoxic action. For consistency the terminology of the list above is followed here.

Cytotoxic chemotherapy

As experience with chemotherapeutic agents and knowledge of cytokinetics increase, more potential roles are found for cytotoxic chemotherapy. Chemotherapy in solid tumours was once restricted chiefly to adjuvant therapy, following reduction of the main bulk of the tumour surgically or by radiotherapy. In particular, it is felt that micrometastases, some of which are possibly induced surgically, can be destroyed in this way. The other traditional place of chemotherapy was as a desperate last measure in uncontrolled and widely disseminated disease after the failure of surgery and radiotherapy. Small wonder that it gained a poor reputation ('hard cases make bad law'). Nevertheless, effective palliation may be possible even in such circumstances.

However, intensive chemotherapy at an earlier stage in the disease, perhaps in association with radiotherapy, can be a highly effective treatment of first choice in certain conditions, such as choriocarcinoma, leukaemia and testicular cancer. Many other tumours are now known to be chemosensitive and chemotherapy is now widely used with increasing success.

Endocrine therapy

Tumours in hormone-dependent tissues, particularly genital tumours, may be inhibited if their growth factors are blocked or antagonized. This is the basis of endocrine therapy. It has the advantage of low systemic toxicity, but because it is cytostatic rather than cytotoxic it can only arrest a tumour or minimize metastasis. Therefore it tends to be used as an adjuvant following tumour minimization by other modes. In this role it can substantially prolong remissions, e.g breast cancer.

Biological, gene and immunotherapy

The greatest successes of recent research have been in this area. As the genomic, intracellular and intercellular controls over cell growth are elucidated, new therapeutic targets become evident and attempts can be made to design appropriate drugs. Such methods are now becoming more widely recognized and recommended, in some cases as primary monotherapy, e.g. *imatinib* in CML.

Multimodal therapy

Adjuvant and neoadjuvant therapy are examples of multimodal therapy. Cancer therapy usually involves a combination of different modalities. One may be used to reduce the bulk of the tumour and another to attempt to eradicate the remainder of the neoplastic cells or prevent the development of metastases. Increasingly, surgery is shown not to be essential at all. For example, the current recommended first-line treatment of anal cancer involves combined radiation and cytotoxic chemotherapy (**synchronous chemoradiation**). Another example is the combined use of biological and cytotoxic agents.

It would be satisfying if the theoretical principles discussed above, when applied rationally to the selection of drugs, produced a high rate of cure in the majority of tumours. Alas, this is not yet true. Certainly the prognosis has improved steadily over the past 20 years and for some cancers 5-year survival is better than 75% (Figures 10.1–10.4). While it is difficult to estimate overall survival for all cancers as a whole, it is clear that there is still a long way to go before we can claim to have 'conquered cancer'. There is still much to be learned about the behaviour and kinetics of neoplastic cells and the design of antineoplastic drugs.

Cytotoxic chemotherapy

Most cytotoxic drug regimens in current use have been devised empirically. Nevertheless, careful application of what knowledge we do have of the behaviour of cancer cells will maximize the chances of success, and this section will illustrate the theoretical basis of common practice in cytotoxic chemotherapy. The combination with other modes of drug therapy will be reviewed later.

Role

Until the introduction of chemotherapy, the sole means of treatment were surgery and radiotherapy, and the prognosis for cancer had improved little in 100 years. Then in the mid-1980s chemotherapy, and more recently screening programmes, started to make an impact, and substantial improvements in survivial were attained.

The high failure rates prior to chemotherapy were usually the result of relapses. Even the most radical surgery or radiotherapy, while it may eliminate the primary tumour, cannot affect metastases. Eventually, in most cases, these metastases brought about a relapse and the resultant widespread dissemination was inoperable. Thus the most that could be expected was remission: cure was generally impossible. Adjuvant chemotherapy has brought about significant improvements in cancer survival rates because of its ability to reach disseminated micrometastases.

Chemotherapy has been gradually refined by:

- Optimization, e.g. combination therapy, dose scheduling.
- Strategies to minimize toxicity.
- Development of more potent and less toxic agents.
- Controlled clinical trials and evidence-based medicine

Nowadays, the prognosis for a small number of malignancies, especially leukaemia, where the growth fraction is high, is excellent. For some others it has improved significantly, e.g. the cure rate for the rare Wilm's renal tumour was only 20% before chemotherapy but now is 80%. Because leukaemia represents no more than 10% of all tumours, such successes have had only a small impact on overall survival. The outlooks for breast and colon cancer have also improved. Yet many malignancies, particularly solid tumours with low growth fractions, remain resistant.

The relative chemosensitivity of common tumours is given in Table 10.13. One potential avenue to explore is a means of assessing the *in vivo* sensitivity and resistance of tumours in individual patients to specific antineoplastic agents, in a manner analogous to antimicrobial sensitivity testing.

Theoretical basis

Two theoretical principles underlie cytotoxic therapy:

- Tumours are often more sensitive to agents that interfere with the biochemistry of cell division, a greater proportion of neoplastic cells being affected than those in normal tissue.
- Tumour tissue usually does not recover as rapidly as normal tissue from such interference.

Cytokinetic differences probably account, in part, for these observations. The first confers a degree of selectivity to cytotoxics; the second limits their toxicity. These differences may be exploited and enhanced clinically, pharmaceutically and pharmacologically by variations in

Table 10.13   Chemosensitivity of different tumours

Very sensitive (usually responsive)	Leukaemias	• chronic lymphoid
		• acute childhood
		• myeloid
	Lymphomas (Hodgkin's, Burkitt's)	
	Choriocarcinoma	
	Testicular teratoma	
	Embryonal tumours	
Fairly sensitive (often responsive)	Breast	
	Ovarian	
	Prostatic	
	Head and neck	
	CNS	
	Lung (rarer 'small cell' form)	
Relatively insensitive (occasionally responsive)	Uterus	
	Skin (melanoma)	
Insensitive (rarely responsive)	Kidney and bladder	
	Liver and pancreas	
	Colorectal cancer	
	Gastric carcinoma	
	Lung ('non-small cell')	

dose scheduling, route of administration, drug combinations, etc.

Selective sensitivity

One reason for the greater sensitivity of neoplastic tissue to cytotoxic action is that it often has a higher growth fraction. There may also be a shorter doubling time, a higher cell loss fraction, or both. The central problem of cytotoxic therapy is that normal bone marrow contains stem cells with comparable growth characteristics to the tumour cells, and so may be affected similarly. (This characteristic is exploited therapeutically when using cytotoxic drugs as immunosuppressants.) Less vital tissues similarly at risk are the gut lining and hair follicles.

Thus bone marrow suppression (**myelosuppression**) is the main constraint on cytotoxic chemotherapy, and most regimens are designed with a view to circumventing or minimizing it. Fortunately, there are often significant quantitative differences between the marrow and tumour stem cell populations. Although marrow stem cells when cycling have a shorter doubling time than many tumours, 80% are usually in the comparatively resistant G_0 resting phase, so bone marrow has a low growth fraction. It also has a low cell loss fraction. Thus, a single dose of a drug has a disproportionately greater effect on the tumour cell population.

Relative recovery

The slow recovery of tumours is partly because resting tumour cells are recruited more slowly into the cycle. The normal response to the death of a substantial number of cells in a tissue is the recruitment of resting stem cells to replenish the deficit. However following cytotoxic damage, tumour doubling time is not markedly reduced, whereas bone marrow tissue recovers, i.e. repopulates, much more rapidly.

Bone marrow recovery
The average lifespan of different blood cells, which is related to the turnover time of their precursors in the marrow, is given in Table 10.14.

Table 10.14	Average lifespans of blood cells
Neutrophils	24 hours
Platelets	7 days
Lymphocytes	Various subpopulations: 10–50+ days
Erythrocytes	120 days

From this it can be seen that if there is a total marrow failure, resistance to infection would be diminished within a few days and coagulation would be compromised within a week but, should the patient survive, anaemia would take 1–2 months to develop. However, if damage is partial, stem cells are rapidly recruited from the resting (G_0) compartment, the doubling rate is accelerated, and ill-effects are minimized. Three weeks is usually sufficient time for marrow recovery following chemotherapy with most agents in most patients. However, this can vary considerably and treatment is closely monitored by frequent blood counts, and levels are allowed to return to normal before the treatment is continued. Different considerations usually apply to haematological malignancies.

Pulsed therapy

Because of the need for time for bone marrow recovery, a typical course of chemotherapy is usually given as a series of cycles of treatment, each of which involves intensive treatment over a few days followed by a rest period. The duration of each cycle of treatment varies considerably depending on the regimen, but is usually 14–28 days, the precise figure being determined empirically in clinical trials.

Figure 10.11 shows various possible outcomes to pulsed therapy depending on the choice of dose, duration of treatment and tumour resistance. One of the many problems of chemotherapy is judging when the tumour has been eradicated. Most commonly, empirical judgements are made on the basis of clinical experience. Alternatively, extrapolations can be made from the rate of response while the tumour was still detectable. This may present the dilemma of having to recommend further treatments with highly toxic drugs,

knowing that for those patients who have already been cured (or responded maximally) these will be superfluous, probably unpleasant and possibly harmful.

Some regimens use a continuous course of therapy rather than pulsing, and this is facilitated where oral administration is possible, e.g *capecitabine* plus *tegafur* in colorectal cancer. *Fluorouracil* is sometimes given as a continuous infusion over a cycle of treatment. In other cases, especially using biological agents, long-term therapy is used, e.g. *imatinib* in CML. These continuous treatments may be combined with pulses of other agents.

Proportional kill effect

Pioneer work on tumour cytokinetics in mouse leukaemia, which is a useful model system because the growth fraction approaches 100%, established two further fundamental principles:

- Cell killing by cytotoxic drugs follows first-order kinetics: the proportion of cells killed varies with the dose, so that higher doses increase the fractional rather than the total kill.
- A viable tumour can develop from a single neoplastic cell.

Thus, equal doses of drugs kill equal proportions of cells. If a certain dose reduces a tumour population from 10^8 to 10^6 cells, the same dose will, in further reducing the size to 10^4 cells, kill a much smaller absolute number of cells. The same dose is needed repeatedly, no matter how small the tumour has shrunk, until every last tumour cell is killed or the tumour mass is small enough to be eradicated by the immune system. This is illustrated schematically in Figure 10.12.

Action

There are two important aspects of the action of the cytotoxic drugs: the biochemical mode of action (pharmacological classification) and the cell cycle phase or phases when active (cytokinetic classification). Both of these guide the design of effective synergistic combinations.

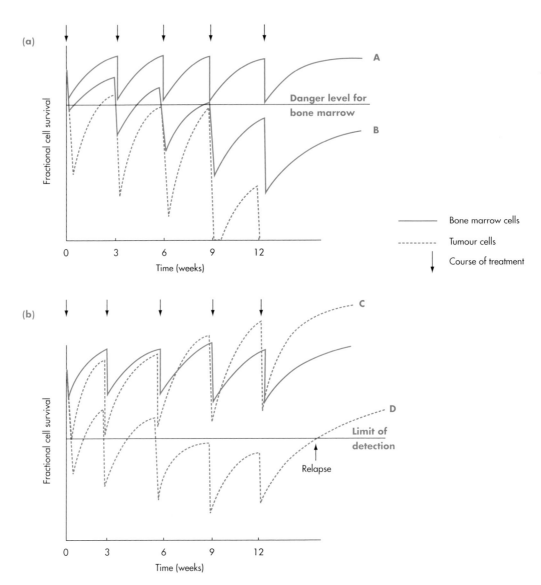

Figure 10.11   Pulsed therapy with marrow recovery phase. (a) Successful tumour eradication, but with differential effect on bone marrow. The figure shows the theoretical effect (expressed as fractional survival) of repeated doses of a cytotoxic regimen on tumour and marrow cell populations. Curve A shows successful chemotherapy: the marrow recovers to give acceptable peripheral blood counts after each treatment while the tumour is progressively reduced. Curve B shows what would happen if the treatment required to reduce the tumour cell population adequately was too intense, so that the cumulative effects produced dangerous marrow depression. (b) Different types of unsuccessful chemotherapy. Curve C shows inadequate dosage; although the bone marrow is spared the tumour regenerates between treatments. Curve D shows what happens if, once the tumour is reduced below the detectable size, treatment is stopped prematurely; eventually there will be a relapse.

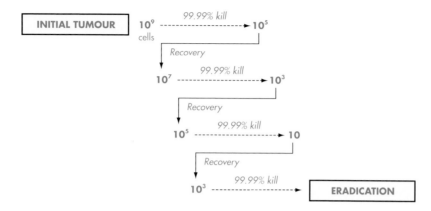

Figure 10.12   Proportional kill effect. The figure shows the theoretical result of successive doses of a particularly effective drug regimen that kills 99.99% of all cycling tumour cells. A reduction in tumour cell number from an initial 10^9 cells occurs after every treatment. However, during the delay between treatments (necessary for marrow recovery) the tumour partially regenerates.

Mode of action

Almost all cytotoxic drugs act within the nucleus to kill cells by interfering with the production or structure of nucleic acid, or occasionally protein. Cell death following exposure to cytotoxic action (and to radiation) is due to the triggering of apoptosis (p. 661).

Cytotoxic drugs are usually classified according to what is believed to be their biochemical mode of action (Table 10.15). The stages in the biochemical sequence of mitosis at which they act are shown schematically in Figure 10.13. Note that additive or synergistic effects might be expected from logical combinations of agents from different groups, combining cytotoxics of different actions and combining cytotoxics with biological agents.

Phase of action

Because the various reactions with which cytotoxics interfere occur at different phases in the cell cycle, different drugs may act at different phases (Table 10.16; Figure 10.14). Unlike most other cytotoxics, **non-specific agents**, e.g. *chlormethine*, act equally on cycling stem cells and non-dividing cells (stem cells resting in G_0 and non-stem cells). Thus, they are highly toxic to normal tissue and are little used nowadays. **Cycle-specific agents**, which potentially act on all phases of cycling cells, but not resting cells, are probably the largest group and generally the most useful. However, the **phase-specific agents**, acting at one particular phase, have uses if appropriately exploited.

Exploiting cytokinetic differences
The full potential of these differences has yet to be realized, but there have been a number of interesting approaches.

Synchronization.   This involves using drugs that arrest the cell cycle at a certain stage, e.g. *dactinomycin* arrests progress from G_1 to S phase; radiotherapy may be used similarly. The drug is then withdrawn and the accumulated cells, which are suddenly 'unblocked', progress to the next phase simultaneously. A drug acting at that next phase is then given, e.g. an antimetabolite acting at S phase. If tumour cells have a different intermitotic time from marrow cells, appropriate timing of the second drug should achieve some selectivity. A further intriguing possibility is to synchronize all marrow cells, and then use an agent that acts at a different phase, thus providing a measure of protection for bone marrow. Conversely, bone marrow colony-stimulating factors (p. 691) might be exploited in leukaemia for their potential to increase the proportion of chemosensitive blast cells in

Table 10.15   Biochemical mode of action of some cytotoxic drugs

Action	Group	Examples
Alkylating agents (cross-link DNA)	Alkyl sulphonate	Busulfan
	Chloroethylamine	Chlorambucil, melphalan, cyclophosphamide, ifosfamide
	Nitrosourea	Lomustine, carmustine
	Heavy metal agent	Cisplatin, carboplatin, oxaliplatin
Antimetabolites (impair nucleotide base incorporation into DNA/RNA)	Purine analogue	Mercaptopurine, tioguanine, cytarabine, fludarabine, cladribine
	Pyrimidine analogue	Fluorouracil, capecitabine, gemcitabine, tegafur
	Antifolate	Methotrexate
	Thymidylate inhibitor	Pemetrexed, ralitrexed
Topoisomerase inhibitors	Camptothecin	Topotecan, irinotecan
	Anthracycline antibiotic	Doxorubicin, daunorubicin, epirubicin, mitoxantrone
	Podophyllotoxin	Etoposide, teniposide
Miscellaneous DNA-RNA inhibitors		Dactinomycin, hydroxycarbamide
DNA scission		Bleomycin
Mitotic spindle inhibitors (tubulin-binding)	Vinca alkaloid	Vincristine, vinblastine
	Taxane	Paclitaxel, docetaxel
Precursor depleter	Enzyme inhibitor	Crisantaspase (asparaginase)
Photosensitizer		Porfimer, temoporfin
Uncertain action	Corticosteroid[a]	Prednisolone

[a] Only cytotoxic in very high doses, possibly by protein synthesis inhibition; lympholytic in leukaemias.
Drugs may act by several mechanisms; it is not always certain which action is responsible for clinical effect.

Table 10.16   Cytokinetic classification of cytotoxic drugs

Phases in which active	Class	Examples
Resting (G$_0$) plus all cycling cells	Non-specific (Class I)	Chlormethine
Cycling cells only		
• certain phases only	Phase-specific (Class II) see Figure 10.14	Antimetabolites Vinca alkaloids Podophyllotoxin Hydroxycarbamide Crisantaspase Taxanes Bleomycin
• all phases	Cycle-specific (Class III)	Alkylating agents Anthracyclines Platinum agents Corticosteroids(?)

Note common synonyms: phase-specific = 'cell cycle stage-specific' (CCSS or CCS); cycle-specific = 'cell cycle stage non-specific' (CCSNS or CCNS).

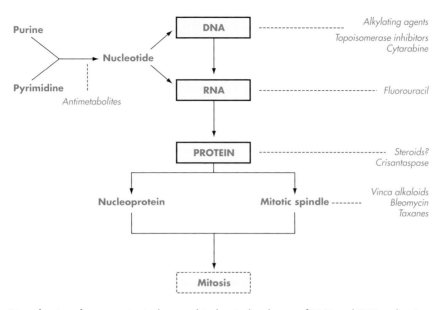

Figure 10.13   Sites of action of some cytotoxic drugs on biochemical pathways of DNA and RNA replication and mitosis.

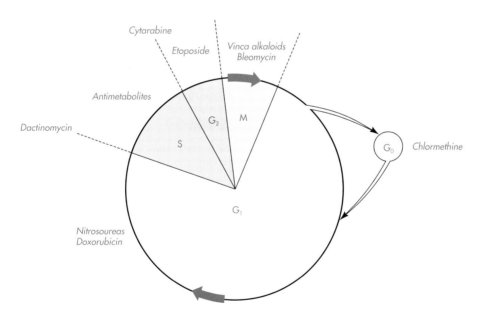

Figure 10.14   Phases of action of some phase-specific cytotoxic agents (Class II).

the marrow by stimulating them to leave the chemoresistant G_0 phase.

Recruitment. Synchronization would have only a limited impact on tumours with a low growth fraction. Instead, a cycle-specific agent might be used to kill all cycling cells; subsequently, many resting cells return to the cycle to be killed by the next treatment. However, this approach is limited by the fact that resting marrow stem cells are also recruited and may eventually be similarly depleted or even eliminated. There have also been experiments in following DNA production through the cell cycle by labelling it with precursor analogues (e.g. *bromodeoxyuridine*) that can be detected by monoclonal antibodies ('flow cytometry'); this could potentially identify which phase a cell is in.

Although some success has been reported with such techniques, e.g. in leukaemia, the difficulty of ascertaining the detailed cytokinetics of tumour cells in specific patients, and the fact that cell populations tend to lose any imposed synchrony, limits their present application.

Differences in dose–response and toxicity

The cytokinetic classification of drugs given above is an oversimplification. Some phase-specific drugs are found to act at more than one phase, and some cycle-specific agents act predominantly at one or two phases only. A distinction of more practical use between the two main classes (II and III, Table 10.16) is made on the basis of their dose–response curves; this also helps ensure their optimal use. Although both classes need to achieve a minimum threshold plasma level, the consequences of further dose increases vary according to the class.

Phase-specific drugs (Class II). Both the therapeutic effect (i.e. the tumour cell kill) and the toxicity (i.e. the marrow cell kill) of this class depend mainly on the duration of therapy, i.e. they are 'schedule dependent'. This is because the dose–response curve rapidly approaches a plateau as all cells in the affected phase are killed by a single dose (Figure 10.15). Continued therapy would then kill cells that had initially been at other phases as they come round to the affected phase. As a result, more cells are recruited from the resting compartment. This process can be exploited to maximize tumour cell kill. However, therapy prolonged beyond one or two neutrophil stem cell cycle times (24–36 h) may prove disastrous as it will deplete the bone marrow stem cell reserve. This is the main constraint when class II drugs are used either alone or in combination. On the other hand, a single very large dose will not be dangerous because the plateau will already have been reached and no further damage, even to the bone marrow, will be possible.

Cycle-specific drugs (Class III). Because these drugs act on all phases, their dose–response curve does not plateau: it is exponential for both tumour and bone marrow (Figure 10.15). Hence, both effectiveness and toxicity are 'dose-dependent', and optimal tumour cell kill is achieved with a single high dose. There is no need to prolong treatment to wait for cells to complete the cycle. However, too high a dose of this class of drug causes excessive myelosuppression. Moreover, if two members of this class are combined the effects will be additive and the toxicity increased, so the doses of each must be reduced.

Non-specific drugs (Class I). With this class of drugs there is very little difference between the effects on bone marrow and on tumour cells (Figure 10.15). Thus, they are potentially very toxic and not used unless absolutely necessary.

Resistance

Development

Although the lack of biochemical specificity is one major drawback with cytotoxic chemotherapy, the development of resistance (i.e. an unusually low tumour responsiveness) is equally important. Theoretically, as long as the tumour remains sensitive, suitable adjustment of dosage should preserve marrow function. However, once resistance develops, the chances of a cure diminish rapidly and when the tumour becomes multi-resistant the therapeutic options become very limited (Figure 10.16).

Unless all tumour cells are killed, resistance will almost invariably develop eventually. Consequently, treatment should be aimed at prompt eradication by early detection and aggressive therapy. Treatment within the 'therapeutic window' before the development of resistance has the best chance of success (Figure 10.17).

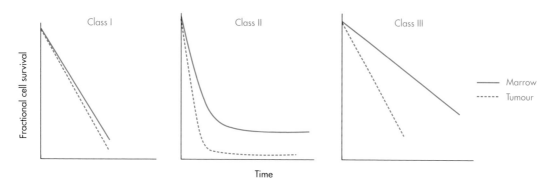

Figure 10.15   Dose–response curves for different cytokinetic classes. Class I drugs (non-specific) show little selectivity for tumour cells and so have a relatively high marrow toxicity. Class II drugs (phase-specific) have non-linear dose–response and dose–toxicity curves, so doses above the minimum effective level are not useful, but prolonged therapy will be. For Class III (cycle-specific) drugs, very high doses may be tolerated, but may not need to be repeated.

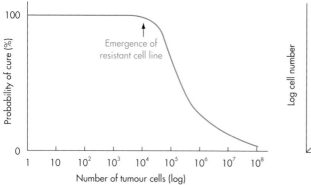

Figure 10.16   Potential survival in relation to tumour cell number. The figure illustrates how the chances of survival fall rapidly once drug-resistant cells have emerged in a typical tumour.

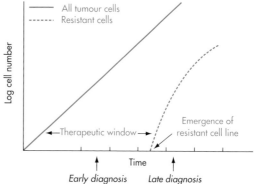

Figure 10.17   Therapeutic window before resistance develops. In most primary tumours there will at first be no resistant cells and early diagnosis and treatment during this phase has the greatest chance of effecting a cure. At some stage, resistant cells emerge and if diagnosis is late there will already be a significant population of resistant cells, dramatically reducing the chances of successful therapy.

Causes

In general, resistance is due either to extra-cellular circumstances that limit drug access to the tumour, or to intracellular pharmacological or biochemical factors that antagonize cytotoxic action (Table 10.17); the latter situation resembles antimicrobial resistance. One of the main aims in devising drug regimens is to prevent or circumvent resistance. Recent studies on the *p53* gene have suggested that treatment resistance may in some cases be associated with

defects in this gene, possibly because cytotoxic drug-induced apoptosis is prevented.

Extracellular resistance

Inappropriate dose scheduling or unwanted interactions may result if cytokinetic factors are not considered. For example, a *methotrexate/crisantaspase* combination is of reduced efficacy because the former arrests cells at the G_1–S boundary, preventing the action of the latter in the S phase. (This is analogous to the potential

Table 10.17 Possible causes of resistance to cytotoxic chemotherapy

Extracellular factors	Drug interaction
	Incorrect/inappropriate dosage schedule
	Immune clearance of antigenic drugs
	Poor access to tumour; sanctuaries
	Poor penetration of tumour
	Low tumour growth fraction, large G_0 compartment
Intracellular biochemical factors	
Quantitative	Reduced cellular uptake
	Increased efflux pump activity
	Reduced prodrug activation
	Increased activity in affected pathway
	Alternative pathway used (block bypassed)
	Increased receptor specificity
	Increased repair of DNA damage
Qualitative (? genetic)	Production of dummy or excess substrate
	Production of drug inhibitors
	Drug inactivation

antagonism of bactericidal antimicrobials by bacteriostatic ones.) Dose spacing that ignores cell cycle times may also reduce effectiveness.

Poor tumour perfusion owing to inadequate vascularization is probably one of the main causes of the resistance of solid tumours to chemotherapy. Poor drug distribution or penetration to micrometastases within **sanctuaries**, e.g. in the brain owing to the blood–brain barrier, also account for some treatment failures. Many of these factors can be minimized by attention to pharmaceutical, pharmacokinetic and cytokinetic aspects of the treatment regimen, e.g. giving a drug intrathecally as 'CNS prophylaxis' in leukaemia if it does not cross the blood–brain barrier.

Intracellular resistance

Neoplastic cells demonstrate a remarkable ability to develop protective mechanisms against cytotoxic drugs. This is one of their few differences from normal proliferating cells, but unfortunately bone marrow cells generally do not become resistant. In some cases cells are intrinsically resistant from the outset. Otherwise, resistance may develop as a result of the increased

mutation rate associated with rapid turnover aided by the inherent mutagenic action of most cytotoxic drugs themselves. Alternatively there may be adaptive changes in metabolism. One adaptation is to produce an excess of the drug's target molecule or a dummy target, in effect mopping up the drug. Chemotherapy exerts a selection pressure that favours the proliferation of resistant cells at the expense of the non-resistant cells, as with antibiotics on microorganisms.

The mechanisms adopted by the tumour cells are often quantitative rather than qualitative metabolic changes, i.e. an inhibited pathway may be avoided or an alternative pathway upregulated. This may be stimulated by negative or positive feedback. For example, normal DNA autorepair mechanisms may be accelerated to make good any damage. Alternatively, chance novel genetic changes may allow the production of specific inhibitors, antagonists or deactivating enzymes.

The principal therapeutic strategies adopted to prevent or overcome resistance are the use of combination therapy in adequate dosage and a prompt change to different drugs when resistance is suspected.

Multiple drug resistance

An individual cell is highly unlikely to develop multiple resistance by several discrete mutations, yet resistance to a range of structurally unrelated cytotoxic agents is quite common and is an extremely serious constraint on chemotherapy. The recent discovery of a non-specific membrane efflux pump for toxins (known as p-glycoprotein or MDR protein) may provide a clue. This appears to pump drugs such as *etoposide, vincristine* and the anthracyclines out of cells. The *mdr* gene coding for this pump has been found in normal cells, and it is presumably expressed when protection is needed from environmental toxins. In multiresistant tumours it may be over-expressed.

Maintenance therapy and resistance

It is instructive to compare pulsed therapy (p. 703) with earlier approaches that were originally modelled on antimicrobial chemotherapy, this being the only model available for early oncologists to emulate. Tumours were then believed to differ from normal tissue exclusively by a more rapid turnover of all cells: at the same time, the toxicity of the cytotoxic agents was greatly feared. The strategy at that time was to attempt to achieve a 'minimum inhibitory concentration' with a single drug, i.e. a constant plasma level that caused minimal toxicity. This was maintained until symptoms disappeared or the tumour was no longer detectable.

We now know that such a regimen would merely keep the tumour at bay and the patient asymptomatic. Eventually, as with antimicrobial therapy, resistance developed (Figure 10.18). A second drug was then used in the same way, and so on, until eventually all possibilities were exhausted and the patient succumbed. Nevertheless, there were a few successes, particularly with leukaemia. Such a strategy is still used for a few tumours that are difficult to eradicate but rarely become resistant. This strategy is also used with schedule-dependent drugs (e.g. *fluorouracil* by continuous IV infusion in colorectal cancer, oral *capecitabine* in breast cancer), but usually in combination with other drugs to limit resistance.

Side-effects

The high incidence of severe adverse effects is another important limitation to the success of cytotoxic chemotherapy.

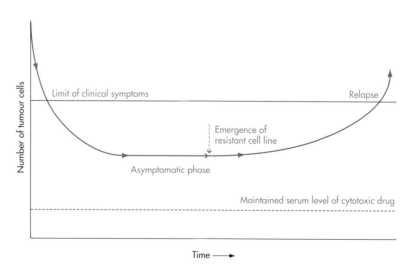

Figure 10.18   Maintenance therapy and resistance. This illustrates the possible effect of maintaining a single cytotoxic drug continuously at a level sub-lethal to tumour cells. Initially the tumour responds, and symptoms disappear, but resistance eventually develops.

Classification

Side-effects can be considered in three main groups (Table 10.18). Almost all agents cause a similar range of cytotoxic and mutagenic effects, a class action that is a direct result of their intended pharmcodynamic action, i.e. impaired cell division. However, the intensity and rate of onset vary between drugs: some are known to be potent myelosuppressants, others frequently cause hair loss, etc. A third group comprises the specific idiosyncratic adverse actions of individual drugs. Examples of the clinical consequences of these toxicities are summarized in Table 10.19.

Cytotoxic action

Myelosuppression. Although bone marrow has a smaller growth fraction than most tumours, the intermitotic times of cycling marrow stem cells are usually much shorter. Thus, the marrow is extremely chemosensitive and almost all cyto-toxics affect it to some extent. There are two general patterns. Most drugs cause rapid falls in peripheral blood count with a nadir for white cells and platelets at 7 days. A few, however, have a more profound but delayed action, with a nadir at 28 days, e.g. nitrosoureas, *melphalan*. There is also a variation in the intensity of the myelo-suppression, e.g. *chlormethine* almost always produces profound falls, *vincristine* has relatively little effect and *bleomycin* (uniquely) almost none.

Different blood cell populations start to decline at different rates depending on the average lifespan of the cells (Table 10.14). The neutrophil count falls first because this is the most labile population with an average life of a day. Platelets are next short-lived. The comparatively long life of RBCs ensures that anaemia from cytotoxic therapy is rare. Lymphocytes are a very heterogeneous population, about which generalizations are not reliable.

Leucopenia (reduced white cell count), especially neutropenia (reduced neutrophils), results in immunosuppression and frequent infections, primarily bacterial. Leucopenia exacerbates the underlying immunodeficiency found in most cancer patients. Thrombocytopenia (reduced platelet count) impairs coagulation, leading to bruising and bleeds, a particular problem because many of these drugs also ulcerate the GIT. Pulsed therapy courses usually do not produce significant anaemia unless prolonged; a notable exception is when platinum-containing agents are used.

Table 10.18   Side-effects of cytotoxics

Cytotoxic action – killing of normal dividing cells

Myelosuppression
Epithelial damage
  • GIT (esp. mouth, colon)
  • urinary bladder
  • hair
  • skin
Infertility (esp. males, esp. alkylating agents)

Mutagenic action – effects of DNA damage

Teratogenicity
Genomic damage
Carcinogenesis

Miscellaneous

General (many or most cytotoxic drugs)
  • emesis
  • extravasation
  • dangers of handling (preparation, reconstitution)
Specific to particular drugs
  • Organ systems: e.g. heart, liver, kidney, lungs, bladder, etc. See Table 10.19.

GIT, gastrointestinal tract.

GIT and bladder. The intermitotic time in gut epithelial cells is not much greater than in bone marrow. Thus, erosion and ulceration are very common, especially in mucous membranes, causing mouth ulcers or diarrhoea, for example. Certain drugs similarly affect the bladder epithelium, causing haematuria. Although usually less serious than myelosuppression, such symptoms may be more immediately disturbing for the patient.

The most common gastrointestinal effects, nausea and vomiting, are not the result of direct cytotoxic action (see below).

Skin and hair. The intermitotic time of skin basal layer cells is about 20 days, and so consid-

Table 10.19   Side-effects of cytotoxic drugs and their clinical consequences

Organ/system affected	Clinical effect	Examples[a]
Bone marrow	Immunosuppression Bleeding Anaemia	Almost all[b]
Chemoreceptor trigger zone	Nausea and vomiting[c] • mild • moderate • severe	 Fluorouracil, methotrexate, etoposide, vinca alkaloids Doxorubicin, cyclophosphamide, high-dose methotrexate Cisplatin, dacarbazine, high-dose cyclophosphamide
GIT	Oral mucositis; ulceration; diarrhoea	Many
Metabolic	Hyperuricaemia; gout; nephropathy	Many
Nervous system	Neuropathy – cranial, autonomic, peripheral	Vincristine
Heart	Cardiomyopathy	Doxorubicin
Liver	Cirrhosis, fibrosis	Methotrexate
Kidney	Nephrotoxicity	Cisplatin
Bladder	Haemorrhagic cystitis	Ifosfamide
Lungs	Pulmonary fibrosis	Bleomycin, methotrexate
Hair follicles	Alopecia	Many

[a] Only limited representative examples given here; see References and further reading.

[b] A few agents have mild or almost absent myelosuppression, especially bleomycin, vincristine.

[c] Occurs to some extent with most cytotoxic drugs; see BNF, Section 8.1.

GIT, gastrointestinal tract.

erably greater than that of marrow; thus serious problems are rare. However, hair loss is quite common and although reversible it is one of the most distressing medium-term complications, especially for women. Regrowth is usually complete once treatment has finished, but the new hair is often subtly different in texture or colour.

Fertility. Spermatogenesis is inhibited and sometimes there may be permanent male infertility, especially from the alkylating agents. Female infertility is less common.

Mutagenesis

Most cytotoxic agents act by damaging DNA, and the effect of the resultant change in the genome depends on whether somatic or germ cells are affected.

Teratogenic action. Cytotoxics are particularly hazardous during the first trimester of pregnancy, i.e. during organogenesis, and the risk seems to be greatest for *methotrexate* and the alkylating agents. There may be spontaneous abortion, prematurity, gross deformity or delayed growth. However, the absolute risk is surprisingly low, and in the later trimesters the risk:benefit ratio, evaluated in consultation with the patient, may favour continuing with therapy. For women of child-bearing age, strict contraceptive precautions are advisable if chemotherapy is planned.

Genomic damage. Heritable defects may be caused if the DNA of spermatozoa or ova is damaged, although most mutations are lethal for the cell. Even exposure *in utero* may affect germ cells, only to be manifested in the subsequent generation. These risks have yet to be fully assessed but are avoided by strict contraception during treatment.

Carcinogenesis. Cytotoxic drugs are one of the many groups of potentially carcinogenic mutagens. Thus neoplastic transformation may, paradoxically, result from cytotoxic therapy, e.g. a second malignancy following *etoposide* therapy. Radiotherapy, which likewise damages DNA, has also been associated with an increased incidence of neoplasms, e.g. up to 2% of ankylosing spondylosis patients treated with X-rays may develop a neoplasm. The long lag time between carcinogenic exposure, mutation and the clinical manifestation of a tumour means that these effects may have been obscured in the past.

Patients on long-term immunosuppressive therapy similarly have a small increased risk of neoplasms, e.g. lymphomas in post-transplant patients treated with *ciclosporin*. This suggests that another possible mechanism for cytotoxic-induced neoplasia is impaired immunosurveillance. Nevertheless, the risk seems to be small. Confirmed cases are few and there is currently no alternative to treating the first tumour as effectively as possible. Patients who achieve long-term survival after successful chemotherapy, e.g. following childhood leukaemia, need careful long-term monitoring for subsequent tumour development that is unrelated to the original disease.

Miscellaneous

Nausea and vomiting. The occurrence of profound nausea, retching and vomiting is what many patients most fear and loathe about chemotherapy. The emetogenic potential of different cytotoxic agents varies considerably (Table 10.19). The effects may last for several days after treatment, are depressing and debilitating, and may even dissuade some patients from continuing with therapy. The symptoms originate partly from direct stimulation of the CTZ (p. 108), which understandably identifies these drugs as highly dangerous and rejects them. There is probably also a local reaction to the damaging effect of cytotoxics on the gastrointestinal epithelium, mediated by 5-HT, which stimulates the CTZ humorally and via nerve endings in the gut.

Modern treatment of nausea and vomiting has substantially reduced the severity and frequency of this problem. Consequently, the 'anticipatory vomiting' occasionally experienced by some patients immediately before their next treatment is rarely seen now.

Other effects. Each drug or group of drugs has its own characteristic adverse effects on major organ systems. Some important examples are given in Table 10.19. A knowledge of these effects is essential in designing cytotoxic combination therapy, to ensure that no one organ system is overexposed to toxicity.

Secondary hyperuricaemia can occur when the large number of cells killed during treatment release nucleic acid bases that are then degraded to produce an excess of uric acid. This can cause gout and uric acid nephropathy (stones), and is most common in the treatment of lymphomas and leukaemias. Treatment of bone tumours (usually metastatic deposits) may release large amounts of calcium, causing hypercalcaemia.

Cytotoxic solutions require care in handling by health workers as they are mutagenic, and some are highly irritant. They are usually reconstituted centrally by hospital pharmacy departments under strict asepsis using laminar flow isolator hoods. For similar reasons, serious local damage to the patient may occur with many cytotoxics if an IV becomes extravasated during administration.

Minimizing side-effects

Numerous strategies have been devised to reduce the damage done to normal tissues by cytotoxic drugs (Table 10.20). The aims are either to reduce discomfort, morbidity or mortality, or to increase the tolerable dose threshold and thus the dose that can be used. Close monitoring is extremely important, especially frequent full blood counts. Other investigations will depend on the

Table 10.20   Strategies for minimizing side-effects of chemotherapy

Side-effect	Method of minimization	Example
Myelosuppression	Transfusions	Blood, platelets Granulocytes Marrow or peripheral stem cells
	Growth factors	Lenograstim, epoietin
	Dose scheduling; careful monitoring	
	Isolation of patient in sterile environment	
Nausea and vomiting	Anti-emetics	
	• 5-HT$_3$ antagonists	Ondansetron
	• dopamine antagonists	Domperidone, prochlorperazine
	• neurokinin inhibitor	Aprepitant
	• cannabinoids	Nabilone
	• benzodiazepines	Lorazepam
	• corticosteroids	Dexamethasone
	• hypnosis; suggestion; relaxation therapy	
Mucositis; mouth ulcers	Oral hygiene	Mouthwashes Palifermin (keratinocyte growth factor)
Subfertility	Sperm banking; in vitro fertilization	
Hyperuricaemia		Allopurinol, rasburicase; hydration
Hypercalcaemia (bony metastases)		Furosemide, hydration
Cardiomyopathy	ECG monitoring	
Hepatotoxicity	Liver function tests (pre and post)	
Nephrotoxicity	Hydration and forced diuresis	
Haemorrhagic cystitis	Hydration and forced diuresis Eliminate bladder-irritant toxic metabolites	Mesna (for ifosfamide and cyclophosphamide)
Alopecia	Minimize systemic access of drugs to scalp Wig	Scalp tourniquet or chilling (ice cap)
Anti-folate induced GI distress/ myelosuppression	Bypass folic acid synthesis block	Folinic acid 'rescue' (for methotrexate)

5-HT$_3$, 5-hydroxytryptamine$_3$

known particular toxicities of the drugs used, e.g. ECG, neurological or liver function tests, etc.

Prevention

Unfortunately, myelosuppression can rarely be completely avoided but is minimized by allowing adequate time for marrow recovery between treatments. Stem cell growth factors, e.g. granulocyte colony-stimulating factor (G-CSF, *filgrastim*),

may be given with chemotherapy to selectively enhance neutrophil proliferation. *Epoetin* can be used for anaemia and *thrombopoietin* is under development for platelets. These agents must be used with caution and close monitoring in haematological tumours, e.g. leukaemia, to avoid stimulating tumour cells.

Forced diuresis is routinely given with nephrotoxic and bladder-toxic drugs to reduce contact time and the urine concentration of drugs. This involves modest over-hydration before therapy followed by a diuretic to maintain a high urine output for at least 24 h following therapy. An osmotic diuretic (e.g. *mannitol*) is preferable to loop diuretics, which are frequently nephrotoxic (e.g. *furosemide*). The haemorrhagic cystitis caused by *cyclophosphamide* and *ifosfamide* is due to the metabolite acrolein, which can be rendered harmless by complexation with *mesna* given concurrently.

No universally effective anti-emetic regimen has been devised (Table 10.20; see also Chapter 3). Some patients seem to benefit more than others, and the emetogenic potential of cytotoxic drugs varies. Delayed reactions are especially difficult to prevent and treat.

Metoclopramide at conventional doses is a dopaminergic antagonist, but when given in high doses acts partly by antagonising 5-HT receptors in the gut and the CTZ. This led to a significant advance in the development of specific 5-HT$_3$ antagonists, e.g. *ondanseteron*, *granisetron*. This group is currently the most effective available and their efficacy is enhanced by combination with corticosteroids. They are now used routinely as first-line anti-emetics with moderately or severely emetogenic cytotoxic regimens.

Dopamine antagonists act both locally and on the CTZ. Traditionally the less potent antipsychotic phenothiazines have been used as anti-emetics, e.g. *prochlorperazine*. *Metoclopramide* has more anti-emetic activity than antipsychotic but still can cause extrapyramidal symptoms or excessive sedation. However, *domperidone* is a dopamine antagonist that does not cross the blood–brain barrier, thereby avoiding these unwanted effects.

Adjuvants that do not have significant anti-emetic action alone but enhance the action of others include benzodiazepines and corticosteroids, or both. Benzodiazepines cause sedation and short-term amnesia, which tends to minimize anticipatory vomiting, and steroids have an additional euphoriant effect. The most recently developed adjuvant is the neurokinin inhibitor *aprepitant*. Cannabinoids have not lived up to their early promise.

Remedy or palliation

Patients who are severely neutropenic, thrombocytopenic or anaemic may be given cell-specific haemopoietic infusions. The short half-life of neutrophils limits their value in this form, but packed platelets and packed RBCs are used routinely.

Autologous bone marrow replacement, in which the patient's marrow is harvested before therapy, is being supplanted by autologous peripheral bone marrow stem cell replacement. In this, the source is the small number of marrow stem cells normally found in blood. This procedure is simpler and engraftment is quicker.

Ingenious ways have been devised to treat the stored marrow stem cell before re-injection, in order to eradicate contaminating neoplastic cells, especially in leukaemias or lymphomas. For example, monoclonal antibodies to receptors expressed on normal immune cells but not neoplastic ones can be used to facilitate their separation. Allogeneic (heterologous) bone marrow transplants from closely matched donors are mainly used in the treatment of leukaemia but may also be used to treat iatrogenic myelosuppression.

Infections in the profoundly immunosuppressed, e.g. after bone marrow transplantation, can be minimized by reverse barrier nursing in sterile conditions. Pharmaceutically, this means that clean precautions have to be observed and original packs used for all drugs.

The use of *folinic acid* salts permits the administration of high doses of *methotrexate*, subsequently 'rescuing' the patient's marrow and other tissues after an appropriate time when a maximal differential neoplastic cell kill has been achieved. In a more general application of the same principle, patients with resistant or widely disseminated disease may be given massive dose chemotherapy, which would normally be fatal owing to myelosuppression. However, patients are subsequently rescued by colony-stimulating factors that promote renewed marrow stem cell activity. This obviously high-risk strategy is only justifiable in certain cases.

For some patients, iatrogenic diarrhoea is antagonized by the opioid analgesics taken for pain control.

Endocrine therapy

The growth of certain tissues, especially the sex organs, is hormone-dependent. In effect these hormones play an analogous role to growth factors in cellular growth, as described above. By manipulating hormone levels the growth of tumours derived from such organs can be reduced, provided that they are still sufficiently differentiated to respond, i.e. they retain hormone receptors.

The effect is cytostatic, suppressing further growth rather than killing cells. Thus, although endocrine therapy can rarely be curative it can provide valuable remissions or can be combined with other treatments to improve their effectiveness. In certain cases (e.g. breast cancer) the remission can be sufficiently long to be classed as a cure. Endocrine therapy may also enable cytotoxic therapy to be avoided or delayed in slowly growing tumours. Further, because metastases usually (but not always) have a similar sensitivity to the primary tumour, this treatment can also be used for disseminated, inoperable disease or to delay the development of secondaries following resolution of a primary tumour. Again this may amount to a cure.

Originally, either the gland secreting the hormone was surgically removed, e.g. the ovaries (oophorectomy), or else a hormone with a naturally antagonistic action was administered, e.g. androgens to women. More recently, specific synthetic antagonists have been developed (Table 10.21) that have far less drastic adverse effects than surgery. Most therapy is based on normal endocrine actions but some is partly empirical. This is especially so in breast cancer and is also evident in the widespread use of corticosteroids. These findings suggest that knowledge of normal hormonal mechanisms is inadequate.

The discussion below briefly outlines the principles of this approach. However, the precise details for different tumours are open to frequent change as evidence mounts and guidelines change. Therefore it is as usual important always to check the latest guidelines.

Table 10.21   Hormone manipulation to influence tumour growth

Strategy	Target hormone	Treatment examples	Tumour
Block synthesis	Steroid	Aminoglutethimide, anastrozole, letrozole	Breast
Block secretion	Androgens	Surgery – orchidectomy	Prostate
	Oestrogens	Surgery – oophorectomy	Breast, uterus
	Steroids	Surgery – adrenalectomy	Breast
	Pituitary hormones	Surgery – hypophysectomy	Breast
	?	High-dose corticosteroid	Various
	Prolactin	Bromocriptine	Breast
	Luteinizing hormone	Gonodotrophin-releasing hormone analogue – goserelin, buserelin	Prostate, breast
	Thyrotropin	Levothyroxine	Thyroid
Block receptor	Anti-androgen	Cyproterone, flutamide, bicalutamide	Prostate
	Anti-oestrogen	Tamoxifen	Breast
Down-regulate	Anti-oestrogen	Fulvestrant	
Physiological antagonism	Androgens	Testosterone	Breast
	Oestrogens	Diethylstilbestrol	Prostate, breast[a]
	Progestogens	Medroxyprogesterone	Uterus, breast[a]

[a] Primarily postmenopausal women.

Thyroid cancer

Levothyroxine has a dual role in patients with disseminated disease for whom thyroidectomy and radio-iodine have proved inadequate. It serves as replacement therapy and also inhibits pituitary secretion of TSH, which may otherwise promote metastatic growth.

Prostate cancer

In advanced disease prostatectomy is of limited value. The surgical techniques originally used to reduce androgen output included orchidectomy (castration), adrenalectomy or hypophysectomy (excision of the anterior pituitary) with predictable serious adverse endocrinological and psychological consequences.

Today 'chemical castration' with progestogens (e.g. *medroxyprogesterone*), anti-androgens (e.g. *cyproterone, flutamide*) or, more rarely, oestrogens (e.g. *diethylstilbestrol*) would be preferred. Subsequently, steroid synthesis inhibitors (e.g. *aminoglutethimide*) can be used. Exogenous corticosteroid therapy is then also needed, to prevent reflex ACTH hypersecretion from overcoming the block and to provide the additional advantage of maintenance corticosteroid replacement. Anti-oestrogens (e.g. *tamoxifen*) have also sometimes been successful. Analogues of gonadotrophin-releasing hormone such as *goserelin* and *buserelin* (Table 10.21) have a paradoxical long-term suppressant effect on natural luteinizing hormone release, thus inhibiting prostatic growth. Cytotoxic therapy, e.g. *docetaxel*, may also have a role, especially if endocrine therapy has failed.

Uterine (endometrial) cancer

Progestogens are used on the assumption that an imbalance between oestrogen and progestogen stimulation, with an excess of the former, may promote endometrial hyperplasia. This has led to some success with metastatic disease.

Breast cancer

Increasing research effort is being directed to finding causes and satisfactory treatments for this, the most common female tumour and the second most common overall cause of cancer death. This complex and much debated topic can only be touched on here and the reader is referred to the References and further reading section for details.

Nearly every mode of endocrine therapy imaginable has been tried, including both oestrogens and anti-oestrogens (Table 10.21). Treatment is usually given as adjuvant therapy following lumpectomy and/or radiation, but maintenance and palliative therapy of metastatic disease are equally important. As with prostatic cancer, the trend is first to use chemical rather than surgical (neo-adjuvant) techniques. Nevertheless radical surgery, e.g. oophorectomy, adrenalectomy or hypophysectomy, is still used in the last resort.

Some idea of the complexity of the problem with breast cancer is seen by considering that oestrogens may induce breast cancer in premenopausal women but inhibit it in the postmenopausal: yet the anti-oestrogens are the most successful agents among the latter group. The explanation lies partly in the fact that after the menopause the adrenals and other tissues still synthesize small amounts of oestrogen so that *tamoxifen*, aromatase inhibitors or adrenalectomy are still useful. Furthermore, in some cases, when a particular hormone therapy stops being successful, withdrawing it will continue the positive response.

Undoubtedly the most useful advance has been the discovery of the importance of oestrogen receptors (ER) in tumour tissue. Found in about 60% of cases (ER+), the presence of these receptors favourably predicts both response to endocrine therapy and prognosis, possibly because such tumour cells are not too regressed. Thus, hormone modulation should be considered in all ER+ patients. Other criteria that determine the suitability and likely success of endocrine therapy include age, menstrual status and the stage of the tumour. Endocrine therapy is most successful in early, localized tumours but may also be helpful as palliative treatment in advanced cases.

Promising results have been reported recently from a US trial of *tamoxifen* for breast cancer prophylaxis in high-risk women (i.e. older age, family history, etc.), although the early cessation of this trial because of its apparent success has been felt in the UK to have prejudiced its overall power.

Corticosteroid therapy

Steroids are used in a wide variety of cytotoxic and endocrine regimens. In addition to useful endocrine activity, they have beneficial effects on some complications and some direct anti-tumour action (Table 10.22). Usually, very high doses are needed but often only for a short time, so that adverse effects are limited.

Other pharmacotherapy

Pharmacotherapy could be optimized if means could be found to limit the action specifically to tumour cells, wherever they were. An early example of targeting was the use of *diethylstilbe-* *strol diphosphate* in the endocrine therapy of prostatic cancer. This ester is an inactive prodrug, allowing high doses with minimal systemic feminizing effects. It is only activated by dephosphorylation within the tumour cells because they have higher concentrations of alkaline phosphatase than normal cells; this releases the oestrogenically active drug, which inhibits prostatic growth. The development of the newer biological therapies continues this concept of exploiting potential biological or biochemical differencies between normal and neoplastic cells.

Biological therapies

Theoretical basis

Following discoveries in molecular biology about the control of cell cycle events it became clear that certain signalling pathways controlling growth and differentiation were excessively activated in various tumours. Although these pathways are part of normal cell growth, and as such are to a certain extent present in all dividing cells including in the bone marrow, they are relatively more prominent in neoplastic cells. This is analogous to the partial selectivity conferred on cytotoxic drugs by the higher growth fractions

Table 10.22   Uses of corticosteroids in cancer therapy

Anti-inflammatory	Symptomatic relief
Euphoriant	Symptomatic relief
Appetite stimulant	
Enhance anti-emetic therapy	
Reduce hypercalcaemia	From bone secondaries
Inhibit secretion of pituitary hormones	ACTH, GTH
Depress DNA/protein synthesis	Antitumour (cytotoxic?) action
Depress haemopoietic cell activity	Antileukaemic action
Inhibit damage from oedema around tumour	e.g. CNS tumours/secondaries; gastrointestinal obstruction

ACTH, adrenocorticotrophic hormone; CNS, central nervous system; GTH, gonadotrophic hormone.

or reduced recovery rates of tumour masses. However, with signalling the disproportion between normal and neoplastic cells seems to be considerably greater, resulting in greater potential selectivity. To further enhance the targeting, many of the agents developed are humanized monoclonal antibodies aimed at specific elements of these signalling processes.

Other characteristics of tumours, such as their propensity to migrate and to encourage neovascularization, are also controlled by similar signalling mechanisms.

Biological therapies offer an increasingly promising line of approach because of the possibility of attaining the holy grail of cancer therapy, i.e. agents that exclusively target neoplastic cells. Few are yet in general use, but many are being investigated. Agents currently available in the UK are listed in Table 10.23 and discussed below; the sites of action of some are

shown in Figure 10.19. Most are used in combination with conventional cytotoxic drugs but some are used as monotherapy.

Sites of action

Growth receptors

By analogy with hormone dependency in genital tumours, the growth of tumours may be dependent on or stimulated by growth factors. In this case the stimuli are not systemic hormones but cytokines. These factors are secreted disproportionately in some neoplastic cells, or their membrane-bound receptors are up-regulated. In up to a third of breast cancers the epidermal growth factor receptor HER2 is amplified. Stimulation of this receptor leads to the expression of an oncogene that promotes further cell and tumour growth, but it can be selectively blocked by the monoclonal antibody *trastuzumab*. The

Table 10.23   Properties of some biological antineoplastic agents

Molecular target class	Receptor	Drug	Action	Indication[a]	Marrow[b] suppression	Route
Interleukin, cytokine		Aldesleukin	Cytostatic	Renal cell carcinoma	Yes	Inj.
		Interferon α,β	Cytostatic	Lymphoma, leukaemia	Yes	Inj.
Growth factor inhibitor	VEGF	Bevacizumab	Cytostatic	Colorectal	Yes[c]	Inj.
Growth factor receptor blocker	HER2	Trastuzimab	Cytostatic	Breast cancer	Yes[c]	Inj.
	EGF	Cetuximab	Cytostatic (cytotoxic?)	Colorectal	No	Inj.
	Retinoid X	Bexarotene	Cytotoxic	Lymphoma	No	Oral
Proteosome inhibitor		Bortezomib	Cytotoxic	Myeloma	Yes	Inj.
Protein-kinase inhibitor	BCR-ABL tyrosine kinase	Imatinib	Cytotoxic	Chronic myeloid leukaemia	Yes	Oral
Lymphocytolytic		Rituxumab, alemtuzumab	Cytotoxic	Lymphoma, leukaemia	Yes	Inj.

VEGF, vascular endothelial growth factor; EGF epidermal growth factor; HER2, human epidermal growth factor receptor 2; BCR-ABL, abnormal tyrosine kinase fusion protein, found in chronic myeloid leukaemia.

[a] Current data; check for recent changes.

[b] Yes = significant, no= not serious.

[c] In combination with cytotoxics.

effect is cytostatic rather than cytotoxic but it can lead to significantly extended remission. A similar effect is seen in colorectal cancer with the epidermal growth factor (EGF) receptor, which can be blocked by *cetuximab*. In cutaneous T-cell lymphoma, *bexarotene* blocks the retinoid X growth receptor.

Despite their selectivity the possibility of bone marrow depression and immunosuppression remains and close monitoring is essential, particularly because experience with long-term use is limited.

Intracellular signalling

Figure 10.19 shows that the signal generated by the stimulation of a cell surface growth factor receptor must be transmitted through the cytoplasm to the nucleus to bring about expression of the gene coding for growth mechanisms. Interfering with signal transduction and second messengers, e.g. protein kinases, offers a method of interfering with gene expression. Protein kinase inhibition has yielded one of the most successful agents to date, *imatinib*. This targets the anomolous protein kinase Bcr-Abl, which is produced as the result of the mutation causing CML. *Imatinib* has transformend the prognosis of CML and is far less toxic than the previous first-line treatment, *interferon alfa*. It is also used in certain gastrointestinal tumours. Similar agents include *erlotinib* for non-small cell lung cancer and *sunitinib* for renal cell cancer.

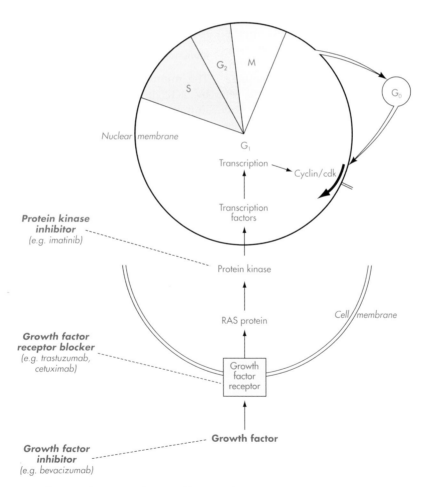

Figure 10.19 Sites of action of some novel targeted biological agents. cdk, cyclin-dependant kinase; M, mitotic phase; G_1, first gap phase; S, synthesis phase; G_2, second gap phase. ‖ Restriction- or check-point.

Angiogenesis

Another approach derives from the observation that many tumours secrete vascular endothelial growth factor (VEGF), a natural stimulant of the development of new capillaries. *Bevacizumab* is a monoclonal antibody against VEGF, denying the growing tumour or its metastases the nutrition essential for further growth. Angiogenesis also facilitates metastatic spread though the circulation so this approach can also limit metastasis. Currently it is used in colorectal cancer. Natural angiogenesis inhibitors such as *angiostatin* and *endostatin* are also being investigated.

By targeting the **proteosome**, the organelle responsible for disposing of effete protein, it is possible to disrupt a number of vital intracellular processes and induce apoptosis. *Bortezomib* is used in multiple myeloma.

Proteases are secreted by tumours to disrupt the extracellular matrix and so promote local invasion, angiogenesis and migration to distant sites. Unfortunately, no matrix metalloproteinase inhibitors (MMPIs, e.g. *maramistat*) have yet proved clinically useful. In order to escape the primary tumour, neoplastic cells must evade cellular adhesion molecules (CAMs and cadherins) tending to hold them to their tissue of origin, and this is an active area of research.

Immunotherapy and gene therapy

Neoplastic transformation involves genetic changes. This change in the genotype, as well as being directly responsible for the changes in growth pattern, may cause tumour cells to differ immunologically from normal cells. For example, they may express abnormal or 'non-self' surface antigens or fail to express 'self' antigens. Indeed, many potential tumours may normally be aborted by immune mechanisms for this reason (p. 652). This suggests a variety of possible therapeutic approaches (Table 10.24), most of which are still experimental. The idea of using the body's own defence mechanisms was perhaps anticipated by George Bernard Shaw's prescient exhortation in The Doctor's Dilemma to 'stimulate the phagocytes'.

Immunotherapy

The immune system could be manipulated either by actively stimulating it or by developing immunoactive substances such as antibodies or immune cells specific for tumour cells (passive immunization; see Chapter 2).

One radical approach being investigated is to infect tumour cells with **'oncolytic'** viruses that

Table 10.24   Potential immunological and genomic treatments for cancer

Method		Example
Immunotherapy		
Active	Non-specific immunostimulation	BCG (Bacillus Calmette-Guérin)
		Levamisole
		Interferon
		Interleukins
	Specific immunostimulation	Killed tumour cells
		Transfected tumour cells
Passive		Monoclonal antibodies
		Polyclonal antibodies
		Sensitized lymphoid cells
Gene therapy		
Immunotherapeutic agent production or stimulation	Implant HLA gene	
	Implant cytokine gene	Interleukin, tumour necrosis factor
Altering neoplastic genotype	Suppress or cancel oncogene	Antisense oligonucleotides
	Replace defective tumour suppressor gene	

selectively damage neoplastic cells rather than normal ones, owing to the defective defences and repair mechanisms of the former.

A vaccine that activates a cell surface molecule on breast cancer cells, making them more susceptible to immune attack, is being investigated, while a vaccine against human papilloma virus (HPV), which is responsible for much cervical cancer, has recently become available. Attempts to stimulate innate immunity have long been used, e.g. Bacillus Calmette-Guérin (BCG) vaccine in leukaemia, *Corynebacterium* in pleural effusions, but are generally unsuccessful; an exception is BCG in bladder cancer. The popularity of the 'immunostimulant' *levamisole* has waxed and waned.

Another approach is to render tumour cells incapable of dividing yet still capable of eliciting a host immune response. This is analogous to the preparation of antimicrobial vaccines using killed or attenuated organisms (active immunization). Irradiated leukaemic cells have been tried, but the lack of success possibly stems from the same reason as the growth of the tumour in the first place – an ineffective host immune response to tumour cells.

A wide variety of natural immunological mediators, usually cytokines (lymphokines), are being investigated and some are in use (Table 10.24). The initial enthusiasm for *interferon* has generally been disappointing, although it is now used successfully in a small number of tumours, e.g. AIDS-related Kaposi's sarcoma and some lymphomas (as well as in immunologic diseases such as hepatitis and multiple sclerosis). Interferons augment T and B cell activity and can inhibit cell division and differentiation.

Interleukin-2 (*aldesleukin*, IL-2), a cytokine produced by T-helper cells, generally enhances T cell and natural killer cell activity against tumour cells. IL-2 has been particularly successful in malignant melanoma and renal cell carcinoma. Most adverse effects are mild, e.g. flu-like symptoms, but occasional hypovolaemia caused by widespread capillary leakage can lead to acute prerenal failure, especially with IV use.

One successful approach has been to develop antibodies against B-lymphocytes, which are involved in lymphomas such as follicular lymphoma and Hodgkin's lymphoma. Both *rituximab* and *alemtuzumab* are classed as **lymphocytolytics**. Both may cause severe allergic-type side-effects resulting from massive cytokine release.

Gene therapy

This involves a fundamental attempt to change the actual genes responsible for the neoplastic process. Cancer is among the first areas of application of this rapidly developing technology, both in facilitating immunotherapy and in changing the neoplastic genome. Cells are being experimentally implanted with a variety of different genes, based on the observation that neoplastic cells may have escaped immunosurveillance because mutation has prevented them from expressing histocompatibility (HLA) antigens. Some tumour cells are implanted (transfected) with appropriate HLA gene sequences and then injected into the patient, to enable a specific immune response to be mounted against the tumour phenotype. Alternatively, genes for cytokines such as interleukins and TNF may be implanted. This bypasses the process whereby HLA normally signals helper T-lymphocytes to recruit cytotoxic lymphocytes by secreting such lymphokines.

More direct genetic manipulation involves either inserting normal tumour suppressor genes or disabling the oncogene responsible for the tumour. One technique undergoing development for the latter purpose is to use antisense oligonucleotides (e.g. *oblimersen*). Nucleotide sequences are synthesized that are complementary to DNA and thus bind specifically to DNA sequences in oncogenes known to be expressed in certain tumours. In this way they can prevent transcription and thus synthesis of the carcinogenic gene product. This technique could also be exploited to block p-glycoprotein synthesis by preventing expression of the *mdr* gene, thus reducing drug resistance. An inversion of this procedure is to transfect normal marrow stem cells *ex vivo* with the *mdr* gene and re-implant them in the patient; this confers on their bone marrow a degree of resistance to cytotoxic damage, thus reducing adverse effects.

An ingenious gene therapy technique for drug delivery is to use a so-called 'suicide gene' or

'Trojan horse vector'. Certain tumours over-express specific abnormal gene products, e.g. AFP in liver cancer. The promoters for some of these genes have been isolated and coupled to promoters for genes expressing enzymes that activate a cytotoxic drug. These enzymes are then preferentially activated in tumour cells. For example, if the enzyme cytosine deaminase is released intracellularly it converts the relatively non-toxic flucytosine, given at the same time, to *fluorouracil*, which then acts as a targeted antimetabolite.

Most of these therapies are still experimental. The main problem is not the identification or preparation of the genetic material itself, nor injection into a genome using retrovirus vectors. The difficulty, as with all gene therapy, is targeting. To be successful, the gene change should be produced in all the neoplastic cells and it is currently not feasible to identify all such cells and to deliver the new gene specifically to each of them. The potential toxicity of any vector used must also be considered.

Complementary medicine

Forms of alternative medicine that complement or enhance orthodox treatment are now widely accepted by cancer care units if requested by patients and not felt to interfere with standard therapy. However, oncologists are sceptical about treatments that claim to produce cures by replacing standard therapy. Numerous dietary interventions, meditation, group therapy and support groups, 'visualization techniques' (in which the patient imagines the tumour, for example, as a physical enemy to be combated) and many others, may have a place for particular patients. However, care must be taken to ensure that they do not raise falsely optimistic hopes nor dissuade the patient from orthodox therapy that could offer a genuine chance of relief or recovery. Cancer patients are especially vulnerable to 'quack' medicine.

However, there is increasing acceptance that psychological factors can influence the outcome of cancer. Stress may increase the likelihood of relapse of breast cancer, but doubts remain about whether psychosocial intervention can significantly improve the chances of remission or cure of cancer in general.

Future developments

Some areas of development in cancer treatment include:

Chronotherapy. There may be predictable diurnal variations in the response of tumours to cytotoxic drugs and the body's response to adverse effects. Efforts are being directed to exploiting this to maximize the former and minimize the latter by careful timing of therapy.

Photodynamic therapy. This involves the use of a photosensitive agent that is selectively accumulated by tumour cells and which is converted to a toxic metabolite or free radical by visible or UV irradiation. This should be distinguished from using cytotoxic drugs to sensitize tumours to radiotherapy.

Prostaglandins. These may be involved in carcinogenesis, possibly through the link with chronic inflammation (p. 652). Chronic *aspirin* intake has for some time been known to reduce the risk of colon cancer, and cyclo-oxygenase has been found to be over-expressed on breast cancer cells. A potential chemopreventative role for NSAIDs, especially cyclo-oxygenase-2-specific inhibitors, is being investigated.

Thalidomide, formerly and notriously used as an antiemetic during pregnancy, is being investigated for its anti-angiogenesis activity, because it inhibits VEGF.

PARP inhibitors. Poly(ADP-ribose) polymerase repairs damaged DNA and if it is inhibited the same repair is normally carried out by BRCA gene products. In breast cancers caused by BRCA1 or BRCA2 mutations this alternative pathway is unavailable, so PARP inhibitors result in cell death and hence tumour regression. However, they should have no adverse effect on normal cells.

Hypoxia. Another approach exploits the fact that solid tumours often have large hypoxic areas, which are chemoresistant. Suitably designed prodrugs such as *banoxantrone* are preferentially activated by cytochome P450 in hypoxic tumour cells, releasing the active cytotoxin.

Differentiation therapy. Because most neoplastic cells are poorly differentiated, stimulating them to differentiate might be expected to abolish their abnormality and re-expose them to normal growth controls and apoptosis. In acute promyelocytic leukaemia (representing about 10% of AML cases) all-trans-retinoic acid (ATRA) blocks the promyelocytic/retinoic acid receptor complex which would otherwise arrest the maturation of promyelocytes, and induces remission in up to 70% of cases.

Rational design of antineoplastic regimens

Many treatment regimens are still derived empirically from clinical experience. Nevertheless, the principles described above do provide a rational basis for designing new regimens, and an explanation for most established ones. The key points are:

- Combine agents with different modes of action.
- Choose agents that are individually effective in the tumour being treated.
- Use the maximum tolerable dose of each.
- Use the most effective means of drug delivery to the tumour.
- Space different drugs to achieve optimum synchronization with the cell cycle.

Combinations

The advantages of combination therapy in cancer are similar to those when it is used in other diseases, especially antimicrobial chemotherapy, but are particularly important with drugs with a such a low therapeutic index. Such combinations have additive or synergistic action, reduced toxicity from individual components because lower doses may be used, and a reduced likelihood of resistance.

Each agent in a combination must have demonstrated action alone against the target tumour, and the components should differ as much as possible in their mode of action. Thus ideally they should have different biochemical actions, come from different cytokinetic classes, act at different phases in the cell cycle, and have different toxicity profiles. The widely used 'CMF' regimen for breast cancer (Table 10.25) illustrates these principles.

Some combinations may reduce toxicity, e.g. *cytarabine* protects against *tioguanine* toxicity by

Table 10.25   CMF combination cytotoxic regimen for breast cancer

Drug	Mode of action	Kinetic class[a]	Main phase of action[b]	Main toxicity[c]
Cyclophosphamide	Alkylating agent	III	All	Bladder
Methotrexate	Antimetabolite – antifolate (anti-dihydrofolate reductase)	II	S	Liver, lung
Fluorouracil	Antimetabolite – pyrimidine analogue (anti-thymidylate synthetase)	II	S	Mucositis, hand–foot syndrome

[a] II, phase-specific; III, cycle-specific.

[b] See Figure 10.14.

[c] Toxicity excluding bone marrow suppression, which all cause to some extent.

preventing its incorporation into DNA, without blocking its therapeutic effect. Other combinations may be antagonistic, e.g. *methotrexate* and *crisantaspase* are both effective individually in leukaemia, but not in combination. Possibly *methotrexate*, by arresting the cells at the G–S boundary, prevents the activity of *crisantaspase* during the S phase.

Dose, scheduling and timing

Opinion varies on the benefits of timing the different components of a combination to take advantage of the different phases at which they act. Some synchronization could be achieved this way. Consider a theoretical combination of *methotrexate + cytarabine + etoposide + vincristine* (specified here solely to illustrate the potential exploitation of cell cycle phases). *Methotrexate* given first will arrest the cells at the G_1–S boundary (see Figure 10.14); then change to *cytarabine* (S–G_2 boundary), followed by *etoposide* (G_2), then finally *vincristine* (M).

Experiments in mice have shown some theoretical justification for this approach, but in man attempts at synchronization have not been successful. The detailed knowledge of the cell cycle times needed to determine the intervals between each drug is often lacking. It is neces-

sary to give each drug long enough for all cells initially at different phases to come to the relevant phase, but this time will vary greatly, both between tumours and between patients.

However, the general principle of consistently high doses for the optimum time has been well established in a similar way to antimicrobial therapy. In an early experiment with leukaemic mice, a 16-day course of *cytarabine* given as a 240-mg bolus every 4 days produced no cure, whereas half that dose given as eight 15-mg injections throughout each fourth day produced a 100% cure. In the second regimen the drug plasma level was high enough for long enough so that all cycling cells reached the S phase and were exposed to it. Similarly, intermittent high-dose *methotrexate* produces better results in human acute leukaemia than continuous low-dose therapy.

Most regimens specify precise intervals. Consider, for example, a regimen used for lung mesothelioma (Figure 10.20). It starts treatment with an infusion containing *magnesium* and *potassium*, to minimize subsequent electrolyte losses caused by *cisplatin*. The antiemetic *granisetron* is given 30 min later and the first cytotoxic, *pemetrexed*, at 1 h. The osmotic diuretic *mannitol* is given 10 min after this, to reduce nephrotoxicity, then *cisplatin* after a further 30 min. Further protective infusions are given after another 2 and 4 h.

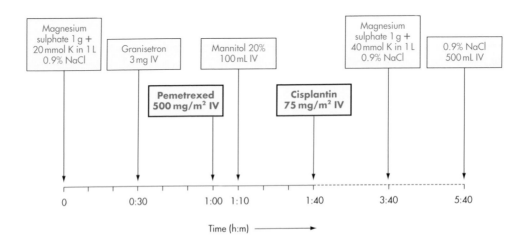

Figure 10.20 A treatment protocol for mesothelioma. (Reproduced with permission from Guys and St.Thomas' NHS Foundation Trust).

Frequency and pulsing

It has already been shown that an interval of 2–4 weeks between courses of treatment is needed to allow normal marrow cell recovery (p. 679).

Clinical pharmacological factors

Pharmacokinetics

Cancer patients often have grossly disturbed metabolic functions with malnutrition and fluid imbalance, which affects plasma protein level and volume of distribution, and liver and renal impairment, affecting drug clearance. Some drugs, e.g. *cyclophosphamide*, require hepatic activation. Patients are also likely to be on several other drugs for complications or symptomatic treatment, so there is considerable potential for pharmacokinetic interactions.

Route of administration and distribution. Cytotoxic drugs are usually given intravenously as a bolus or continuous infusion. This provides predictable plasma levels, whereas oral absorption in cancer patients may be impaired by the effects of chemotherapy such as gut damage or nausea and vomiting. Moreover, oral cytotoxics are often poorly tolerated. Because the usual aim of chemotherapy is the eradication of systemic metastases, methods for selective local administration to a tumour to minimize systemic toxicity are not as useful as might at first be expected. Intra-arterial infusion with the intention of delivering high local drug concentrations into large poorly perfused solid tumours is rarely successful. It causes frequent injection site damage, requires cumbersome arrangements if infusion is to be continuous, and has limited action on metastases. Occasionally, intrathecal administration is used for hydrophilic drugs that do not cross the blood–brain barrier, e.g. *methotrexate* for potential CNS metastases in leukaemia. Where malignant effusions are troublesome, e.g. in the pleural or abdominal cavities, intracavity instillation may be used palliatively, e.g. with *bleomycin*.

Table 10.26   Principles of cancer chemotherapy

Decision	Principle	Rationale
Treat or not?	• Decide realistic goal • Assess risk against potential benefit	Prolong life, improve quality of life
When?	Early – when tumour load smallest	Minimize remaining cell number Minimizes resistance Still vascularized Least chance of metastasis
Which drugs?	• Drugs with established activity • Use effective combinations	Synergistic – reduced toxicity and resistance
How much?	Use maximum tolerated doses	Exploit differential sensitivity (tumour/bone marrow) Reduce resistance
How long?	For short pulses	Minimize marrow damage
How often?	• Allow time for normal (marrow) cells to recover • Repeat treatment as often as necessary or tolerable	Exploit differential recovery Proportional kill effect
What cautions?	• Monitor blood counts closely • Use appropriate strategies to minimize toxicity • Use appropriate supportive therapy	Minimize bone marrow toxicity

Clearance. The pharmacokinetics and cytokinetic class of the drugs used need to be considered when deciding dose and duration of therapy (Figure 10.15). For drugs with such a narrow chemotherapeutic index, which nevertheless need to achieve adequate levels to be effective, more than usual care is needed.

Principles of chemotherapy: summary

A brief summary of the principles described in this section is given in Table 10.26.

References and further reading

Bradley J, Johnson D, Rubenstein D (2001). *Lecture Notes on Molecular Medicine*, 2nd edn. Oxford: Blackwell.

Corrie P (2004). Cytotoxic chemotherapy: clinical aspects. *Medicine* **32(3)**: 25–29.

Danaei G, Hoorn S V, Lopez A D, *et al*. (2005). Causes of cancer in the world: comparative risk assessment of nine behavioural and environmental risk factors. *Lancet* **366**: 1784–1793.

Hart I R (2004). Biology of cancer. *Medicine* 2004; **32(3)**: 1–5.

Jell G, Bonzani I, Stevens M (2005). Stem cells in regenerative medicine. *Pharm J* **275**: 695–698.

Johnston S R D, Gore M E (2004). Biology of cancer: clinical applications. *Medicine* **32(3)**: 6–10.

Lind M J (2004). Principles of cytotoxic chemotherapy. *Medicine* **32(3)**: 20–24.

Pecorino L (2005). *Molecular Biology of Cancer*. Oxford: Oxford University Press.

Pelengaris S, Khan M (2006). *The Molecular Biology of Cancer*. Oxford: Blackwell.

Souhami R, Tobias J (2005). *Cancer and its Management*, 5th edn. Oxford: Blackwell.

Tannock I F, Hill R P, Bristow R G, Harrington L (2005). *The Basic Science of Oncology*, 4th edn. New York: McGraw-Hill.

11

Haematology

Anaemia occurs when the level of functional haemoglobin in the blood falls below the reference level appropriate to the sex and age of an individual. Alternatively, anaemia can be defined as a reduction in red blood cell count or in the packed cell volume.

Anaemia is a major world public health problem, due to poor diet, chronic diseases, wars and famine: this chapter considers the more common causes. It does not deal with anaemia due to sudden bleeding.

Bone marrow failure is discussed briefly, as a basis for understanding the use of new biological agents. The clotting system and the management of anticoagulation is covered in the final section.

Some other aspects of haematology (e.g. leukaemias) are covered in Chapter 10, clotting problems affecting the cardiovascular system in Chapter 4 and some aspects of blood transfusion in Chapter 2.

Red blood cell production and function

Erythpoiesis

Mature red blood cells (RBCs, erythrocytes) are biconcave discs 7.5 μm in diameter containing haemoglobin (Hb), which comprises about a third of the cell mass. This shape provides a large surface area for oxygen diffusion into the cell.

The erythrocytes are derived from the same common pluripotent stem cells as all the other formed elements of the blood (see Chapter 2, Figure 2.1) and ultimately from lineage-specific bone marrow cells under the influence of cytokines (primarily interleukins and granulocyte-macrophage colony stimulating factor, GM-CSF) and, finally, *erythropoietin* (EPO). The latter is a hormone produced in peritubular kidney cells, and to a lesser extent in the liver, in response to anaemia and reduced tissue oxygen levels that together stimulate erythroid precursors to divide and mature. This mechanism balances RBC production precisely to their loss through haemorrhage and senescence, etc.

Chronic renal disease (see Chapter 14), many other chronic diseases and haemodialysis cause EPO deficiency, which are treated with recombinant human *epoetin* (EPO). However, some patients develop antibodies to this and repeated twice- or thrice-weekly IV or SC injections are required (SC injections are contra-indicated in chronic renal failure). Many *epoetin* analogues and mimetics are being explored with a view to minimizing these problems (see References and further reading).

Maturation into erythroid colony-forming units (CFU-E) is promoted by an erythroid colony-stimulating factor (CSF-E). As the cells mature in the bone marrow they become increasingly sensitive to EPO and there is progressive loss of ribosomal RNA and mitochondria and increased synthesis of cytoplasmic Hb. In parallel with this, the nucleus becomes condensed and is finally lost, forming **reticulocytes**.

Reticulocytes are released into the circulation after about 1–2 days in the bone marrow: nucleated RBCs are not normally present in blood. Reticulocytes normally retain some ribosomal RNA and continue to synthesize Hb for a further 1–2 days in the circulation, during which time the RNA and mitochondria are lost completely and the mature, enucleate erythrocyte is formed. The process of erythpoiesis is summarized in Figure 2.1 (p. 27). The reticulocytes normally form about 1% of the total erythrocytes, but this proportion is increased if there is loss of red cells, e.g. due to traumatic bleeding or haemolysis, because increased numbers of reticulocytes are released into the blood as a normal response, to recover oxygen-carrying capacity.

Because the mature erythrocyte does not contain any DNA or RNA it is not a true cell and has often been described as a 'corpuscle'. However, it has a well-defined, stable structure and its description as a 'red blood cell' is universally used. Erythrocytes have a strong, deformable cytoskeleton that enables them to pass through the smallest blood vessels without damage. The cytoskeleton is composed of several interlinked proteins, i.e. alpha- and beta-spectrins, actin, ankyrin and proteins 4.1, 4.2 and 4.9. The latter proteins are identified by numbers corresponding to their relative positions on electrophoresis.

About 0.8% (100%/120) of the original cell population is lost per day and this is normally balanced by a reticulocyte gain. If erythropoiesis fails completely, e.g. in aplastic anaemia (Table 11.6), the red cell and reticulocyte counts decline by about 6% per week, with no compensatory reticulocyte gain. Successful treatment in this situation increases the proportion of reticulocytes to above normal levels in the short term, until normal function is achieved.

Although RBCs lose their ability to synthesize protein and carry out oxidative metabolism they retain some crucial metabolic capacity. This includes the anaerobic Embden–Meyerhof glycolytic pathway, which provides four functions:

- Production of energy via ATP.
- Maintenance of the red cell membrane and cell architecture.
- Formation of NADH to maintain the iron of haem in the ferrous state.
- Production of 2,3-diphosphoglycerate (2,3-DPG) that modulates Hb function (see below).

There is also a hexose monophosphate shunt, which provides NADPH to preserve the sulphydryl groups of HbA and so maintain Hb tertiary structure. This metabolism is essential to protect the cells from oxidative stress and yield the normal erythrocyte life span of about 120 days. These pathways are outlined in Figure 11.1.

The survival of RBCs and the sites of destruction of senescent RBCs, primarily the liver and the spleen, can be determined by radiolabelling with ^{51}Cr and monitoring the change in radiation levels with time and the sites of concentration of radiation, measured with an external gamma-camera.

Table 11.1 lists normal values for some haematological and biochemical parameters.

Haemoglobin synthesis and function

Haemoglobin (deoxygenated haemoglobin, Hb) is the component of the erythrocyte that transports oxygen from the lungs to the tissues and

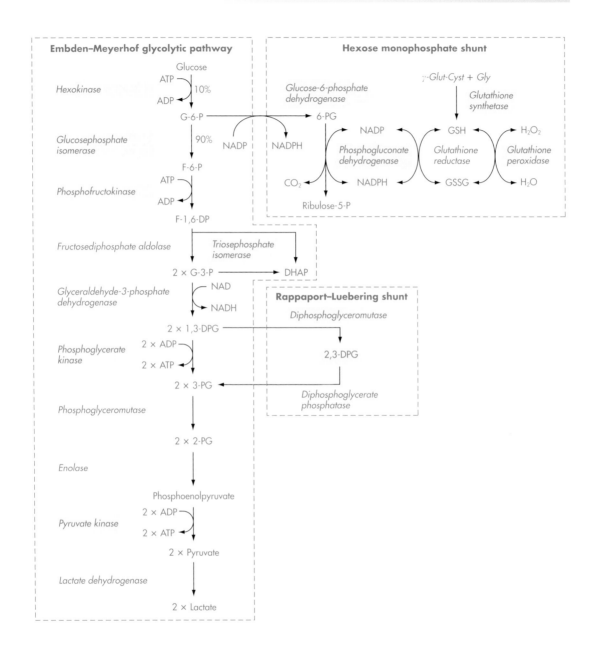

Figure 11.1 Pathways of glucose metabolism in erythrocytes. Emden-Meyerhof glycolytic pathway. Notes: 1 The hexose monophosphate shunt generates NADPH for the production of glutathione, thus maintaining sulphydryl bonds in their reduced state and membrane integrity. 2 The Rappaport–Luebering shunt produces 2,3-diphosphoglycerate, which stabilizes deoxyhaemoglobin and so aids oxygen liberation in the tissues. 3 There is a net gain of two molecules of ATP per molecule of glucose metabolized, thus providing energy to the red blood cell. Named enzymes (italics) are those for which there are known hereditary deficiency diseases: other enzymes have been omitted. The commonest enzyme deficiency is that of glucose-6-phosphate dehydrogenase (G6PD), causing deficient reducing power, followed by pyruvate kinase (PK), causing a loss of energy (ATP) provision (both in bold italics). ADP, adenosine diphosphate; ATP, adenosine triphosphate; cyst, cysteine; DHAP, dihydroxyacetone phosphate; DP, diphosphate; DPG, diphosphoglycerate; F, fructose; G, glucose; Glut, glutamyl; gly, glycine; GSH, reduced glutathione; GSSG, oxidized glutathione; NADP, nicotinamide adenine dinucleotide phosphate; NADPH, reduced NADP; P, phosphate; PG, phosphoglycerate.

Table 11.1   Normal values for some haematological parameters[a]

	Males	Females
Haemoglobin (g/dL)	13.5–17.7	11.5–16.5
RBC count ($\times 10^{12}$/L)	4.5–6.5	3.0–5.6
Packed cell volume (PCV, haematocrit, L/L)	0.4–0.54	0.37–0.48
Mean cell volume (MCV, fL)	80–96	80–96
Mean cell haemoglobin (MCH, pg)	27–34	27–34
Mean cell haemoglobin concentration (MCHC, g/dL)	31–37	31–37
RBC distribution width (RDW; see text)	10.5–14.5	10.5–14.5
RBC mass (mL/kg)	24–35	20–30

	Males and Females
Total blood volume (mL/kg)	64–85
Plasma volume (mL/kg)	40–50
Serum vitamin B_{12} (pm/L)	150–675
Serum folate (nm/L)	3–40
RBC folate (nm/L)	100–600
White blood count (WBC, $\times 10^9$/L)	
Total	4–11
Basophils	0.02–0.1
Eosinophils	0.04–0.4
Lymphocytes	1.0–4.0
Monocytes	0.2–1.0
Neutrophils	2.0–7.5
Platelet count ($\times 10^9$/L)	150–400

[a] Values vary considerably in different texts and those given here are the approximate means of published data. Local laboratory values may differ and should be consulted.

RBC, red blood cell.

fL, femtolitre; pg, picogram; pm, picomol; nm, nanomol.

some carbon dioxide from the tissues to the lungs. Hb is produced in the mitochondria of the developing red cells. In adults, most of it is HbA, an allosteric protein composed of two alpha polypeptide chains and two beta polypeptide chains, i.e. $\alpha_2\beta_2$, the remainder comprising about 3% of HbA_2 ($\alpha_2\delta_2$) plus HbF (fetal Hb). HbF is slightly different from the adult form, being $\alpha_2\gamma_2$, which binds oxygen more strongly than HbA. Each globin molecule binds one molecule of the iron-porphyrin haem, so the complete Hb molecule contains four molecules of haem.

Also present in the red cell is 2,3-diphosphoglycerate (2,3-DPG), formed by red cell glycolysis (Figure 11.1), which binds the beta chains and stabilizes the Hb in a tense conformation that has a lower affinity for oxygen than the relaxed conformation produced when Hb binds oxygen to form oxyhaemoglobin (HbO_2). This has implications for Hb function. The 2,3-DPG is formed in the RBCs mostly under the relatively anaerobic conditions in the tissues and its binding promotes the release of oxygen there. In the aerobic conditions in the lungs less 2,3-DPG is produced, thus favouring the relaxed conformation that promotes oxygen uptake to form HbO_2. The differing pH and carbon dioxide concentrations between the lungs and the tissues reinforce these reactions, thus favouring oxygen uptake by Hb in the lungs and HbO_2 dissociation to release oxygen in the tissues.

Under normal conditions about 98.5% of the oxygen is transported as HbO_2 and the remainder is dissolved in the plasma. Carbon dioxide, being very soluble, is carried mostly (70%) as bicarbonate in the plasma, 23% is combined with Hb as carbaminohaemoglobin ($HbCO_2$) and about 7% is carried dissolved in plasma which, in equilibrium with the bicarbonate, forms a pH buffering system.

The Hb from effete red cells is broken down into iron, porphyrins and amino acids, which are recycled.

Iron metabolism

The dietary iron intake is matched very closely to iron losses. There is no specific mechanism for transport into the gut and iron lost in this way, e.g. by shedding of enterocytes, is highly conserved. The normal average daily diet in the UK contains about 15–30 mg of ferric iron, mostly from iron-fortified breakfast cereals, less than 10% of which is absorbed in the duodenum and jejunum. The factors affecting iron absorption are listed in Table 11.2.

Before this iron can be absorbed it must be reduced to the ferrous state. Specialized cells in the mucosal crypts of the gut migrate to the luminal surface, where they produce a ferri-reductase and a divalent metal transporter (DMT1) in the villi of the enterocyte brush border. The DMT1 then carries the ferrous iron across the cell membrane by an active transport process. Iron is stored in the cells as **ferritin** or transferred into the plasma by another transporter via the enterocyte base.

Three control mechanisms are involved. After an iron-rich meal a dietary regulator makes the villi resistant to further iron absorption for some days. The 'memory' of the iron status of the body at the time of their formation then regulates iron transport into the enterocytes. Finally, there is a means of signalling the level of erythropoiesis to the enterocytes. Further iron is lost from ferritin stores in the enterocytes when these are shed into the gut lumen.

There is also some dietary haem iron from animal meat, and some from Hb breakdown, which is more readily absorbed than elemental iron.

Iron transport and storage

Most of the total body iron is transported in the plasma as Hb. However, the serum contains about 11–30 μmol/L, bound to the specific transporter **transferrin**, which is synthesized in the liver: the higher levels occurring in the morning. Each molecule of transferrin binds two atoms of ferric iron derived mostly from RBC breakdown in reticuloendothelial macrophages and oxidized in arterial blood. The iron–transferrin complex binds to specific receptors on erythroblasts and

Table 11.2 Some factors influencing iron absorption from the gut

Factors increasing absorption	Factors reducing absorption
Ferrous state	Ferric state
Reducing agents, e.g. ascorbic acid	Oxidizing agents
Gastric acid	Alkalis (antacids)
Inorganic state	Organic state
Hereditary haemochromatosis (causes excessive iron storage in various body organs) as haemosiderin	Sequestration by phytate and phosphate in the diet (untreated bran)
Iron deficiency (low iron body stores)	Iron overload (high iron body stores)
Increased erythropoiesis	Reduced erythropoiesis
Alcohol	

reticulocytes in the bone marrow, where the iron is released and recycled into haem.

About a third of the total iron load is stored in the hepatocytes, reticuloendothelial cells and skeletal muscle, mostly as ferritin and normally about a third as **haemosiderin**. The latter is an insoluble protein–iron complex found in the liver, spleen and bone marrow, where it can be visualized by light microscopy after staining, unlike ferritin.

Persistence of haemosiderin in erythroblast mitochondria occurs in **sideroblastic anaemia** (see below), which may be inherited or acquired (Table 11.2). It is due to a failure of haem synthesis, which may reflect poisoning of enzymes by drugs, e.g. *isoniazid*, or toxins, e.g. alcohol or lead.

Useful indicators of iron status include serum iron, ferritin level and total iron-binding capacity (TIBC).

Anaemia

The unqualified use of the term 'anaemia' means simply that the level of functional Hb in the blood falls below the reference level appropriate to the sex and age of an individual. The WHO defines these lower levels arbitrarily as 13 g/dL in adult males (normal range (N) = 13–17) and 12 g/dL in adult females (N = 12–16). Children of both sexes below 14 years of age have lower levels, the cut-off for anaemia being 11 g/dL in those aged 6 months to 6 years and 12 g/dL in the 6–14 age group. Levels are normally measured at sea level. These values may differ between populations and at altitudes where the partial pressure of oxygen is low, causing increased RBC and Hb production. However, many apparently normal individuals have Hb levels below these arbitrary values.

Defined in this way anaemia is the common outcome of many different pathologies, i.e. it is a secondary condition, and it is important to diagnose the underlying cause, so that specific treatment can be given. Thus some forms of anaemia have an adjectival prefix that describes the underlying disorder, e.g. pernicious anaemia, aplastic anaemia (p. 725), leucoerythroblastic

anaemia, due to space-occupying lesions of the bone marrow, e.g. leukaemia.

Anaemia is a very common blood disorder and is believed to affect about 30 million people worldwide but the true figure is unknown because of poor data from deprived areas with poor nutrition and unknown levels of intestinal parasites causing blood loss.

It is convenient to discuss anaemia under three headings:

- Normocytic, normochromic.
- Microcytic, hypochromic.
- Macrocytic.

Investigation of anaemia

It is not possible to diagnose anaemia by observation, e.g. by unusual pallor of complexion or of the inner surface of the lower eyelid. However, if there are other symptoms or signs that may be explicable by anaemia these features may prompt investigation. Anaemic patients often complain of non-specific conditions (tiredness, reduced exercise tolerance and shortness of breath), but these are more usually due to very common conditions (being overweight, inadequate exercise and unfitness, depression, and CVD).

The results of simple laboratory tests, obtained with automated blood cell counters, which give rapid results, include:

- Mean cell volume (MCV, in femtolitres [fL]).
- RBC distribution width (RDW), a measure of the variability of MCV.
- Mean corpuscular Hb (MCH, in picograms/RBC [pg]).
- Mean cell Hb concentration (MCHC, in g/dL).

Secondary parameters derived from these, e.g. the MCV/MCH ratio, are also used. However, the microscopic examination of a stained blood film permits an examination of red cell morphology which, considered with other laboratory and patient data, usually gives the diagnosis. Even if these data are not conclusive they will guide further testing for specific conditions, e.g. microscopy of bone marrow to investigate cell morphology or after a trephine with a special large needle to obtain a sample of bone to observe bone marrow architecture and the presence of abnormal cells. These samples are usually obtained from the posterior iliac crest. The trephine biopsy has to be processed as a tissue sample, so the result is available only after several days.

Normocytic, normochromic anaemias

One group in this category, i.e. those with a normal or low reticulocyte count and normal bone marrow morphology, are often described as **secondary anaemias**, because there is always an underlying condition (Figure 11.2). Diagnosis then depends on tests to identify the latter and exclude serious pathology, e.g.

- Bleeding, destruction of RBCs (haemolysis), especially in the acute stage.
- Leukaemias and bone metastases (secondary deposits) from primary cancers elsewhere in the body (see Chapter 10).
- Aplastic anaemias or abnormal cell production.
- Renal failure, causing failure of erythropoietin production.
- The early stages of the anaemia of chronic disease (see below).

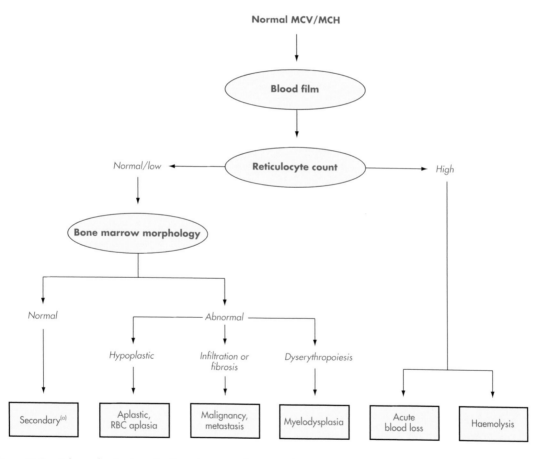

Figure 11.2 Scheme for the investigation of normocytic, normochromic anaemia. Text in bold type indicates investigations. MCV/MCH, mean red blood cell volume/haemoglobin; RBC, red blood cell. [a]Due to e.g. inflammation, hepatic/renal disease. (Modified from Fig. 5 in Parker-Williams EJ. Investigation and management of anaemia. Medicine 2004; **32**(5):18, with permission from The Medicine Publishing Company and Elsevier Ltd).

Haemolytic anaemias

The body can respond up to eightfold by increasing RBC production and by increasing the amount of active marrow. Provided the rate of loss is less than the capacity of the marrow to respond, higher than normal RBC destruction does not always cause anaemia. However, the proportion of reticulocytes is increased, and there may be spherical or other abnormally-shaped RBCs or red cell fragments. The many possible causes of haemolytic anaemia (see below) are listed in Table 11.3.

Extravascular haemolysis

Most haemolytic anaemias result from RBC breakdown by reticuloendothelial macrophages,

---

Table 11.3　Possible causes of haemolytic anaemia

Inherited RBC defects

Membrane defects
- Hereditary elliptocytosis
- Hereditary spherocytosis

Metabolic defects
- Glucose-6-phosphate dehydrogenase deficiency (G6PD, see Table 11.4)
- Pyruvate kinase deficiency

Haemoglobin defects
- structural – abnormal haemoglobins (HbS, HbC, HbE)
- defective synthesis – thalassaemia syndromes

Acquired RBC abnormality

Blood group incompatibility
- Haemolytic blood transfusion reaction; ABO, Kell, Rh (haemolytic disease of the newborn)
- Autoimmune haemolysis; warm or cold antibody, drug-induced

Not immunological
- RBC fragmentation
  - Thrombotic thrombocytopenic purpura
  - Haemolytic uraemic syndrome
  - Pre-eclamptic toxaemia (pregnancy)
  - Disseminated intravascular coagulation (see Chapter 2)
  - Meningococcal septicaemia (see Chapter 8)
  - Prosthetic heart valve
- Infections
  - *Mycoplasma pneumoniae*
  - Infectious mononucleosis (glandular fever)
  - *Clostridium perfringens*
  - *Plasmodium falciparum* malaria
- Drugs and chemicals
  - In G6PD (see Table 11.4)
  - Burns
  - Paroxysmal nocturnal haemoglobinuria

Modified from Figure 7 in Parker-Williams EJ. Investigation and management of anaemia. *Medicine* 2004; **32**(5):19, with permission from Elsevier Ltd.
RBC, red blood cell.

notably in the spleen, i.e. extravascular haemolysis. These are often the result of inherited RBC membrane defects.

In **hereditary spherocytosis (HS)** the RBC membrane is weakened and poorly supported by the cytoskeleton, resulting in somewhat spherical cells that are more rigid than the normal biconcave disks. The abnormal cells cannot negotiate the small vessels of the spleen and are broken down there. The inheritance is usually autosomal-dominant and affects about 1/5000 northern Europeans, though it may skip a generation, but may be due to a recessive pattern of inheritance, or new random mutations in some cases.

There is a wide variation in the age at presentation, some babies being jaundiced at birth whereas others may be hardly affected. Chronic haemolysis causes pigment gallstones (see Chapter 3), splenomegaly, and folate deficiency.

Affected neonates require repeated blood transfusions until they are old enough for splenectomy, which is usually curative. However, splenectomy carries a life-long risk of serious infection so is indicated only if justified by the severity of the patient's condition. Multiple immunizations and antibiotic prophylaxis are required.

Hereditary elliptocytosis is about twice as prevalent as HS and is somewhat similar, though milder. Less than 10% have significant haemolysis and splenectomy is required only occasionally.

Intravascular haemolysis
In all haemolytic anaemias the RBC survival is reduced, but the survival time is determined only rarely.

Destruction of RBCs within the circulation releases Hb. Some of this is bound by plasma protein, but excess is filtered at the renal glomeruli and most appears in the urine, though some is reabsorbed by the tubular cells in which it is deposited as **haemosiderin** and can be detected in the urine. Part of the plasma Hb is oxidized to **methaemoglobin**, which cannot function as an oxygen carrier and breaks down to globin and ferrihaem. The latter is usually bound in the plasma, but excess binds to albumin as methaemalbumin, which can be detected in the plasma photometrically: this is the basis of the Schumm test. All of the HbA and its products are metabolized in the liver and recycled into Hb.

The consequences of intravascular haemolysis include:

• High serum unconjugated bilirubin, high urinary urobilinogen and raised serum lactic dehydrogenase, which are indicators of RBC breakdown.
• Indicators of increased erythropoiesis, e.g. increased proportion of reticulocytes.

In some haemolytic anaemias there may also be abnormally-shaped RBCs or red cell fragments (see below).

Abnormal red cell metabolism
The RBC has very restricted metabolic capacity, the principal systems being the Embden-Meyerhof pathway and the connected hexose monophosphate shunt (see Figure 11.1). There are two main enzyme deficiencies that may occur, one each in each of these pathways.
Glucose-6-phosphate dehydrogenase (G6PD) deficiency. This is the most common of the enzyme deficiencies. There are numerous isoforms of the enzyme, the genes for which are X-linked. Heterozygous females may have two different populations of RBCs and may appear to be clinically normal but all females homozygous for the mutant are affected. The enzyme is involved in the production of NADPH (see above) and is crucial for the maintenance of glutathione, and so the flexibility and integrity of the RBC. Its absence causes RBC rigidity and leakage and the oxidation of Hb to methaemoglobin, which is deposited on the inner surface of the membrane. The result is haemolysis in the spleen. Over 100 mutant forms are known.

G6PD deficiency involves millions of people in central Africa, the Mediterranean borders, the Middle East and South-East Asia. In some areas up to 40% of the population may be affected, especially males.

The reduction of enzyme activity renders the RBCs very sensitive to oxidative stress. There may be:

• Neonatal jaundice.
• Chonic haemolytic anaemia.

- Acute haemolytic episodes due to:
  - Drugs (Table 11.4).
  - Bacterial and viral infections and diabetic ketoacidosis.
  - Ingestion of fava beans.

Diagnosis may be difficult because the RBC count is normal between attacks. However, there will be evidence of haemolysis, especially during attacks, though this may be self-limiting because the older, more affected RBCs are damaged selectively. Many RBCs will have irregular margins, with 'bites' taken out of the membrane where deposited methaemoglobin has been removed in the spleen. Direct assays for G6PD are available.

Treatment involves avoidance of any causative drugs, treatment of infections (see Chapter 8) and proper management of diabetes mellitus (see Chapter 9). Blood transfusions are often essential and splenectomy may help, but this is unlikely.

Pyruvate kinase (PK) deficiency is the second most common of the enzyme deficiencies, but much less so than G6PD. It causes low levels of ATP and increased levels of 2,3-DPG (see Figure 11.1), and so energy-starved and rigid RBCs. The high levels of 2,3-DPG (see above) minimize the severity of anaemia, by increasing oxygen unloading in the tissues. The blood film shows 'prickle cells' and reticulocytosis. The most prominent signs are anaemia, jaundice and splenomegaly. Exchange blood transfusions are required in infancy, pregnancy and infections, throughout life. Aplastic crises may occur. In severe cases, there may be bone changes similar to those seen in thalassaemia (see below).

Splenectomy may be helpful and may reduce the need for frequent blood transfusions. Folic acid supplementation is needed (see Figure 11.4). **Abnormal Hb synthesis.** These conditions may cause abnormal globin chain production

Table 11.4 Some drugs and chemicals that may cause haemolysis in glucose-6-phosphate dehydrogenase deficient individuals[a]

Antimicrobial agents
4-Aminosalicylic acid (PAS)[b], chloramphenicol, dapsone and sulphones, doxorubicin, furazolidone, nalidixic acid, nitrofurantoin, nitrofurazone, quinolones (see Chapter 8), most sulphonamides including co-trimoxazole

Antimalarials (may have to be tolerated in acute malaria)
Chloroquine, mepacrine, pamaquin[b], primaquine, pyrimethamine, quinine

Antiparasitic agents
Niridazole[b]

Analgesics
Amidopyrine[b], aspirin (>1 g daily), paracetamol (acetaminophen), phenacetin[b], phenazopyridine[b,c]

Vitamins
Menadione, menadiol sodium phosphate

Antiarrhythmics
Procainamide, quinidine

Other agents
Acetanilide[b], chlorate, dimercaprol, hydroxychloroquine, levodopa, methylthioninium chloride, naphthalene, probenicid[b], trinitrotoluene, toluidine blue

[a] Individual sensitivities may vary considerably because of the numerous enzyme isoforms or may only occur in association with infections, acidosis, etc., or in some ethnic groups.
[b] Not marketed in the UK.
[c] May cause haemolysis in normal subjects.

(**thalassaemias**) or abnormal globin chain conformation (**sickle-cell anaemia**).

Thalassaemias occur in a wide arc, stretching from Spain to Indonesia but may occur in any population. The name comes from the Greek word for sea: all the countries with affected populations have extensive sea borders. They are the result of differing relative rates of production of the alpha and beta chains, or a complete absence of one of these.

Beta-thalassaemias are caused by a complete or relative absence of beta-globin chains, and affect all races. The excess of alpha-chains combines with gamma and delta Hb chains, producing very low levels of normal HbA and increased levels of HbA_2 and HbF (see above). Mutations in the beta-globin gene cause the production of unusable forms of Hb. **Alpha-thalassaemias** mostly affect Orientals and those of Middle Eastern origin. **Thalassaemia minor** (thalassaemia trait) is an asymptomatic or mildly symptomatic heterozygous state. **Thalassaemia major** is the result of beta-chain gene mutations giving a homozygous state, or doubly heterozygous state, i.e. the H6 genes from each parent are mutated in different ways. There is severe anaemia from the age of 3–6 months, when there is normally a switch from the gamma-chain production characteristic of fetal Hb (HbF, $\alpha_2\gamma_2$), to beta-chain production, characteristic of normal adult Hb ($\alpha_2\beta_2$). However, HbF synthesis continues beyond this point and most patients have some HbF. The liver and spleen are enlarged, sometimes grossly, and the erythropoietic bone marrow extends abnormally into bones that are not normally haemopoietic, e.g. in the face and hand, causing facial, and sometimes hand, deformities. The anaemia is severe and regular blood transfusions are required, but if these are needed frequently splenectomy is indicated (see above).

Frequent transfusions lead to **haemosiderosis**, i.e. iron overload from deposition of haemosiderin in tissues, causing widespread organ damage if it is not corrected. This requires removal by venesection (i.e. regular bleeding), provided that the patient has a functional bone marrow to replace the leucocytes that are lost. Regular folic acid supplementation and ascorbic acid are also required. The latter enhances iron excretion by keeping the excess iron in the more soluble ferrous state.

Complexing with *desferrioxamine mesilate*, an iron chelating agent that binds tissue stores rather than Hb iron, is an alternative to venesection. It is given as an overnight SC infusion, or by syringe driver, 3–7 times a week according to need. *Desferrioxamine* may also be given at the same time as a blood transfusion, but must not be mixed with the blood or given via the same infusion line: administration via the same cannula when the transfusion is complete is convenient. Iron excretion is again enhanced by giving ascorbic acid.

Deferiprone is a newer, orally active iron-chelating agent for use if *desferrioxamine* is contra-indicated or is not tolerated. However, fertile women should take strict contraceptive precautions because *deferiprone* is a known teratogen and is embryotoxic. Blood dyscrasias, notably agranulocytosis, have also been reported, so weekly neutrophil counts must be done and patients and their carers warned to report immediately any signs of infection, e.g. fever or sore throat. *Filgrastim* may be required (see Chapter 10). Care is required if there is any renal or hepatic impairment.

Deferiprone also complexes zinc, so plasma zinc concentrations also need to be monitored. Joint pain may occur.

As usual with complex medications the manufacturers' literature should be consulted on the use of both of these agents.

Alpha-thalassaemias have a more complex inheritance because alpha-chain synthesis is controlled by two pairs of structural genes, one pair from each parent. Because there are four alpha genes, there are four possible conditions:

- Single gene deletion confers the carrier state, and subjects are haematologically normal.
- Deletion of two genes causes a mild hypochromic microcytic anaemia (see below), i.e. **thalassaemia trait**.
- Deletion of three genes results in **HbH disease**. There is a variable degree of anaemia, splenomegaly and the RBCs are typical of thalassaemia (see above).
- Deletion of all four genes is incompatible

with life and babies are stillborn with features similar to those of severe beta-thalassaemia.

Women at risk who wish to bear a child are identified on the basis of racial and geographical origin and personal or family history and are usually offered antenatal diagnosis. If they carry a genetic abnormality, and their partner also carries thalassaemia genes, the mother is normally referred for fetal genetic diagnosis, and offered termination of the pregnancy if the fetus is severely affected.

Sickle-cell syndromes

These inherited Hb defects affect people mostly in central Africa (25% population carriage of the defective gene) and parts of the Middle East and India. Afro-Caribbeans are commonly affected. There is often co-inheritance of the sickle cell gene with those for beta-thalassaemia and other abnormal Hb conditions. The condition may be homozygous, giving HbSS and causing **sickle-cell anaemia**, or heterozygous (HbAS), causing **sickle-cell trait**.

The deoxygenated HbS is insoluble, and polymerizes in the RBC. This is initially reversible, but the cells finally take on their characteristic, rigid sickle shape. These cannot negotiate the microcirculation and there is clotting and tissue infarction, often in the bones. Because HbS releases its oxygen more readily than normal Hb, patients usually feel well, but a sickling crisis may be triggered by hypoxia.

The heterozygous condition (HbAS) is initially mild, because infants produce fetal Hb (HbF) for 3–6 months. Symptoms then become apparent, due to a change from producing HbF to HbS, in place of the normal HbA. High levels of HbF tend to prevent sickling and many Middle Eastern and Asian people co-inherit increased HbF levels and have relatively mild disease because fetal Hb is a more efficient oxygen carrier than HbA.

Complications are the result of anaemia and circulatory impairment. Although patients are often generally well, they suffer chronic anaemia and repeated painful **sickling crises**, caused by a variety of stressors, e.g. infection, dehydration, acidosis, exposure to cold and anaesthetics. Crises cause severe pain and opioid analgesics

(see Chapter 7) may be required. Special care is needed if anaesthesia is contemplated.

Renal impairment is common in late stage disease and may progress to renal failure. Infections, especially pneumococcal disease, are common and need immunization and prophylactic antibiotics. Aseptic bone necrosis, *Salmonella* osteomyelitis and chronic leg ulceration occur. Pulmonary hypertension occurs, due to RBC sequestration in the lungs and ischaemic liver cirrhosis, and a severe pulmonary syndrome may occur. Excess bilirubin production causes pigment gallstones (see Chapter 3). Strokes are relatively common.

Between crises, patients require regular folic acid and prompt treatment of infections. Crises that cannot be managed with analgesics require hospital admission. Blood transfusion is required only if their Hb level falls significantly below their norm. Transfusion also aborts a sickling crisis if the proportion of sickle cells is reduced to less than about 30%. Exchange tranfusion, i.e. withdrawal of the same volume of the patient's blood as is transfused, may be required to avoid excessive blood viscosity and so reduced microvascular blood flow, especially in severe pulmonary involvement.

Autoimmune haemolytic anaemias are described on p. 723.

Microcytic, hypochromic anaemias

The RBCs have a MCV of <78 fL due to some disturbance of iron metabolism, and there is a low MCV/MCH ratio. Following this observation, examination of the blood film usually permits rapid diagnosis. Figure 11.3 presents an algorithm for the investigation and diagnosis of this condition.

There may be:

- Iron deficiency.
- Impaired availability of iron, in the anaemia of chronic disease.
- Defective globin chain synthesis in thalassaemias.
- Defective haem synthesis in sideroblastic anaemia.

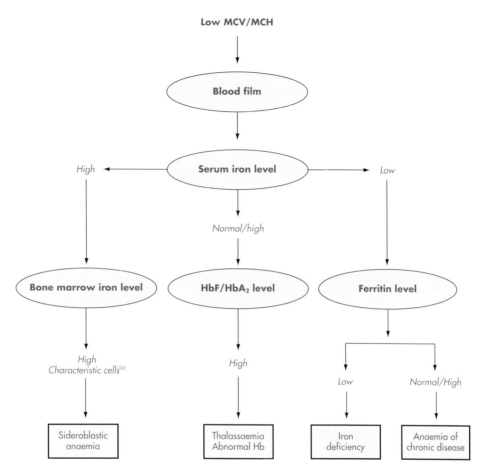

Low MCV/MCH

Blood film

Serum iron level

High ← → Low

Normal/high

Bone marrow iron level   HbF/HbA$_2$ level   Ferritin level

High
Characteristic cells[a]   High   Low   Normal/High

Sideroblastic anaemia   Thalassaemia Abnormal Hb   Iron deficiency   Anaemia of chronic disease

Figure 11.3   Scheme for the investigation of microcytic, hypochromic anaemia. Text in bold type indicates investigations. HbF, fetal haemoglobin; HbA$_2$, a form of haemoglobin normally comprising about 2% of total haemoglobin in adult blood; MCV/MCH, mean red blood cell volume/haemoglobin. [a]Ring sideroblasts, due to defective haem synthesis, giving iron granules around nucleus. (Modified from Fig. 1 in Parker-Williams EJ. Investigation and management of anaemia. *Medicine* 2004; **32**(5):15, with permission from The Medicine Publishing Company and Elsevier Ltd).

Indicators of iron status in anaemias are shown in Table 11.5.

Iron deficiency anaemia

It will be seen from Table 11.5 that the **ferritin** level distinguishes between simple iron deficiency and the anaemia of chronic disease. Ferritin is a soluble form of storage iron that is a good index of total body iron level. Examination of a stained blood marrow film is conclusive if there is any doubt. Determination of the percentage of transferrin saturation may also be useful.

Anaemia of chronic disease. A low-grade anaemia is common in chronic inflammatory states, e.g. RA and the connective tissue diseases (see Chapter 12), chronic infections, e.g. tubercular osteomyelitis and some fungal infections, and thalassaemia trait (see above).

Sideroblastic anaemia is due to abnormal bone marrow stem cells and may be inherited. Because it is X-linked, it is transmitted through the female line. There is defective haem synthesis and characteristic cells in the bone marrow show a ring of iron deposits (ring sideroblasts). The acquired form may be caused by toxins, including drugs, e.g. alcohol abuse, *isoniazid* and lead

Table 11.5 Test for the evaluation of iron status in anaemias

Test	Iron deficiency anaemia	Anaemia of chronic disease	Sideroblastic anaemia	Thalassaemia trait
Serum iron	↓	↓	↑	N/↑
Total iron-binding capacity	↑	↓	N	N
Percentage saturation	↓	↓	↑	N/↑
Ferritin	↓	N/↑	↑	N/↑
Bone marrow iron stores	Absent	N/↑	↑	N/↑
Sideroblasts	Absent	Absent	'Ring' sideroblasts	Present
Soluble transferrin receptor	↑	N/↑ [a]	N	N/↑ [a]

[a] Raised when iron deficiency complicates the anaemia of chronic disease or in thalassaemia trait.
Modified from Figure 2 in Parker-Williams EJ. Investigation and management of anaemia. *Medicine* 2004; **32**(5): 15, with permission from Elsevier Ltd.

toxicity. The anaemia may be severe and refractory to treatment. There is usually a bimodal distribution of RBC size, with both microcytic and mildly macrocytic cells. Patients with generally poor production of all cell types (pancytopenia) have a poor prognosis and may progress to **acute myeloblastic leukaemia (AML)**.

The thalassaemias are described above.

Macrocytic anaemias

Classification, aetiology and diagnosis

There are megaloblastic, non-megaloblastic and haemolytic types.

Megaloblastic macrocytic anaemias result from impaired DNA synthesis and nuclear matu-

Table 11.6 Some causes of folic acid and vitamin B_{12} deficiencies

Folic acid deficiency	Vitamin B_{12} deficiency
• Poor intake: poverty, elderly, infancy, poor diet, alcohol abuse • Increased demand: *Physiological* – prematurity, pregnancy, lactation *Pathological* – haemolytic anaemia, high erythropoietic activity, malignancy, renal dialysis • Increased loss: urinary (acute liver disease, heart failure), malabsorption states (see Chapter 3): coeliac disease[a], severe Crohn's disease or ulcerative colitis, dermatitis herpetiformis • Infection: tropical sprue • Antifolate drugs – methotrexate, pyrimethamine (prolonged use), trimethoprim, co-trimoxazole, anticonvulsants	• Inadequate intake: vegan diet • Intrinsic factor deficiency: pernicious anaemia, total or partial gastrectomy, hereditary • Malabsorption states (see Chapter 3): small intestine disease – coeliac disease, Crohn's disease, resection of terminal ileum, tropical sprue, severe pancreatic disease, drugs (nitrous oxide, colchicine, neomycin) • Infection:HIV/AIDS, small intestine (*E. coli*, *Bacteroides fragilis*, tapeworm)

[a] Unlikely effect.
Modified from Figure 4 in Parker-Williams EJ. Investigation and management of anaemia. *Medicine* 2004; **32**(5):17, with permission from Elsevier Ltd.

ration. RNA and protein synthesis continues after nuclear development has ceased, causing a relatively large immature RBC with a high cytoplasmic mass (megaloblasts). Megaloblasts can be observed in bone marrow smears as unusually large RBC progenitor cells with dispersed nuclear chromatin and several nucleoli. Because the factors causing defective erythropoiesis also affect all other bone marrow cell lines, thrombocytopenia and leucopenia also occur, usually in the later stages. Characteristic large leucocytes may also occur.

Non-megaloblastic macrocytic anaemias are usually due to toxic agents, non-bone marrow organ failure, e.g. alcoholic liver disease and hypothyroidism, or aplastic anaemias (bone marrow failure; see below). RBC agglutination produces large clumps of cells that may be reported erroneously as macrocytosis by automated blood analysers.

Megaloblastic macrocytic anaemias may be due to:

- Deficiency of vitamin B_{12} or folic acid (Table 11.6 and Figure 11.4), or abnormal metabolism of these.
- Therapy with drugs interfering with DNA synthesis, e.g. *azathioprine, cytarabine, cyclophosphamide, fluorouracil, hydroxycarbmide, mercaptopurine, tioguanine* and *zidovudine.*

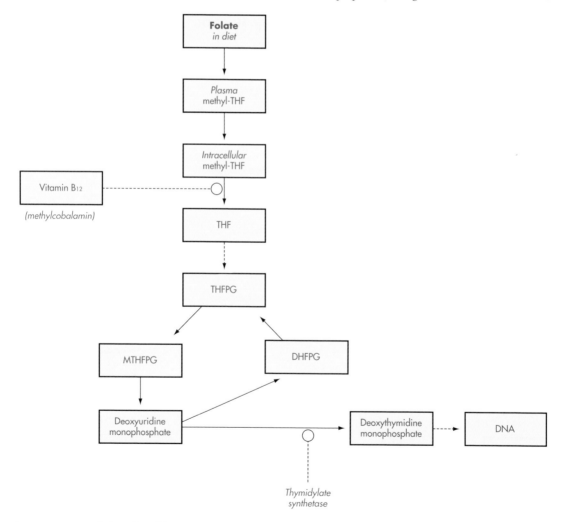

Figure 11.4   Metabolic roles of folate and vitamin B_{12}. DHFPG, dihydrofolate polyglutamate; DNA, deoxyribonucleic acid; THFPG, tetrahydrofolate polyglutamate; MTHFPG, 5,10-methylene THFPG; THF, tetrahydrofolate; – – O, promotes.

Aciclovir and *ganciclovir* may also cause megaloblastosis.
• Deficiency of enzymes essential for DNA synthesis.

Diagnosis and aetiology

A scheme for the diagnosis of macrocytic anaemia is given in Figure 11.5.

Because reticulocytes are larger than normal RBCs, any situation causing significant blood loss, e.g. trauma or haemolysis, will result in the release of reticulocytes from the bone marrow, causing a reticulocytosis and macrocytosis, at least in the short term, until treatment corrects the abnormalities.

Deficiencies of vitamin B_{12} or folic acid are usually of dietary origin, e.g. strict vegans, malnutrition, gastrointestinal problems (e.g. malabsorption, see Chapter 3), excessive alcohol intake, medication history, gastric carcinoma and gastrointestinal surgery. These potential causes need to be investigated. Hypothyroidism may be associated with pernicious anaemia and smoking may also cause vitamin B_{12} deficiency.

Folate deficiency occurs in malabsorption, pregnancy, neoplastic diseases associated with a high cell turnover, including severe infections.

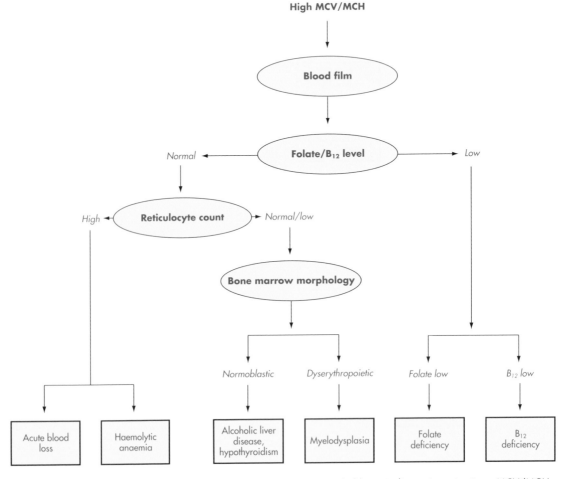

Figure 11.5   Scheme for the investigation of macrocytic anaemias Text in bold type indicates investigations. MCV/MCH, mean red blood cell volume/haemoglobin. (Modified from Fig. 3 in Parker-Williams EJ. Investigation and management of anaemia. *Medicine* 2004; **32**(5):16, with permission from The Medicine Publishing Company and Elsevier Ltd).

Antifolate medication, e.g. *methotrexate* and *trimethoprim*, anticonvulsants, e.g. *phenobarbital*, *phenytoin* and *primidone*, causing increased demand, and loss of folic acid in peritoneal dialysis and haemodialysis (see Chapter 14) may also contribute to low blood folate levels. An acute onset may occur in those with marginal folate stores.

Heavy menstrual losses in women and haemolytic anaemias (see above) also cause deficiencies.

Clearly, assays for vitamin B_{12} and tests to establish the reasons for low levels are required, e.g. absorption tests (Schilling test and antibodies to parietal cells, intrinsic factor and thyroid tissue), and establishment of the origin of folate deficiency are required.

Macrocytosis occurring with a normal RDW usually indicates heavy alcohol consumption and this is confirmed by a high serum level of gamma-glutamyl transpeptidase (GGT), a marker of liver damage.

Management of anaemias

This must be based on specific therapy and thus depends on accurate diagnosis. Effective treatment should give an increased reticulocyte count within 10 days. If this response does not occur, or if the Hb level does not improve, the diagnosis should be reviewed. Clearly, if anaemia is due to an underlying disease state, e.g. the anaemia of chronic disease, treatment must involve correction of that condition, in addition to the application of appropriate specific therapy.

Blood transfusion may be indicated if there has been a sudden fall in the erythrocyte count or Hb concentration, e.g. in acute drug- or infection-induced haemolytic crises in G6PD and pyruvate kinase deficiency (see Figure 11.1 and pp. 713 and 714) and inherited RBC disorders. It is also the mainstay of treatment in thalassaemias and in sickle-cell disease (see above). Transfusion is hazardous in elderly patients because the rapid increase in blood volume raises the blood pressure and this, together with the associated increase in venous return stresses the heart. Both of these are undesirable in those with compromised cardiac func-

tion (see Chapter 4). Cardiac stress is also caused if the recipient's cell count is near normal, due to increased blood viscosity. Further, the procedure carries the risks of infection and immunological errors, despite rigorous protocols. Repeated transfusions of whole blood cause **transfusion haemosiderosis** (iron overload), with liver, pancreas, heart muscle and endocrine gland damage. This usually requires treatment with the iron-chelating agent *desferrioxamine* (see above).

The alternative, orally active chelating agent *deferiprone* is licensed for use in patients with thalassaemia major (see above) in whom *desferrioxamine* is contra-indicated, or are intolerant of it. However, it may cause serious blood dyscrasias.

Erythropoietin

Darbepoetin and *erythropoietin alfa* and *beta* are useful only in the anaemia of chronic disease, especially renal disease, notably those on dialysis (see Chapter 14), and in those receiving cancer chemotherapy (see Chapter 10). They are also used in patients with moderate anaemia, i.e. Hb 10–13 g/dL, who are awaiting major surgery likely to involve major blood loss, e.g. hip replacement, to minimize the need for blood transfusion.

Iron therapy

Iron deficiency is often difficult to treat. The preferred treatment is to use ferrous sulphate tablets (1 tablet = 65 mg Fe^{2+}), one before breakfast, because it is better absorbed on an empty stomach. Further, diets that include bran, muesli or wholemeal bread contain phytates, which may interfere with iron absorption. Twice-daily dosing may be needed if there is continuing blood loss, but the commonly prescribed three times daily regimen is usually excessive and is needed only rarely. However, iron may cause gastrointestinal side-effects (see below) that cause patient non-adherence, so after-meal dosing may have to be accepted.

Ferrous fumarate may be a suitable alternative if a patient is intolerant of *ferrous sulphate* and the 200-mg tablet provides the same amount of iron as a *ferrous sulphate* tablet. There are several liquid dosage forms that are suitable for infants and young children.

Treatment is continued for 2–4 months after the Hb level has been normalized, to replenish iron stores.

Injections of *iron dextran* or *iron sucrose* are rarely required, but may be needed if a patient is intolerant of oral iron, and if there is malabsorption (see Chapter 3) or continuing bleeding.

There is no good evidence to support the use of slow-release or compound oral products. Although they are less likely to cause gastrointestinal upset, this is possibly because only a small proportion of the dose is absorbed.

Iron and folic acid tablets are given prophylactically to pregnant women at risk of the combined deficiency. However, the amount of folic acid in these is too low for the prevention of neural tube defects in the fetus (see below) and for the treatment of megaloblastic anaemia.

Tolerability is the determining factor in the choice of product. Nausea and epigastric pain are common and are dose-related, but this does not seem to hold for diarrhoea or constipation, though dose reduction may help. *Ferrous gluconate* tablets containing 35 mg Fe^{2+}, i.e. about half the amount in *ferrous sulphate* tablets, or one of the liquid preparations, will be needed for this. Oral iron may exacerbate diarrhoea in patients with IBD (see Chapter 3) and this occurs more commonly with modified-release forms that are released lower in the GIT. Also, care must be exercised in those with bowel stricture (narrowing) and diverticular disease (see Chapter 3). Constipation is especially likely in older patients and may lead to faecal impaction.

Correction of vitamin B_{12} and folate deficiencies

Vitamin B_{12} deficiency. *Hydroxocobalamin* is given intramuscularly, 1 mg on alternate days for 5–6 doses to replenish normal body stores, mainly in the liver, of 3–5 mg. An alternative regimen is to give the 1-mg dose on 3 days a week for 2–3 weeks. Because daily losses are normally very small, this is sufficient to maintain requirements for 2–4 years' normal metabolism. Due to the long persistence of *hydroxocobalamin*, a maintenance dose of 1 mg is then given every 2–3 months, usually for life. Clinical improvement is rapid (<48 h) and a maximal reticulocyte response occurs in about 7 days. However, existing long-standing CNS damage, a result of vitamin B_{12} deficiency, is irreversible.

Cyanocobalamin is no longer used because it is excreted more rapidly than *hydroxocobalamin* and requires monthly injections. It is now known that giving a 2-mg dose PO daily is also effective, but only 50-µg tablets are available. The use of low-dose oral preparations as a 'tonic' is irrational. However, they are prescribable under the UK NHS for vegans and others with a dietary deficiency, both for prevention and treatment of vitamin B_{12} deficiency, though this is inferior to *hydroxocobalamin* treatment.

Isolated **folate deficiency** should not be corrected unless vitamin B_{12} levels are adequate, because the latter is essential for correct folate metabolism and giving folate makes extra demands for vitamin B_{12} (see Figure 11.5). This may produce frank vitamin B_{12} deficiency in a patient with a marginal vitamin B_{12} level and so may cause widespread neurological damage. For this reason, multivitamin products, e.g. vitamins capsules, do not contain folic acid. Low levels of vitamin B_{12} also prevent full folate metabolism, so the folic acid is not available for normal purposes. If folate needs to be given and the patient's vitamin B_{12} status is suspect or unknown, both folic acid and vitamin B_{12} should be given.

The normal therapeutic dose is 5 mg of folic acid daily, the same as is used in chronic haemolytic disease. Women trying to conceive should take a prophylactic dose of 200–400 µg daily, or 400–500 µg daily for those at risk of a first neural tube defect, e.g. if either wife or husband has a neural tube defect. However, 4–5 mg daily until the 12th week of pregnancy is needed to prevent a recurrence of a neural tube defect.

Folic acid may reduce the plasma concentrations of antiepileptics (see Chapter 6), i.e. *phenytoin*, *phenobarbital* and *primidone*.

Acquired haemolytic anaemias

Inherited haemolytic anaemias, including those due to congenital metabolic defects, are discussed on pp. 712–716.

Non-immune haemolytic anaemias

These are one type of acquired haemolytic anaemia. There are numerous non-immune causes of intravascular haemolysis, for example:

- Mechanical RBC damage caused by excessive turbulence or shear in the circulation:
    - Calcified heart valve stenosis and malfunctioning mechanical heart valves (see Chapter 4).
    - Martial arts or prolonged running, which damage RBCs in the circulation of the feet.
    - Microangiopathic haemolytic anaemia, caused by severe hypertension (see Chapter 4).
    - Infection, e.g. disseminated intravascular coagulation (see Chapter 2).
    - Inflammatory conditions, e.g. polyarteritis nodosa (see Chapter 13).
- Paroxysmal nocturnal haemoglobinuria is due to a rare RBC membrane defect causing extreme sensitivity to complement C3 (Chapter 2). As the name implies, the haemoglobinuria is increased during sleep.

These non-immune causes of intravascular haemolysis are not discussed further in this text. However, most haemolysis is extravascular and results from RBC destruction in the phagocytic cells of the reticuloendothelial system in the liver, bone marrow and, especially, the spleen. If the bone marrow is able to respond, so that RBC replacement is able to keep pace with destruction, i.e. there is compensated haemolysis; the condition does not require treatment. Pharmacotherapeutic or surgical intervention is appropriate only if the condition causes respiratory or cardiovascular limitation or there is a serious underlying condition.

Autoimmune haemolytic anaemias

These are due to the production of anti-RBC autoimmunoglobulins (auto-Igs; Chapter 2). They are detected by a positive direct Coomb's test (Figure 11.6) and can be divided into two types. That in which the reaction with the auto-Igs occurs strongly at body temperature is the 'warm' type and is due to IgG autoagglutinins. Reactions that occur below 37°C (often <30°C) characterizes the 'cold' type and involve IgM autoagglutinins (Table 11.7; see Chapter 2).

The distinction is important because it affects management. The cold type responds poorly to treatment (see below), and patients with cold-type disease develop symptoms only in a cold environment.

Pathology. No primary pathogenic aetiology has been identified for either condition, but associated diseases are listed in Table 11.7.

Autoagglutinins (IGMs) that activate the complement cascade (see Chapter 2) cause intravascular haemolysis. However, IgGs often do not activate complement, but cells coated with IgG autoagglutinins may be either completely phagocytosed in the spleen or their cytoskeleton is damaged so that they become spherical (spherocytes) and continue to circulate until they too are trapped in the spleen and phagocytosed. Thus IgG autoagglutinins usually cause extravascular haemolysis.

Investigation. Results with electronic analysers usually give spuriously low RBC and Hb levels and a high MCV, all of these being due to RBC agglutination. Results with the cold type usually revert to approximate normality if the sample is warmed. The warm type gives nearly normal results in usual laboratory conditions. However, agglutination is best observed by microscopy, which also shows spherocytes.

Anaemia is usually mild, >7.5 g/dL of Hb, but severe haemolysis may occur rarely.

Clinical features – warm type haemolytic anaemias. These are more frequent in middle-aged women than men, but otherwise can occur in both sexes at any age. They tend to follow a relapsing–remitting course, but folate deficiency and infections may cause severe haemolysis. The commonest associations are with drugs that act as haptens (see Chapter 2), e.g. *methyldopa* and penicillins, and rheumatic and related diseases (Table 11.7; see also Chapter 12). Lymphomas, e.g. Hodgkin's disease and non-Hodgkin's lymphoma, and chronic lymphocytic leukaemia (see Chapter 10) are also associated. Autoagglutinins against Rhesus antigens (see Chapter 2) may be present. The spleen is enlarged proportionately to the severity of the haemolysis and is palpable below the left rib cage.

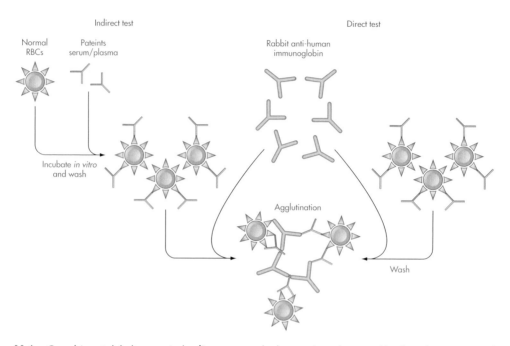

Figure 11.6   Coomb's antiglobulin tests. In the **direct test**, washed patient's erythrocytes (that have been sensitized *in vivo* by reaction with the patient's autoantibodies) are mixed with anti-human globulin (produced in rabbits or other animals), causing agglutination of the erythrocyte–autoantibody complexes. This demonstrates the presence of anti-erythrocyte autoantibodies, or sometimes complement components (usually C3), on the patient's RBCs. The test is used to diagnose or confirm haemolytic transfusion reactions, haemolytic disease of the newborn (HDN; see Chapter 2), autoimmune haemolytic anaemia, and drug-induced immune haemolytic anaemia, etc. However, other considerations, e.g. the temperature at which the reaction occurs and the class of autoantibody involved, are necessary to give a complete diagnosis. In the **indirect test**, normal erythrocytes are sensitized *in vitro* by reaction with the patient's plasma or serum, containing anti-erythrocyte antibodies, to produce erythrocyte–antibody complexes. The washed complexes are reacted with anti-human globulin, to crosslink the erythrocyte–antibody complexes, causing their agglutination, as in the direct test. The indirect test detects free anti-erythrocyte antibody in the patient's plasma or serum and is used in cross-matching potential donor and recipient's blood prior to transfusion and for antibody screening, etc. RBCs, red blood cells, erythrocytes.

Table 11.7   Principal features of autoimmune haemolytic anaemias

	Warm type	Cold type
Temperature at which antibody binds most strongly to RBCs	37°C	<37°C, usually <30°C
Class of antibody	IgG	IgM
Direct Coomb's test result (see Figure 11.6)	Strongly positive	Positive
Underlying disease state	Autoimmune disorders, e.g. systemic lupus erythematosus Lymphomas, e.g. Hodgkin's disease Chronic lymphatic leukaemia Carcinomas Drugs, e.g. methyldopa, penicillins	Infections, e.g. *Mycoplasma pneumoniae*, infectious mononucleosis (glandular fever) Lymphomas Paroxysmal cold haemoglobinuria

RBC, red blood cell.

Management. Any underlying disease should be treated and alternatives used to replace any drugs that are implicated, but haemolysis may continue for more than 3 weeks even though the drug is completely eliminated.

Patients should not normally receive blood transfusions, because autoagglutinins are widespread in donor serum, and careful cross-matching at 37°C is required if transfusion is essential. Washed red cells carry very little donor serum, but cross-matching of donor RBCs with the recipient's serum is essential to avoid lysis of donor RBCs.

High-dose *prednisolone* is effective in about 80% of patients and reduces the production of autoagglutinins, by suppressing B and T cell activity. It may also suppress RBC destruction in the spleen. If there is no response, or if relapse occurs when the dose is reduced, splenectomy is required. However, even this may be inadequate and immunosuppression, e.g. with *azathioprine* or *cyclophosphamide* (see Chapter 10), is then required.

Clinical features – cold type haemolytic anaemias. In about 50% of patients no cause can be found, especially in the older age group. This form is usually associated with a gradual onset of chronic haemolysis. Infections, e.g. infectious mononucleosis ('glandular fever', due to Epstein–Barr virus), *Mycoplasma* pneumonias, and cytomegalovirus infections are the commonest cause in the remainder, with an acute presentation. This latter form may be severe. Acrocyanosis, e.g. Raynaud's phenomenon (see Chapter 12) and similar blanching of the skin in the feet, occurs in cold conditions.

Management. Apart from treating any associated conditions, e.g. infections, and avoidance of cold conditions, little can be done. None of the treatments used for warm type disease, i.e. *prednisolone*, splenectomy and immunosuppression, is usually effective.

Neutropenia and agranulocytosis

Neutropenia is defined as a neutrophil count $<1.5 \times 10^9$/L. An almost complete absence of neutrophils is agranulocytosis, because they form about 85% of the total granulocyte count, i.e. neutrophils, eosinophils and basophils, and the factors that underlie neutropenia also affect other granulocytes.

Aetiology

- Inherited: ethnic (more common in non-white races), numerous rare inherited defects.
- Treatment of neoplastic disease with cytotoxic drugs (see Chapter 10).
- Following stem cell transplantation.
- Aplastic anaemia, i.e. bone marrow failure, which may be:
  - congenital;
  - due to drugs or chemicals, e.g. penicillins, cephalosporins, *chloramphenicol*, gold salts, antiepileptics (*phenytoin*, *carbamazepine*), oral hypoglycaemic agents, NSAIDs, *quinine*, volatile aromatic hydrocarbons ('glue sniffing');
  - result of infections, e.g. Epstein–Barr virus, hepatitis, HIV/AIDS, TB, typhoid fever;
  - due to bone marrow infiltration with neoplastic cells, e.g. in leukaemias and lymphomas.
- Megaloblastic anaemia (see above).
- RA, Felty's syndrome, SLE, Sjögren's syndrome (see Chapter 12).

Symptoms

These are primarily infections that increase in frequency and severity as the neutrophil count falls. Below 0.5×10^9/L life-threatening pneumonia and septicaemia are likely. Chronic tiredness may be regarded as a minor condition, thus delaying diagnosis and treatment.

Children are usually diagnosed at about 4–6 months of age, but the course of the disease is fairly benign and in most cases remits spontaneously after 6–24 months.

Diagnosis

This depends on a low neutrophil count, examination of a bone marrow trephine, demonstration of antineutrophil antibodies and the detection of other autoimmune conditions.

Pharmacotherapy

Any implicated drugs should be stopped and associated conditions treated. Prompt treatment of infections with parenteral broad-spectrum antibiotics, e.g. *ceftazidime* plus *gentamicin*, plus *flucloxacillin* if *Staph. aureus* is suspected. This may be modified according to local guidelines and re-evaluated according to the patient's progress and laboratory guidance.

Granulocyte-colony stimulating factor (rhG-CSF), i.e. *filgrastim*, *pegfilgrastim* (increased duration of action) or *lenograstim*, may help in a severe infection that is responding poorly to antibiotics. Like other new biological agents it should be used under specialist supervision, because it can have serious side-effects, e.g. malaise, bone and muscle pain, exacerbation of arthritis, sudden onset of severe agranulocytosis, urinary abnormalities, hepatic enlargement and spleen enlargement with a risk of spleen rupture.

Immunosuppressive agents, e.g. *azathioprine*, *cyclophosphamide*, *ciclosporin* and antilymphocyte globulin, if the condition has an autoimmune basis.

Corticosteroids are a second-line option because the response to them is very variable and they increase the risk of fungal and viral infection.

Haemostasis, fibrinolysis and anticoagulation

Haemostasis is a vitally important and highly organized and regulated homeostatic mechanism. Its function is to secure the optimal flow of blood to organs and cells under physiological conditions and to respond rapidly to disturbances, e.g. bleeding caused by tissue damage, and restore normality. There are four major components that co-operate sensitively to achieve this result:

- Vascular endothelium and intima.
- Platelets.
- Components of the coagulation system.
- Fibrinolytic system.

Common investigations into the clotting cascade are given in Table 11.8.

Vascular endothelium and intima

The endothelium (see Chapter 4) is much more than an elegant smooth inner lining of the vessel wall that separates the blood from reactive components of the intima and minimizes turbulence in the blood, though it does both of these. In the following discussion, the locations and functions of individual components of the clotting and thrombolytic pathways are described first and these are then drawn together when the clotting cascade is described.

Under normal conditions, it prevents thrombosis (clotting), partly by repelling cellular components of the blood by its surface charge. It also has direct anticoagulant properties due to:

- Production of nitric oxide, which inhibits platelet adhesion and aggregation and causes vasodilatation, thus maintaining a patent blood vessel.
- Production of epoprostenol (prostacyclin), which inhibits platelet aggregation, also preventing vascular blockage.
- Presence of heparan and dermatan sulphates, which are direct anticoagulants.
- Exoenzymes that break down platelet activators, e.g. ADP.
- Thrombomodulin on the surface provides a high affinity, specific thrombin binding site and the thrombomodulin–thrombin complex activates protein C 1000-fold (PrCa). PrCa acts as an anticoagulant.

When the endothelium is damaged:

- **Tissue factor (TFr)** is exposed and remains located at the site of damage.
- **Von Willebrand factor (vWF)** in the plasma binds collagen and platelets together via their GP1b binding sites or collagen binds platelets via their GP1a binding site.
- Reduced thrombomodulin production results in less PrCa, which gives reduced anticoagulant activity to limit thrombin generation, and so prevents runaway coagulation. Protein S acts to bind PrCa to the endothelial surface.

Table 11.8   Common investigations of blood coagulation[a]

Investigation	Procedure	Comments
Platelet count	Automated analyser	N = 150–400 × 10^9/L
Activated partial thromboplastin time (APTT)	Add kaolin (or other surface activator), phospholipid, Ca^{2+}[b], phospholipid (platelet substitute), to patient's plasma	N = 30–50 s (depends on exact method used). Best for deficiencies of factors VIII: C[b], IX, XI, XII, antiphospholipid antibodies (see above) and to monitor heparin and heparinoid treatment
Prothrombin time (PT)[a]	Add tissue thromboplastin (as animal brain extract or recombinant product) to patient's plasma	N = 30–50 s Best for deficiencies of factors V, X, XII, warfarin treatment, liver disease (less suitable for I, II, VII)
International normalized ratio (INR)[c]	The patient's PT divided by the PT with normal blood, using international (WHO) standard reagents	N = 1.0–1.3, see Table 11.10 for target values Should be reproducible worldwide
Thrombin time	Add thrombin to patient's plasma	N = 12 s Prolonged for fibrinogen deficiency, abnormal fibrin function, or their inhibitors, e.g. heparin, fibrin degradation products (fragments X, Y, D, E, N)
Skin bleeding time	Apply sphygmomanometer cuff to arm, inflate to 50 mmHg, make two cuts with jig to forearm, each 1 mm deep by 40 mm long; blot every 30 s	N = 2.5–9.5 min

[a] Factor numbers and names are as follows (see also Figure 11.7; not all factors have been named).

I	Fibrinogen	VII	Proconvertin	XI	Plasma thromboplastin antecedent
II	Prothrombin	VIII	Antihaemophilic globulin A	XII	Hageman factor
III	Tissue thromboplastin	IX	Antihaemophilic globulin B	XIII	Fibrin stabilizing factor
V	Proaccelerin	X	Stuart-Power factor		

The end-point is clotting in all tests other than skin bleeding time. Corrections can be made for various conditions.

[b] Blood samples are collected in citrated vials to bind calcium and prevent clotting in transit.

[c] INR is determined from PT.

- **Tissue type plasminogen activator inhibitor** is released, which blocks activation of tissue plasminogen, thus preventing clot lysis and maintaining clot stability.

Platelets

These are derived from the (myeloid) mega-karyocytes and are an essential component of haemostasis. They are normally confined to the vascular lumen by a mutually-repulsive static charge between them and the vascular endothelium, by the production of nitric oxide and epoprostenol by the endothelial cells and the high-velocity laminar flow in the core of the lumen. However, when the endothelium is damaged, vWFr is exposed and binds the platelets to collagen, even under conditions of high flow. However, this binding is not permanent and the platelets dissociate and roll slowly along the endothelium. In this situation the platelets become activated and the platelet GpIIb-IIIa receptors bind both the vWFr and fibrinogen, platelet adhesion becomes irreversible and aggregation occurs, resulting in propagation of the primary clot. When flow is reduced, fibrinogen, fibronectin (a large glycoprotein adhesion molecule) and collagen may initiate platelet adhesion without the intervention of vWFr.

Von Willebrand's disease (p. 731) is an autosomal-dominant condition, causing either a deficiency or an abnormal function of vWFr.

Platelet activation

This is caused by the binding of arachidonic acid, thromboxane A_2, ADP, fibrinogen and collagen. The level of cAMP is reduced and phopholipase C is activated. The phopholipase generates inositol triphosphate, which mobilizes calcium, triggering several calcium-dependent reactions, e.g. secretion of the contents of platelet granules.

Activation is accompanied by morphological change, the platelets become spherical with large pseudopodia, followed by contraction of the cytoskeleton, clot shrinkage and platelet plug formation (see Chapter 2).

Platelet dysfunction

It is unsurprising from the central role of platelets in clotting that a deficiency of them, i.e. **thrombocytopenia** ($<100 \times 10^9$/L, normal 100–500 $\times$ 10^9/L), will lead to bleeding problems, e.g.

- Moderate haemorrhage after injury.
- **Purpura**, i.e. spontaneous bleeding into the skin, usually in the form of a petechial rash, caused by numerous small bleeds, which occurs at platelet counts of 20–50 $\times 10^9$/L (N = 150–400 $\times 10^9$/L). This type of rash does not blanch under pressure, unlike inflammatory rashes, and also accompanies meningococcal meningitis (see Chapter 8).
- Easy bruising, epistaxis (nose bleeds), conjunctival haemorrhage, blood blisters in the mouth and blood oozing from gums and menorrhagia (heavy periods).

- In severe disease ($<20 \times 10^9$/L) there may be brain and retinal haemorrhage.

Thrombocytopenia may be due to:

- Inherited abnormalities of platelet function, e.g. von Willebrand's disease (see above).
- Reduced platelet production, e.g. infiltration of the bone marrow in leukaemias and lymphomas. **Gaucher's disease** is a lysosomal storage disease, due to abnormal lipid metabolism, in which large amounts of lipoids are deposited in bone marrow and spleen cells, causing splenomegaly and so excessive platelet destruction. It is particularly common in Jews of Eastern European origin (1 in 2000–3000 live births).
- Excessive peripheral destruction, due to, e.g.
  - Autoimmune platelet destruction, sometimes with drugs acting as haptens (see Chapter 2). It may also occur in neonates by a process similar to that causing haemolytic disease of the newborn (HDN; see Chapter 2).
  - Heparin therapy (rarely; see below).
  - Non-immune platelet destruction, e.g. in hypersplenism, with or without splenomegaly, due to alcoholic cirrhosis, acute and chronic infections, e.g. hepatitis (see Chapter 3), pregnancy, renal failure, endocarditis (see Chapters 4 and 8), malaria and syphilis, and systemic inflammatory diseases, e.g. SLE, RA and Sjögren's syndrome (see Chapter 12).

    Other causes may be drugs, e.g. cephalosporins, penicillins, *quinine*, *ciclosporin*, *mitomycin*.

Management of thrombocytopenia includes:

- Stop any drugs that may be implicated.
- Diagnose and treat any underlying or associated diseases, e.g. *H. pylori* infection, hepatitis C, cytomegalovirus and HIV infections. Treatment of Gaucher's disease may include high-dose steroids, infusion of *alglucerase* and splenectomy.
- High-dose *prednisolone*, i.e. 1 mg/kg/day for 4 weeks, reducing slowly to zero if possible. About 70% of patients respond, about half of whom have a long-lasting remission. High-

dose pulsed *dexamethasone* has also been used.

- Immunosuppressive agents may help in refractory disease, e.g. *azathioprine, mycophenolate mofetil, ciclosporin, danazol* and *vincristine*.
- *Alemtuzumab* or *rituximab* (unlicensed indications) are monoclonal antibodies, given by IV infusion, that cause lysis of B-lymphocytes. They may help in patients with refractory autoimmune disease. Although *rituximab* has been used with minimal side-effects, these agents may cause severe anaphylaxis (see Chapter 2) and should be used under specialist supervision with full resuscitation facilities available.
- **Splenectomy** is used as a last resort, especially in the elderly who may be unfit for major surgery, but this exposes the patient to recurrent severe infections.
- Children are treated only if there is significant bleeding. *Prednisolone* is the first-line therapy (see above). Chronic disease requires long-term steroids (with the risk of growth retardation), IV Ig, or ultimately splenectomy, with a life-long risk of infection. Treatment clearly poses considerable problems.

IV immunoglobulin (IV Ig) gives a prompt but temporary (3-week) increase in the platelet count. It is therefore used only in the acute treatment of serious haemorrhage, usually with corticosteroids, or to increase the count prior to splenectomy, and so prevent intra-operative bleeding. There is a risk of unsuspected viral transmission.

Platelet transfusions are not usually beneficial, because they are destroyed rapidly. However, they are used acutely to control life-threatening bleeding, e.g. brain haemorrhage.

Antiplatelet agents

Most anticoagulants affect the venous circulation and have little effect on clotting in the arteries. Antiplatelet agents reduce platelet aggregation and may inhibit thrombus formation in the arteries, and so are beneficial in those conditions in which arterial thrombosis is the prime cause, e.g. MI (see Chapter 4) and some strokes. They are also useful in embolic diseases, i.e. vascular blockage caused by clots or clot fragments, e.g. pulmonary embolism (PE), retinal vein occlusion and some strokes.

Aspirin

This is readily hydrolysed at blood pH (7.4) to release acetic acid. *Aspirin* irreversibly acetylates a serine residue near the active centre of platelet cyclo-oxygenase (COX) and therefore prevents the formation of thromboxane (TX A_2), a vasoconstrictor and potent initiator of platelet activation. Because platelets have no synthetic ability, the effect is permanent as long as *aspirin* is being taken.

For the secondary prevention of thrombotic IHD and stroke, 150–300 mg is given as soon as possible after the initial event and this is followed by 75 mg daily (low-dose) for lifelong maintenance.

The use of low-dose *aspirin* for primary prevention is appropriate only in those in whom the estimated 10-year risk of CVD and stroke, nonfatal and fatal, is ≥20% (see BNF and the References and further reading section), provided that any hypertension is controlled adequately. In the remainder, the possible benefit is outweighed by the potential side-effects, e.g. gastrointestinal bleeding. Other uses are in atrial fibrillation, provided there are no other risk factors for stroke, angina pectoris (AP) and intermittent claudication (cramping pain in the legs due to ischaemia, induced by exercise and relieved by rest).

Glycoprotein IIb-IIIa ihibitors: abciximab

This monoclonal antibody to GpIIb-IIIa receptors on platelets is used as an adjunct to *heparin* and *aspirin* for the prevention of ischaemic complications in high-risk patients:

- Those undergoing percutaneous transluminal coronary intervention (PTCI), e.g. angiography or angioplasty (see Chapter 4).
- Those with unstable angina pectoris (AP) for the prevention of MI in those scheduled for PTCI. An IV injection is given initially, followed by an IV infusion started 10–60 min before the procedure and continuing for 12 h.

It should be used only once during the procedure because the serious side-effect of bleeding, possibly complicated by hypotension, bradycardia, chest pain, fever, thrombocytopenia and hypersensitivity reactions, are enhanced by repeat dosing.

It is contra-indicated if the patient already has active bleeding, a bleeding tendency, or thrombocytopenia, has had major surgery, intracranial or intraspinal surgery or trauma in the previous 2 months, stroke within 2 years, an intracranial neoplasm, arteriovenous malformation, aneurysm, severe hypertension or hypertensive retinopathy, or is breastfeeding.

In view of this long list of potential hazards, it is not surprising that it must be used under specialist supervision.

In 2002 NICE published guidance on the use of GpIIb-IIIa inhibitors for ACS (Table 11.9).

Glycoprotein IIb-IIIa ihibitors: eptifibatide and tirofiban

These are licensed for use with *aspirin* or *heparin* to prevent MI in patients with unstable AP, or those who have non-ST-segment elevation MI. They have generally similar side-effects and contra-indications to *abciximab*. However, *eptifibatide* should be used within 24 h of the last episode of chest pain and *tirofiban* within 12 h. *Tirofiban* may cause a reversible thrombocytopenia.

Both agents are given by IV infusion, under specialist supervision, but *eptifibatide* requires an initial IV loading dose.

Other antiplatelet agents

The thienopyridines, *clopidogrel* and *ticlopidine*, have similar actions, contra-indications and side-effects. *Ticlopidine* is not licensed in the UK.

Clopidogrel is used as a prophylactic oral anti-coagulant in patients with a history of symptomatic ischaemic disease. It is also licensed for use combined with low-dose *aspirin* in acute coronary syndrome without ST-segment elevation (see Chapter 4). In the latter circumstances, the combination is given for at least 1 month, but not usually for longer than 9–12 months. Readers are directed to the BNF for further details of interactions, etc. Although *clopidogrel* should be initiated only in hospital inpatients, several trials have reported it to be a safe and effective alternative to *aspirin*.

Dipyridamole is used as an adjunct to other oral anticoagulation for the prevention of thromboembolism associated with prosthetic heart valves. Modified-release preparations are licensed for the secondary prophylaxis of ischaemic stroke and TIAs. There is no good evidence for the benefits of its long-term use with low-dose *aspirin* in the prevention of serious ischaemic cardiovascular events. However, there is evidence from one trial that this combination reduces the risk for non-fatal stroke, though gastrointestinal side-effects were more troublesome and more people withdrew from the combination than from *aspirin* alone.

Table 11.9 NICE guidance on the use of GpIIb-IIIa inhibitors (September 2002)

Abciximab, eptifibatide and tirofiban should be considered in the management of unstable angina pectoris and non-ST-segment-elevation MI.

They are recommended for patients at high risk of MI or death when early PTCI is desirable but does not occur immediately. Either eptifibatide or tirofiban is recommended in addition to other appropriate drug treatment.

A GpIIb-IIIa inhibitor is indicated as an adjunct to PTCI[a]:
- When early PTCI is indicated but is delayed.
- In patients with diabetes.
- If the procedure is complex.

[a] Currently, only abciximab is licensed for use in PTCI (author's comment).

MI, myocardial infarction; PTCI, percutaneous transluminal coronary intervention.

Epoprostenol (prostacyclin) may be used in renal dialysis patients, either alone or with *heparin*. Because it is a potent vasodilator it causes flushing, headaches and hypotension. Its half-life is only about 3 min, so it has to be given by continuous IV infusion, but with these patients it can be added conveniently to the existing return dialysis line.

Clotting cascade

Haemostasis

This resembles the complement cascade in that factors are split to form enzymes or factors with other activity (see Chapter 2) that act sequentially, thus giving massive amplification of the initial reaction. It has been conventional to consider the clotting pathways as composed of two separate routes, intrinsic and extrinsic, similar to the situation with complement. However, the two pathways are now known to be integrated *in vivo*, forming a unified whole. A summary of these reactions is shown in Figure 11.7. Because there has been confusion in nomenclature, most of the various elements are now designated by roman numerals, but these are not numbered in sequence. Activated forms are denoted by the suffix 'a'.

Tissue factor (TFr) is a glycoprotein that is expressed constitutively on fibroblast surfaces and is inducible in endothelial and other cells by IL-1, TNF and endotoxin, especially if the cells are damaged. It acts as a co-factor with **Factor VII (FrVII)** to initiate the cascade. The **FrVII–TFr complex** activates **FrIX** and **FrX**, forming **FrIXa** and **FrXa**. The latter acts with **FrVa** to form the **tenase complex (FrXa–FrVa)** that converts prothrombin to thrombin, in association with phospholipid and Ca^{2+}. Thrombin has the key role in the process and converts:

- FrV $\rightarrow$ FrVa, to generate additional tenase complex.
- Fibrinogen $\rightarrow$ fibrin.
- FrXIII $\rightarrow$ FrXIIIa, which in turn crosslinks the fibrin fibres, forming a stable clot matrix.
- FrXI $\rightarrow$ FrXIa, which then converts FrIX $\rightarrow$ FrIXa and FrVIII $\rightarrow$ FrVIIIa. The FrVIIIa–FrIXa complex converts FrX $\rightarrow$ FrXa, providing an

additional source for the tenase complex that is required because it elicits the production of a tissue factor pathway inhibitor (TFrPI) and inactivates FrVIIa–TFr. The TFrPI is one of the components that serves to limit excessive coagulation. The conversion of FrXI $\rightarrow$ FrXIa may also occur by auto-activation.

FrVIIa is known to bind to platelets independently of TFr and causes the release of thrombin at sites of vascular injury. Although there have been only a few randomized trials, recombinant FrVIIa has been reported to be effective in the management of haemorrhage due to trauma or surgery, e.g. upper gastrointestinal bleeding (see Chapter 3), liver transplants and acute intracerebral haemorrhage, but these are unlicensed indications. In the latter case, it produced improved outcome and reduced mortality. It is presently licensed for the treatment of haemophilia (see below) and inherited disorders of platelet function.

Inherited coagulation disorders: haemophilias and von Willebrand disease

The haemophilias are X-linked genetic disorders of haemostasis that are due to deficiencies of coagulation factors. There are two forms: the most common is due to a deficiency of FrVIII:C, its procoagulant form, which circulates in the plasma in association with vWFr (see above) and causes **haemophilia A**. FrIX deficiency causes **haemophilia B**. Because the conditions are X-linked all affected women are carriers and their sons have a 50% chance of haemophilia and daughters have a 50% chance of being a carrier. However, it is estimated that up to one-third of mutations in the FrVIII gene may be spontaneous and so not inherited from a parent. Because almost all haemophiliacs are male, and the defective gene is X-linked, all of their daughters are carriers but all of their sons are normal, unless the mother is a carrier. A very small number of women are haemophiliacs, due to inactivation of the normal chromosomal allele, a process known as **lyonization**, very early in embryo development.

The prevalence of haemophilia A is about 1 per 5000–10 000 and haemophilia B is about one-fifth as common.

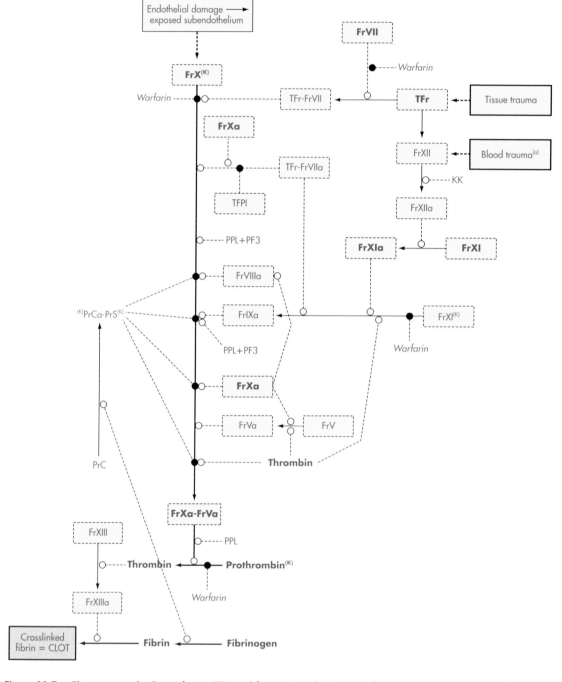

Figure 11.7 Clotting cascade. Tissue factor (TFr) and factors V and VIII are co-factors and have no enzymic function. FrXa-Va is known as the tenase complex. Note the central roles of TFr and FrX in the early stages and of thrombin in the final stages. Fr, factor; KK, kallikrein; PPL, phospholipid. Hyphens indicate complex formation. —O, promotes; —●, inhibits. [a]Blood trauma includes septicaemia (see Chapter 2), some malignant neoplasms, some patients with heparin-induced thrombocytopenia (p. 740), patients with antiphospholipid syndrome, protein C and protein S deficiencies (see Figure 11.8), or Factor V Leiden disease. [K]Vitamin K-dependent factor. Vitamin K is a cofactor for the modification of glutamate residues of prothrombin, FrVII, FrIX, FrX, PrC and PrS, to enable them to bind Ca^{2+}. Without calcium binding, clotting does not occur.

The FrVIII gene is very large (186 kilobases) and numerous mutations have been identified that may produce a range of levels of functionality, the normal range of FrVIII level being 50–200% of the mean. The FrIX gene is much smaller (33 kilobases) and is inherited similarly to FrVIII, though recessive forms also occur. Some mutations give rise to the 'Leyden' phenotype that disappears after puberty.

Deficiency of vWFr, the functions of which are described on p. 726, also causes a bleeding tendency that may vary from mild to severe. They are much more common than the haemophilias and the prevalence of mild von Willebrand disease (vWD) is estimated to reach 1% in some populations. This high frequency is a reflection of its dual roles in FrVIII:C carriage and platelet binding to vascular endothelium. There are three forms of vWD, the genes for which are located on chromosome 12, two genes being inherited as autosomal dominant alleles, and the other recessive.

Clinical features. All of these conditions confer a haemorrhagic tendency, and bleeding may be spontaneous, e.g. epistaxis or bleeding from the gums and mouth, or occur after minor trauma, e.g. dental treatment, or surgery.

Haemophilia A and B cannot be distinguished clinically. Children with haemophilia are usually healthy at birth, though excessive cord bleeding and heavy bruising due to birth trauma may occur. Symptoms develop towards the end of the first year, especially bruising, but spontaneous bleeds become less frequent in adults. The popular idea that patients 'bleed to death' after minor trauma is incorrect, though intracranial haemorrhage may be life-threatening. The major problem is bleeding into muscles and weight-bearing joints (**haemarthrosis**) and recurrent joint bleeds may cause serious damage there. Patients should not be given IM injections. Bleeding after trauma usually requires therapeutic intervention.

Both sexes are affected in vWD. Mucosal bleeding and bleeding after trauma or surgery are the principal problems but, unlike haemophilia, bleeding into joints and muscles occurs only rarely. Menorrhagia may present problems in fertile women. Patients with milder disease may not present until their third or fourth decade.

Management of haemophilia.   Genetic counselling is an essential component of the care of affected families, and genetic analysis is available for the detection of carriers. Antenatal diagnosis is also used to detect those who have slipped through the net, especially recent immigrants.

Management involves detection of the particular clotting factor deficiency and its replacement. In the 1980s and 1990s, freeze-dried factor concentrates were prepared from large donor pools, but these transmitted unsuspected viral infection to some patients, especially hepatitis and HIV. This was countered by careful donor selection, viral inactivation by irradiation and immunization against hepatitis. However, there was still concern about the possibility of transmission of variant Creutzfeld-Jakob disease, and **recombinant human FrVIII and FrIX** (rhFrVIII, rhFrIX) are now available and have replaced concentrates from plasma.

Unfortunately, inhibitory antibodies to FrVIII are formed in about 10% of treated patients and has required desensitization treatment in specialized centres (see Chapter 2). These inhibitors are active against both endogenous factors and those given therapeutically and cause severe problems in treatment. The problem has been exacerbated by the administration of rhFrVIII because it is not complexed with its carrier molecule (vWFr) and consequently is more immunogenic. Inhibitor formation occurs only rarely with FrIX. Recombinant activated FrVII overcomes the inhibitor problem in both types of haemophilia, because it bypasses the reactions that require FrVIII and FrIX in the clotting cascade (Figure 11.7). It is licensed for the treatment of haemophilia patients in whom inhibitors have developed.

Vasopressin, the ADH, and its more potent, longer-acting analogue *desmopressin* stimulate the release of FrVIII (and vWFr) from endothelia and WBCs and are used in mild to moderate haemophilia A to reduce the need for exogenous FrVIII. *Vasopressin* is used with an anti-fibrinolytic agent, e.g. *tranexamic acid*, which boosts its effect. The latter is also used to control bleeding due to minor procedures in haemophiliacs, e.g. dental extractions, but are not used with FrIX because of the thrombotic risk. Antifibrinolytic agents (see below) are also used with rhFrVIII to assist in the control of external bleeding.

Modulation of haemostasis – intrinsic anticoagulant pathways and fibrinolysis

These are an integral part of the clotting cascade and provide for control of haemostasis, to prevent excessive coagulation that could compromise the circulation, and for the removal of the clot when it has fulfilled its functions of preventing haemorrhage and providing a support matrix for vascular wall repair.

Intrinsic anticoagulant pathways include:

- TFrPI, mentioned above.
- **Antithrombins (serpins)**, which block the activation of FrV, FrVIII, FrXI and the conversion of fibrinogen to fibrin.
- **Heparin**, which potentiates the action of **antithrombins** against FrXa and thrombin, the activity of antithrombins being increased 2000-fold.
- **Thrombin** probably binds to **thrombomodulin** that is bound to endothelial cell surfaces. When bound, thrombin loses its procoagulant properties and is transformed into a highly active anticoagulant.
- The thrombin–thrombomodulin complex vastly increases the activation rate of **protein C (PrC)**. The PrCa breaks down FrVa and FrVIIIa and so inhibits additional thrombin production.
- The PrCa, together with its co-factors **protein S (PrS)** and Ca^{2+}, binds to phospholipid on cell surfaces and so prevents the conversion of prothrombin to thrombin by the tenase complex.
- FrXIIIa binds alpha$_2$-antiplasmin to fibrin and may protect the clot from fibrinolysis.

Fibrinolysis

Solution of the platelet–fibrin clot is an essential sequel to clotting and removes the clot when vascular repair has occurred and the clot is no longer needed. **Tissue type plasminogen activator (tPA)** is secreted from endothelial cells and, bound to fibrin, converts plasminogen to **plasmin**, which activates tPA by splitting it into a double-stranded molecule. Plasmin also hydrolyses FrV, FrVIII, FrXIII, fibrinogen and fibrin. The latter yields fragment X, which inhibits thrombin, and fragments Y, D and E, which inhibit fibrin polymerization. Alpha$_2$-antiplasmin and tPA are inhibited, thus preventing undue fibrinolysis, fibrinogen consumption and haemorrhage.

A diagram of the fibrinolytic pathways is given in Figure 11.8.

It is apparent from the foregoing account that the numerous steps and counteracting factors involved in the haemostatic and fibrinolytic pathways enable the processes to be controlled with exquisite sensitivity to produce a response tailored precisely to the requirements of local situations.

Recombinant tissue-type plasminogen activator (rt-PA, *alteplase*) is used for clot dissolution in acute myocardial infarction (AMI) (see Chapter 4), pulmonary embolism (PE, see Chapter 5) and, under the supervision of a specialist neurological physician, for acute ischaemic stroke. It is administered by IV injection, followed by IV infusion. *Alteplase* treatment for AMI (see Chapter 4) must be given within 3 h to be of maximal benefit, the earlier the better to minimize permanent myocardial damage. *Reteplase* and *tenecteplase* are also licensed for use in AMI and have the advantage of being given by IV injection only, without the need for IV infusion. Fibrinolytics are especially beneficial in those with ST segment elevation or bundle branch block (see Chapter 4).

Reteplase is licensed for the thrombolytic treatment of AMI and should be given within 12 h. *Heparin* and *aspirin* are administered both before using *reteplase* and afterwards, to minimize the risk of re-infarction.

Immediate MRI/CT imaging will distinguish between thromboembolic and haemorrhagic strokes. Serious exacerbation of bleeding results if lytic agents or anticoagulants are used in unsuspected haemorrhagic stroke. Imaging will also demonstrate the presence of occult pathology, e.g. a tumour or rapidly enlarging aneurysm, and trauma, which are contra-indications to the use of *alteplase*, etc. Other exclusion criteria are recent major surgery, recent MI and bacterial endocarditis (see Chapter 8).

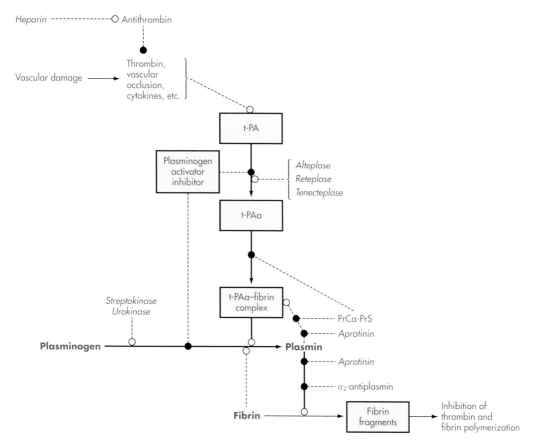

Figure 11.8 Fibrinolytic system. This is an integral part of the clotting system (see text and Figure 11.7). Drugs affecting fibrinolysis in italics. Urokinase is no longer available (unlicensed) in the UK. PrC, protein C; PrCa, activated PrC; PrS, protein S; t-PA, tissue type plasminogen activator; t-PAa, activated t-PA; —●, inhibition; —O, stimulates.

Streptokinase, another plasminogen activator prepared from streptococci, is used for MI, PE, DVT, acute arterial thromboembolism and central retinal artery or vein thrombosis. Although much cheaper than the other agents, it has the disadvantage that it produces a persistent allergic state and cannot be used repeatedly in a patient without special precautions. Anaphylaxis and Guillain-Barré syndrome are serious side-effects.

Many patients with branch retinal vein thromboembolism do not require thrombolytic therapy and do well with no treatment or *aspirin* antiplatelet therapy and end up with only minor retinal scarring.

The sites of action of these agents are shown in Figure 11.8.

Antifibrinolytic agents may be used to prevent excessive blood loss in surgical procedures. The use of *tranexamic acid* in haemophilia is referred to above. It is given by slow IV injection in prostatectomy and orally in menorrhagia and hereditary haemorrhagic telangiectasia. The latter is a rare, autosomal-dominant condition in which there are widespread collections of dilated capillaries and arterioles that bleed easily. They are visible as a skin rash that blanches under pressure and in the mouth, lips, nasal mucosa and on the tips of the fingers and toes. Recurrent profuse epistaxis and gastrointestinal bleeding cause anaemia, but the first presentation may be an embolic TIA or stroke. *Tranexamic acid* is contra-indicated in severe renal disease and thromboembolic states and should be used with caution in severe haematuria because it may cause ureteric clotting and obstruction.

Aprotinin is a proteolytic enzyme inhibitor that acts on plasmin and kallikrein. It is given by slow IV injection or infusion in major surgery, e.g. open heart surgery, tumour resection and following thrombolytic therapy (see above). Its use in liver transplantation is unlicensed.

Etamsylate is another antifibrinolytic agent that is licensed for the prevention of blood loss in menorrhagia. It reduces capillary bleeding if there is a normal platelet count, probably by correcting abnormal platelet adhesion to endothelium.

Procoagulable states – antiphospholipid syndrome

This is an autoimmune, connective tissue type disorder (see Chapters 2 and 12) that is characterized by antibodies against cell membrane phospholipids. It is sometimes associated with SLE (see Chapter 12). Because of this, and because the antibodies also react with the artificial antibody cardiolipin that was used in the old Wasserman test for syphilitic antibodies, they have been called 'lupus anticoagulant' and 'anticardiolipin'.

Aetiology, clinical features and pharmacotherapy

The autoantibody target is **beta$_2$-glycoprotein (β_2-GP1)**, sometimes known as apolipoprotein H. The autoantibodies are known to reduce the levels of annexin V, a surface adhesion protein that occurs in vascular endothelium and the placenta.

Clinical features. There are recurrent arterial and venous thromboses, causing about 20% of strokes occurring before the age of 45. Adrenal gland thrombosis may cause Addison's disease. Placental clotting is responsible for about 30% of miscarriages in women who have suffered two or more spontaneous abortions.

There is the paradoxical situation of a pro-thrombotic state *in vivo* and antibodies that have an anticoagulant effect *in vitro*, the reason for which is unknown. Other features are migraine,

epilepsy and other CNS effects, heart valve disease and the skin rash, livedo reticularis, a net-like pinkish rash surrounding pale areas of skin, showing the pattern of the blood supply in the epidermis.

Investigations. The antibodies are detected by enzyme-linked immunosorbent assay. The ESR and antinuclear antibody tests (ANA; see Chapter 12) are usually negative. The direct Coomb's test (Figure 11.6) is positive.

Treatment is with *aspirin*, if mild, or *warfarin* if moderate to severe (see below). *Heparin* has to be substituted for *warfarin* in pregnancy, which should be managed by a gynaecological specialist.

Therapeutic anticoagulation

The purpose of this treatment is to prevent:

- Venous and arterial clotting and clot propagation, e.g. in antiphospholipid syndrome (see above).
- Clotting in the cardiac chambers or coronary circulation, e.g. in atrial fibrillation and on prosthetic heart valves.
- Embolization from these clots, e.g. causing stroke or PE. Clotting in the brain.

Patient assessment

Relative contra-indications include:

- Recent major surgery or traumatic injury, a bleeding tendency, active bleeding, e.g. from a peptic ulcer (see Chapter 3), or a family history of excessive bleeding.
- Inadequately controlled hypertension (see Chapter 4).
- Severe hepatic or renal dysfunction. Liver disease causes a deficiency of erythropoietic factors and important clotting proteins. Both liver and kidney diseases result in deficiencies of erythropoietin and thrombopoietin (see Chapter 2).
- Drug abuse, if injections are used.
- Alcohol abuse, which may cause gastric bleeding and dementia and damages the liver.

- *Heparin* may cause a hypersensitivity reaction and is unsuitable in thrombocytopenia because it reduces the platelet count.

Many of these conditions are amenable to treatment and anticoagulation should not be initiated until appropriate therapy has been given or until wounds are healed.

A medication history must be taken and any potential interactions considered, e.g. are the drugs essential or can alternatives be used? This is particularly important if *warfarin* therapy is contemplated because its activity may be enhanced or reduced by a very large number of other agents, including *aspirin* and NSAIDs, alcohol, herbal remedies (e.g. St John's wort) and dietary changes (appropriate references should be consulted for a comprehensive listing).

Although analgesic doses of *aspirin* are contra-indicated in those taking *warfarin*, low-dose *aspirin* (75 mg/day) is acceptable in those at risk of thromboembolism, provided that the dose of warfarin is determined (see below) while the patient is taking the *aspirin*. It should be remembered that clotting changes occur both when starting *aspirin* and if it is stopped.

Warfarin is a potent teratogen and causes severe fetal deformity, especially if taken in weeks 6–12 of gestation, when organogenesis is occurring. However, the use of all antiplatelet drugs at any stage of pregnancy may cause miscarriage or some degree of fetal malformation. Heparins do not cross the placenta but may cause undesirable problems in the mother, e.g. a reduced platelet count, hyperkalaemia due to inhibition of aldosterone secretion, skin necrosis, hypersensitivity reactions including anaphylaxis and osteoporosis. Low molecular weight heparins are safer, but their use with prosthetic heart valves has been contentious.

Preliminary investigations are listed in Table 11.9.

Warfarin management

Pharmacology. *Warfarin* is the standard coumarin oral anticoagulant in the UK. *Acenocoumarol* (nicoumalone) is used occasionally, as is *phenindione*, a non-coumarol.

Warfarin inhibits the carboxylation of the vitamin K-dependent clotting factors, i.e. FrII, FrVII, FrIX and FrX, and the coagulation inhibitor proteins, i.e. PrC and its cofactor PrS (see above).

It is readily absorbed, the peak plasma level is achieved at about 1.5 h, and the onset of action is at about 48 h (24–72 h). Because of its once-daily dosing, steady-state levels are not reached for about 5 days. Accordingly a loading dose is given for the first 4 days of treatment. It is 97% bound to plasma proteins, displacement being the basis of its interactions with other acidic drugs. The half-life is very variable between individuals, being in the range 24–72 h.

Therapy is monitored using the **international normalized ratio (INR**; Table 11.8), which is the ratio of the patient's prothrombin time (PT) to that of a normal control, using standardized reagents. Recommended target levels for various conditions are given in Table 11.10.

Induction. The initial loading dose is determined according to the baseline PT and should be reduced if this is prolonged (normal values: PT 12–16 s, INR 1.0–1.3), if the patient's liver function tests are abnormal, if the patient is elderly or in cardiac failure, is on parenteral feeding, has a low body weight and is taking drugs known to potentiate *warfarin* activity. Although the normal initial loading dose is given in the BNF as 10 mg/day for 2 days, the British Guidelines on Oral Anticoagulation (see References and further reading, p. 741) recommend 5 mg/day for 4 days. All recommendations here are based on these guidelines.

High loading doses produce rapid reductions in the levels of the anticoagulant proteins C and S (see above and Figure 11.8) and may cause SC thrombosis and skin necrosis. Accordingly *heparin* (see below) is given to patients at high risk of thromboembolism before initiating *warfarin*, e.g. in atrial fibrillation (see Chapter 4) or if there is a personal or family history of venous thrombosis. This should be continued until the INR is >2 for 2 days. In such cases the starting dose of *warfarin* should not exceed 5 mg/day.

Maintenance dosing. The average is 3 to 9 mg/day, but this varies very widely (0.5 to >25 mg/day, and the required dose is managed on a 'sliding scale', e.g. Table 11.11.

Table 11.10   Target levels of INR recommended for various conditions

Indication	Target INR[a]
Venous thromboembolism	
• DVT or PE prophylaxis (maintain >2.0 if high risk)	2.0
• Treatment of first episode or recurrence off warfarin	2.5
• Treatment of recurrence on warfarin	3.5
• Antiphospholipid syndrome	3.5[b]
Cardiac indications	
• Atrial fibrillation (maintain INR >2.0 for 4 weeks pre-cardioversion and post-cardioversion)	2.5
• Dilated cardiomyopathy	2.5
• Mural thrombus post-MI	2.5
• Rheumatic mitral valve disease	2.5
• Mechanical heart valves	3.75

[a] All target values have a range of ± 0.5, except that for mechanical heart valves, which is ± 0.75 (read together with the text and Chapter 4).
[b] Level varies with clinical condition of patient.
DVT, deep-vein thrombosis; MI, myocardial infarction; PE, pulmonary embolism.
Modified from Shannon MS. Anticoagulation in practice. *Medicine* 2004; **32**(5): 33–37, new data supplied by Dr Shannon (personal communication) and Guidelines of British Committee for Standards in Haematology, with permission from Elsevier Ltd.

Problems with warfarin. Most serious bleeds occur at the target INR and the bleeding risk increases exponentially with INR values >5. Treatment of bleeds depends on their site and severity. For major haemorrhage the following are appropriate.

• Stop warfarin and determine a baseline INR. Determine and treat the cause of bleeding, e.g. unsuspected renal, hepatic or gastro-intestinal problems.
• Give prothrombin concentrate (FrII + FrVII + FrIX + FrX) up to 50 units/kg, depending on the INR, or fresh frozen plasma (FFP) 15 mL/kg.
• Give *phytomenadione* (vitamin K_1) 5–10 mg by slow IV injection and repeat after 24 h if the INR is still high. The degree of reversal is determined by the severity of the bleed. It is preferable not to reverse anticoagulation completely, because *warfarin* resistance may then occur, and it may be advisable to halve the starting dose of *phytomenadione*.
• When bleeding has been controlled, monitor the INR and resume *warfarin* at a lower dose.

For minor bleeds, e.g. epistaxis, sub-conjunctival haemorrhage, bruising and mild haematuria, it is sufficient to stop or reduce *warfarin* until the bleeding is controlled.

For a high INR without bleeding, the Guide-lines recommend:

• INR >8: stop *warfarin* until INR <5. Give *phytomenadione* PO if there are any risk factors for bleeding, e.g. liver or kidney dysfunction, uncontrolled peptic ulceration or hyper-tension, a personal or family history of bleed-ing problems, or a non-concordant patient. However, *phytomenadione* is oil-soluble and oral dosing is not suitable for people with malabsorption (see Chapter 3). Slow IV injec-tion of a micellar formulation is suitable in these patients.
• INR 6–8: stop *warfarin* for 1–2 days and recommence at a lower dose.
• INR <6 but more than 0.5 above target level: stop or reduce *warfarin* until INR <5 and recommence at a lower dose.
• INRs within ± 0.5 of the target level are acceptable and do not require action.

Table 11.11   Partial table for initiating warfarin in atrial fibrillation and maintenance doses according to INR levels – the 'Sliding Scale'

Day	INR	Warfarin dose (mg/day)	
1–4		5	
5 – Check INR	• ≤1.7	5	
	• 1.8–2.2	4	
	• 2.3–2.7	3	
	• 2.8–3.2	2	
	• 3.3–3.7	1	
	• >3.7	0	
6–7 (no INR check)	As day 5	As day 5	
		Previous dose (mg)	Dose from day 8 (mg)
8 onwards until INR is stable.	• ≤1.7	5.0	6.0
Check INR, then:	• 1.8–2.4		5.0
	• 2.5–3.0		4.0
	• 3.0		3.0 for 4 days
	↓	↓	↓
	↓	↓	↓
	↓	↓	↓
	• ≤1.7	1.0	2.0
	• 1.8–2.4		1.5
	• 2.5–3.0		1.0
	• 3.1–3.5		0.5 for 4 days
	• >3.5		Omit for 2 or more days

Modified from Shannon MS. Anticoagulation in practice. *Medicine* 2004; **32**(5): 33–37, with permission from Elsevier Ltd.

- Cancer patients and those who have had a venous thromboembolism (VTE) are at significant risk of further thrombosis despite appropriate *warfarin* treatment. Trials have shown that low molecular weight heparins (LMWHs) halve the risk of recurrent VTE compared to *warfarin*, with no increase in mortality or bleeding episodes. The BCSH guidelines state that LMWHs are superior to *warfarin* in cancer patients.

Because of these problems and the costs and inconvenience of *warfarin* management there have been numerous unsuccessful attempts at producing an oral *warfarin* replacement that is more predictable in use and so does not require close monitoring. The only agent that was intro-duced, *ximelagatran*, has been withdrawn permanently due to its potential to cause severe liver damage.

All patients taking oral anticoagulants should be issued with a **treatment booklet** that gives the patient advice on their treatment and provides a diary of all doses that have been used. This should be carried at all times as an alert to doctors in the event of trauma requiring hospital treatment.

Heparins

Pharmacology of heparin. Unfractionated *heparin* is a glycosaminoglycan produced by mast cells that is extracted from porcine mucosa. It is therefore unsuitable for strictly observant Jews and Muslims. Heparan sulphate is a related compound found in the extracellular matrix of most eukaryotic cells.

Heparin has a rapid onset of action and a short duration of effect. It consists of heterogeneous chains of molecular weight 2–30 kDa. Most preparations can be given by IV or SC injection, but *Calciparine* (a proprietary *heparin* product) can be used only by the SC route. Some indications for *heparin* use are given in Table 11.12.

An important side-effect of *heparin* use, including LMWHs (see below), is immune-mediated heparin-induced thrombocytopenia (HIT) that normally occurs after 6–14 days' treatment and causes a paradoxical thrombosis. Thus platelet counts should be done for patients in whom heparins are to be used for >5 days. A platelet count of ≤50% of normal requires immediate withdrawal of the *heparin*. If continued anticoagulation is required, it should be replaced with a heparinoid or lepirudin (see below).

Rapid reversal of *heparin* activity requires the administration of *protamine sulphate*, a specific antidote. LMWHs are reversed only partially by *protamine sulphate* and their duration of action is longer.

Inhibition of aldosterone secretion by heparins may result in hyperkalaemia (see Chapters 2, 4 and 5), with adverse cardiac effects, so prolonged therapy requires serial plasma potassium measurements. Mild to moderate hyperkalaemia can be treated with a polystyrene sulphonate ion exchange resin, but glucose plus insulin is needed if a more rapid reduction in potassium level is required (see Chapter 9).

LMWHs, i.e. *bemiparin, dalteparin, enoxaparin, reviparin* and *tinzaparin*, are produced from unfractionated *heparin* by depolymerization and have a molecular weight of 3–6 kDa. They are generally as effective and safe as unfractionated *heparin* for the prophylaxis of venous thromboembolism and are probably more effective

Table 11.12   Indications for the use of heparin, low molecular weight heparins (LMWHs)[a] and heparinoids

Drug and group	Indications
Unfractionated heparin, bemiparin, reviparin and tinzaparin	Prophylaxis of DVT and PE, moderate risk Prophylaxis of DVT and PE, high risk[b] Treatment of DVT and PE[b] Prevention of clotting in extracorporeal circuits, e.g. in haemodialysis[c] (not reviparin)
Dalteparin and enoxaparin	As above **plus** Treatment of unstable coronary disease, including non-ST segment-elevation MI (see Chapter 4)
Danaparoid sodium (heparinoid)	Prophylaxis of DVT in general and orthopaedic surgery Thromboembolic disease in patients with a history of heparin-induced thrombocytopenia

[a] Doses in BNF and manufacturers' literature are expressed as units of antifactor Xa activity, but doses of enoxaparin are also given in milligrams. Once-daily SC dosing is usual. Unfractionated heparin may also be given as an IV bolus, followed either by IV infusion or 12-hourly SC bolus injections. In the latter case, daily laboratory monitoring is essential

[b] Weight-banded dosing is available in manufacturers' literature.

[c] See Chapter 14.

DVT, deep-vein thrombosis; MI, myocardial infarction; PE, pulmonary embolism.

Modified from data supplied by Dr Muriel S Shannon (personal communication) with permission. This is an updating of her article "Anticoagulation in practice" in *Medicine* 2004; **32**(5): 33–37.

than unfractionated *heparin* in orthopaedic surgery. Some indications for their use are given in Table 11.12.

Because they have a longer duration of action than unfractionated *heparin* they are given conveniently by once-daily SC injection.

Heparin activity is monitored using the **activated partial thromboplastin time (APTT)**, but this is not needed if heparins are used in well-defined standard prophylactic regimens.

Other antithrombotic agents

Danaparoid sodium is a heparinoid that is licensed for the prevention of DVT in general surgery and in patients with HIT (see above). However, it is not clear whether there is a cross-reaction with heparins.

Bivalirudin and *lepirudin* are recombinant hirudins, i.e. they are the biogenetic analogues of *hirudin*, the anticoagulant that enables leeches (*Hirudo medicinalis*) to maintain blood flow when feeding on animals. Their use is monitored by APTT, not INR.

Bivalirudin is licensed for use in patients undergoing percutaneous coronary angiography and angioplasty (see Chapter 4). The Scottish Medicines Consortium have approved it for restricted use in patients undergoing percutaneous coronary interventions who would have been considered for treatment with unfractionated *heparin* plus a platelet GPIIa-IIIb inhibitor, i.e. *abciximab*, *eptifibatide* and *tirofiban*. *Lepirudin* is licensed only for use in patients with HIT.

Fondaparinux sodium is a new synthetic pentasaccharide FrXa inhibitor that is licensed for the prophylaxis of venous thromboembolism in medical patients, those undergoing abdominal surgery and major orthopaedic surgery of the legs.

References and further reading

British Committee for Standards in Haematology (2005). Guidelines on oral anticoagulation (warfarin) (update). *Br J Haematol* 132: 277–285.

Claster S, Vichinsky E (2003). Managing sickle disease. *BMJ* 327: 1151–1155.

Gordon-Smith T, Marsh J, eds (2004). Haematology Part 1. *Medicine* 32(5): 1–45.

Hardman S M C, Cowie M R (1999). Anticoagulation in heart disease. *BMJ* 318: 238–244.

McDougal I C, Eckardt K-U (2006). Novel strategies for stimulating erythropoiesis and potential new treatments for anaemia. *Lancet* 368: 947–953.

Provan D, ed. (2003). *ABC of Clinical Haematology*, 2nd edn. Oxford, Blackwell.

Tait R C, Cefcick A (1998). A warfarin induction regime for outpatient anticoagulation in patients with atrial fibrillation. *Br J Haematol* 101: 450–454.

Internet resources

http://www.bcshguidelines.com (British Committee for Standards in Haematology – includes numerous guidelines).

12

Rheumatology: musculoskeletal and connective tissue diseases

There are over 200 rheumatological disorders, producing about 25% of the average GP's workload. Some disorders are primary joint problems, but muscles, tendons and ligaments may also be affected. Systemic diseases may present as a joint problem and trigger a rheumatological referral. Our progressively ageing population, with prolonged joint stresses and poor working practices may cause persistent problems, increasing the workload.

Many patients imagine that 'rheumatism' leads inexorably to chronic disability. This does not reflect current practice, but derives from times when life and work were much harder than now and good medical care was generally unavailable. Most patients are now treated effectively by their GP or paramedical staff and counselling can relieve inappropriate anxiety, but the drugs used can have serious side-effects.

Rheumatic fever is covered in Chapter 8.

Introduction

This chapter describes the principal rheumatological conditions to aid an understanding of
their treatment and to assist recognition of those
non-joint signs, e.g. facial or other rashes,
conjunctivitis, bowel problems, etc., which may
indicate significant underlying disease and the
need for prompt referral. The term 'rheumatism'
is used loosely by laypeople to describe any form
of pain or dysfunction associated with the joints
or muscles. This covers a wide range of conditions (Table 12.1). None of the many attempts at
classification is wholly satisfactory, because the
aetiology of most of the diseases is obscure. Joint
disease (arthropathy) and joint inflammation
(arthritis) frequently accompany a variety of
diseases whose principal effects are elsewhere
than on the joints, e.g. diabetes mellitus, psoriasis and UC, so careful diagnosis is essential.
Only the principal disease states in this group are
discussed below. Table 12.1 also gives the disease
abbreviations used most frequently throughout
this chapter.

In this chapter, the terms 'rheumatoid' and
'arthritis' are used only for inflammatory joint
conditions: 'rheumatic' and 'rheumatism' apply
non-specifically to all types of pain or abnormality involving the joints, muscles, tendons and
associated structures, e.g. in SLE (p. 798) or
rheumatic fever (p. 564).

Specialization in this field is especially important because of the large variety of diseases and
drug toxicities. NSAIDs are widely used and
cause the largest proportion of adverse reaction
reports of any drug group (see p. 775). Some of
the other drugs used may also cause severe side-
effects. Unless the condition is acute and severe,
most patients are self-medicating when they seek
advice, increasing the risk of drug interactions.

Anatomy and physiological principles of the musculoskeletal system

Two types of joint are affected by rheumatic
disease, **synovial** and **fibrocartilaginous**. The
former allows a wide range of free movement

and so includes all the hinge joints of the limbs.
The latter allows only limited movement and
include primarily those joints of the vertebral
column and the hip girdle, including the
sacroiliac joints and the pubic symphysis (the
anterior joint between the two pubic bones).

Disease of fibrocartilaginous joints is primarily
degenerative and traumatic, whereas problems
in synovial joints tend to be inflammatory.

Synovial joints

This is the type of joint found in the legs, arms,
hands and feet. From the generalized diagram
given in Figure 12.1 it can be seen that the ends
of the two opposing bones are covered with a
firmly attached layer of **hyaline (articular)
cartilage**. This is about 6 mm thick in young
adults but only 1–3 mm thick in the elderly. The
cartilage is radiolucent and avascular, giving the
appearance of a joint space on X-ray (Figure
12.2(a); see also Figure 12.6(a)), though the two
layers of cartilage are normally in close contact.
The bearing surfaces of the cartilage are
lubricated and supplied with nutrients by a
small volume (<2 mL in a knee joint) of a
viscous, colourless **synovial fluid** containing
a hyaluronate–protein complex, albumin and
some white cells, electrolytes, etc. The whole is
surrounded and stabilized by a tough, **fibrous
capsule** that may be thickened in places and by
ligaments, which further strengthen the joint.
However, joint stability depends largely on the
strengths of the attached and surrounding
muscles, and one of the objects of physiotherapy
is to strengthen the muscles and so reinforce the
joints. Some joints have additional structures,
e.g. the tough, fibrous cartilage of the **menisci** in
the knee joint (Figure 12.2(a)) that helps to
absorb stresses and further improve stability, and
bursae (see below).

The synovial fluid is produced by the
surrounding **synovial membrane** that contains
the cells that secrete the fluid, and phagocytic
cells. This membrane is not flat and featureless:
it has numerous folds, which allow for wide-
ranging joint movement, and fat pads and
inner projections together fill much of the joint
cavity. These internal projections ensure good

Table 12.1   Some diseases and conditions that may give rise to rheumatic diseases and joint pain

Pathological class and examples	Abbreviation
Inflammatory arthritides	
Rheumatoid arthritis	RA
Juvenile idiopathic arthritis	JIA
Seronegative arthritides	
Ankylosing spondylitis	AS
Psoriatic arthritis (see Chapter 13)	
Enteropathic arthritis (see Chapter 3)	
'Degenerative' joint disease	
Osteoarthritis; primary, secondary	OA
Crystal deposition arthropathies (metabolic disorders)	
Gout	
Pyrophosphate arthropathy (pseudogout)	
Systemic connective tissue diseases (collagen-vascular diseases)	
Systemic lupus erythematosus	
Systemic sclerosis (scleroderma)	SLE
Vasculitides:	
• polyarteritis nodosa	PAN
• giant cell arteritis	GCA
• polymyalgia rheumatica	PR
• Wegener's granulomatosis	WG
Reactive arthritis	
Rheumatic fever	
Reiter's syndrome	
Arthritis secondary to systemic disease	
Amyloidosis	
Sarcoidosis	
See also Table 12.3	
Joint infections	
Septic arthritis	
Localized and traumatic conditions	
Back and neck pain	
Carpal tunnel syndrome	
Tendonitis and tenosynovitis	
Fibrositis and fibromyalgia	
Enthesopathies and sports injuries	
Tennis elbow, golfer's elbow	
Iatrogenic arthritides	
Drug-induced: lupus-like syndromes, arthralgias due to drugs, vaccines and sera	
Chronic haemodialysis (see Chapter 14)	

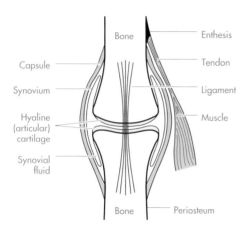

Figure 12.1   Generalized diagram of a synovial joint. The joint is stabilized by the ligaments and muscles (only one of each is shown). The enthesis is the point of attachment of the tendon to the bone. The periosteum is the specialized connective tissue, with bone-forming potential, that covers all bones.

distribution of the synovial fluid and provide some cushioning against mechanical shock to the joint. The synovial fluid does not normally clot but, if there is inflammation, fibrinogen enters the fluid, which is then able to clot like normal inflammatory exudates (see Chapter 2). The increased volume and pressure of fluid within the joint (due to inflammation) and any clotting, limit joint movement.

Joint pain derives primarily from the stretching and inflammation of the fibrous structures (capsule and ligaments) and the periosteum, the thin layer of tissue that covers all bones in the body: sensation in the synovial tissues is poor. Inflammation often results in joint deformity because there is a variable amount of inflammatory exudate, causing swelling, and the limb is held unconsciously in a position that provides the maximum joint volume, to accommodate the increased volume of synovial fluid and so reduce the pressure and pain. Chronic inflammation may lead to permanent joint damage.

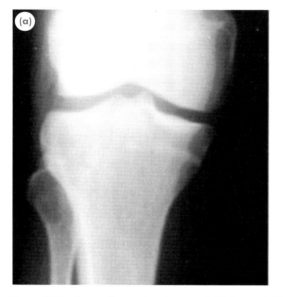
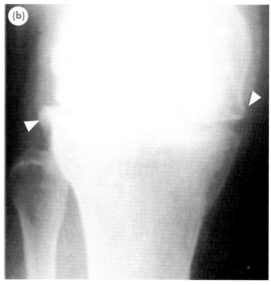

Figure 12.2   X-rays of normal and osteoarthritic knees. (a) Normal: note the smooth bone margins and the well-defined joint 'space', occupied by radiolucent cartilage. In the knee, this space is large, being occupied by the cartilage covering the bone and two pads of cartilage (the menisci, one on either side), which absorb the shocks occurring during exercise. (b) Osteoarthritis: showing loss of joint space (owing to cartilage destruction and failure of cartilage repair), and osteophytes at the bone margins (arrows). (Reproduced with permission from Dr AC Keat, Northwick Park Hospital, London, UK.)

Fibrocartilaginous joints

The arrangement of the joints in the vertebral column is illustrated in Figure 12.3. The vertebrae are covered with a thin layer of hyaline cartilage, similarly to synovial joints, but there is no capsule and associated synovium or synovial fluid. However, there is a very small amount of extracellular fluid that gives some lubrication. The vertebrae are separated by **intervertebral discs**, which consist of a strong fibrous capsule filled with a proteoglycan gel that provides an effective shock absorber.

Synovial sheaths and bursae

These occur where closely opposed structures move relative to each other, and especially where skin or tendons need to move freely over bony surfaces. **Bursae** are enclosed clefts of synovial membrane that are supported by dense connective tissue, the synovium sometimes being continuous with that of an adjacent joint. The central potential space is normally filled with a capillary film of synovial fluid that permits free movement to occur between the two layers of bursal synovium. Thus the

prepatellar bursa lies between the skin and the lower half of the **patella** (kneecap). It provides free, smooth movement when the knee is flexed and prevents damage to the skin and the tibial head by the tendons. Similarly, the **olecranon bursa** prevents friction between the skin and the point of the elbow. Inflammation of these bursae (bursitis) causes the accumulation of synovial fluid, with swelling, tenderness, pain and restriction of movement and the conditions of 'housemaid's knee', 'students' elbow' or 'miner's elbow'.

Synovial sheaths occur around tendons that pass under ligaments or through fibrous tunnels, e.g. the **carpal tunnel** (see Figure 12.11) in the wrist. The sheath consists of a closed, double-walled synovial cylinder enclosing a capillary film of interwall synovial fluid. The inner wall is attached loosely to the tendon, and the outer wall to the bones, ligaments or other adjacent structures. This arrangement again permits free movement of the tendon through surrounding tissues, similarly to the bursae, and inflammation of the sheaths (tendonitis) causes similar problems to bursitis.

'**Ganglia**' are synovial herniations (bulges) from a tendon sheath or joint and should not be confused with nerve ganglia.

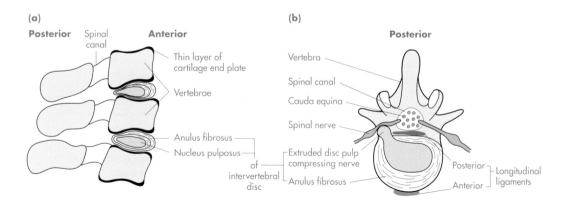

Figure 12.3 Diagram of fibrocartilaginous joints in the lumbar region of the vertebral column and the result of disc prolapse ('slipped disc'). (a) General arrangement (sagittal section). (b) Disc prolapse (transverse section): because the annulus fibrosus of the disc is thicker anteriorly and the rear of the disc is restrained by the posterior longitudinal ligament, the pulp (nucleus pulposus) tends to be extruded posteriorly and laterally under pressure, compressing a spinal nerve on one side and causing unilateral symptoms.

Joint nutrition, maintenance and repair

The synovial membrane is supplied with blood and nutrients from the underlying vascular connective tissue. Nutrients for the **chondrocytes**, which are responsible for synthesizing all of the components of the joint cartilage, diffuse from the blood supply of the synovium through the synovial fluid. The latter also returns waste products from the avascular cartilage covering the bone back to the circulation.

There is normally a slow continuous turnover of joint cartilage, which contains largely a unique type of collagen (type II) plus highly hydrophilic proteoglycans. The latter bind the structurally important type IX and XI collagens, which are present in only small amounts but are crucial for cartilage stability.

When collagen is compressed, the structural water, held by hydrogen bonding, is released from the proteoglycans and is regained when the force is removed. This mechanism temporarily increases the synovial fluid volume and makes it less viscous, thus cushioning stresses and facilitating movement. In adults the chondrocytes do not normally replicate, but repeated trauma reactivates their division. The resultant increased metabolism accelerates the dismantling and regeneration of damaged cartilage, but the effect is not a true replacement but a remodelling, which may result in an imbalance between cartilage degradation and synthesis, and so inappropriate replacement.

In **osteoarthritis** (a degenerative joint disease; p. 754), the composition and size of the proteoglycan molecules is altered, and the type II collagen fibrils are replaced with the more common, less suitable type I collagen that is characteristic of skin and tendons. Changes also occur in the underlying bone.

The immune system and rheumatic diseases

Genetic aspects

There are clear associations between human leucocyte locus A (HLA) genes and rheumatic diseases, especially inflammatory ones. It will be recalled that the HLA system consists of a series of closely linked genetic loci located on the short arm of chromosome 6, and forms part of the major histocompatibility complex (MHC; see Chapter 2). Certain of the HLA antigens occur more frequently in patients with some rheumatic diseases than in general populations of the same ethnic origin (Table 12.2). For example, HLA-DR4 tends to be associated with severe RA and the presence of a nucleotide sequence in the allele coding for a detectable pentapeptide in the HLA-DRβ1-1 gene that, in association with the presence of rheumatoid factor, indicates a 13 times increased risk of development of bone erosions (see below).

However, although associations between rheumatic diseases and HLA antigens are valuable pointers to pathogenesis, few of these are of diagnostic value and they do not currently influence management. The genetic status of an individual merely indicates an increased likelihood of suffering a rheumatic disease: the development of symptoms requires exposure to a currently unknown environmental trigger. Further, tissue typing is a complex and expensive process and does not help in prognosis, except in certain limited situations. The principal reason for pursuing these genetic relationships is the hope that better understanding of the fundamental mechanisms involved may lead to more effective, less toxic treatments and to better

Table 12.2 Some associations between HLA antigens and rheumatic diseases

HLA antigen	Disease	Risk[a]
DR4, Dw4	Rheumatoid arthritis (adult)	6
Dw14	Rheumatoid arthritis (adult)	5
DR2, DR3	Systemic lupus erythematosus	3
DR3	Sjögren's syndrome	6
DR4	Polyarticular juvenile arthritis	7
B27	Ankylosing spondylitis	90
	Reiter's syndrome	40
	Inflammatory bowel disease, psoriatic arthritis, and spondylitis	10

[a] Approximate values relative to general population.

diagnostic and prognostic tests. This has occurred already to some extent, leading to the very successful introduction of anti-cytokine antibodies in treatment.

Osteoarthritis

A mutation in the COL2A1 gene causes the production of a variant form of type II collagen and is associated with the occurrence of premature osteoarthritis (OA). Further, the risk of needing a hip replacement for OA in siblings of a patient who has had the operation is three times that in the general population. **Aggrecan**, a protein–chondroitin–keratan sulphate macromolecule, is important in load dispersal in joints, and genetically determined variants are associated with hand OA in elderly men.

These and other similar considerations have led to the estimate that about two-thirds of OA has a genetic basis.

Rheumatoid arthritis

The concordance rate for monozygotic (identical) twins, i.e. the risk of one contracting RA if the other has the disease, has been estimated as 12–30%. This is four to five times the risk in dizygotic (non-identical) twins. The general risk to other siblings is about eight times that in the general population.

Overall, about 40% of RA is linked to the possession of specific HLA antigens, especially DR4 and Dw4. This clearly points to RA being an autoimmune disease, or at least having an autoimmune component. The presence of HLA-DR4 is associated with the severity of RA and, in decreasing order of disease severity, its prevalence is 90% in Felty's syndrome (p. 767), 70% in patients referred to rheumatologists, and 40% in general practice patients with RA.

Other HLA-DR antigens are implicated in the occurrence of RA in particular geographical and ethnic groups, e.g. DR1 in most of Southern Europe, DR10 in Spaniards, Indians and Jews, and DR14 in some North American Indians.

Interestingly, the likelihood of the occurrence of some side-effects to *gold* or *penicillamine* (p. 772) is also genetically linked, e.g. nephrotic syndrome with HLA-DR3.

Ankylosing spondylitis

The association of ankylosing spondylitis (AS, p. 788) with HLA-B27 is the strongest for any rheumatic disease and carries a 200 times increased risk. HLA-B60 carries only a threefold risk. Thus, the concordance rate for HLA-B27-positive monozygotic twins, one of whom has AS, is 75%. In a general group of dizygotic twins this risk falls to only 12%. Taking all genes into account, the chance of inheriting AS is about 90%, so inheritance far outweighs environmental factors as a risk factor for the condition.

The association is confirmed if we compare the prevalences of HLA-B27 and AS in different population groups: in some native North Americans these are 50% and 8%, respectively; in Northern Europeans these levels fall to 8% and 0.3%; and in indigenous Australians to <0.5% and zero.

Environmental factors and other genes are also important for the disease to occur. It seems likely that the HLA-B27 gene requires additional genes, plus an environmental determinant, to cause rheumatic symptoms: no disease results if an additional gene is absent, even in the presence of the environmental trigger.

Tissue typing may be useful in prognosis in certain limited situations. Young patients with inconclusive symptoms and signs who are HLA-B27 positive need to be watched for the onset of significant disease, some of them being more likely to develop AS than typical juvenile chronic arthritis. Also, young male patients with low back pain who are HLA-B27 negative and do not have IBD (see Chapter 3) or psoriasis (see Chapter 13) are unlikely to have AS.

Cytokines

Many of these small protein autacoids are involved in inflammation (see Chapter 2) and have been implicated in rheumatic diseases, though their precise roles are uncertain. They may be **autocrines**, acting on the cell that secretes them, **paracrines**, acting on neighbouring cells, or they may have endocrine properties and act on remote tissues, e.g. erythropoietin.

Tumour necrosis factor alpha (TNF-α) is a potent pro-inflammatory agent, released by macrophages, that induces **interleukin-1 (IL-1)** production by T cells. IL-1 in turn promotes the hepatic production of acute-phase proteins (see Chapter 2), in association with IL-6, and is found in the synovial fluid associated with several types of arthritis. IL-1 has been implicated in stimulating the release of lysosomal enzymes, producing joint erosions in RA, and collagen degradation in OA. Excessive production of IL-1 may be responsible for maintaining a chronic inflammatory reaction in damaged joints.

The major treatment development for RA in recent years is the introduction of anti-TNFα monoclonal antibodies, i.e. *adalimumab, etanercept* and *infliximab* (see below). These are used to treat RA that has not responded adequately to conventional disease-modifying agents. There is also one anti-IL-1 agent (*anakinra*) that is currently used primarily in clinical trials.

Interleukin-2 (IL-2) is crucial in promoting antigen elimination, and a deficiency of it has been demonstrated in RA and SLE (p. 798). This deficiency may also contribute to the maintenance of joint inflammation, owing to a failure to clear antigens completely. **Interferons (IFNs)** are produced by several types of cell, and IFN-gamma may also be involved in joint pathology.

A deficiency of T helper cell production of erythropoietic interleukins (IL-3 and IL-5) may be implicated in causing the anaemia often seen in RA (p. 751). Finally, trials of IL-1 inhibitors, IFN-gamma and IL-2 for treating a variety of arthritides are in progress.

Examination, investigation and assessment

History and examination

Many diseases can give rise secondarily to muscular or joint pain (Table 12.3), and patient misconceptions may lead them to give misleading descriptions of pain that they ascribe to joint disease. It is therefore important to regard the patient as a whole and to decide whether there is actually an arthropathy or other related problem that falls within the speciality of rheumatology. The relevant details of the history and examination are given in Table 12.4.

Investigation

Although a wide range of investigations might be carried out, only those that are commonly performed are dealt with briefly below. They are discussed in this section only in general terms, the specific indications being dealt with under the various disease headings.

Haematology

Acute-phase proteins

These are a family of about 30 proteins produced by the liver in response to cytokines released from macrophages and other cells at the site of inflammation (see Chapter 2). Some of these can be used as indicators of acute rheumatic disease activity, e.g. CRP, SAA, (pp. 751, 807) serum ferritin and fibrinogen. The fibrinogen is not

Table 12.3   Some non-rheumatic diseases that may give muscular or joint pain

Infections
Bacterial: endocarditis, dysentery, gonorrhoea, hepatitis, meningitis, rubella, salmonellosis, streptococcal sore throat, tuberculosis.
Fungal; protozoal

Metabolic and endocrine
Acromegaly, diabetes mellitus, hyperlipoproteinaemia, osteoporosis, osteomalacia, Paget's disease, parathyroid disease, thyroid diseases

Systemic diseases
Chronic renal failure, haemophilia, hypogammaglobulinaemia, inflammatory bowel disease, leukaemias, myelomas, neuropathy (loss of joint sensation), respiratory (e.g. bronchiectasis, fibrosing alveolitis)

Skin diseases
Erythema nodosum, psoriasis

Table 12.4 Aspects of the history and examination relevant to rheumatic diseases[a]

History

Age, sex, race

Occupation

Pain
- now: location, severity, duration
- pattern of onset, joint involvement, periodicity
- precipitating, aggravating and relieving factors

Associated symptoms
- stiffness, joint swelling
- skin, gastrointestinal, eye and respiratory

Presenting complaint (see Table 12.5)

Past medical history (see Table 12.6)
- medication history: drugs used, dose, period, effectiveness, side-effects

Family history

Social history

Ability to cope; patient's attitudes, e.g. expectations of outcome from the consultation and treatment, interpretation of symptoms and emotional response to them

Examination

Joints
- swelling, inflammation, pain or tenderness, deformity, symmetry of involvement
- surrounding abnormalities, muscle wasting
- movement: range, noises or grating
- stability
- functional capacity

The whole patient
- appearance, posture, gait
- nodules: subcutaneous, lung, eyes, etc.
- finger clubbing
- fever
- neuropathies (loss of sensation)
- systemic review of all organ systems

See also Chapter 1, Table 1.2. Items here are aspects of special relevance to rheumatic diseases.

measured directly, its concentration being reflected in the ESR. The increased blood protein causes an increase in blood and plasma viscosity, but this effect is outweighed by red cell clumping.

Erythrocyte sedimentation rate (ESR) is a non-specific indicator of inflammation anywhere in the body. However, because the test is easily performed at the bedside, it is widely used as a rapid and simple screening test. The sedimentation rate increases owing to increased levels of fibrinogen and Igs that increase RBC clumping, thus increasing sedimentation, and so apparently causing a mild anaemia. Very low ESR values may be due to serious underlying disease, e.g. multisystem disorders (pp. 798–807), certain infections, or malignancy. Unfortunately, changes in RBC size or morphology that occur in some severe anaemias (see Chapter 11) can also affect the ESR.

C-reactive protein (CRP) is another non-specific indicator of inflammation, which is normally present in low concentration in plasma. The protein, so-called originally because it reacts with *Streptococcus pneumoniae* type C polysaccharide, is synthesized in the liver and its concentration rises within 6 h of fever, inflammation, tissue damage or necrosis. This is a much more rapid response than the ESR, and CRP is the marker of choice in the diagnosis of inflammatory diseases. However, it is less useful than ESR and plasma viscosity for monitoring the progress of chronic inflammatory states.

Serum amyloid-A protein (SAA) is the precursor of one type of amyloid, the fibrous protein that is characteristic of amyloidosis (p. 807) and is present in some patients with RA. SAA levels, similarly to CRP, are modestly raised in SLE, but may be high in RA and Still's disease, and RA is the most common cause of secondary amyloidosis.

Anaemia

Many chronic inflammatory diseases cause a mild, normocytic anaemia, related to reduced erythropoiesis (see Chapter 11). This may reflect the level of inflammatory disease activity, as also do ESR and CRP, and reduced levels of IL-3 and

IL-5. Hb levels lower than about 10 g/dL in males and 9 g/dL in females may indicate other possible causes (for example, iatrogenic gastro-intestinal blood loss due to drugs used to treat rheumatic disease, e.g. NSAIDs, which irritate the GIT and also inhibit the production of gastroprotective PGs).

Leucocytes

Leucocytosis (raised white cell count) may result from infection, severe exacerbations of RA, or treatment with corticosteroids. The condition may also be an indication of serious systemic inflammatory disease, notably polyarteritis nodosa (PAN; p. 807). **Neutropenia** (see Chapter 11) may indicate the presence of SLE (p. 798), or Felty's syndrome (p. 767) in a patient with RA, but may also reflect drug-induced myelo-suppression (bone marrow depression), e.g. due to *sodium aurothiomalate*, *penicillamine* and immunosuppressive drugs.

Platelets

The platelet count may be raised (**thrombocytosis**) in active inflammatory diseases or after an acute bleeding episode. The converse, **thrombocytopenia**, may indicate Felty's syndrome or iatrogenic bone marrow toxicity. In both neutropenia and thrombocytopenia, immediate drug withdrawal is essential because fatal bone marrow depression may follow.

Biochemistry

Serum phosphatases. Raised **serum alkaline phosphatase (ALP)** may be used to detect those patients whose bone pain is due to metabolic bone disease, e.g. Paget's disease and osteo-malacia. High levels of **serum acid phosphatase (ACP)** in older men indicate the possibility of backache being due to metastatic deposits from prostatic carcinoma.

Creatine kinase (CK). This is a useful screening test in patients who may have muscle damage in **polymyositis** or **dermatomyositis**. It is also a feature of heart muscle damage in MI and sometimes in myositis caused by statins (see Chapter 4).

Serology

Rheumatoid factors (RFs). These are autoanti-bodies against the Fc fragment of IgG (see Chapter 2). The tests routinely employed primarily detect IgMs, though some RFs are IgGs. Normally, the IgG molecule is folded and protected, but reaction with antigens exposes reaction sites so that flocculation can occur. Patients whose serum contains significant levels of RFs are described as '**seropositive**', and the RF titre roughly reflects disease activity. Some laboratories use the **differential agglutinating test**, which gives a titratable measure of RFs in the serum, but the test has poor specificity. RFs are present in the serum of only about 75% of RA patients and are also found in those with SLE, some chronic infections and in some of the elderly-well.

A recent advance is based on the detection of antibodies to **cyclic citrullinated peptide (CCP)**, which has been shown to perform better than the test for RFs. Anti-CCP assays are about 85% sensitive for RA and can detect about a third of patients who are RF-negative, but have RA.

Complement. Raised levels of complement components (see Chapter 2) occur in many of the significantly inflammatory rheumatic diseases. Low levels of complement components, especially C3 and C4, reflect disease activity in SLE, because they indicate immune complex formation: decreasing levels imply deterioration in the patient's condition.

Fluorescent antinuclear antibody test (ANA or ANF). This is used as a rapid preliminary, non-specific screening test for diseases in which autoantibodies to cell nuclei occur, e.g. in SLE and mixed connective tissue disease.

DNA binding test. This radioimmunoassay detects antibodies against native (normal), double-stranded DNA. The level of DNA binding indicates disease activity in SLE, though the test is rather insensitive. It is usually used only in patients who are strongly positive in the ANA test.

Extractable antigens. A wide range of autoantibodies against soluble nuclear and cytoplasmic antigens detected by counter-immunoelectrophoresis are used to contribute to diagnosis in a variety of systemic connective tissue disorders, e.g. SLE, Sjögren's syndrome and systemic sclerosis.

Anti-streptolysin 'O' titre (ASO). Levels of this antibody indicate recent streptococcal infection and may be used to confirm a diagnosis of rheumatic fever.

Tissue typing. Detection of the presence of the histocompatibility antigen HLA-B27 may occasionally help in the diagnosis or exclusion of seronegative arthropathies (p. 789).

Synovial fluid

This is normally present as a small volume of a clear, pale yellow, viscous fluid. It may be examined for the following:

- Protein (high in inflammatory arthritis).
- Leucocytes (see Chapter 11; high in RA, neutrophil counts are high in septic arthritis).
- Microorganisms (septic arthritis).
- Crystals of urate (gout) and pyrophosphate (pseudogout).

Urinalysis

This may give clues to the origin of symptoms, e.g.:

- Glycosuria: frozen shoulder and tendon contractures are associated with diabetes (Chapter 9).
- Microscopic haematuria: Reiter's syndrome (p. 809), or metastatic bone pain caused by urinary-tract carcinoma.
- Proteinuria: multiple myeloma as a cause of back pain.
- Sterile pyuria: TB causing bone and joint pain. *Mycobacterium tuberculosis* will not grow in the medium used for the normal bacteriological examination of urine (see Chapter 8).

Imaging

Radiology

X-rays are invaluable in revealing joint damage (Figure 12.2(b); see also Figure 12.6(b)) and for monitoring the progress of joint disease. Radiography is also useful in distinguishing between OA and RA, and as an aid in the diagnosis of AS and pseudogout. Occasionally, it may be necessary to use more specialized techniques, e.g. CT, MRI, arthrography (with radio-opaque contrast media injected into the joint) or arthroscopy (see below), and radionuclide bone scanning, when X-ray findings are negative or equivocal. CT and MRI scans can provide greater information on changes that are difficult to visualize using normal techniques, e.g. intervertebral disc prolapse (Figure 12.3 and p. 812).

Arthroscopy

An endoscope (a thinner version of that shown in Chapter 3, Figure 3.5) can be inserted into a joint to examine it, and this is a relatively safe and simple procedure. Arthroscopy is particularly valuable in the knee, where it permits complete examination of the cartilage, synovium and ligaments. Biopsies can be taken, synovial fluid aspirated and loose fragments or torn sections of cartilage can be removed with minimal trauma.

In scintiscanning, technetium-99m-labelled *disodium etidronate* and similar agents are occasionally used to detect bone lesions.

Ultrasound scanning

This is rapidly becoming a first-line procedure for detecting musculoskeletal problems and can be used to guide injection into joints, etc. and to measure bone density in the feet. High-resolution ultrasonography is more sensitive than radiography for detecting synovitis and bone erosions. It can also visualize periarticular structures.

Tissue biopsy

Biopsy is only occasionally helpful, as a confirmatory test, in some diseases associated with rheumatic symptoms, e.g. giant cell arteritis (temporal arteritis, p. 805), SLE (kidney, p. 798), and some myopathies.

Functional capacity

The principal components of a detailed assessment of functional capacity are listed in Table 12.5. However, a simpler approach is used for most clinical purposes:

- Grade 1: completely independent.
- Grade 2: needs aids and appliances, but is still independent.
- Grade 3: needs help with daily tasks, e.g. bathing, dressing, cooking.
- Grade 4: needs considerable and constant help; confined to a wheelchair or to bed.

The Stanford Health Assessment Questionnaire (Disability Index) is widely used in patients with

RA and the WOMAC index in those with OA (see References and further reading.

Table 12.5	Components contributing to the assessment of functional capacity

Duration of morning stiffness

Grip strength

Functional questionnaire: e.g. ability to dress, walk, open doors, turn taps, pick up small objects

Degree of joint movement: e.g. fingers, arms, hips, knees; chest expansion, spinal extension when stooping

Ability to perform activities of daily living: e.g. work-related tasks, maintaining the home, child care

Principal arthritic diseases

Osteoarthritis

Description and epidemiology

Osteoarthritis

Osteoarthritis (OA, osteoarthrosis) is the most common cause of arthritis, the most common disease of synovial joints, and is a major cause of disability, but it does not have a simple definition. OA is characterized by:

- Changes in the structure of joint cartilage, sometimes with calcification, and cartilage loss.
- Loss of joint 'space' on X-ray, which also shows **osteophytes**, i.e. bony outgrowths from the margins of the affected bones, and hardening (sclerosis) of the bone adjacent to an affected joint. Note that the apparent joint 'space' is normally occupied by opposing layers of cartilage.
- The larger joints are the most affected, i.e. hip, knee and ankle, but the wrist, finger, foot and spinal joints may also be involved.

- Inflammation is a minor primary feature and may be secondary to irritation of the soft tissues surrounding affected joints, e.g. by osteophytes. A variable degree of secondary inflammation is very common, but does not cause increases in the ESR and CRP.

These features contrast with those of RA (see below).

As in all mechanical bearings, wear tends to occur in joints after a long period of use, and some degree of cartilage damage is almost universal in the elderly. This may affect the synovial joints (**osteoarthrosis**) or the fibro-cartilaginous joints of the vertebral column (**spondylosis**). The term **osteoarthritis** implies inflammation, which is secondary to joint damage, unlike RA (see below) in which inflammation is the primary condition. Thus the neutral term osteoarthrosis is better terminology, but osteoarthritis is almost universally used.

OA is often called 'degenerative joint disease', but this is inaccurate because symptoms are probably due to an imbalance between damage and repair. Inappropriate repair (remodelling) secondary to joint damage also occurs. This remodelling process should be contrasted with the situation in RA (see below), where the underlying pathogenetic mechanism is a maladaptive immune response.

OA and soft tissue rheumatism (p. 809) together are responsible for most of the primary care rheumatological workload. They are the cause for most prescriptions for NSAIDs, but this is likely to change (pp. 759, 772). Although OA occurs worldwide and most Caucasians over 60 show radiological evidence of OA, hip involvement is less common in Black Africans and Chinese.

Classification

Osteoarthritis is classifiable into two groups:

- **Primary (idiopathic)** is of unknown origin, and may be localized to a single joint or involve three or more groups of joints.
- **Secondary** to other conditions. These are:
  - Excessive joint stress, e.g. overloading in obesity and manual labour.
  - Consequent on trauma, overuse, joint misalignment, joint surgery, etc., or bone disease, e.g. Paget's disease.
  - Congenital or developmental.
  - Inherited: e.g. metabolic disease, acromegaly, Gaucher's disease.
  - Neuropathic, e.g. Charcot's arthropathy.

Pathology and aetiology

Primary osteoarthritis

This comprises a cluster of conditions affecting the cartilage and bone of mostly the hip, spine, hand and knee synovial joints. Important risk factors for primary OA are:

- **Age**. Although OA is a very frequent condition in the elderly, being present in >70% of 75-year-olds, it is not universal and so cannot be considered as a normal feature of the ageing process.
- **Wear and tear**. The subchondral bone (immediately underlying the cartilage) is known to undergo microfractures in normal use, and repeated fracture and healing results in bone changes that reduce its ability to absorb shocks and increase the fracture risk. Further, muscle weakening with lack of exercise, due to joint pain, and advancing age results in loss of adequate joint support, thus allowing abnormal joint movement which causes further cartilage damage. The cartilage is softened and there is separation of the collagen fibrils.

Although wear and tear does not, by itself, necessarily cause OA, lengthy involvement in weight-bearing work or sports increases the risk of knee and back OA, and continual occupational lifting of heavy loads increases the incidence of hip OA five times.

Joint surgery, e.g. menisectomy (removal of the semilunar cartilage in the knee) predisposes to OA of the treated joint.

Local **biochemical factors** in individual joints may contribute and acute exacerbations may be due to **calcium pyrophosphate deposition disease** (p. 798).

The composition and size of the proteoglycan molecules of the joint cartilage is altered and the rate of repair no longer keeps pace with that of degradation. Further, the type II collagen fibrils are replaced with the more common, less suitable type I collagen that is characteristic of skin and tendons. There is synovitis with production of IL-1 and TNFα, which recruit the metalloproteinases that cause collagen breakdown. IL-1 inhibits the production of new collagen II. Changes also occur in the underlying bone, with new bone formation occurring at the margins of the articular cartilage, to form the osteophytes (Figure 12.2(b)), and in the subchondral bone, which is denser, but weaker, than normal. Mutant genes (see below), producing abnormal collagen, may also be involved.

The persuasive argument that increased weight or obesity imposes additional stresses and wear on joints fails to explain why the ankle joint is usually spared. However, in middle-aged women, every 5-kg increase in weight increases the risk of OA of the knee by 30%. Knee OA causes considerable morbidity and disability in 10% of those affected over 50 years of age.

There is a **genetic predisposition** – it is estimated that about 50% of OA is the result of inherited factors. In **primary generalized OA (PGOA)** there is widespread early joint involvement. It is sex-linked, being three times more common in women, and tends to run in families, as does the development of **Heberden's nodes**, i.e. bony enlargement of the **distal interphalangeal joints** (DIP; terminal finger joints; Figure 12.4). Less common are the similar **Bouchard's nodes** at the **proximal interphalangeal joints** (PIP joints). Symptoms tend to start at about the time of the menopause and there is a low-grade inflammatory component. Involvement of the first metacarpophalangeal joint (MCP; thumb) causes swelling and gives the hand a squarish appearance. The nodes are the readily visible results of osteophytes. The spine also tends to be affected (spondylosis), especially in the neck (cervical) region. PGOA is unusual in Black populations, but is particularly common in people of British descent, with about 30% of white North American and Northern European adults having some osteoarthritic features. PGOA is not related to climatic or environmental factors, and there is no association with HLA antigens. Any genetic effect is likely to be polygenic.

Secondary osteoarthritis

Accelerated wear due to joint damage or malfunction, e.g. obesity and sports injury, may lead to impaired or inappropriate repair mechanisms, e.g. osteophyte formation causing Heberden's nodes (see above). A listing of some common causes is given in Table 12.6.

The condition may develop insidiously over up to 50 years, and may be due to the production of an abnormal collagen structure that is less able to withstand the applied stresses.

Immunodeficient patients (e.g. those with AIDS and hypogammaglobulinaemia) are particularly susceptible to the complication of an episode of septic arthritis (joint infection), which leads to OA.

Clinical features

The frequently used and weight-bearing joints (hands, hip, knee, spine; Figure 12.2(b)) are principally affected and contribute to disability. Unlike RA, there is no systemic (extra-articular) involvement (p. 766) in OA. The predominant features are:

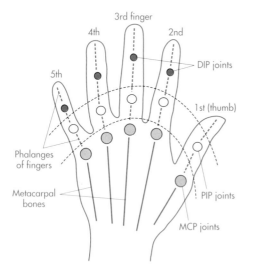

Figure 12.4   Joints and bones of the hand. DIP, distal interphalangeal; MCP, metacarpophalangeal; PIP, proximal interphalangeal. The joints of the foot corresponding to the MCP joints are the MTP (metatarsophalangeal) joints. The foot bones corresponding to the metacarpals are the metatarsals.

Table 12.6   Some conditions that commonly predispose to secondary osteoarthritis

---

Trauma
Obesity, fractures, dislocation, sports injuries, joint surgery (including arthroscopy)

Genetic and congenital
Conditions affecting joint alignment, joint hypermobility, haemophilia, acromegaly, hyperparathyroidism, chondrocalcinosis, ochronosis

Post-inflammatory
Rheumatoid arthritis, gout, pseudogout, septic arthritis

Bone disease
Paget's disease

Drugs
Corticosteroid therapy causing bone necrosis, injection of insoluble agents into joints

---

- **Pain**. Onset is gradual, occurring initially after exercise, i.e. exacerbated by use, but later also at night and at rest, with tenderness on pressure.
- **Stiffness**. This may be severe after a period of rest, but is transient, and although patients often complain of stiffness on rising ('morning stiffness'), this usually lasts less than 15 min. This should be contrasted with the situation in RA in which morning stiffness may be severe and prolonged.
- **Loss of function**. This is extremely variable and may occur early, even though the pain is slight. Conversely, even gross joint changes may not be accompanied by significant functional impairment, though there may be some limitation of movement.
- **Joint swellings**. These are usually hard (Heberden's and Bouchard's nodes; see above), due to osteophytes (sidewards outgrowths at the bone ends, Figure 12.2(b)), or they may be softer and partly due to inflammation. This differs from RA, in which the swellings are 'boggy' and tender. Inflammation and tenderness may occur in the early stages and during the acute exacerbations, and last a few weeks. These conditions occur without apparent cause, notably if joints are over-used.

The joints most commonly involved are:

- DIP joints, normally spared in RA.
- PIP joints, less common.
- The feet, especially the first metatarsophalangeal (MTP) joint (large toe), which takes the heaviest loading.
- The knees (Figure 12.2(b)), hips, cervical and lumbar spine.

The joints most commonly spared, unless the damage results from repetitive occupational trauma (e.g. road drill operators and motorcycle dispatch riders), are the shoulder, elbows, wrists, MCP joints (usually affected in RA) and ankle.

The course of OA is highly variable, and 25–30% of patients with established features may show no clinical or radiographic deterioration over long periods.

Investigation

X-radiography is an important aid in differential diagnosis and assessment of OA. Table 12.7 contrasts the principal radiographic features in OA and RA, which are illustrated in Figures 12.2(b) and 12.6(b). There is a correlation between radiographic features and the reporting of pain, though not with pain severity. Ultrasonography is used increasingly.

All other tests are usually normal in OA, though there may occasionally be an increase in ESR during an acute inflammatory exacerbation.

Management

Aims

Because OA is not reversible, except by surgical interventions such as joint replacement, the aims of management are to:

- relieve pain;
- maintain mobility and function;
- prevent further joint damage;

Table 12.7   Comparison of the principal radiographic features in osteoarthritis and rheumatoid arthritis[a]

Feature	Osteoarthritis	Rheumatoid arthritis
Joint space	Reduced	Reduced
Erosions	No	Yes
Osteophytes	Yes	No
Bone density at joints	Increased (sclerosis)	Reduced (porosis)
Bone cysts	Yes[b]	No

[a] This table should be read in conjunction with Figures 12.2 and 12.6.

[b] Although bone density is increased it is weaker than normal bone and cysts form under the cartilage, possibly because some of the increased synovial fluid, containing enzymes, is forced into exposed bone.

- improve the patient's mental health and quality of life.

The modes used in management include patient education and counselling, physiotherapy and occupational therapy, the correction of any exacerbating factors, drugs, and surgery.

Patient education and counselling

Many patients fear that their condition will develop into crippling arthritis, so it is important to reassure them and stress that disease progression is very gradual and that function is usually well maintained. Even if severe deterioration of major joints occurs, e.g. in the hips, knees or hands, surgery is very effective.

Because the problem is an imbalance between the wear and repair of joints, patients should understand that it is essential for them to follow proper physiotherapist guidance on exercises, which are designed to maintain muscle strength without undue joint stress, e.g. swimming. Unwise exercise causes further damage to joints that are already compromised. However, rest is not advisable except during an acute exacerbation because it may lead to loss of muscle power and to excessive stiffness: patients need controlled exercise. Attaining an ideal weight reduces joint stress in overweight patients.

Research has demonstrated that mental health improves with effective treatment and thus reflects disease activity.

Physical therapies

Physiotherapy (PT) and **occupational therapy (OT)** have an important role to play in maintaining muscle strength, and so increasing joint stability, in giving the patient additional confidence to manage independently, and in maintaining mobility and independence as far as possible. The modes used include the following.

Exercises to maintain and restore muscle power and function are effective, especially after surgery. The power of the quadriceps muscles in the thigh must be sufficient to preserve general mobility, balance and the ability to rise from chairs, etc. Muscle power should be improved before a patient undergoes elective surgery as this greatly aids recovery: any period of bed rest causes a rapid loss of muscle mass and power. Isometric exercises, in which muscles are exercised against fixed resistance with minimal joint movement and change in muscle length, improve muscle power without joint wear. Swimming and hydrotherapy (exercising in a warm pool against water resistance) are also excellent forms of exercise, because the weight of the body is supported by the water, thus reducing joint stress.

Occupational assessment and training, i.e. advice on alternative methods of carrying out tasks at home and at work, or retraining by occupational therapists to minimize joint trauma includes the following:

- Provision of aids and appliances, and modifications of the home to improve mobility and ease tasks, e.g. splints, easy-turning taps, specially adapted implements and, in exceptional circumstances, widening doors and providing ramps for wheelchair access.
- Local heat, diathermy, ultrasound, etc. are widely used, but provide only temporary relief.
- Physiotherapists, osteopaths and chiropractors can help by mobilizing and realigning joints and relieving associated muscle spasm.

Correction of exacerbating factors

The effects of OA may be exacerbated by a variety of conditions, some of which are potentially correctable, at least in part. Corrective measures include:

- Weight reduction.
- Treatment of any concurrent disease.
- Surgical or other orthopaedic correction of anatomical abnormalities that place abnormal stresses on other joints. For example, unequal leg length causes wear both to the leg joints and to those of the pelvis and vertebral column.
- Maintenance of physical activity and general fitness.
- Wearing of correct footwear and use of appropriate walking aids.
- Encouraging a positive outlook.

Pharmacotherapy

Medicines have in the past had only a limited role in the treatment of OA patients, the aims being symptomatic relief , i.e. reduction of pain and discomfort; inflammatory exacerbations; depression and anxiety.

However, good control of all of these is now possible and should give an acceptable quality of life. Although complete abolition of pain may not be possible without undue side-effects, some residual pain is a useful reminder to patients that they should exercise cautiously.

Analgesics and non-steroidal anti-inflammatory drugs

Opinions differ as to which of these groups is most appropriate. **Simple analgesics** (see Chapter 7) are widely used, but there is considerable variation in their tolerance and efficacy between patients. Most patients are maintained on a single product (*paracetamol* (acetaminophen), occasionally *codeine, dihydrocodeine* or *tramadol*, depending on pain severity, taken regularly. Combinations of *paracetamol* with *codeine* or *dihydrocodeine* (*co-codamol* and *co-dydramol*, respectively, in the UK) are widely used but may not be more effective than *paracetamol* alone and can cause opioid dependence and severe constipation.

The *paracetamol-dextropropoxyphene* combination (*co-proxamol* in the UK) will be withdrawn completely, because it is no more effective than *paracetamol* alone and is the most common suicide agent there (see Chapter 7). Normal analgesic doses (600–900 mg) of *aspirin* are effective but are rarely used because of gastric toxicity.

NSAIDs are discussed more fully under the treatment of RA (pp. 772–8), but some points are relevant here. Although NSAIDs are popular, there have been reports that some, e.g. *ibuprofen* and *naproxen*, may accelerate cartilage damage or prevent its repair. However, although the clinical significance of this is unclear it may be more appropriate to use a drug that is alleged to promote cartilage repair, e.g. *aceclofenac*. However, NSAIDs, especially the COX-2 selective agents, which have significant adverse cardiovascular effects, are usually not justified unless there is a significant inflammatory component.

Elderly patients, the group most likely to be affected by OA, are particularly sensitive to NSAID toxicity (pp. 774–8). *Naproxen* probably has the best balance between efficacy and toxicity.

It is reasonable to use NSAIDs only for the occasional painful exacerbation, e.g. when OA is accompanied by joint deposition of apatite (p. 798). Several NSAIDs seem to be unsuitable in OA on grounds of toxicity (e.g. *indometacin* and *ketoprofen*), because treatment is usually lifelong. *Tolmetin*, which is not licensed in the UK, belongs in this group.

Meloxicam, the first 'second-generation' NSAID to be marketed as a relatively selective cyclooxygenase 2 inhibitor (see Figure 12.9), is licensed for the short-term treatment of exacerbations of OA, and existing NSAIDs, e.g. *diclofenac, etodolac, nabumetone, naproxen* and *piroxicam*, are also partially COX-2-selective and are licensed similarly. These agents do cause less gastrointestinal distress than other non-selective NSAIDs and may be suitable in the older group of patients involved.

Some of the 'third-generation' NSAIDs, the highly selective COX-2 inhibitors, may cause severe cardiovascular problems and *rofecoxib* has been withdrawn in the UK. NICE advice is that, until further research data are obtained, the COX-2 inhibitors are appropriate for patients at high risk of gastrointestinal complications, such as gastric or duodenal ulcer (see Chapter 3), perforation and bleeding. The patients principally affected include:

- those over the age of 65;
- patients who have taken non-selective NSAIDs and have peptic ulceration or epigastric pain, with bleeding or are regular or chronic users of antacids or antisecretory drugs (see Chapter 3) or have ceased treatment due to gastrointestinal side-effects;
- people who are regular smokers or alcohol consumers;
- those who have any concurrent chronic disease and take associated medications.

COX-2 selective NSAIDs are contra-indicated in patients with IHD or cerebrovascular disease.

Until definitive information is available, patients taking NSAIDs require careful monitoring for adverse gastrointestinal and cardiac signs. Those prescribed older NSAIDs or highly selective COX-2 inhibitors should be told to report immediately any new epigastric or chest pain, breathlessness or exercise limitation. Presumably the prescriber will do this and pharmacists should reinforce the advice. However, the need for this type of medication clearly requires review, especially in older patients and those with adverse cardiovascular and cerebrovascular risk profiles.

Despite this evidence, the absolute risk of a serious cardiovascular event is small and a decision should be taken with the active involvement of patients as to whether they are prepared to accept the risk in view of the benefit they receive from an NSAID. None of this has a bearing on the occasional short-term NSAID use, e.g. for gout (see below), sports injury and headaches. Further, some patients obtain relief from topical NSAID treatment, to which the above considerations presumably do not apply, because of the very low systemic absorption of drug.

Other drugs

Slow-acting antirheumatic drugs (SAARDs; see Table 12.13 and p. 770) and systemic corticosteroids have no place in the treatment of OA. However, a severely affected joint that is inflamed, or in which there is a fluid effusion, may respond well to an intra-articular corticosteroid injection, though this is controversial, and the benefit is usually only temporary. Because there is the possibility of long-term joint damage with repeated injections, owing to suppression of protein (cartilage) synthesis, this should be done only occasionally.

Intra-articular injections of *sodium hyaluronate*, given weekly on three to five occasions, is reported to be more beneficial than a steroid injection, and hyaluronic acid derivatives are now available to supplement that in synovial fluid. These products are mentioned in the BNF but do not have a formal entry.

There have been several reports of the beneficial effect of glucosamine sulphate, 750–1500 mg twice daily, taken over at least 3–6 months. One international group found that this abolished cartilage loss from synovial weight-bearing joints, e.g. the knee, over a period of 3 years and have proposed that this agent should be regarded as a disease-modifying agent for OA. Treatment will have to be life-long because otherwise cartilage loss will resume at a similar rate to previously when the medication is stopped. The question of whether glucosamine sulphate should be taken prophylactically by all elderly people has not been addressed in research, but is clearly a point of interest. About one-third of patients withdrew from the trial, mostly because of side-effects (20%) or lack of efficacy (3%), but this is similar to withdrawal in the placebo group. The beneficial effect may take 6 months or more to be noticeable, so perseverance is required. Glucosamine is not licensed as a medicine in the UK and is not prescribable through the NHS.

Levels of the pain transmitter **substance P** (see Chapter 7) are raised in OA and this causes increased synovial levels of PGs and collagenase. Reduction of the substance P level is therefore desirable and this can be done using topical *capsaicin* cream. This product is thus a logical second-line agent after a simple analgesic, or as an adjunct to systemic treatment. However, it is very irritant and must not be used on inflamed or broken skin, and the hands should be washed thoroughly after application, to avoid eye and facial contamination.

Antidepressants are used to alleviate the depression associated with chronic pain and may improve the analgesic response (see Chapter 7).

Women receiving hormone replacement therapy (HRT) have been shown to be less likely to develop OA, especially of the knee, and HRT can also be euphoriant. The benefit on the knee, which is lost if HRT is stopped, may be related to the prevention of osteoporosis and so to the maintenance of bone density adjacent to joints. However, many women have stopped taking HRT, or refused to start it, because of the perceived cancer risk. A bisphosphonate is a suitable alternative to HRT if osteoporosis has been documented by dual energy X-ray absorptiometry.

Surgery

Severe, uncontrolled pain or serious loss of function may necessitate surgery. **Arthroplasty** (joint replacement) is especially successful for the hip, the pain relief being excellent and mobility usually being returned close to normal, provided that the operation is carried out before joint damage is too severe and collateral damage, e.g. to the joints of the vertebral column, has not occurred. Knee and finger joint replacement are slightly less successful and that of other joints still less so, though techniques and results are improving continually.

Arthroscopic debridement. Joint lavage with physiological saline benefits some patients, possibly by removing debris or inflammatory mediators from the joint space.

Other operations to fix joints permanently (**arthrodesis**) or to remove osteophytes (e.g. for bunions) may be undertaken occasionally for particular patients. In those for whom arthroplasty is inappropriate, **osteotomy**, i.e. cutting the bone or removing a section of bone near a joint, with or without re-alignment, may be successful for pain relief in disease of the knee or hip joints. The reasons for this are poorly understood, but correction of misalignment of the limbs clearly relieves stresses on associated joints. Also, diversion of metabolic activity to the surgically produced wound away from the adjacent joint, and may reduce further inflammation and cartilage damage there.

Rheumatoid arthritis

Introduction

Unlike OA, which is a local, generally non-inflammatory disease, rheumatoid arthritis (RA) is usually a chronic, progressive, inflammatory, systemic disease that primarily affects synovial joints (see above).

The most common extra-articular features are anaemia, soft tissue nodules (p. 767), vasculitis, sicca syndrome (p. 802) and fibrosing alveolitis.

Epidemiology and aetiology

In the UK, about 1% of the population is affected, with a 1:2 male:female premenopausal sex ratio, although among the elderly the incidence is equal in both sexes: this points to a hormonal influence. Although RA often remits in pregnancy (75% of patients), use of the combined contraceptive pill does not reduce the overall risk of developing RA, but may delay its onset. It has also been suggested that changes in sex hormone levels may modulate T cell responses by suppressing IL-2 production, a promoter of T cell proliferation and cytolytic killer cells.

The incidence of RA seems to be decreasing. In the UK, the prevalence in women aged 45–64 years halved over a recent 30-year period and the incidence in Pima (North American) Indians fell by about 60% over 17 years, to about 0.5% annually. Although the global prevalence is about 1%, with only minor racial and geographical variations, RA is almost unknown in rural Africa. The peak period of onset of RA is between 35 and 55 years of age, though it can start at almost any age.

The concordance in monozygotic twins gives a heritability of 50–60%, partly due to the genes encoding HLA-DRB1 class II molecules (see Chapter 2). Also, HLA-DRB1 in first-degree relatives gives a six times increased risk. HLA-DR4 and DR1 are also involved, but these genes probably determine disease severity and persistence rather than causation. Patients with an allele of the HLA-DRB1 gene who are seropositive for RFs (see below) have a 13 times increased risk of having bone erosions after 1 year.

The trigger factors and the basis of the prolonged, intense inflammatory process of RA are largely unknown: despite extensive research and our much greater understanding of immunopathology, current explanations are speculative. The concept of RA as an autoimmune disease is popular, and there are large numbers of mature memory T cells (CD45RO) in rheumatoid joints, derived from CD4+ (TH) cells (see Chapter 2). These promote Ig production by B cells, and there is no negative feedback, hence the production of **rheumatoid factors** (RFs, a class of autoantibodies; see above).

The presence of CD45RO cells implies prior exposure to antigen. However, the experimental use of anti-CD4 Igs does not affect the course of the disease. Further, although infection with HIV specifically targets CD4+ T cells, HIV/AIDS does not seem to affect the incidence or course of RA. However, some HIV-positive patients do have a polyarthritis, which is believed to be a reactive arthritis (p. 809).

It has been suggested that there is a persistent antigenic stimulation by Epstein–Barr virus, the cause of glandular fever. Retroviruses have also been suspected in experimental animal models, but no virus has been implicated to date. Bacterial causes, e.g. *Proteus mirabilis*, are also disputed, but infection followed by incomplete clearance of microbial nucleic acid is a possible persistent stimulus. There is a high incidence of HLA-DR1, DR4 and Dw4 genes in RA patients. DR4 carriers have a high reactivity to *M. tuberculosis* and, interestingly, T cells cloned from the synovial fluid of RA patients seem to react with tubercular antigens. There may also be an association between DR4 and T cell receptor genes.

The temporary ablation of B cells induces remission, suggesting the important role of RFs in maintaining inflammation. Also, the benefit derived from the use of antiproliferative immunosuppressants and anti-cytokine antibodies (see below) emphasizes the central importance of immunological processes in RA pathogenesis.

It is possible that RA was introduced into Europe in the 18th century by contact with Native Americans, implying an infectious aetiology.

A low socioeconomic status is predictive of a poor outcome, but this is a common finding in many diseases and is probably associated with an adverse lifestyle, e.g. a diet high in saturated fats and with low fish consumption, and under-utilization of medical resources. Further, it is known that smoking confers an increased risk, and is greater in population sectors with a low socioeconomic status.

Course

The onset of classical RA is normally insidious, polyarticular (i.e. several joints are affected) and symmetrical (i.e. the same joints are usually affected on both sides of the body at any one time). The small joints (PIP, MCP, MTP, wrists) are affected first, although a monoarticular onset, usually in the knee or the wrist, occurs in some 20% of patients (Table 12.8). Fatigue and malaise may precede joint symptoms by several months.

In about 20% of patients there is an abrupt onset with marked systemic symptoms. This acute form is alleged to have a better prognosis, but the eventual outcome is probably not affected. Following recovery, it may be many years before another attack occurs.

Even less common is a **palindromic onset**, with acute episodes affecting one joint for up to 48 h, followed by remissions and exacerbations affecting other joints at intervals of days to months. About 50% of patients who experience this type of onset will suffer typical chronic RA after a very variable period, sometimes lasting several years.

Disease activity has been reported to wax and wane unpredictably and spontaneously, so patients who experience a remission while taking or using some product will naturally, though often mistakenly, attribute their improvement to that use. However, spontaneous remission is unlikely in those who have synovitis and high levels of inflammatory markers at 12 weeks after initial diagnosis. This is the basis of the move to early diagnosis and early aggressive treatment (see below).

Natural variation in disease activity is one of the principal problems in the evaluation of new anti-rheumatoid drugs: large numbers of patients have to be used in very well-designed trials over long periods in order to obtain statistically meaningful results.

Patients with severe disease have significant morbidity and mortality. Of those referred to hospital consultants only about 50% are likely to be working after 10 years of active disease and women have a 5-year reduced life expectancy and men 7 years, or were severely disabled. However, these data are over 12 years old and the situation has since improved. Moreover, RA is not necessarily relentlessly progressive (see below).

Poor prognostic factors include:

• Inadequately controlled polyarthritis with a high ESR/CRP and high levels of RFs.

- Structural joint damage leading to disability.
- Genetic susceptibility, indicated by the presence of HLA-DR4, and/or a family history of RA.
- Low socioeconomic status and educational attainment and heavy manual labour.

RA is rare in men under 30 years, and reaches a peak at about age 65. In women, the incidence rises progressively from about age 25 to a broad peak at 45–75 years.

Pathology

Inflammation of the synovial membrane is the cardinal initial feature (Figure 12.5) and RA has been grouped with other immune-mediated inflammatory diseases (IMIDs; see Chapter 2) that share a common inflammatory pathway. The cells lining the synovium multiply, the surface becomes thickened and covered with villi, and fibrin is deposited from the inflammatory exudate. In severe cases the synovium may be 1 cm thick, normally being less than 1 mm.

The deeper layers become infiltrated with lymphocytes and plasma cells, the latter producing RFs. Most patients become seropositive within a year of symptom onset and may show high RF titres, and most joint damage occurs in the early stage after diagnosis.

However, there are few neutrophils in the synovium, though they are the commonest cells in the synovial fluid. Phagocytosis of the immune complexes formed in the fluid results in an increase in oxidative metabolism, liberating damaging free radicals and lysosomal enzymes that attack joint tissues.

As the inflammation proceeds, the synovial margin develops outgrowths of metabolically active **pannus** that invades and dissolves underlying cartilage and bone to produce the characteristic **erosions** (Figures 12.5 and 12.6(b)). With severe disease progression, the supporting ligaments and tendons are weakened and the joint will **sublux**, i.e. become partially or completely dislocated (Figure 12.6(b)), and eventually the associated limbs are deformed and non-functional. Finally, the joint may become ankylosed, i.e. fibrosed and calcified and thus stiff and non-functional, but pain-free. This progression of changes is illustrated in Figure 12.5. Tendons and tendon sheaths undergo changes similar to the synovial changes.

The mechanisms responsible for these changes are unknown, but activation of T cells by macrophages and unidentified antigens cause cytokine release. Cytokines are also produced by synovial fibroblasts. Thus TNFα and IL-1, IL-2, IL-4 and IL-8 are important in the initiation and maintenance of inflammation and cartilage and bone damage and synovitis, so the use of

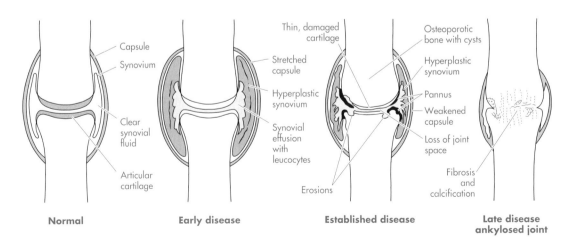

Figure 12.5 Progression of joint damage in untreated rheumatoid arthritis. The end result in severe disease is an ankylosed (rigid), painless, non-functional joint.

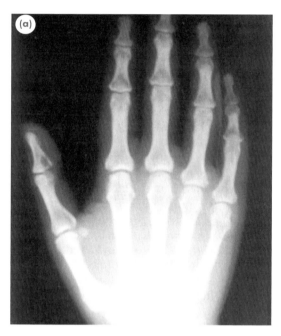 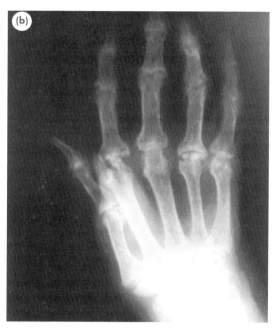

Figure 12.6   X-ray of the hand in rheumatoid arthritis. (a) Normal: note the clearly defined joint 'spaces' in both the hand and the wrist. (b) Severe rheumatoid arthritis: note the loss of joint space owing to cartilage destruction and substantial erosions of the heads of the metacarpal bones (see Figure 12.5) and the carpal (wrist) bones. The first metacarpal (thumb) has subluxed under the second and there is slight ulnar deviation (see Figure 12.7). Most of the finger bones are osteoporotic (showing grey = radiolucent). (Reproduced with permission from Dr AC Keat, Northwick Park Hospital, London, UK.)

cytokine inhibitors in treatment is logical (see below). It has also been suggested that deposition of iron in the synovial tissues, which does occur, promotes free radical damage. Hence chelating agents are being investigated to treat some patients with severe RA.

Clinical features

Articular features

These are outlined in Table 12.8. The most characteristic form of onset involves:

- **Symmetrical small joint polyarthritis** commencing in the MCP and PIP joints of the hands (Figure 12.6(b)), the wrists and the corresponding joints in the feet. Affected joints are very hot, swollen, red and tender, and are often shiny.
- **Morning stiffness.** Initially, morning stiffness lasts >15 min and may persist for >1 h before

maximal relief. With disease progression, morning stiffness increases, becoming prolonged and disabling, and it may eventually take a patient some 2 h to dress. Almost any joint may be affected, especially the wrists and the upper cervical spine. Wrist and PIP involvement (Figure 12.6(b)) always suggests a diagnosis of RA, because these are usually spared in OA.

Despite this catalogue of potential disability, it is important to appreciate that the majority of patients have only mild to moderate disease and are treated adequately by GPs: 25% recover partially, but few remit completely. A minority, perhaps 10%, is referred to hospital consultants and about 50% of these, i.e. only some 5% of the total, suffer serious disability. Most GPs will have one or more significantly disabled patients.

More advanced disease may produce characteristic hand deformities, resulting in a progressive loss of function that manifests as:

Joints involved and frequency[a]

Hands, 90; wrists, 85; knees, 80; feet, 70; shoulder, 60; hip, 10

General features

Inflammation	Any joint may be involved, but DIP[b] joints of the hands and feet tend to be spared.
Muscle wasting	Associated with disuse of any joint.
Joint deformity	Hands, especially MCP joints[c]; feet, especially MTP joints[c]; wrists[c], knees. The shoulder and hip joints are relatively spared.
Joint erosions	At any joint actively affected.
Other lesions	Hands, tendons; feet, bunions; wrists, carpal tunnel syndrome (p. 809); knees, Baker's cysts (p. 766), bursitis (p. 811).

[a] Numbers are the approximate percentages of patients affected.
[b] DIP, MCP, MTP, joints of the hands and feet (Figure 12.4).
[c] Subluxation may occur (see text).

- **Subluxation** of the MCP joints, so that the proximal phalangeal heads slip partly under the metacarpal heads.
- **Ulnar deviation** (Figure 12.7(a)), in which the hand is tilted laterally away from the thumb.
- **Boutonnière** and **swan neck** deformities of the fingers (Figure 12.7(b)) due to damage to joint ligaments.

Changes in the upper cervical spine may cause serious instability, because ligament damage may allow subluxation of one or more vertebrae, producing kinking and compression of the spinal cord (Figure 12.8), resulting in reduced neck mobility and occipital, neck, shoulder and arm pain, or sensory loss. In particular, subluxation of the atlas on the axis may allow the dens to compress the upper cervical spine, and traumatic injury in this area, e.g. caused by a whiplash effect in a motor accident, may even cause death, though this is fortunately rare. Similarly, manipulation of the cervical spine in RA may result in permanent disability, even tetraparesis (partial or total paralysis of all four limbs), so physiotherapy or other manipulation of this area is usually totally contra-indicated in RA unless investigation demonstrates normal anatomy there.

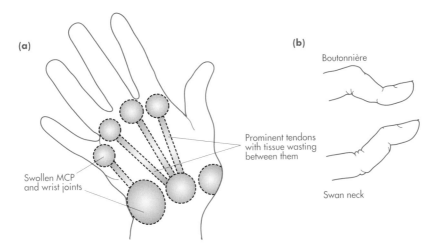

Figure 12.7   Hand in severe rheumatoid arthritis. (a) The hand shows ulnar deviation and the thumb is subluxed under the palm. (b) Types of finger deformity. MCP, metacarpophalangeal.

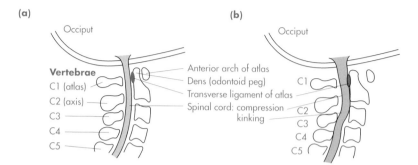

Figure 12.8   Cervical spine and the effects on it of severe rheumatoid arthritis. (a) Normal: the spinal cord and the vertebrae lie on a smooth curve, and the dens is held firmly by the transverse ligament of the atlas. The atlas is so-called because it carries the weight of the 'globe' (the head). The axis is the vertebra on which the head and atlas rotate. (b) Severe rheumatoid arthritis: weakening of the ligaments has allowed the vertebrae to sublux forwards so that they lie on a stepped curve causing kinking and compression of the spinal cord. The weakened transverse ligament of the atlas has allowed the dens to move away from the anterior arch of the atlas, compressing the spinal cord.

Periarticular features

These changes are those associated with the joints, but not arising from within the joint. Pain and stiffness within a joint may result in wasting of the associated muscles. Because tendon sheaths resemble synovium, **tenosynovitis** (p. 811) may occur with pain and diminished joint movement. Tendons may be extensively damaged and may even rupture. Swelling of the tendon sheaths within the restricted confines of the carpal tunnel often causes **carpal tunnel syndrome** (p. 809). **Raynaud's syndrome** (p. 804) and carpal tunnel syndrome may appear before the joint symptoms.

Bursitis (p. 811) is also common, especially in the feet, with resultant bunion formation.

In the knees, high intra-articular pressure may cause the synovium to balloon out into the popliteal fossa to form a **Baker's cyst**. If this ruptures, due to increased pressure occurring in the joint during knee flexion, synovial fluid is forced into the calf muscle, causing severe pain, mimicking a DVT (see Chapter 11).

Extra-articular features

These are sometimes described as complications of RA (see below), but because RA is a systemic disease, signs and symptoms, often inflammatory, may occur almost anywhere in the body (Table 12.9).

Haematological abnormalities are common. **Anaemia** is the most frequent of these, and is an almost invariable accompaniment to active disease. Iron-deficiency anaemia is common in patients being treated with NSAIDs, due to upper gastrointestinal bleeding, and this may be superimposed on the normochromic, normocytic type associated with many chronic diseases, caused by bone marrow hypoplasia (see Chapter 11). **Splenomegaly** is common, occurring in some 5% of patients (Table 12.10).

Table 12.9	Principal extra-articular (systemic) features and complications of rheumatoid arthritis
General	Malaise, tiredness, depression, fever
Skin	Nodules, sweaty palms, palmar erythema, nail fold infarcts
Blood and lymphoid system	Anaemia, lymphadenopathy, splenomegaly, Felty's syndrome (see Table 12.10)
Cardiovascular	Raynaud's syndrome, pericarditis, myocarditis, heart nodules, vasculitis
Eye	Keratoconjunctivitis sicca, episcleritis, scleritis
Neurological	Nerve entrapment, peripheral neuropathies
Respiratory	Lung nodules, pleurisy, pulmonary fibrosis

Table 12.10   Principal features of Felty's syndrome

Seropositive rheumatoid arthritis

Splenomegaly, causing pancytopenia, especially
neutropenia, causing infections and
thrombocytopenia, causing bleeding

Haemolytic anaemia

Skin pigmentation, leg ulcers

Most of the other types of blood abnormality
that occur are associated with drug therapy and
include leucopenia, thrombocytopenia and,
infrequently, aplastic anaemia.

Involvement of the lymphoid system is
common and **lymphadenopathy** (enlarged,
rubbery, non-tender 'glands') occurs in some
30% of patients, usually in association with
active disease.

Felty's syndrome is an uncommon, late
feature of seropositive RA. It occurs in 1% of
patients with severe RA, and is characterized by
splenomegaly and neutropenia, though widespread haematological and other signs may
occur (Table 12.10). The syndrome runs an
unpredictable course, with severe neutropenia
predisposing to serious infections. In rare cases,
systemic corticosteroids and splenectomy are
required.

Rheumatoid nodules are painless, often SC,
granulomas (see Chapter 2), 0.5–3 cm in diameter. They usually occur near the elbow but may
occur in bursae, tendons or tendon sheaths at
any pressure site. They may also occur internally,
e.g. in the lungs or heart or, fortunately rarely,
in the eye. If the nodules occur in the lungs,
then bronchoscopy with biopsy is indicated to
distinguish them from bronchial carcinoma or
tubercles (see Chapters 2 and 5). If bronchoscopy is not readily available, the nodules are
usually removed surgically, to provide a certain
diagnosis and protect the patient from the
possibility of bronchial carcinoma, as far as
possible. Although nodules usually occur in
seropositive RA and are virtually diagnostic, they
are also found in a few patients with SLE (see p.
798 and Chapter 13).

RA is associated with a reduced lifespan,
largely due to an increased incidence of infection, progressive systemic disease and amyloidosis. Nodules may form in the myocardium,
usually associated with high titres of RFs.

Investigation and diagnosis

Classic criteria

A diagnosis of definite RA requires at least four of
the following criteria, developed by the American
College of Rheumatology (ACR) and revised in
1988. The following are expressed more briefly
than the ACR criteria. To satisfy criteria 1 to 4,
symptoms or signs must be present continuously
for at least 6 weeks.

1. Morning stiffness for ≥ 1 h.
2. Arthritis of three or more joints and soft tissue
   swelling.
3. Arthritis of hand joints (wrist, MCP or PIP
   joints).
4. Symmetrical arthritis.
5. Rheumatoid nodules.
6. Serum RF (positive in <5% of normal control
   subjects).
7. Radiographic changes. Hand X-ray changes
   typical of RA must include erosions or
   unequivocal bony decalcification.

Strict formal application of these criteria is
helpful in doubtful cases, but most doctors would
make a provisional diagnosis on less rigid ones.

Investigation

Typical results of some common investigations
in patients with RA are given in Table 12.11. The
general picture is that of a chronic inflammatory
disease, primarily affecting the joints, with an
immunological component.

The anaemia is typical of that which accompanies many chronic diseases (see Chapter 11), and
serum iron studies may be unhelpful in diagnosis. In particular, **serum ferritin** is an acute-
phase reactant (see Chapter 2), and levels may be
elevated in RA. Confirmation of the nature and
extent of anaemia may therefore require bone
marrow examination. Another common cause of

Table 12.11   Typical results of investigations in rheumatoid arthritis

Haematology			Serology	
ESR	↑		RFs	Present (75%)
CRP	↑		Complement	N/ ↑
Hb	↓		Immunoglobulins	↑ (often)
TIBC	↓ /N		**Synovial fluid (changes are not specific)**	
Serum iron	↑		Translucent or opaque	
			Viscosity	↓
			Protein	↑
			Radiology	
White cell count	{ Usually N ↑ (severe episodes) ↑ (infection) ↑ (steroid therapy)		Early disease: osteoporosis, marginal bone erosions Established disease: loss of joint space, bone erosions, subluxation or dislocation, ankylosis?	
Platelets	{ Usually N ↑ (in active disease and acute bleeding)			

↑ , ↓ , increased or decreased level; CRP, C-reactive protein; ESR, erythrocyte sedimentation rate; Hb, haemoglobin; N, normal; RFs, rheumatoid factors; TIBC, total iron binding capacity.

anaemia in RA is drug-induced gastrointestinal bleeding (p. 775), and this may complicate the interpretation of haematological data.

The WBC count is usually normal, but **leucocytosis** and **thombocytosis** may be associated with severe exacerbations. Conversely, **neutropenia** and **thombocytopenia** may occur in Felty's syndrome, and may also be caused by iatrogenic myelosuppression, predisposing to infections and a bleeding tendency.

Plasma viscosity is usually increased, due to increased levels of acute phase proteins, notably fibrinogen, complement, gamma globulins and RFs.

Diagnosis

Although full-blown RA is unmistakable, many patients show only certain features and, because there is no pathognomonic test, the diagnosis is sometimes revealed with certainty only after some time. The occurrence of early morning stiffness, symmetrical painful polyarthritis, high RF titre and joint erosions, i.e. ACR criteria 1, 2, 4, 6 and 7, is usually conclusive. The occurrence of certain features may make a diagnosis particularly difficult, namely:

• Mono-articular involvement.
• Lack of erosions after several years of disease.
• Seronegativity.
• High antinuclear antibody titre (p. 799).
• Involvement of the lumbar spine, skin, kidneys or CNS.

The significance of these is discussed later in this chapter.

Functional assessment

Regular functional assessment (see Table 12.5) is essential in charting the progress of the disease and the effectiveness of treatment.

Complications

Complications of RA fall into four groups (see Table 12.9).

Inflammatory

Eye involvement is common:

- **Sjögren's syndrome** (p. 801) may affect about 20% of patients, 85% of them female and mostly seropositive. The syndrome causes dry eyes and a dry mouth, resulting from lymphocytic infiltration of the lachrymal and salivary glands. Other exocrine glands, e.g. in the digestive tract and the sweat glands, may also be affected. This syndrome may also occur in association with related diseases, e.g. SLE, systemic sclerosis and polymyositis.
- **Episcleritis**, causing a localized or diffuse hyperaemia of the sclera (white of the eye) is less common.
- **Severe scleritis**, which involves the deeper layers of the sclera, is uncommon but more serious.

Arteritis (vasculitis) may cause widespread obstructive vascular lesions and is an indication of severe disease. Together with the formation of myocardial nodules it is also the principal cardiovascular problem. Arteritis usually presents as **nail fold (periungual) infarcts**, i.e. small areas of black or brown dead tissue around the nail margins. The involvement of larger vessels may result in leg ulceration or peripheral neuropathies.

Respiratory complications reflect diffuse inflammation and include **fibrosing alveolitis** and, especially in men, **pleurisy** and **pleural effusions** ('rheumatoid lung').

Infective

Septic arthritis, due to joint infection by *Staphylococcus aureus* (in adults and children) or *Haemophilus influenzae* (mostly in children), is a rare but important complication. The latter is now unusual, since the introduction of Hib vaccine. Debilitated and immunosuppressed or immunodeficient patients, e.g. those with AIDS and hypogammaglobulinaemia, are particularly susceptible.

Secondary to abnormal metabolism

Mild anaemia occurs in about 80% of cases. More severe anaemia is usually iatrogenic and may require treatment (see Chapter 11).

Osteoporosis may lead to bone fractures. **Amyloidosis** (p. 807), the widespread deposition in tissues of abnormal amyloid protein, may occasionally cause clinical problems, notably nephrotic syndrome (see Chapter 14).

Iatrogenic

Adverse reactions to medication are very common and are discussed below in the section on pharmacotherapy.

Management

Objectives and strategy

The aims are to:

- relieve pain and discomfort and ameliorate symptoms;
- arrest or limit disease progression and, if possible, reverse pathological changes;
- maintain mobility and function, and promote the best possible quality of life.

These are achieved by a holistic approach, considering the patient's functional, medical, social and economic problems. The modes used are:

- Patient education and counselling.
- Physical: physiotherapy, osteopathy, occupational therapy, appliances, etc.
- Social: domestic assistance, modification of the home environment, financial support.
- Pharmacotherapy: analgesics, anti-inflammatory agents (i.e. NSAIDs, anti-cytokine drugs and corticosteroids), slow-acting ('disease-modifying') anti-rheumatic drugs (i.e. immunoregulators and antiproliferative immunosuppressants).
- Appropriate management of anaemia and other complications. Psychiatric support (see Chapter 6).
- Surgery: synovectomy, arthroplasty and other joint surgery.

Patient education and counselling

Because of the wide range of symptoms and their severity, and because patients almost inevitably fear that they will be completely crippled, it is important for them to comprehend as fully as possible the nature of the disease and the various procedures that may be used for management. An optimistic, but realistic, approach by all medical and paramedical staff is helpful, because only a small proportion of patients have serious disability and effective new treatments are being introduced.

Patient education underpins all subsequent management. Useful information is given in the patient leaflets provided by the NHS and the UK's Arthritis and Rheumatism Council, but these can only supplement authoritative verbal information. Such patient education needs to be an ongoing process because of the need to respond to the development of new symptoms and because there is a large amount of information to assimilate, which is impossible to convey in one or two sessions.

Depression may be sufficiently severe to require psychiatric intervention.

Physical methods

Rest may be valuable in an acute episode. Complete bedrest is occasionally used for a minority of patients but if not properly supervised, with adequate physiotherapy, this may lead to permanent disability owing to joint disuse and muscle wasting.

Physiotherapy is very valuable, and includes the use of splints or support bandaging to rest particular joints or to correct deformity. A carefully planned series of exercises, e.g. swimming and isometric exercises, is important in maintaining muscle power without over-stressing damaged joints. Other widely used methods, e.g. the application of heat wax baths, cold, short wave therapy, etc., may provide some short-term relief of pain and stiffness.

Occupational therapy is an essential component of management.

Monitoring

The ACR has recommended the following criteria for defining improvement. There should be demonstrable improvement in:

- The number of swollen and tender joints.
- At least three of the following measures of disease activity:
  - Patient assessment.
  - Physician assessment.
  - Pain score.
  - Disability score.
  - Serum levels of acute-phase reactants, e.g. CRP, ESR, plasma viscosity.

An appropriate goal for treatment is a better than 50% improvement in these criteria.

Pharmacotherapy: introduction

The drug treatment of RA is summarized in Table 12.12. Early drug management for mild disease is similar to that used in OA (p. 759), although anti-inflammatory drugs (mostly NSAIDs) are used, with an increased risk of adverse reactions. Inadequate relief or control, more severe symptoms or a definite diagnosis of seropositive RA leads to the use of slow-acting antirheumatic drugs (SAARDs), also described as 'disease modifying anti-rheumatic drugs (DMARDS)'. However, the extent to which any of this group of drugs significantly modifies disease progression in the long term is arguable. The term SAARD defines the principal characteristic of this group, that they take about 4–6 months' treatment to achieve their maximum therapeutic effect.

Although the inflammation responds to current treatments, the destructive process due to

Table 12.12   The management of confirmed rheumatoid arthritis[a]

Step	Criterion	Action[b]
1	All patients	Education Physiotherapy, controlled exercise
2	Very mild symptoms	Simple analgesics
3	At any stage	3.1 Inadequate pain relief: 'top-up' simple analgesics, increase dose of NSAID 3.2 A few painful joints: rest, e.g. splinting; intra-articular corticosteroid 3.3 Surgery: e.g. synovectomy, arthroplasty, arthrodesis
4	Mild to moderate moderate disease	NSAIDs[c] 4.1 Ibuprofen or diclofenac 4.2 Change to naproxen or meloxicam or piroxicam 4.3 Morning stiffness >1 h: change to indometacin 4.4 Trial of others
5	Moderate to severe or aggressive disease	SAARDs[d] 5.1 SSZ or MTX or hydroxychloroquine 5.2 Azathioprine 5.3 Gold or penicillamine 5.4 Immunomodulators: leflunomide or ciclosporin 5.5 Cyclophosphamide 5.6 Cytokine inhibitors: adalimumab, etanercept or infliximab
6	Severe presentation **or** exacerbation **or** elderly	Corticosteroid[e]
7	Significant functional impairment of a few joints	Surgery: e.g. synovectomy, arthroplasty, arthrodesis

[a] This is an example of common usage and does not represent a firm recommendation of one drug or course of action over another. Patients vary widely in disease presentation and response to treatment and prescribers have individual approaches.

[b] Numbers represent a possible sequence at each step.

[c] NSAIDs should be tried for 2 weeks at the minimum appropriate dose, unless contraindicated. If relief is inadequate, the dose should be increased for a further 2 weeks. If still ineffective, a change should be made to a different chemical class (Table 12.14) or a more potent drug. All patients aged over 65 years and younger patients who develop epigastric discomfort should also take an H_2-antagonist or proton pump inhibitor.

[d] With moderate to severe or progressive disease, a SAARD should be introduced as soon as a definite diagnosis of RA has been made because joint damage may commence early. All take some time before their full effect is obtained.

[e] A severe presentation or exacerbation should be treated promptly with prednisolone. Corticosteroids provide prompt relief, but the dose should be reduced to the minimum required to control symptoms, preferably nil, once control has been gained. Low doses may be needed until SAARDs take effect. Patients aged over 65 years tolerate NSAIDs poorly and may be better off with prednisolone, despite the adverse effects.

SAARD, slow-acting anti-inflammatory drug; MTX, methotrexate; NSAID, non-steroidal anti-inflammatory drug; SSZ, sulfasalazine.

pannus (p. 763) is less amenable. However, TNFα blockade (see below) does reduce the irreversible joint erosions that cause much disability.

Anti-inflammatory drugs include:

- NSAIDs.
- Corticosteroids.
- High-dose *aspirin* and salicylates are rarely used nowadays, except in some Third World countries where drug cost is an overriding consideration.

In comparison, the SAARDs (Table 12.13) include:

- Immunomodulators, i.e. immunosuppressants; e.g. *methotrexate, ciclosporin* and *leflunomide*.
- Cytokine inhibitors, e.g. inhibitors of:

  - TNFα, i.e. *adalimumab, etanercept* and *infliximab*
  - IL 1, i.e. *anakinra*.
- *Sulfasalazine (SSZ)*.
- Gold compounds, *penicillamine* and antimalarials.

Pharmacotherapy: anti-inflammatory drugs and analgesics

Non-steroidal anti-inflammatory drugs

NSAIDs have been the drugs of first choice for the treatment of mild RA for many years because they possess both analgesic and anti-inflammatory properties, and many are available (Table 12.14). They are also used as

Table 12.13   Slow-acting antirheumatic drugs (SAARDs)

Drug		Cautions, contra-indications and side-effects	Monitoring procedures
All	CCI:	Increase dose slowly to minimize adverse reactions (except antimalarials) Elderly Pregnancy Hepatic or renal disease	Generally[a]: careful examination of the patient and inquiry for adverse reactions (especially bleeding or bruising tendency, fever, sore throat or mouth[b]; also kidney and liver damage, rashes); regular full blood counts[b]
	SEs:	Gastrointestinal disturbance (oral forms[c]) Blood dyscrasias[b]	
Sulfasalazine	CCI:	G6PD deficiency Porphyria	Regular liver function tests for first 3 months
	SEs:	Hypersensitivity to salicylates or sulphonamides	
Gold (auranofin and sodium aurothiomalate)	SEs:	Pruritus (may herald severe skin disease), pulmonary fibrosis, kidney damage	Annual chest X-ray
Penicillamine	SEs:	SLE, hypersensitivity reactions	
Hydroxychloroquine	CCI:	Psoriasis[d]	Regular eye checks (see text, retinopathy very unlikely at low doses)
	SEs:	Headache, myopathy, retinopathy	

[a] These are additional to the specific requirements listed for individual drugs.

[b] Indicators of possible blood dyscrasias (rare with antimalarials).

[c] All are orally administered, except sodium aurothiomalate (IM).

[d] May severely exacerbate existing psoriasis. There are numerous other contra-indications (see BNF).

CCI, cautions and contra-indications; G6PD, glucose 6-phosphate dehydrogenase; SEs, side-effects; SLE, systemic lupus erythematosus (p. 798).

an adjunct to SAARDs if symptomatic support is required until benefit is obtained.

Patient response to NSAIDs and tolerance of them is very variable, so it may be necessary to try several products to determine which has the best combination of efficacy and tolerability. The basis for this inter-patient variability is unclear, but it is likely to be more related to disease activity than to drug pharmacokinetics or anti-PG activity. These drugs have a rapid onset of action but the full analgesic and anti-inflammatory effect may not be apparent for a week or so, largely dependent on dose frequency and the consequent time to reach steady state. If adequate relief is not obtained within 2–3 weeks at full dosage, a change to another product is indicated. However, relief of pain and early morning stiffness is often incomplete at tolerable doses.

Mode of action

The activity of NSAIDs is ascribed to their inhibition of **cyclo-oxygenase** (COX) activity and thus of PG synthesis. COX exists in two isoforms that may be expressed constitutively, i.e. they are always produced, in only a limited range of tissues. COX-1 is constitutive in the stomach, kidneys, intestines and platelets, while COX-2 is inducible by inflammation in joints, the brain, kidney, vascular endothelium and reproductive tract.

Activation of COX-1 leads to the formation of autacoids, e.g. protective prostacyclins, in the gastric mucosa and vascular endothelium, PGE_2 in the kidney and thromboxane (TXA_2) in the platelets. COX-2 is involved in fever, the central modulation of pain and the initiation of uterine contractions and fetal expulsion in childbirth, but its physiological roles are not fully defined.

Although COX-2 may play a role in ulcer healing in animals and occurs around human gastric ulcers, the clinical significance of this is unknown. COX-2 is mostly inducible by cytokines and other pro-inflammatory stimuli that cause an inflammatory response localized to the site of production, e.g. in joints (Figure 12.9).

COX-2 differs from COX-1 only by the substitution of isoleucine by valine in the active site. This produces a larger NSAID binding site, which is the rationale for the development of the COX-2 inhibitors.

Aspirin and most of the older NSAIDs inhibit both COX isozymes but the relative effects differ considerably between drugs, and most of the older NSAIDs are relatively selective for COX-1 inhibition. This may be clinically significant because selective inhibition of leukotriene (LT) production by COX-2 induction should therefore spare distant, uninflamed sites, e.g. the stomach. Because COX-1 is not inhibited by the selective COX-2 agents, its normal actions in the stomach and kidney will still produce the eicosanoids

---

Table 12.14   Chemical classification of non-selective[a] non-steroidal anti-inflammatory drugs

Anthranilic acids	Mefenamic acid, flufenamic acid[b], meclofenamate sodium[b]
Arylalkanoic acids	Arylacetic acids: aceclofenac[c], diclofenac, tolmetin Arylbutyric acids: fenbufen Arylpropionic acids[c]: ibuprofen, fenoprofen, flurbiprofen, ketoprofen, naproxen
Alkanes	Nabumetone
Enolic acids (oxicams)	Piroxicam, meloxicam, tenoxicam
Indole and indene acetic acids	Etodolac, indometacin, acemetacin, sulindac
Salicylates	Diflunisal[c], (aspirin)

[a] Agents with relatively greater COX selectivity have recently been introduced but are liable to cause cardiovascular problems (see text).

[b] Not licensed in the UK.

[c] Aceclofenac, diclofenac and diflunisal have similar properties to the arylpropionic acids

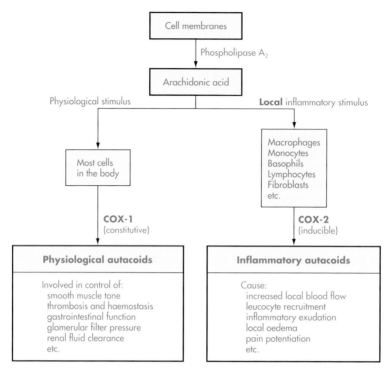

Figure 12.9   Simplified scheme for physiological and inflammatory autacoid formation by cyclo-oxygenase (COX) isozymes. Non-selective NSAIDs inhibit COX-1 and COX-2: selective NSAIDs inhibit COX-2 preferentially.

necessary for normal gastrointestinal and renal functions, so COX-2 inhibition spares the harmful effects on these organs caused by the non-selective agents.

Differing relative potencies and selectivities against COX-1/COX-2 are alleged to account for the differences between NSAIDs. It has been suggested that inhibition of COX-1 causes most of the side-effects of NSAIDs, while that of COX-2 is principally responsible for the anti-inflammatory action.

It is still unclear whether these alleged benefits of selective COX-2 inhibitors (coxibs) are translated fully into clinical superiority. *Etodolac*, now known to be a coxib, has been in use for many years and its side-effect profile does not seem to be markedly different from that of non-selective NSAIDs.

The large RCT (VIGOR) with *rofecoxib*, the first coxib to be licensed as such, confirmed its gastrointestinal safety relative to *naproxen* (relative risk (RR) 0.4). However, there was a relative fivefold increase in the risk of MI (see Chapter 4).

The subsequent APPROVe trial, in which participants were allowed to take daily *aspirin*, found an RR of 1.92 for MI or cerebrovascular events (stroke) with *rofecoxib*, and an increased risk of heart failure. This increased cardiovascular risk has been confirmed by case-control studies. Consequently, *rofecoxib* has been withdrawn by the manufacturer.

Other coxibs (*celecoxib, valdecoxib* and *parecoxib*) have also produced an increased cardiovascular risk. *Valdecoxib* has been withdrawn because of severe skin problems and *parecoxib* is licensed only for the short-term relief of acute post-operative pain. Cardiovascular problems with *etoricoxib* are similar to those with *diclofenac*, although *etoricoxib* does not differ from placebo in causing headache, nausea and diarrhoea.

It has been suggested that the basis for these observations is that the selective COX-2 inhibitors significantly reduce levels of prostacyclin (PGI_2), an inhibitor of platelet aggregation, and do not affect thromboxane (TXA_2, a potent vasoconstrictor) formation by COX-1. There is therefore an increased tendency for vascular obstruction.

Although the incidence of serious upper gastrointestinal damage does appear to be less with selective COX-2 inhibitors, a 2006 systematic analysis concluded that these drugs and high-dose non-selective COX inhibitors other than *naproxen* are associated with about a 45% increased risk of adverse cardiovascular events (MI, stroke or vascular death; see Chapter 4). This does not appear to apply to high-dose *naproxen*.

The UK's CSM and the European Medicines Evaluation Agency (EMEA) therefore recommend that COX-2 inhibitors are contra-indicated in patients who have:

- IHD.
- Cerebrovascular disease.
- Moderate to severe heart failure (NYHA II–IV; see Chapter 4)
- Significant risk factors for cardiovascular events, i.e. diabetes mellitus, hyperlipidaemia, hypertension and smoking, or for peripheral artery disease.

If a patient taking a coxib has a significant cardiovascular risk profile, or develops such a risk, they should be switched to alternative medication.

Coxibs should only be used in preference to non-selective NSAIDs when specifically indicated, i.e. in those who are at particular risk of gastroduodenal ulcer, with perforation or bleeding (see Chapter 3), and after a careful assessment of a patient's cardiovascular and overall risks.

Although Commission on Human Medicines (CHM) recommends that the lowest effective dose of *any* NSAID should be prescribed for the shortest possible time, this is hardly meaningful for many of those needing NSAIDs, because the principal conditions for which they are used e.g. osteoarthritis, RA and ankylosing spondylitis are of long duration. For most of the current coxibs that have been introduced, the cardiovascular risks outweigh their beneficial gastroprotective and anti-inflammatory effects.

However, this presumably does not affect short-term coxib use for treating or preventing dental, post-operative and other pain, though prescribers may prefer well-tried simple analgesics in the light of current information.

The new selective COX-2 inhibitor *lumiracoxib* was licensed in 2003 but was withheld pending review of its adverse effects. It was marketed in 2005 for the treatment of osteoarthritis. The large TARGET trial showed it to have a gastroprotective effect compared to non-selective NSAIDs in patients with OA.

Further, a meta-analysis of *lumiracoxib* osteoarthritis trials showed that, for a combined end-point of MI, ischaemic and haemorrhage stroke and cardiovascular death there was a slightly lower incidence of adverse cardiovascular events than with non-naproxen NSAIDs, but about a 40% increased risk compared with *naproxen*. Despite all this, as this text was about to go to press it was announced that the MHRA has suspended approval for *lumiraroxib* because an unacceptable number of patients taking standard doses for a short period have exprienced severe liver damage.

Interestingly, the results of this scrutiny of *lumiracoxib* safety, provoked by the findings with other coxibs, indicates that *naproxen* has rather different characteristics from other non-selective NSAIDs and has a relatively low incidence of adverse cardiovascular events, including small reductions in both diastolic and systolic blood pressure. However, the concomitant use of *aspirin* probably counteracts these benefits.

Side-effects

NSAIDs are responsible for the largest number of 'yellow card' reports to the CSM of any drug group, reflecting both their numerous side-effects and interactions (Table 12.15) and their frequency of use. Most adverse drug reactions (ADRs) are minor, but the principal adverse reaction, **gastric ulceration**, may lead to significant bleeding and severe anaemia, even perforation. Taking NSAIDs increases the risk of these reactions in RA patients about three times, with a sixfold increase in the risk of perforation of the gut. Patients do not become tolerant to this effect and the incidence of hospital admission due to gastrointestinal haemorrhage is increasing.

Table 12.15 Possible side-effects, interactions, cautions and contra-indications of non-steroidal anti-inflammatory drugs

Side-effects[a]	
Gastrointestinal	Gastric discomfort, nausea, diarrhoea, bleeding (occasionally severe), peptic ulceration, rectal irritation (suppositories)
Neurological	Headache, dizziness or confusion, vertigo, tinnitus, psychiatric disturbance, eye problems
Dermatological	Rashes, photosensitivity
Hypersensitivity reactions	Asthma, angioedema
Haematological	Purpura
Fluid retention	May precipitate heart failure or exacerbate hypertension, renal failure (rare)

Some important interactions[b]	
Warfarin[c]	May enhance anticoagulant effect
Diuretics	Antagonism of diuretic effect, increased risk of hyperkalaemia with potassium-sparing diuretics
ACEIs	Antagonism of hypotensive effect, increased risk of hyperkalaemia and renal failure
Digoxin	Increased serum concentration of digoxin, antagonism of effect on heart failure (due to fluid retention)
Ciclosporin	Increased risk of nephrotoxicity
Methotrexate	Increased risk of toxicity
Lithium	Increased serum concentration of lithium, possibly toxicity
Probenecid	Reduced excretion of indometacin, ketoprofen and naproxen
Quinolone antibiotics	Risk of convulsions

Cautions	
Elderly, respiratory disease, asthma, allergic disorders, peptic ulceration, renal, cardiac or hepatic impairment, pregnancy, breastfeeding, dehydration, diuretic therapy, haemorrhoids (suppositories), children (see text)	

Contra-indications	
Gout, children (see text), anticoagulant/antiplatelet therapy (especially with aspirin), hypersensitivity to aspirin or any NSAID	

[a] Side-effects vary in severity and frequency between drugs and, especially, between patients. See the BNF and manufacturers' literature.
[b] Only the most important interactions are listed: indometacin is the most likely to interact with other drugs. See BNF Sections 10.1 and 10.1.1 and manufacturers' literature.
[c] Potentially life-threatening interaction.
ACEI, angiotensin-converting enzyme inhibitor; NSAID, non-steroidal anti-inflammatory drug.

Factors that increase the risk of serious gastrointestinal side-effects by at least 50% include the following:

- Age >65 years.
- History of gastrointestinal problems, e.g. recent upper abdominal pain, active peptic ulcer and regular or recurrent use of antacids or antisecretory drugs.
- Previous NSAID intolerance or cessation of treatment due to gastrointestinal disturbance.
- Cigarette smoking.
- Alcohol consumption.

- Any concurrent chronic disease and associated medications.

NSAIDs may also cause deterioration in renal function, with fluid retention and oedema. This is particularly important in the elderly and in patients in whom renal function is already compromised, e.g. creatinine clearance <30 mL/min. All NSAIDs tend to cause fluid retention, resulting in acute cardiac decompensation in patients with heart failure and limited cardiac reserve. There is one Australian report suggesting that 29% of the hypertension cases found among the elderly Australian population are due to NSAIDs.

Other side-effects are rashes, notably with *diclofenac*, *fenbufen* and *sulindac*.

All NSAIDs cause premature closure of the ductus arteriosus if used regularly during pregnancy, delay childbirth and increase the duration of labour.

Minimizing gastrointestinal side-effects

The gastric side-effects of NSAIDs are due to a combination of local irritation and systemic mechanisms, but antisecretory agents (e.g. H_2-RAs and PPIs) help to protect against NSAID-induced gastric ulceration.

Also *misoprostol*, a 'cytoprotective' PGE_1 analogue, is marketed for co-administration with NSAIDs to minimize gastric damage, and fixed combinations with *diclofenac* and *naproxen* are available. *Misoprostol* may be slightly more effective than the H_2-RAs in preventing gastric ulcers, but both types of drug are equivalent in protecting against duodenal ulceration. However, *misoprostol* may cause severe diarrhoea and other gastrointestinal, central nervous and gynaecological side-effects, which may necessitate withdrawal.

These agents are intended to overcome the damaging gastrointestinal effects of NSAIDs, while permitting the anti-inflammatory benefits to continue. Although the coxibs may make it possible to minimize the use of antisecretory and other gastroprotective drugs in a particular patient, it is likely that prescribers will now avoid coxib use.

It has been alleged that NSAIDs increase **cartilage damage** in the long term. They are known

to suppress bone formation, and have been used to prevent undesirable ossification following total hip replacement. The clinical significance of this in treating RA is unclear.

There is a continuous turnover of articular cartilage throughout life, and the glycosaminoglycan (GAG) matrix turns over considerably more rapidly than the fibrillar collagen. This remodelling has been reflected in the regression of joint pathology in some arthritic patients. Changes in chondrocyte activity affect this process and may be the pathological basis of OA and some other arthritides. Local cytokine release, notably IL-1, may interfere with natural repair mechanisms and we know that human cartilage is more sensitive than animal tissue: this emphasizes the need for caution when interpreting the results of experiments with animal models of rheumatic diseases. Further, it is known that some NSAIDs modulate IL-1 activity, e.g. *indometacin* increases it seven times.

One short-term *in vitro* study with human osteoarthritic and normal cartilage has shown that NSAIDs probably fall into three groups on the basis of their effects on GAG synthesis: i.e. stimulatory (e.g. *aceclofenac*); no effect (e.g. *aspirin*, *diclofenac*, *tiaprofenic acid*) and inhibitory (e.g. *ibuprofen*, *indometacin*, *naproxen*). This result with *indometacin* may reflect its known effect on IL-1 levels.

The effects of *aspirin* and *diclofenac* appear to depend on individual cartilage metabolism. *Ketoprofen* and *piroxicam* may stimulate GAG synthesis in young cartilage but not in adults.

Although these laboratory results were obtained at NSAID concentrations similar to the plasma levels achieved with normal dosing, it is notoriously difficult to extrapolate from short-term *in vitro* studies to the clinical situation. These findings provide some rational basis for NSAID selection, at least in OA, and may be unimportant if, for example, *indometacin* is used for the short-term treatment of acute gout (see below). However, they may be significant if long-term use is contemplated in patients with demonstrable cartilage damage. The effects are quite distinct from the analgesic properties of this drug group.

It must be concluded that, despite the advantages and wide use of NSAIDs, there is an obvious need to develop safer alternatives to the present generation of these agents.

Selection

NSAIDs are often classified by their chemical structures (see Table 12.14), but this is generally unhelpful in choosing a product for a patient except to select a chemically unrelated drug if an ADR, e.g. hypersensitivity, dictates a change of medication. The main differences between the approximately 20 available NSAIDs are their *in vitro* potency and the incidence of side-effects. However, the potency differences do not translate into increased clinical effectiveness at recommended dosages and there is nothing to choose between any of the current NSAIDs in this respect. Thus the principal criterion for choice is patient acceptability, i.e. minimal side-effects:

- *Ibuprofen* has a relatively low incidence of side-effects and so is a common first choice for patients with mild symptoms, but it has relatively weak anti-inflammatory properties.
- *Naproxen* is more potent, has a reasonable effectiveness/toxicity balance and is conveniently taken twice daily: it is probably the first-line drug for those with moderate symptoms.
- Modified-release forms of *diclofenac* and *ketoprofen* are widely used alternatives.
- *Nabumetone* has been shown to produce less endoscopically proven gastric lesions than many other NSAIDs.

Although the coxibs are no longer regarded as a first-line choice, *meloxicam* is licensed for the treatment of pain and inflammation in rheumatic diseases generally, though the BNF does not currently list a lower incidence or smaller range of side-effects. It may cause serious skin and gastrointestinal reactions. *Tiaprofenic acid* may cause severe bladder irritation.

Unfortunately, effectiveness and toxicity seem to be associated with the current range of non-selective NSAIDs, of which *naproxen* seems to be preferable (see above and Table 12.15).

Because the products will be taken for long periods, compliance is aided by the use of drugs or products with convenient dosing patterns, i.e. once or twice daily. However, the differences in the pharmacokinetic properties of the drugs has been blurred by the introduction of modified-release versions of those with a short half-life.

A procedure used by some rheumatologists is to give a patient a 14- or 21-day supply of each of three products, to be taken consecutively, and allow the patient to choose the most acceptable. If none of the first group chosen is acceptable, a further selection can be tried. Some 50% of patients are likely to respond to the first agent tried, and a further 30% to the second. Approximately 5% fail to derive satisfactory benefit from any of this group of drugs.

However, NSAIDs are probably over-prescribed. They are the principal cause of drug-related problems in the elderly and are often used when there is no evidence of inflammation and a simple analgesic would suffice.

Restrictions on specific NSAIDs

Azapropazone

The UK CSM has restricted its use to RA, AS and acute gout only when other NSAIDs have been tried and failed. It is contra-indicated in patients with a history of peptic ulcer. The maximum daily dose has been reduced to 600 mg for those with RA and AS aged over 60y, and those with impaired renal function.

Piroxicam

The Committee on Human Medicinal Products (CHMP) has advised that:

- Piroxicam should be initiated only by physicians experienced in treating inflammatory and degenerative rheumatic disease.
- Piroxicam should not be used as a first-line treatment.
- In adults, use of piroxicam should be limited only to the symptomatic relief of OA, RA and AS.
- Piroxicam dose should not exceed 20 mg daily.
- Piroxicam should no longer be used for the treatment of acute painful and inflammatory conditions.
- Treatment should be reviewed 2 weeks after initiating piroxicam, and periodically thereafter.

- Concomitant administration of a gastro-protective agent should be considered.

Note Topical preparations containing piroxicam are not affected by these restrictions.

Piroxicam is not recommended for the treatment of acute musculoskeletal disorders in children (author's comment).

Corticosteroids

These are the most potent anti-inflammatory agents available and are also immunosuppressive. They produce a dramatic response. Some studies have suggested the prevalence of use of corticosteroids in RA to be as high as 80%, accounting for about 25% of all steroid usage. Although it used to be generally believed that corticosteroids have little effect on the underlying disease process, they may limit the extent of joint damage if used in early RA (see below), and during severe inflammatory episodes.

Mode of action

Corticosteroids down-regulate the production of LTs, PGs, complement components, interferons, other cytokines and histamine. However, they are not myelosuppressive because they act on mature immune cells to prevent B cell and T cell clone proliferation. In contrast, the antiproliferative immunomodulators (see below) act on immune cell precursors in the bone marrow, and incidentally on all other haemopoietic cells.

Side-effects

Even patients given relatively low doses, e.g. 5 mg *prednisolone* daily, over long periods may show significant side-effects, and these are more frequent at higher doses, as usual. The effects seen include:

- Fluid retention and hypertension.
- Weight gain (additional to fluid retention).
- Loss of bone density (osteoporosis) and increased risk of fracture.
- Increased susceptibility to infections, e.g. shingles, chickenpox may be fatal.
- Reduced glucose tolerance.
- Cataract formation and glaucoma.
- Impaired wound healing.
- Loss of SC tissue.

- Proximal myopathy.
- Steroid psychosis.
- Cushing's syndrome.
- Suppression of the hypothalamic-pituitary-adrenal axis.

Interactions

Corticosteroids reduce blood levels of salicylates. Thus, the introduction of steroids in a patient taking *aspirin* as an analgesic is illogical. Further, if a patient is taking an effective dose of *aspirin* plus a steroid, withdrawal of the steroid may precipitate *aspirin* toxicity. However, use of this combination has a high risk of gastrotoxicity and is undesirable.

They have many other interactions that are not relevant to antirheumatic drugs, and the reader is directed to the BNF and standard texts for information on these.

Uses

Because of these well-known side-effects, the corticosteroids have a strictly limited role in the treatment of RA. They are invaluable when serious complications occur, e.g. intolerable pain, uncontrolled loss of function, and especially vasculitis (p. 805). High doses, i.e. 60–100 mg of *prednisolone* daily PO, or an equivalent IV or IM injection of *methylprednisolone*, may be used in the short term for severe uncontrolled rheumatoid disease or for serious systemic complications, e.g. vasculitis. Pulsed high doses, e.g. up to 1 g of IV *methylprednisolone* on three consecutive days, are sometimes used to avoid the corticosteroid dependence that occurs with gradual progressive or prolonged regimens. Corticosteroids also have a place in the prompt, short-term relief of severe exacerbations, and possibly as an adjunct to early SAARD treatment, to give rapid relief and to prevent early joint damage, until the SAARD effects are manifest. However, this application is usually met with NSAIDs. A few RA patients who are intolerant of other treatments derive adequate benefit from low-dose oral *prednisolone*, i.e. 5.0–7.5 mg/day.

It has been shown that the early introduction of 7.5 mg/day of *prednisolone* following diagnosis, in addition to other treatments, retards joint erosion over a 2- to 4-year period. Withdrawal of the steroid in the third year may result in the initiation of joint damage in some patients and its resumption in those with joint damage at the start of corticosteroid use. This anti-erosive dose should be reduced gradually to zero after 2–4 years, in order to avoid long-term ADRs.

In very elderly patients, corticosteroids may be used for the maintenance of already limited mobility and function, when their advantages, including an increased sense of well-being, may outweigh their long-term disadvantages.

Local corticosteroid treatment. Water-insoluble corticosteroids, e.g. *triamcinolone hexacetonide* or *methylprednisolone acetate*, may be injected into a particular joint, with aspiration of excess synovial fluid, to control a local flare-up there. Provided the injection is placed correctly in the joint, and leakage does not occur, periarticular SC atrophy should not be a problem. Intra-articular injections provide periods of relief that vary from a few days to months, but such injections should not be used more than three times annually, in order to avoid further joint damage. If greater frequency is indicated, an alternative treatment should be sought. Corticosteroid joint injections must always be carried out with scrupulous aseptic technique to avoid the possibility of infection. Joints must not be injected if infection is suspected, as the steroid is likely to exacerbate the problem.

Tendons and bursae may also be injected. However, it is essential to inject the tendon sheath and not the tendon itself, otherwise tendon rupture is likely. Because the Achilles tendon (in the heel) does not have a proper sheath it should not be injected. Corticosteroid eye drops are essential for the control of serious eye complications (Table 12.9).

Analgesics

Simple and compound analgesics, e.g. *paracetamol* (acetaminophen) and *codeine-* and *dihydrocodeine*-based products (see Chapter 7) are used at any stage as 'top up' therapy if additional pain control is required. However, because inflammation is central to RA, analgesics are inappropriate as monotherapy.

Pharmacotherapy: slow-acting anti-rheumatic drugs (SAARDs)

Introduction

Patients with mild disease are treated satisfactorily with NSAIDs. Those with moderate to severe disease, or if there is a progression from mild to moderate symptoms or signs, need a SAARD (see Table 12.13). If a SAARD is effective and tolerated in a particular patient, any of these second-line agents will improve both the joint problems and any extra-articular symptoms and will abolish the need for corticosteroids, or spare the steroid dose. Patients usually require an NSAID in the early stages, if they are not already taking one, to provide symptom relief until the SAARD is fully effective. If there is no objective evidence of benefit with a SAARD after 6 months, it should be discontinued and an alternative sought.

Irreversible joint damage and impairment of function tend to occur early in the course of the disease, especially in the 2 years following diagnosis, so SAARDs should be used immediately a firm diagnosis of RA has been made, i.e. much earlier than previously recommended and certainly within the first 2 years, to achieve maximal benefit. Careful monitoring for both effectiveness and toxicity is essential, especially in the early stages of treatment. It may be important to try to identify those patients in the subset who are likely to suffer more aggressive disease.

Some patients may benefit from combination SAARD therapy, especially if they have responded partially to monotherapy, but the response is very variable. One small North American study found that *methotrexate–SSZ–hydroxychloroquine* triple therapy gave at least a 50% improvement in symptoms over single agents, with no evidence of excessive toxicity. In a Dutch trial, an intensive regimen with *methotrexate–SSZ–prednisolone* gave significant improvement over *SSZ* alone, but this benefit disappeared when the *prednisolone* was withdrawn. Patients who respond well but incompletely to *methotrexate* may benefit from the addition of *ciclosporin*.

The modes of action of most of these agents in RA are uncertain, but they are all mildly or significantly cytotoxic and should suppress lymphocyte activity and so the inflammatory response (see Chapter 2).

Antiproliferative immunomodulators

These are arguably the most effective of the second-line agents, but they have a relatively high incidence of ADRs (see also Chapters 10 and 14) and there are hazards associated with long-term immunosuppression. They are therefore used only for patients with proven, moderate or severe or progressive disease that is not adequately controlled by NSAIDs, or who cannot tolerate other products. This is especially important with RA because, although distressing, it is rarely fatal and requires prolonged treatment.

Use is usually restricted to specialized units with adequate monitoring facilities, particularly for undesirable myelosuppression while causing desirable damage to immune stem cells, producing immunosuppression. In contrast, corticosteroids act on mature immune cells and so do not cause myelosuppression.

All antiproliferative (cytotoxic) drugs are teratogenic and may have side-effects on spermatogenesis. They are therefore avoided, used with great care, or may be absolutely contraindicated, in women of child-bearing age and those who are breastfeeding. Exceptionally, they may be considered for the control of a severe exacerbation in a woman who is already pregnant: this is a matter for discussion and cooperation between rheumatologist and gynaecologist, and possibly a specialist in cytotoxic chemotherapy (see Chapter 10 for a more detailed discussion).

Methotrexate
Methotrexate is a dihydrofolate reductase inhibitor, and so blocks folate synthesis. *Methotrexate* is licensed for the treatment of moderate to severe active RA that is unresponsive to 'conventional' therapy. It is relatively well tolerated at the lower doses (5–25 mg weekly) used in rheumatology. It is currently the first choice of many rheumatologists and is increasing in popularity because it has a simple once-weekly dosage regimen: severe adverse reactions have resulted from daily dosing, so

pharmacists need to take special care when dispensing *methotrexate*. However, its drop-out rate after 1–2 years is only about 40–50% of that found with other SAARDs. Nevertheless, *methotrexate* must be used with great care if there is any evidence of renal or hepatic impairment (it may cause liver cirrhosis) or of the pulmonary complications of RA. Renal impairment may lead to the accumulation of toxic levels. The UK's CSM advises a full blood count, and also that renal and liver function tests be made initially and weekly until patients are stabilized, and then at 2- to 3-month intervals thereafter. Patients should promptly report any occurrence of sore throat or fever, and any other signs of infection.

Methotrexate is unsuitable for the treatment of RA in pregnant women (it has been used as an abortifacient), and contraceptive precautions must be taken both during and for 6–12 months after therapy. *Methotrexate* also damages spermatozoa, and there should not be any attempt made at conception by men within 6 months of its use.

Azathioprine
This agent is a prodrug, being metabolized slowly to *6-mercaptopurine*, a purine antagonist. Like *methotrexate*, *azathioprine* is widely used, but it has a slower onset of action.

In addition to their use in treating RA, these two drugs are used to treat severe, progressive psoriatic arthropathy (see Chapter 13). In this setting, *azathioprine* seems to be the more effective for the arthritic symptoms, and *methotrexate* for the skin lesions.

Cyclophosphamide
This nitrogen mustard is an effective DNA alkylating agent, with a rapid onset of action, though it causes a very high incidence of side-effects (90% of patients). *Chlorambucil* is chemically related to *cyclophosphamide*, but tends to produce fewer short-term side-effects.

Azathioprine, *cyclophosphamide*, and sometimes *chlorambucil*, are usually used as reserve agents.

Other immunomodulators

One promising development is the use of low-dose *ciclosporin* (see Chapter 14), which can improve all clinical parameters in severe RA. *Ciclosporin* inhibits T cell activation and cytokine production, and so is immunosuppressive, but is not myelosuppressive. Because long-term treatment is required, careful determinations of drug blood levels and serum creatinine are essential to avoid nephrotoxicity. This does not appear to be as significant a problem with the low-dose regimens that have been used in RA as in those used for immunosuppression in organ transplantation. However, *ciclosporin* is usually reserved for non-responders or those intolerant of other drugs. Two formulations with very different oral bioavailabilities are available, so extra care is needed in prescribing and dispensing.

Leflunomide is a reversible inhibitor of dihydro-orotate dehydrogenase, an enzyme believed to be involved in the autoimmune processes leading to RA. It appears to reduce the symptoms and signs of RA significantly and retards joint damage. However, it may cause severe hepatotoxicity, so patients' liver function should be monitored regularly, especially in the first 6 months of use. It has a very long half-life, partly due to its active metabolite. Because it has serious effects on germ-line cells, its long persistence means that fertile women must take strict contraceptive precautions before starting, during, and for at least 2 years after stopping treatment. Men are also affected, but the restriction period after their treatment is reduced to at least 3 months. Plasma level monitoring is required throughout. The long half-life also means that any serious ADRs will also be prolonged. A washout procedure using *colestyramine* or *activated charcoal* for 11 days is available (see the manufacturer's literature) to limit side-effects and to reduce the waiting period before attempting conception.

Sulfasalazine (SSZ)

This was introduced for the treatment of inflammatory bowel disease (IBD; see Chapter 3). In RA, *SSZ* is as effective as *penicillamine*, and slightly less so than *gold*, but has significant advantages over both of these. It has a faster onset of action than the other agents and is less toxic, and so has emerged as a first-line drug, like *methotrexate*, if NSAIDs are ineffective or are not tolerated, or if symptoms are moderate to severe.

Adverse effects (see Table 12.13) are more likely to occur in older patients, those who have previously used other disease-modifying agents and in slow acetylators. The most serious ADRs are due to myelosuppression, e.g. occasional leucopenia, neutropenia and thrombocytopenia, rarely agranulocytosis and aplastic anaemia, and hypersensitivity reactions, e.g. anaphylaxis, Stevens–Johnson syndrome and exfoliative dermatitis. Thus full blood counts, including differential white cell and platelet counts, should be performed before starting treatment and at monthly intervals for the first 3 months. Liver function tests should be carried out at the same time. The UK's CSM recommends that patients taking *SSZ* should be advised to report any unexplained bleeding, bruising, purpura, sore throat, fever or malaise. Those with glucose-6-phosphate dehydrogenase deficiency may develop haemolytic anaemia.

The UK product licence in RA is only for the enteric-coated tablets, because trials were carried out with that dosage form. It was felt that patients who had been taking NSAIDs for some time might be more susceptible to gastrointestinal disturbance, though this has not been established, and the benefits of enteric coating have been challenged for patients with IBD. Though these points require confirmation, it is reasonable to proceed more cautiously in patients who have experienced gastrointestinal problems or have been taking other SAARDs and to increase the dose at 14-day intervals, rather than the recommended 7, up to the normal maximum of 2–3 g daily. However, as many patients may withdraw from *SSZ* treatment as from *gold* and *penicillamine*, mostly in the first few months.

Patients should be warned that the urine may be coloured orange-yellow and that extended-wear contact lenses may be stained.

The activity of *SSZ* in RA, and its side-effects, appears to be related primarily to the sulfapyridine moiety and not to the salicylate component, which provides the benefit in IBD. This finding has prompted a re-investigation of the possibility of a bacterial aetiology for RA. As antimicrobials, the sulphonamides are competitive antagonists of *p*-aminobenzoic acid, thus inhibiting folate synthesis. Because human cells are unable to synthesize folate, this cannot be the basis of its anti-inflammatory action. Thus its mode of action is unknown.

Other SAARDs

Like most other SAARDs, these agents (*gold, penicillamine* and antimalarials) have a slow onset of action (unlike the NSAIDs), and it make take 4–6 months for their effectiveness to be fully apparent.

Modes of action in RA. These are mostly unknown and several different mechanisms are likely. *Gold salts* may inhibit the activation and maturation of phagocytic and T cells, but their anti-inflammatory activity in conditions other than RA is minimal. The only certain activity of *penicillamine* is as a chelating agent for heavy metals, but this is not the basis for its action in RA, in which it causes a marked reduction in the levels of RFs (IgMs), by unknown mechanisms. Antimalarials are known to have mild cytotoxic activity.

Clinical activity. Up to 70% of patients may show improvement in both symptoms and the objective indicators of disease activity, e.g. ESR, CRP, RFs and anaemia, though the extent of such improvement is very variable. Older SAARDs are usually reserved for patients who are unresponsive to *methotrexate*, *SSZ* or *ciclosporin*, or who are intolerant of these. Because SAARDs are not curative, drug administration is necessary for as long as active disease persists and side-effects are tolerated.

Toxicity. SAARDs are significantly more toxic than NSAIDs, and so are used only in moderate to severe and progressive disease. They require careful monitoring with full haematological and other tests as appropriate (see Table 12.13). It is thus essential that patients are counselled carefully to ensure they appreciate fully the possible advantages and disadvantages of treatment with these drugs, and that they are prepared to co-operate in the regular monitoring procedures required.

Gold salts

These are available as both oral and IM formulations. The most common side-effect with the oral form is diarrhoea, but the range of toxicities of the oral and IM agents is otherwise similar, though the injectables are more troublesome.

Sodium aurothiomalate (gold sodium thiomalate) is the only injectable gold salt available in the UK and is equivalent to others that are available elsewhere, e.g. *aurothioglucose*. It is given by deep IM injection, followed by gentle massage at the injection site. Therapy is initiated with one or more small test doses to minimize the possibility of a major idiosyncratic adverse reaction. *Aurothiomalate* is continued with weekly doses until clinical improvement is apparent, usually at 2–4 months, about 300–500 mg cumulative dose, or there are significant side-effects (e.g. rashes, blood dyscrasias, renal or hepatic toxicity). If a favourable response is seen, maintenance is continued with a lower 2- to 4-weekly dose, as long as the drug is tolerated, for up to 5 years after complete remission. If relapse occurs, treatment is stepped up to the initial dose level until control is regained. Complete relapse must be avoided, if possible, because second courses of *gold* are usually ineffective. Treatment is stopped if no benefit occurs when a total dose of 1 g is reached, usually after about 6 months.

Because of its toxicity, careful monitoring is mandatory, especially with *sodium aurothiomalate* (see Table 12.13).

Auranofin is the orally active agent. The initial twice-daily dose is increased by 50%, to three daily doses, after 6 months if the response is inadequate. The bioavailability is about 25%, but when steady-state serum concentrations are reached after about 10 weeks, less than 1% of the ingested dose is retained in the body. However, serum levels do not correlate with activity or side-effects. Patients can be transferred from parenteral *gold* to *auranofin* directly, without overlap or washout. However, *auranofin* is relatively little used.

Penicillamine

This oral agent is slightly less active than *gold* and has a similar spectrum of side-effects, though it is somewhat better tolerated. The daily dose is increased every 4–8 weeks until clinical improvement occurs, and the maintenance dose is then held at that level. Administration is usually stopped if it has not produced benefit after 1 year or if unacceptable side-effects or toxicity occur.

Side-effects may occur in up to 50% of patients, but often respond to dose reduction or to temporary withdrawal of the drug (see Table 12.13). Minor side-effects, e.g. taste disturbance and nausea, usually clear with continued use.

Antimalarial drugs

Chloroquine and *hydroxychloroquine* are relatively weak antirheumatic agents that are used in rheumatology at about five times the dose used for malaria prophylaxis. Although they are often taken as antimalarials for prolonged periods without problems occurring, the combination of the increased dose, possible greater susceptibility of rheumatoid patients and the fact that antirheumatic treatment is likely to be very prolonged, greatly enhances the possibility of significant side-effects (see BNF, Section 10.1.3), notably rashes, myopathy and retinopathy.

Although retinopathy is rare in patients with normal renal and hepatic function, fear of blindness has limited the use of these drugs. *Chloroquine*, which is significantly the more toxic to the retina, is used to treat RA only if treatment with all other drugs has failed. The BNF advises that retinal toxicity is very unlikely with doses of *hydroxychloroquine sulphate* up to 4 mg/kg daily, calculated on the basis of lean body weight in obese patients. However, the maximum dose is 6.5 mg/kg daily, not exceeding a total of 400 mg/day. Early retinopathy appears to be reversible: this places a premium on patient counselling to ensure that they appreciate the importance of stopping treatment immediately they are aware of any visual impairment, and of prompt ophthalmological referral. The Royal College of Ophthalmologists gives the following advice, updated 2004:

• Baseline assessment should include:

 – Establishment of normal renal and hepatic function.
 – Enquiry for visual impairment not corrected by glasses.
 – A recording of near visual acuity (with glasses if used) by a reading test.
 – A check by an optician if there is any visual impairment.
• If no abnormality is detected, commence treatment with *hydroxychloroquine sulphate*. The annual evaluation should comprise a simple enquiry about vision and repetition of the reading test.
• Patients should:
 – Be referred to an ophthalmologist if any visual impairment or eye disease is detected at baseline assessment.
 – Stop treatment and consult the prescriber immediately if any change in visual acuity or blurred vision develops.
 – If long-term treatment is required, an ophthalmologist should be involved in regular monitoring.

These drugs have rather complex pharmacokinetics, with a wide variation in elimination half-life between patients. The route of excretion is mainly renal. The drugs are widely distributed in the body and are very strongly bound in the melanin-containing tissues of the skin and the eye. They are very persistent; indeed, *chloroquine* has been reported to be detectable in the retina 16 years after stopping treatment!

There are anecdotal reports of benefit from normal antimalarial doses, which are smaller than those used in RA, when patients with RA travel to malarious areas and some patients with mild disease may benefit from such doses, with their preferable safety profile.

An advantage of these drugs is that they can be continued in pregnancy, but breastfeeding should be avoided if it is essential to continue with this treatment.

Mepacrine is a former antimalarial agent that has been superseded by more effective drugs. However, it is occasionally used to treat RA unresponsive to other agents, discoid lupus erythematosus (p. 800) and the protozoal infection giardiasis (see Chapter 8).

Cytokine inhibitors

Currently three inhibitors of TNFα, a potent pro-inflammatory agent, are available. These are *adalimumab*, *etanercept* and *infliximab*. *Anakinra* inhibits interleukin-1 (IL-1) activity (Table 12.16).

Use

Adalimumab and *etanercept* are licensed for use in severe active and progressive RA in patients who have not been treated with *methotrexate* and have failed to respond adequately to other SAARDs. It is normally used together with *methotrexate*, but if the latter is inappropriate it may be used alone.

Anakinra is licensed for use in combination with *methotrexate* in patients who have not responded to *methotrexate* alone. However, NICE guidance is that it should not be used for the routine management of RA, but only in patients participating in a controlled long-term clinical trial. Further, it is not recommended by the Scottish Intercollegiate Guidelines Network.

There are special British Society for Rheumatology and NICE guidelines for the use of these agents and a special Biologics Registry has been established by the British Paediatric Rheumatology Group.

TNFα inhibitors

All of these agents are potent immunosuppressives and may trigger latent infections by *Mycobacterium tuberculosis* and varicella-zoster virus (VSV, see Chapter 8). Patients should therefore be checked for infections, especially latent or active TB, before treatment commences. Any active infection is a contra-indication until effective antimicrobial treatment has been instituted and the disease is controlled. Further, patients should be monitored for infections during and after treatment and should be instructed to report any signs of infection, e.g. persistent

Table 12.16 Properties of cytokine inhibitors used in rheumatology

Cytokine inhibited and drug	Indications	Cautions and contra-indications	Side-effects[a]
Tumour necrosis factor α Adalimumab[c] Etanercept[c] Infliximab[b,c]	RA, AS, PsA: moderate to severe active disease when response to SAARDs is inadequate or they cannot be used	Pregnancy, breastfeeding Severe infections Heart failure Hepatic[d] or renal impairment Demyelinating CNS conditions	Infections, possibly severe (TB and septicaemia) Cardiovascular, CNS, gastrointestinal, respiratory, arthritic, eye, skin, urinary and metabolic problems
Interleukin-1 Anakinra[c,e]	RA	Prone to infections Pregnancy, breastfeeding History of asthma Neutropenia	Injection site reactions Neutropenia Infections Headache

[a] For details see text and BNF.

[b] May also cause severe hypersensitivity reactions.

[c] Normally used with methotrexate, or without if methotrexate is contra-indicated.

[d] Not etanercept.

[e] Not for routine use (see text). Not recommended by Scottish Medicines Consortium.

AS, ankylosing spondylitis; CNS, central nervous system; PsA, psoriatic arthritis; RA, rheumatoid arthritis; SAARD, slow-acting antirheumatic drug; TB, tuberculosis.

cough, weight loss or fever for TB. If VSV infection is likely, varicella-zoster Ig is appropriate. If there are severe side-effects with these agents (Table 12.16) or no response within 3 months, treatment should be discontinued.

Other drugs and treatments

Many other approaches, mostly immunomodulatory, have been used in an attempt to control RA, but all of these procedures remain experimental.

The bisphosphonate *disodium pamidronate* has been shown to be effective in AS (see below), and may prevent joint erosions in psoriatic arthropathy (see above and Chapter 13), if used early enough. Other bisphosphonates may act similarly.

Thalidomide (unlicensed drug) has marked anti-inflammatory and immunomodulatory properties, suppressing superoxide and hydroxyl free radical formation. It has shown good results in RA within a few weeks, and remission may last for years in some patients, though others may relapse 2 months after stopping the drug. Some patients may remain symptom-free with low-dose maintenance treatment. The most common side-effects are drowsiness, constipation and leg oedema, with no evidence of neuropathy. The well-known teratogenicity of *thalidomide* restricts its use to males and postmenopausal females. It is available through the named patient procedure, and its application in RA should only be undertaken under the supervision of a specialist experienced in its use.

Intra-articular injection of *osmium tetroxide* (osmic acid, preceded by a local anaesthetic plus *methylprednisolone*) has been used for synovial ablation, as an alternative to surgical synovectomy. About 70% of patients with severe refractory joint problems may benefit, but pain may recur. Complete regeneration of both synovial membranes and nerve endings occurs after a variable period.

Epoetin, or *darbepoetin* (longer-acting), may correct the resistant anaemia of active disease. Any iron, vitamin B_{12} or folate deficiency requires correction before commencing *epoietin* treatment. In addition to haematological improvement these agents also reduce the ESR and improve well-being. Use in RA is an unlicensed indication.

As in asthma (see Chapter 5), LT antagonists are under investigation for use in the arthritides. *Tenidap* appears to have multiple actions: it inhibits COX and 5-lipoxygenase and also IL-1 formation and action. Injection of IL-1 receptor antagonist protein (IRAP, IL-1ra) has improved symptom scores in patients with active severe RA, with minimal side-effects, though it is likely to be immunogenic. A liposomal formulation of the latter has been proposed for injection into joints, but no products have yet been marketed.

Evidence is accumulating that synovial macrophages and fibroblasts may be more important than T cells, and this is an active research area.

One limitation of the biological agents is that they are themselves immunogenic, so they need to produce long-lasting results with a single short course of treatment: repeat courses are unlikely to succeed. However, because immunogenicity is highly specific, treatment with another biological agent may be possible. Further, although many of them are human, or humanized, recombinant products they still have numerous side-effects. For example, *adalimumab*, *etanercept* and *infliximab* can cause blood pressure abnormalities, gastrointestinal disturbances, skin rashes, respiratory and central nervous problems. *Epoetin* may produce severe hypertension, thromboembolism, RBC aplasia and skin reactions. These agents should be used only by specialists experienced in their use.

Levamisole, an immunostimulant ascaricide used against roundworm infections, is available on a named patient basis, and *dapsone*, which has both immunosuppressive and pro-inflammatory properties, have also been used. Both are unlicensed indications.

Yttrium-90 radiocolloid has been injected into inflamed joints as a local cytotoxic and immunosuppressive agent, with variable success.

Tetracycline antibiotics, e.g. *minocycline*, have been used on the hypothesis that RA is caused by mycoplasma infections, or is associated with them. Although some success has been achieved it is unclear whether this is due to their antimicrobial or immunomodulatory properties or to inhibition of phospholipase A2 and collagenases.

It has also been suggested, but unproven, that selenium supplementation is beneficial. Selenium is an essential trace element and a component of glutathione reductase, but the recommended daily allowance should not be exceeded because it is very toxic in overdose. This is difficult to manage because the selenium content of drinking water varies widely with the locality, so the local water supply utility should be consulted. Selenium supplements are available only via 'health food' suppliers.

Fish oil supplements, e.g. *Maxepa*, may help some patients with RA, but not OA.

Surgery

Orthopaedic surgery has a great deal to offer in the management of local problems when medical management has failed to give adequate control. However, it is important for surgery to be performed before joint damage is so far advanced that good function cannot be restored. The most successful procedures are:

- Arthroplasty.
  - Total hip replacement (success rate >95%).
  - Total knee replacement (success rate > 90%).
- Removal of metatarsal heads, for eroded, subluxed MTP joints.
- Elbow synovectomy and removal of the radial head.

Other procedures include hand and wrist surgery, especially for tendon release, and fusion of the cervical spine if instability causes spinal cord compression. Arthroplasty of the PIP joints has successfully restored hand function. Operations on other joints are less common. Arthrodesis and osteotomy (p. 761) are used occasionally.

Juvenile idiopathic chronic arthritis

Definition and epidemiology

Juvenile idiopathic chronic arthritis (JIA) is the neutral, catch-all classification of conditions that used to be called juvenile chronic arthritis, juvenile RA and Still's disease. In only about 5% of patients does the condition resemble adult RA. In the remainder it is clinically and pathologically distinct from RA, although there are certain similarities.

It may be defined as persistent joint swelling starting before the age of 16, other diseases being excluded. However, some rheumatologists define it more tightly as synovitis occurring in at least 1–4 joints persisting for at least 6 weeks, or a lesser number of joints confirmed by biopsy. Additional joints may become involved after some months. The condition is variable in presentation and its true nature may become apparent only some time after the first appearance of symptoms.

The UK incidence is about 1 in 10 000, with a prevalence of 1 in 1000, making it one of the commonest chronic childhood diseases, and JIA is a major cause of childhood disability.

Aetiology and clinical features

The condition often presents as swelling of a large joint, e.g. knee, ankle or wrist joint, in that order of frequency. Arthritis of a single small joint is unusual, but the fingers, toes, hip, shoulder, spine and jaw may become involved, usually assymmetrically (see RA, p. 764). Knee involvement may sometimes be associated with a Baker's cyst (see p. 766).

Fever, lethargy, weakness and discomfort often occur, but significant pain is unusual, though young children often cannot give a good history.

Diagnosis, management and prognosis

Diagnosis may be difficult unless the clinician is familiar with normal musculoskeletal development in children.

The five or so disease states encompassed by JIA are currently classified according to the pattern of clinical presentation, but the boundaries between the various groups are difficult to define. These groups are classified by the European League Against Rheumatism as given below.

- **Systemic onset:**
  - 20% of patients.
  - Usually starts in early childhood, but onset is possible up to the age of 17.
  - Often infection-associated.
  - High fever, systemic symptoms and rash that often remit after a few weeks.
  - May be oligoarticular or widespread. Children with polyarthritis have poor prognosis.
- **Persistent oligoarticular:**
  - One to four joints involved.
  - 50% of patients, mainly girls under 5 years, F:M = 5:1.
  - Associated with HLA-B27 in older boys, but this may be an early indication of AS (p. 789). Other HLA-DR associations suggest the possibility of UC (see Chapter 3). Antinuclear antibodies (ANA) are present in about 75% of this group, but may also suggest the possibility of SLE (p. 798). Most develop one of the seronegative spondyloarthritides (see below) and possibly IBD (see Chapter 3).
  - Probable increased risk for anterior uveitis (20% of patients in this group). Early diagnosis and treatment are essential to avoid sight problems or blindness.
- **Extended oligoarticular**, i.e. starts as oligoarticular and progresses to further joint involvement with anterior uveitis. Prognosis is poorer than in the persistent oligoarticular group.
- **Polyarticular (RF negative).** 25–30% of patients, usually girls under 5 years, with symmetrical arthritis of upper and lower limbs. Eye and growth problems may be significant.
- **Polyarticular (RF positive).** Presents in older children and resembles adult RA, but erosions occur rapidly (see above).
- **Psoriatic juvenile onset arthritis.** Similar arthritic pattern to the extended oligoarticular group, which may precede psoriasis by many years (see Chapter 13).
- **Enthesis-related arthritis.** This is probably a precursor to adult AS (see below). It mostly affects boys over 8 years, and initially affects

the feet and knees. The characteristic pelvic and spinal symptoms of AS may appear later.

The diagnosis and management of JIA is normally carried out in specialist centres, with the involvement of a multidisciplinary team. Diagnosis is made solely on clinical grounds and may initially be difficult because of the variety of systemic diseases that can cause joint symptoms (see Table 12.3). However extensive investigation, although not required for diagnosis, may be needed to exclude these possibilities, especially septic arthritis. Marked systemic symptoms, e.g. fever, weight loss, bone and night pain, may indicate an alternative diagnosis. A single inflamed joint requires joint aspiration to exclude the possibility of infection or crystal deposition disease (p. 791).

Generally, the outlook is better than in adult RA of comparable joint involvement, and about 75% of patients have no significant residual disability. Occasionally, amyloid disease (p. 807) and eye involvement may be severe.

The principal aim of management is to ensure that there is a minimum of physical, educational and social disability while the symptoms are present and when the disease eventually becomes inactive.

Pharmacotherapy

This resembles that in adult RA, with appropriate allowance for the fact that children are particularly vulnerable to blood dyscrasias and developmental abnormalities. *Aspirin* must not be used in children and adolescents under 16 years old because of the risk of Reye's syndrome until an unequivocal non-febrile diagnosis has been made. *Paracetamol* (acetaminophen) is preferred. NSAIDs (usually *diclofenac, ibuprofen, naproxen* or *piroxicam*) are the usual basis of treatment.

Corticosteroids, *methotrexate* and *hydroxychloroquine* are used as a last resort in severe systemic disease, but corticosteroids may be used to manage symptoms until *methotrexate* gives relief. The anti-TNF agent *etanercept* (p. 785) is the only anticytokine that is licensed for use in JIA.

Seronegative spondarthritides

This group of inflammatory diseases has two features in common. As the name implies, they affect the spine and rheumatoid factors are absent. Other common features are:

- Sacroiliitis, causing buttock pain.
- Enthesitis, i.e. inflammation of the points of insertion of tendons or ligaments into the bones (Figure 12.1).
- Associations with:
  - Psoriasiform skin lesions (see Chapter 13).
  - IBD (see Chapter 3).
  - Eye inflammation, i.e. conjunctivitis and iritis.
  - Reactive arthritis (see below).

They include:

- Ankylosing spondylitis.
- Reiter's syndrome (p. 809).
- Psoriatic arthritis (see Chapter 13).
- Enteropathic arthritis, associated with IBD (see Chapter 3).

Ankylosing spondylitis

Definition and epidemiology

Ankylosing spondylitis (AS) is a seronegative, chronic spondyloarthritis, i.e. it is an inflammatory disease, primarily involving the spine, eventually leading to fusion of the vertebrae. Young adult males are the most likely to have significant symptoms.

The disease affects about 15/10 000 of UK Caucasian populations with a male:female ratio for incidence of about 4:1 for moderate to severe disease, though mild disease is more common in women, the overall M:F ratio being about 2:1. AS is less common in East Asians and Blacks, with a prevalence about half that in Caucasians. Onset is mostly in the 20–40-year age group, the principal age of onset being 20–25 years, but the inflammatory symptoms may remit in older patients. However, residual joint damage persists. Some 10% of first-degree relatives also have AS, and there is a familial association with the other diseases mentioned above (see Table 12.2).

Aetiology

This is unknown, but HLA-B27 occurs in more than 95% of Caucasian patients with uncomplicated AS showing no other symptoms, whereas its prevalence in the general population is about 6%. HLA-B27 occurs infrequently in Black races and Japanese, who rarely suffer from AS, and the frequency of this gene in patients suffering from both AS and psoriasis or IBD is reduced to 60%. If HLA-B2 occurs in Blacks it confers an increased risk. There are more than 10 variants of the HLA-B27 gene, some of which clearly confer a predisposition to develop these diseases, though others seem to be protective. However, AS appears to be a multigenic condition, with other MHC associations.

There is an environmental component, probably an unidentified infective agent. HLA-B27 has an important role in antigen presentation to T cells. One small trial has indeed shown the presence of cytotoxic (CD8+) T cells that recognize arthritogenic bacteria (e.g. *Salmonella*, *Yersinia*) and possibly also auto-antigens in arthritic joints, and kill infected cell lines. A suggestion that *Klebsiella pneumoniae* is implicated has been disputed.

Pathology

The hallmark of AS is bilateral inflammation of the non-synovial sacroiliac joints at the base of the spine. The inflamed areas are infiltrated with mature lymphocytes, including plasma cells. The **synovitis** that occurs at other joints is similar to that in RA, but **enthesopathy** (inflammation of the points of attachment of tendons to bone) is a prominent feature. The intervertebral ligaments are especially affected. There is a high tendency for ankylosis and calcification, usually a variable ascending spinal ankylosis, and the whole spine may become rigid in patients with advanced disease.

Clinical features, diagnosis and complications

Onset is usually insidious, initially with episodic low back pain and stiffness, especially in the morning. Much of this arises from pelvic joint inflammation, especially the sacroiliac joints, causing moderate to severe pain and stiffness in the buttocks and lower back. The pain may alternate between the two sides. Systemic malaise, tiredness, anorexia and weight loss also occur, but are less severe than in RA. Some 20% of patients, usually the younger ones, present with peripheral joint problems.

Diagnosis is based primarily on the clinical features and X-rays.

Plantar fasciitis, i.e. inflammation of the enthesis of the plantar fascia, the long, tough ligament that supports the arch of the foot and connects the calcaneum (heel bone) and the metatarsal bases. It is subjected to considerable stress, because it has to stretch with each take-off from the ball of the foot when walking, running or jumping. It is commonly associated with a plantar spur, an outgrowth from the forward edge of calcaneum, due to excessive traction on the enthesis. Plantar fasciitis is common in runners whose shoes do not have adequate cushioning, in people with flat feet who are standing for most of the day and in AS.

Spinal rigidity compromises posture and movement, and respiration becomes wholly diaphragmatic if the rib articulations in the thoracic spine are severely affected. Serious spinal fractures can occur in patients with rigid spines.

Iritis (anterior uveitis) may occur in 25% of patients, the severity being unrelated to that of the arthropathy.

Management

The aims of management are the relief of pain, with anti-inflammatory analgesics, and the minimization of stiffness and deformity, by physiotherapy.

Early diagnosis and forceful education about the value of a regular programme of morning exercises, to prevent the formation of calcified bridges between vertebrae, are the basis of successful management. Plantar fasciitis is treated by relieving pressure on the enthesis with a suitable pad and ensuring suitable footwear. Rest and a local injection of corticosteroid may also help.

However, without good pain management it may be impossible to maintain an effective exercise regimen.

NSAIDs are the mainstay of symptomatic treatment and are very effective if used in full dosage. *Aceclofenac* and *meloxicam* are licensed for the treatment of AS and are probably the drugs of first choice. *Indometacin*, one of the most potent, is often used, though any NSAID that is tolerated will usually be satisfactory. A COX-2 inhibitor that has relatively low cardiovascular toxicity, e.g. *lumiracoxib* (see above), may be preferable if a patient is at risk of gastrotoxicity and it proves effective.

Once improvement has occurred, the dose is stepped down to the minimum necessary to give reasonable control of symptoms, and this level should be maintained as a permanent prophylactic dose, regardless of apparent disease activity, provided that side-effects are not too obtrusive.

A long-acting NSAID (see above), or a modified-release formulation, taken at night may reduce the morning stiffness.

A bisphosphonate, e.g. standard-dose monthly IV *disodium pamidronate*, has been shown to be effective in patients who do not respond to NSAIDs. The bisphosphonates are used widely to treat osteoporosis because they inhibit bone resorption and so reduce bone turnover. This approach is logical to prevent the development of osteophytes and the abnormal bone growth that leads to spinal ankylosis. Any of the other bisphosphonates, e.g. *alendronic acid* or *risedronate sodium*, should act similarly, but are not yet proven to be effective. However, this is likely, and they would obviate the need for repeated IV infusions. This advance in pharmacotherapy is very welcome, though the benefit demonstrated so far is modest. These are unlicensed indications.

Cytokine (TNFα) inhibitors, e.g. *adalimumab*, *etanercept* and *infliximab*, have been shown to give significant improvement (see above; also in psoriatic arthropathy), but *etanercept* and *infliximab* are the only ones licensed for use in AS. They are approved for adult patients with severe symptoms that have not responded to conventional agents. Cost, and the necessity for repeated SC injections (*etanercept*) or IV infusions (*infliximab*) are significant problems. The development of antibodies limits their utility (see above). They should be discontinued if there is no response within 6 weeks of the initial injection or infusion.

SAARDs, e.g. *gold* and *penicillamine* (see above), are not generally useful. *SSZ* or *methotrexate* may help to control any associated peripheral arthropathy, but have little effect on spinal inflammation.

Local corticosteroid injections may also be helpful for peripheral joint problems or enthesopathies.

Active physiotherapy, with a planned morning exercise programme, is invaluable for the minimization of spinal rigidity, the maintenance of function and to prevent spinal deformity. Swimming is especially recommended because the increased body buoyancy permits exercise but minimizes joint stress. Rest and immobility, e.g. splinting, increase the risk of deformity.

Surgery (arthroplasty, especially total hip replacement) may be necessary for severe hip involvement, and to manage the vertebral fractures that occur in a rigid and osteoporotic spine. Other spinal procedures are hazardous.

A single course of spinal radiotherapy is used occasionally, and is anti-inflammatory within the radiation target area. Repeat courses are contra-indicated because they produce a high incidence of leukaemia and soft tissue tumours.

The prognosis is relatively good: at least 80% of patients are able to maintain employment and there is a normal lifespan.

Crystal deposition arthropathies

Common features and pathology

The diseases in this group share the feature of deposition of crystals of metabolites in the joints, with consequent inflammation and joint damage. Their principal characteristics are given in Table 12.17.

It is not known what factors promote the deposition of crystals in the synovial fluid. Once there, the positively-charged crystals become coated with negatively-charged proteins, especially IgG and phospholipids, thus enhancing phagocytosis by macrophages. This results in the liberation of lysosomal and cytoplasmic enzymes, which attack the synovial membrane,

and promote the release from neutrophils of a specific pro-inflammatory glycoprotein. Injection of this glycoprotein into joints produces symptoms that are indistinguishable from those of gout. Chemotactic factors are also released and promote leucocyte recruitment, thus multiplying the effect.

Similar effects can be produced by a variety of crystals or other substances introduced into the joint space, e.g. cholesterol and corticosteroid suspensions injected to relieve joint inflammation. Exacerbations of osteoarthritis may be due to microcrystals of hydroxyapatite released from the bone, causing a similar effect.

Table 12.17   Some features of crystal deposition arthropathies

Disease	Metabolite deposited	Crystal shape	Joints involved	Prevalence[a]
Gout	Monosodium urate	Needle	Peripheral, small	1%, mostly males 40–50 years of age
Pseudogout (pyrophosphate arthropathy)	Calcium pyrophosphate	Rhomboidal	Large (knee)	0.4%, M:F = 3:2, 60–80 years of age

[a] Approximate international statistics.

Gout

Gout is an arthropathy resulting from the deposition of crystals of monosodium urate in the joints and surrounding tissues.

Aetiology and epidemiology

Gout is the result of **hyperuricaemia**, though it is difficult to define the latter satisfactorily because there is a continuous normal distribution of serum urate levels. The solubility of uric acid in serum is about 0.38 mmol/L (6.3 mg/dL). The 95% population limits are 0.18–0.42 mmol/L (3.0–7.0 mg/dL) for men and 0.13–0.34 mmol/L (2.2–5.7 mg/dL) for women. Consequently, the serum is supersaturated with urate in about 3% of UK men and gout is overwhelmingly a male problem (90–95% of cases). Fortunately, only a minority of men with high serum urate levels show clinical symptoms, but it is not clear why this is so. Further, some patients with gout have relatively low urate levels. However, clinical symptoms are overwhelmingly associated with hyperuricaemia.

A simplified outline of uric acid metabolism is given in Figure 12.10, which shows that hyperuricaemia may result either from excessive production of uric acid or from reduced renal elimination, the latter being the most common cause. In **primary gout** there are numerous factors operating on a background of genetic predisposition to produce clinical symptoms. The causes of **secondary hyperuricaemia** and **gout** are given in Table 12.18. Treatment with thiazide diuretics often causes some degree of

hyperuricaemia, but fortunately does not often cause an attack of gout. However, diuretics are a relatively common cause of gout in elderly women.

The prevalence of gout varies widely, being about 0.3% in the UK and about 2% in France. In Maoris, who have a strong genetic predisposition, it is about 10%.

Pathology

If hyperuricaemia results in the crystallization of monosodium urate in synovial fluid, small, needle-shaped crystals can also be seen within the leucocytes, causing the release of lysosomal enzymes.

If untreated, gout leads initially to the deposition of urate crystals on the surface of the cartilage, with subsequent cartilage damage and finally to the deposition of masses of urate crystals within and around the joints, producing extensive joint destruction. Nodular accretions of monosodium urate (**tophi**) may occur. A characteristic site for these is the cartilaginous margin (**helix**) of the pinna of the ear, but they occur also on tendons and in bursae associated with the affected joints. Tophi are granulomatous structures, containing the urate crystals in a protein–lipid–polysaccharide matrix, which eventually become calcified. In **long-standing chronic gout**, joint erosions occur that contain calcified deposits. Urate deposition tends to occur in peripheral joints where the temperature is lower than the core body temperature, resulting in reduced urate solubility: cartilage is avascular, and so has no warming blood supply,

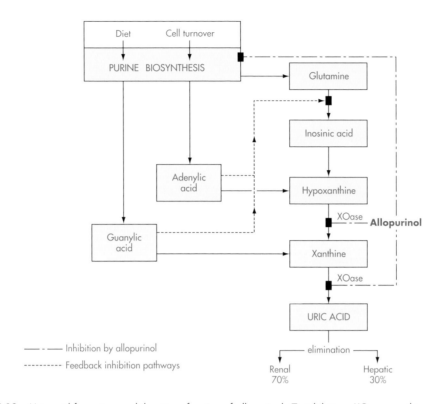

Figure 12.10   Uric acid formation and the sites of action of allopurinol. ■, inhibition; XOase, xanthine oxidase.

and the affected joints are normally cool in unaffected individuals.

The precipitation of monosodium urate from urine within the kidney, or of uric acid under acid conditions, may result in the formation of renal stones, possibly causing urinary-tract infection and obstruction and renal failure (see Chapter 14).

Clinical features

Acute gout

In some 75% of cases a first attack affects the big toe, and this form is called **podagra**. Other common sites are the ankles, knees, elbows, wrists and fingers. An attack often starts overnight or a few hours after an acutely stressful episode, e.g. MI or major surgery. The joint becomes exquisitely painful and inflamed and the overlying skin may flake over the next few hours: this sign plus the symptoms is almost conclusive. The attack subsides spontaneously over a few days or weeks, though most sufferers seek treatment. There may be no recurrence, or a second attack may follow after a variable period ranging from days to years.

Attacks tend to be more severe in younger patients, aged under 30 years.

Chronic gout

This is uncommon, except in patients who are non-compliant with medication, or those with a metabolic abnormality. Acute episodes occur with increasing frequency, leading to tophus formation and permanent joint damage. Renal impairment increases with time and this is aggravated in about one-third of patients by associated hypertension, though the latter is

Table 12.18   The aetiology of secondary hyperuricaemia

| | Factors causing uric acid | |
	Under-excretion	Overproduction
Iatrogenic	Diuretics, especially thiazides[a] Low-dose aspirin or fructose administration Ciclosporin (due to renal toxicity)	Cytotoxic drugs, radiotherapy (increased cell destruction)
Self-inflicted (poor lifestyle)	–	Obesity, excessive consumption of alcohol or purines (meat)
Renal	Renal failure Hypertensive nephropathy Sarcoidosis Lead poisoning	–
Cardiovascular	Heart failure	–
Metabolic	Ketosis (diabetes mellitus) Starvation Myxoedema	Inherited enzyme defects
Other conditions	Hypercalcaemia	High cell turnover (neoplastic diseases, psoriasis)

[a] Probably the most common cause of secondary gout.

probably a reflection of the kidney damage, rather than a cause.

Diagnosis

This is based on the symptoms and signs outlined above, and the finding of a high serum urate level. However, the association of the latter with joint pain does not necessarily imply a diagnosis of gout: because 90% of people with hyperuricaemia do not have gout; there may be a coincidental association of hyperuricaemia with a different arthritic problem. However, gout is very unlikely if the serum urate level is <3 mmol/L (5 mg/dL).

The principal diagnostic confusion occurs with septic arthritis. The diagnosis can be confirmed unequivocally only by the microscopic demonstration of urate crystals in the synovial fluid of the affected joint, but this is necessary only in doubtful cases and it may be difficult to obtain a sample. Aspiration of small joints is impossibly painful during an attack.

Three-quarters of patients with gout have features of the **metabolic syndrome** (formerly called 'syndrome X'; see Chapter 9), i.e.:

- Glucose intolerance.
- Hyperinsulinaemia and insulin resistance.
- Central obesity (waist circumference $\geq$94 cm (37 in) in men, $\geq$80 cm (32 in) in women.
- Hypertriglyceridaemia.
- Low HDL level.
- Hypercortisolaemia.
- High small dense, LDL cholesterol levels.

This is linked to the 'western' lifestyle, with a high saturated fat diet and inadequate physical activity, though genetic factors are thought to be responsible for about 70% of the variance in fat distribution.

The implication is that patients should aim for a healthy lifestyle, regular physical activity (walking rapidly for at least 30 min daily), healthy weight (BMI 21–22 kg/m^2) and waist circumference <94 cm in men, <80 cm in women.

Those with a familial history of gout should therefore be educated at an early age to comply with these principles.

Management

Aim

The aims of management of gout are:

- The prompt relief of pain in an acute attack and its rapid termination.
- To eliminate secondary causes, if possible.
- The prevention of recurrence and complications (e.g. renal stones and renal failure, joint damage and the formation of tophi) in chronic sufferers by correction of hyperuricaemia.

General measures

Acute attacks
The approach is to:

- Rest the affected joint (splinting may help in the severe acute stage).
- Maintain a high fluid intake to reduce hyperuricaemia and prevent renal urate stone formation.

Chronic gout
The approach is to:

- Maintain a high fluid intake, to prevent urate crystallization in the kidney.
- Lose weight if obese, to reduce tissue mass and so urate production and to reduce loading on joints (see above).
- Provide dietary advice:
  - Avoid alcohol, which reduces urate solubility in the serum, and especially beer, which is high in purines.
  - Reduce carbohydrate intake, which is protein-sparing and so promotes protein build-up in the tissues.
  - Avoid foods rich in purines, e.g. offal, shellfish, spinach.
- Endoscopic shock wave lithotripsy etc. (see Chapter 14) for urate kidney stones.

However, even a strict low-purine diet has only a small effect, reducing the serum urate level by about 10–15%.

Pharmacotherapy

Acute attacks
Immediate initiation of treatment is important, and NSAIDs are given as early as possible, unless these are contra-indicated (see below). High-dose *indometacin* is often the drug of choice, e.g. 75 mg immediately, 50 mg 6- to 8-hourly on the first and second days, 25 mg four times daily on the third day, then slowly tapering to zero over 10–14 days. Symptoms usually remit completely after 5–7 days. In the elderly, or if *indometacin* is contra-indicated or is not well tolerated, a choice may be made from *naproxen*, *acelofenac*, *diclofenol*, *etoricoxib*, *ketoprofen* and *sulindac* at clinically comparable dosage, depending on acceptability to the patient. *Azapropazone* may be needed if other agents are ineffective.

Etoricoxib is the only COX-2 inhibitor licensed for the management of acute gout and is given only once daily. Because of the relatively short period of treatment, the risk of cardiovascular problems is much reduced. Because it is more liable than other NSAIDs to cause hypertension, or exacerbate it, *etoricoxib* should not be prescribed to patients with uncontrolled blood pressure. If *etoricoxib* is nevertheless considered advisable, because of its relatively low incidence of upper gastrointestinal side-effects, full blood pressure monitoring should be carried out.

Occasionally, moderately potent opioids (see Chapter 7) may need to be added to control intolerable pain.

If NSAIDs are not tolerated, or if there is renal impairment (which may accompany gout), a history of peptic ulceration, hypertension or heart failure, or if the patient is taking *warfarin*, the action of which is potentiated by NSAIDs, then *colchicine* is indicated. This is very effective: it suppresses macrophage recruitment and multiplication and specifically inhibits production of the pro-inflammatory glycoprotein. The pain normally starts to remit in 12–24 h and may be completely controlled in 2–3 days. However, *colchicine* is more toxic than NSAIDs and tends to cause diarrhoea and vomiting: these side-effects are often used as an index of adequate dosage. *Colchicine* has been used at the outset as an aid to diagnosis, but a prompt response to it is not specific. **Pseudogout**, which is less common (see

below), tendon calcification and other conditions with symptoms similar to gout, which may
cause diagnostic difficulty, also respond.

In resistant cases, systemic injections of *corti-
cotrophin* or a corticosteroid may be used.
Steroids may also be injected into an affected
large joint (unlicensed indication) in the course
of aspiration for diagnostic purposes, but this
may be impossibly painful.

Cytokine inhibitors (see p. 785) have not yet
been shown to be effective, and cost would be a
problem, but this may be acceptable in the
short term for a very severe attack. *Aspirin* and
salicylates have no place in the treatment of
gout because they reduce urate excretion and
antagonise the action of uricosuric agents.

Paradoxically, *allopurinol* or a uricosuric agent
(see below) must not be started during an acute
attack because they will often worsen and
prolong symptoms, probably by mobilizing
urate from deposits. It is known that sudden
changes in serum urate levels tend to precipitate
attacks. *Allopurinol* also interferes with uric acid
excretion. If an acute attack occurs during
existing urate-lowering treatment, the treatment
should be maintained, and the acute attack
treated normally.

Interval control

This is management of the patient in the
intervals between attacks. It includes:

- Control of precipitating and aggravating
  factors, e.g. diet, alcohol intake, obesity and
  drugs, especially thiazide diuretics: these
  must be dealt with regardless of possible
  pharmacotherapy.
- Evaluation of the need for pharmacotherapy,
  e.g. management of hyperuricaemia, other
  antigout drugs.

An isolated attack is not an indication for
prophylactic pharmacotherapy unless the serum
urate level is consistently very high (it is usually
high, >0.60 mmol/L [>10 mg/dL]) in an acute
attack), there is evidence of urate nephropathy
or there are tophi. The disadvantages of long-
term prophylaxis need to be weighed carefully
before lifelong treatment is initiated.

Infrequent attacks are best managed by
general measures and high-dose NSAIDs, as in an
acute attack, because otherwise therapy needs to
be lifelong. Continuous low-dose *colchicine* is
used occasionally, though it is contra-indicated
in pregnancy (it is an antimitotic agent) and if a
mother is breastfeeding. *Colchicine* must be used
cautiously in the elderly and if there is any suspicion or evidence of gastrointestinal, cardiac,
hepatic or renal impairment.

Management of hyperuricaemia

If there are specific indications, i.e. more than
two attacks in a year, tophi, joint or renal damage,
or if the patient insists on treatment, lifelong
prophylactic pharmacotherapy is considered at
least 3 weeks after an initial attack has subsided;
earlier treatment may prolong the attack. Urate-
lowering drugs are used, two methods being available: either by reducing urate production or by
increasing renal urate excretion.

The target serum urate level is about
0.25 mmol/L (4.2 mg/dL), maintained over long
periods to achieve regression of tophi. Because
rapid reduction of serum urate levels tends to
provoke attacks of gout, prophylactic *colchicine*
or NSAID cover should be given for the first
3–6 months of both treatment modes, continued
if necessary until urate levels are normalized.

Reducing urate production. *Allopurinol* is
currently the drug of choice for this purpose. It
is a xanthine oxidase inhibitor (Figure 12.10)
that also inhibits purine biosynthesis. Treatment
should be initiated at a low dose, increasing
gradually until urate levels are normalized. An
adequate fluid intake (2–3 L/day) should be
maintained to minimize the possibility of kidney
stone formation. Because *allopurinol* is excreted
renally the dose has to be reduced if renal function is impaired. The dose required is based on
the creatinine clearance. In severe hyperuricaemia and normal renal function the daily dose
may be as high 700–900 mg, but in severe renal
failure (see Chapter 14) this may have to be
reduced to 100 mg three times per week.

Allopurinol also reduces the formation of
calcium oxalate renal stones.

A new non-purine xanthine oxidase inhibitor,
febuxostat, is in a late stage of development.

Although apparently well tolerated in the short term, it remains to be seen whether it will prove sufficiently non-toxic to be taken over many years: treatment of hyperuricaemia is normally life-long.

Secondary hyperuricaemia. *Allopurinol* may also be used to prevent the acute hyperuricaemia caused by the rapid breakdown of abnormally high numbers of leucocytes when cytotoxic treatment is instituted for treating leukaemias and lymphomas (see Chapter 10).

The recombinant urate oxidase, *rasburicase*, oxidises uric acid to allantoin, which is water soluble and so is excreted readily via the kidney, is used similarly. It acts rapidly, e.g. in a phase III study the plasma concentration fell by 86% in 4h, and steady state is achieved in 2–3 days.

Treatment with these agents should be commenced **before** cytotoxic treatment or radiotherapy is initiated, if possible, because both treatments may cause rapid tissue and leucocyte breakdown, leading to increased urate production.

Side-effects and interactions. *Allopurinol* is usually well tolerated, the most common side-effects being rashes, sometimes with fever. The dosage should be reduced in renal or hepatic impairment. In the former case an active metabolite, oxypurinol, may accumulate and precipitate the potentially life-threatening **allopurinol hypersensitivity syndrome**. Thus if rashes occur, treatment must be stopped immediately, because they may herald a potentially severe reaction. Treatment may be restarted cautiously following a mild skin reaction, but **recurrence is an absolute contra-indication** to further use, as is an initially severe reaction. Gastrointestinal discomfort may be reduced by taking *allopurinol* after meals. Because the metabolism of xanthine is suppressed, high concentrations of the latter may be excreted and may crystallize in the urinary tract, hence the need for a high fluid intake, especially in the early stages of treatment.

The activity of the cytotoxic purine analogues *azathioprine* and *mercaptopurine* is potentiated by the use of *allopurinol*, which also inhibits their metabolism, so if these drugs are being used their dose should be reduced to one-quarter if *allopurinol* is used concurrently.

The action of oral anticoagulants may also be potentiated, so particular attention needs to be paid to prothrombin time/INR measurements (see Chapter 11). However, the clinical significance of this interaction is doubtful.

Because hydrogen peroxide is produced, *rasburicase* may produce haemolytic anaemia and methaemoglobinaemia in patients with G6PD deficiency or hereditery anaemia (see Chapter 11). Consequently *rasburicase* treatment should be supervised by an experienced haematological oncologist. Otherwise, *rasburicase* is well-tolerated, sometimes causing fever and, less commonly, gastrointestinal disturbances. Because it is a protein, it may cause allergic reactions.

Increased renal excretion is achieved with the **uricosuric agent**, *sulfinpyrazone*. This inhibits renal tubular reabsorption of uric acid, and so is ineffective if renal function is impaired. Although used less nowadays because it is more toxic than *allopurinol*, it retains a place for patients intolerant of the latter. Initiation of treatment is undertaken with the same precautions as for *allopurinol*. *Sulfinpyrazone* may also be used in addition to *allopurinol* if the latter provides inadequate control of serum urate levels.

Although *probenecid* has been used similarly to *sulfinpyrazone*, and is included in the BNF in the 'gout' section, it is now available only on a named-patient basis for the prevention of nephrotoxicity associated with the antiviral drug *cidofovir*.

Side-effects and interactions. *Sulfinpyrazone* is generally well tolerated, but should be used carefully if patients have peptic ulceration or renal impairment, because it may cause gastrointestinal distress and its action depends on adequate renal function. It must not be given with *aspirin* or salicylates, which antagonize its action in the renal tubules. The urine should be alkalinized, e.g. with citrates, if the uric acid level is high, to give the maximum solubility of uric acid and prevent urate stone formation. A night-time dose of *acetazolamide*, a carbonic anhydrase inhibitor and weak diuretic, has also been used to alkalinize the urine (unlicensed application). Gastrointestinal disorders occur most commonly, but hypersensitivity reactions and blood dyscrasias may also occur: regular blood counts are advisable with *sulfinpyrazone*.

A new uricosuric agent, *benzbromarone*, has the advantage that it retains its activity in moderate renal impairment. It is not currently licensed in the UK, but importation is available through the named-patient procedure.

Research is under way to see whether it is possible to increase urate excretion by antagonizing the urate transporter-1 (URAT1) molecule that is responsible for the tubular reabsorption of urate in the kidney.

Pyrophosphate arthropathy

Pyrophosphate arthropathy, also known as calcium pyrophosphate deposition disease, CPPD, pseudogout or chondrocalcinosis, results from the excessive deposition of calcium pyrophosphate in joints. Minor deposits are common and are usually asymptomatic. The aetiology is usually not identified, but some genetic and predisposing factors, e.g. age and hyperparathyroidism, are known. CPPD is about one-third as common as gout.

The calcium pyrophosphate crystals probably form initially in cartilage and are shed into the synovial fluid. Thus microscopic examination of the latter gives a clear diagnosis. It is probable that acute exacerbations of osteoarthritis are due to calcium pyrophosphate shedding from damaged cartilage.

The disease may present acutely, resembling acute gout, or as a degenerative chronic arthritis, sometimes with intermittent acute episodes.

Management resembles that of osteoarthritis, but *colchicine* is as effective in CPPD as in gout. Otherwise there is no specific treatment: NSAIDs are effective in acute attacks and intra-articular injections of corticosteroids are highly beneficial.

Autoimmune connective tissue disorders

There is currently no satisfactory classification for this group of chronic, progressive inflammatory diseases, formerly called 'collagen-vascular diseases' or 'multisystem disorders'. A possible grouping is given in Table 12.19. They share the following features:

- Widespread inflammation of organs and systems throughout the body, notably causing vasculitis and arthritis.
- Autoimmune features, with circulating auto-antibodies and immune complex deposition.
- Unknown aetiology.

Two types of antineutrophil cytoplasmic antibodies (ANCA) are seen in the systemic vasculitides: cytoplasmic, proteinase 3 ANCA (PR3-ANCA, formerly cANCA) and perinuclear, myeloperoxidase ANCA (MPO-ANCA, formerly pANCA). Both are anti-enzyme antibodies, so causing an autoimmune state. There is an association with HLA class II antigens and the production of IgG autoantibodies (see Chapter 2). Mixed connective tissue diseases are strongly associated with the HLA-DR4 genotype.

Patients often show features of more than one of these diseases. The syndrome described as '**mixed connective tissue disease**' may be a distinct entity, but is possibly a variant of scleroderma.

Because fever and arthralgias are common presenting symptoms, patients are usually referred to rheumatologists.

Systemic lupus erythematosus

Definition and epidemiology

This non-organ-specific, multisystem, autoimmune disease primarily affects young women.

Table 12.19   Multisystem disorders and associated diseases

Disease grouping	Examples
Chronic autoimmune diseases	Systemic lupus erythematosus (SLE)
	Sjögren's syndrome
	Scleroderma and systemic sclerosis
	Raynaud's syndrome
Systemic vasculitides	
Large vessel vasculitis (aorta and main branches)	Giant cell arteritis (GCA)
	Polymyalgia rheumatica
Medium vessel vasculitis (main visceral arteries, e.g. renal, hepatic, coronary, mesenteric)	Polyarteritis nodosa (PAN, small arteries also involved, but less so)
Small vessel vasculitis (distal vessels connecting with arterioles	Wegener's granulomatosis
Other multisystem disorders	Amyloidosis, sarcoidosis

Systemic lupus erythematosis (SLE) occurs worldwide, and may affect up to 0.5% of Black women in North America and the West Indies and women in the Far East. There are over 30 000 diagnosed patients in the UK.

Aetiology

There is an inherited tendency for SLE, the concordance rate for monozygotic twins being about 25%, whereas that for dizygotic twins and first-degree relatives of patients is about 3%. In Caucasians, this is linked to an increased frequency of HLA-B8 and DR3 genotypes, and in Japanese with DR2.

Inherited deficiencies of a number of components of the complement system occur, e.g. of C2, C4a and C4b in 83% of patients, these being linked to the HLA type.

There is a defect in T cell regulation of the immune response, associated with B cell activation and a failure to clear the resultant immune complexes.

Sex hormone status is also involved, because oophorectomy (ovary removal) or treatment with androgens has relieved lupus-like symptoms in experimental animals. Also males with Klinefelter's syndrome, who are genetically XXY or XXYY, are prone to SLE.

Pathology and diagnosis

SLE damages a wide range of tissues. Damage to cells is known to release DNA, and this may provoke the formation of anti-dsDNA antibody. Plasma DNA has a high affinity for the collagen in the glomerular basement membrane, so binding of DNA in this region may be expected to lead to the formation of immune complexes (ICs), triggering local inflammation. These observations provide an explanation for two of the features of SLE: the presence of antinuclear antibodies (see below) and renal involvement. A further reason for glomerular involvement in SLE is local glomerular hypertension, which promotes extravasation of cells and nuclei from the circulation, which can then attach to the basement membrane.

Fluorescent antibody studies show widespread IC deposition in cellular basement membranes. This probably accounts for most of the manifestations of the disease, especially the vasculitis in the arterioles and capillaries. Although these ICs may be formed in all individuals, SLE sufferers may be unable to clear them because of complement deficiencies, notably C2 and C4.

The standard screening test is the **fluorescent antinuclear antibody test** (ANA; ANF, antinuclear factor), which detects antinuclear antibodies and is positive in virtually all patients with SLE. However, the ANA test is not specific (some 3% of the population is ANF-positive, but only about 3% of these have SLE) and so is used only as a routine screening test. More confidence can be placed in **dsDNA binding tests**, though some 15% of patients are falsely negative in these, especially in early or mild disease. Because this test is applied only to patients who are strongly positive in the ANA test this type of result does not give rise to ambiguities.

Despite the inflammation, the CRP is not raised, though the ESR is usually high in concordance with disease activity. The criteria for diagnosis are given in Table 12.20.

Some people have the immunological markers of SLE but do not have overt disease.

Drug-induced SLE

Many drugs are capable of producing a lupus-like syndrome (Table 12.21), but this is usually relatively mild, rarely provoking renal involvement, and tends to remit when the drug is withdrawn. It is doubtful whether this is related to true SLE.

Drugs may trigger attacks only in susceptible subjects, and all pharmacotherapy in SLE

patients needs careful supervision. A history of drug allergies is common in patients with drug-induced SLE.

Clinical features

SLE may affect almost any organ, though the liver is rarely involved. The approximate percentage frequencies of the principal organs involved are: joints, 95%; skin, 80%; CNS, 60%; kidneys, 50%; lungs, 40% and heart, 40%. Fever, arthralgias and myalgias are common, accompanied by headaches, depression, malaise and tiredness.

There is often a symmetrical facial 'butterfly'-shaped rash, giving a wolf-like appearance; hence the name 'lupus'. The occurrence of the rash may be triggered by sunlight, with or without photosensitizing drugs. If rash is the principal presenting symptom, patients may be referred initially to a dermatologist.

Although an episodic course is usual, some patients have chronic disease with exacerbations and complete remissions occurring over a very variable time period. The pattern of established disease is usually apparent in its early stages. SLE used to be represented as a relentlessly progressive, fatal condition, but the 10-year survival rate is now about 90%. Severe problems are unlikely if they have not devel-

---

Table 12.20   Criteria for the diagnosis of systemic lupus erythematosus (SLE)

For a diagnosis of SLE, at least four of the following criteria need to be present simultaneously, or serially, during a period of observation:

Malar (facial) rash
Discoid rash (see p. 801)
Photosensitivity
Oral or nasopharyngeal ulcers
Serositis
Non-erosive arthritis involving two or more peripheral
    joints
Pleuritis or pericarditis
Renal disease (persistent heavy proteinuria)
Fits or psychotic features
Haemolytic anaemia or thrombocytopenia or
    leukopenia
Antinuclear and other auto-antibodies

Table 12.21   Some drugs that may cause a lupus-like syndrome

Cardiovascular drugs
Beta-blockers, hydralazine, methyldopa, procainamide, quinidine

Antimicrobial agents
Griseofulvin, isoniazid

Antiepileptics
Ethosuximide, phenytoin, primidone

Antipsychotics
Chlorpromazine, lithium carbonate

Others
Oral contraceptives, penicillamine, propylthiouracil

oped within this time: most patients now do reasonably well.

Management

General

Because of the potential widespread and diverse nature of symptoms, patients need to be counselled carefully and told to report any new symptoms as they occur. Reassurance is appropriate for most. They should be warned of the need to protect themselves from bright sunshine, because of photosensitivity, and of the potential for drug allergies.

Pregnancy is not contra-indicated, except in severe disease, but specialist gynaecological care is essential.

Pharmacotherapy

Corticosteroids

These are the mainstay of treatment, using high doses in acute severe episodes and low-dose maintenance therapy in most patients. Their well-known side-effects make it important to step down the dose to about 7.5 mg/day of *prednisolone*, or less if possible, once symptoms are controlled. However, not all patients need continuous maintenance therapy.

Immunosuppressants

Azathioprine or *cyclophosphamide* are often used for their steroid-sparing effect and to control renal involvement or severe symptoms. Other treatment is supportive and symptomatic, e.g. renal dialysis.

Mild disease confined to the joints can usually be controlled with NSAIDs. *Hydroxychloroquine* is useful if these are inadequate and for the control of skin lesions.

Chronic discoid lupus erythematosus

Clinical features and pathology

Chronic discoid lupus erythematosus (CDLE) is a benign, chronic, episodic, erythematous skin disorder that mostly affects the face, although the scalp, hands and feet may also be affected. The rash may be symmetrical (like SLE) or asymmetrical. The lesions are sharply defined, slightly scaly, erythematous discs about 5–10 mm in diameter, sometimes slightly larger. If a scale is removed, the underside will show a 'hairy' appearance due to the adherent pilosebaceous plugs that filled the underlying hair follicles: this sign is pathognomonic. Older lesions tend to heal with scarring and hair loss. Pigmentation may occur in white skin and depigmentation is common in coloured skin. Usually, there are no systemic features with CDLE, but about 5% of patients eventually develop SLE.

Similarly to SLE, the lesions are caused by the deposition of ICs, in this case in the basal layer of the skin, causing cell destruction. There may be a high ESR and cells usually associated with SLE or similar diseases (LE cells) occur in the serum.

Pharmacotherapy

High protection factor sunblock preparations are used for photosensitivity. CDLE is one of the few indications for the use on the face of potent or moderately potent corticosteroids, e.g. *clobetasol*: intralesional injections are sometimes used.

If this does not achieve control, antimalarials may be helpful, as in SLE. Antimycobacterial drugs are sometimes used because they have anti-inflammatory properties. The antileprotic drug *clofazimine* is preferred to *rifampicin*, so as not to prejudice the use of the latter for TB.

Monoclonal antibodies against the CD40 ligand (see Chapter 2) are undergoing trial.

Sjögren's syndrome (keratoconjunctivitis sicca)

Definition

Classically, Sjögren's syndrome is defined as a triad of:

- Xerophthalmia (dry eyes).
- Xerostomia (dry mouth).
- A connective tissue or rheumatoid disease, usually RA.

If only the first two of these symptoms occur, this is described as the 'primary' form, sometimes called '**sicca syndrome**', which also causes symptoms resembling mild SLE. It is not known whether this represents a complication of occult connective tissue disease or whether the two conditions are triggered by a common agent. There is an association of sicca syndrome with lymphoid hyperplasia and high levels of circulating antibody, suggesting the presence of a distinct autoimmune disease.

However, Sjögren's syndrome is usually secondary, occurring in about 20% of those with other autoimmune and connective tissue diseases, e.g. RA, SLE or systemic sclerosis (see below).

Overall, about 0.5% of adult females are affected, the female:male ratio being 9:1.

A similar condition occurs in association with HIV infection, so investigation needs to exclude this possibility.

Pathology

This is a chronic autoimmune disease causing destruction of exocrine glands, due to lymphocytic infiltration. The aetiology is unknown, but there is an association with an HLA-DR3 and other HLA genotypes.

There is also hyperactivity of B cells, shown by auto-antibodies, e.g. RFs and antibodies to small RNA-protein complexes. Levels of IgG are very high.

Clinical features

The general drying up of exocrine secretions may cause effects on many organ systems, though in most patients the disease remains a minor mouth and eye problem. These effects include:

- Eyes: grittiness, irritation, morning lid stickiness and conjunctivitis.
- Mouth: there is difficulty in chewing and swallowing food; inability to speak continuously; a smooth, erythematous, sensitive tongue;

greatly increased dental caries and parotid gland enlargement. Candidal infection is common.
- Respiratory tract: the failure of secretion predisposes to infection.
- Genital tract: atrophic vaginitis and **dyspareunia** (difficult or painful coitus) in premenopausal women.
- Kidneys: some patients develop nephritis, but major renal pathology is rare.
- Raynaud's syndrome (in 25% of patients; see below).
- Non-erosive **arthritis** (33%).
- **Vasculitis**, causing purpura and sometimes glomerulonephritis.

Other features may be seen, e.g. leg ulceration and an increased tendency to hypersensitivity reactions. Patients with persistent parotid gland enlargement may develop **non-Hodgkin's B cell lymphoma**, but this can be predicted by the presence of circulating cryoglobulins (IgMs precipitated at low temperatures).

Management

In secondary disease this consists of managing the underlying condition, plus symptomatic relief as in the primary syndrome.

Treatment of primary Sjögren's syndrome is solely symptomatic, and focuses on replacement of secretions, thus minimizing discomfort and any damaging effects. Treatment includes:

- Eye drops: frequent use of preparations containing *hypromellose, polyvinyl alcohol* or *acetylcysteine* ('artificial tears').
- Mouth problems:
  - Scrupulous attention to dental hygiene to minimize premature, gross dental caries.
  - Mouthwash solution tablets, compound sodium mouthwash or more potent antiseptic mouthwashes, e.g. *chlorhexidine gluconate*, if toothbrushing is painful.
  - Commercial 'artificial saliva' preparations, and sugar-free demulcent pastilles, to alleviate dryness; *pilocarpine* may also help.

- *Fluconazole* or *itraconazole* for oropharyngeal candidiasis.
- *Hydroxychloroquine* for joint problems.
- Corticosteroids or cytotoxic immunosuppressants, e.g. *cyclophosphamide*, for severe systemic problems, e.g. vasculitis.
- Lymphoma; normal treatment (see Chapter 10).

Diuretics and anticholinergic drugs aggravate the lack of secretions and should be avoided.

Systemic sclerosis and scleroderma

Definition

Scleroderma is characterized by widespread tissue fibrosis. There is a dense hardening of skin collagen, especially of the hands and face, giving a tense, shiny appearance to the affected skin and puckering around the mouth. Vascular abnormalities and degenerative changes also occur.

If the internal organs are affected, the term **systemic sclerosis** is more appropriate, but the terms tend to be used interchangeably. Systemic sclerosis may lead to renal, pulmonary or cardiac failure. Dermal collagen is also normal.

Clinical features and pathology

The disease is uncommon (UK annual incidence about 10 per million, USA slightly higher) and occurs principally in women aged 30–50 years, with an overall female:male ratio about 3:1.

The symptoms described above are the result of three features:

- **Vascular damage**: Raynaud's syndrome (see below) occurs in nearly all patients, often months or years before other symptoms. This, and finger joint arthropathy, are common presenting features.
- **Fibrosis**: from the deposition of collagen and adhesive proteins (e.g. fibronectin), produced by fibroblasts. This causes oesophageal

dysfunction and sometimes a rapidly progressive visceral involvement.
- An **activated immune system**: the active fibroblasts are associated with TH (CD4+) lymphocytes, macrophages and degranulation of mast cells. About 75% of systemic sclerosis patients have antinuclear Igs, e.g. antinucleolar or anticentromere.

A genetic susceptibility has been mapped to MHC genes. Intriguingly, nucleic acid similarity between the target of some antiscleroderma auto-antibodies, DNA topoisomerase-1, and some mammalian retroviruses raises the possibility that scleroderma is triggered by viral infection. However, exposure to industrial chemicals (e.g. vinyl chloride and trichloethylene) and *bleomycin* (a cytotoxic antibiotic) may cause a similar syndrome.

Some 60% of sufferers have a limited cutaneous form of scleroderma that starts with Raynaud's syndrome, sometimes years before other symptoms appear. In the other 40% the systemic symptoms appear either at the same time as the Raynaud's syndrome or shortly afterwards.

The disease follows a chronic, highly variable course. Acute renal hypertension, lung fibrosis and hypertension, and cardiac problems may occur.

Management

Management of scleroderma is primarily symptomatic. Corticosteroids may be used to suppress synovitis. Cytotoxic immunosuppressants and antithymocyte globulin, if given early enough, may be helpful. They also help to spare the steroid dose. ACEIs have vastly improved the morbidity and mortality from renal involvement (see Chapters 4 and 14), and the usual cause of death is now pulmonary fibrosis. *Penicillamine* and *IFN-gamma* have been used experimentally to stem fibrosis.

The survival rate at 7 years after diagnosis is about 50%, but in some patients the disease stabilizes or regresses at about this time. In limited cutaneous disease the comparable survival is about 75%.

Raynaud's syndrome

Definition and epidemiology

The nomenclature of this condition is confused. The primary (idiopathic) form, which occurs without any underlying rheumatoid or connective tissue disorder, has been called 'Raynaud's disease', that secondary to other diseases being called 'Raynaud's phenomenon'. This division seems artificial, not least because Raynaud's disease may precede the onset of symptoms of an underlying disease by many years and is then seen to be a prodrome of that disease. In this text the neutral term 'Raynaud's syndrome' is preferred for both. However, the distinction is important because it is essential to identify any underlying disease state and institute appropriate treatment.

Primary Raynaud's syndrome, which especially affects young women, is due to spasm of the arterioles and small arteries, especially in the fingers and toes, resulting in intermittent blanching of the overlying skin. Occasionally other extremities (e.g. the nose, tongue and ears) may be involved. About 5% of people are affected.

The secondary form (Table 12.22) may reflect local nerve damage (e.g. in miners and dispatch riders), similarly causing vasospasm, or the use of vasospastic drugs, but may be due to inflammation, e.g. vasculitis.

Clinical features

The primary form causes intermittent, reversible attacks, precipitated by exposure to cold or emotional upset. The hands are most often affected, but attacks rarely involve the thumb. The affected fingers go white and may even become cyanosed and finally red as rewarming occurs. Paraesthesias, e.g. numbness, tingling or burning are common, and pain may be severe during circulatory recovery.

The primary disease is a common condition that affects 5% of the population. It usually causes bilateral symptoms whereas secondary disease may produce unilateral, irreversible ones, the affected area being permanently sensitive to adverse conditions, especially cold.

Recurrent severe episodes may eventually cause small infarcts in the affected digits, but the condition is usually non-progressive.

Diagnosis

The symptoms described above are pathognomonic. However, attacks of secondary Raynaud's syndrome may precede the onset of symptoms due to the underlying disease, e.g. RA, scleroderma or carpal tunnel syndrome (p. 809), by months or years. It is thus essential to look carefully for the markers of any underlying disease.

Management

General measures

In secondary Raynaud's syndrome, treatment is that of the underlying disease. The most useful basic approaches, whether or not the condition is primary are:

- To avoid:
  - Cold; keep warm locally and generally.
  - Peripherally vasoconstricting drugs, e.g. *ergotamine*, beta-blockers.
  - Smoking.

Table 12.22   Some causes and associations of Raynaud's syndrome

Cause	Examples
Idiopathic	Genetic, mostly young women
Trauma	Pneumatic drill workers, motorcycle dispatch riders
Secondary	Arteritis, mixed connective tissue disease, myxoedema, progressive systemic sclerosis, rheumatoid arthritis, Sjögren's syndrome, systemic lupus erythematosus
Drug-induced	Beta-blockers, ergotamine, methysergide

- To be scrupulous about hand hygiene, cuts, etc. and skin care.
- Physiotherapy needs to be started at the onset and performed regularly to promote good circulation.

Pharmacotherapy

Drugs are widely used, but most drug use is empirical. The following may help.

- **Vasodilators**:
  - Calcium channel blockers (see Chapter 4) are sometimes effective. *Nifedipine* is the only one licensed for this purpose in the UK, but *nicardipine*, and possibly *amlodipine* and *felodipine*, may also be useful. They tend to cause headache, flushing and dizziness and tachycardia. Reports of efficacy are somewhat contradictory.
  - Other vasodilators (see Chapter 4) may help, such as ACEIs (e.g. *captopril* and *enalapril*). *Naftidofuryl* and *inositol nicotinate* are other possibly helpful agents but may cause postural hypotension and the side-effects described for CCBs.
  - *Cinnarizine, moxisylyte, pentoxifylline* and *prazosin* have not proved to be useful.
  - *Epoprostenol*, an antiplatelet drug, is also a potent vasodilator and has been used if there are seriously compromised ischaemic areas. It must be given by continuous IV infusion because of its very short half-life of 3 min. *Epoprostenol* may cause severe flushing, headache and hypotension and so its use must be supervised closely. It is unsuitable for patients with IHD because the vasodilatation diverts blood from ischaemic areas and aggravates the problem. Its more stable analogue *iloprost* may be preferred if *epoprostenol* is not tolerated (unlicensed use).
- **Other agents**: *gamolenic acid*, in evening primrose oil, and halibut liver oil have been reported to be helpful.
- Nitric oxide, generated topically by mixing sodium nitrite and ascorbic acid gels, has been reported to improve the microcirculation.

Surgery

This may help, for example to relieve median nerve compression in associated carpal tunnel syndrome (p. 809). Sympathectomy has been used if there is a risk of digital gangrene, but the long-term outcome is uncertain.

Vasculitides

Vasculitis is inflammation of blood vessel walls. Because of the prime importance of blood vessel function these conditions may have serious, widespread effects. The classification is debated: that used here is widely accepted. The features of the primary conditions and some associated ones are given below. There is overlap between the types.

Antineutrophil cytoplasmic antibodies (PR3-ANCA and MPO-ANCA) are found in some of the acute vasculitides. PR3-ANCA is present in the serum of 90% of patients with Wegener's granulomatosis (see below). MPO-ANCA antibodies occur in up to 60% of other vasculitides, other rheumatic diseases and IBD (see Chapter 3).

Large-vessel vasculitis

Giant cell arteritis

Clinical features

Giant cell arteritis (GCA) usually involves only the carotid arterial tree. Patients present with fever, severe malaise, weight loss, facial pain and jaw pain on chewing that forces rest (claudication). **Polymyalgia rheumatica** (see below) is a frequently associated condition. Most patients are over 60 years of age, and women are affected more than men. Severe, localized headache is common, usually unilateral (temporal or occipital), with marked tenderness of the temple or scalp, e.g. when combing the hair, hence the alternative names **temporal** (or **cranial**) **arteritis**. Doubtful cases may be resolved by temporal artery biopsy, but this is performed only occasionally.

The ESR is very high, 50–120 mm/h (normal <20 mm/h), as is the CRP level. One very serious complication is sudden, reversible or irreversible, unilateral or bilateral blindness (25% risk). Rarer complications include ischaemia of the brainstem, cranial and peripheral nerves, and major arteries.

Pharmacotherapy

High-dose corticosteroids, e.g. 60–100 mg *prednisolone* daily, are essential to prevent blindness, and should be commenced immediately the diagnosis is suspected. The dose may be reduced after 1 month, depending on the condition of the patient and the reduction in ESR. Some consultants favour lower starting doses of 40 mg. The headache usually remits within 48 h of the first dose, and this rapid response may be helpful diagnostically.

The disease usually remits within 24–36 months' treatment in about 75% of patients, but the remainder require maintenance low-dose steroids, e.g. 10 mg *prednisolone* daily, because the risk of visual loss persists for several years. Recurrence of symptoms, or increased ESR or CRP, at any stage, dictate a return to full steroid dosage.

Patients need to be taught to manage their disease and to increase the corticosteroid dose immediately according to an agreed protocol if their condition deteriorates. They should then see their doctor as soon as possible. A prompt reaction to deterioration may pre-empt the need for more aggressive treatment later.

Polymyalgia rheumatica

Aetiology and epidemiology

Polymyalgia rheumatica (PMR) is defined by its clinical features. Some cases are associated with GCA, though most show quite distinct features and more widespread arteritis. PMR occurs mainly in the elderly, with two-thirds of patients being aged over 60 years, and is uncommon before the age of 50 or above 80. The female:male ratio is 2:1.

PMR is more common in Northern Europe. There are marked seasonal variations in incidence (about 70 per 100 000 in the over-60s), and these have prompted a search for infective causes, but without success. Because PMR is

unusual in patients' partners, environmental factors are unlikely to be implicated.

Clinical features

The principal symptoms are stiffness and aching, principally in the shoulder and pelvic girdles, e.g. the neck, shoulders, upper arm, buttocks and thighs. There is prolonged and severe early morning stiffness lasting more than 1 h, malaise, depression and weight loss. Onset may be sudden and dramatic (e.g. overnight), but in most cases occurs gradually over about 2 weeks. In the latter case, it may all too easily be dismissed as part of 'ageing'.

Pharmacotherapy

Symptoms respond rapidly to moderate doses of *prednisolone*, e.g. 15–25 mg daily. If there is any evidence of vasculitis, the higher doses used for GCA should be used because of the risk of sudden blindness (see above). The dose is gradually reduced to the minimum required to control symptoms and normalize the ESR. It is possible to withdraw steroids completely in about 75% of patients within 2–3 years. In the remainder, disease duration may be 7–10 years and the risks of prolonged corticosteroid treatment have to be weighed against those associated with the disease, notably blindness.

Azathioprine is often used for its steroid-sparing effect, and *dapsone*, *cyclophosphamide* and antimalarials have also been used.

The same considerations apply to patient self-management as in GCA.

Medium- and small-vessel vasculitis

Polyarteritis nodosa

This intense inflammation of the small and medium arteries, e.g. in coronary, pulmonary, kidney, muscular and mesenteric arteries, commonly occurs at the junctions of vessels, causing characteristic aneurysms that are visible in the retina. The widespread distribution of the lesions leads to correspondingly extensive and severe symptoms.

Polyarteritis nodosa (PAN) is a rare disease that affects middle-aged men more than women (male:female ratio about 2.5:1). In about 20% of patients PAN is associated with hepatitis B infection. A small number of cases appear to be associated with hypersensitivity reactions to penicillins and sulphonamides. These observations point to the possibility of the inflammation being triggered by immune complex deposition in arterial walls (see Chapters 2 and 14). However, the aetiology is generally unknown.

There is infiltration of all the layers of the affected arteries by inflammatory cells, leading to degeneration of the arterial walls, and to ischaemia. Inflammation and thrombosis may lead to tissue infarction in almost any organ.

The clinical features are the result of widespread ischaemic organ damage, involving the skin, cardiovascular and nervous systems, kidney and lungs, associated with non-specific symptoms, e.g. polyarthritis, myalgia, fever, weight loss and malaise. The ESR and CRP are raised. Such extensive symptoms clearly indicate a severe and alarming disease. Joint involvement is common, but is rarely serious. The disease runs a very variable course from a mild cutaneous vasculitis to severe, life-threatening involvement of major organs.

Management is with high-dose corticosteroids, immunomodulators, e.g. *azathioprine* or *cyclophosphamide*, and appropriate symptomatic support.

Wegener's granulomatosis

This rare disease mostly affects adults over 40 years of age, causing widespread small vessel granulomatous arteritis. Pulmonary, renal and sometimes eye lesions occur. The initial symptoms may be severe rhinorrhoea, cough and pleuritic pain, so patients usually present to chest clinics. Some 85% of patients have nephritis (see Chapter 14) that is rapidly progressive without prompt diagnosis and treatment, and is a sign of widespread systemic disease. The ESR is raised and MPO-ANCAs are usually present.

The aetiology is unknown, but it has been suggested that drugs may be involved, though no consistent associations have been demonstrated.

Pharmacotherapy

The condition, once uniformly fatal, responds well to high-dose *prednisolone* plus *cyclophosphamide*. The latter is given as pulsed intermittent IV therapy or as continuous low-dose oral treatment. When remission has been achieved, at about 3–6 months, the *cyclophosphamide* is usually replaced with *azathioprine*, to minimize toxicity.

Other multisystem diseases

Amyloidosis

This is the deposition of abnormal, extracellular, fibrous protein in various tissues throughout the body. The proteins include Ig fragments and precursors of normal serum proteins and are resistant to proteolysis *in vitro*. The deposits may be localized or widely distributed. Several different forms are distinguished, depending on the structure of the protein chains. It may be inherited or acquired.

The commonest inherited form is due to autosomal-dominant mutant genes coding for variants of the protein transthyretin. This is the retinol-binding and thyroxine-binding transport globulin that is mostly synthesized in the liver. Over 50 different amino acid substitutions are known. Other forms of amyloid are derived from fibrinogen and lysozyme chains.

Because many organs may be involved, patients may present with any of a diverse range of symptoms, e.g. heart failure, nephrotic syndrome, purpura, peripheral neuropathy and weight loss.

In secondary amyloidosis the deposits are formed from abnormal serum amyloid A (SAA), an acute phase protein. It may be associated with dialysis arthropathy, diabetes mellitus, Alzheimer's disease (the commonest form of senile dementia), Creutzfeldt–Jakob disease, RA, JIA and any of the systemic connective tissue diseases (see above). It usually presents with renal syndromes (proteinuria) or heart failure. In the Third World it may accompany TB and other chronic infections. The primary disorder must be identified and treated, if possible.

Once regarded as relentlessly progressive, many patients can now be managed effectively, e.g. with *prednisolone*, the alkylating agent *melphalan* (see Chapter 10), *colchicine* (for familial Mediterranean fever, triggered by rickettsial infection), or combinations of these. Transplantation of almost any affected organ, especially the liver, may be curative. Patients who respond to treatment show gradual regression of amyloid deposits. Transplant patients do little worse than others without amyloid, but surgery may be complicated by haemorrhagic problems and poor wound healing.

Sarcoidosis

Epidemiology and clinical features

This is a relatively common (UK prevalence about 20 per 100 000) granulomatous disorder, mostly affecting young adults aged 20–40 years, with widespread non-caseating granulomas in lymph nodes, liver, lungs, eyes and skin. They are less common in the joints, muscles, heart and CNS. Eye lesions occur in 25% of cases and skin lesions in about 10% (see below). Afro-Caribbeans usually have a more severe form of sarcoidosis, but it is less common in Asians.

It usually presents with a restrictive lung defect (see Chapter 5) and bilateral hilar lymphadenopathy, often detected on routine X-ray, or small joint, tendon and associated soft tissue swelling, occurring in about 5% of patients. The picture may strongly resemble RA, but this frank arthritis is usually associated with lung problems or **erythema nodosum** (a florid, painful, dusky red rash on the lower limbs, espe-

cially in the lower shins and ankles). Cardiac symptoms may occur rarely, in isolation.

The underlying abnormality appears to be the sequestration of T-lymphocytes in the lungs, causing depression of T cell function, but there is no evidence of CMI involvement (see Chapter 2). Spontaneous recovery is common.

Löfgren's syndrome is characterized by the abrupt onset of malaise, fever, large joint arthritis, erythema nodosum and lung symptoms.

Management and pharmacotherapy

About 65% of patients do well simply with NSAIDs. Those with Löfgren's syndrome usually respond similarly, though symptoms may take up to 3 months to resolve, and lung lesions up to 18 months.

Corticosteroids are the mainstay of treatment for lung, cardiac, CNS, liver and spleen involvement. They may also help for hypercalcaemia, but if this is severe ample IV fluids, and sometimes *disodium pamidronate*, are required. Severe disease may necessitate the use of second-line drugs, e.g. *methotrexate* or *hydroxychloroquine*, as in RA. *Ciclosporin* has been used experimentally but its value has been disputed, so it is usually reserved for non-responders to conventional treatment.

Eye problems (uveitis) are usually treated with topical corticosteroids, e.g. *dexamethasone* or *clobetasone* (lower risk of glaucoma), but also require mydriatics, e.g. *cyclopentolate*. They may be severe enough to require systemic corticosteroids.

Combined heart–lung and kidney transplantation has been used in end-stage non-responders, but the disease is likely to affect the transplanted organs subsequently.

Other rheumatic disorders

Reactive arthritis

This is an ill-defined entity, but the term is usually used to describe arthritis that follows an identifiable infection, often rheumatic fever or enteric infections, e.g. *Campylobacter* infection, dysentery, *Salmonella* food poisoning, AAC (see Chapter 8), and some sexually-acquired infections.

Reiter's syndrome

Definition

This multi-system disorder is usually characterized by:

- Urethritis.
- Seronegative spondarthritis (p. 789).
- Conjunctivitis.
- Skin lesions.

These may follow sexually transmitted diseases, e.g. non-specific urethritis or cervicitis. The acronym 'SARA', Sexually Acquired Reactive Arthritis, has been coined for this condition, about 50% of cases being associated with *Chlamydia trachomatis* or *Ureaplasma urealyticum* 'non-specific' urethritis. Gut infections, e.g. bacillary dysentery, may also be involved.

This is largely a male problem (80–95%), with most patients aged 16–35 years. There is a strong association with HLA-B27 (between 60% and 95% in various reports) that suggests the existence of a genetic susceptibility to an infection-triggered, immune-mediated disease.

Clinical features

Typically, there is a low-grade fever, conjunctivitis, arthritis and urinary-tract symptoms. The arthritis tends to affect a few joints asymmetrically, primarily in the lower limbs, and usually remits after a few weeks or months. Sacroiliitis and spondylitis can occur at any stage, usually in

severe cases associated with sexually-acquired infection. About 50% of patients experience a single episode, but recurrences occur in the remainder over a period of years, probably following repeated gastrointestinal or urinogenital infections. Repeated attacks lead to joint damage, which is sometimes severe.

Management

Management of Reiter's syndrome involves:

- Physiotherapy to reduce possible ankylosis.
- Early, aggressive treatment of any infection, e.g. tetracyclines for most urinogenital infections, including *Chlamydia*, may reduce arthropathy.
- NSAIDs.
- Corticosteroids for severe systemic complications, or for injection into isolated, badly affected joints.
- Aspiration of badly swollen joints.
- Surgery in late disease, as for AS (p. 789).

Soft tissue rheumatism

This section describes briefly the most common minor non-arthritic soft tissue lesions. They are relatively common and treatable. Topical therapy with creams and liniments is popular (p. 811). Physical treatments, e.g. physiotherapy, osteopathy, chiropractic and acupuncture, are widely used, and help to relieve pain and associated muscle spasm.

Carpal tunnel syndrome (CTS)

Definition

This entrapment neuropathy is the result of compression of the median nerve at the wrist, where it passes between the tendons and the transverse ligament (Figure 12.11).

Aetiology and epidemiology

CTS may be idiopathic or occur in association with many diseases or conditions, e.g. RA, Raynaud's syndrome, fluid accumulation (pregnancy, premenstrual or postmenopausal), tenosynovitis (e.g. sports injury, overuse of the wrist, repetitive strain injury and local trauma), obesity, diabetes mellitus, hypothyroidism, amyloidosis and acromegaly. The condition may occur at any age, mostly in women.

Clinical features

These include:

- **Paraesthesias**, e.g. tingling, sensory loss and numbness in the first three-and-a-half digits of the hand (Figure 12.11(a)), i.e. in the area of distribution of the median nerve, although symptoms may be rather diffuse. The patient often wakes at night and hangs the arm over the bedside or wrings the hand to obtain relief.
- **Pain** in the hand, wrist or forearm.
- **Weakness** of the hand and wasting of the ball of the thumb.

Management

This comprises:

- Management of any underlying disease or predisposing condition.
- Local injection of corticosteroids.
- Splinting.
- Nerve decompression by surgical division of the transverse ligament of the wrist. However, a precise diagnosis is an essential prerequisite; this procedure will give no benefit if the root of the problem lies elsewhere, e.g. nerve compression at the elbow, neck or shoulder.

Tendonitis and tenosynovitis

Tendonitis is tendon inflammation. It is rarely diagnosed precisely in general practice, and many syndromes are **enthesopathies**. The aetiology is uncertain but may be associated with

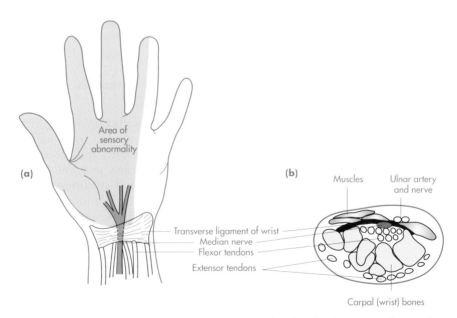

Figure 12.11 Carpal tunnel syndrome and the associated anatomy of the hand and wrist. (a) Left palm showing the usual area of sensory abnormality in carpal tunnel syndrome, i.e. the area served by the median nerve. (b) Section through the wrist showing the median nerve lying immediately under the transverse ligament, in the 'carpal tunnel' formed by the ligament and the carpal (wrist) bones.

an inflammatory arthropathy or minor repetitive trauma. The most common lesions include:

- **Supraspinous tendonitis**, characterized by pain on straight arm raising.
- **Frozen shoulder**, a more serious condition, occurring at any age in adult life, but mostly in older patients; it may cause restriction of shoulder movement and severe pain, especially at night.
- **Tennis elbow**, with pain occurring over the lateral (outer) aspect of one elbow joint.
- **Golfer's elbow** causes pain on the medial (inner) side of an elbow.
- **Achilles tendonitis**, behind the ankle.
- **Plantar fasciitis** gives pain in the sole of the foot.

Tenosynovitis is inflammation and swelling of the tendon sheaths. It is commonly caused by trauma and overuse injury, but it is also a frequent accompaniment to RA and other inflammatory arthropathies. Type II hyperlipoproteinaemia (see Chapter 4) is a predisposing factor.

The use of quinolone antibiotics (see Chapter 8) has occasionally been associated with **tendon rupture**, especially in the Achilles tendon, but also in the shoulder and hand. This rare side-effect has also been reported in those taking corticosteroids and may occur within 48 h of starting treatment. Elderly patients are more prone to tendonitis. Patients should be warned that if they experience any tendon pain or discomfort, especially of the Achilles tendon, they should stop taking the antibiotic and see their doctor immediately.

Management

Rest and the application of heat or cold, as the patient finds most effective, and NSAIDs are used. Local injection of corticosteroids is used in resistant cases, under consultant supervision, because it is important not to inject the tendon itself: injection into a tendon may itself cause rupture. Physical therapies are used progressively as the condition improves, and are helpful for preventing adhesions. Surgery to divide tendon sheaths or remove calcified deposits may be needed in persistent cases, and may be curative.

Topical NSAIDs are popular, partly because when patients rub in the product they feel that they are contributing to their own treatment and because the massage also stimulates local blood supply and interferes with pain signal transmission, so contributing to healing. Penetration into joints has been demonstrated and a meta-analysis found that topical forms of *diclofenac*, *ibuprofen*, *ketoprofen* and *piroxicam* gave at least 50% pain reduction in acute soft tissue trauma, sprains and strains. Similar benefits were seen in chronic conditions, e.g. tendonitis and osteoarthritis. Although they avoid the gastrointestinal side-effects associated with oral dosing, the use of large amounts of topical products and occlusive bandaging may cause excessive penetration and systemic effects, e.g. renal impairment, especially in older patients, and those with inflammatory skin problems. These POM products are unlikely to be beneficial in RA, but may give some benefit to those with OA (see above) and soft tissue rheumatism.

They should be applied with gentle massage only, not used on abraded skin or large areas and should not be occluded. Women who are pregnant or breastfeeding should avoid these products.

OTC products may contain an NSAID or salicylate plus a rubefacient and should not be used overenthusiastically, as above.

Bursitis

This is inflammation of a bursa, the most common sites being the large toe (bunion), shoulder, lower pelvis ('tailor's bottom'), knee ('housemaid's knee', shop workers' knee, from kneeling on hard floors), and elbow ('miner's or 'students' elbow').

The aetiology is often unknown but is usually the result of trauma. Other possible causes are inflammation of adjacent joints, gout or infection.

There is pain and local tenderness, and swelling is a feature of the last two conditions mentioned above. Occasionally, chronic bursitis may follow repeated trauma, e.g. from shoes (bunions), unresolved infection or gout.

Management includes rest, with or without splinting, and high-dose NSAIDs plus local injection of corticosteroids in severe or persistent cases: NSAIDs alone are of limited value. Physical therapies are used progressively as the pain and inflammation subside.

Inflamed bursae sometimes continue to enlarge and require surgical dissection, with excellent results.

Fibrositis and fibromyalgia

This is a group of non-specific conditions presenting with diffuse pain, tenderness and stiffness of muscles and their connective tissues, with local tender points. Pain is felt most frequently in the back, neck, shoulders, chest and buttocks.

There is no specific disease entity. It is assumed to be due to trauma, exposure to cold, viral infection or stress. Management is purely symptomatic with analgesics, and topical and physical treatments.

Low back pain

Definition

This is pain in the lower lumbar, lumbosacral and sacroiliac regions. It is sometimes accompanied by **sciatica**, which is neurological pain occurring in the distribution of the sciatic nerve, i.e. in the buttocks and the lateral (outer) aspect of the leg and the foot. It can be very severe and incapacitating.

Aetiology

The pain is mostly the result of 'degenerative' joint disease (OA) and so is very common in the elderly (50% of the 60+ age group). However, buttock pain in younger patients may be due to AS (see above). A first attack of mechanical low back pain is unusual below 20 years of age or after 50 and raises the possibility of an organic cause.

A common cause is a **prolapsed intervertebral disc** (PID, 'slipped disc'), when the capsule of an intervertebral disc ruptures or herniates under strain (e.g. lifting, bending stress, sports

trauma and sneezing) and the nucleus pulposus (pulpy centre) is extruded into the spinal canal to press on a nerve root. A strong longitudinal vertebral ligament usually prevents the extruded pulp pressing directly on the spinal cord, so pressure is normally directed to one side to give unilateral symptoms (see Figure 12.3(b)). There is associated muscle spasm, which exacerbates the condition. A new PID is uncommon in the elderly.

One iatrogenic cause is prolonged systemic corticosteroid therapy, leading to osteoporosis and collapse of one or more vertebrae (crush fractures), often causing bilateral nerve root compression and severe pain.

Pregnancy or obesity may also cause strain and low back pain.

Diagnosis

Frequently, no abnormality can be demonstrated with X-rays, so it may be difficult to make a precise diagnosis, unless there is a fracture, dislocation or PID. MRI scanning is the preferred procedure and is justified if symptoms are severe. A full blood count, ESR or blood biochemistry are appropriate if an inflammatory lesion, a metabolic origin or malignancy are thought to be likely.

More invasive investigations are rarely justified. However a **myelogram** (i.e. X-ray following injection of a radio-opaque dye to visualize the spinal cord) may be done in difficult cases to determine the extent of spinal cord damage, though MRI is less invasive and will usually show this. This is important if there is evidence of neurological deficit, e.g. leg paraesthesias or loss of control of bladder or bowels, or to direct possible surgery.

Management

Acute back pain

Management is conservative because most patients recover completely in 6–8 weeks of partial rest with warmth, plus analgesic support. However, excessive rest is undesirable, causing muscle wasting and delaying recovery. If pain is severe, recovery is prolonged or there are neurological signs, active treatment is indicated, including:

- Local injections of *pethidine* (meperidine), local anaesthetics or a long-acting corticosteroid, if there is severe, acute pain. Oral *pethidine* is ineffective (see Chapter 7).
- Muscle relaxants, e.g. *diazepam* or *meprobamate*, to relieve muscle spasm.
- Manipulation, provided it is certain that there is no PID or fracture, otherwise serious neurological damage may be caused.
- Traction and surgery may occasionally be indicated for persistent motor weakness, and as a matter of urgency if there is loss of control of bladder or bowel function.
- NSAIDs are often used in the community but are seldom superior to simple or opioid analgesics.

Chronic back pain

No generally satisfactory treatment is available. Orthodox management includes:

- Weight reduction.
- Treatment of any underlying disease.
- Analgesics appropriate to pain severity.
- Patient education on the avoidance of back strain and poor posture, including advice on working conditions and suitable seating.
- Carefully graded exercises and physiotherapy to strengthen the back muscles and so improve joint stability.
- Spinal supports (corsets, belts) in an acute exacerbation, but prolonged use is undesirable because muscle tone, and therefore support, is lost.
- Occasionally, surgical removal of the disc (**discectomy**, usually percutaneously) or a vertebral arch (**laminectomy**). Enzyme injections are sometimes used to dissolve the disc pulp (**chemonucleolysis**, e.g. with *chymopapain* from the papaya plant), but are less satisfactory because of allergic reactions.
- Spinal fusion is undertaken rarely.

Other physical modalities, e.g. osteopathy, chiropractic, are of undoubted benefit to many sufferers, who tend to seek a variety of 'alternative' medical treatments, sometimes in desperation at the unsatisfactory outcome of orthodox medical treatment.

References and further reading

Abdel-Nasser A M, Rasker J J, Valkenburg H A (1997). Epidemiological and clinical aspects relating to the variability of rheumatoid arthritis. *Semin Arthritis Rheum* **27**: 123–140.
Anonymous (1998). Modifying disease in rheumatoid arthritis. *Drug Ther Bull* **36**: 3–6.
Arthritis and Rheumatism Council (UK) Patient leaflets and booklets, Practical Problems series, Student Handbook, Topical Reviews Series. (www.arc.org.uk)
Clarke A K, Hart F D (1993). *Clinical Problems in Rheumatology*. London: Martin Dunitz.
Creamer P, Hochberg M C (1997). Osteoarthritis. *Lancet* **350**: 503–509.
Dingle J T (1996). The effect of NSAIDs on human articular cartilage glycosaminoglycan synthesis. *Eur J Rheum Inflamm* **16**: 47–52.
Edwards C J (2005). Immunological therapies for rheumatoid arthritis. *Br Med Bull* **73–74**: 71–82.
Griffiths I D, Kelly C, eds (2006). Rheumatology (2 parts), Medicine (Parts 9 and 10): 331–437.
Hakim A, Clunie J G A, Haq I (2006). *Oxford Handbook of Rheumatology*. Oxford: Oxford University Press.
Han T S, Lean M E J (2006). Metabolic syndrome. In: Lean M E J, ed. Nutrition. *Medicine* **34** (Part 12): 501–560.
Klippel J H, Dieppe P A (1995). *Practical Rheumatology*. London: Mosby International.
National Prescribing Centre (1996). Second line drugs in rheumatoid arthritis. *MeReC Bulletin* **7**: 9–12.
National Prescribing Centre (1997). Topical non-steroidal anti-inflammatory drugs: an update. *MeReC Bulletin* **8**: 29–32.
Pincus T (1995). Long term outcomes in rheumatoid arthritis. *Br J Rheumatol* **34** (Suppl. 2): 59–73.
Rains C P, Noble S, Faulds D (1995). Sulfasalazine: A review of its pharmacological properties and therapeutic efficacy in the treatment of rheumatoid arthritis. *Drugs* **50**: 137–156.
Reginster J Y, Deroisy R, Rovati LC, *et al.* (2001). Long-term effects of glucosamine sulphate on

osteoarthritis progression: a randomized, placebo-controlled clinical trial. *Lancet* **357**: 251–256.

Sambrook P, Schreiber L, Taylor T, Ellis A (2001). *The Musculoskeletal System*. Edinburgh: Churchill Livingstone (Harcourt).

Smith W L (1992). Prostanoid biosynthesis and mechanism of action. *Am J Physiol* **268**: F181–F191.

Snaith M L, ed. (1995). *ABC of Rheumatology*. London: BMJ Publishing Group.

Spilker B (1990). *Quality of Life Assessments in Clinical Trials*. New York: Raven Press.

Streiner D L, Norman G R (2003). *Health Measurement Scales: A Practical Guide to their Development and Use*, 3rd edn. Oxford: Oxford Medical Publications.

Van Ryn J, Pairet M (1997). Selective cyclooxygenase-2 inhibitors: pharmacology, clinical effects and therapeutic potential. *Expert Opin Invest Drugs* **6**: 609–614.

13

Skin diseases

The skin is the largest single organ of the body, with an area of about 1.75 m^2 for an average adult. Because the skin is visible and accessible and gives the first impression from which we judge people, patients are self-conscious about any perceived abnormality. They may expect faster, more complete resolution of a superficial lesion than an invisible, internal one. The unique skin symptom, itch, can lead to sleep loss and irritability if severe, and can cause emotional problems if associated with a visible, possibly disfiguring lesion.

Dermatological problems comprise about 10% of a GP's case load, and probably more for pharmacists. Diagnosis and treatment leave much to be desired and pharmacists need to learn to diagnose and advise patients confidently. This requires knowledge and experience. Further, the incidence of atopic dermatitis and skin malignancies has doubled over the past 20 to 30 years and these conditions need to be recognized early.

This chapter deals primarily with eczema and dermatitis, psoriasis, acne, rosacea and urticaria, which comprise most of the dermatological case load and discusses the special drug classes used (corticosteroids and retinoids). It concludes with brief discussions of drug side-effects on the skin and of transdermal absorption, an important, developing drug delivery system.

There are 16 full colour plates (between pp. 822 and 823) to aid recognition and some of the specialist books listed in the References and further reading section give further assistance with this.

Skin anatomy and physiology

Functions

The skin has five principal functions:

- To **protect** the underlying organs from physical, chemical and mechanical injury.
- To **control fluid loss** from the body (the skin contains nearly 20% of the total body water).
- To assist in **controlling the body temperature** by sweating and radiation from the surface.
- To act as an important **sensory organ** for touch, pain and external temperature etc.
- To act an **organ of emotional expression**, as it exhibits feelings by its colour, e.g. flushing and blanching, and sweat and odour production.

Anatomy

There skin consists of three principal layers (Figure 13.1): the epidermis, the dermis and the subcutaneous tissues.

Epidermis

This is the main protective layer of the skin, and therefore of the entire body.

Structure

The epidermis is composed of four subsidiary layers (Figure 13.1), most of which (95%) are derived from the **keratinocytes**. These comprise:

- The basal **(germinal) layer**, the deepest part, normally consists of a single sheet of cycling stem cells, most of which divide progressively and mature to form the other three layers of the epidermis. There is a small proportion of resting stem cells that can be recruited into growth to repair damage (see Chapter 2). The basal cells are joined by intercellular bridges, desmosomes and hemidesmosomes, that enhance strength and distribute mechanical stresses more evenly through the skin. Desmosomes join adjacent skin cells, hemidesmosomes join the basal layer to dermal tissue.
- The **prickle cell layer**, composed of cells also joined by intercellular bridges, is just above the basal layer and contains cells in intermediate stages of development into the granular layer. The prickle cell layer also contains Langerhans cells, which are immunologically important dendritic cells that are APCs, express class II MHC antigens and have receptors for complement (see Chapter 2).
- The **granular layer** comprises a few rows of cells containing granules derived from their degenerating nuclei. These cells gradually

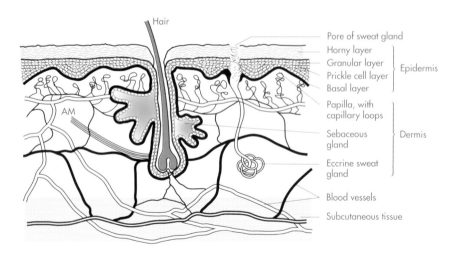

Figure 13.1 The anatomy of the skin. The arrector pili muscle (AM) is shown pulling the hair into the erect position, a reaction to fright or cold: this produces 'gooseflesh' in less hairy areas.

migrate towards the surface and finally form the outermost **horny layer**.

- This horny layer (**stratum corneum**) consists of keratinized, enucleate cells that are shed continuously as small scales from the surface.

There is thus a continual replacement of the hard, keratinized, horny layer from the basal cells. The horny layer varies considerably in thickness, being very thick on those areas that are subject to wear and pressure. i.e. the palms and soles of the feet, and thinnest in the flexures, e.g. axillae and eyelids. Keratin, an insoluble fibrous protein, is the principal constituent of the horny layer and the skin appendages, the nails and hair, and the organic matrix of tooth enamel.

All of these structures, together with the oily secretions of the glands (see below), serve to protect the underlying tissues, the **dermis** and deeper tissues, from mechanical damage and to control undue water and heat loss.

The **nails** are extensions of the horny layer and consist of solid plates of translucent keratin. Finger nails grow at the rate of approximately 0.1 mm daily, taking 4–5 months for complete replacement. Toe nails grow at about half this rate, so treatment of toe nail conditions needs to be more prolonged than for finger nails.

Melanocytes form about 5% of the basal layer. They are dendritic cells, forming an irregular network that is very variable in extent. The **melanin** that they synthesize is transferred through their dendrites to other epidermal cells. Exposure to sunlight or ultraviolet (UV) radiation promotes melanin synthesis, the concentration of which in the epidermis influences the basic skin pigmentation of individuals. However, skin colour also depends on the extent of dilatation of the skin capillaries, the relative proportions of oxidized and reduced Hb in them, and on the presence of yellow carotene pigments in the blood vessel walls and surrounding tissues. Carotenes are present primarily in fatty tissue and are precursors of vitamin A. Dark-skinned people have the same proportion of melanocytes in the basal layer as do the fair-skinned, but they synthesize melanin at a faster rate.

Associated features

These include the hair and the apocrine, eccrine and sebaceous glands. The **hair** arises in tubular downgrowths from the epidermis into the dermis, the **hair follicles**. At the base of the hair follicle is a bulb containing the root and the **papilla**. The latter is a projection of the dermis into the bulb and contains blood vessels, nerves and melanocytes. There are three types of hair:

- The long hairs of the scalp, beard, moustache, axillae and pubic areas.
- Vellus (downy) hair occurring on the rest of the surface.
- A small amount of short, stiff hairs on the eyebrows and eyelids, in the nostrils and ear canals and the face in males.

Growth of the long and stiff hair is under androgenic control, so hair growth varies with sex, age, during pregnancy, etc. The hair follicles are formed naturally only during embryonic growth and the number is therefore fixed at birth, so hair loss due to follicular degeneration cannot normally be restored. However, it has been reported that the expression of two compounds in mouse epithelial cells, beta-catenin and LEF-1, causes adult epithelial cells to revert to an embryonic state and produce new hair follicles. Two problems remain to be solved before this discovery can be translated into treatment for hair loss: whether the results are applicable to humans and elucidating the control mechanisms for this process, to prevent excessive hair growth and the possible formation of (benign) follicular tumours.

Loss of hair (**alopecia**) or its abnormal increased production (**hirsutism**) may thus be an indicator of endocrine abnormality, systemic disease (Table 13.1) or autoimmunity. All visible hair is dead, and no medical treatment can affect it once it has been formed, though its appearance may be improved (or harmed) cosmetically. Scalp hairs grow continuously for some 2–6 years at the rate of about 10 mm per month before falling out. They are replaced by regrowth or by activation of dormant follicles. All treatments for hair loss are unsatisfactory, though topical *minoxidil* will promote the growth of vellus hair for as long as it is used. High-potency topical or intralesional corticosteroids (see Table 13.11)

Table 13.1   Some causes of hair disorders

Hair loss

Diffuse

Male-pattern baldness (androgen-dependent)

Telogen effluvium, i.e. excessive rate of hair loss due to iron-deficiency anaemia, infections, post partum and stress

Hair shaft defects

Endocrine deficiency: hypothyroidism, hypopituitarism, hypoparathyroidism

Systemic lupus erythematosus

Syphilis

Drugs, e.g.:

- cytotoxics: cyclophosphamide, mercaptopurine, doxorubicin, epirubicin, colchicine
- anticoagulants: heparin, coumarins
- antithyroid: thiouracils, carbimazole
- tuberculostatics: ethionamide
- vitamins: vitamin A
- synthetic retinoids, especially etretinate, less common with isotretinoin

Localized

Alopecia areata

Fungal infections

Discoid lupus erythematosus

Lichen planus

Harsh treatments, e.g. dyes, permanent waves, bleaches and traction

Hirsuitism

Endocrine: adrenal, pituitary, ovarian, menopausal

Congenital abnormalities

Idiopathic (hair follicle hypersensitivity to androgens?)

Drugs: androgens, minoxidil, corticosteroids, ciclosporin

and *ciclosporin* may induce regrowth, but regression occurs on withdrawal of all treatments. Oral photochemotherapy (PUVA, p. 847) has been reported to be successful in up to 30% of patients.

There are two types of **sweat glands**. The **apocrine glands** are large glands that open mostly into the hair follicles in the axillae, scalp, anogenital area and around the nipples. They produce a milky secretion containing carbohydrates, proteins, fatty acids etc., the production of which is stimulated by emotions such as pain, fright and sexual excitement. These glands develop at puberty and are therefore part of the secondary sexual characteristics.

Eccrine glands occur all over the skin, though their concentration varies enormously with the site, and they play an important role in temperature regulation. Eccrine glands occur as coils of cells in the dermis and open via invisible pores onto the surface where they discharge the sweat, a watery fluid containing 0.5–1% of chlorides, lactic and other acids and nitrogenous compounds, mostly urea.

The **sebaceous glands** are present all over the body, except the palms and soles. They are especially common on the scalp, face, forehead, chin, chest and back, opening into the hair follicles. They do not have ducts, but the cells break down to release the waxy **sebum**. The function of sebum is uncertain, though superficial spread of its waxy component influences water movement out of the skin and its retention there. The skin also produces large amounts of a mixture of substances, known collectively as **natural moisturising factor**. Because sebum production is partly under hormonal control, its odour presumably has a sexual role. Modified sebaceous glands produce wax (**cerumen**) in the ears and form the **meibomian glands** of the eyelids. The latter occasionally become blocked, forming small, benign, irritant cysts (**chalazion**): if these are troublesome they are removed surgically. Chalazion should not be confused with **styes**, which are infections of the hair follicles.

Dermis

The outermost papillary part of the dermis lies immediately under the epidermis and rises irregularly into it, producing the **dermal papillae**, which contain blood vessels and nerve elements. The deeper part of the dermis contains a variety of elements:

- Connective tissue, e.g. collagen and elastic fibres, which supports the epidermis, confers elasticity and helps to maintain skin hydration
- Cellular elements: migratory, i.e. a few leucocytes (histiocytes) that are phagocytic and also form reticulin fibres, and fixed, i.e. fibroblasts and mast cells. These cellular elements are important, since they control the differentiation and function of the overlying epidermal epithelium, resistance to infection and reactions to environmental allergens.
- Blood vessels, which nourish the skin and help to regulate local temperature.
- Smooth muscle fibres, which erect the hairs and cause 'gooseflesh'.
- Nerves, which are sensory (touch, pain, temperature) and autonomic (controlling the blood vessels and hair follicles).
- Lymphatic vessels, for drainage of intercellular fluid.

Subcutaneous tissue

Below the dermis is a layer of loose, **areolar connective tissue**, containing adhesion proteins, nerves and fat, plasma cells (see Chapter 2) and mast cells, embedded in a semi-solid matrix. This layer has important functions:

- Storage of water and fat, helping to maintain dermal and epidermal hydration.
- Insulation against excessive heat loss or gain.
- Provision of an access route for nerves and blood vessels to muscles and the dermis.
- Protection of underlying tissue.

Clinical features of skin diseases

Histopathology

The pathological changes that occur in skin due to disease are often not diagnostic, unless invading microorganisms can be recognized. However, there may be characteristic changes in the epidermis in diseases such as **psoriasis** (p. 838) or **pemphigus**, or in the dermis, e.g. in **scleroderma** (see Chapter 12). The structures of some types of lesions are illustrated in Figure 13.2, and common pathological changes are listed in Table 13.2.

Many skin conditions are inflammatory or have inflammation (see Chapter 2) as a significant component.

Diagnosis

History

The important aspects of the dermatological history (see also Chapter 1) are:

- Where did it start? (Figure 13.3).
- Duration.
- What changes have occurred in the severity?
- The extent when seen, and in the past, i.e. changes over time, distribution (Figure 13.3).
- Features (Tables 13.3 and 13.4): wet or dry, colour, size, itch (pruritis).
- Interference with sleep, work, leisure and social contacts.
- Aggravating or relieving factors, e.g. treatments, diet, clothing, light, temperature, seasonal variation, emotional stress, medicines.
- Family history, e.g. allergies and atopic conditions, eczema (p. 849) and psoriasis (p. 838).
- Medication history.

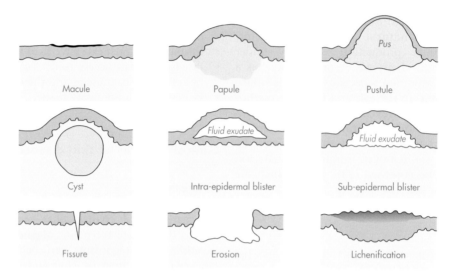

Figure 13.2   Some types of skin lesions (diagrammatic).

Table 13.2   Changes that may occur in the skin due to disease

Descriptive term	Pathology	Examples
Epidermal changes		
Acantholysis	Separation of the epidermal cells from each other, causing splits, vesicles and bullae	Herpes zoster, drug eruptions
Acanthosis	Increased depth of the prickle cell layer	Psoriasis, warts
Hyperkeratosis	Excessive production of the horny layer	Corns, ichthyosis
Inflammation	T cell recruitment, increased blood flow and intercellular fluid	Eczema, psoriasis
Parakeratosis	Incomplete keratinization, with nuclei in the horny layer	Psoriasis
Spongiosis	Intercellular oedema of the prickle layer	Eczema
Dermal changes		
Capillary	Lymphocytic infiltration	Systemic lupus erythematosus
	Sclerosis and obliteration	Scleroderma
Collagen	Sclerosis	Scleroderma
degeneration	Atrophy	Age, corticosteroid treatment
Fibrosis	Hypertrophy	Keloid scars
Inflammation	T cell recruitment, increased blood flow and intercellular fluid	Eczema, psoriasis

• Occupation and hobbies.
• Cosmetic usage, including hair dyes, perfumes, aftershave lotions, and creams, etc.

The last two of these categories, and the patient's own observation, may provide valuable clues as to the cause of **contact dermatitis** (p. 852). The emotional response of the patient may also be very important because visible lesions may cause considerable distress even though they are benign, and the associated emotions may aggravate the condition.

Inspection and identification of the types of skin changes and of lesions (Figures 13.2 and 13.3, the Plates and Tables 13.2–13.6) require a good light and sometimes magnification.

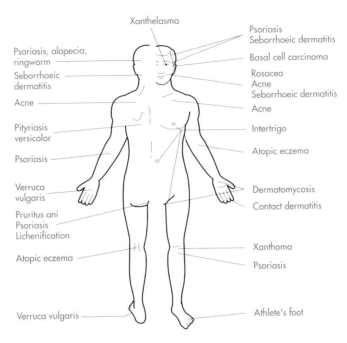

Figure 13.3   Principal sites of occurrence of some common dermatoses.

Table 13.3   Principal features of some common localized lesions

Clinical features	Disease state
Non-pigmented lesions	
Pearly sheen, often facial, slowly enlarging, usually raised margin with central ulcer, patients usually >50 years of age	Basal cell carcinoma[a] (rodent ulcer)
Usually firm, hyperkeratotic, pin-head to pea-sized, often on hands or soles of feet, epidermal ridges disrupted, pain on lateral pressure	Warts
Firm or hard, deep set, often below knees, patients usually >50 years of age	Histiocytoma
Pigmented lesions	
Collections of blood vessels	
• raised in children, usually paler and flatter in adults; clotting may give bluish pigment	Angiomas, naevi
• solitary, raised red, shiny or eroded, bleeds readily, often presents acutely	Pyogenic granuloma
Uniform, static, even surface, pale to very dark brown	Mole
Light or dark brown, raised often whitish markings, warty, greasy, patients >50 years of age	Seborrhoeic warts
Usually pigmented (not always), enlarging slowly or rapidly, development of satellite lesions, ulceration or bleeding	Malignant melanoma[a]

[a] Malignant, the remainder are benign

Table 13.4 Some features of scaly rashes

Clinical feature	Possible disease state
Non-inflammatory	
Mild	Effects of weather, social habits[a]
Present from childhood	Ichthyosis
Adult onset	May indicate systemic disease
Pigmented, ovoid, localized on exposed surfaces, usually elderly	Solar keratoses
Localized, progressive lesions or change in a previously static lesion	Possible malignancy
Inflammatory	
Localized	
Non-pigmented, mild to moderate itch	Infestations, tinea, intertrigo, stable plaque psoriasis
Non-pigmented, very itchy	Contact dermatitis
Generalized	
Raised, commonly discrete 'salmon pink' plaques, slightly itchy, scaling	Psoriasis
Very itchy	Dermatitis/eczema
Discrete lesions, raised border, paler centre	Tinea
Child or young adult, sudden onset with single 'herald patch', mildly itchy, usually on trunk, upper arms and legs, remits without treatment	Pityriasis rosea
Itching slight to severe, papules up to 5 mm diameter, shiny violaceous to brown, commonly on wrists, waist, thighs, inside mouth	Lichen planus

[a] Excessive washing, harsh detergents, etc.

Psychological features

Patients with skin diseases tend to be more disturbed by their condition, relative to its severity, than are those with other types of illness. This is particularly true of visible lesions. Many common skin diseases, although potentially disfiguring, are completely benign and non-transmissible, e.g. naevi, dermatitis, psoriasis and acne. Patients often experience what has been called the 'leper complex', being at least somewhat rejected by their families, friends and acquaintances, or expecting to be so, and thus becoming miserable and reclusive.

Itching, a common accompaniment to many dermatoses, may make patients restless during the day and sleepless at night, leading to tiredness, irritability, demoralization and social difficulties.

A clear diagnosis and simple explanation will often help patients enormously. A readiness to touch non-infectious lesions, demonstrating the conviction of the healthcare worker or carer that the disease is benign and non-transmissible, can be a very effective way of reducing anxiety.

Examination

General aspects

In community pharmacy it may be difficult to gain a sufficiently broad experience, over a long enough time, to be able to recognize even some common skin lesions readily. It is certainly impracticable to learn to do so adequately as a student, though there are several well-illustrated books that can be of great help (see References and further reading). Prior self-treatment, especially with corticosteroids, may alter the appearance of lesions dramatically. There is a temptation to proceed directly to examination of the patient and to form a diagnosis on that basis, because patients often present by showing a readily visible lesion and asking for advice. Although skin symptoms and signs may be pathognomonic, e.g. in acne or stable plaque psoriasis, the history is usually of prime importance, because the skin has only a limited repertoire of symptoms with numerous possible causes. Also, the characteristics and severity of lesions may vary widely, even in the same patient with the same disease at different times.

Some general symptom groups and the features which may make it possible to identify the nature of the problem and come to a diagnosis are described below, but the details of the most common diseases are described later in this chapter.

Allergic conditions
These are usually very itchy (itch arises solely in the epidermis). Localized lesions may be due to **contact dermatitis** (Plate 1), **atopic dermatitis** (Plates 13 and 14 and p. 852) or **urticaria** (p. 864).

Rashes
These are temporary skin eruptions, varying from small spots to larger areas.

Facial rashes. These are often due to environmental factors, e.g. weather or sunlight, or may be readily recognizable, e.g. acne. If they are due to atopic dermatitis there is often a fairly characteristic appearance: dry, finely scaling skin, facial pallor, swelling or creasing around the eyes and, possibly, a 'creased' pigmentation on the neck. Lesions localized to the eyebrows and perinasal area are usually due to **seborrhoeic dermatitis** (p. 853), while those around the eyes or mouth may be a contact dermatitis (p. 852) from cosmetics, cleansers or medicated creams. Fluorinated corticosteroid creams (see Table 13.11), which should never be used on the face, are one

regrettable, avoidable cause or aggravator of **perioral dermatitis** (Plate 3).

Areas of inflammation that flush with heat, foods or stress and that tend to become papular are usually due to **rosacea** (Plate 4 and p. 863). Aggravating factors, e.g. corticosteroids, vasodilators, alcohol, hot drinks and hot sunshine, should be avoided. There is possible confusion between acne (p. 856) and rosacea, but there are no comedones (blackheads) with rosacea. If acne is mild it may be left untreated, but topical antibiotics (*metronidazole* or *tetracycline*) are usually effective. Oral *tetracycline*s, or even a retinoid (p. 835) may be necessary in resistant disease: eye involvement requires specialist management.

Other common causes of facial rashes are seborrhoeic dermatitis and infections, especially in children and teenagers, e.g. **herpes simplex** and **impetigo** (see Chapter 8).

SLE (see Chapter 12) is a potentially serious disease that may present with a butterfly-shaped rash over the cheeks and bridge of the nose, though accompanying symptoms, e.g. arthralgia and fever, are usual. A benign form, **discoid lupus**, causes more limited, well-defined, erythematous plaques on the cheeks.

Scaly rashes. An approach to the identification of scaly rashes is outlined in Table 13.4. Serious problems may arise for the patient if large areas of skin are affected moderately or severely, because temperature and water regulation mechanisms may then be impaired. In severe cases this may lead to hypothermia and dehydration.

Acute generalized rashes. It is to be hoped that patients with lesions of this type (Table 13.5) will consult their doctors promptly. However, patients are frequently reluctant to do this or fail to realize the severity of their condition.

Generalized rashes, especially in childhood, are often caused by infections, when there will be associated systemic symptoms, e.g. sore throat, fever, aches and joint pains, possibly with a history of recent case contact. **Guttate psoriasis** (p. 840), with widespread small lesions, may also be triggered by mild infections, especially sore throats.

Table 13.5   Some causes of acute generalized rashes

Cause	Examples
Infections	Measles (rubeola), German measles (rubella), chickenpox (varicella), glandular fever (infectious mononucleosis)
Drugs	Antibiotics (especially penicillins), antirheumatics (e.g. gold), antithyroids, diuretics, morphine-type alkaloids, oral hypoglycaemic agents, psychotropics
Purpura[a]	Drugs, clotting defects, infections
Psoriasis	Following sore throats; relapse of psoriasis after corticosteroid treatment
Autoimmunity	Blistering rashes, e.g. pemphigus, bullous pemphigoid

[a] A rash due to bleeding into the skin (see text).

Erythroderma (widespread inflammation of the skin) may occur as a complication of eczema and psoriasis. Nearly the whole skin becomes dry, dusky red and there is profuse scaling, hence the term '**exfoliative dermatitis**', accompanied by pitting oedema (see Chapters 4 and 14) and grossly enlarged lymph nodes. The increased blood flow through the skin stresses the heart and this extra load may precipitate heart failure (see Chapter 4). Temperature regulation is compromised and patients may become seriously hypothermic. Further, gut function is impaired, due to diversion of blood from the intestines, and may cause malabsorption (see Chapter 3). The condition occurs mostly in males and in the elderly, and is potentially life-threatening. If it occurs without a prior skin disease, a search must be made for possible underlying disease, e.g. HIV infection or neoplastic disease (lymphoma or leukaemia).

Localized lesions
The diagnosis of these should always be approached carefully because, although the majority are benign, they are occasionally malignant, especially in older patients and if they are isolated. The most common cutaneous malignancy is the **basal cell carcinoma** (BCC, Plate 5), which is much more common in fair-skinned races, especially if there has been prolonged skin exposure in sunny climates. Patients often regard the lesion as a minor, benign 'sore', but must be strongly encouraged to see their doctor as soon as

possible, without alarming them unduly, because they metastasize late and early treatment carries an excellent prognosis, whereas delay can lead to severe damage to underlying tissues.

Moles and **warts** are common and are usually recognized readily, but any change in them should be regarded very seriously. If there is any doubt about the nature of an isolated lesion, prompt medical referral without causing undue alarm is mandatory, though patients are often reluctant to see their doctors. The characteristics of some localized lesions are given in Table 13.3.

Special signs
Koebner's sign is the occurrence of lesions along the track of a skin injury, e.g. a scratch, sunburn or chickenpox lesions, and may be a feature of psoriasis, lichen planus or warts.

Nikolsky's sign is the easy separation of apparently normal epidermis from the dermis by pinching or rubbing. It occurs in **pemphigus vulgaris**, a blistering disease in which there is a loss of cohesion of the more superficial epidermal cells, though the basal layer remains attached to the dermis.

Investigation

Patch tests for contact dermatitis are done by sticking a strip of a non-allergenic carrier, impregnated at intervals with solutions or gels of different suspected compounds, to a patient's back or arm and observing the occurrence of a reaction after 48 h (Figure 13.4). Such reactions may persist for 4–7 days. **Prick (scratch) tests** may occasionally be used to identify systemic allergens in atopic subjects, though such procedures carry the risk of severe generalized reactions and should only be carried out where full resuscitation facilities are available.

Other tests include microscopical examination of skin, hair and nails, or scrapings from the bases of vesicles; blood counts and pathogen culture, serology, etc., the biopsy of chronic lesions, especially if there is a possible malignancy and inspection under Wood's light (365 nm UV), to observe hair fluorescence in some types of **tinea**.

The **radioallergosorbent test** (RAST, see Chapter 5, Figure 5.16) is used to determine the presence and titre of reaginic antibodies (IgE; see Chapter 2) when investigating atopic conditions, e.g. dermatitis and urticaria.

Various techniques of **ultrasonography**, which provide a two-dimensional picture through the skin, are now being used in specialized units.

The skin and systemic disease

The association of skin lesions with systemic symptoms may indicate the presence of severe underlying disease and must always be taken seriously. Conditions in this group include thyroid and kidney diseases, renal failure, diabetes mellitus, hyperlipidaemias and malignancies (Table 13.6).

Common associated systemic features include general malaise, muscle weakness, joint pains, fever and weight loss. The dermatological features that may be warning signs of serious disease include the following:

- Acute onset, especially over 50 years of age, e.g. cancer, etc.
- Progressive symptoms, e.g. cancer, chronic diseases.
- Blistering and widespread urticaria.
- Erosion of tissue, e.g. venous ('varicose') ulcers, cancer.
- Generalized itching, unrelated to local lesions, in liver and renal disease.

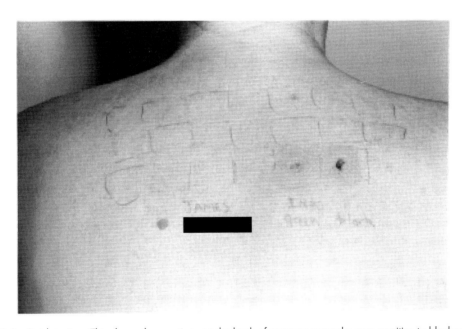

Figure 13.4   Patch testing. This shows the reactions on the back of a young man who was sensitive to black and green printing inks. Reproduced with permission Dr J J R Almeyda, Enfield Health District, London, UK.

Table 13.6   Some dermatological manifestations of systemic disease[a]

Disease	Clinical features
Hyperthyroidism	Hyperhidrosis (sweating); pruritus; production of fine scalp hair, occasional alopecia; pretibial myxoedema (raised red nodules on the legs, often associated with successful treatment for hyperthyroidism)
Hypothyroidism	Coarse, broken scalp hair; hair loss; pruritus; dry skin
Renal disease	Pruritus (due to uraemia); erythema multiforme
Diabetes mellitus	Pruritus; bacterial and fungal skin infections, especially boils; granuloma annulare; necrobiosis lipoidica (firm reddish-yellow skin plaques, which may precede the onset of diabetes); leg ulcers, consequent on diabetic ischaemia and glucose-promoted infection
Cushing's syndrome	Acne vulgaris; hirsutism; striae (stretch marks due to corticosteroid-induced thinning and weakening of dermal and SC tissue)
Addison's disease	Increased pigmentation of gums, new scars and palmar creases
Gastrointestinal disease	Perianal ulceration and pyoderma gangrenosum (with Crohn's disease, liver disease, some blood malignancies); malabsorption; dermatitis herpetiformis (with gluten enteropathy)
Musculoskeletal disease	Rheumatoid arthritis, systemic lupus erythematosus
Hyperlipidaemias	Xanthomata; xanthelasma (see text)
Hepatic porphyria	Photosensitivity; hyperpigmentaion; hypertrichosis; blistering
Graft vs host disease	Widespread rashes (papular, epidermal necrosis and sloughing)
Neoplastic disease	Lymphomas: pruritus, urticaria, herpes zoster, exfoliative dermatitis, ichthyosis (thickening of the skin) Leukaemias: purpura, blistering, ulceration, pruritus, herpes zoster Carcinoid syndrome: flushing Various: skin nodules, adult dermatomyositis

[a] See text and Plates 6 and 7 for further detail.

- Recurrent boils (diabetes mellitus).
- Xanthomas (yellowish plaques of cholesterol deposition, often around the elbows and knees, indicative of hyperlipidaemias; see Chapter 4), especially in young adults. When these occur around the eyelids, usually in middle-aged patients, the condition is known as xanthelasma (Plate 6).

A widespread rash following treatment of a sore throat with *ampicillin* is virtually pathognomonic for glandular fever. **Purpuras** are rashes due to bleeding into the skin and always require urgent medical referral. They may be distinguished from rashes that are inflammatory in origin because they do not blanch under pressure: a clear plastic spatula or a drinking glass pressed onto the skin compresses dilated blood vessels and so causes temporary blanching of inflammatory rashes but not of purpuric ones. Purpuras may be caused by allergic reactions to drugs, resulting in platelet destruction and clotting failure (Plate 7; Chapter 11), to other clotting or vascular defects (Chapter 11), or to infection, e.g. meningococcal meningitis. Because drugs are a common cause, a medication history may give important clues.

General management of skin diseases

Basic approach

There are two essential considerations:

- Reassurance of the patient and the reduction of anxiety (see above).
- Avoidance of actual or potential irritants and precipitants.

The range of the latter is very wide and includes soaps, detergents, cosmetics, perfumes, clothing, foods, plastics, rubber, metals (jewellery), lubricating oils, cement, drugs, components of vehicle bases of medicaments, etc. This important aspect requires considerable detailed attention.

An example of the problems involved is provided by the use of rubber gloves: they often do not give adequate protection and are prone to leakage and internal contamination, causing contact dermatitis. If rubber gloves are used, they should be disposable or they should be turned inside out, washed and dried to remove contaminants, preferably after each occasion of use. Further, plasticizers and other additives in glove materials may cause similar trouble, and extensive trials of different manufacturers' gloves may be needed to find an acceptable brand for an individual. It may also be necessary to wear cotton gloves inside the rubber gloves. These problems affect professionals, e.g. doctors, dentists, pharmacists working in production units handling cytotoxic drugs and making additions to IV infusions, as well as housewives and kitchen workers. When handling cytotoxic drugs there is the additional problem of drug penetration through the gloves.

Intensity of treatment

There is a considerable danger of over-treatment and the application of medicaments that are known to have serious potential side-effects, e.g. potent corticosteroid creams and ointments (Table 13.11). Products may contain unsuspected allergens, e.g. the drug itself, lanolin, antiseptics or antioxidants, and may aggravate the original condition or add further problems. If the condition deteriorates while using a product of known effectiveness against it, an adverse reaction should always be suspected, rather than drug resistance. Further, excessively frequent or vigorous application of medicaments, or their removal from damaged skin, may further harm sensitive areas. Minimal treatment with the simplest and mildest effective product should be the rule.

There are five basic target groups of conditions, for each of which a different degree of intervention is appropriate:

- Lesions from which the skin will usually recover spontaneously with minimal intervention, e.g. contact dermatitis, many occupational skin diseases, mild acne.
- Conditions which require protection of the skin by the application of emollients, barrier creams or 'inert' preparations, e.g. mild nappy rash.
- Conditions which will respond to active treatment, e.g. psoriasis, acne and eczema.
- Infections and infestations which require specific antimicrobial or antiparasitic treatment, e.g. impetigo and scabies.
- Those conditions in which little can be done currently to influence their course, e.g. cutaneous scleroderma.

Medical management is essential in the following situations:

- Lesions affecting more than 10% of the body surface area (BSA; see Table 13.7).
- Conditions with associated systemic features.
- Progressive lesions, increasing in severity or size.
- Ulcerating lesions or those that are breaking down centrally.
- Pigmented lesions, other than static ones which are clearly warts or moles.
- Any lesion which has recently changed in character.
- Conditions in which there is a significant inflammatory component.
- Blistering lesions, unless they are known to be due to a minimal insult, e.g. an insect bite, and the patient is otherwise well.
- Conditions which markedly interfere with the patient's lifestyle or occupation.

Table 13.7 Fractions of the body surface area[a] and the approximate amounts of topical product required for application to them

Part of body	Fraction of BSA (%)[a]	Weight[b] for 1 week	Part of body	Number of fingertip units[c]
Scalp (hair)	4	15	Face and neck	2.5
Face	4	15	Arm and forearm	3
Each arm	9	30	Hand	1
Each hand	1	4	Leg and thigh	6
Each leg	18	60	Front of trunk	7
Chest plus abdomen	18	60	Back of trunk	7
Whole of back	18	60	Foot	2
Genitalia	1	4		

[a] BSA, body surface area, approximate figures.

[b] Approximate weight of product (g) required to cover the body part, when applied by a trained operator or patient, assuming two applications per day. The approximate maximum 'safe' weekly doses of topical corticosteroids (p. 832) are as follows: moderate/mild potency (see Table 13.11), 50 g; potent, about 30 g; very potent, about 15 g. Use of a high-potency steroid (Group I) for more than 7 days should be undertaken only under the supervision of an experienced dermatologist.

[c] One 'fingertip unit' (FTU) is 'the amount of ointment expressed from a tube with a 5 mm diameter nozzle applied from the distal skin crease to the tip of the index finger.' (Long CC, Finlay AY, *Clin Exp Dermatol* 1991; **16**: 444–447.) Figures in the table are expressed to the nearest half-unit. One FTU covers approximately 312 cm^2 (adult males) and 257 cm^2 (adult females) and is roughly 0.5 g. The hand area (fingers closed) represents 0.76% of the BSA in men and 0.70% in women (Long CC, Finlay AY, *BMJ* 1996; **313**: 690).

Note: The information on the left-hand side of the table does not read across to that on the right-hand side.

• Any unidentified lesion which arises acutely in the middle-aged or elderly.

Selection of treatment

Clinical features

Clearly the choice of treatment will depend on:

• The nature, extent and severity of the lesions.
• Whether they are visible and consequently cause the patient considerable anxiety.
• The duration and progression of the condition.
• What is known about the natural history of the condition, i.e. whether it is likely to remit or to have serious sequelae.
• Patient preference, e.g. for a particular formulation or type of emollient.

The patient's perception of their condition is important because steps must be taken to relieve their distress, even though it may be known that the disease is benign and self-limiting: a holistic approach is required.

The general treatment of target symptoms is outlined in Table 13.8.

Type and amount of product

There is sometimes confusion as to whether to use ointments or creams, but the simple rule is 'wet on wet, dry on dry'. Thus oil-in-water (o/w) creams are usually used on moist lesions (ointments will not stick anyway), and ointments or w/o creams on dry or scaly lesions, which also aid skin rehydration. This may need to be modified according to patient acceptability and the site, e.g. lotions and gels are usually preferred on the scalp.

Table 13.7 gives an indication of the proportion of the BSA represented by various parts of the body, and the approximate amounts of product required for treatment. However, the amounts used, even by specially trained dermatology nurses, may vary considerably. A simpler

Table 13.8   The general treatment of dermatological target symptoms

Target symptom	Type of treatment	Examples
Dryness	Hydration	Ointments, oily creams, occlusive dressings
	Emollients	Aqueous cream, emulsifying ointment
Exudation	Astringents	Aluminium or zinc salts, potassium permanganate
		Wet dressings
	Absorption of exudations	Pastes, cellulose/pectin gel, impregnated bandages
	Prevention of adhesion	Paraffin gauze and other non-adherent dressings
Local heat	Cooling	Wet dressings, especially alcoholic solutions, calamine lotion (possibly); cooling is by evaporation
Tenderness	Emollients	Aqueous cream; barrier products, e.g. dimeticone creams
	Lotions, creams	Calamine (?)
Irritation/itch (pruritus)[a]	Antipruritic	Astringent lotions, calamine products (?), crotamiton, local anaesthetics[b], local or oral antihistamines[b]
Infection	Antimicrobials	Imidazoles, systemic or topical antibiotics[c]; antivirals, e.g. aciclovir; topical antiseptics, e.g. povidone-iodine, potassium permanganate
Sweating	Astringents	Aluminium salts
Localized lesions	Non-spreading	Stiff ointments and pastes
	Highly localized	Very stiff pastes, e.g. Lassar's paste

[a] Persistent generalized pruritus not associated with rashes should provoke a detailed search for underlying systemic disease, see also Table 13.10.

[b] May cause skin sensitization in some patients.

[c] Topical antibiotics may encourage microbial resistance and cause skin sensitization.

[?] Calamine is of doubtful efficacy and is now little used.

approach is to use the **fingertip unit** of Long and Finlay. Patients using grossly more than the amounts indicated are likely to be using the product excessively.

It is important to remember that virtually any product used in treatment may itself be irritant or allergenic for some patients due to components of the base, additives or medicaments. Even *hydrocortisone* cream has been known to cause rashes. If the condition fails to respond or deteriorates, this may be the result of inappropriate treatment or some component of the medicament.

Targeting symptoms

Dryness

Emollients are invaluable in the management of dry skin conditions, whether they are primary, or secondary to other diseases such as eczema, and are the fundamental basis of dry skin treatment. They leave an oily film that prevents evaporation of water and thus maintains skin hydration: adding external water provides only transient hydration that is lost rapidly.

Emollients may give substantial relief when used alone and will at least reduce the need for potent medication. A useful routine is given below, but this needs to be tailored flexibly to patient preference to achieve the desired result:

- Avoid soaps and household detergents, which may be irritant or allergenic and promote drying by removing the film of natural moisturizing factor (see below).
- Use emulsifying ointment, or aqueous cream or a commercial alternative, to wash and bathe, or a bath oil or gel, as the patient prefers.

Table 13.9   Characteristics[a] of some emollients

Product	Heaviness	Greasiness
Emulsifying ointment	+++	+++
Hydrous ointment	++	+++
Commercial paraffin-based ointments e.g. DiproBase ointment	++	++
Unguentum Merck	+	++
Hydrous ointment	+	++
Arachis oil-based creams[b], e.g. Oilatum	+	++
Urea-based, e.g. Aquadrate	+	++
Calmurid	+	+
E45	+	+
Paraffin-based creams, e.g. DiproBase, Ultrabase	+	+
Bath additives, e.g. Alpha Keri, Balneum, Oilatum Emollient	+	+

[a] The terms 'heaviness' and 'greasiness' are subjective, and are meant to convey how the products feel when applied to the skin. These impressions will differ considerably between patients. (Modified with permission from Graham-Brown R, *Update* 1986; **33**: 539–544.)

[b] May cause severe allergic reactions in sensitive subjects. + → +++, property increases.

- Use a 'light' emollient cream, i.e. relatively non-greasy and readily absorbed (Table 13.9), after bathing or washing, over the entire affected area. However, in dry skin conditions a greasier product ('heavy cream') may be preferable, because it gives better skin hydration, though it is very uncomfortable if large areas of skin are covered with an oily film. If this cannot be tolerated by the patient, a compromise has to be found. Emollients may also relieve skin tenderness.
- A barrier cream (see BNF Section 13.2.2) may be used on the hands before work, but may cause its own problems (p. 827).

The skin produces large quantities of a complex mixture of substances, known collectively as **natural moisturizing factor (NMF)**, which is believed to be intimately involved in the maintenance, repair and hydration of the epidermis. Some inherited dry skin conditions, e.g. ichthyosis, are presumably the result of an inadequate production of NMF. One component of NMF is *sodium pidolate*, a potent humectant used in some commercial emollients.

Pruritus (itching)

Itch is a symptom that is unique to the skin, and may be caused by a variety of diseases and conditions (Table 13.10). The natural response is to scratch the affected site, but this provides only temporary relief and the itch returns, to be followed by more scratching. If this 'itch–scratch–itch cycle' persists, the skin may become lichenified, i.e. thickened and roughened, or even excoriated, i.e. scratched sufficiently to cause bleeding, and the skin may become infected or be permanently damaged.

Topical treatment.   *Aqueous cream* with 1–2% *menthol*, and *physiological saline* are widely used to relieve minor itching, and some commercial bath oils, e.g. Balneum Plus and Dermalo, have antipruritic properties. Lotions may be cooling, protective, astringent and antipruritic and are often used on inflamed and weeping skin. Although previously used widely, *aluminium acetate lotion* and *calamine lotion*, sometimes with *ichthammol*, are now uncommon. *Crotamiton lotion* may be preferred by some patients, although there is little objective evidence of effectiveness. *Coal tar* products may also help to reduce itching. Calamine lotion may be too drying and should not be used for scaling dermatoses, for which the oily preparation is preferable. Calamine preparations are rarely used nowadays, because they are ineffective.

Table 13.10 Some causes of pruritus

Pruritic skin lesions

Dermatitis/eczema
Psoriasis
Drug reactions
Allergic reactions, urticaria
Lichen planus
Parasitic infestations, e.g. lice, scabies
Helminth infections
Viral and fungal dermatoses, e.g. chickenpox
Dermatitis herpetiformis[a]
Psychogenic

Generalized pruritus without skin lesions

Anaemia
Pregnancy
Diabetes mellitus
Thyroid disease
Haematological disease
Anorexia nervosa
Old age
Chronic renal failure
Liver disease
Hodgkin's disease and other neoplasms

Anogenital pruritus

Contact dermatitis, e.g. clothing
Diabetes mellitus
Anal discharge or leakage, faecal soiling
Postmenopausal
Parasitic infestations, e.g. lice, scabies, threadworms
(mostly children)
Psychogenic

[a] See Chapter 3.

Provided that there is no infection, occlusive medicated bandages, e.g. *zinc paste* with *coal tar* or *ichthammol*, covered with stockinette or crepe bandage, can be left in place for a week or more. This helps to break the itch–scratch–itch cycle and so allows the skin to heal. Some of these are particularly easy to remove without damaging the skin.

A cream formulation of the tricyclic antidepressant *doxepin* is licensed for treating pruritus in dermatitis. However, it may cause local discomfort and systemic antimuscarinic effects if it is significantly absorbed, e.g. urinary retention, drowsiness, dry mouth etc. (see Chapter 6).

Systemic treatment. Antihistamines should be given orally as antipruritics and not used topically, because they may cause sensitization. Although many patients use topical antihistamines without any side-effects, the patients who need them most are those most likely to be sensitized by them, so they are preferably avoided.

The sedative antihistamines, e.g. *hydroxyzine*, *promethazine* and *alimemazine*, are preferred, with appropriate warnings about drowsiness, driving, etc., and are especially useful at night, when their sedative effect is beneficial in preventing restlessness and scratching during sleep. A particular advantage of *hydroxyzine* is its anxiolytic action.

Because the antipruritic effect tends to accompany sedation, the newer, non-sedating antihistamines may be less useful for this purpose. However, these effects are relative and non-sedating antihistamines are often used during the day and sedating ones at night. It should be noted that although the newer antihistamines are relatively non-sedating, e.g. *acrivastine, fexofenadine* and *mizolastine* this does not mean that they are safe under all circumstances and they may not be suitable for use in children.

They have antimuscarinic effects and must be used cautiously in patients with prostatic hypertrophy, urinary retention and glaucoma, all of which tend to be common in the elderly. They may also cause severe hypersensitivity reactions. These drugs should be avoided if there is significant hepatic impairment, hypokalaemia or other electrolyte disturbance. Further, many antihistamines must not be used with anti-arrhythmic agents, e.g. *amiodarone, disopyramide, procainamide* and *quinidine*, because serious arrhythmias have occurred (see the BNF and manufacturers' literature). Syncope (fainting) in patients taking these antihistamines may indicate an arrhythmia and should be investigated.

Broken and weeping skin
The best initial treatment is still the traditional astringent, mildly antiseptic, potassium permanganate soaks (1/8000). Unfortunately, the skin

and clothing will be stained brown and some patients find this cosmetically unacceptable. Once the skin starts to heal, other medications can be applied. Alternatively, *physiological saline* soaks may be useful. If the area is infected, systemic antibiotics will be required: like the antihistamines, most topical antibiotics are liable to cause skin sensitization and should be avoided.

Non-adherent dressings should be used if the area needs to be covered, and oily preparations, e.g. compound zinc oxide creams and ointments, are preferred on weeping skin to avoid crusting and the adherence of dressings: this is an exception to the normal 'wet on wet' rule.

There is a large range available of new breathable dressings with good adherence and flexibility. These protect the area, allow oxygen penetration and control moisture loss, so they can be left in place for long periods. They are very useful for incipient pressure sores, though good nursing care will avoid their occurrence.

Routes of administration

Topical treatment

Topical treatments are only of value in superficial (epidermal) dermatoses. If lesions are deep-seated, any agent applied to the surface that reaches the dermis will be removed rapidly in the circulation. Consequently, dermal disorders require systemic therapy.

Although topical corticosteroids have revolutionized the treatment of many skin diseases the older products still have a place in the first-line treatment of mild to moderate disease. Thus *coal tar* products are still used in the management of mild **psoriasis**, e.g. 5% crude *coal tar* in a suitable base, or tar paint (pp. 843–4) and may also be helpful in chronic atopic eczema (p. 852), e.g. 15% *coal tar* solution in emulsifying ointment applied before bathing. However, newer products are more acceptable cosmetically. Commercial products are more elegantly formulated than the equivalent official formulary ones and so are usually more acceptable to patients. A *coal tar + salicylic acid + sulfur + coconut oil* ointment is very useful in treating **scalp psoriasis**, although it is very greasy.

Intertrigo, i.e. dermatitis of the skin folds under the breasts or in the axillae, often macerated and infected with *Candida albicans*, is treated with dry, non-staining antimicrobial agents, e.g. an imidazole gel, which are preferable and more acceptable cosmetically than creams. The site is occluded by the opposing skin folds, so it may be necessary to separate infected skin folds with an antimicrobial-impregnated dressing, to promote healing. Care must be taken that patients are not sensitive to the products, notably iodine, because patients with skin problems tend to be more liable to develop skin sensitization than the general population. In all situations, the simplest treatments are best and safest, especially if there is any doubt.

Systemic treatment

This may be required in a variety of situations:

- If there are associated systemic symptoms, e.g. psoriatic arthropathy.
- To control serious conditions, e.g. erythroderma (p. 824) and angioedema (a severe urticarial reaction; p. 864).
- When local treatment might cause skin sensitization, e.g. antibiotics or antihistamines.
- When topical treatment is ineffective or inappropriate, e.g. the use of systemic cytotoxic drugs, corticosteroids, antibiotics and some retinoids.

Corticosteroids

Topical corticosteroids are widely used in dermatology. This merits special consideration because their indications, cautions, side-effects, etc. differ in important respects from those experienced with systemic corticosteroid use.

Topical use

Selection

This depends primarily on four considerations:

- The severity of the condition: clearly, the more severe the damage the greater the potency needed, but this must be tempered by the knowledge that the greater the damage or inflammation, the greater will be the systemic absorption through that site.

- The site of application: sites particularly sensitive to their side-effects are the axillae, under the breasts, behind the ears and the genital area, i.e. wherever there are skin folds and delicate skin. It should be clear that greater care needs to be exercised if the face or other exposed areas are to be treated, because any side-effects (see below) will then be obvious and very important to the patient.
- The nature of the condition, e.g. they are contra-indicated in rosacea, perioral dermatitis and untreated bacterial, fungal and viral infections, because they are likely to be exacerbated.
- Patient characteristics, e.g. the very young and very old.

Potency

These products are classified in the BNF into four different potency groups (Table 13.11). However, this classification must be regarded as approximate because formulation has a considerable influence on potency. Further, percutaneous absorption will be greater with a more extensive area of application, a greater degree of skin inflammation and with occlusion of the site.

The concentration of drug used will influence the relative potency. Prescribers frequently order dilutions of commercial products, but the advantages of this are questionable, because it should be possible to choose a properly formulated product of lower potency. Further, extemporaneous dilution has several disadvantages: the product is no longer sterile, it may not be adequately preserved, and injudicious manipulation may impair the

Table 13.11   The approximate potencies of some topical corticosteroids[a]

Corticosteroid	Concentration (%, w/w)	Corticosteroid	Concentration (%, w/w)
Very potent			
Clobetasol propionate	0.05	Halcinonide	0.1
Diflucortolone valerate[b]	0.3		
Potent			
Beclometasone dipropionate[b]	0.025–0.05	Fluprednidene acetate[c]	0.1
Betamethasone valerate[b]	0.1	Fluticasone propionate	0.005–0.05
Desoximetasone[b]	0.25	Hydrocortisone butyrate	0.1
Diflucortolone valerate[b]	0.1	Mometasone furoate	0.1
Fluocinonide	0.05	Triamcinolone acetonide[d]	0.1
Fluocinolone acetonide[b]	0.025		
Moderate potency			
Alclometasone dipropionate	0.05	Fluocinolone acetonide	0.00625
Betamethasone valerate	0.025	Fluocortolone and esters	0.25
Clobetasone butyrate	0.05	Fludroxycortide	0.0125
Desoximetasone	0.05	Hydrocortisone with urea[e]	1.0
Mild potency			
Fluocinolone acetonide	0.0025	Hydrocortisone base/acetate[f]	0.1–2.5

[a] Based on the BNF classification.

[b] Potency depends on concentration; lower concentrations may be in moderate/mild groups.

[c] Available only with miconazole as an antifungal agent.

[d] Available only with antimicrobial agents.

[e] Different formulations may vary widely in potency.

[f] Includes all products containing an antimicrobial agent.

uniformity of a carefully formulated and manu-factured product. For example, some potent corticosteroid ointments are dispersions of a *propylene glycol* solution of drug in the base, and excessive manipulation or warming of the product may cause the dispersed droplets to coalesce. A non-uniform product results, even though the correct diluent is used.

Side-effects

These will vary with the potency, the amount applied, the area covered, frequency of applica-tion and whether the site is inflamed, occluded or particularly sensitive. Side-effects may be local or systemic and are often related to the cytostatic properties of steroids. Repeated application of potent steroids leads to wasting of SC tissue, due to inhibition of fibroblast maturation and conse-quent failure of collagen repair in the dermis, similar to what happens in the normal ageing process. This results in thinning of the skin and **telangiectasis**, i.e. a reddening resulting from the disclosure and expansion of the small blood vessels in the dermis, because they are no longer adequately supported (Plate 16). If this effect is severe, the larger vessels will also become promi-nent and the capillaries will become fragile, so that minor trauma leads to substantial bruising (**ecchymosis**). A similar underlying process may also produce **striae**, permanent disfiguring stretch marks as the dermis and SC tissues lose elasticity.

Suppression of local non-specific defence mechanisms (see Chapter 2) by corticosteroids may occur due to inhibition of macrophage and neutrophil activity, resulting in delayed healing and the aggravation of skin infections, notably herpes simplex. Topical corticosteroids are therefore contra-indicated if there is any suspi-cion of bacterial, viral or fungal infection unless formulated or used with an effective antimicro-bial agent. The combination of their cytostatic effects and the suppression of local defence mechanisms means that they are usually contra-indicated for the management of skin ulcers, because they may delay healing and promote infection.

Use of the more potent synthetic steroids may result in local erythema, contact dermatitis (Plate 12) and perioral dermatitis (Plate 3). It is not clear whether the latter condition is due to a true sensitivity to the drug, whether the steroid triggers a latent erythematous tendency or is a variant of rosacea (p. 863). Corticosteroids will aggravate rosacea and, being comedogenic, may exacerbate acne (p. 856). Mild skin depigmenta-tion may also occur, due to depressed melanocyte activity.

Systemic absorption may be significant, depending on the factors mentioned above. Thin skin areas, e.g. behind the ears, and the genitalia, hairy areas and inflamed and damaged skin permit greater drug penetration than normal skin. Occlusion of a treated area, by folds of skin or dressings also enhances pene-tration. The potent and very potent products (see Table 13.11) are all capable of producing significant percutaneous **adrenal suppression**, so they must be used with great care, especially in children, whose skin is thinner and whose surface area to body weight ratio is greater than that of adults. Absorbed steroid may also cause some degree of **immunosuppression** due to inhibition of lymphocyte multiplication and maturation.

Patients must therefore be counselled carefully on how to use these products, the major criteria being that they are applied sparingly to the specific lesions and usually not massaged into the skin or occluded. The approximate amounts of products needed for application to various parts of the body are given in Table 13.7. Patients must also be warned that these products are prescribed for treatment of the condition presented, and must not be hoarded to use as panaceas for all skin ailments, or loaned to friends or relatives.

Both patients and some prescribers are wary of steroid use, so that the preparations used may be too weak to control symptoms adequately. A short burst of a potent agent is usually quite safe: it will often be more effective, and safer in the long run, to control symptoms rapidly with a potent agent and then reduce the potency, rather than to titrate the dose upwards.

Precisely placed **intralesional injections** of poorly soluble forms may be more effective than potent topical products for severe localized lesions, e.g. keloid scars (fibrous, raised and enlarging).

Systemic use

The best estimate of oral corticosteroid usage in the UK is that there are about 250 000 patients, taking an average of 8 mg/day of *prednisolone*, though most of this is not dermatological. Most users are in the 60- to 80-year age group.

In dermatological practice, systemic steroids are indicated only for severe dermatoses. The normal rules for steroid therapy should be followed, i.e. the minimum dose needed to control the condition should be used, and this should be reduced as rapidly as possible on a sliding scale to the minimum maintenance dose required, preferably nil. However, daily doses of *prednisolone* <7.5 mg, or the equivalent of other products, are unlikely to produce significant adrenal suppression and other major side-effects in adults. If adrenal suppression does occur during long-term therapy it may be prolonged after the cessation of treatment, so corticosteroids must never be withdrawn abruptly after 3 weeks or more of continuous use. Because the physiological demand for corticosteroid is increased in stressful situations, e.g. serious illness, accidents and major surgery, the dose needs to be increased in these circumstances. Patients using long-term corticosteroids need to learn how to manage their dose in these conditions.

Injudicious use of corticosteroids may permanently stunt children's growth. At the other end of life, perimenopausal and postmenopausal women, and some elderly men, are at risk of osteoporosis, the physiological bone loss being increased in proportion to the cumulative dose of corticosteroid. This may lead to peripheral bone fractures following falls, particularly of the neck of femur and wrist, and vertebral crush fractures. Only about 14% of patients receive preventative treatment, which should be based on bone density measurement. In postmenopausal women, hormone replacement therapy (HRT) manages the symptoms of the climacteric as well as the osteoporosis, but has fallen out of favour because of the associated cancer risk. Otherwise, the best strategy is to ensure an adequate calcium intake (about 1.5 g/day), with vitamin D if sun exposure is limited, plus a bisphosphonate, e.g. *alendronate*, cyclical *etidronate* or *strontium ranelate*.

In the occasional very frail elderly patient, an **anabolic steroid**, e.g. *nandrolone*, may be appropriate because it has beneficial effects on both bone density and muscle, but has many side-effects and the deep IM injection of its oily solution may be poorly tolerated.

Retinoids

These compounds are related chemically to vitamin A (retinol). The vitamin derived from natural sources is a mixture of isomers of which the most active is all-trans-retinol, the form produced synthetically.

Retinol is essential for normal skin formation and keratinization and for proper cell maturation and differentiation generally. However, it has only a moderate activity and an unfavourable therapeutic ratio, high doses causing serious side-effects on the skin, mucous membranes, liver and CNS. The synthetic retinoids are more potent and have a better therapeutic ratio, though they are still rather toxic compounds with an extensive list of side-effects (Table 13.12). Synthetic retinoids should be used only if there are adequate haematological, hepatic and other monitoring facilities available.

The more recently developed 'second-generation' compounds, e.g. *acitretin*, tend to have less serious side-effects, especially neurological and hepatic. 'Third-generation' polyaromatic agents, the arotinoids, e.g. *arotinoid ethyl ester*, are some 100–1000 times as potent, but none of these is yet available.

Mode of action

Retinoids bind to inducible nuclear retinoic acid receptors (RARs; vitamin A receptors) that interact with the promoter regions of specific nuclear genes that control the maturation and development of a variety of tissue cells and so regulate their transcription. Three types of RAR are known, only two of which (RAR-alpha, RAR-gamma) are expressed in human skin. RAR-alpha is present primarily in the basal layer, and its concentration declines progressively as the cells migrate towards the surface. Conversely,

Table 13.12   Some side-effects and contra-indications of systemic retinoids[a]

Tissue or organ affected	Side-effect
Mucous membranes	Dryness and cracking of lips, dryness of mouth, nasal bleeding, hoarseness
Skin	Dryness and hyperfragility, especially palms and soles; dermatitis; erythema; pruritus; shiny, smooth, 'sticky' (sweaty) skin; hyperpigmentation; photosensitivity; exacerbation of acne
Hair	Diffuse alopecia (mild)
Nails	Thinning, fragility, paronychia
Eyes	Dryness, irritation, pain, conjunctivitis, abnormal night vision, colour blindness (expert referral required)
Hyperlipidaemia[b]	LDLs increased, especially VLDL and triglycerides; HDL cholesterol decreased
Musculoskeletal	Bone abnormalities in children (not suitable for prolonged treatment), arthralgia, myalgia
Liver	Acute hepatitis
CNS (occasionally)	Nausea; headache; malaise; drowsiness Possibly irreversible depression, suicidal thoughts, anxiety, aggression (rare, expert referral required)

Contra-indications

Pregnancy, breastfeeding (absolute contraindications)
Hepatic or renal impairment
Hyperlipidaemia
Avoid vitamin A supplementation, UV radiation, excessive exposure to sunlight

[a] See also the BNF and manufacturer's literature
[b] (V)LDL/HDL, (very) low-density/high-density lipoproteins.

RAR-gamma predominates in the granular layer. Binding of retinoids to these RARs produces specific actions on keratinocyte differentiation.

They also possess antiproliferative and anti-inflammatory actions. They thus have four therapeutic actions:

- Promotion of normal keratinocyte differentiation in the epidermis.
- Blockade of excessive cell proliferation and epidermal growth by down-regulation of ornithine decarboxylase, which is involved in hyperplasia and hyperproliferation.
- Suppression of excessive sebum production.
- Anti-inflammatory, due to inhibition of PG synthesis and the consequent production of pro-inflammatory agents, e.g. HLA-DR and lipoxygenase products and interleukin-6, and modification of both humoral and cellular immune responses.

Apart from their effects on the epidermis, these drugs have powerful effects on general cell maturation. In acute promyelocytic leukaemia (see Chapter 10) there is a failure of promyelocytes to differentiate into mature granulocytes. *Tretinoin* and other retinoids cause dose-dependent rapid maturation of these immature cells and may be used as maintenance treatment following cytotoxic chemotherapy to induce remission.

Pharmacokinetics

The retinoids are lipophilic and have a relatively low oral bioavailability, so oral dosage forms should be taken with meals to enhance absorption. The currently available compounds cross the placenta and are highly teratogenic. They are excreted in breast milk and cause skeletal abnormalities in breastfed infants.

Etretinate is a highly lipophilic aromatic retinoid. There is a large interpatient variation in bioavailability after oral use and it has a very long persistence because it is stored in body fat. The effective terminal half-life ($t_{1/2}$) is about 90 days. Although the blood levels of *etretinate* after stopping are therapeutically inadequate, they may still be teratogenic: it is detectable in plasma up to 2–3 years after chronic dosing has ceased. *Acitretin*, a metabolite of *etretinate*, has a $t_{1/2}$ of only 2 days and does not accumulate in the tissues. However, because it is esterified to *etretinate* in the liver this benefit is partly nullified.

Isotretinoin is an isomer of *tretinoin*, the acid form of vitamin A, and has a bioavailability of about 25% following oral administration. Peak blood levels are reached in 1–4 h and the elimination $t_{1/2}$ following chronic dosing is of the order of 10–20 h, steady-state blood levels being reached in 3–4 days. Its major active metabolite, 4-oxo-isotretinoin, has a similar terminal $t_{1/2}$ because its formation is rate limited. The shorter $t_{1/2}$ of *isotretinoin* makes it safer than *etretinate*.

Acitretin and *isotretinoin* should be used systemically only under the supervision of a consultant dermatologist. Prescribing of *acitretin* is limited to consultants and it is available to hospital and named community pharmacies only.

Tazarotene is an esterified prodrug of the active agent, tazarotenic acid, to which it is hydrolysed in the skin. Although used topically, it penetrates skin significantly. In short-term topical use the $t_{1/2}$ is about 18 h. End metabolism of tazarotenic acid yields inactive compounds and appears to be autoinducible: peak plasma levels after 3 months are about 10% of those seen after 13 days.

In the epidermis, all of these compounds bind to both RAR-alpha and RAR-gamma. Vitamin A is transported in the blood by a specific retinol binding protein (RBP). *Isotretinoin* is almost completely protein-bound, but to serum albumin and not to RBP.

The potent aromatic retinoid, etretin, is a major metabolite of *etretinate* and has interesting pharmacokinetics. Although its terminal $t_{1/2}$ is about 50 h, so that it persists as long as *etretinate*, isomerization to its inactive cis-analogue occurs readily. Thus it is very unstable and very difficult to formulate, and aromatic retinoids have not yet produced useful therapeutic agents.

Adapalene is a synthetic polycyclic, lipophilic retinoid derived from naphthoic acid. Although structurally unrelated to other current retinoids, *adapalene* is somewhat similar in structure to the arotinoids, and is very stable. It binds preferentially to epidermal RAR-gamma and, because skin penetration is very low, it is undetectable in plasma, urine and faeces.

Indications

The retinoids are a potent and interesting group of drugs with great potential. Although there are currently only a few licensed indications, they are known to have beneficial effects in other diseases (Table 13.13) and there are many more for which there is evidence of potential benefit. Further development of this group of drugs may have a profound influence on our understanding of skin diseases and their treatment and of cell maturation processes in general.

Acne. *Tretinoin* and *isotretinoin* are used topically for all grades. *Isotretinoin* is licensed for the treatment of both inflammatory and non-inflammatory lesions. *Adapalene* is a topical treatment for mild to moderate acne. Oral *isotretinoin* is used for severe, refractory disease.

Psoriasis. *Tazarotene* is used topically to treat mild to moderate disease limited in area. *Acitretin* is used orally for the treatment of severe, resistant or complicated psoriasis and for some other disorders of keratinization.

Photodamage. Topical *tretinoin* gives slow improvement over 3–4 months of hyper-pigmented, wrinkled skin caused by chronic excessive sun exposure.

Table 13.13   Some indications for the use of retinoids[a]

Licensed indications[b]

Moderate to severe acne
Psoriasis (all forms)
Congenital disorders of keratinization
Photodamaged skin, including hyperpigmentation
Induction of remission in acute promyelocytic leukaemia

Indications for which benefit has been demonstrated

Rosacea
Hydradenitis suppurativa (inflammation of abnormal sweat glands)
Lichen planus
Neoplastic skin diseases: basal cell carcinoma, squamous cell carcinoma, chemoprophylaxis of skin cancer in predisposed patients

Potential indications

Chronic discoid lupus erythematosus
Pemphigus (an autoimmune blistering disorder)
Cutaneous manifestations of Reiter's syndrome
Generalized granuloma annulare
Cutaneous sarcoidosis (a chronic, granulomatous disease)
Basal cell carcinoma

[a] Modified from David M, Hodak E, Lowe NJ, Med Toxicol 1988; 3: 273–288, and others.
[b] Licensed in the UK.

Other uses.   Because of toxicity, oral *tretinoin* is no longer used for the treatment of psoriasis that, although disfiguring, is rarely life-threatening. However, it is used as a first-line treatment to induce remission in acute promyelocytic leukaemia, after relapse and in resistance to standard chemotherapy. Low-dose *acitretin* has also been reported to reduce skin cancer incidence in renal transplant patients who are on long-term immunosuppressive treatment.

Further details relevant to specific treatment are discussed under the diseases concerned.

The side-effects are dealt with Table 13.12.

Psoriasis

Psoriasis is a hereditary chronic skin disorder, usually characterized by scaly plaques or papules, and often distributed on areas exposed to frequent minor trauma.

Pathology

Psoriasis is characterized by increased turnover of the basal skin cells. Their doubling time is reduced from some 20–30 days to about 2–3 days, and there is an increased growth fraction (see Chapter 10). Further, the three lowest layers of the epidermis are involved in cell germination instead of the normal, single basal layer. Because the resultant cell production considerably exceeds the rate of cell differentiation, the epidermis is thickened (Figure 13.5) and nucleated cells are present throughout the entire thickness, i.e. the normal granular layer is absent. Even the horny layer contains cells with degenerate nuclei instead of being composed of amorphous keratin.

This increased metabolism causes a full-thickness inflammation of the skin. There is infiltration of neutrophils and activated lymphocytes that release growth-stimulating cytokines. Dilated, tortuous capillaries are present high in the dermis and these occur even in the apparently normal skin of patients with psoriasis.

Psoriatic arthropathy (Plate 8) is the consequence of a synovitis that, though very similar to that of RA (see Chapter 12), is believed to be a distinct entity. The condition affects about 7% of patients with psoriasis.

One current theory is that there is an inherited defect of keratinization resulting in abnormal keratinocyte surface antigens. If immunocytes encounter these, e.g. following minor skin trauma, an immunological response is triggered, with consequent stimulation of the basal layer. This is supported by the finding that initiation of psoriasis is accompanied by an influx of CD4+ (helper) T cells into lesions (see Chapter 2). Further, CD8+ T cells (cytotoxic) are responsible for the maintenance of lesions. It has also been suggested that there are genetically abnormal

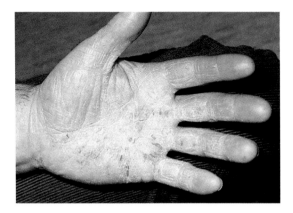

Plate 1 Contact dermatitis. The hands are a common site because they are exposed to a wide range of potential irritants, e.g. detergents and lubricating oils.

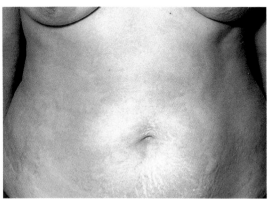

Plate 2 Urticaria. This is a very florid reaction. The raised, itchy weals are surrounded by areas of inflammation. The cause of this reaction was never determined, but common causes are medicines, food additives, animals and plants.

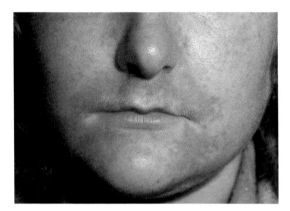

Plate 3 Perioral dermatitis. Note the sparing of the skin immediately around the lips. This reaction was due to a synthetic steroid used to treat an initial reaction caused by cosmetics.

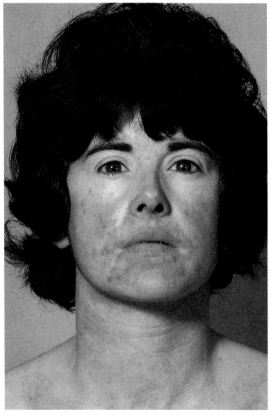

Plate 4 Rosacea. The rash is usually milder and more localized than in this patient. This florid reaction was the result of aggravation by a steroid cream.

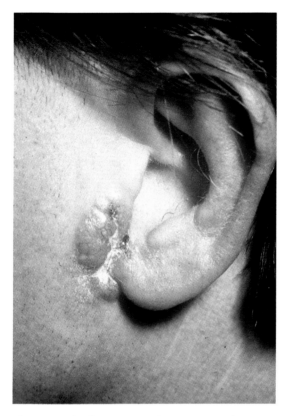

Plate 5 Basal cell carcinoma. This is in a typical site, i.e. areas exposed to sunlight. Note the raised, pearly margin, with veins coursing over the surface. Small lesions are uniform but central ulceration may develop with enlargement, as in this example. This patient is rather young, lesions being uncommon under age 40 years.

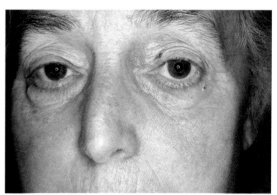

Plate 6 Xanthelasma. Note the large yellowish plaques (cholesterol deposits) on both upper eyelids near the nose and the smaller plaques elsewhere.

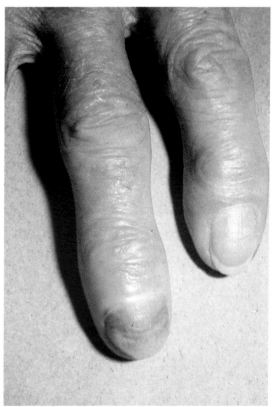

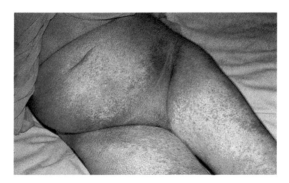

Plate 7 Purpura. This is a florid example of Henoch-Schoenlein purpura, an anaphylactoid reaction often due to medicines or following streptococcal throat infection. In this case, a woman known to be penicillin sensitive took some of her bronchitic husband's amoxicillin capsules.

Plate 8 Psoriatic nails and finger joint arthropathy. Note the pitting, darkening and separation (onycholysis) of one nail. The terminal (DIP) joints are inflamed, swollen and painful whereas they are normally spared in rheumatoid arthritis (see Chapter 8, p. 482).

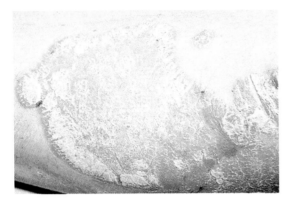

Plate 9 Plaque psoriasis. Note the raised margin and heavy scaling on a pinkish-red ground.

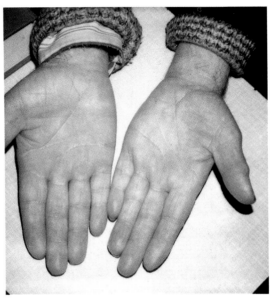

Plate 11 Hyperlinearity of the palms. This is a mild contact dermatitis reaction. Subjects with this sort of skin are particularly liable to react badly to irritants.

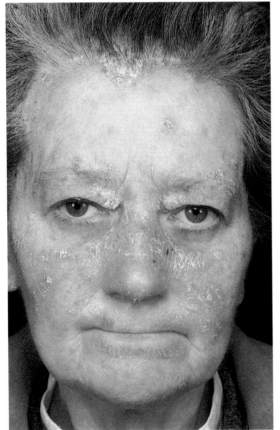

Plate 10 Scalp and facial psoriasis. This chronic rash was particularly noticeable in the hair. Scalp psoriasis does not usually spread far beyond the hair margin and when mild is often mistaken for dandruff.

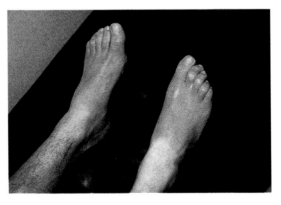

Plate 12 Allergic contact dermatitis. Reactions on the feet may be due to dyes or chrome tanning agents in leather. Plastic footwear may aggravate the problem due to plasticizers or to moisture trapping, giving high humidity and skin maceration. The well-demarcated reaction may subsequently spread widely.

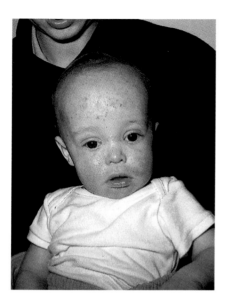

Plate 13 Infantile atopic eczema. The face, especially the forehead, scalp and trunk are usually affected. In older children, the area behind the ears and the flexions of the wrists and knees are often involved symmetrically.

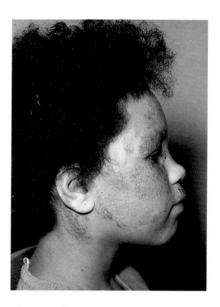

Plate 14 Chronic atopic eczema. This teenager shows the typical dry, scaly, pustular skin and thinning of the outer margin of the eyebrow. Depigmentation may occur in dark skinned patients.

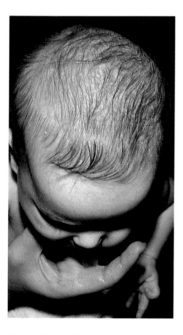

Plate 15 Cradle cap in an infant (3 months of age). This is characterized by coarse, yellowish, greasy, scalp scales. Some children also develop non-irritant erythema and scaling in the body flexures, especially the napkin area, but are otherwise well.

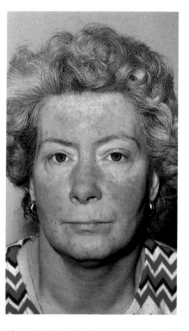

Plate 16 Facial telangiectasis. This irreversible damage was caused by the chronic application of a moderately potent corticosteroid cream. The effect is due to the superficial blood vessels showing through the thinned skin.

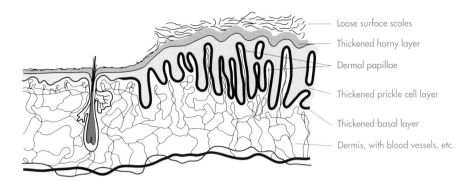

Loose surface scales
Thickened horny layer
Dermal papillae
Thickened prickle cell layer
Thickened basal layer
Dermis, with blood vessels, etc.

Figure 13.5   Comparative anatomy of normal and psoriatic skin. The diagram shows a section through the edge of a psoriatic plaque. The plaque (on the right) shows increased thickness of the basal, prickle cell and horny cell layers, large amounts of surface scale, greatly elongated dermal papillae and increased vascularity/inflammation in the dermis.

fibroblasts that fail to control keratinocyte proliferation. There is overexpression of transforming growth factors alpha and beta and levels of TNF alpha are also raised, the latter being a potent proinflammatory agent (see Chapter 2).

Aetiology

The precise cause of these changes is not clear. However, there is a polygenic inherited tendency to develop psoriasis. There is an association with certain histocompatibility antigens (HLA-B13, B17, Bw57 and Cw6). HLA-DR7 is associated with both skin and joint disease and HLA-DR4 with the latter only (see Chapter 12). HLA-B27, which is strongly associated with (seronegative) AS (see Chapter 12), is also linked to psoriatic joint disease and the severe pustular form of psoriasis. HLA-B28 is associated with a particularly severe form of psoriatic arthritis.

Environmental factors are implicated in addition to the strong genetic component. Psoriasis occurs more frequently in colder climates in the winter. Known **trigger factors** include:

- Trauma: skin laceration, pressure from belts, brassieres, etc.
- Infections: streptococcal tonsillitis, especially in children; HIV.
- Stress, e.g. marital, bereavement.
- Hormone status: there is an increased incidence in pregnancy and at puberty and the menopause.

- Sunburn or excessive exposure to the sun is harmful in 10% of patients, although sunshine may benefit others, and its lack predisposes to attacks.
- Drugs: alcohol, antimalarials, beta-blockers, chlorpropamide, *lithium*, smoking.

Infants may develop napkin psoriasis, which usually responds readily to treatment.

Epidemiology

Psoriasis is very common and affects about 2% of Caucasians, though many more have mild disease for which they do not seek medical treatment. About 30% of patients have a first-degree relative who is also affected. Siblings have a 17% risk, and patients' children have a 25–50% risk if one or both parents respectively are sufferers. Identical twins have a concordance rate of about 50%, so environmental factors are clearly important.

The incidence is similar in both sexes. About 75% of cases occur between the ages of 15 and 25 years, but it is unusual for lesions to appear before the age of 10. The condition tends to appear earlier in females than in males. The potential to develop the disease persists throughout life, though the skin may appear normal, so children may develop symptoms before these appear in their parents. The remaining 25% develop symptoms in their mid-fifties.

The disease is less common among Asians, Blacks and Eskimos, and is almost unknown in Native Americans. The situation with Eskimos has been taken as circumstantial evidence for an important role of essential fatty acids, present in fish oils, in maintaining epidermal integrity.

Clinical features and diagnosis

Onset of psoriasis is usually gradual. In classical **plaque psoriasis** the skin lesions are well defined, raised, reddish ('salmon pink'), slightly itchy plaques of tissue which are covered with large amounts of loose, silvery scales (Plates 9 and 10), surrounded by completely normal-looking skin. In dark-skinned people the underlying colour may be much darker, even purplish.

Acute attacks occur most often in childhood and may be triggered by streptococcal tonsillitis. They often start as evenly scattered small discoid lesions (**guttate psoriasis**) that tend to clear spontaneously within 4 months. This is **erythrodermic psoriasis** (see below). A few of these patients develop chronic disease at about 5–7 years of age, when it occurs as large, symmetrically located plaques, e.g. affecting both knees or elbows, though it may spread to affect 80% of the skin surface. The lesions sometimes heal spontaneously, starting in the centre, and may thus be confused with ringworm.

In **pustular psoriasis** sterile, yellow pustules occur, often at the edges of plaques in severe disease, but sometimes associated with flexural lesions. This form is often very resistant to treatment and is potentially life-threatening if widespread, because fluid loss and temperature control are compromised. Chronic brownish pustules on the palms and soles are strongly associated with smoking.

The most common sites, in approximate descending order of frequency, are the elbows, knees, scalp, lower back, chest, face, abdomen and genitalia: all areas exposed to mild trauma from clothing and physical activity. Scalp psoriasis (Plate 10) may easily be mistaken for severe dandruff if mild, or for seborrhoeic dermatitis (see below). Diagnostic features are that the plaques on the scalp are raised, as on other areas, and usually isolated, so the margins are palpable

and well-defined: the lesions tend to spread somewhat beyond the hair line.

The course of the disease is very variable. Psoriasis is normally a chronic, mildly irritant condition. Some patients have a single episode followed by complete and prolonged remission. Otherwise it is usually non-progressive, with occasional unpredictable exacerbations. Severity may either increase or decrease with time.

The combination of 'thimble' nail pitting, distal interphalangeal (DIP) arthropathy and nail discoloration (see below) is pathognomonic. If the scales are scratched off, the underlying skin is inflamed and they leave small bleeding points, because the capillaries are near the surface. This sign is very strongly suggestive for the condition.

Complications

The nails are affected, usually symmetrically, in about 25% of cases (Plate 8), usually in long-standing psoriasis. They show thimble-like pitting and later thickening, ridging and separation from the nail bed (**onycholysis**). An orange to brown discoloration of the distal lateral margins of the nail bed is characteristic and may be mistaken for tobacco stains.

Joint pain, i.e. psoriatic arthropathy, occurs in about 7% of patients. This tends to be asymmetrical, affecting the larger joints and the DIP finger joints (see Chapter 12, Figure 8.5) adjacent to affected nails. Psoriatic arthropathy is seronegative (see Chapter 12) and may precede or follow the skin changes. In contrast, RA usually spares these joints and is characteristically symmetrical and seropositive (see Chapter 12). Psoriatic arthropathy occasionally leads to severe joint damage and disability.

Erythrodermic psoriasis is a severe, widespread, inflammatory form of the disease. The cause is usually unknown, but it may be triggered by injudicious treatment with potent steroids. If the condition is extensive, serious and possibly life-threatening hypothermia and dehydration may result, because there may be a loss of 90–95% of the normal horny layer. High-output cardiac failure (see Chapter 4) may be precipitated in patients with compensated heart failure, owing to the extensive skin inflammation and consequent increased dermal blood flow.

Management

The two prime objectives are to:

- Produce a complete clearing of the affected areas: if this is attained, the disease-free intervals between relapses are increased, even in very chronic conditions.
- Reduce distress: if lesions are visible, the disfigurement is particularly distressing to juveniles and young adults because it is interpreted by the lay public as a serious and highly infectious disease. However, it is benign except in its severest forms and is certainly not transmissible. Thus, it is important to reduce stress and to reassure patients: a willingness to touch the plaques helps to convince the sufferers of the harmless nature of their condition.

The specific treatment aims are to:

- Promote normal maturation of epidermal cells, with vitamin D derivatives and retinoids.
- Reduce epidermal cell turnover, using cytotoxic or cytostatic agents, e.g. *dithranol*, corticosteroids, *methotrexate*, phototherapy and retinoids.
- Reduce inflammation, with corticosteroids and immunosuppressants.
- Remove scale using keratolytics, e.g. *salicylic acid*, *coal tar*.
- Hydrate the skin and reduce itch, with emollients.

While this treatment classification is convenient, there is an inevitable overlap between the classes of drugs used. Cytotoxic or cytostatic drugs are also anti-inflammatory, e.g. *methotrexate*, and corticosteroids are anti-inflammatory, immunosuppressive and cytostatic.

Factors influencing treatment selection are:

- Age.
- Form of psoriasis, i.e. plaque, guttate, pustular or erythrodermic.
- Site and extent (localized or generalized) of skin involvement.

- Prior successful and unsuccessful treatment.
- Concurrent disease, e.g. HIV.

Although the course of the disease is highly unpredictable and relapses are common, modern treatments may be very effective and so an optimistic, sympathetic attitude should be maintained. Mild psoriasis may need only the liberal use of emollients and the patient should be reassured that it is a benign condition. Many patients will need long-term maintenance medication with occasional intensive treatment for exacerbations. However, there is considerable variation in response to different treatments, and in one patient at different times with the same treatment.

Widespread unstable plaque psoriasis, and the guttate or erythrodermic forms, should be managed by a dermatological consultant.

A general outline of treatment of psoriasis is given in Table 13.14. Careful counselling is necessary for all patients, regardless of the treatment mode, to ensure that they understand the lifelong nature of their condition, how to use the treatment, the side-effects of treatment, and what to do in an exacerbation and if side-effects are troublesome. Carers and family members need to be fully involved, to ensure that they understand the problems and to apply products to lesions that are not accessible to the patient.

Topical pharmacotherapy

Tar preparations, *dithranol* and *salicylic acid* have been used safely and successfully for many years, but have largely been replaced by the vitamin D analogues and retinoids, which do not smell or stain skin and clothing.

Promotion of normal cell maturation

Vitamin D analogues
Calcipotriol (calcipotriene) and *tacalcitol* are vitamin D analogues that reduce excessive epidermal cell proliferation, improve cellular differentiation and strongly inhibit T cell activation by interleukin-1. Unlike vitamin D itself, these agents do not usually affect calcium

Table 13.14   Management of psoriasis

Aim	Mode	Drugs and techniques used[a]
Promote normal cell growth and maturation	Vitamin D analogues Retinoids	Calcipotriol (calcipotriene), tacalcitol Tazarotene, acitretin
Reduce cell turnover	Cytotoxics Antiproliferative drugs	Methotrexate, hydroxycarbamide Dithranol (anthralin): high concentration/short time, Ingram regimen Vitamin D analogues: calcipotriol (calcipotriene), tacalcitol Phototherapy[b]: PUVA, tar + UVB (Goeckerman regimen), RePUVA Retinoids: tazarotene, acitretin (Tar products)
Reduce inflammation	Corticosteroids, immunosuppressants	Corticosteroids[c]: hydrocortisone, clobetasone butyrate Methotrexate, ciclosporin
Remove scale	Keratolytics	Salicylic acid Propylene glycol Tar products
Hydrate the skin	Emollients (p. 829)	Aqueous cream, DiproBase, etc.
Reduce itch	Antipruritics	Antihistamines: Daytime: e.g. acrivastine, astemizole, cetirizine Night-time: e.g. azatidine, hydroxyzine, alimemazine Crotamiton

[a] Also see text. Some drugs fall into more than one class: cytotoxics are also immunosuppressants and both are anti-inflammatory.

[b] Includes photochemotherapy. PUVA, psoralen + long-wavelength ultraviolet radiation (UVA); RePUVA, retinoid + PUVA; UVB, short-wavelength ultraviolet radiation.

[c] Used only under specific circumstances, not as a general treatment (see text).

metabolism significantly. Nevertheless, they should be used cautiously in patients with disorders of calcium metabolism. Caution is also necessary in pregnancy and if they are used to treat patients with generalized pustular or erythrodermic psoriasis, because the widespread inflammation in these latter conditions allows greater skin penetration, so they are more likely to cause hypercalcaemia. Similarly, they should not be used under occlusive dressings. In common with most drugs, hepatic impairment reduces the metabolism of the vitamin D analogues and renal impairment reduces their elimination, so patients with these conditions are at greater risk of hypercalcaemia. Because the ratio of skin surface to body weight is greater in children, and their skin is thinner than in adults, there is a greater risk of local reactions and systemic absorption, and so of hypercalcaemia

and abnormal bone formation. They are unsuitable for use in young children.

They are as effective as *betamethasone* in clearing mild to moderate plaque psoriasis. They are less likely to cause skin irritation than other forms of vitamin D, and seem to be relatively free from significant side-effects, especially *tacalcitol*, and are more acceptable to patients than short-contact *dithranol* (see below). However, they should not be used for the more inflammatory forms of psoriasis, nor during an inflammatory exacerbation of otherwise stable disease, because of the increased risk of systemic absorption. They may exacerbate the psoriasis, but this is rare. It is important to wash the hands thoroughly after use, to avoid transfer to the eyes and other sensitive areas.

Calcipotriol and *tacalcitol* are licensed in the UK for treating any grade of plaque psoriasis, but only if affecting not more than 35–40% of the skin surface. They should be used under the supervision of a dermatological unit and treated areas should not be occluded, though this may be difficult to achieve.

Calcipotriol is available as a cream, ointment and scalp lotion. The manufacturers advise liberal application once or twice daily, avoiding the face. However, the maximum weekly dose is limited to 5 mg of *calcipotriol* in adults, in any mixture of the three products. Because absorption is greater through the scalp, the amounts of the scalp lotion are less than those of the cream and ointment. Suitable amounts in adolescents 12–18 years are about 75% of the adult dose and this is reduced to about 50% in children aged 6–12 years. It is not recommended for use in younger children.

There is also a *calcipotriol-betamethasone* ointment for use in adults only. The *betamethasone* is present in a low concentration to minimize irritation by the *calcipotriol*, but see the comments on the use of corticosteroids in psoriasis below.

Calcitriol (1, 25-dihydroxycholecalciferol) is an active form of vitamin D that is licensed for use in mild to moderate plaque psoriasis. Because of its greater potency it is more likely than the products described above to cause side-effects, but the ointment has a much lower concentration of drug than is used with *calcipotriol*. The maximum dose of the ointment equates to about one tenth of the weekly dose of *calcipotriol*. It should be used with caution in hepatic or renal impairment and in pregnancy and breastfeeding.

Tacalcitol ointment is used similarly to the *calcitriol* product, but is applied once daily at night, avoiding the eyes (maximum 10 g daily because of its greater potency). If used with UV radiation (see below), the UV exposure should be given in the morning and the *tacalcitol* ointment applied at night.

All vitamin D analogues may cause hypercalcaemia, so they should not be used if there is any abnormality of calcium metabolism, nor if there is sufficient inflammation or skin damage to permit excessive absorption of the drug. They must be used with caution in pregnancy.

Retinoids

Tazarotene is used for the topical treatment of mild to moderate plaque psoriasis affecting up to 10% of the skin surface (see Table 13.7) in adults (over 18 years). There are insufficient data on the treatment of younger patients and larger areas.

This topical drug reduces basal cell hyperplasia via RAR-alpha binding and promotes normal basal cell maturation and progression to granular cells. Improvement may be seen within a week and a good response occurs in 65% of patients after 12 weeks. The benefit may be maintained for at least 12 weeks after stopping, so pulsed treatment may be appropriate.

As with other retinoids (p. 835), *tazarotene* must be used with great care and is suitable primarily for the non-intertriginous areas of the trunk and limbs, provided that the skin is not inflamed, eczematous or covered with hair. In hairy areas, skin penetration is enhanced via the hair follicles. Exposure to the sun, UV light or solaria must be strictly limited. Other precautions include washing hands immediately after use, avoidance of contact with the eyes, face, scalp and eczematous or inflamed skin. Pregnancy and breastfeeding are absolute contra-indications, because of teratogenicity.

The common side-effects, which occur in 10–20% of patients, are skin irritation, erythema, burning, contact dermatitis, skin pain and worsening of psoriasis, and are related to concentration and duration of treatment. If severe, these should be managed by cessation of therapy and use of emollients. Irritation can be avoided by applying the ointment sparingly and carefully to the plaques only, avoiding unaffected skin, and emollients and cosmetics should not be applied within one hour of product application.

Tazarotene is unsuitable for treating pustular and erythrodermic psoriasis.

Keratolytics, antipruritics and skin hydration

Salicylic acid

Creams and ointments containing 2% of *salicylic acid* are used primarily as mild keratolytic agents to remove excessive skin scales. It also helps to stabilize *dithranol* and can be used to remove *dithranol* staining (see below).

Coal tar

This has mild keratolytic, antimitotic and antipruritic actions and is thus effective only in mild cases. Although tar is a recognized carcinogen, there are no reports of associated skin tumours over more than 40 years of pharmaceutical use. The crude forms of tar are more effective than refined ones, especially as antipruritics, but the latter and the numerous commercial preparations are more acceptable cosmetically and cause less staining. *Coal tar* is used in the form of creams, ointments, pastes, lotions and bath emollients in a range of concentrations, often prepared from *coal tar* solutions. Some older tar preparations may be unsuitable for use on the scalp or face where they may be irritant or cause folliculitis, and specially formulated commercial shampoos are available. Tar preparations should not be applied to infected areas.

Coal tar is sometimes combined with *salicylic acid* or *hydrocortisone*, adding additional keratolytic and anti-inflammatory effects. It may also be used with UVB radiation (see also PUVA, below), when it presumably acts as a skin sensitizer. *Coal tar and salicylic acid ointment* has been used for many years. Because this is cosmetically unattractive and difficult to prepare, it has largely been replaced by commercial products.

Propylene glycol (50% aqueous solution) is also mildly keratolytic. Further information on emollients and antipruritics is given above (p. 830).

Reducing cell turnover

Dithranol (anthralin)
This is a synthetic agent that has been a mainstay of psoriasis treatment for over 80 years. Although effective, it is now giving way to less irritant and more cosmetically acceptable drugs, e.g. the vitamin D analogues.

Its mode of action is not known precisely, but *dithranol* inhibits thymidine incorporation into DNA, mitochondrial DNA replication and repair, and ATP supply in epidermal cells. It also uncouples oxidative phosphorylation. The combined effects of these leads to inhibition of cell growth.

The principal side-effects are a local burning sensation, discomfort, soreness and moistness, which may need discontinuation of treatment.

Contra-indications to *dithranol* treatment are spreading of a lesion which is anything other

than gradual and it must not be used immediately following topical steroids.

If reactions occur, a bland emollient preparation, should be used for 14 days before recommencing treatment with a lower concentration of *dithranol* and building up slowly once more to the highest tolerated concentration. A moderate-potency corticosteroid, e.g. *betamethasone valerate* 0.025% cream, may be used for *dithranol* burns. Reactions following corticosteroid use (p. 834) are similarly managed with weaning and emollients.

Major problems with *dithranol* are that it is very irritant and chemically unstable, so the extemporaneous preparation of pastes and ointments is unwise. Further, without suitable milling equipment it is difficult to prepare the very fine dispersions that are required for low irritancy, though hospital manufacturing units are usually suitably equipped. Poor dispersions result in highly localized irritation from large particles. Production staff must be made aware of the hazards involved in handling *dithranol* powder, especially if it gets into the eyes. They must wear suitable protective clothing and wash thoroughly after use.

Dithranol is readily oxidized to brown or purplish pigments, especially under alkaline conditions, which stain skin and fabrics and are difficult to remove. *Salicylic acid* has been used for stain removal. This chemical instability means that concentrations less than 0.05% are not normally practicable, due to significant loss of potency. The triacetate ester is more stable, because the hydroxyl groups are protected by esterification, the ester being hydrolysed to *dithranol* in the skin. The ester is used occasionally, being less irritant than *dithranol* but also less active.

Commercial products provide well-formulated, stable preparations that are cosmetically very acceptable to patients. This has the additional benefit of encouraging patient compliance, thus improving control and hastening the response.

Phototherapy
Both natural (sunlight) and artificial UV radiation may be beneficial and are often used after tar or psoralen baths. UVB, i.e. short wavelength, 290–320 nm radiation, responsible for sunburn, is used either alone or with emollients as required.

Alternatively UVA, i.e. longer wavelength, 320–365 nm, is used with a psoralen: this is **photochemotherapy** (PUVA).

Once the lesions have cleared, mild UV exposure may prolong the period of remission, but over-exposure and burning must be avoided. Patients are usually tested for UV sensitivity by graduated exposure. Although sunlight helps some patients it may trigger attacks in others. Further, hot climates often exacerbate the condition because sweating readily leads to skin maceration. The procedure aggravates erythrodermic and pustular disease.

Anti-inflammatory treatment

Corticosteroids are potent anti-inflammatory agents and have cytostatic effects that reduce cell proliferation in the basal layer, but they have only a limited role in the treatment of psoriasis. Although there is an inflammatory element in psoriasis, and potent steroids may produce a dramatically rapid symptomatic improvement, there may be a substantial rebound effect on withdrawal and subsequent difficulties in treatment. If used as a first-line treatment, corticosteroids may so modify symptoms as to make a definitive diagnosis very difficult. If rebound occurs there may need to be a prolonged weaning period, using progressively less potent preparations and finally an emollient. This may take from 4–8 weeks, depending on the severity of the symptoms, during which time *dithranol* must not be used.

However, a low- or medium-potency product with low toxicity, e.g. *hydrocortisone* or *clobetasone butyrate* creams, are useful under careful supervision on sensitive sites such as the flexures, ears, face and genital areas, where many other agents are too irritant. Treatment should be short-term and more potent products avoided, because permanent skin damage may occur rapidly. Scalp lotions may also be useful for short-term treatment if *coal tar* or *coal tar-salicylic acid* shampoos are ineffective, or if the scalp preparations referred to above are not cosmetically acceptable.

There are combined preparations in which *coal tar* is occasionally combined with *dithranol* (anthralin). However, they are incompatible: the *dithranol* reacts with tar bases and undergoes

a rapid free radical oxidation. Nonetheless, there is one commercial tar ointment that contains both *dithranol* and *salicylic acid*: presumably, the *dithranol* is protected by the non-aqueous environment and the *salicylic acid*.

Topical treatment modes

Scale removal

If the scaling is very thick, e.g. on the elbows and knees, it will hinder the penetration of drugs, so it may be helpful initially to remove excess scale by using 2% *salicylic acid* ointment on its own for a week or so. *Propylene glycol* is also used.

Coal tar

Provided that the psoriasis is mild and not too extensive, a correspondingly mild therapeutic approach is appropriate. Ointments or creams containing *coal tar* may be used, in association with tar baths, until the lesions have cleared. Treatment should be started with the weaker preparations, probably those including *salicylic acid* to help remove excess scale. However, the vitamin D analogues are simpler to use and cosmetically more acceptable than *coal tar*, but are considerably more expensive and are POM products. Tar preparations are available OTC, but the formulary products are increasingly difficult to obtain.

Scaling on the scalp may be especially thick, so this area can be treated with the *coal tar and salicylic acid ointment*, which may be applied once or twice daily, usually for 1 h and shampooed out. This is very greasy and many patients do not find this cosmetically acceptable. A similar commercial product (Cocois) is available OTC and is used daily initially, if the scaling is severe, and is then used once weekly. These treatments are unsuitable for young children and children 6–12 years using this should be supervised medically. The commercial *coal tar* shampoos are also very useful. *Calcipotriol scalp solution* is cosmetically more acceptable, but is not recommended for children under 12 and there is a restricted total weekly dose (see above).

The **Goeckerman regimen** involves the use of topical tar preparations, especially baths, followed by UVB radiation. *Coal tar* may also be used in conjunction with *dithranol* (the **Ingram**

regimen, see below), though retinoids are probably the single agent of choice for most patients.

Dithranol

Dithranol has often been used as a first choice, with excellent results, especially if the condition is mild to moderate. It is also used if *coal tar* treatment has not been successful.

The older preparations were rather messy ointments or, for more severe cases, consisted of *dithranol* in *Lassar's paste*. The purpose of the latter is to provide a stiff vehicle that prevents *dithranol* spreading from the site of application onto surrounding skin, because it stains and irritates normal skin. This formulation also contains *salicylic acid*, which helps to minimize oxidation of the *dithranol*. The *dithranol* concentration used normally varies between 0.1% and 0.5%, depending on the tolerance of the patient's skin (fair skins are more sensitive) and the response. Although concentrations in the range 0.05% to 4%, even up to 10%, have been used, the higher concentrations require inpatient day care management, at least initially.

The paste is applied precisely to the areas of the lesions, usually by a trained nurse using a spatula. Treatment commences with the lowest concentration and the contact time is increased every 3–4 days if there is a response and there are no significant side-effects. If a response is not obtained, a higher strength is used. The approach is to find the contact time/strength balance that gives a satisfactory response without burning the skin.

This procedure normally produces some response within 1 week, and many patients will be completely clear, i.e. no palpable lesions, in 2–3 weeks, though chronic cases may take 6 weeks. The purple-brown skin staining that develops indicates that the lesions are responding to the medication. This does not require treatment because it usually clears spontaneously within a further 2 weeks, to leave 'normal' skin, though the psoriatic potential remains. Patients need to be counselled about this. *Dithranol* products are generally unsuitable for application to sensitive areas, i.e. the face, ears, flexures and near the genitalia (but see below). These areas are often treated with steroid creams, with or without *coal tar*.

Clearly, pastes are unsuitable for application to the hair.

The **Ingram regimen** is a common procedure often used in severe cases as an intensive inpatient routine. It involves:

- Initial patch testing with 0.1% *dithranol* in Lassar's paste, to determine skin tolerance.
- Soaking in a bath containing *coal tar* (coal tar solution or a commercial equivalent) to remove scale and sensitize the lesions.
- Exposure to UVB radiation to give a slight erythema, i.e. a dose that mildly damages the basal layer.
- Application of *dithranol* in Lassar's paste at the desired concentration, leaving for 24 h, removing with oil and bathing as before. The paste is normally powdered over with talc and covered with a tubular bandage. A top-up may be necessary after 8–12 h.

Dithranol creams are more acceptable cosmetically than pastes or ointments and are generally less irritant, though they act more slowly. They are more suitable for use by patients at home and can be used on the scalp. Because the scalp skin is very thin and sensitive, all products used there have a limited contact time. The product has to be washed of with copious warm water and soap must not be used because it enhances skin penetration.

Intensive short contact time regimens have been the major advance in *dithranol* treatment, i.e. '30-minute therapy', rather than the 24 h of the Ingram regimen. These involve the application of higher concentration *dithranol* creams before bathing at night. This has proved to be similarly effective to conventional treatment, though the lesions may take slightly longer to clear, up to one month as against 3 weeks. However, there are substantial advantages:

- Less interference with the patient's life.
- Better patient acceptability and compliance.
- No need for hospital inpatient or day care treatment.
- Less staining of clothes and bed linen.

Higher concentrations of *dithranol* have been introduced in commercial preparations to suit the short contact time approach, with up to 2%

being used in the community. Concentrations up to 8% are sometimes used in hospital.

The lower-strength creams are also suitable for application to delicate areas such as the flexures, provided that no burning or undue local reaction occurs. Shorter contact times may be preferred here. The apparently normal skin at scalp margins and behind the ears must be avoided, because it is very sensitive. Concentrations other than those prepared by the manufacturers are sometimes requested by prescribers, but commercial preparations should not be diluted without careful inquiry because the precise formulation may be critical. Rather than attempt extemporaneous preparation it is preferable to use a weaker preparation for a longer contact time or a more concentrated one for a shorter time, depending on patient tolerance.

Phototherapies

PUVA treatment is used for widespread involvement of the trunk. This involves treating the patient with *methoxsalen* (8-methoxypsoralen), a phytochemical photosensitizing agent. Patients bathe in a solution of the drug before irradiation in a cabinet with a bank of UVA tubes; alternatively an oral dose is taken 2 h before UVA irradiation. Higher UV doses (longer exposure times) are more effective than lower ones, but cause increased side-effects (see below).

This approach is more effective than the Ingram regimen. *Trioxysalen* (trioxsalen, 4,5′, 8-methoxypsoralen) is a similar drug that is not licensed in the UK but is used in North America.

Dark goggles should be worn during the treatment and for a further 8 h, to minimize the risk of cataract formation.

Combination treatment with a retinoid (Re-PUVA) has been used for resistant psoriasis, and is probably the most effective modality. However, the UVA dose must be very carefully controlled.

Many patients will experience long periods of remission with PUVA regimens. The methods are technically simple and can readily be used on an outpatient basis, usually twice weekly for about 5 weeks. They are liked by patients because they avoid the use of messy topical products.

Some patients experience nausea and headaches, and burns may occur, even with careful

calculation of the UV dose. In the long term, there is premature skin ageing and a slightly increased risk of skin malignancies, especially **squamous cell carcinoma**, so patients under 40 should not be treated unless other approaches are ineffective. Most consultants use PUVA routinely, though it is usually confined to specialist centres in the UK.

Narrow band UVB phototherapy appears to be as effective as PUVA and avoids the need for psoralens.

Systemic pharmacotherapy

Acitretin

This retinoid, a metabolite of *etretinate* (p. 837), is the only member of this group licensed in the UK for the systemic treatment of severe psoriasis unresponsive to other treatments. It is especially useful for pustular disease. Because of its toxicity, *acitretin* is reserved for use under the supervision of hospital consultants. *Acitretin* interacts with both RAR alpha and RAR gamma receptors (see above).

There is considerable interpatient variation in absorption and metabolism, so the dose must be individualized for each patient. *Acitretin* is usually given with other treatments and is sometimes given in one year cycles comprising nine months of treatment followed by a three month rest period. Some dermatologists use the drug in low dosage as an adjunct to *dithranol* or PUVA treatments, if these give inadequate control.

Mucocutaneous side-effects of *acitretin* are common, e.g. dryness of the skin, cracked lips and dry eyes. Generalized pruritus, nail problems, nosebleeds and hepatotoxicity may occur, as does slight transient alopecia. *Acitretin* can cause a rise in plasma lipids and serum triglycerides, and may exacerbate diabetes mellitus, so they must be monitored regularly. Concurrent use with vitamin A, *tetracyclines* and *methotrexate* must be avoided, because of cumulative toxicity. Because *acitretin* is highly teratogenic, meticulous contraception must be initiated for 1 month before treatment and maintained throughout, and for at least 2 years after stopping treatment. Those taking *acitretin* must not donate blood for 1 year after treatment cessation because of the possibility of terato-genicity in pregnant recipients. Hepatic and renal impairment are other contra-indications. The drug is rarely used in children because it may cause growth impairment, due to prema-ture closure of the epiphyses, the growth plates at the ends of the bones.

There is a long list of other side-effects and precautions and the BNF and the manufacturer's literature should be consulted.

Immunosuppressants, immunomodulators and cytotoxics

These potentially very toxic agents are used in psoriasis in lower doses than are used to treat neoplastic disease (see Chapter 10) and to prevent rejection of organ transplants (see Chapter 14). Because skin diseases are rarely life-threatening there must be careful individualized evaluation of the risk–benefit balance before these drugs are prescribed.

Methotrexate

Methotrexate is a very effective antifolate agent but is reserved for the treatment of severe exacer-bations or intractable cases because of poten-tially serious side-effects. *Methotrexate* must be used extremely carefully in the elderly, is unsuit-able for children, and is therefore restricted to use by specialists only.

In psoriasis, *methotrexate* is usually given orally in low dosage, i.e. 10–25 mg once weekly. This dosage frequency must be strictly adhered to: there have been serious blood dyscrasias, liver cirrhosis and even death, with more frequent dosing. The UK's CSM has advised that:

* A full blood count and renal and liver func-tion tests be carried out before starting treat-ment, and repeated weekly until therapy is stabilized. Patients should then be monitored carefully every 2–3 months.
* Patients should be told to report all symptoms and events occurring during treatment, especially sore throat.

Blood dyscrasias may occur abruptly and *calcium folinate* rescue (see Chapter 10) may be required. Abnormal liver function tests are a contra-indication to starting or continuing treat-ment, and liver biopsies should be taken if liver function tests (see Chapter 3) fail to return to normal after stopping *methotrexate* treatment.

Renal function tests (see Chapter 14) are also required because *methotrexate* is nephrotoxic and accumulates in renal failure.

Analgesics reduce the excretion of *methotrexate* and death has occurred with concurrent use of NSAIDs, so such combinations are preferably avoided in psoriatic arthropathy and patients warned about the risks of self-medication with products containing NSAIDs. This is not an absolute contra-indication, but special care is needed if a patient needs analgesic anti-inflammatory treatment. Other drugs which may increase toxicity include penicillins, *phenytoin*, *pyrimethamine* (antimalarial) and *trimethoprim* (another antifolate agent).

Methotrexate is teratogenic and is absolutely contra-indicated in pregnancy and during breastfeeding. Conception should be avoided for at least 6 months after use in either sex.

Hydroxycarbamide (0.5–1 g daily) has been used in patients who are intolerant of *methotrexate* or in whom the latter is contra-indicated, but it is also myelosuppressive.

Ciclosporin

This is a calcineurin inhibitor that was origi-nally introduced to prevent rejection of kidney transplants (see Chapter 14). It has been used for the treatment of psoriasis (low-dose; 2.5 mg/kg daily, rising to 5 mg/kg daily) unre-sponsive to other treatments, and a very high proportion of patients respond. It is also very useful for erythrodermic disease.

However, the renal toxicity of *ciclosporin* means that it should only be used under expert supervision and patients must be moni-tored for renal function and hypertension. Exposure to UV radiation, e.g. UVB or PUVA (see above), and excessive exposure to sunlight should be avoided. Its potent immunosuppres-sant effects mean that special care is required if infections or neoplastic disease are present, or possible, and no alternative treatment is suitable.

The antirheumatoid drug, *leflunomide* (see Chapter 12), is also used for treating active psoriatic arthritis (see Chapter 12).

Biological agents

Efalizumab, *etanercept* and *infliximab* are licensed for use in psoriasis. *Efalizumab* is a monoclonal antibody that inhibits T cell activation and so the production of pro-inflammatory cytokines (see Chapter 2). It is licensed for the treatment of moderate to severe chronic plaque psoriasis, in patients who have not responded to at least two other systemic treatments and photochemotherapy (PUVA), or who are intolerant of such therapy. It is given weekly by SC injection.

Side-effects include exacerbation of psoriasis and the possible development of other forms, e.g. psoriatic arthritis, and if this occurs treatment must be stopped. Treatment should also be stopped if there is no response after 12 weeks. Other side-effects are influenza-like symptoms, joint pain, leucocytosis and, more rarely, thrombocytopenia and injection-site reactions. These reactions make it unsuitable for treating children and adolescents, but these rarely suffer psoriasis.

It should be used with caution in hepatic or renal impairment and in patients with low platelet counts. The latter should be checked before treatment commences, then monthly for three months and, if the condition responds, three monthly.

Contra-indications include immunodeficiency, severe infections, active TB, a history of neoplastic disease, pregnancy and breastfeeding.

The **TNFα antagonists** *etanercept* and *infliximab* have evidence of benefit and have been used to treat moderate to severe chronic plaque psoriasis. These are also licensed for psoriatic arthritis (see Chapters 2 and 12). They are contra-indicated in pregnancy and in breastfeeding women. They should be used with caution in immunosuppressed individuals, in those exposed to varicella-zoster infection, patients with a history of cardiovascular disorders, ischaemic syndromes, renal impairment, seizures, demyelinating diseases, e.g. multiple sclerosis and Guillain-Barré syndrome, dyspnoea and bone fracture.

Further information on the biological agents is given in Chapter 12.

Antipruritics

Oral antihistamines are occasionally used if itching is troublesome, the sedating side-effects of the older drugs being useful at night. Anxiolytics may also be useful in some patients to relieve associated stress and anxiety, so *hydroxyzine*, which has sedative, anxiolytic and antihistaminic properties, is often used. However, the most effective approach is adequate counselling and reassurance and effective treatment of the psoriasis.

Other treatments

Corticosteroids are sometimes injected into lesions, to control chronic plaques resistant to other treatments.

Experimental treatments

There is limited evidence that *dimethylfumaric acid* and *monoethylfumaric acid* improve chronic plaque psoriasis, but there was a high rate of withdrawal due to flushing and gastrointestinal effects. There is no evidence on their suitability for long-term maintenance treatment, so routine use of these agents requires further evidence of efficacy and safety.

Improvements in psoriasis have been reported in patients treated with *IFN alfa* and the anti-arrhythmic drug *amiodarone*. The somatostatin analogue, *octreotide*, also has anti-psoriatic activity, possibly because the increased epidermal cell growth is influenced by human growth hormone. However, it is too early to say whether any of these will find a place in routine therapy.

Treatments combining two of the widely used modalities described earlier have been used, but there is insufficient evidence to justify their routine use. There are likely to be increased side-effects due to a summation of the side-effects of the regimens used.

Rarely, surgical removal of troublesome plaques has been used and has produced a local cure.

Eczema and dermatitis

Definition and classification

Eczema is an inflammatory, highly itchy, usually chronic, eruption of the epidermis and outer dermal layers.

The terms eczema and **dermatitis** are often used synonymously, but it has been conventional to use the term dermatitis to describe skin reactions due to external agents, and eczema for reactions to endogenous factors in atopic individuals. However, this is an artificial distinction because in many of these conditions there is an interaction between genetic and environmental factors. Current British practice tends to use the term dermatitis plus a qualifying adjective, e.g. atopic dermatitis and seborrhoeic dermatitis. A classification and some of the characteristics of dermatitis are given in Figure 13.6.

This group of diseases comprises the largest single group seen in skin clinics and is responsible for about 25% of all dermatological referrals to consultants.

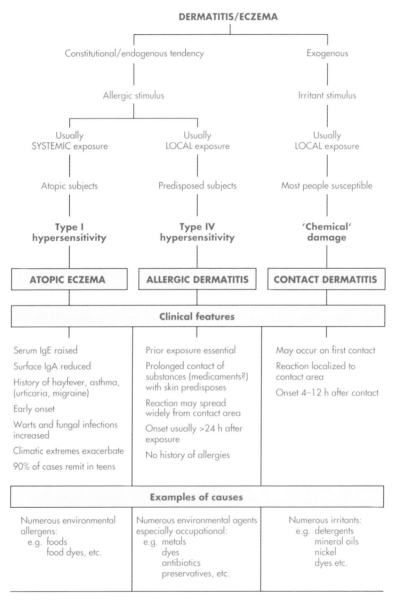

Figure 13.6   Classification of the principal forms of eczema and dermatitis.

Aetiology and pathology

Essential fatty acid metabolism

An interesting discovery has been that essential fatty acids (EFAs) are important in the maintenance of epidermal integrity (an example of their nomenclature is arachidonic acid, which is a 20:4n-6 acid, i.e. it consists of a 20-carbon chain with four double bonds, the first of which links carbons 6–7). The composition of the plasma phospholipids is significantly changed in patients with atopic dermatitis compared with controls, the level of cis-linoleic acid being increased, whereas those of its metabolites (including arachidonic acid) are substantially reduced. Because linoleic acid is the major dietary n-6-EFA, this points to a metabolic defect, probably a reduced activity of delta-6-desaturase. This enzyme converts linoleic acid to gamma-linolenic acid, a rate-limiting step. There is also a reduction of alpha-linoleic acid metabolite concentrations in atopic respiratory disease and the same enzyme may be involved. However, the oral administration of linoleic acid and gamolenic acid in the form of evening primrose oil is not regarded as beneficial, but this is available as an emollient cream via the UK NHS.

Modification of n-3 metabolite levels would require the administration of fish oils, and circumstantial evidence from the study of Eskimo populations indicates that this may be beneficial in some skin diseases, notably psoriasis. However, it is likely that the benefit of halibut liver oil is due to its vitamin A content, which is important for epidermal maturation (see retinoids; p. 835).

Because abnormal levels of serum fatty acids have also been observed in patients with allergic respiratory disease it seems possible that abnormal fatty acid metabolism is a fundamental feature of atopy, though whether this is a cause or effect remains to be elucidated.

Reactions to environmental agents

Dermatitis is inflammation of the epidermis. **Contact (irritant, toxic) dermatitis** is usually the result of mechanical or chemical disruption of the horny layer of the skin. Sensitivity varies greatly, and dermatitis is more likely in individuals with an excessively dry skin, in the elderly, and after childbirth. Atopic subjects have drier skin than normal, even if there is no active dermatitis. However, almost anyone can develop this form of dermatitis if the insult is sufficiently severe or prolonged. An indication of a tendency to develop such reactions is given by the presence of thin dry skin showing numerous fine furrows on the palms and palmar surfaces of the fingers (hyperlinearity, Plate 11), which is a mild reaction to chronic irritants.

In some patients there is a more severe reaction, with erythema, severe irritation, swelling, vesicle formation and exudation. This may be due to **allergic dermatitis** (Plate 12, Figure 13.6), in which external agents penetrate the horny layer through minute abrasions or the hair follicles and ducts of the sweat glands. This skin penetration may be allowed by low levels of IgA (surface-protective antibody; Chapter 2). The allergens bind to antigen-presenting Langerhans cells in the middle layer of the epidermis, which then migrate to the local lymph nodes and activate T cells. Because these activated TH2 cells migrate to all areas of the body via the blood, the entire skin surface becomes sensitive. After a very variable period (days to years), and usually after repeated reinforcement, subsequent contact with the same agent elicits a type IV (delayed) hypersensitivity reaction that may take 24–72 h to develop (see Chapter 2).

Almost any substance can sensitize the skin, but the most common agents include:

- Irritants:
  - Soaps and detergents, the commonest cause of hand dermatitis.
  - Plants: e.g. Compositae, primulas.
  - Solvents, e.g. lubricating oils and petrol, which remove protective lipids and may contain irritant additives.
  - Plasticizers in rubber and plastics, e.g. rubber gloves.
- Allergens and haptens (see Chapter 2):
  - Dyes: e.g. hair dyes and in clothing and shoes.
  - Fragrances and preservatives, now included widely in household products.
  - Medicines: e.g. antibiotics, topical antihistamines and anaesthetics, wool alcohols,

preservatives and antioxidants and some corticosteroids.
• Metals: e.g. nickel, chromium and cobalt, e.g. in jewellery.

Endogenous reactions

In **atopic eczema** (Figure 13.6) there is a skin reaction to presumed systemic antigens. This occurs only in genetically predisposed (atopic) subjects and is associated with a personal or family history of atopy, i.e. allergic rhinitis (perennial or seasonal), asthma and, occasionally, urticaria and migraine. It has been estimated that some 10% of the population is susceptible to this form of dermatitis, though only about half of these actually develop the skin reaction. The fundamental mechanism appears to be a reduced T-suppressor cell activity, and levels of circulating IgE may be increased 10-fold. This results in a type I (immediate type) hypersensitivity reaction when the antigen is encountered. Levels of surface-protective antibody (IgA) are low, and this may account for the ability of allergenic substances to penetrate mucous membranes and produce systemic sensitization.

It is possible that in skin carriers of *Staphylococcus aureus* the bacteria produce superantigens that activate large numbers of T cells and so cause the widespread release of inflammatory cytokines and excessive IgE production.

About 10% of sufferers also have a tendency to develop chronic **lichen simplex**. This causes well-defined areas of dry, roughened, itchy, hyperpigmented skin. The problem starts with attacks of itching provoked by minor stimuli. Scratching causes lichenification and the area becomes very liable to itch, thus provoking a reflex itch–scratch–itch cycle, often leading to excoriation. Infection of the damaged skin is then common. The back of the neck, legs, outer forearms, groin, anal and genital areas are most frequently involved.

Food allergies are commonly blamed, though these are far less common than is popularly believed. Such allergies cannot be tested for simply, so the only approach is the use of a rigid, often unacceptable, exclusion diet with gradual replacement of individual foods or food components. This requires dedicated persistence by

clinician, nutritionist and patient over a long period. Breastfeeding reduces the incidence of the disease, though it is unclear whether this results from the delayed introduction of artificial foods or is a consequence of the protective effect of maternal antibodies.

Clinical features

Contact and allergic dermatitis

The affected area is always itchy and there may be anything from mild inflammation to severe swelling and vesiculation. In **contact dermatitis** (Plate 11) the reaction is initially confined to the area exposed to the damaging agent, but limited local spread may occur. With chronic insult the horny layer disintegrates and the skin becomes thickened, dry and scaly. This leads to loss of the water-retaining property of the skin.

In **allergic dermatitis** the reaction is initially similarly confined to the contact area and is sharply demarcated (Plate 12), but the reaction may spread widely from the original site, especially in the chronic condition.

Continuing exposure, excoriation or infection may result in the establishment of a chronic state in both conditions, which are very common. They affect 10–20% of occupationally exposed workers, and occur in twice as many women as men.

Atopic eczema

This is a genetically determined allergic skin condition that often starts in the first year of life (about 75% of cases; Plate 13), usually in the third or fourth months. However, it may appear for the first time in older children or adults. In infants it usually affects the face, scalp and extensor surfaces of the limbs, but in later years it may become more localized and chronic (Plate 14). Lesions always itch, often severely. The course is unpredictable, with occasional or frequent exacerbations and remissions up to 30–40 years of age, or sometimes throughout life, because atopy is determined genetically. In about 50% of children there is a slow improvement throughout childhood, with complete remission by puberty.

There is usually a personal or family history of hay fever, urticaria (see below) or asthma, i.e. other forms of atopy. In some unfortunate individuals all four conditions may coexist.

Older children and adults often have localized, cracked areas in the flexures behind the knees, elbows, on the eyelids, neck and wrists. The skin tends to be very dry in most patients, and scratching may lead to chronic lichen simplex, i.e. thickened, rough skin confined to areas of scratching, and infection. Severe scratching leads to weeping lesions (excoriation), frequently aggravated by bacterial infection.

The condition follows a relapsing/remitting course and infantile eczema tends to clear in 3–5 years and a small proportion may recover within 18 months. Exacerbations may be caused by primary irritants, stress, climatic changes and clothing, especially wool. There is an increased susceptibility to skin infections, notably warts and dermatomycoses, and herpes simplex infections may cause serious generalized illness. Long-standing sufferers tend to develop cataracts in early adult life.

Seborrhoeic dermatitis (seborrhoeic eczema)

This is an acute or chronic eruption that principally affects the scalp, face and the skin over the sternum and between the shoulder blades, i.e. the areas with large numbers of sebaceous glands. It may also affect intertriginous areas, i.e. armpits, navel, groin and below the breasts. Despite its name, there is no clear association with sebum flow. This is a genetically determined condition that predisposes the skin to respond with seborrhoeic reactions to almost any form of skin damage.

It occurs in two quite distinct age groups. In infants this occurs as **cradle cap** (Plate 15), with thick, yellowish, encrusted lesions on the scalp and a papular, red eruption of the face. It may also affect the napkin area.

The adult form appears to be unrelated to the infantile one. Onset is gradual with grey to yellowish scaly lesions and dandruff. It may be otherwise asymptomatic, though there is often a varying degree of itch. The rash occurs mainly on the trunk, but in severe cases the perinasal area, hair line, similar to Plate 10, and sternal area may

be affected. Facial lesions mostly occur in men. Very rarely the condition may become more generalized and this form has been ascribed to poor diet and hygiene. Eruptions may be associated with upper respiratory tract and pyogenic infections (see Chapter 8).

Seborrhoeic dermatitis can be distinguished from atopic eczema in difficult cases because IgE levels and the RAST test are usually normal in seborrhoeic dermatitis and raised in atopic eczema.

Dandruff is a mild form, associated with colonization with the yeast *Pityrosporum (Pityrosporon) ovale*, though whether this is causative or is an opportunistic invader of damaged skin is unclear. However, eradication of the yeast improves the condition.

Discoid (nummular) eczema

In this relatively uncommon condition, chronic, widespread discoid lesions occur, consisting of confluent vesicles, which ooze and crust. Lesions are more common on the extensor aspects of the arms and legs and on the buttocks.

Pompholyx

This is sometimes called dishydrotic dermatitis or vesicular palmar eczema. As the latter name implies, the condition has a restricted skin distribution, affecting only the hands (80%) and feet, primarily the palms, sides of the fingers and soles. The term 'dishydrotic' is misleading because there is no abnormality of the sweat glands. Pompholyx usually occurs in young adults aged 12–40 years and may be acute, with no previous history of atopy or skin conditions, chronic or recurrent. Some cases are due to an allergic reaction to active skin disease elsewhere on the body, e.g. **tinea pedis** and **scabies**, with which it may be confused.

Initially there is an intensely itchy or burning vesicular rash. If untreated, the vesicles coalesce to form large, fluid-filled bullae (blisters) that may rupture and become infected, causing pain and possibly cellulitis and lymphadenopathy. The chronic condition is marked by crusts and dry, cracked skin. Heat or emotion, causing sweating, and hot, humid weather may precipitate attacks.

'Varicose eczema'

This is also known as **stasis**, **gravitational** or **asteatotic** eczema. It is not a true eczema, because the underlying condition is neither allergic nor irritant, but due to poor peripheral circulation causing pooling of the blood in the lower legs, with resultant oedema. This causes capillary damage, pericapillary deposition of fibrin and poor tissue perfusion. The poorly nourished skin is hyperpigmented and is very friable and readily liable to damage by contact irritants or minor trauma. Varicose dermatitis is essentially a problem of elderly patients and, because smoking impairs the peripheral circulation, these are mostly men.

The condition responds poorly to treatment, especially because the circulation in the area is so poor. Steroids are largely ineffective, support stockings and occlusive tar bandages or modern absorptive or 'breathable' dressings are usually more useful. Bioengineered skin is now available and gives good healing. There is a tendency to chronic ulceration and infection. If poor circulation is due to atheroma of the femoral or iliac arteries, angioplasty or arterial by-pass grafting may improve the circulation substantially, and with it the skin condition.

Complications

Apart from the hazard of opportunistic infection, the most serious complication of dermatitis is **exfoliative (erythrodermic) dermatitis**, in which there is a gradual onset of widespread inflammation and scaling. This occurs mainly in middle-aged men. Patients feel generally unwell with hypothermia and rigors due to impairment of temperature regulation consequent on extensive skin damage.

Diagnosis

The diagnosis is usually made clinically. A careful history and examination (p. 819) is essential to identify any possible allergen or irritant. Patch tests may be used to identify or confirm contact allergens in allergic dermatitis. Intradermal prick tests with suspected allergens and, especially, the **RAST procedure** (see Chapter 5, Figure 5.16), to determine IgE levels, may help in doubtful cases but patients are often allergic to multiple agents.

Because of the limited repertoire of skin reactions there is a possibility of confusion with other skin diseases and, especially, with reactions to serious systemic conditions (p. 825; Table 13.6) such as lymphomas, SLE (see Chapter 12) and skin infestations, e.g. scabies.

Management

Aims

The aims of management are:

- Patient education and reassurance.
- Avoidance of identifiable precipitating or aggravating factors and prevention of recurrence and chronicity.
- Relief of troublesome symptoms, e.g. itch, dry and fissuring skin, moist or weeping and infected lesions, sleep loss.
- Control of the disease process.

General principles and pharmacotherapy

Patient education and reassurance
Because there is no specific, curative pharmacotherapy patients have to learn to manage their symptoms over a long period. A positive, encouraging outlook on the part of the doctor, nurse and pharmacist is important. Patients should also be made aware that a tendency for atopic reactions to recur persists throughout life and of what it is reasonable to expect from treatment.

Avoidance of precipitants
These include especially soaps and detergents, airborne allergens, plants, medicaments and occupational triggers. Vigorous washing in hot water, which dries the skin by removing sebum lipids should be minimized: patients should wash and bathe in warm water using an emollient, e.g. aqueous cream or emulsifying ointment as a soap replacement (see Table 13.9). Complete avoidance is often difficult or impossible, but career choice, e.g. avoiding hairdressing, nursing or contact with lubricating oils, may be important.

Finding a suitable emollient and using it freely is the cornerstone of dermatitis management, and will minimize the need for corticosteroids. An emollient alone, used freely, may be adequate in mild disease.

Control itching

The liberal use of emollients (see Table 13.9) is fundamental to management, especially for dry skin, and systemic antihistamines, e.g. *hydroxyzine*, which is also sedative and helps with sleep problems. Bland topical antipruritics (p. 830) may also help.

Moist or weeping lesions

Astringent (drying) lotions, e.g. 0.01% potassium permanganate solution or aluminium acetate lotion. If large areas are affected, potassium permanganate baths can be used (see Table 13.8). However, most patients find potassium permanganate unacceptable because of the brown staining of the skin.

Control inflammation

Use the mildest possible product. *Coal tar* is used occasionally. However, topical corticosteroids (p. 833) form the essential component of active dermatitis treatment, used in the most appropriate pharmaceutical dosage form, i.e. cream, gel, lotion or ointment, for the shortest possible time. A potent preparation may be needed initially (see Table 13.11) and is safe for short-term use, e.g. 7–10 days, but must not be used on the face or in the flexures, i.e. the groin, armpits and under the breasts. In these situations apposition of the skin surfaces causes occlusion of the site, causing increased absorption of the steroid and skin damage. Only mild preparations are suitable for application to these areas. Potent corticosteroids are also unsuitable for use in young children.

Once the symptoms have come under control the potency should be reduced gradually to the mildest that will control symptoms. Exacerbations may need a return to the potent product used initially, and patients should be given guidelines on self-management of their condition.

Corticosteroids should be applied only to inflamed areas and not to uninvolved skin.

However, it should be remembered that significant systemic absorption may occur if there are large areas of inflamed skin, so widespread corticosteroid treatment may cause adrenal suppression, especially with potent preparations. Liberal emollient use should be continued.

In severe disease with marked systemic symptoms, high doses of oral corticosteroids may be required for a short time to gain control rapidly. The treatment can then be stopped abruptly if it has been used for less than 3 weeks and relapse is unlikely. Alternatively, the dose can be stepped down rapidly to about 7.5 mg *prednisolone* (or its equivalent) daily and then more slowly. Careful supervision is needed to avoid relapse. The objective is to move progressively to minimal use of a mild topical corticosteroid, or to complete discontinuation if symptoms are episodic. If treatment has been more prolonged, follows a longer course within the preceding year or doses greater than 40 mg *prednisolone* daily have been used, more gradual dosage reduction is necessary. If withdrawal is too abrupt, acute glucocorticoid insufficiency (Addison's disease) may result.

High-dose corticosteroid use may precipitate post-primary TB, which may be prevented by suitable prophylactic treatment, or shingles (see Chapter 8). The latter may be interpreted as an exacerbation of the eczema and inappropriate use of corticosteroid creams will cause widespread skin lesions that need prompt treatment with oral *aciclovir*, *famciclovir* or *valaciclovir* (see Chapter 8).

The immunomodulator *ciclosporin* (see above and Chapter 14) is licensed for short-term use, i.e. <8 weeks, in severe atopic dermatitis when conventional therapy has been ineffective or is contra-indicated. At least two full dermatological and physical examinations are required before initiating treatment, including blood pressure and renal function tests. It is contra-indicated if renal function is abnormal, if there is malignancy and if hypertension or any infections, especially herpes simplex, are not under control. The serum creatinine level should be monitored fortnightly during therapy (see Chapter 14).

Pimecrolimus and *tacrolimus* are used topically if maximal topical corticosteroid therapy has not given adequate control or has caused severe side-effects. They should not be used near the eyes and mucous membranes and excessive exposure to sunlight or UV radiation should be avoided.

NICE has recommended that *pimecrolimus cream* is appropriate for the (short-term) control of mild to moderate atopic eczema and to prevent or treat exacerbations of disease. It has also been used in children aged 2–16 y. Topical *tacrolimus* is licensed for treating moderate to severe disease in adults (0.1% ointment) and children aged 2–15 years (0.03% ointment).

These agents are still under evaluation for safety and therapeutic role and should not be used as first-line agents unless there are specific reasons against the use of topical corticosteroids. They should be used under the supervision of dermatological consultants.

Unlicensed treatments for severe refractory dermatitis include the systemic use of *azathioprine* or *mycophenolate mofetil*.

Infection control

Skin hygiene requires careful attention. Infections should be controlled promptly with systemic antibiotics, after taking swabs for sensitivity testing. Multi-resistant *Staphylococcus aureus* (MRSA; see Chapter 8) and beta-haemolytic streptococci may be implicated. An antiviral agent (see above) is necessary for herpes simplex infections, which may be severe.

Other treatments

It is difficult to be more precise about treatment, because patients vary very widely in their symptoms and in the ways in which they react to medication. Most patients with chronic disease eventually settle down to a particular regimen of emollients and topical corticosteroids that they find suits them best, more vigorous treatment being used to treat exacerbations, as appropriate. A *lithium/zinc ointment* is available for the treatment of seborrhoeic dermatitis and appears to be effective, largely non-irritant and suitable for facial use. However, it must not be used near the eyes or on mucous membranes.

Second- and third-line therapies include:

- Hospital admission for intensive or systemic therapies.
- Phototherapy or PUVA (see p. 847).

- Use of the immunomodulators mentioned above. Other antagonists of proinflammatory cytokines, e.g. *etanercept*, have not found a place in this context.

Gamolenic acid, used orally, is no longer considered to have a role, but may possibly be beneficial in a few patients at any stage as an adjunct to other therapy, but this is controversial. It is not without side-effects, e.g. headache and gastrointestinal discomfort, and may even cause pruritus, and must be used cautiously in pregnancy and if there is a history of epilepsy. It is used in one emollient cream.

Exfoliative dermatitis

This is a life-threatening complication. Rest, a high-protein diet to replace the serum proteins lost through the extensively damaged skin, and the use of high-dose systemic steroids comprise the normal treatment mode, plus the specific management of any underlying cause, if one can be identified. All nonessential drugs should be withdrawn.

It may also complicate psoriasis, lymphomas and leukaemias.

Acne

Definition

Acne is a hormone-associated disorder of the pilosebaceous (hair) follicles and is characterized by excessive sebum production, **comedones** (blackheads), papules and pustules (whiteheads). The lesions occur primarily on the face, but the upper chest, back and arms, etc. may be affected in severe cases, i.e. any area where pilosebaceous follicles occur. Only the palms and soles are spared completely.

Epidemiology

Acne affects adolescents in industrialized societies, females being affected at a slightly earlier age (10–17 years) than males (14–19 years). The condition is rare in infancy, but the incidence rises sharply with the onset of puberty, and about 80% of the 12–18-year age group is affected to some extent. Some 70% of cases remit spontaneously after about 5 years, and most of the remainder improve slowly thereafter. However, acne occasionally persists into late adulthood, affecting five times as many women (5%) as men, though men tend to be more severely affected because of their higher androgen levels. Hirsute females are more liable than other women to suffer acne and this should provoke a search for an endocrine abnormality.

Although it is more common in cold climates and industrialized areas, acne may be aggravated by hot, humid conditions once established.

Pathology and aetiology

The underlying problem seems to be an exaggerated response of the pilosebaceous units to normal levels of circulating androgens, causing increased production of a modified sebum.

Because the composition of the sebum is altered, there is hyperkeratosis in the mouth of the follicular duct and outflow of sebum is blocked, causing gross enlargement of the pilosebaceous follicles. Saprophytic bacteria, notably *Propionibacterium acnes*, are trapped in the follicle and their metabolism produces inflammatory substances from the sebum, so that the follicles become surrounded by inflammatory (polymorphonuclear and lymphoid) cells. Excessive production of free fatty acids in the sebum may initiate blockage of the follicles and maintain the inflammatory response.

Oxidation of tyrosine at the surface of the trapped sebum by oxygen and tyrosinase produces **melanin**, staining the sebum to give the characteristic black comedone: 'blackheads' are not due to dirty skin. Although bacterial activity exacerbates the condition there is no evidence that acne is infective in origin. In some cases rupture of comedones releases their contents into the underlying tissues, causes an intense dermal inflammation (**cystic acne**).

There is a genetic predisposition with a familial association, and the condition is aggravated by stress, hormones (premenstrually) and a hot climate. Certain drugs may aggravate acne or cause an acneiform reaction as a side-effect (Table 13.15). An environmental or iatrogenic

---

Table 13.15   Some iatrogenic and environmental causes of acne-like eruptions

Iatrogenic
Hormones: corticosteroids, corticotrophins, androgens, anabolic steroids, gonadotrophins
Halogenated drugs: e.g. halothane, hexachlorophane, hyoscine butylbromide, ipratropium bromide, propantheline bromide, bromocriptine (rarely)
Some antitubercular drugs: e.g. isoniazid, rifampicin
Some anticonvulsants: e.g. phenytoin, phenobarbital, troxidone
Psychotropic drugs: e.g. lithium, maprotiline, chloral hydrate
Sulphur-containing drugs: e.g. disulfiram, thiouracils
Miscellaneous: dactinomycin, antibiotics[a], cyanocobalamin, ciclosporin, quinine

Environmental, occupational, etc.
Cosmetics, especially 'heavy' or oily products
Oily sunscreens
Mineral oils
Creosote, pitch, tar
Chlorinated aromatic compounds[b], polychlorbiphenyls, herbicides, preservatives

[a] Due to colonization of lesions with resistant bacteria or *Candida albicans*.

[b] Cause chloracne.

cause is probable whenever acne occurs in an older patient or in an unusual facial distribution.

It has been alleged that acne is due to a poor, fatty diet, but this is without foundation.

Clinical features

Acne is so common and usually has such a characteristic appearance that the diagnosis is seldom in doubt. Onset is gradual, initially with blackheads and whiteheads, progressing to inflamed nodules. The skin and scalp are greasy and dandruff is usually present.

Pustules and deep cysts occur in some patients if the condition is not controlled. Cysts cause intense local inflammation and eventually heal to leave permanent, characteristic depressed scars. Cystic acne, which is aggravated by a hot climate, may be very resistant to treatment and improve only with a move to more temperate conditions.

Because the onset usually coincides with the period of increased sexual awareness, and the lesions are visible and often unsightly, there is always emotional and psychological distur-bance, sometimes severe. This may lead to aggressive or reclusive behaviour.

Occasionally there may be confusion with:

- Rosacea (see below).
- Perioral dermatitis (Plate 3), sometimes caused by the inappropriate use of topical steroids around the mouth, may also give an inflamed, pustular eruption but comedones and a greasy skin are absent.
- Atopic dermatitis (p. 852).
- Seborrhoeic dermatitis (p. 853).

Because the management of these differ from that of acne a firm diagnosis is essential.

Management

Aims

The aims of management are to:

- Encourage an optimistic outlook and ensure perseverance and compliance with therapy.
- Prevent disfiguring scarring.
- Unblock the ducts of the sebaceous glands by:
  - Reducing sebum production.

Table 13.16 Pharmacotherapy of target features of acne

Aim	Mode of action	Class of agent	Examples
Reduction of:			
Scarring	Loosening of keratin plugs	Keratolytic	Benzoyl peroxide, salicylic acid/sulphur preparations
		Retinoid	Tretinoin
Hyperkeratinization of sebaceous follicles	Antiproliferative	Retinoid	Isotretinoin
		Corticosteroid[a]	Hydrocortisone, methylprednisolone
Inflammation	Reduce skin flora	Antimicrobial	Benzoyl peroxide, clindamycin, erythromycin, tetracyclines, potassium hydroxyquinoline sulphate
Sebum production	Hormonal regulation	Anti-androgens plus oestrogen	Co-cyprindiol
	Regulation of cell activity	Retinoids	Isotretinoin, tazarotene, tretinoin

[a] Topical corticosteroids should not normally be used for acne, though commercial preparations containing them are available.

- Reducing keratinocyte activity in the duct.
- Loosening the keratin plugs, thus achieving a free flow of sebum.
• Suppress the growth of bacteria that produce inflammatory substances.

General measures

The types of treatment used are outlined in Table 13.16, and a flow chart for the treatment of acne is given in Figure 13.7.

Patients should be advised sympathetically of an optimistic outcome, because acne can be treated very successfully, though not necessarily cured, with safe medication. Complete healing occurs in most cases. However, rapid improvement must not be expected, and successful treatment requires at least six months' therapy. The improvement rate is approximately as follows:

• 4–6 weeks, some improvement.
• 2–3 months, 40% improvement.
• 6 months, 75% improvement.

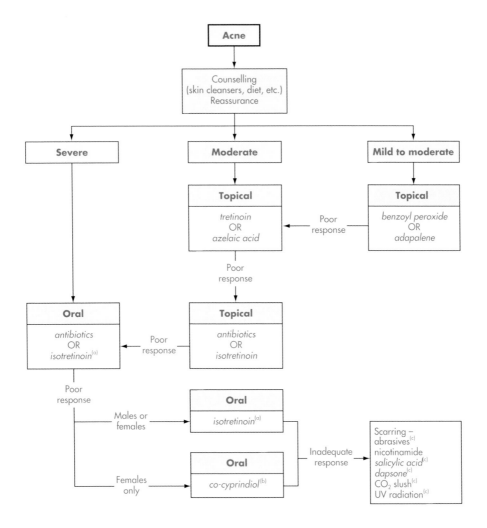

Figure 13.7   Flow chart for the treatment of acne. [a]Oral isotretinoin is highly teratogenic. Strict contraceptive precautions are essential. [b]Acts as a contraceptive. [c]These agents are not recommended for general application. They are suitable only for specialist use.

Patients should be taught appropriate self-management. Because most of them tend to have rather sensitive skins, any new treatment should be initiated cautiously at the lowest available concentration. Detergent washes may help by reducing greasiness, but excessively frequent or vigorous treatment is undesirable. Greasy make-up should be avoided.

Good compliance is essential for success, most failures being associated with lack of perseverance or non-adherence to the correct method of use of medication. Initially, once-daily use on a restricted area for 4–5 days will detect the possibility of a severe reaction, before using twice-daily over the whole area. The intensity of treatment can then be increased stepwise.

Patients should avoid squeezing comedones, because this may cause or exacerbate permanent scarring by forcing infected sebum into surrounding tissue, causing intense inflammation. Exposure to sun and wind may be helpful, by promoting skin peeling, but may aggravate reactions to medications.

Topical pharmacotherapy

Skin reaction to treatment

Some degree of inflammation and scaling is inevitable with most treatments, except *adapalene*, and is desirable because it indicates efficacy. However, inflammation should not be too severe and it is advisable to have a 1- to 2-day 'drug holiday' after a moderate reaction, before recommencing treatment. An area larger than that currently affected should be treated, but the area around the eyes must be avoided.

Patients using *benzoyl peroxide* or the vitamin A derivatives *tretinoin* or *isotretinoin* (gels or lotions are preferable to creams because they are non-greasy), should avoid bright sunshine and exposure to UV 'sun' lamps, which may produce photosensitive reactions, and there is a remote possibility of an increased incidence of skin tumours with topical retinoids. Both of these retinoids are available with *erythromycin* (see below).

The use of a retinoid in the morning and *benzoyl peroxide* at night may be more effective, but this is inappropriate if the *benzoyl peroxide* produces significant peeling. Peeling due to the prior use of *benzoyl peroxide* should be allowed to heal before using a topical retinoid.

Inflamed comedonal lesions

Benzoyl peroxide. This mildly bactericidal keratolytic agent is one of the most effective treatments for mild disease. It is available in a variety of formulations in concentrations of 2.5–10%. Patients with sensitive skins should start with 2.5% once daily, otherwise the 5% products are satisfactory: a test patch is desirable before full area usage. The aim is to build up to use of the 10% product twice daily, if tolerated. The skin irritation is believed to be associated with the activity of the drug and often subsides as treatment proceeds.

No benefit has been shown for preparations with added sulfur, though products with added antimicrobials, e.g. *erythromycin, hydroxyquinoline, miconazole*, are available (see below).

Patients should be warned that *benzoyl peroxide* may bleach clothing.

Azelaic acid. This very well-tolerated dicarboxylic acid appears to act by interfering with the mitochondrial function in melanocytes and, presumably, in other basal layer and pilosebaceous cells. It also has antimicrobial properties and is similarly effective to *benzoyl peroxide* and, additionally, may prevent post-inflammatory hyperpigmentation in dark-skinned patients.

It is not normally used in pregnant or breast-feeding women, and should not be used near the eyes.

Antibiotics. Topical antimicrobial treatment is popular because it avoids the problems associated with long-term systemic use. However, skin sensitization may occur (*neomycin* is no longer used for this reason) and they may encourage the emergence of resistant strains. Because of this, it is preferable to use *benzoyl peroxide, azelaic acid* or *adapalene* first. Further, topical antimicrobials are not usually used for longer than 10–12 weeks, though if a response occurs the course may be repeated after a gap of 3–4 weeks, to minimize resistance, which is an increasing problem. They produce reduction of local inflammation by reducing infection and recruitment of pro-inflammatory cells and by a mild cytotoxic effect.

Lotions containing *erythromycin*, *clindamycin* and *tetracycline* are useful for mild to moderate inflammatory acne. Combinations of *erythromycin* with *benzoyl peroxide*, retinoids or *zinc acetate* may help to minimize antibiotic resistance.

Retinoids. *Adapalene* is a retinoid-like topical agent, formulated as a 3- to 10-μm microcrystalline suspension in a gel base. This particle size gives good penetration into the pilosebaceous follicles. *Adapalene* achieves most of the aims of treatment, having four clinical effects: it is comedolytic, it loosens the keratin plugs and reduces sebum production and the inflammation caused by the irritant effect of sebum and microbial action on damaged tissue. The specificity of *adapalene* results in good tolerance. Although it seems to provide a faster response than *tretinoin*, the overall outcomes of the two drugs appear similar. The contra-indications are similar to those for *tretinoin*. Treatment should be stopped if it causes severe irritation.

Adapalene is licensed in the UK for treating mild to moderate acne.

An important advantage of retinoids over antibiotics is that retinoids do not induce *Pr. acnes* resistance. Further, *adapalene* does not interact with other treatments and is very stable.

Mild to moderate comedonal acne

Because retinoids (p. 835) normalize development of follicular keratinocytes, they are used when there are numerous comedones. *Tretinoin* is comedolytic and keratolytic and is available as a cream, gel or lotion in concentrations of 0.01% and 0.025%. The lower of these should be used for patients with sensitive skins, or as a starter dose.

Because it causes photosensitivity reactions, *tretinoin* should not be used with UV lamps, and exposure to sunlight should be minimized. Some patients do better by using this in the morning and *benzoyl peroxide* at night, but both products should not be applied simultaneously. If the latter has been used for some time, causing skin peeling, topical retinoids should not be used until the skin has healed completely.

Tretinoin is contra-indicated in pregnancy (contraceptive precautions should be taken in women of child-bearing age), eczema, on broken or sunburned skin and if there is a history of cutaneous malignancy.

Isotretinoin is an isomer of *tretinoin* with similar properties. It is available as a 0.05% gel, with or without *erythromycin*, and is also used systemically (see below).

Retinoids should not be used in severe acne involving large areas. Contact must be avoided with the eyes, mucous membranes, i.e. nostrils and mouth, and eczematous, sunburned or damaged skin. They should be used with care on sensitive skin, e.g. the neck and behind the ears, and concentrations should not be allowed to build up in the angles of the nose. Retinoids should not be applied until the skin has recovered fully from the effects of damaging treatments, e.g. peeling agents, UV radiation, abrasive skin cleansers, astringent lotions or cosmetics. Finally, strict precautions should be taken to avoid exposure to UV radiation or sunlight: high protection factor sun creams or protective clothing should be used.

Severe acne should be managed by consultant dermatologists.

Other topical treatments

Nicotinamide gel promotes skin peeling and may be useful. It tends to cause dryness and irritation, and the frequency of application should be reduced if these reactions are not tolerated.

UV radiation is occasionally used to promote skin peeling in resistant acne, but it must be used cautiously if there is any evidence of photosensitivity; in addition, the eyes must be protected. All topical treatments irritate the skin to some extent and make it particularly UV sensitive.

Exfoliation has also been achieved using glycolic acid or by swabbing with a solid carbon dioxide–acetone slush.

Corticosteroids are not recommended for use in acne treatment because the fluorinated agents aggravate the condition, and the more potent steroids may cause irreversible skin damage (p. 834; Plate 16). Further, *sulfur* and *salicylic acid* preparations, and debridement with mild abrasives, are not considered to be helpful and should no longer be used. However, the large cysts that occur in severe acne may respond to intralesional injections of *hydrocortisone sodium phosphate* or *sodium succinate*.

Superficial facial damage has been treated with exfoliating agents and laser therapy and deeper scarring with injections of collagen, but a year should be allowed after comedone clearance before scars are assessed.

Systemic pharmacotherapy

This is required in moderate to severe acne unresponsive to topical treatment and for difficult to reach areas. It may be advisable to continue topical therapy for 1–2 years, concurrently with systemic treatment: exceptional cases may need continued topical therapy for some 10–12 years, though this should not be necessary if retinoids or full doses of antibiotics are used.

Antibiotics
If topical antibiotics fail to give significant improvement after 2 months, systemic antibiotics are used.

For optimal effect, *erythromycin*, *doxycycline* or other tetracyclines should be used at normal antibiotic doses until the lesions have resolved completely. This may take at least 6 months, the dose then being tapered to zero over the ensuing month or two (see Chapter 8). Although doses lower than those used for normal antibiotic use are common, they are less effective and run the risk of failure due to resistance, although there is less risk of side-effects. Antibiotics may occasionally exacerbate acne due to colonization of the lesions with resistant microorganisms, usually Gram-negative bacteria or *Candida albicans*, which need appropriate treatment (see Chapter 8). Repeat courses of antibiotics may be needed and do not appear to be commonly associated with problems of bacterial resistance or excessive side-effects (see Chapter 8).

Tetracyclines should be used with the usual precautions regarding timing of doses in relation to food and other medications. If compliance is a problem, *doxycycline* (once-daily) or *minocycline* (twice-daily) may be preferred; in fact, the latter has been reported to be more effective than *tetracycline*, possibly because of fewer resistance problems. However, *minocycline* may cause a lupus-like syndrome and a bluish/brown skin discoloration: the drug should be stopped immediately if either of these reactions occurs. Tetracyclines are unsuitable for children under 12 years of age because it is deposited in the teeth and bones, causing undesirable tooth discoloration, and may reduce tooth and bone growth.

If there is no response after 2 months, or if there is deterioration or a recurrence during treatment, a change should be made to a second-line antibiotic, e.g. *clindamycin* or *trimethoprim*. Alternatively, if treatment has been initiated in community practice the patient should be referred to a specialist clinic.

Hormone therapy
If an oral contraceptive is being used, a change to one with a higher oestrogen content may be helpful (if tolerated), on order to increase the anti-androgenic activity.

Resistant acne in females may be treated with *co-cyprindiol*, a *cyproterone–ethinylestradiol* combination, which reduces sebum secretion by 30% and acts as a hormonal contraceptive. A clear improvement is usually apparent after several months. The product must not be used in males.

Isotretinoin
Patients with pustules or severe cystic acne, or who are unresponsive after 2 months of antibiotic treatment, may need hospital referral. Late-onset acne, at 30–50 years, is also usually resistant to antibiotics. Acne unresponsive to other agents usually responds dramatically to *isotretinoin* (p. 837), often with lasting improvement. *Isotretinoin* causes a marked inhibition of sebum gland activity and complete or nearly complete remission in about 12–16 weeks. Sebum production may remain at low levels for up to a year or so after stopping treatment. Consequently, many acne patients experience long periods of remission with *isotretinoin*, though men under 25 years of age are more likely to relapse. There is also a secondary anti-inflammatory effect.

There is a long catalogue of side-effects associated with *isotretinoin* (see Table 13.12). Because of its toxicity, long-term *isotretinoin* administration may be unjustified for treating a minor disease state such as acne, although the condition is admittedly potentially disfiguring. Repeat courses are inadvisable. The oral form is available in the UK only through hospital consultants, and through them to named community pharmacies. Sore eyes, cracked lips and dry, peeling skin are common and can be managed with hypromellose eye drops and emollients, respectively. Keratolytics (*salicylic acid*), abrasives and laser treatment must be avoided. Because *isotretinoin* is highly teratogenic, fertile women must take strict contraceptive measures, starting 1 month before initiating treatment and continuing for at least 1 month after stopping. Fertile women should be tested for pregnancy 2–3 days before menstruation is expected and treatment started on day 2 or 3 of the cycle.

Isotretinoin is contra-indicated if pregnancy is possible and in patients with hyperlipidaemia or abnormal liver function.

Other treatments

A small trial of the antigout drug *colchicine* in antibiotic-resistant acne (unlicensed indication) has been reported to produce up to 70% improvement, especially in severe cystic nodular disease. This is the subject of further trial, which will need to demonstrate tolerance of this rather toxic drug, notably the absence of diarrhoea.

Dapsone is used occasionally if other treatments fail (unlicensed indication). There are potentially severe side-effects, including *dapsone* syndrome, i.e. rash with fever and eosinophilia, which requires immediate cessation of treatment. Other blood dyscrasias also occur.

Rosacea

Definition and epidemiology

Rosacea is a chronic inflammatory condition, characterized by reddish, acneiform lesions of the face and forehead and telangiectases, but without comedones (see Plate 4). Although less common than acne, rosacea affects about 1% of dermatological outpatients in the UK. In contrast to acne, rosacea is much more common in women, especially during and after the menopause.

It is possible that perioral dermatitis (p. 823; Plate 3) is a variant form of rosacea, although it has also been ascribed to cosmetic allergy. It may be important to identify which of these is causing a rash around the area of the mouth because treatment is different. Corticosteroids aggravate both rosacea and perioral dermatitis (see below).

Aetiology and clinical features

The pathology of rosacea is unknown, but it may be a familial condition. It is provoked by anything causing persistent flushing of the face. The flushing correlates with:

- Perimenopausal incidence, especially if the climacteric is prolonged.
- Ingestion of alcohol, hot drinks and spicy foods.
- Exposure to bright sunshine and high winds (there is a high incidence in outdoor workers).

Flushing usually starts on the forehead. Unlike acne, rosacea usually affects the face only and the 30–50-year age group. Although there are no comedones, there are closed papules, more generalized inflammation and the skin is dry, despite sebaceous gland hypertrophy. The latter may cause rhinophyma, with a disfiguring, bulbous, reddened nose, primarily in male alcoholics. The ears and eyelids may occasionally be similarly affected. New facial capillaries develop and these may dilate to form telangiectases. Ocular involvement is a serious complication requiring specialist ophthalmological care.

Pharmacotherapy

Mild rosacea may not require treatment unless it is causing psychological distress. Mild to moderate disease is treated empirically with topical *metronidazole* gel or cream, or any of the topical antibiotics used for acne. However, preparations with an alcoholic base may aggravate flushing. Emollients may be useful.

Moderate to severe rosacea and resistant disease requires the use of high-dose antibiotics; e.g. 1–2 g/day of *erythromycin*, 1 g/day of *tetracycline* or 100–200 mg/day of *minocycline*, for

3–6 months. Topical antibiotics should be continued. The benefit of antibiotics is probably due their mild toxicity to epidermal structures. Severe disease unresponsive to antibiotics may require *isotretinoin*: 100–200 µg/kg of body weight/day is normally sufficient but higher doses may be needed. *Isotretinoin* is a very toxic drug and the usual precautions and contra-indications must be observed (see above). This is an unlicensed indication.

Antibiotics may be ineffective against erythema and flushing: a beta-blocker can help with the former and, paradoxically, 4% topical *nicotinamide* with the latter, but this may be very irritant. Low-dose *clonidine*, e.g. 25 µg twice-daily, may also help to control flushing, but has potentially serious side-effects, notably intractable, severe depression. This is clearly undesirable in a patient who is already depressed because of their condition.

Ocular involvement requires specialist oph-thalmological management. Rhinophyma is dealt with by plastic surgery, nowadays usually by high-frequency diathermy or laser therapy, which may give long-term benefit.

Corticosteroids are contra-indicated in rosacea and perioral dermatitis. If the latter is thought to be due to an allergic reaction to cosmetics it should be treated by cessation of use and oral antihistamines. If the rash is resistant to anti-allergic therapy, it is likely that it is due to perioral dermatitis, so the temptation to use *hydrocortisone cream*, which may be requested by patients, should be resisted.

Urticaria

Definition

The condition involves transient, pruritic, chronic or recurrent inflammatory weals, plaques and papules. It is also known as nettlerash and, mostly in North America, as hives. The weals are raised, oedematous lesions, that are very variable in size and extent.

Hereditary angioedema (angioneurotic oed-ema) involves larger areas of the SC tissues and dermis, producing gross swelling.

There is an arbitrary distinction between acute and chronic urticaria. The acute form persists for less than 30 days before remission occurs, with recurrences after variable periods, whereas chronic urticaria involves episodes lasting for longer than 30 days.

Pathology and aetiology

The condition can have various causes (Table 13.17):

- Immunological, mediated by IgE, comple-ment components or immune complexes (see Chapter 2).
- Physical, caused by several external agents, including drugs.

Whatever the mechanism, the final result is gross dilatation of the skin capillaries, allowing the escape of fluid, and sometimes leucocytes and less frequently erythrocytes, from the circu-lation into the dermis, i.e. localized oedema. The escape of erythrocytes causes a purpuric rash (p. 826) that may leave residual pigmentation.

Acute urticaria is usually due to a type I (allergic) reaction in atopic subjects, which releases histamine from mast cells. Possible stimuli are given in Table 13.17.

The underlying mechanisms in chronic urticaria are unknown in 80–90% of cases, but may be:

- Immune complex disease (see Chapter 2) coupled with a defective complement cascade, e.g. lack of inhibition of C3a by carboxypeptidase B permits an ongoing reaction.
- Abnormalities of the arachidonic acid–eicosanoid pathway (see Chapter 12), evidenced by sensitivity to salicylates and *indometacin*.
- Chronic infection, e.g. *H. pylori* (see Chapter 3).
- Autoimmune disease:
- IgG auto-antibody reacting with IgE cross-linked to receptor sites.

There is a linkage between autoimmune mast cell disease and autoimmune thyroid disease in about 15% of patients, so thyroid function tests may be indicated.

Table 13.17   Aetiology of urticaria

Immunological reactions

Hypersensitivity: Mediated by IgE
Foods: meat, shellfish, eggs, nuts (especially peanuts), wheat gluten, strawberries, additives (benzoates, tartrazine)
Environmental allergens: house dust (mites), feathers
Drugs releasing histamine: especially aspirin and salicylates; indometacin; codeine; morphine; penicillins; iodinated radiocontrast media, e.g. sodium diatrizoate
Parasitic infestations (helminths, fleas, lice)
Chronic diseases: infections (sinus, urinary), thyrotoxicosis, systemic lupus erythematosus, lymphomas

Mediated by complement (especially hereditary angioedema)
Antibodies (sera, immunoglobulins), blood products

Physical

Cold, heat, sunlight, pressure (clothing), rubbing, vibration, vigorous exercise

Psychogenic, idiopathic

Some patients with SLE and Sjögren's syndrome (see Chapter 12) have an urticarial vasculitis.

Hereditary angioedema is a severe, episodic, autosomal-dominant inherited disorder that affects the face, larynx, extremities and gut. It is associated with an abnormal or deficient C1 esterase inhibitor (see Chapter 2), allowing excessive bradykinin formation. The condition is sometimes associated with perivascular leucocytosis and eosinophilia in the area of lesions. Chronic urticaria may coexist with angioedema.

Clinical features and diagnosis

Acute urticaria is defined by the symptoms. There are transient pruritic weals, possibly lasting for hours, which may vary in size from 1–2 mm to 10–80 mm or be widespread; these may be oval, annular or may follow bizarre shapes and patterns. The weals are usually pink, though larger lesions have a light central area with an erythematous margin, somewhat resembling tinea. The weals occur commonly on pressure areas, hands, feet and trunk, especially exposed areas.

Hereditary angioedema affecting the lips, tongue, larynx and neck, is one of the few derma-

tological emergencies because it may compromise respiration. The weals characteristic of other forms of urticaria do not occur, but tissue swelling may be moderate to gross, and in some cases the patient becomes completely unrecognizable. Abdominal involvement causes severe pain. Chronic urticaria may coexist with angioedema.

About 25% of sufferers have chronic urticaria. This occurs in the age range 10–50 years, most commonly in the 20–40-year age group, and about twice as many women as men are affected. The symptoms are similar to those of the acute form, though some patients have symptoms lasting 20 years or more. Patients tend to be intolerant of salicylates and benzoates. Some aetiologies can be determined by simple challenge tests:

- Cold: application of an ice cube for 10 min gives a weal within 5 min of removal.
- Solar: exposure to an UV or powerful sun lamp for 30–120 s gives weals within 30 min.
- Cholinergic: a hot shower produces weals on the neck, limbs and trunk.
- Pressure: firm pressure perpendicular to the skin, e.g. excessively tight clothing, gives a persistent weal after 1–4 h.

Apart from pressure-related forms, these tend to be associated with angioedema, so prompt emergency treatment needs to be available (see below).

Management

The management of urticaria involves:

- Avoidance of known precipitants.
- Oral antihistamines (both H$_1$ and sometimes H$_2$ blockers), non-sedating during the day, e.g. *acrivastine*, *cetirizine*, *desloratadine*, *fexofenadine* or *mizolastine*, and a sedating antihistamine at night (see p. 831 for side-effects), e.g. *alimemazine*, *hydroxyzine* or *promethazine*. *Ranitidine*, an H$_2$ blocker, may also help. *Doxepin* has both antihistaminic and antidepressant properties and is useful for patients depressed by their condition.
- Corticosteroids:
  - A moderate-potency topical steroid for most patients (see Table 13.11).
  - Oral *prednisolone*: for severe reactions, especially angioedema. The very severe throat swelling of those suffering from hereditary angioedema needs IV *hydrocortisone* and SC *adrenaline* (epinephrine).
- Severe resistant urticaria may respond to *ciclosporin* or to human normal immunoglobulin.
- *Danazol* may be helpful for the long-term treatment of hereditary angioedema (unlicensed indication in the UK).
- Whole fresh plasma, C1 esterase inhibitors and plasmapheresis: these methods are successful with the immune complex form of urticaria because they remove circulating antigen–antibody complexes.

Drug-induced skin disease

Skin eruptions are one of the most common manifestations of systemic or topical drug therapy (Table 13.18). Probably every pharmaceutical product has the potential to cause dermatoses, even topical steroids, though this is very unlikely with *hydrocortisone*. The reactions may be immunological in character and cover the whole range of skin manifestations.

Table 13.18   Some side-effects of drugs on the skin[a]

Side-effect	Examples of drugs which may cause the adverse reaction
Exanthematous eruptions (erythemas or widespread macular rashes)	Amitriptyline, barbiturates, diuretics, gold salts, sulphonylureas, penicillins (especially ampicillin), penicillamine, sulphonamides
Urticaria	Antisera, aspirin, cephalosporins, penicillins, X-ray contrast media
Fixed drug eruptions	Barbiturates, chlordiazepoxide, metronidazole, phenolphthalein, sulphonamides
Acneiform reactions	Androgens, antiepileptics, antitubercular drugs, bromides, corticosteroids, halides
Photoallergic and phototoxic reactions	Antibiotics; phenothiazine antipsychotics, especially chlorpromazine; sulphonamides; sulphonylureas; thiazides
Eczematous reactions	Anaesthetics (local), antibiotics, antihistamines (topical), methyldopa
Exfoliative dermatitis	Carbamazepine, gold salts and heavy metals, isoniazid, phenindione, streptomycin
Purpuras	Indometacin, quinine, sulphonamides, thiazides

[a] Systemic use, except where indicated. Excludes reactions to vehicles, antioxidants, preservatives, etc.
See also Table 13.15.

The systemic use of drugs may cause various types of lesions:

- Bullous or vesicular, e.g. sulphonamides.
- Erythematous, e.g. antisera.
- Lichenoid, e.g. antimalarials, *gold*, *phenothiazines*.
- Photosensitive, e.g. *chlorpromazine*, sulphonamides.
- Pruritic, e.g. tetracyclines.
- Purpuric, e.g. barbiturates, chloramphenicol, *aspirin*.
- Urticarial (see above).

One rather unusual type of response is the fixed drug eruption, which is characterized by a skin reaction in the same localized sites on each occasion that the drug is taken. If the reaction occurs repeatedly, there may be persistent pigmentation of the site, even in the absence of the drug and of an overt skin reaction. Common causes are barbiturates and phenolphthalein, but phenobarbital is used nowadays only for the treatment of epilepsy (see Chapter 6).

Serious systemic reactions may also occur, such as Stevens–Johnson syndrome, with a severe rash, high fever, joint pains and painful involvement of the mucous membranes. This needs expert diagnosis and management, using rest, antibiotics and high-dose corticosteroids.

Reactions to topical treatments include any of those described on p. 851.

The skin as a route for systemic drug delivery

Transdermal (percutaneous) administration is a technique for delivering drugs systemically at a controlled rate over a relatively prolonged period: it is not used for the topical treatment of skin diseases.

The principal barrier to drug penetration of the skin is the horny layer. 'Shunt routes' through the hair follicles and sweat glands are significant in the early stages after application, but only for some electrolytes and highly polar corticosteroids and antibiotics, which penetrate keratin poorly. These shunt routes are important because they are probably the principal routes of penetration and systemic absorption of the topical corticosteroids, though they contribute only marginally to the steady-state flux across the epidermis for many agents. Once past the horny layer, the drug molecules rapidly penetrate the living tissues of the epidermis and dermis and are swept away into the circulation.

The skin also acts as a drug reservoir, due to:

- Binding by proteins in the horny layer, giving a persistence of up to 2–3 weeks after application has ceased.
- Concentration of lipophilic agents in the fatty tissues in the dermis, from which they leach gradually into the circulation. However, this mechanism contributes little to any effect that the product may have on most skin problems, which are generally epidermal in origin.

Factors relevant to penetration include:

- Concentration of the drug.
- Formulation of the product.
- Mode of use (occlusion and greasy vehicles enhance skin penetration).
- Contact time.
- Site of application, e.g. the skin behind the ears is very thin and may be the preferred site, and the presence of hair follicles and sweat glands.
- Patient age: young children and the elderly have readily penetrable skin.
- Features of the disease state, e.g. inflammation and excoriation enhance drug penetration.

Factors affecting the likelihood of side-effects are the skin type (fair-skinned people are more likely to suffer an adverse reaction) and the potential of the formulated product to cause skin problems, e.g. rashes due to the drug, preservatives, adhesives, plastics, etc.

Further details of this subject concern the formulation pharmacist and are not pertinent here (see References and further reading).

References and further reading

Brown R G, Burns T (2002). *Lecture Notes on Dermatology*, 8th edn. Oxford: Blackwell Science.

Chien Y W (1992). Transdermal drug delivery and

delivery systems. In: Chien Y W, ed. *Novel Drug Delivery Systems*. New York: Marcel Dekker.

Fitzpatrick T B, Johnson R A, Wolff K, *et al.* (1997). *Color Atlas and Synopsis of Clinical Dermatology*, 3rd edn. New York: McGraw-Hill.

Hallworth R B (1998). Prevention and treatment of postmenopausal osteoporosis. *Pharm World Sci* **20**: 198–205.

Marks R (2003). *Roxburgh's Common Skin Diseases*, 17th edn. London: Arnold.

14

Renal system

Renal disease and its ultimate consequence – renal failure – represent important issues in the health debate. Although it is now technically feasible to relieve or reverse renal failure, limits to what can be done in practice arise from ethical issues surrounding the allocation of healthcare resources and the organization of organ donation, issues that are under constant debate.

Chronic renal failure is potentially fatal and may condemn a patient to years of dialysis with a substantially reduced quality of life. Successful renal transplantation provides an almost complete solution and now has an extremely good outcome; however, society has not yet fully adjusted to the implications of organ donation. Regular controversies on the persistent vegetative state and 'brain death' testify to this.

This chapter first reviews the normal function of the kidney. Subsequently, the consequences of impairment of these functions, i.e. homeostatic imbalances and renal failure, are explained. Finally, the common clinical conditions that cause these abnormalities are discussed.

Physiological principles of the renal system

The kidney is both structurally and functionally complex, and plays a central role in homeostasis. Thus, many possible forms of renal malfunction can cause a wide range of clinical conditions. Manifestations of renal disorder include fluid, electrolyte and pH imbalances, haemodynamic imbalance, the accumulation of drugs, toxins and waste metabolic products, loss of essential metabolites, and endocrine abnormalities such as anaemia and bone disease.

Pathological processes such as infection, inflammation, auto-immunity, neoplasia and toxins can cause structural damage to the glomeruli, the tubules or the urinary tract. Systemic or local circulatory insufficiency can also seriously compromise renal function. The most common pathologies are glomerular inflammation, urinary-tract infection and drug-induced nephrotoxicity. In this section we review the physiological principles of normal renal function, so that abnormalities of the renal system may be better understood.

Anatomy

The gross anatomy of the renal system is shown in Figure 14.1. It is important to distinguish between the kidneys, which are structurally complex, and the urinary tract, the function of which is essentially the storage and transport of urine. Three main regions are distinguished within the kidney: the **cortex**, the **medulla** and the **pelvis**. The cortex contains the glomeruli and the proximal and distal tubules, and the medulla contains the loops of Henle. Glomeruli in different areas have different-length loops of Henle to permit differential control over urine concentration. The loops of the juxtamedullary nephrons (nearest the medulla) extend almost to the pelvis, the area into which the formed urine drains from the collecting ducts. Throughout the kidney there are interstitial cells, probably concerned with endocrine functions.

Although kidney disorders are almost always serious, disorders in the lower urinary tract are seldom serious in themselves but often symptomatically troublesome. However, chronic obstructive problems in the lower urinary tract may eventually cause damage to the kidneys.

The importance of the kidneys may be judged from the fact that although they together weigh just 500 g (less than 1% of body weight) they receive 25% of the cardiac output. Thus renal blood flow is about 1.2 L/min. Like many other organs, the kidneys are modular, each having about 1 million functional subunits or nephrons, each of which performs all the major renal functions and which together provide a total filtration area of 1 m². This represents

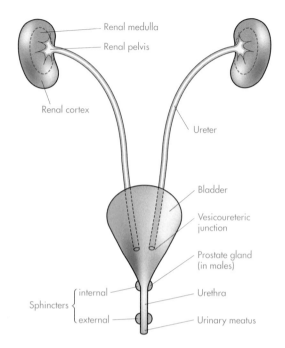

Figure 14.1   Anatomy of renal system.

considerable functional over-capacity because life can continue quite normally with one-half of a single functioning kidney, i.e. only 25% of nephrons functioning. Thus when the kidneys are diseased, serious symptoms do not appear until there has been over 90% damage; more-over, such damage is often irreversible, making treatment difficult.

Summary of renal functions

The kidney is the body's key organ of overall homeostatic control and its functions may be considered in three main groups (Table 14.1). Elimination of waste is usually the main function associated with the kidney, but the regulatory functions are equally important, and the kidneys are also involved in several major endocrine systems.

Table 14.1   Functions of the kidney

Elimination of waste/surplus	Carbohydrate-derived Nitrogenous Other	Water, acid Urea creatinine, uric acid, guanidine, amines, etc. Sulphate, phosphate, exogenous toxins, etc.
Regulation of fluid and electrolyte balance	Total body water Plasma osmotic pressure, pH Na, K, Ca, Mg, etc. Chloride, bicarbonate, phosphate, etc.	
Endocrine homeostasis	Blood pressure Calcium and bone metabolism RBC production	

RBC, red blood cell.

Elimination

The potentially toxic by-products of metabolism must be excreted, along with excess nutrients and any exogenous toxins absorbed from the gut and their subsequent metabolites. Generally, elimination is passive, although certain substances are actively secreted.

Carbohydrate metabolism, the major energy pathway of the body, produces carbon dioxide and water. Most carbon dioxide is eliminated passively by the lungs, but the kidneys have far more control in secreting it, in small but crucial amounts, as acid. Although much of the water produced by metabolism, along with that taken in the diet, is lost through sweating, respiration and insensible losses, once again the kidney exercises selective control to maintain water balance.

The predominant nitrogenous waste product is **urea** from protein metabolism and its level in the blood provides a useful approximate index of renal function. Nucleic acid breakdown produces **urate**, which is actively secreted, and muscle metabolism produces **creatinine**, which is also used as an index of kidney function. Some sulphate and phosphate are also released by protein metabolism. Urea is not as harmful as is commonly believed, guanidine, amines and other metabolites (phenols, hydroxyacids, etc.) being more toxic.

The kidney also has a role in the catabolism of peptides, notably insulin.

Fluid and electrolyte balance

The kidney plays a crucial, active role in maintaining the correct ionic, osmotic, pH and fluid balances throughout the body. It detects imbalances, secretes local regulatory hormones, and actively excretes or retains substances as necessary. One of the drawbacks of its interaction with so many different systems is that there may occasionally be conflicting demands, which can be resolved only by compromises. For example, chloride may be variously regarded as an anion, an acid or simply an osmotically active particle, depending on circumstances. Controlling chloride to preserve electrical neutrality or osmotic balance may compromise pH balance.

Water balance
The body is normally in positive water balance, the kidney adjusting for varying intakes and losses by altering water clearance. Certain irreducible constraints enforce a minimum average daily intake of about 1 L (Table 14.2). The kidneys require at least 500 mL of water to excrete the average daily load of osmotically active waste products at maximal urinary concentration, i.e. under maximal ADH stimulation. This is just about balanced by the water produced from the metabolic oxidation of carbohydrates. Thus the minimum dietary intake needed is that which will replace insensible losses in breath, faeces and perspiration (excluding additional or exertional perspiration).

Table 14.2   Approximate average daily water balance (mL)[a]

Obligatory losses		Sources of replacement	
Kidneys[b]	500	Metabolism of glucose	500
Skin[c]	500	Diet	1000
Lungs[c]	400		
Faeces[c]	100		
TOTAL	1500		1500

[a] Only minimum values given (mL); there are considerable daily variations.

[b] Normally, daily urine output is about 1000 mL greater than this obligatory minimum, owing to increased dietary intake.

[c] 'Insensible losses'.

Fluid compartments

The main fluid compartments of the body are given in Figure 14.2. The intravascular and extravascular components of the extracellular fluid (ECF) are in equilibrium by free diffusion, except that plasma proteins cannot usually leave the blood. Although water diffuses across cell walls passively under osmotic forces, there are membrane pumps effecting the flow of most other substances to and from the intracellular fluid (ICF). However, the activity of these pumps is largely dependent on concentration gradients. Thus the kidney, by controlling ECF composition, influences all compartments.

There is a complex and subtle interplay between the maintenance of ECF osmotic pressure, mainly through control of sodium concentration, and the total volume and relative distribution of fluid between the compartments.

The kidney also controls the plasma potassium level and thus total body potassium. By selectively varying the secretion of hydrogen ions and reabsorption or regeneration of bicarbonate the kidney can significantly alter plasma pH, and thus body pH.

Endocrine functions

The kidney is involved in three important systemic hormonal systems.

Blood pressure

Renal involvement in blood pressure control operates via a number of mechanisms (p. 880). This is partly 'enlightened self-interest' because the kidney cannot operate without an adequate perfusion pressure, but it also contributes to the systemic blood pressure control mechanisms.

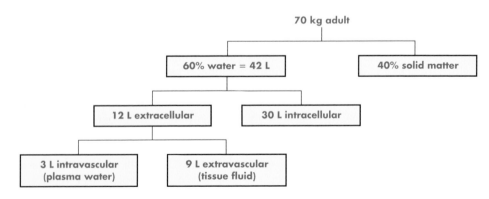

Figure 14.2   Body fluid compartments. Plasma water, volume of water in blood (i.e. excluding cells and colloidal protein).

Calcium

The kidney is vital to calcium and bone metabolism. In addition to being a target organ for vitamin D and parathormone, the kidney is responsible for the final stage in the activation of vitamin D by hydroxylating 25-hydroxycholecalciferol to 1,25-dihydroxycholecalciferol. An overview of vitamin D metabolism is given in Chapter 3, p. 150.

Erythropoiesis

In response to hypoxaemia, the kidney secretes erythropoietin, which promotes RBC production in the bone marrow. Without erythropoietin, erythropoiesis cannot proceed efficiently and Hb levels stay below 6–8 g/100 mL, producing anaemia. In certain less common renal diseases, e.g. polycystic kidney and renal tumour, there is erythropoietin over-production, with consequent polycythaemia.

It can now be appreciated why renal failure is so serious. In acute renal failure (ARF) it is mainly elimination and fluid/electrolyte regulation that are affected. The patient suffers particularly from retention of excess water, acid and potassium. In chronic renal failure, endocrine malfunction adds other problems, including hypertension, bone disease and iron-resistant anaemia.

Mechanisms of elimination

The kidney goes about elimination in a seemingly perverse and inefficient manner. Instead of selectively excreting unwanted substances it filters almost everything, and then selectively reabsorbs what needs to be conserved. About 10% of the total renal blood flow, i.e. 120 mL/min, is filtered at the glomeruli, along with most low-molecular weight constituents: this is the glomerular filtration rate (GFR). Some 99% of this 180 L/day is then actively reabsorbed, leaving an average daily urine volume of only about 1.5 L. (This system may be a relic of the aquatic era of the evolution of life, when the large amounts of fluid and sodium that were lost could easily be replaced.)

There are three main phases of elimination (Figure 14.3):

- Size-elective but otherwise indiscriminate ultrafiltration across the glomerular membrane from plasma into the tubular lumen to produce filtrate.
- Active reabsorption into plasma of useful substances in bulk, mostly from the proximal tubule.
- Selective secretion from plasma or reabsorption into plasma of certain critical substances in small amounts to maintain the fluid and electrolyte balances, mainly in the distal tubule and collecting duct.

To understand how certain diseases affect renal function, the factors that affect filtration and the patterns of reabsorption and secretion must be briefly reviewed. This simple discussion will not distinguish between the cortical and juxtamedullary nephrons; unless otherwise stated, the former are usually implied.

Filtration

During glomerular ultrafiltration blood cells and colloidal macromolecules, i.e. plasma proteins, are retained but smaller molecules (crystalloids) are carried through the glomerular basement membrane (GBM) under hydrostatic pressure by solvent drag (convection). Substances with a molecular weight <5000 Da pass freely. Passage decreases with increasing molecular size, especially above about 25 kDa; only 3% of Hb (64 kDa) would pass if it were free in plasma, and less than 1% of albumin (minimum size approx. 70 kDa) passes. Anions pass less easily than cations because the GBM is negatively charged, but again this effect is only significant for larger molecules.

Factors affecting glomerular filtration rate

The GFR is the key index of renal function because if there is no filtration then none of the regulatory mechanisms that act on the filtrate can operate. Figure 14.3 is a functional diagram of a nephron, which identifies the sites where factors which influence the GFR operate. Table 14.3 summarizes the clinical conditions under which these factors can become altered. This usually happens due to changes in filtration pressure (especially the systemic arterial

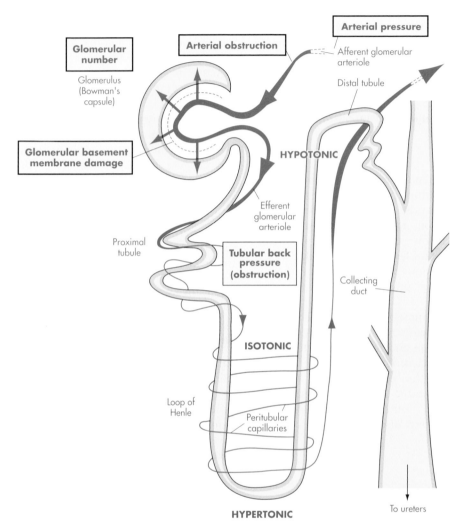

Figure 14.3   Diagram of single nephron showing main functional components and factors that influence filtration (boxed).

pressure). The integrity of the basement membrane is another important factor.

Perfusion. The kidney strives to maintain systemic arterial blood pressure, but failing that, filtration pressure at the glomerulus is defended by intrarenal mechanisms. Probably the most common cause of ARF is when such mechanisms are overwhelmed by severe systemic hypotension, e.g. from haemorrhagic or cardiogenic shock. Long-term damage to renal arteries, e.g. arteriosclerosis and/or atherosclerosis from untreated hypertension, can cause chronic renal failure.

Renal autoregulation maintains renal blood flow, filtration pressure and GFR over wide variations in renal perfusion pressure, principally by alterations in the calibre of afferent and efferent glomerular arteries. The afferent arterioles are dilated by intrarenal PGs, while the efferent ones are constricted by intrarenal angiotensin. In this way the transmembrane hydrostatic pressure, and hence GFR, is defended. One input to this system is tubulo-glomerular feedback. If the GFR

Table 14.3   Factors that can reduce glomerular filtration rate

Factor	Clinical condition where altered
Impaired renal perfusion	
Reduced systemic blood pressure	Heart failure, shock (e.g. myocardial infarction, haemorrhage)
	Drugs, toxins, etc.
Renal arterial obstruction	Renal thrombosis, atherosclerosis
	Untreated hypertension
Damaged glomerular basement membrane	Inflammation (glomerulonephritis)
	Connective tissue disease (e.g. systemic lupus erythematosus)
	Diabetic nephropathy
	Nephrotoxic drugs (e.g. penicillamine)
Reduced glomerular number	Ageing, chronic renal failure, nephrectomy
Increased tubular back pressure	Urinary-tract obstruction (e.g. stones, tumour)
	Tubular inflammation ('tubular nephropathy')
	Tubular infection (pyelonephritis)

is altered, the consequent changes in the solute load of the glomerular filtrate are detected in the distal tubule by the juxtaglomerular apparatus (p. 879), which is involved in intrarenal hormone systems.

Another important intrarenal regulatory mechanism is the potentially confusingly named **glomerulotubular balance**. This is a second line of defence if GFR is compromised beyond the ability of the primary compensatory mechanisms to cope. It serves to preserve excretion of water, sodium and other solutes in the face of reduced GFR. It thus provides one aspect of renal reserve, delaying the onset of symptomatic uraemia if renal function declines chronically.

The operation of these control mechanisms is illustrated by the adverse effect of ACEIs in patients with obstructive lesions in both renal arteries (bilateral renal artery stenosis), or patients in whom renal perfusion is otherwise compromised by hypovolaemia (low blood volume) or cardiac failure. In such cases optimal renal perfusion is being maintained partly by raised levels of angiotensin originating from the renal response to the hypoperfusion. Angiotensin maintains renal blood flow by causing intrarenal efferent arteriolar constriction and also, possibly, by elevating systemic BP. ACEIs, by blocking this protective mechanism, may precipitate renal failure by causing a signif-

icant reduction in renal perfusion. Similarly, PG inhibitors, e.g. NSAIDs, can have an adverse effect on renal haemodynamics, causing renal impairment and fluid retention.

Glomerular basement membrane. The GBM is a sensitive structure that is exposed to high flow rates and high concentrations of potential toxins and mediators. It can be damaged by numerous pathological processes, and this underlies many chronic renal diseases. If the GBM is damaged, its permeability to large particles, especially smaller colloids such as albumin, may be increased, causing proteinuria. In more severe cases there may also be, paradoxically, retention of water and sodium owing to a degree of renal impairment (reduced GFR).

Simple variations in pore size cannot account for these changes; porosity may be partly related to a loss of the negative membrane charge, which normally repels the similarly charged plasma albumin. Normally some proteins smaller than about 60–100 kDa are filtered, but almost all are completely reabsorbed. However, the reabsorptive capacity is low and soon exceeded if there is an increase in tubular protein concentration. The catabolism of filtered protein within the renal tubules, which is normally minimal, may be increased in the presence of proteinuria to compensate.

Glomerular number.   In chronic renal failure, diminishing renal function is believed to result from a reduced number of fully active nephrons rather than to a general decline in the function of all nephrons (the 'intact nephron hypothesis'). A progressive loss of functional nephrons is the main reason why the elderly have reduced renal function – a process that continues throughout adult life. Normally about half of the nephrons are lost by the age of 80 years.

Tubular back pressure.   Obstruction anywhere along the urinary tract will inhibit filtration by increasing the pressure within the tubule, which reduces the filtration pressure across the GBM. Such obstruction can occur within the tubules themselves if they are damaged; in the renal pelvis (in pyelonephritis and some forms of nephrotoxicity); or in the lower urinary tract (owing to the presence of a ureteral stone or bladder outflow obstruction).

Reabsorption and secretion

Clinically, the important features here are the consequences of the interlinked exchange mechanisms that the kidney employs.

Overall pattern through nephron

Proximal tubule.   The glomerular filtrate contains essential nutrients as well as waste matter. Most of the former are returned to the circulation by reabsorption from the proximal tubule into the peritubular capillaries (Figures 14.3 and 14.4). There are specific pumps for most substances, such as sodium, potassium, bicarbonate, amino acids, glucose, etc. Water follows osmotically and chloride electrochemically. These pumps have a maximum transport capacity, and if the filtrate concentration of a substance exceeds the capacity of the pump the substance appears in the urine. The plasma concentration of the substance is then said to exceed its renal threshold. The most common example of this is glycosuria in diabetes mellitus.

Most nutrients, and about 70% of the filtered water and electrolytes, are reabsorbed proximally. Reabsorption depends largely on uncon-

trolled bulk transport, necessitated by the profligacy of glomerular filtration. Osmotic diuretics act in this region by increasing the osmotic pressure of the filtrate, which inhibits water reabsorption.

Some substances, especially acids and bases, are actively secreted in the opposite direction, from the peritubular capillaries into the proximal tubule, e.g. uric acid and many toxins and drugs. This increases the clearance of molecules that have escaped filtration.

Loop.   The main function of the loop of Henle is not to reabsorb water and electrolytes but to generate an osmotic gradient between the renal cortex (hypotonic) and the medulla (hypertonic) by a countercurrent mechanism. This enables the collecting ducts, which pass through this gradient, to adjust urine concentration under the influence of ADH. No more than 10–15% of sodium, chloride and water are reabsorbed here. The powerful loop diuretics, e.g. *furosemide*, act by inhibiting this mechanism, preventing subsequent attempts at concentration by the collecting ducts.

Distal tubule.   In the distal tubule, and to a lesser extent in the collecting ducts, there is the potential for fine adjustments. Although the total amounts of solutes reabsorbed are not great – no more than the final 10% of sodium and water – this is where the kidney exerts its main control of electrolyte balance. The thiazide diuretics inhibit this mechanism.

Selective control in distal tubule

The distal tubule is crucial to the homeostasis of several important systems. If body sodium, blood volume or blood pressure is low, the distal reabsorption of sodium, with chloride or bicarbonate and some water, can be increased by the action of the mineralocorticoid aldosterone. Here, sodium does not carry with it an iso-osmotic load of water, so the immediate effect is a net increase in plasma osmotic pressure.

Aldosterone also inhibits the secretion of potassium into the urine, in response to body requirements, reabsorbing it in exchange for sodium. The aldosterone-antagonist (potassium sparing) diuretics, e.g. *spironolactone*, act here. Potassium secretion is closely linked to that of

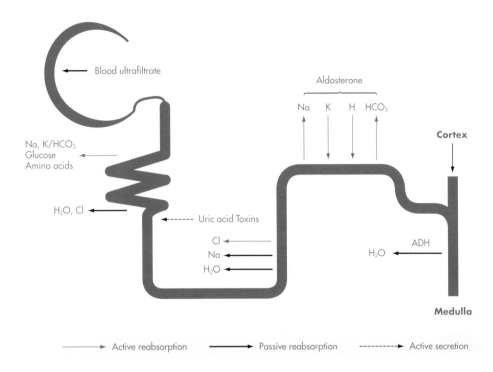

Aldosterone

Na   K   H   HCO₃

Cortex

Blood ultrafiltrate

Na, K/HCO₃
Glucose
Amino acids

H₂O, Cl

Uric acid Toxins

Cl
Na
H₂O

ADH

H₂O

Medulla

Active reabsorption   Passive reabsorption   Active secretion

Figure 14.4   Reabsorption patterns in the renal tubule. HCO_3, bicarbonate; Cl, chloride; Na, sodium; H, acid; ADH, antidiuretic hormone.

acid (hydrogen ions) because the same transport mechanism is used for both. However, acid secretion is under a different, and therefore potentially conflicting, control mechanism. This is triggered by variations in plasma pH, which affects the activity of tubular carbonic anhydrase, thereby altering acid production and secretion in the tubules (p. 881).

Total body water. If the body is fluid-depleted or relatively hypertonic, ADH is secreted. This hormone permits passive diffusion of water from the glomerular filtrate in the distal tubule and collecting duct back into the peritubular capillaries. This is possible because the ducts pass through the hypertonic region of the renal medulla. Conversely, when the body is relatively hypotonic or fluid overloaded, ADH secretion is inhibited, water is prevented from leaving the ducts and a dilute urine is produced. In diabetes insipidus ADH secretion is deficient, resulting in severe polyuria.

Consequences of tubular exchanges

There will be occasions when conflicting demands on the kidney mean that one adjustment needs to be compromised to allow another. Usually the maintenance of osmotic pressure is paramount, but in severe hypovolaemia the defence of blood pressure by fluid retention takes precedence. Three consequences of the main exchange mechanisms need to be emphasized, because they have important implications for electrolyte imbalance and its management (Figure 14.5):

1. Sodium is reabsorbed with either chloride or bicarbonate (to preserve electrical neutrality).
2. Sodium is exchanged for either acid (hydrogen ions) or potassium in the distal tubule (cation exchange to preserve electrical neutrality).
3. All acid secreted results in an equivalent amount of bicarbonate being reabsorbed (equimolar amounts, generated by carbonic anhydrase).

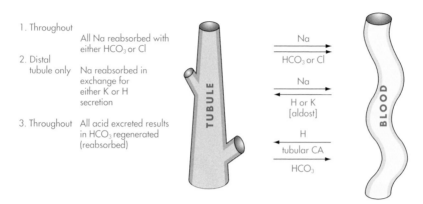

1. Throughout   All Na reabsorbed with
                either HCO₃ or Cl
2. Distal
   tubule only   Na reabsorbed in
                 exchange for
                 either K or H
                 secretion
3. Throughout   All acid excreted results
                 in HCO₃ regenerated
                 (reabsorbed)

Figure 14.5   Important exchanges between blood in the peritubular capillaries and the filtrate in the renal tubules. Aldost, aldosterone; CA, carbonic anhydrase; Cl, chloride; H, acid; HCO₃, bicarbonate; Na, sodium; K, potassium.

Potassium and pH balance

The amount of potassium that can be reabsorbed in the distal tubule, where fine control is exercised, is related to the amount of acid secreted (Figure 14.5 (2)). To secrete acid in exchange for sodium, the tubule must forgo the secretion of potassium because potassium and acid use the same transport mechanism; at the same time the tubule must also reabsorb bicarbonate (Figure 14.5 (3)). Thus, as far as the kidney is concerned, potassium moves with alkali (this is easy to remember if one associates K with KOH). Therefore, when the body requires alkali, in the form of bicarbonate, it tends to accumulate potassium and when it wants to eliminate excess alkali, potassium tends also to be lost.

Ordinarily this causes no problems, but the transport mechanism may become saturated if the demand is excessive. Competition between potassium and acid then forces a compromise to be made so that dyskalaemias (potassium imbalances) are frequently associated with pH imbalances. Thus, for example, if hypokalaemia is not corrected alkalosis will eventually occur as the kidney attempts to retain potassium by using this exchange pump and in doing so it secretes acid. Conversely, acidosis is often complicated by hyperkalaemia.

Chloride and pH balance

Because alkali conservation (bicarbonate reabsorption) is linked to chloride excretion, in effect chloride moves with acid. However, plasma pH is determined primarily by the carbon dioxide/carbonic acid/bicarbonate equilibrium (p. 881), the only anion here being bicarbonate. Thus, if bicarbonate is displaced from the plasma by another anion, such as chloride, the resulting fall in bicarbonate will cause acidosis.

Similarly, if there is a high tubular load of chloride then it may be used non-specifically as the anion to accompany the reabsorption of important cations, which compromises bicarbonate reabsorption and produces a loss of alkali (Figure 14.5 (1)). Hence the tendency to hyperchloraemic acidosis when chloride intake is abnormally high.

This has important implications for fluid therapy with 0.9% sodium chloride solution (physiological saline). Compare its ionic composition with extracellular fluid, e.g. plasma:

- *Physiological saline*:   Na, 150 mmol/L; Cl, 150 mmol/L (approx.).
- *Extracellular fluid*:   Na, 150 mmol/L; Cl, 100 mmol/L (approx.).

Thus 0.9% NaCl is by no means 'normal', and the term 'normal saline' is now outmoded. Although iso-osmotic, it is relatively chloride-rich and prolonged IV administration, in the standard 3 L/day regimen, eventually produces hyperchloraemic acidosis. Conversely, prolonged diuretic therapy, by increasing chloride loss, may produce hypochloraemic alkalosis (in addition to a hypokalaemic alkalosis). Conversely, a benefit of simple physiological saline infusion is that it will correct mild metabolic alkalosis, so that acidic solutions, e.g. ammonium chloride, are rarely needed.

Sodium, potassium and pH

In a similar way, sodium imbalance is also likely to be associated with both pH imbalance and dyskalaemia (Figure 14.5 (2)). The rationale for these associations is left to the reader to elucidate, applying the same principles as used above.

Homeostasis

Total body water and osmotic pressure

Control

The mechanisms for the control of fluid volumes and extracellular osmotic pressure are complementary and interdependent. The volume of water in the body (total body water, TBW) is determined by the total amount of osmotically active substances. Normally, water clearance is adjusted to maintain a uniform osmolar concentration approximately equivalent to twice the plasma sodium level. Sodium levels are controlled by the renal regulation of tubular reabsorption. The distribution of water between the intracellular and extracellular compartments (plasma plus tissue fluid) is also primarily determined by osmotic forces, the osmotic pressure within cells normally being about the same as that of plasma.

Because TBW is usually distributed optimally, it is only necessary for the body to monitor one compartment for it to regulate all. Blood volume is the most 'accessible' because this is reflected in blood pressure. This is monitored in several ways with feedback to renal control mechanisms (p. 880).

The inter-relationship between adjustments of plasma osmolarity and body water is shown in Figure 14.6. Note that aldosterone controls sodium reabsorption, but does not affect blood pressure directly. Aldosterone serves only to change plasma osmotic pressure, because the sodium reabsorption under aldosterone control is not accompanied by an iso-osmotic amount of water. The feedback loop is completed by ADH, which adjusts water reabsorption as appropriate.

Thus volume imbalance causes changes in electrolyte reabsorption via aldosterone, whereas osmotic imbalance causes changes in water reabsorption via ADH. This interdependence of the two systems permits very fine control.

Imbalance

The juxtaglomerular apparatus (JGA) is an area of specialized tissue strategically located between the afferent and efferent glomerular arterioles and beginning of the distal tubule in each nephron, and in contact with all three (Figure 14.6). The JGA can thus detect changes in pressure in the afferent arteriole (usually proportional to systemic arterial pressure) and consequent changes in tubular filtrate flow and concentration. It can then attempt to rectify any fall in BP by the secretion of renin, which causes the activation of both systemic (plasma) angiotensin and local mechanisms involving intrarenal angiotensin and vasodilatory PG.

In order to see how this system functions, consider the consequences of haemorrhage or severe diarrhoea. The iso-osmotic volume loss (hypovolaemia) causes a fall in BP. In response, the JGA secretes renin, aldosterone increases sodium reabsorption, and plasma osmotic pressure rises. This promotes ADH secretion, increasing tubular water reabsorption and restoring TBW. Conversely, in hyponatraemia the osmotic imbalance initially causes reduced water reabsorption and increased urine volume (via ADH), tending to normalize osmotic pressure at the expense of TBW, blood volume and BP. Subsequently the systems once again interact gradually to restore all parameters.

Thirst is a relatively crude mechanism for replenishing both electrolyte and fluid loss, because there is little control over the composition of intake. This loosely controlled process requires the kidney to make the appropriate fine adjustments.

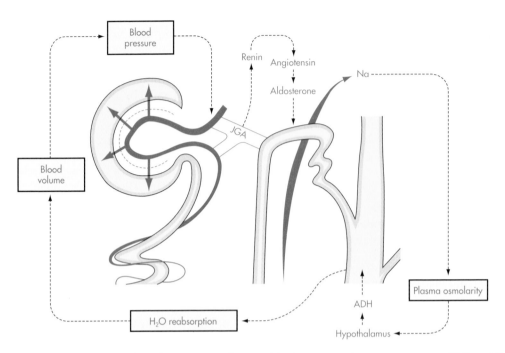

Figure 14.6   Inter-relationship of mechanisms controlling total body water and osmotic pressure. ADH, antidiuretic hormone; JGA, juxtaglomerular apparatus.

Blood pressure control

The main ways in which the kidney is involved in maintaining BP are briefly summarized here and discussed fully in Chapter 4.

Simple pressure natriuresis

If BP changes, a complex interplay of autoregulatory variations in glomerular blood flow and/or tubular reabsorption makes compensatory changes in urine volume. Thus, a fall in BP will cause an automatic fall in urine volume, the fluid retained tending to restore BP. Generally the GFR is maintained constant so as not to compromise excretory functions; the principal mechanism for this is a change in tubular reabsorption.

Renin/angiotensin/aldosterone and the osmoreceptor/antidiuretic hormone systems

These are discussed above.

Atrial natriuretic factor

Rises in blood volume can be detected by increased pressure in the atria of the heart, which secrete a peptide, atrial natriuretic peptide (ANP) that acts in the kidney to promote water loss (by preventing reabsorption). ANP seems to play a role in unloading the heart in heart failure (see Chapter 4).

Acid–base balance

Acid generated by metabolism, plus dietary intake, means that the body is in strongly positive acid balance. This presents three problems: elimination of the excess, defence of pH in plasma and throughout body water, and the ability to adjust for unexpected variations in acid or alkali input or loss. The vast bulk of the excess is eliminated by the lungs; blood buffers defend pH; and the kidney adjusts for variations.

Respiratory compensation

Most of the carbon dioxide produced by the aerobic metabolism of carbohydrate is eliminated routinely by the lungs (about 15 000 mmol of acid per day; Figure 14.10). Yet despite their massive capacity, the lungs can only be used temporarily to adjust for unwanted changes in acid level. If excess acid is produced, prolonged fast breathing to eliminate it is exhausting, and the extra energy used produces yet more carbon dioxide. Conversly, to compensate for alkalosis by reducing respiration cannot be achieved without causing hypoxaemia. Moreover, the net effect of respiratory adjustments is to produce absolute increases or falls in blood buffering capacity. Nevertheless, the lungs provide important rapid primary respiratory compensation. This can be judged from the fact that, in the absence of initial pH imbalance, if respiratory rate were reduced to 25% of normal, blood pH would soon fall to 7.0. Indeed, this is the pathogenesis of respiratory acidosis, which occurs when a respiratory abnormality impairs elimination of carbon dioxide.

Renal compensation

It is the kidney that makes the long-term adjustment for abnormal changes in pH (assuming it is not itself the primary cause of the problem) by appropriate changes in acid secretion and complementary bicarbonate regeneration. The kidneys normally secrete only a small, but crucial, amount of acid: on average about 100 mmol per day. However, this can be varied considerably to compensate for dietary or metabolic imbalance or respiratory impairment. This secondary renal compensation is delayed and slow, but can work indefinitely. A consequence is that in renal failure, metabolic acidosis is a major problem.

Control of this important process is essentially autonomous and passive. Carbonic anhydrase in the tubular cells is simply responding to the law of mass action: as the plasma level of carbon dioxide rises, more is hydrolysed and consequently more acid is secreted and bicarbonate regenerated. There is no central or humoral control but the proper functioning of the tubules is of course essential. Respiratory function on the other hand is very tightly controlled by medullary receptors sensitive to pH. However, pH is used by the respiratory centre merely as an index of carbon dioxide accumulation: the principal role of this mechanism is the maintenance of blood oxygen level.

Plasma pH

Plasma pH is determined by the ratio of bicarbonate to total carbon dioxide (free carbon dioxide plus carbonic acid):

$$pH \propto \frac{[\text{bicarbonate}]}{[\text{carbon dioxide}]} \qquad (14.1)$$

This ratio is determined by the equilibrium position of the hydration of carbon dioxide, which is catalysed by carbonic anhydrase in kidney tubules and all body cells:

$$CO_2 + H_2O \underset{\text{anhydrase}}{\overset{\text{carbonic}}{\rightleftharpoons}} H_2CO_3 \rightleftharpoons HCO_3^- + H^+$$

Although other ions, e.g. phosphate and ammonium, are involved, this hydration is essentially the process that occurs in the tubules as acid is secreted and bicarbonate reabsorbed or, more correctly, regenerated. Further, both fat metabolism and the anaerobic metabolism of carbohydrate produce ketoacids (acetoacetate, lactate, etc.) and protein metabolism results in the production of sulphate and phosphate. These non-volatile acids must also be eliminated by the kidney.

Maintaining pH homeostasis

To maintain blood pH at 7.4 ± 0.05, the mechanisms described above work in concert, as follows:

- Small natural changes (most commonly falls) are initially countered by the blood buffer system.
- If this is insufficient, the respiratory centre responds rapidly by altering respiratory rate to increase the retention or elimination of carbon dioxide, thereby adjusting the bicarbonate/acid ratio and returning pH to normal. This happens whether or not the initial cause was actually a change in carbon dioxide level.
- Finally, renal compensation will slowly restore the absolute as well as the relative levels of acid and bicarbonate.

Clinical features and investigation of renal disease

The clinical features of renal dysfunction are either changes in urine flow and composition, or systemic features secondary to failure of renal mechanisms. The spectrum of clinical features in renal failure in particular are considered in detail when this topic is covered below (p. 897).

Symptoms

Patients readily associate symptoms arising in the lower urinary tract as renal in origin. However, as a consequence of the imbalances caused by renal malfunction, symptoms may arise in any body system and may at first be obscure and seem unrelated to the renal system.

Urinary symptoms

Some of the common urinary symptoms and their possible clinical implications are summarized in Table 14.4. While micturition abnormalities usually result from the lower urinary tract, persistent abnormalities of urine volume imply a more serious aetiology. Oliguria is defined as less than 500 mL of urine per day. This is because it is the minimum volume required to carry the average daily osmotic load of waste matter at maximal urine concentration; any less implies a degree of malfunction. However, the precise value for an individual will vary somewhat depending on diet, body size and fluid intake.

Systemic features

Volaemic and osmotic imbalance

Fluid and electrolyte imbalance commonly result from renal impairment. Fluid imbalance generally has haemodynamic consequences with cardiovascular features such as changes in BP, oedema, shortness of breath, etc. Osmotic imbalance usually results in neurological features, e.g. drowsiness, convulsions, because of changes in the intracranial pressure; (see below).

'Uraemia'

This term, implying high levels of blood urea, is a traditional synonym for renal failure; another is azotaemia (high levels of nitrogenous products). Sometimes the former term is used more specifically for the clinical picture and the latter for the biochemical picture. These contribute to the general malaise, lethargy, pruritus, cramps, peripheral tingling, nausea, vomiting and anorexia of which patients frequently complain. However, the clinical consequences of renal failure extend far beyond the immediate effects of high blood levels of urea or other nitrogenous metabolic waste products. In addition, pH imbalance and abnormalities of sodium, potassium

Table 14.4   Urinary symptoms

Abnormality	Symptom	Definition	Possible causes
Micturition	Dysuria	Painful	Urinary-tract infection/inflammation
	Hesitation	Difficulty in starting	Outflow obstruction (e.g. prostatitis, stone)
	Frequency		Stress, polyuria, infection, prostatitis
	Incontinence	Difficulty in preventing	Stress, neuromuscular
	Nocturia	Frequency at night	Polyuria, heart failure, diabetes
Urine volume	Polyuria	>2.5 L/day[a]	Diet, climate
			Renal tubular disease
			Chronic renal failure
			Diabetes (mellitus or insipidus)
	Oliguria	<500 mL/day[a]	Obstruction, renal failure
	Anuria	<100 mL/day[a]	Obstruction, renal failure

[a] Urine output.

and other substances cause specific symptoms that will be discussed in the appropriate sections below.

Signs, examination and investigation

Urine

Much information on kidney function can be inferred by looking for evidence of the consequences of suspected malfunction. This is generally easier, less invasive and often more sensitive than examination of the kidneys directly. Useful qualitative and semi-quantitative information is given by microscopic or chemical examination of the urine. Simple biochemical urine tests, valuable for preliminary screening, can nowadays be done using dipsticks, and should be part of a routine clinical examination (Table 14.5).

Renal function

More accurate measurements are required for the diagnosis, staging and monitoring of serious disease, or when drug dosage adjustment is required.

Filtration and clearance

Because the principal function of the kidney is filtration, the rate at which this occurs is a crucial measure of its efficiency. However, direct measurement of this rate is difficult and so the concept of clearance is utilized. Clearance is defined as a hypothetical volume of blood from which a substance would be completely removed by filtration in 1 min. It is calculated by measuring the blood or plasma concentration of the substance, urine flow rate (usually measured over 24 h to minimize collection errors) and the urine concentration of the substance. The clearance is given by:

$$\text{Clearance} = \frac{\text{Urine concentration} \times \text{Urine flow rate}}{\text{Plasma concentration}}$$

We know that approximately 120 mL of filtrate is normally produced each minute. If a substance were completely filtered at the glomerulus and subsequently neither reabsorbed from the tubules nor secreted into them, then the equivalent of 120 mL of blood would be completely cleared of the substance each minute and its clearance would be 120 mL/min. Inulin fulfils these criteria, but it is usually more convenient to exploit creatinine, a natural body constituent, which very closely does so. Creatinine clearance is thus the usual index of GFR. (Creatinine is actually secreted to a small extent in the tubules, so its clearance gives a slightly high estimate of GFR; fortuitously however, current laboratory measurement

Table 14.5   Simple semi-quantitative examination of urine

Test	Significance/implication
Specific gravity	Urine concentrating ability (tubular function)
pH (indicator method)	Generally not very helpful; a failure to acidify urine (renal tubular acidosis) requires detailed assessment
Abnormal constituents	
Protein (proteinuria; albuminuria)	Glomerular disease; vigorous exercise (transient)
Blood (haematuria)	Infection/inflammation/tumour
Haemoglobin	Haemolytic anaemia
Pus (pyuria)	Renal or urinary-tract infection
Leucocytes	Urinary-tract infection
Nitrite	Urinary-tract infection
Crystals (crystalluria)	Depends on identity of crystals
'Casts'	Clumps of protein and blood cells; often in glomerulonephritis or pyelonephritis

slightly overestimates plasma creatinine, tending to cancel this out.)

Creatinine clearance measurement involves a tedious and error-prone 24 h urine collection. Hence, a single serum creatinine measurement will often suffice because the serum creatinine level depends on the balance between production (which is dependent on muscle mass, gender and age and is normally constant for an individual) and renal output (which is directly proportional to filtration rate). Creatinine clearance can be calculated from the serum creatinine level alone by correcting for age, sex and weight using tables or a simple formula:

$$\text{Creatinine clearance} = K \times \frac{(140-\text{Age}) \times \text{Weight}}{\text{Serum creatinine}}$$

where age is in years, weight is ideal body weight in kg, serum creatinine in micromol/L and the correction factor K is 1.04 for females and 1.23 for males. This is the Cockroft and Gault formula. Creatinine clerance normally falls with age as nephrons are lost, and it is lower in females because of lower muscle mass. Thus, for example, a normal value for a 75-year-old female would be about 50 mL/min, whereas for a 25-year-old male it would be 100–120 mL/min. Because of the population sample from which the formula was originally derived, it is not applicable to those under 18, obese, oedematous, pregnant or with severly reduced muscle mass (e.g. undernourished or cachexic). Creatinine levels can also be affected by external factors (Table 14.6) and there are also ethnic variations. Other formulae have been devised to allow for ethnicity or diet, avoiding using weight as a parameter, e.g. the 'modification of diet in renal disease' (MDRD) formulae, which gives a direct estimate of GFR.

Unfortunately, serum creatinine does not start to rise significantly until there is serious renal impairment, so early renal disease is easily missed if this method is relied upon. This is because early renal damage is often compensated by hypertrophy and hyperfiltration of remaining nephrons, which maintains clearance. Furthermore, the serum creatinine level is inversely related to GFR, and the effect of this reciprocal relationship, illustrated in Figure 14.7, is that quite large early falls in GFR will cause relatively small absolute rises in creatinine. For example, when the GFR has fallen to 50% of normal (60 mL/min), creatinine level doubles to only about 200 micromol/L, not far outside the normal range. Subsequently it starts to rise sharply, e.g. fourfold normal when GFR falls to 25% and 10-fold normal when GFR fall to 10%.

Thus serum creatinine cannot be relied upon to detect moderate renal impairment. Its main value in renal disease lies in monitoring the

Table 14.6   Factors affecting creatinine and urea levels

Creatinine	Urea
Raised by	
High muscle bulk	High protein diet
Red meat meal	GI bleeding
Severe muscle damage (rhabdomyolosis)	Catabolic state, e.g. cachexia (wasting)
	Dehydration; reduced GFR
Drugs reducing tubular secretion (cimetidine, trimethoprim, probenecid, K-sparing diuretics)	Drugs (tetracycline, corticosteroid)
Lowered by	
Low muscle bulk	Protein deficient diet/starvation
Pregnancy	Liver failure
	Pregnancy

GFR, glomerular filtration rate; GI, gastrointestinal.

decline in renal function of a known sufferer from chronic kidney disease, following a single initial full creatinine clearance measurement to establish the relationship to serum creatinine in that particular patient. Progression can best be followed by plotting the reciprocal of creatinine clearance: the slope of the resulting straight line indicates the rate of decline of renal function. Any change in this slope requires investigation. Furthermore, an extrapolation can be made to indicate the time when GFR will fall below 10 mL/min, and thus to predict when a patient will probably require some form of renal replacement therapy (Figure 14.7).

Blood urea measurements suffer from similar but more diverse limitations. Blood urea levels are affected acutely by dietary variations in protein intake, by skeletal muscle damage and by catabolic states, e.g. fever or starvation. It is therefore less reliable than creatinine in reflecting GFR. Nevertheless, blood urea is a traditional general index and first approxima- tion of renal function and malfunction (the routine 'urea and electrolytes' or 'U and E's').

Other markers that are cleared without reab- sorption or secretion (e.g. Iohexol, cystatin C) are being investigated but are not yet in routine use. Radioisotope clearance may also be used,

e.g. labelled EDTA. If precision is required, inulin clearance can be determined by serial measure- ment of the fall in plasma concentration at timed intervals following a bolus injection; this pharmacokinetic method avoids urine collection errors.

Tubular function

Urine concentrating ability can be tested by subjecting the patient to water deprivation. Inability to conserve water, manifested clinically as polyuria, may be an early sign of chronic renal disease. ADH can be used to establish whether it is of pituitary origin, e.g. diabetes insipidus, or is nephrogenic, e.g. tubular disease, nephrogenic diabetes insipidus. Giving an acid or base load can be used to test the kidney's ability to secrete or conserve acid, i.e. its urine acidifying ability.

General secretory function is tested with a substance that is completely cleared in one pass through the nephron owing to maximal tubular secretion, e.g. para-amino hippuric acid (PAH). The secretion of specific metabolites can if neces- sary be tested by giving known loadings. This might be helpful, e.g. in distinguishing diabetes mellitus from renal glycosuria, a rare condition of reduced glucose threshold.

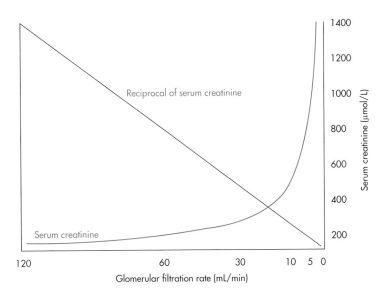

Figure 14.7 Changes in serum creatinine concentration and reciprocal creatinine concentration correlated with glomerular filtration rate.

Blood chemistry

The above tests can give precise measures of discrete renal functions, but in practice it is the consequences of impaired function that are clinically important. The best indices are thus the plasma levels of the metabolites and toxins normally cleared renally. In addition to urea and creatinine, routine measurement of plasma sodium, potassium, bicarbonate, calcium, phosphate and pH is vital in estimating and monitoring renal function, although of course the plasma levels of these substances may be altered by other factors and disorders.

Imaging

Ultrasound will show the size and position of the kidneys and bladder; this technique has replaced plain abdominal X-ray and IV contrast radiography (urography) as the first-line investigation because it is cheaper and less invasive. Enlargement of both kidneys suggests polycystic disease, while unilateral enlargement implies obstruction. Shrunken kidneys imply, non-specifically, advanced chronic renal disease. Calcified deposits (stones) in the kidney or ureters will also be visible. Doppler ultrasound can be used to visualize arterial supply and intrarenal blood flow; this is less invasive than the alternative, angiography, although the latter gives much more reliable and complete information. CT and MRI scanning are also used to examine intrarenal structures.

An IV excretory urogram (IVU; formerly intravenous pyelogram or IVP) uses an X-ray contrast medium to produce a series of images which will show any inequality of perfusion between the kidneys, the rate and extent of renal filling, internal renal structural abnormalities, e.g. cysts, and the patency and completeness of voiding of the lower urinary tract. However, patients may react badly to iodine-containing contrast media. Isotope urography yields similar information and is potentially less toxic, although less readily available. In antegrade urography a needle is introduced into the renal pelvis (nephrostomy) and contrast medium injected, giving a picture of the whole urinary outflow pathway.

The lower urinary tract can be visualized by retrograde urography to investigate possible obstruction; the contrast medium is administered via a urethral catheter. There is a significant risk of introducing infection, but the technique may still be used if the patient cannot tolerate IV contrast media. The lower urinary tract may also be investigated with a fibre-optic cystoscope, which also permits biopsy samples to be taken. However, biopsies of the renal mass must be taken percutaneously. They are particularly useful in the differential diagnosis of nephritis and in assessing transplant rejection.

Fluid and electrolyte imbalance

Only a general outline of the principles of this complex topic are given here. The References and further reading section lists some excellent specialist texts.

Volume and osmotic imbalance

Because control of total body water and plasma osmolarity are closely linked there are often coexisting imbalances. There is seldom a simple loss or excess of either water or sodium, but if so the result would be a mixed disorder, e.g. primary (pure) water depletion would cause hypovolaemia with hypernatraemia. Moreover, a patient's observed biochemical status may be due to the primary problem, to inadequate or incomplete compensation, or to treatment. For example, water and sodium loss from excessive sweating, over-compensated by drinking hypotonic fluid (e.g. pure water) will at some stage cause both hypervolaemia and hyponatraemia.

Aetiology

Some of the possible combinations of volume and osmotic imbalance and their possible primary causes are summarized in Table 14.7.

Water imbalance
Water depletion occurs either through excessive losses or deficient intake. As water depletion causes severe thirst, it will usually only become serious when thirst cannot be satisfied. The

Table 14.7   Disorders of osmotic and water balance

Imbalance	Possible causes	Comment
Hypervolaemia		
Hyperosmolar	Excess Na intake, (e.g. HCO_3)	Rare
Normo-osmolar	Excessive intake	True hypervolaemia
	• diet	Excessive IV infusion
	Fluid retention	
	• renal failure	
	• drugs	e.g. corticosteroids
	• aldosteronism	Cushing's disease, heart failure
Hypo-osmolar	Excessive hypotonic fluid intake	Water intoxication
	• excessive thirst, beer intake	
	• excessive IV infusion	Especially dextrose 5%
	Impaired water clearance	
	• inappropriate ADH secretion	
	• prostaglandin inhibition (NSAIDs)	
Normovolaemia		
Hypo-osmolar	'Dilutional' hyponatraemia	
	• excessive hypotonic fluid intake	e.g. beer
	• dehydration + hypotonic replacement	Net Na loss
	'Sick cell syndrome'	Na-pump problem (severe illness)
Hypovolaemia		
Hyperosmolar	Predominant water loss	Primary water depletion
	• hyperventilation	
	• sweat, e.g. hot climates, fever ⎱	GI fluids and sweat are hypotonic
	• GI fluids (vomit, diarrhoea) ⎰	
	• osmotic diuresis	
	– hyperglycaemia (diabetes mellitus)	
	– mannitol	
	• reduced ADH secretion/action	
	– diabetes insipidus	
	– drugs, e.g. alcohol, lithium	
	Reduced intake	
	• coma, dysphagia, post-operative	
Normo-osmolar	Excessive isotonic fluid loss	Dehydration
	• as above with partial compensation	
	• burns, haemorrhage	
	• polyuric chronic renal failure ⎱	
	• diuretic phase of acute renal failure ⎰	See pp. 901 and 908
	• excessive diuretic use	

ADH, antidiuretic hormone; GI, gastrointestinal; NSAID, non-steroidal anti-inflammatory drug.

degree of associated hypernatraemia will depend on salt intake and the effectiveness of renal compensation by fluid retention. The main causes of water excess are renal, although excess fluid intake may produce a hypervolaemic, hypo-osmolar state.

Sodium and osmotic imbalance

Sodium imbalance is rarely the direct result of either excess or deficient sodium intake. More usually it reflects either compensated primary water imbalance or a renal sodium handling defect.

Plasma sodium concentration gives a valuable index of the relative excess or deficit of sodium and water and thus of the underlying cause of any fluid or electrolyte imbalance. However, the plasma sodium level must always be interpreted in association with the haemodynamic status and haematological parameters. Thus hypovolaemia from isotonic fluid loss (e.g. from burns) would not cause a sodium imbalance, but would raise packed cell volume, whereas predominant water depletion (e.g. from vomiting) would lead to hypernatraemia. Net sodium loss, e.g. dehydration and inappropriate (hypotonic) replacement, would result in hyponatraemia.

Generally, sodium imbalance implies an osmotic imbalance. However, in some circumstances other osmotically active substances can first appear in the plasma in abnormal amounts and the sodium level will then be adjusted accordingly. For example, in diabetic hyperglycaemia or severe uraemia, sodium will effectively be displaced from the plasma by glucose or urea, giving a secondary or appropriate hyponatraemia. Thus, abnormal plasma sodium measurements may reflect neither abnormal sodium balance nor true plasma osmolarity. Further complications can arise in hyperlipidaemia or hyperproteinaemia when the aqueous fraction of plasma is reduced. This is not taken into account by the usual sodium measurement techniques, and so the sodium level will appear low even though it is actually in isotonic concentration in the plasma water; this is termed 'pseudohyponatraemia'.

Pathophysiology

The consequences of fluid or osmotic imbalance are far-reaching, which is why the body defends normal balances so strongly. In general, fluid imbalance has haemodynamic consequences while osmotic imbalance causes neurological complications (Figure 14.8).

Volume imbalance

Even small changes in the intravascular (blood) volume can affect BP, cardiac performance and tissue perfusion. In contrast, the intracellular and the extracellular (extravascular tissue) spaces can tolerate quite large changes. The tissues most affected will be those under least external pres-

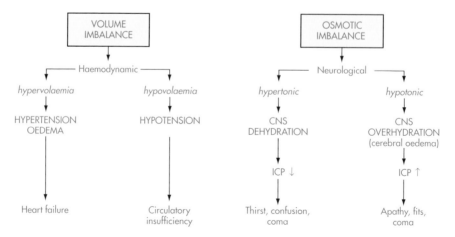

Figure 14.8 Pathophysiological consequences of volume and osmotic imbalance. CNS, central nervous system; ICP, intracranial pressure.

sure opposing fluid redistribution. These include soft tissues and areas where hydrostatic forces increase diffusion from the capillaries into the tissues, e.g. in dependent areas such as the ankles. This is one mechanism of oedema formation. Usually, oedema is without ill effect, except in the lungs, where pulmonary oedema is always dangerous.

Isotonic changes in total body water will usually be restricted to the ECF, i.e. plasma and tissue fluid, because sodium movement into cells across cell membranes is restricted. Changes in free water, e.g. excess of hypotonic fluid, or water with a solute such as glucose which is normally diffusible across cell membranes, will be distributed throughout all body fluid compartments. Thus in either case, but especially in the latter, the haemodynamic consequences will be buffered, delayed and less severe: even if the water is initially in the plasma (e.g. over-infusion, renal retention) most of it will diffuse out into the extravascular space. Moreover, most intravascular water will be accommodated by the capacitance vessels, i.e. the veins, so the effect on BP and cardiac loading will be reduced (Chapter 4). Nevertheless, hypervolaemia is a common cause of cardiovascular problems, e.g. decompensated heart failure.

Osmotic imbalance

If there is an acute osmotic imbalance between the extracelular and intracellular compartments, water will diffuse passively under osmotic forces. Plasma and tissue fluid that is hypertonic relative to ICF will draw water from all body cells, causing intracellular dehydration. Conversely, hypotonic ECF will overload cells with water. Small changes in the intracellular volume of most tissues are of little consequence, but the brain is an exception. Because the brain is contained within the rigid skull, small changes in volume will alter intracranial pressure, and quite small alterations in this pressure can have serious neurological effects, potentially resulting in coma or death.

These effects only occur after acute changes; compensatory mechanisms eventually tend to correct the imbalance. Aldosterone and ADH will restore extracellular osmotic pressure by adjusting sodium clearance, and brain cells

threatened with dehydration can manufacture osmotically active substances intracellularly to retain water.

If plasma oncotic (colloid osmotic) pressure is reduced owing to hypoproteinaemia, there will be a disproportionate loss of water to the tissues. Although the absolute osmotic differences are relatively small the resultant oedema can sometimes be gross, as in nephrotic syndrome (p. 939).

Clinical features

The combination of signs and symptoms presented by a patient will depend on the primary cause, the main volaemic (haemodynamic) or osmotic (neurological) consequences and secondary effects or compensations. The acute effects before compensation are summarized in Table 14.8.

Management

Degree and speed of intervention

The first step is to ascertain the cause of osmotic imbalance. If the situation is not critical, i.e. there are no severe neurological problems or pulmonary oedema, correction of the cause will often be sufficient. If there is no underlying renal disease the body is able to reverse most imbalances eventually. Otherwise, minimal intervention with the very simplest of corrections may suffice. More specific measures usually need be taken only when there is renal impairment.

Great care is needed, even with simple correction. All interventions, whether by the oral or the parenteral route, initially alter only the volume or concentration of the plasma. Equilibration between intravascular and extracellular fluid occurs quite rapidly, but several hours are needed for equilibration between the extracellular and intracellular compartments. Thus, too rapid a correction will cause a disproportionate, potentially dangerous initial change in plasma osmolarity or blood volume and result in an overshoot, e.g. hyponatraemia treated too vigorously with hypertonic saline may cause an equally harmful hypernatraemia.

Conversely, if therapy is too delayed, compensation will have already been initiated –

Table 14.8   Clinical features of volume and osmotic imbalance

Hypervolaemia	Hypertension Heart failure ('high output') Oedema (especially pulmonary) Oliguria (if renal impairment is cause) Increased intraocular pressure, visual problems Weight gain
Hypovolaemia	Thirst, dry mouth, sunken cheeks Reduced intraocular pressure, visual problems Pale cold skin, with loss of turgor (dehydration of dermis) Low cardiac output, tachycardia (Postural) hypotension, collapse, shock Oliguria, incipient pre-renal failure Weight loss
Hypernatraemia/hyperosmolar	Confusion, hallucinations, convulsions, coma Muscular jerks Oliguria or polyuria (depending on cause)
Hyponatraemia/hypo-osmolar	Anorexia, nausea and vomiting Lethargy, apathy, confusion Headache, convulsions, coma Reduced intraocular pressure (osmotic loss), visual problems

particularly in the brain – and correction may then have an opposite effect. For example, if plasma is hypertonic for too long, brain cells will also become hypertonic. At that stage, rapid attempts at correction with hypotonic fluids may then cause CNS over-hydration and raised intracranial pressure.

Fluid dose estimation and monitoring

Various formulae are available for calculating fluid and electrolyte deficits and the amounts needed for correction from electrolyte measurements. However, these can only be used for initial guidance. Subsequently, it is far more important to observe the effect of initial therapy and make appropriate adjustments according to the patient's physical signs and haemodynamic and biochemical status.

The main measures used in monitoring water balance and general hydration, which must be considered together, are:

• Sodium concentration.
• Blood pressure (or preferably CVP).
• Packed cell volume.

Secondary considerations include:

• Urine volume.
• Possibility of pH imbalance.

Specific therapy

Dehydration and hypovolaemia.   Mild volume deficit, especially of gastrointestinal origin, may be corrected with glucose-electrolyte oral rehydration salt solutions if the patient is able to drink. Severe volume depletion with circulatory insufficiency requires IV therapy, and physiological saline is usually satisfactory. Restoration of urine output is the best index of success. Physiological saline infusion should not be continued unnecessarily because it can lead to hyperchloraemic acidosis (p. 878).

Hypernatraemia.   If neurological involvement is threatened, the logical treatment would be a sodium-reduced fluid. Sodium chloride 0.45% or weaker solutions are available, but dextrose 5% is probably better. This is isotonic on injection but yields pure water once the dextrose is metabolized. Dextrose 4% plus sodium chloride 0.18%

('dextrose saline') is similar but provides some sodium. Nevertheless, sodium chloride 0.9% is often adequate if renal function is unimpaired. Because the aim is a gradual reduction of osmotic pressure, the small diluting effect produced is temporarily beneficial until the kidneys can make the necessary compensation.

Hypervolaemia.   If mild, this can be treated by simple water restriction. In severe cases with pulmonary oedema or threatened cardiac failure, a diuretic is needed.

Hyponatraemia.   Mild hyponatraemia can be treated orally with sodium chloride, but more aggressive action is needed if cerebral oedema develops. Temporarily, a poorly diffusing osmotic diuretic such as mannitol may be infused to elevate plasma osmotic pressure. Corticosteroids such as *dexamethasone* are also advocated but neither the mechanism nor the benefit is clear. Such cases may be treated – very cautiously – with hypertonic sodium chloride, with a concentration of up to 5% being used.

Inappropriate secretion of ADH can be treated with demeclocycline. The treatment of diabetes insipidus is not considered here.

Potassium imbalance

Pathophysiology

Distribution of body potassium
Most body potassium (K^+) is either within the cells or in bone (Figure 14.9). Extracellular fluid K^+, as measured in the plasma, represents only a very small proportion of total body load. Yet it is that which has the greatest physiological importance, being involved in maintaining the membrane potential of all cells. Changes in plasma K^+ of more than $\pm$ 2 mmol/L can have serious effects on nerve and muscle function, especially in the heart. The terms hypokalaemia

and hyperkalaemia refer specifically to plasma level abnormalities, and say little about total body potassium balance.

Bone potassium is exchanged very slowly and so plays little part in acute changes. The ICF acts as a reservoir and buffers plasma potassium so that considerable variations in total body potassium can occur before the plasma level changes: up to 200 mmol can be lost from the cells with no appreciable change in plasma K^+. Despite plasma level being a poor index of potassium status it is the only easily accessible direct measure available. Any related pH imbalance must also be taken into account when interpreting plasma K^+ levels.

Homeostasis
Extracellular K^+ is in equilibrium with the ICF, an unequal distribution across the cell membrane being maintained by the sodium (Na^+-K^+ exchange) pump. Cellular uptake of K^+ is promoted by an alkaline plasma (pH >7.4), aldosterone, adrenaline (epinephrine) via beta-receptors, and insulin.

A rise in plasma K^+ causes insulin release, which promotes the uptake of glucose and K^+ by cells. Whether this is a co-transport mechanism or simply the supply of extra energy for the pump itself is not known, but it provides a useful therapeutic strategy in hyperkalaemia. Conversely, acidic conditions, lack of insulin, beta-blockers and the absence of aldosterone, inhibit K^+ uptake and may cause hyperkalaemia.

These factors have a special significance in renal tubular cells where they control not only the intracellular/extracellular distribution but also total body potassium. When the filtrate reaches the distal tubule almost all potassium has been reabsorbed. If plasma K^+ is too high, aldosterone causes the distal tubule cells to remove K^+ from the plasma and secrete it into the tubular fluid (urine), in exchange for Na^+. Further, as has been shown (p. 878), because

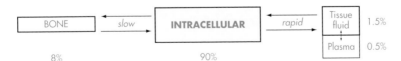

Figure 14.9   Distribution of body potassium.

this same transport mechanism mediates acid secretion, secondary acid-base imbalances can arise.

Aetiology

Gross abnormalities in total body potassium, which may or may not be reflected in plasma level changes, must be recognized in addition to clinically significant hypokalaemia or hyper-kalaemia. Because K^+ is not metabolized, total body imbalance arises from abnormalities in either intake or loss (Table 14.9). Acute changes will affect the plasma level, but more protracted changes will at first be compensated by the intra-cellular pool. Acute plasma potassium imbal-ances may also arise from disturbed intracellular/extracellular distribution, with no net change in total body K^+.

Hypokalaemia
Normally the body is in positive potassium balance. Daily renal, faecal and sweat losses rarely exceed 40 mmol, and a healthy diet provides 50–100 mmol. However, a diet which is deficient in fresh fruit and vegetables can cause potassium deficiency.

Most diuretics cause some potassium loss, partly by presenting more filtered sodium to the distal tubule. The kidney tries to compensate for the enforced natriuresis by reabsorbing more Na^+, and in doing so exchanges it for K^+. Although neither diet nor diuretics alone usually cause clinically significant hypokalaemia, the combination may be serious, especially in the elderly.

Alkalosis affects the plasma potassium level in two ways. It directly promotes cellular uptake of K^+ and it causes the kidney to conserve acid by reabsorbing it distally in preference to K^+. This increases K^+ loss and can exacerbate the hypokalaemia.

Aldosteronism (excess mineralocorticoid activity) can present in various ways, e.g. Cushing's disease, Conn's syndrome, cortico-steroid therapy, heart failure or hypopro-teinaemia (e.g. from hepatic disease or nephrotic syndrome). In the last two conditions, reduced BP and/or circulating fluid volume activate the RAAS, causing excess aldosterone secretion with Na^+ retention and K^+ loss.

Gastrointestinal secretions contain relatively high levels of K^+, and laxative abuse is sometimes a hidden cause of hypokalaemia. Liquorice,

Table 14.9 Causes of potassium imbalance

	Hypokalaemia	Hyperkalaemia
GI intake	Poor diet	Excess K salts/supplements
GI output	Laxative abuse Vomiting, diarrhoea Fistula, stoma	
Renal clearance	Drugs • loop and thiazide diuretics • osmotic diuretics • corticosteroids Alkalosis Aldosteronism	Renal failure Drugs • K-sparing diuretics • aldosterone antagonists Acidosis Adrenal insufficiency
Distribution	Alkalosis Beta-adrenergic agonists, SNS Theophylline Insulin	Acidosis Tissue trauma, exercise Diabetes mellitus (uncontrolled)

GI, gastrointestinal; SNS, sympathetic nervous system.

which is sometimes used as a laxative, has an aldosterone-like action.

Hyperkalaemia

Potassium excess (hyperkalaemia) is less common than hypokalaemia, but harder to treat. Renal failure is probably the most common cause of hyperkalaemia, and this is one of the main problems in managing renal patients. Dietary causes are rare, but over-zealous use of potassium salts, e.g. potassium citrate mixture in the self-treatment of cystitis, can be responsible. Over-use of potassium supplements is only a remote possibility, given patients' well-known lack of enthusiasm for the common slow-release forms. More subtly, potassium-retaining diuretics, e.g. amiloride and spironolactone, can lead to excessive inhibition of K^+ secretion, especially in combination with the ACEIs. This situation can be exacerbated in the elderly, who usually have impaired renal function.

Clinical features

Dyskalaemias disturb the transmembrane ionic balance and the membrane potential, so muscle and nerve cells are particularly susceptible.

Hypokalaemia, depending on its duration and severity, can cause numbness, weakness, paralysis, low cardiac output, tachyarrhythmias and heart failure. The myocardial toxicity of *digoxin* is also enhanced. In the longer term, renal damage can occur, while inhibition of gastrointestinal activity can lead to bowel obstruction. Renal attempts at compensation with potassium conservation and acid loss leads to metabolic alkalosis, as occurs with long-term diuretic overuse. Chronic severe hypokalaemia can impair renal concentrating ability, leading to ADH-resistant polyuria and polydipsia.

Hyperkalaemia, although more dangerous, causes fewer symptoms and indeed may be silent until cardiac arrest occurs. A characteristic ECG change of a spiked T-wave may be observed. Acidosis is a further complication.

Management

Correction of abnormal plasma levels is the immediate therapeutic target in potassium imbalance. Oral therapy is adequate for mild imbalances but severe dyskalaemia (<3 or >6 mmol/L) needs urgent attention, mainly to protect the heart. However, the total body excess or deficit will be many times larger than the simple correction of plasma level would imply.

For example, a plasma level of 2.5 mmol/L requires 2 mmol/L to restore a normal level of 4.5 mmol/L. For an average plasma water volume of 3 L this requires $3 \times 2 = 6$ mmol of K^+ (less than half a standard oral potassium tablet). But most of the administered potassium will be distributed extravascularly, diffusing rapidly into the tissue fluid (9 L) and then more slowly, over 24 h, into the cells (30 L). The plasma will retain less than one-fifteenth of the administered dose. However, because of the time this takes to occur, attempts at rapid correction with the calculated total body deficit (in this case, $6 \times 15 = 90$ mmol) would cause acute hyperkalaemia. Conversely, too rapid a reduction in raised plasma K^+ by dialysis will cause hypokalaemia. Gradual adjustment with frequent monitoring of plasma level is important.

Hypokalaemia

Generally speaking, it is easier to get potassium into a deficient body than it is to extract an excess.

Mild hypokalaemia. Dietary correction is preferred. The routine prescription of potassium supplements with diuretics is no longer thought necessary and should preferably only follow plasma level measurement of K^+.

Most potassium salts have an unpalatable, saline taste. Effervescent formulations disguise the taste, but they usually contain bicarbonate, which is often contra-indicated because of the associated alkalosis. Liquid preparations of the chloride are perhaps underused. Very large oral slow-release forms are perhaps the least complied with of all medication, and there is the additional possibility of gastrointestinal irritation, ulceration or obstruction.

Fixed-dose combination preparations, e.g. diuretic and potassium, used to be popular but need particular care. In addition to the usual problems of preformulated combinations (inflexibility of individual component dosage, possible confusion over adverse effects, etc.), these preparations seem particularly likely to cause severe gastrointestinal lesions. They have now been superseded by potassium-sparing diuretics.

Severe hypokalaemia.   This needs parenteral potassium usually by IV infusion. Because of the time needed for equilibration it must not be injected too rapidly or in too high a concentration. Acceptable maxima are a 40 mmol/L solution given at no more than 20 mmol/h, with an 80 mmol daily maximum.

Hyperkalaemia

Mild hyperkalaemia.   It is possible to reduce plasma potassium level slowly by binding it in the gut lumen with a cationic ion exchange resin such as polystyrene sulphonate, used as the calcium or sodium salt. This is unpalatable and it can be given rectally, but neither route is very efficient at potassium removal.

Severe hyperkalaemia.   The immediate need is to correct the plasma level: the overall body excess is less urgent. Calcium (10 mL of 10% calcium gluconate) is injected to provide a temporary physiological antidote to the cardiotoxic effect. This is followed, in the absence of renal impairment, by infusion of up to 200 mmol of sodium bicarbonate (depending on the degree of acidosis), insulin (20 units) and glucose (50 g). This stimulates potassium uptake into all body cells, reducing the plasma level, but of course does not correct the total body excess. In non-diabetic patients the insulin may not be needed because the glucose will stimulate its release. Beta-adrenergic agonists may also be used, e.g. nebulized or injected *salbutamol*. The effect may be additive to that of insulin and glucose.

 Measures to reduce body potassium level then follow. An ion exchange resin treatment is started, but dialysis may be necessary if plasma levels cannot be controlled satisfactorily. Otherwise, renal compensation is given time to work.

Acid–base imbalance

This potentially confusing topic will be dealt with here in a simplified way, to enable imbal-

ances and therapy to be understood in principle. One common problem with the terminology can be readily clarified. Any pH imbalance resulting from respiratory disorder is termed 'respiratory' (either acidosis or alkalosis); all other forms are 'metabolic', whether or not they are caused by a apparently genuine metabolic defect. Thus the ingestion of battery acid is as 'metabolic' as lactic acidosis, although 'non-respiratory' is a preferable term.

Aetiology

Acid–base imbalance may be conveniently visualized by considering the normal and possible abnormal routes for the intake, production and output of acid and bicarbonate in relation to the equation that controls pH (Figure 14.10). Over-activity or under-activity of any of these pathways can cause pH imbalance (Table 14.10).

 Because the body is normally in positive acid balance, acidosis is more common than alkalosis. Respiratory acidosis is usually predictable because of associated cardiorespiratory disease; respiratory alkalosis is rare. Among the vast number of possible non-respiratory disturbances, gastrointestinal causes are common and acidosis is also a major problem in renal failure. The accumulation in the blood of lactate, ketoacids or acidic drug metabolites is another major cause. Biguanide-induced lactic acidosis is now rare.

Investigation and diagnosis

The first priority is to identify and correct the underlying cause. Initially this involves measurement of blood CO_2, $H_2CO_3^-$ and pH, and a simplified guide is given in Figure 14.11. The precise biochemical picture will depend on the nature and degree of compensation. Complex mixed disorders are possible, e.g. metabolic and respiratory acidosis in a poorly controlled diabetic with COPD.

Anion gap
Normally total plasma cations (mainly Na^+ and K^+) exceed the measured anions (mainly Cl^- and HCO_3^-) by about 15 mmol/L. The difference,

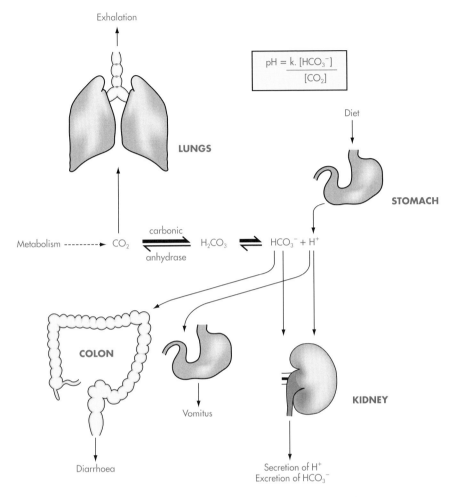

Exhalation

$$pH = \frac{k. [HCO_3^-]}{[CO_2]}$$

Diet

LUNGS

STOMACH

Metabolism --------→ CO_2 $\rightleftharpoons$ H_2CO_3 $\rightleftharpoons$ $HCO_3^- + H^+$

carbonic anhydrase

COLON

Vomitus

KIDNEY

Diarrhoea

Secretion of H^+
Excretion of HCO_3^-

Figure 14.10 Normal and abnormal intake and output of acid and bicarbonate, related to the normal acid–base balance equation. H^+, acid; HCO_3^-, bicarbonate; H_2CO_3, carbonic acid; CO_2, carbon dioxide.

called the anion gap, is made up by phosphate, sulphate, protein and other organic acids:

$$\text{Anion gap} = ([Na^+] + [K^+]) - ([Cl^-] + [HCO_3^-])$$

In acidosis caused by the accumulation of endogenous or exogenous toxic organic acids (e.g. lactate, salicylate), these anions displace bicarbonate and the anion gap is increased. Conversely, in acidosis from simple acid accumulation (e.g. renal failure) or bicarbonate loss (e.g. diarrhoea), the bicarbonate is replaced by chloride so the gap is normal. Lactic acidosis is sometimes further subdivided into type A caused

by tissue hypoxia and type B caused by abnormal production of acids, e.g. in uncontrolled diabetes mellitus.

Clinical features

The effects of pH imbalance are profound but non-specific, and diagnosis is usually made biochemically. Most systems in the body are affected (Table 14.11) but the main clinical problems are cardiovascular. Acidosis reduces cardiac contractility, an effect potentiated by beta-blockers, and dilates arteries and constricts veins; all have adverse

Table 14.10   Possible causes of pH imbalance

Acidosis (pH <7.2)	Alkalosis (pH >7.6)
Carbon dioxide gain Respiratory failure Obstructive airways disease Respiratory depression (inc. drugs)	**Carbon dioxide loss** Hyperventilation (panic attacks)
Bicarbonate loss Diarrhoea Carbonic anhydrase inhibitors Renal tubular acidosis Aldosterone deficiency Hyperkalaemia Hyperchloraemia	**Bicarbonate gain** Antacid overuse (Sodium bicarbonate) 'Milk alkali syndrome' Potassium citrate mixture Aldosteronism Hypokalaemia Hypochloraemia Diuretics

Acid gain
Renal failure
Ketoacidosis
  • starvation
  • diabetes mellitus
Lactic acidosis
  • exercise
  • shock
  • hypoxia
  • biguanides
  • fructose/sorbitol IV
Salicylate poisoning
Reye's syndrome
Ammonium chloride overuse
	Acid loss
	Vomiting, pyloric stenosis
	Aldosteronism
	Hypokalaemia

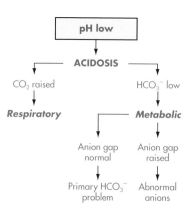
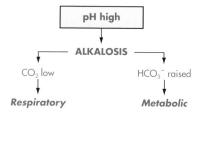

Figure 14.11   Biochemical parameters of pH imbalance. CO_2, carbon dioxide, HCO_3^-, bicarbonate; H_2CO_3, carbonic acid.

haemodynamic effects. Oxygen dissociation from Hb is increased, which may improve tissue oxygenation but impairs pulmonary oxygen uptake.

The CNS is depressed by acidosis, but nerve and muscle excitability are increased by alkalosis, leading to seizures and tetany. In non-respiratory disorders the respiratory rate is altered to compensate for this. Urinary acid secretion is changed appropriately, with consequences for potassium balance.

The distribution and clearance of acidic and basic drugs is affected. This is the basis of forced diuresis for treating poisoning. Alkali loading causes an alkaline urine which encourages the clearance of acids such as salicylate. Conversely, acid will encourage the clearance of bases, e.g. many psychotropic agents, such as amphetamine.

Management

Unless the severity of the imbalance is causing cardiovascular or CNS problems or the cause is irreversible, e.g. chronic renal failure, the best general strategy is simply to remove the cause and allow the body to carry out normal correction at its own pace.

Acidosis

Chronic moderate acidosis can be treated orally with sodium bicarbonate. In acute severe metabolic acidosis specific correction is avoided if the patient can be expected to recover spontaneously. The use of bicarbonate infusion is easily misjudged, causing an equally serious 'alkaline overshoot'.

Various strengths of bicarbonate injection are available. The preferred 1.26% preparation is isotonic (300 mmol/L) and provides about one-sixth of a mmol/mL of bicarbonate. For urgent cases more concentrated solutions are available as boluses, but these must be injected very slowly. An 8.4% solution provides 1 mmol/mL, which facilitates dose calculation but is very hypertonic (six times physiological). Intermediate strengths are also available. Lactate is no longer used because it acts indirectly and some acidotic patients may not be able to metabolize it to its active form (bicarbonate).

The total dose needed is usually 100–200 mmol of bicarbonate. An estimate in mmol can be made empirically from the patient's body weight (kg) and the measured plasma bicarbonate:

Bicarbonate dose = ⅓ Body weight ×
(Normal plasma HCO_3^- − Measured HCO_3^-).

However, as with K imbalance, frequent monitoring and adjustment are better guides.

In respiratory acidosis the cause must be treated directly, if necessary by ventilation. Simple bicarbonate correction is inappropriate.

Alkalosis

Metabolic alkalosis can usually be treated with simple infusions of 0.9% sodium chloride (p. 878). Sometimes, however, direct infusion of acid is required. Hydrochloric acid has been used, but the hydrochlorides of ammonium, lysine or arginine are preferred. Ammonium chloride may be given orally.

Respiratory alkalosis is very rare and is almost invariably a temporary self-correcting condition (e.g. during childbirth). Rebreathing from a bag, which limits carbon dioxide loss, may speed recovery.

Renal failure

Renal failure denotes a global loss of renal function, but it occurs to different degrees. The body can maintain normal homeostasis with renal function reduced to about half the normal GFR, particularly if the decline is slow, and even then symptoms may not be seriously troublesome. Different sources vary in their definitions of

Table 14.11   Clinical features of pH imbalance

Acidosis	Alkalosis
Hyperventilation	Hypoventilation
Impaired consciousness	Seizures, tetany
Hyperkalaemia	Hypokalaemia
Cardiovascular	
• reduced cardiac output	
• arrhythmias, arrest	

degrees of renal failure, and there are also different systems depending on whether acute or chronic failure is being discused. A generic grading, based on reduced GFR, assuming a normal GFR of 120 mL/min in a healthy young male, would be:

• Renal impairment: 100–60 mL/min
• Mild renal failure: 60–30 mL/min
• Moderate to severe renal failure: 30–10 mL/min
• End-stage renal failure: <10 mL/min.

Like heart failure, renal failure is not a specific disease but a complex syndrome with many possible causes but a fairly uniform clinical presentation. In ARF the impairment of regulatory and excretory functions predominates: in the chronic form (chronic renal failure, CRF) there is also an endocrine abnormality.

ARF most commonly occurs secondary to generalized circulatory failure. The condition develops rapidly and has a high mortality but is reversible if treatment is provided early enough: if the patient survives there may be no permanent sequelae. CRF by contrast has an insidious onset and is usually caused by direct damage to the renal tissue. The large natural renal reserve and the slow progression of CRF mean that considerable irreversible damage has usually occurred by the time the patient reports symptoms. There is then an inexorable decline towards end-stage renal failure, which is fatal without renal replacement therapy, i.e. dialysis or transplantation. However, the rate of decline varies with the underlying cause, and can be slowed by treatment.

Classification and aetiology

The many factors which can impair renal function may be divided into three groups, depending on whether the primary fault is in renal perfusion, the kidney tissue itself or urinary outflow (Table 14.12).

Pre-renal failure

The kidney relies on a continuous supply of blood at sufficient pressure to maintain the glomerular filtration, and endeavours to maintain systemic or intrarenal perfusion pressure by numerous homeostatic feedback mechanisms. However, severe hypovolaemia and/or hypotension, owing usually to fluid depletion, cardiac failure or other shock states, overwhelmingly compromise this, and ARF commonly follows.

Intrinsic renal failure

The kidney is especially prone to immunological or toxic damage. This is probably because in its excretory role the kidney accumulates high concentrations of the products of the immune system (e.g. immune complexes) and of metabolism, and its high blood flow exposes the renal tissues to potential toxins to a far greater extent than most organs. Nephrotoxicity is a common cause of renal failure, and a medication history is essential in investigating any unexplained renal impairment.

The glomeruli and the tubules and interstitial tissues may be affected independently by different causes, although some conditions affect both, e.g. ischaemia following circulatory failure. Intrinsic damage is usually a chronic process but toxic or ischaemic nephropathy can be acute.

Post-renal failure

Obstruction anywhere from the renal pelvis to the urethra is a less common and often reversible cause of renal failure. Back pressure is raised in the tubules and this reduces the glomerular filtration pressure and hence the GFR. The obstruction is usually within the urinary tract, but external pressure from an abdominal mass may also be responsible.

Post-renal failure is usually chronic. Occasionally, acute forms may cause anuria. A common cause of this in elderly men is prostatic hypertrophy obstructing bladder outflow.

Acute tubular nephropathy (ATN)
This term describes acute reversible tubular damage and is sometimes called, somewhat inaccurately, 'acute tubular necrosis'. It can be an important consequence of acute pre-renal failure following circulatory insufficiency that is not rapidly reversed. Thus ARF and ATN frequently

Table 14.12   Aetiology of renal failure

General pathology	Examples
Pre-renal	
Circulatory shock	Hypovolaemia (burns, dehydration, haemorrhage)
	Cardiogenic (myocardial infarction)
	Septicaemia/septic shock
	Liver disease, pancreatitis
	Obstetric (septicaemia, haemorrhage)
Intrinsic renal	
Glomerular	Autoimmune (e.g. glomerulonephritis)
	Connective tissue disease (e.g. SLE)
	Diabetic nephropathy
Tubular	Acute tubular nephropathy (vasomotor, nephrotoxic)
	Interstitial nephritis
Renovascular	Renal thrombosis, infarction
	Hypertension: essential, malignant
	Connective tissue disease (polyarteritis, etc.)
Infection	Pyelonephritis, malaria
Nephrotoxicity	Glomerular (e.g. penicillamine, heavy metals)
	Interstitial (e.g. penicillin, NSAID)
Metabolic	Hypercalcaemia, hypokalaemia
	Hyperuricaemia
Congenital	Polycystic disease
Post-renal	
Stones	Usually oxalate
Structural	Tumour, stricture, prostatitis
Nephrotoxicity	Analgesic nephropathy (e.g. phenacetin)
	Crystal uropathy (e.g. sulphonamides)
	Urate deposition (cytotoxics, gout)
Outside the urinary tract	Abdominal tumour (e.g. ovarian)
	Retroperitoneal fibrosis (e.g. methysergide)

NSAID, non-steroidal anti-inflammatory drug; SLE, systemic lupus erythematosus.

coexist and, confusingly, the terms are sometimes used synonymously. ATN may also be the result of renovascular, glomerular or tubular disease or toxic damage.

What difference is there, for the kidney, between renal ischaemia resulting from renovascular obstruction, nominally 'intrinsic ATN', and general systemic circulatory collapse (pre-renal)? The conventional distinction, made on clinical grounds, is that pre-renal failure is rapidly corrected by restoration of circulation whereas once ATN has supervened recovery is usually much slower.

The precise pathology of ATN is complex and incompletely understood. An important component is intense intrarenal vasoconstriction, which inhibits filtration because of the reduced afferent glomerular artery pressure. The nephrotoxicity of PG inhibitors, e.g. NSAIDs, is due to a similar effect. The vasoconstriction may simply be a response to injury, or it may be a maladaptive attempt to maintain renal perfusion pressure. In either case the subsequent ischaemic damage is counterproductive. Moreover, it may be perpetuated even after perfusion has been restored, owing to glomerular damage or tubular obstruction with inflammatory or necrotic debris.

Pathophysiology

The loss of renal function has multiple complex and serious consequences. One useful distinction, which helps to account for the clinical pictures found in different types and stages of renal failure, is between glomerular and tubular dysfunction. Although both structures may be damaged, the trauma is often predominantly to one or other, e.g. glomerulonephritis primarily causes glomerular damage whereas *aminoglycoside* nephrotoxicity is mainly tubular. In pre-renal failure both types occur at different stages.

Glomerular dysfunction

The principal causes of this are pre-renally impaired perfusion, intrinsic glomerular inflammation and post-renal obstruction. As the main function of the glomeruli is filtration, there is a fall in GFR with retention of those substances usually cleared by filtration, including water (Table 14.13).

The consequent reduced volume of filtrate and slower tubular flow permits increased proximal tubular reabsorption, which reinforces these effects. Furthermore, the reduced amounts of sodium delivered to the tubules means that less is available for the distal exchange mechanism involved in acid and potassium secretion.

In some types of glomerular damage, despite a reduced GFR, there may be an apparently paradoxical increased protein loss (proteinuria; discussed below).

Tubular dysfunction

The main function of the tubules is the selective reabsorption of water, electrolytes and other

Table 14.13   Consequences of glomerular dysfunction

Clinical feature	Cause
Oliguria Hypervolaemia Uraemia Hyperkalaemia Hyperphosphataemia Hyperuricaemia	Reduced filtration plus increased reabsorption
Hyperkalaemia Acidosis	Reduced secretion owing to reduced distal [Na]

useful substances. Thus, the main consequence of tubular failure is the voiding of large volumes of dilute urine (polyuria) of low specific gravity, along with electrolytes and nutrients (Table 14.14).

If the loop of Henle fails to generate an adequate intrarenal concentration gradient in the medulla, urine cannot be concentrated and passive reabsorption is compromised by the consequently increased tubular flow rate. Because of the proximal tubular failure there is a vast increase in potassium loss, which completely swamps the limited potassium retention that would be caused by the impaired distal sodium–potassium–acid exchange pump. On the other hand, the failure in distal acid secretion is significant and acidosis results.

Table 14.14   Consequences of tubular dysfunction

Clinical feature	Cause
Polyuria	Reduced countercurrent and reduced Na/water reabsorption
Hypokalaemia Glycosuria Phosphaturia; hypophosphataemia Aminoaciduria	Reduced reabsorption
Acidosis	Reduced exchange/ secretion

Summary

Predominant glomerular damage results in reduced urine volume, retention of water, acid and electrolyte, and possibly protein loss. This is the syndrome of oliguric renal failure. Tubular damage leads to acidosis, urine of low specific gravity and, if the GFR is adequate, to polyuria with fluid and electrolyte depletion.

Acute renal failure

Aetiology and prognosis

Although most of the conditions listed in Table 14.12 can cause ARF, pre-renal causes such as hypovolaemia or shock are by far the most common (75% of cases). Less common are intrinsic causes such as nephrotoxicity and acute glomerulonephritis (20%). ARF as a result of post-renal obstruction is uncommon (5%).

ARF is a serious medical emergency that can develop very rapidly and has a high mortality. It may be defined as a sudden fall in GFR to below about 15 mL/min. Without treatment, survival is less than 10%, which shows the crucial role of correct renal function. With treatment in a specialist unit, mortality can be reduced to below 50% but oliguric forms have a poorer prognosis. These outcomes reflect the seriousness of the conditions that precipitate ARF and the rapidly progressive nature of the subsequent multi-organ failure caused, rather than inadequacy of management. With the increased availability of renal dialysis, the outlook for ARF has improved, and death now rarely results from biochemical derangement.

Course

Whatever the primary cause, untreated ARF usually follows a fairly well-defined and predictable course (Figure 14.12). Onset is frequently associated with oliguria, which continues for up to a month if the patient survives. Urine flow then recovers and the patient may become polyuric (up to 5 L per day) for 5–10 days. During the final recovery phase, which may last several months, urine flow and renal function gradually return to normal.

A simplified explanation of these phases is as follows:

- The early **oliguric** phase is caused by poor glomerular perfusion or tubular obstruction. Both result in a predominant pattern of glomerular dysfunction with reduced renal clearance and fluid and electrolyte retention. Any tubular impairment is masked by the reduced glomerular filtrate.
- In the **polyuric** ('diuretic') phase the glomeruli have recovered somewhat and are again producing filtrate, although the GFR remains low. However, tubular dysfunction persists, causing failure to concentrate and loss of fluid and electrolytes. The initial diuresis may be partly due to the accumulated fluid and osmolar load, but this could not alone account for the prolonged pattern sometimes seen.
- In the **recovery** phase the tubule cells slowly regenerate.

After recovery there is usually no overt residual renal damage. Although sensitive measures of clearance will almost certainly detect some degree of permanent impairment, this is well

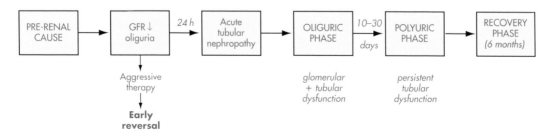

Figure 14.12   Typical clinical course of acute renal failure. GFR, glomerular filtration rate.

within the renal reserve. The effect of a single episode of ARF resembles a small acceleration of renal ageing, with additional nephrons having been lost prematurely.

In pre-renal ARF, ischaemia rapidly produces ATN. Intrinsic toxic tubular damage has the same effect. ATN is a serious complication which usually accounts for the oliguric phase, but may be avoided if the circulation is promptly restored or the offending toxin, usually a drug, is withdrawn (Figure 14.12). Similarly, early and aggressive immunosuppression can minimize the seriousness of some types of acute glomerulonephritis.

Clinical features

In the more serious oliguric phase the clinical problems are mainly of fluid and electrolyte overload and accumulation of metabolic by-products. Secondary or indirect complications such as infection, pericarditis and bleeding may also occur. Other symptoms will depend on the initial cause and the stage at which treatment is started. For example, even though hypovolaemia may have caused pre-renal failure it could be masked by subsequent fluid retention. Table 14.15

summarizes most possible features, which are unlikely to occur simultaneously, along with a brief outline of their conservative management.

In the polyuric phase, dehydration and electrolyte depletion are possible, but are rare nowadays. Modern treatment has reduced the frequency with which ARF occurs, and may prevent it entirely.

Management

There is no specific remedy for ARF. Management is aimed at eliminating the cause and keeping the patient alive until the kidney function recovers naturally. Thus the aims are to:

- Discover and reverse or remove cause.
- Correct fluid and electrolyte imbalances.
- Minimize renal complications, i.e. ATN.
- Support the patient through the acute oliguric phase.
- Avoid fluid and electrolyte depletion in the later phases.
- Avoid nephrotoxic drugs

Many of these aims are met by renal dialysis, but conservative management may be adequate and is discussed first.

Table 14.15   Clinical features and conservative management[a] of oliguric acute renal failure

Pathology	Clinical finding[b]	Management[b,c]
Hypovolaemia	Hypotension Low cardiac output (Shock)	Plasma, dextran, saline (Inotropes)
Oliguria	Fluid overload	Fluid/Na restriction (Osmotic or high-dose loop diuretic?) Bladder catheter
Hyperkalaemia	Arrhythmias	See p. 894
Acidosis	Low plasma bicarbonate	Bicarbonate infusion
Uraemia	Nausea, vomiting Diarrhoea Pruritis	Protein restriction?
Non-specific azotaemia	Tiredness, lethargy	Adequate non-nitrogenous caloric intake

[a] Without dialysis.
[b] Parentheses indicate less common findings or treatments.
[c] See text.

Discovering the cause

The cause of ARF, particularly if pre-renal, will usually be evident from clinical examination, but a medication history should always be sought. Nephrotoxicity is an increasing cause of renal dmage, especially among the elderly. Table 14.16 summarizes the common drugs responsible, with an indiction of how they damage the kidney. Intrinsic renal damage may be more obscure as may some indirect forms of obstruction. A plain abdominal X-ray and an ultrasound scan are usually carried out if there is anuria. If the failure is advanced, supportive and symptomatic treatment are more important than immediate definitive diagnosis.

It is essential to ascertain if the episode is unique or is possibly an acute exacerbation of a steadily deteriorating chronic renal failure, so-called 'acute-on-chronic' failure. The patient's history and general clinical status should establish this quite easily.

Restoration of function

In pre-renal failure, the first priority is prompt fluid or blood replenishment and restoration of the cardiovascular function, with monitoring of CVP; this can prevent ATN from developing. If sudden anuria suggests urinary tract obstruction (e.g. cardiovascular function seems unimpaired) the patient can be catheterized, which also enables accurate assessment of urine output. A number of techniques formerly used have been invalidated by recent evidence: these include osmotic or high-dose loop diuretics, bolus fluid challenge and low-dose *dopamine* infusion.

Fluid and electrolytes

A careful balance must be struck between the repletion of any volume deficit which might have first caused the failure, and the prevention of accumulation from subsequent oliguria. The patient's fluid balance and haemodynamic status must be evaluated precisely before resorting to diuretics, which might cause further volume depletion and exacerbate the condition. Similarly, diuretics are inappropriate in obstruction, e.g. in prostatic hypertrophy, and surgery or cautious catheterization are more appropriate. During the oliguric phase, sodium and fluid are restricted and fluid balance is monitored closely by weighing and meticulous charting of intake/output.

The choice between crystalloid or colloidal fluid replenishment ('plasma expansion') is still debated. The theoretical advantage of the latter, e.g. albumin, dextran, hydroxyethyl starch or gelatin, is in preventing water loss from the intravascular compartment to the tissue fluid and cells. Crystalloid solutions risk causing pulmonary oedema and ascites with a reduced gain in restoring circulation. However, the advantages of colloids have not been borne out by careful trials and they are now not generally recommended except where specifically indicated by the nature of the loss that originally precipitated the ARF, e.g. haemorrhage.

Hyperkalaemia is managed as usual (p. 894). Acidosis may be cautiously treated with sodium bicarbonate, taking care to avoid fluid and sodium overload.

Dialysis

If oliguria persists or ATN has supervened, or if plasma urea, creatinine or potassium are rising rapidly, patients are dialysed for short periods as required. This solves most of the problems and has the advantage of allowing a near-normal diet. Continuous arteriovenous haemofiltration is the preferred technique (p. 920), espeially in haemodynamically unstable patients, and minimises fluid restriction. Haemodialysis or peritoneal dialysis (PD) may also be used. Dialysis facilitates parenteral nutrition if it is needed.

General measures and support

Some protein restriction may be needed if gastrointestinal or cutaneous uraemic symptoms are severe (Table 14.15). However, over-zealous protein restriction is avoided as it can retard recovery, especially as patients may be hypercatabolic, with increased protein breakdown and weight loss. If protein is restricted, caloric intake must be maintained by increasing carbohydrate and fat intake. Parenteral feeding may be needed in the early stages. Daily fluid intake is restricted to the daily urine output plus 500 mL to replace insensible losses (Table 14.2).

Infection is common. All drug therapy, including antibiotics, must be carefully evaluated to avoid toxic accumulation of renally

Table 14.16   Common drugs causing nephrotoxicity[a]

Drug		Glomerulonephritis	Interstitial nephritis	Tubular necrosis	Obstructive uropathy	Other
Antimicrobial	Penicillin	+	++			
	Cephalosporins		+	++		
	Tetracycline					+
	Aminoglycoside		+	++		
	Co-trimoxazole		+			
	Sulphonamides	+	+	+	+	
	Erythromycin		+			
	Vancomycin			+		
	Amphotericin			+		
	Rifampicin	+	+			
Analgesic/antirheumatic	Phenacetin		+		++	
	Paracetamol[b] (acetaminophen)		+		+	
	NSAID[c]	+	++			
	Gold	++	+	+		
	Penicillamine	++				
Diuretic	Loop		++			
	Thiazide	+	+			
Radiocontrast media				++		
Cytotoxic	Many				+	
	Methotrexate			+		
	Doxorubicin	+				
	Cisplatin			+		
Heavy metals	Lead, mercury, etc.		+	+		
Antihypertensive	ACEI[b]	+	+			
	Methyldopa			+		
	Hydralazine	+				
	Propranolol		+			
Miscellaneous	Ciclosporin, tacrolimus			++		
	Lithium		+	+		
	Allopurinol	+	+		+	+
	Phenytoin		+			
	Interferon		+			
	Methysergide				+	

[a] This list is neither comprehensive nor exclusive, but serves to illustrate likely problems with common drugs.

[b] In overdose.

[c] Also cause intrarenal glomerular blood flow 'dysregulation'.

+ damage; ++ serious damage

ACEI, angiotensin-converting enzyme inhibitor; NSAID, non-steroidal anti-inflammatory drug.

cleared drugs or their sodium salts. Specialist clinical pharmacists have an important role here.

Recovery

After the critical phase has passed, patients are soon discharged. They will need to be instructed about maintaining an adequate fluid and electrolyte intake and keeping a fluid balance chart.

For most patients the first episode of ARF will be their last. Survivors make an apparently complete recovery, but a few will develop CRF, the first attack representing an acute-on-chronic decompensation against a background of progressive renal disease.

Chronic renal failure (chronic kidney disease)

CRF presents a very different picture from ARF. It usually has different causes, is insidious in onset, follows a slowly progressive course and is irreversible. In addition to azotaemia and fluid and electrolyte problems there are serious endocrine abnormalities. On the other hand, there is usually time to consider the best management options before the patient reaches end-stage renal disease (ESRD) and the range of treatments available can provide the vast majority of patients with a reasonable quality of life.

Aetiology

It is difficult to quantify the relative frequencies of different causes of CRF. Patients usually present very late, with kidneys so shrunken and fibrosed that retrospective diagnosis is impossible. Table 14.17 gives one estimate of the distribution of probable causes among Europeans, but it is approximate, and there are geographical, ethnic and racial variations. For example, hypertensive nephropathy is more common among Afro-Caribbeans, and diabetic nephropathy more common among South Asians, and this accounts partly for higher ESRF rates among these populations. In developing countries, as usual infectious causes are far more prominent.

Generally CRF is due to intrinsic renal disease, often glomerular in origin. Diabetes (the prevalence of which is rising) is an increasing

Table 14.17   Causes of chronic renal failure

Cause	Approximate frequency (%)
Glomerulonephritis	10–15
Diabetes[a]	20–35
Multisystem disease, tumour, miscellaneous[b]	10–15
Hypertension/renovascular	15
Pyelonephritis	10
Congenital (including polycystic)	10
Drug nephrotoxicity	5–10
Interstitial nephritis	5
Unknown	5–15

[a] Frequency as cause of renal disease varies with ethnic group.

[b] Including systemic lupus erythematosus, polyarteritis, scleroderma, haemolytic-uraemic syndrome, gout, tuberculosis, sickle cell disease, etc.

problem, as is iatrogenic disease, especially among the elderly, and the various multisystem disorders as advances in treatment prolong survival. Hypertension is now usually recognized earlier and treated better than previously. Renal neoplasms are uncommon.

Few preventative measures can generally be recommended because the uncertain aetiologies of the more common causes, such as glomerulonephritis and pyelonephritis. Nevertheless, there is no excuse for the lack of vigilance that permits most iatrogenic renal disease to occur, especially in the elderly. Further, in diabetes, improved control and the use of ACEIs slow the rate of progression of CRF and reduce the prevalence of end-stage diabetic nephropathy. Fortunately, the management of advanced renal failure is relatively uniform, regardless of the aetiology.

Epidemiology

Because of national and regional differences in diagnosing, reporting and treating ESRD, figures for incidence and prevalence are elusive or highly variable. Most available data derive from analyses of patients considered for renal replacement therapy and so are skewed by treatment policies. For the UK, the approximate most recently available data are given in Table 14.18.

The significance of some of this information will become clearer when discussing renal replacement therapy.

There are national and racial differences in incidence, doubtless reflecting both environmental and genetic differences. While in the UK the annual incidence is 100 per million population (pmp), in Europe it is 135 pmp and in the US 335 pmp. The US figure is made up of an incidence among whites of 256 pmp and among blacks of 980 pmp. In Australia figures are overall much lower but show a similar racial disparity (94 pmp vs 420 pmp).

Course

The slow decline in the number of functional nephrons, GFR and renal reserve may take decades to pass from normal to end-stage, although the progression tends to accelerate as end-stage is approached. Several staging systems have been used to to chart this progress, and a recent one is given in Table 14.19. Patients often first present with a history of several months of vague ill health, with tiredness, pruritus, sickness and loss of appetite and weight. Hypertension is often found and patients may have been ignoring moderate urinary symptoms, usually

---

Table 14.18   Statistics of renal replacement therapy, UK 2004[a]

Numbers awaiting, entering or undergoing treatment

End-stage renal disease, new cases, 2004[b]	6000 (*100 pmp[c]*)		
		Dialysis 54%	HD 75%
			PD 25%
Total in RRT programmes	40 000 (*600 pmp*)		
		Transplant 46%	Living donor 25%
			Cadaveric 75%
Awaiting transplant	5000		
Annual donations/transplants	2000 (*30 pmp*)		

Survival figures

Graft survival at 1 year – live donor	95%
– cadaveric donor	88%
Graft survival at 5 years – live donor	82%
– cadaveric donor	70%
Patient survival at 1 year	Transplant 97%
	Dialysis 84%

[a] Rounded figures, from UK Renal Registry and UK Transplant.
[b] Entering renal replacement programme.
[c] Per million population.
RRT, renal replacement therapy; HD, haemodialysis; PD, peritoneal dialysis.

polyuria, for some time. Another common presentation is ARF following abnormal stress on the already impaired kidneys (acute-on-chronic renal failure).

Following diagnosis, declining function is monitored by regular serum creatinine measurement, which correlates inversely with GFR (Figure 14.7). Careful management during this stage can minimize complications and may delay the onset of the end-stage decline. The patient then has time to review and discuss with the physician the ultimate treatment options, and to prepare psychologically.

Whatever form of renal replacement therapy patients undergo, there is a reduced life expectancy. The greatest mortality is from CVD, mainly IHD and heart failure. Following transplantation there may be complications resulting from long-term immunosuppression, e.g. infection and neoplasia.

Pathology

In CRF there is usually a complete and permanent failure of increasing numbers of nephrons. This contrasts with ARF where there is usually a uniform reversible partial impairment of all nephrons. Consequently, in CRF the residual intact nephrons come under increased loading. Changes in intrarenal haemodynamics cause compensatory glomerular hypertension and temporary increases in filtration rates (hyperfiltration). However, these are maladaptive, eventually causing or accelerating glomerular sclerosis and tubular atrophy, and the kidneys gradually shrink. One important exception is polycystic disease, where gross enlargement occurs, although functional tissue is similarly reduced.

Renal reserve consists of there being far more nephrons than are needed to sustain life, but numerous adaptations and compensations operate when the number is so reduced as to threaten renal function. Adaptation to maintain water, acid, sodium and potassium levels is good, so serious hypervolaemia, acidosis and changes in plasma electrolyte levels may be prevented until the GFR falls below 5–10 mL/min, which determines the onset of the end-stage. However, both urate and phosphate will accumulate before then. Urea and creatinine levels also rise, in inverse proportion to the fall in GFR, because there are no compensation mechanisms for these molecules. This results in various symptoms.

Before end-stage, the patients' reduced renal reserve makes them prone to decompensation if additional demands are made on the kidneys. These extra demands can produce an exacerbation or an acute-on-chronic crisis that may be the first indication of severe renal disease: they include infection, surgery, fluid depletion (e.g. severe diarrhoea or vomiting), trauma, certain drugs (e.g. tetracyclines) and excess potassium (e.g. potassium-retaining diuretics, foods with high potassium content).

Table 14.19   Progression and nomenclature of chronic renal failure (based on UK National Kidney Foundation)

Stage	Description	Alternative description	GFR[a] mL/min	Symptom prevalence	Urine production
1	Normal	Diminished renal reserve	120–90	–	Normal or mild polyuria
2	Early CRF	Renal impairment	90–60	+	Usually polyuria
3	Moderate CRF	Early renal failure	60–30	+ +	Oliguria
4	Severe CRF	Pre-end stage renal failure	30–15	+ + +	Oliguria
5	End-stage renal failure		<15	+ + + +	Oliguria/anuria

[a] Assumes normal GFR = 120 mL/min.

CRF, chronic renal failure; GFR, glomerular filtration rate.

Pathophysiology and clinical features

A summary of the main clinical problems of CRF is given in Table 14.20, with their presumed pathogenesis and the measures taken to retard progression or limit symptoms. When ESRD is reached, many of these features are mitigated or reversed by renal replacement therapy.

Fluid and electrolyte imbalance
Urine concentrating ability is often diminished in the early stages, causing dilute polyuria and the risk of dehydration and electrolyte depletion, as in the polyuric phase of ARF. This is partly the result of an osmotic diuresis induced by raised urea levels in the tubular filtrate of the remaining intact nephrons.

In the later stages urine volume falls and the consequent retention of sodium and water is the main cause of the hypertension usually found in CRF patients. Other potential complications of hypervolaemia are oedema, including pulmonary oedema, and heart failure. At the onset of end-stage failure the patient may become anuric.

Uraemia
The major biochemical problems do not result from the accumulation of urea itself but of various electrolytes and miscellaneous other mainly nitrogenous toxins. Nevertheless, urea can cause troublesome gastrointestinal symptoms and may be responsible for the capillary fragility and purpura (bruising) seen in renal patients. Uraemia also damages platelets, increasing the bleeding tendency.

Although urate levels are raised, clinical gout is rare. Various other 'middle molecules' (500–5000 Da, nitrogenous and otherwise) may contribute to the variety of non-specific symptoms. Continuous ambulatory peritoneal dialysis (p. 920) is particularly efficient at clearing these substances, leading to an improvement in well-being.

Potassium and acid
These are not retained in dangerous amounts until end-stage. Before that, renal patients seem to tolerate mild hyperkalaemia and acidosis, or adapt to them. However, along with water reten-

tion these are the most serious acute problems at end-stage.

Metabolic features
There are several inter-related changes in lipid and carbohydrate metabolism (Table 14.20). The kidneys normally catabolize several hormones, including about one-third of all natural insulin, and this mechanism is diminished. Conversely, glucose tolerance is reduced, so the effects are unpredictable, especially in diabetics. Dyslipidaemia results in a raised, atherogenic lipid profile.

Cardiovascular disease
Hypertension is almost universal and there is an increased incidence of IHD and heart failure. Numerous factors contribute. Hypertension results from fluid retention and possibly renin/angiotensin abnormalities. Dyslipidaemia and hypertension accelerate atherosclerosis, which is a common feature. Heart failure is multifactorial, involving hypervolaemia, hypertension, ischaemia and anaemia. Cardiomyopathy is part of a generalized myopathy caused by calcium and phosphate imbalance, with ectopic calcification (p. 910) in the heart as well as the coronary arteries. Pericarditis sometimes occurs. CVD accounts for almost half of all deaths in renal failure patients.

Anaemia
The major cause of anaemia in renal patients is marrow hypoplasia due to reduced or absent erythropoietin (see also Chapter 11). The iron-resistant, initially normocytic, normochromic picture resembles that seen in many chronic diseases (though for a different reason). Hb levels rarely exceed about 8 g/dL (normal = 12–18 g/dL). Iron and folate deficiencies are often superimposed owing to anorexia, dietary restrictions, a bleeding tendency, and losses from haemodialysis and frequent blood testing. There are also gut losses due to stress ulceration. Thus later iron deficiency may cause a microcytic, hypochromic picture. Renal anaemia significantly reduces the quality of life of renal patients, producing poor exercise tolerance and increasing the risks of cardiac failure and exposure to multiple transfusions.

Table 14.20   Clinical features of chronic renal failure

Cause	Clinical feature	Conservative management
Retention		
Sodium/water	Hypertension Oedema, general and pulmonary Heart failure	Na/water restriction, diuretics, antihypertensives
Potassium	Hyperkalaemia, arrhythmia	Dietary restriction
Nitrogenous		
• urea	Nausea, vomiting, purpura	Protein restriction
• urate	Hyperuricaemia, gout	
• creatinine	?	
• others?	Lethargy, anorexia, etc.	
Middle molecules[a]	Lethargy, anorexia, etc.	
Phosphate	Renal osteodystrophy	Dietary restrictions, phosphate binders
Acid	Metabolic acidosis, dyspnoea	Oral bicarbonate
Melanin, etc.	Skin pigmentation	
Endocrine		
Vitamin D and calcium deficiency	Renal osteodystrophy (see text)	Vitamin D analogues, calcium phosphate binders
Hyperphosphataemia	Myopathy	
Metastatic calcification	Peripheral neuropathy, cramps Pruritis	
Erythropoietin deficiency	Anaemia	Erythropoiesis-stimulation agents
Other		
Glucose tolerance ↓	Hyperglycaemia; hyperlipidaemia?	Care with diabetics
Insulin metabolism ↓	Hypoglycaemia	
Lipoprotein lipase ↓	Hyperlipidaemia, atherosclerosis, ischaemic heart disease	Dietary fat restriction; lipid-lowering agent (statin)
Immunodeficiency	Infections	Antibiotics
?	Pericarditis	
Platelet defect	Impaired coagulation	
Stress ulceration		Histamine (H_2) antagonist
Problems with drug therapy	(see text)	

[a] Various metabolites in the 500–5000 Da range (see text); ?, uncertain.

Renal bone disease

The syndrome of renal osteodystrophy involves complications secondary to vitamin D failure, with consequent disturbed calcium and phosphate metabolism. Together they form perhaps the most serious group of chronic clinical problems because of their prevalence, their widespread, multisystem secondary effects and the difficulty of treatment.

The pathophysiology of osteodystrophy includes impaired bone mineralization (osteomalacia or 'renal rickets'), bone demineralization (osteitis fibrosa) and extraskeletal deposition of calcium phosphate, especially in blood vessels, joints and muscle (metastatic or ectopic calcification). Figure 14.13 shows a simplified account of the pathogenesis of these features in relation to normal calcium homeostasis.

The clinical consequences are fractures, bone pain, deformity, arthritis, (cardio)myopathy and arteriosclerosis with regional ischaemia (especially in coronary vessels). In addition, abnormal calcium and/or phosphate levels may contribute to pruritus, anaemia, anorexia, muscle cramps, tetany and peripheral neuropathy.

Other features

The immune system is compromised. Impaired metabolism and/or urinary clearance of melanin and other pigments often gives a characteristic brown skin pigmentation. Abnormal plasma constituents may affect erythrocytes and coagulation factors, causing haemolysis and a haemorrhagic tendency that results in bruising, nose bleeds, gastrointestinal bleeding, etc. Some of these problems are ascribed to the retention of 'middle molecules'. Gastrointestinal stress ulceration is common.

Lethargy, fatigue and general malaise occur more in patients who are poorly managed or who are less compliant with their treatment regimens or fail to comprehend them.

Drug-related problems

The way in which renal impairment affects drug use is dealt with separately (p. 914).

Management

The general management strategy and conservative treatment of the patient before ESRD are considered first. Renal replacement therapy is considered on pp. 916–929.

Aims and strategy

The aims in managing CRF are:

- Early detection.
- Identification and removal of cause.
- Retard deterioration in renal function.

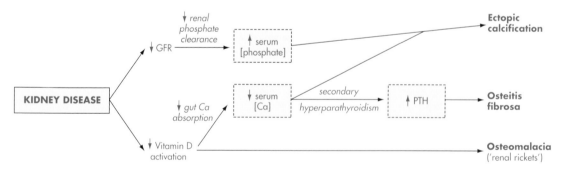

Figure 14.13 Pathology of renal osteodystrophy. Renal disease causes both phosphate retention and impaired vitamin D activation. Calcium levels fall owing to reduced vitamin D failing to facilitate Ca absorption. The abnormal Ca/phosphate levels stimulate the parathyroids. Osteomalacia (impaired mineralization) results from reduced vitamin D, from raised PTH and from low serum calcium levels. Eventually the serum phosphate level rises sufficiently to cause the solubility product ([Ca] × [phosphate]) to be exceeded, resulting in ectopic calcification. The parathyroid gland attempts to correct both ionic abnormalities by secreting excess PTH (secondary hyperparathyroidism). The subsequent increase in calcium gut uptake and reduced calcium renal reabsorption, with the opposite effects on phosphate, together with resorption of both from bone (demineralization), normalizes levels temporarily. As the GFR falls renal phosphate clearance eventually becomes impossible and phosphate levels rise. Ca, calcium; PTH, parathyroid hormone.

- Identification and management of complications.
- Preparation of the patient for renal replacement therapy.

Early detection of CRF is unusual, and often a primary cause cannot be identified because the disease is advanced by the time it is detected. However, certain groups of patients with particular susceptibility need special monitoring. This includes patients with hypertension, diabetes, a chance finding of proteinuria or a family history of renal disease.

Once CRF has been diagnosed, potential aggravating factors such as untreated hypertension, urinary tract obstruction and the use of nephrotoxic drugs must first be eliminated. 'Acute-on-chronic' exacerbations in patients not yet at end-stage, resulting from infection, fluid depletion or overload, etc., must be treated promptly. Complications such as anaemia, hyperphosphataemia and secondary hypertension must be minimized; as well as their direct problems, they contribute to progression of renal decline. Precise dietary recommendations remain controversial, but appropriate dietary control may also slow the progression of the renal damage.

Regular measurements of serum creatinine provide a reliable index of the decline in function and enable the onset of end-stage to be predicted. The rate of decline varies greatly between patients but is generally constant for a given patient. Patients must be encouraged to come to terms psychologically with the fact that they have an irreversible illness that eventually will require artificial support or surgical intervention. How this idea is introduced will depend on the clinician's assessment of the patient's resilience. The family should also be involved and encouraged to be supportive.

As patients approach end-stage they will, unless unsuitable, be tissue typed and entered on the transplantation register. Their home may be assessed for the suitability of home dialysis, and a SC arterio-venous fistula may be fashioned in preparation for haemodialysis.

The situation does not remain static once end-stage has been reached: the treatment mode needs regular re-assessment. Patients may need to switch between different forms of dialysis, in and out of hospital, according to circumstances. Should a transplant prove unsuccessful, they must return to dialysis.

Fluid and electrolytes
Daily fluid intake is restricted to urine output plus 300–500 mL. Such restriction can be extremely unpleasant in the later stages because thirst is so troublesome. When there is severe oliguria or complete anuria, a restriction of total fluid intake to 500 mL including drinks, sauces, fruit, cleaning teeth and liquid medication may be almost impossible to maintain. However, the swift symptomatic penalties of incipient heart failure or pulmonary oedema are salutary correctives.

Salt intake is restricted, with low-salt foods and no added salt. High-potassium foods, such as fresh fruit and vegetables, chocolate, etc. (the very ones that non-renal patients on diuretics are encouraged to seek) are avoided. As this becomes less effective, gastrointestinal ion exchange resins may be added to reduce potassium absorption. Uncontrolled hyperkalaemia is one of the prime indications for starting dialysis.

Acidosis can be managed with oral sodium bicarbonate, but calcium carbonate is needed when sodium restriction is critical; the calcium may also benefit bone disease. The usual care is needed if bicarbonate infusion is used to treat acidosis (p. 897), and persistent severe acidosis is another indication for dialysis.

Diet
Adequate nutrition with high-quality protein in reduced amounts (40–50 g/day) will prevent a negative nitrogen balance and protein malnutrition, and may also slow the disease progression. However, high-protein diets are thought to encourage hyperfiltration, thus accelerating renal decline. Very low-protein diets in the early stages have their advocates.

When the GFR falls below about 50 mL/min protein must be restricted to minimize uraemic complications. Low protein diets have the beneficial side-effect of reducing phosphate, potassium and acid intake, and this might account in part for their apparent effect in some trials of reducing degeneration of renal function.

It is important, whatever course is adopted with regard to protein, that patients have an adeqauate caloric intake, because the nausea and anorexia symptomatic of renal disease tend to lead to poor nutrition. Adequate caloric intake is provided by increasing carbohydrate and unsaturated vegetable fats or oils, using dietary supplements. The lower the protein content of the diet, the more important that it should be of high biological value, so essential amino acid (EAA) supplements may be needed. A further way of minimizing nitrogen catabolism while maintaining protein synthesis is to include ketoacid analogues of EAAs in the diet, as these can be transaminated and thus provide EAAs without additional nitrogen intake.

Vitamin supplementation should not be needed, but many patients, even before dialysis, are given water-soluble multivitamins and iron to compensate for possibly poor nutrition and the loss of blood in frequent blood tests. Dietary compliance, including with electrolytes and especially with fluid, tends to be poor and the involvement of a renal dietician is highly recommended. The summation of the different restrictions can be difficult for a patient to comprehend, and malnutrition, anxiety or guilt may occur. Dietary restriction may be partially relaxed once the patient has started on dialysis.

Hypertension and other cardiovascular problems

Control of BP is a key factor in reducing the progression of CRF. Careful attention to fluid and sodium intake may at first be sufficient to control the hypertension that most patients suffer. ACEIs are the drugs of choice because they have the additional benefit of retarding the progression of CRF, possibly by causing intrarenal vasodilatation and thus reducing glomerular hypertension. Of course, the potential nephrotoxicity of ACEIs in the presence of renovascular disease must not be forgotten. ACEIs may be supplemented with diuretics while the patient is still producing urine. A non-DHP CCB, e.g. *diltiazem*, is the preferred additional drug if BP is not adequately controlled with ACEIs. Thereafter, any of the usual antihypertensives may be added. ACEIs are particularly beneficial in minimising type 1 diabetic nephropathy, but in type 2 diabetes ARAs are the drugs of choice.

Diuretics are needed for pulmonary oedema and heart failure, and temporary dialysis may be necessary if these are unsuccessful. If dietary modification fails, hyperlipidaemia may require HMG CoA reductase inhibitors (statins). The clearance of statins is less affected by renal impairment than other lipid-lowering agents.

Anaemia

Any iron or haematinic vitamin deficiency must first be treated in the usual way (Chapter 11) but this never restores the normal Hb level. Before the availability of *epoetin* the use of multiple transfusions was the only recourse in the anaemia of CRF. This could depress erythropoiesis and also cause iron overload. Moreover the wide range of antibodies that the patient raises against the pooled blood received in this way throughout his or her illness could sensitize them against a future transplant, although this was minimized by using washed packed RBCs.

The advent of genetically engineered erythropoiesis-stimulation agents (ESAs) has solved this. *Epoetin* and *darbepoetin* are recombinant forms of human erythropoietin, the natural red cell growth factor secreted by the normal kidney and acting on the bone marrow. The improved Hb levels that can now be consistently achieved significantly improve the quality of life of CRF patients.

Epoetin as biosynthesised occurs in two different levels of glycosylation, as alfa and beta forms, but these are clinically equivalent. *Darbepoetin* is even more glycosylated and this confers a significantly longer half-life. Numerous other ESAs are under development.

Indications and use. ESA therapy is mainly used in renal patients. Initially reserved for those on haemodialysis, its indications have broadened as the cost has reduced. PD patients, and now increasingly pre-dialysis CRF patients, are offered it if their Hb is sufficiently low and not managed by haematinics. ESAs are also used for anaemia following chemotherapy-induced bone marrow depression and to facilitate the collection of autologous transfusion blood prior to surgery. Care must be taken to follow the precise dosage guidelines, which vary according to indication and also specify titration and maintenance protocols. *Epoetin* is usually injected 3 times weekly; the longer half-life of *darbepoetin* permits once-weekly dosing. For stabilized patients less frequent dosing of both agents appears to be adequate and is quite common.

The target Hb level for each patient needs careful assessment, but a Hb no greater than 13 g/dL is usually aimed for, and about 12 g/dL if the patient has any CVD. ESA therapy must be matched by appropriate iron intake, and iron supplementation is usually required. This is usually given intravenously to accommodate the increased iron requirement generated by the *epoetin*, especially in haemodialysis patients. Moreover, careful optimization of iron status can reduce the demand for *epoetin*, thus conferring considerable economies.

Adverse effects and cautions. The main potential problem is potentiation of hypertension, possibly causing encephalopathy with convulsions. Also, thromboses may obstruct vascular catheters used for haemodialysis access. The reason for the conservative Hb targets is that if complete normalization of the Hb level were attempted, cardiovascular complications could arise owing to the resulting polycythaemia (excessive RBC count) causing increased blood viscosity, blood volume and blood pressure. A rare adverse effect of *epoetin alfa* is an immunologically-mediated pure red cell aplasia, which if it occurs precludes furthur use of any erythropoietin derivative, This effect seems to be associated with SC use and so IV administration only is currently recommended.

Renal bone disease

Osteodystrophy is difficult to manage because it changes during the course of the illness and thus requires different treatments at different times. Renal bone disease is one of the complications that is least improved by dialysis. The related metastatic calcification of the aorta and coronary arteries contribute significantly to CVD in renal patients.

For hypocalcaemia in the absence of hyperphosphataemia, raising the plasma calcium level will improve osteomalacia (Figure 14.13). Initially, calcium supplements may be used, *calcium carbonate* being the most suitable as it will also counteract acidosis and complex some phosphate in the gut. Later, vitamin D analogues *calcitriol* or *alfacalcidol* are needed, neither of which rely on renal hydroxylation for activation (as does natural vitamin D, *colecalciferol*). They tend to elevate the plasma calcium level, so close monitoring of this is essential, otherwise this could exacerbate metastatic calcification.

Hyperphosphataemia is treated initially with phosphate restriction, but this is extremely difficult to achieve because phosphate occurs widely in foods, e.g. dairy products, many fish, eggs, liver, many vegetables, chocolate, nuts. Eventually, oral phosphate binders are required, to prevent dietary phosphate and any phosphate in gastrointestinal secretions being absorbed. Formerly, *aluminium hydroxide* was the standard therapy: this forms insoluble aluminium phosphate in the gut, which is lost in the faeces. Aluminium hydroxide is given in dry capsule form, e.g. 'Alu-Cap', the more usual antacid mixture being unsuitable for fluid-restricted patients. However, significant aluminium absorption occurs in renal patients who clear it inefficiently, and long-term use is associated with dementia and anaemia; it will actually also cause a form of osteodystrophy. This was exacerbated in certain areas by exposure to aluminium in dialysis fluids derived from the local water supply.

Current practice favours *calcium carbonate* tablets with the incidental benefits mentioned above, though large doses are needed. Magnesium and *lanthanum* salts have also been used, and do not produce hypercalcaemia as may *calcium carbonate*. Close monitoring of plasma phosphate and calcium are vital because doses are easily misjudged and dietary mismanagement by the patient may undo the most careful adjustment. The newer ion-exchange resin *sevelamer* offers advantages in reducing arterial calcification but is expensive so currently is used only in combination with oral calcium.

If secondary hyperparathyroidism is troublesome and refractory to medical management, then partial or total parathyroidectomy may be indicated. Calcimimetics, e.g. *cinacalcet*, are currently being tested; these stimulate the calcium sensor on the parathyroid, thereby reducing PTH secretion.

Other problems

Some of the miscellaneous problems such as neuropathy, gastrointestinal upset, pruritus, etc. may resolve if the above methods are successful, particularly protein restriction and calcium and phosphate control. Others may need to await dialysis, which almost invariably produces a notable improvement in general well-being.

Drug use in renal impairment

There are several important questions to be asked when considering drug therapy in patients with renal impairment. This applies to all drugs, whether used for the renal disease itself or for a co-morbidity.

- Is the drug nephrotoxic?
- Is the drug essential?
- What is degree of renal impairment?
- What proportion of drug is cleared by kidney?
- Does drug have narrow therapeutic index?
- Is the drug's action or toxicity altered in renal impairment?

If a drug is potentially nephrotoxic, it should be avoided if possible because these toxic effects, even if only mild or rare, are likely to be of more significance in the presence of renal impairment. Is an alternative drug of comparable clinical action but more favourable pharmacokinetic profile available? If not, then the initial drug will need to be used with care and following appropriate dosage adjustment. The degree of renal impairment, measured quantitatively, will indicate whether and to what extent the dose will need to be reduced. This calculation will have to be further refined by consideration of what proportion of the drug dose is normally cleared by the kidney; many drugs have more than one route of clearance.

Another important point is the drug's therapeutic index. If this is narrow, even small reductions in clearance, giving small rises in serum level, could cause toxicity. We also need to know if rapid achievement of therapeutic serum level is important, because attainment of steady state may be delayed in renal impairment. These

factors will be discussed briefly; see also References and further reading.

Nephrotoxicity

Adverse drug effects on the kidney are well documented by the BNF, in both Appendix 3 and individual monographs. A summary was given in Table 14.16.

Renal clearance

In order to judge whether or not a drug will be renally cleared, some general pharmacokinetic principles need to be reviewed (see Chapter 1) In renal impairment we are primarily concerned with drugs that are water soluble i.e. polar or hydrophilic, which are normally predominately cleared by the kidney, e.g 98% for *gentamicin*. We are less concerned about hydrophobic drugs (i.e. lipid-like, non-polar or fat-soluble), which rely on hepatic metabolism for clearance, e.g. *theophylline*, *phenytoin* or *warfarin*. Exceptions are when the hepatic metabolite is renally cleared, clinically active or more toxic that the original drug; in such cases accumulation in renal impairment may be important, e.g *codeine* metabolised to *morphine*. Other drugs are cleared partially by both routes, e.g. *digoxin* (15% hepatic, 85% renal). It is only the renal component that is altered in renal impairment; usually the other route is unaffected, and this must be taken into account in dosage adjustment.

The change that occurs to the renal component of clearance means that the drug is cleared more slowly. The same dose will be retained longer, i.e. the half-life will increase, and thus with regular dosing the plasma level will be higher. These changes will be in proportion to the fall in GFR or creatinine clearance. Consider, for example, a patient who has a creatinine clearance of 60 mL/min, taking a drug that is cleared 100% renally. Assuming the normal creatinine clearance is 120 mL/min, the dosage reduction to give normal plasma levels should be 50%. But if the drug is only half cleared by the kidney, the dose reduction would need to be only half that, i.e. 25%.

Therapeutic index

Even if a drug does accumulate to a limited degree, this may be of little consequence if the therapeutic effect, and especially the toxic effect, are not closely related to the plasma level. Thus some accumulation of most penicillins is usually of little consequence and can be tolerated, so dosage adjustment of oral penicillins is very rarely necessary, even though most are cleared mainly be the kidney.

Loading dose

Because in renal impairment half-lives are increased, it will take longer for a drug to achieve its steady state plasma level. Steady state following the regular dosing of any drug occurs after about five half-lives, whatever the dose or renal function. In some cases it may not be acceptable to wait this long in a renally impaired patient, e.g. with antibiotics or *digoxin*, especially if the dose has been reduced because of the impairment. In such cases, a loading dose may be given to achieve therapeutic concentrations quickly. Calculation of a loading dose is not dependent on clearance (only on dose and volume of fluid in the body) so the normal loading dose is given, or possible higher if there is severe oedema, even if subsequent dosage is to be reduced.

Drug handling

When the renal function is impaired there is more to consider than reduced clearance. A number of consequences follow from the metabolic and biochemical abnormalities secondary to the renal impairment, which could effect drug action or handling.

Oedema and volume of distribution
In renal impairment, fluid retention with oedema is usual, which would tend to increase the volume of distribution of hydrophilic drugs.

Counteracting that however is the fact that the kidney will not be clearing hydrophilic drugs so efficiently. Thus the net effect of these two opposing trends is difficult to predict and means that careful observation and/or therapeutic drug monitoring may be necessary.

Uraemia and drug binding
Some of the metabolites that accumulate in uraemia, including urea, may displace a drug from its plasma protein binding sites, raising the plasma level, e.g. *phenytoin*, *diazepam* and *theophylline*. By analogy with a drug interaction, this is only likely to be of significance if the urea level is high and the protein binding of the drug is normally high (>90%). Moreover, the rise in free plasma level will increase the clearance of the displaced drug (especially if it is usually cleared hepatically), reducing adverse consequences. Furthermore, renal patients tend to have hypoproteinaemia owing to proteinuria, poor diet and chronic illness, further reducing binding.

Reduced drug metabolism
Normally, insulin is partially metabolised in the kidney; thus, renal impairment could alter the control of diabetes. To avoid hypoglycaemia, insulin dose may need to be reduced. We have already noted that metabolic activation of vitamin D is reduced in renal impairment.

Pharmacodynamic changes
In addition to these pharmacokinetic effects, there can also be pharmacodynamic changes in the actions of some drugs. The blood–brain barrier is less effective in renal failure patients, so some centrally acting drugs such as benzodiazepines might have exaggerated effects. Renal patients are more prone to upper gastrointestinal bleeding and ulceration and so are more sensitive to the gastro-erosive effects of NSAIDs.

Dosage adjustment

Considering all these possible influences on drug action and clearance, drug selection and dosing in renal impairment is problematic. It requires experience and judgement as well as access to specialised formularies, such as that produced by the UK Renal Pharmacists Group, giving the changes in drug parameters such as half life or proportion of renal clearance in different degrees of renal impairment. The advice of a renal pharmacy specialist should always be sought.

Assuming it is essential to give a drug the clearance of which will be affected by renal impairment, pharmacokinetic calculations can be made to show how clearance will be reduced. These can be done effectively by programs on hand-held computers. However, it still needs judgement to decide how the dosage reduction will be implemented. Suppose it is calculated that the clearance is reduced by 50%. Does this require half the normal dose at the same interval or the same dose at double the normal interval? Either would compensate for the reduced clearance.

It will depend, among other things, on the plasma level profile required. If a roughly constant plasma level with small peaks and troughs is required (e.g. with anticonvulsants, *lithium*), dose reduction is indicated; in such cases, initialising therapy may need a loading dose. If a pronounced peak or a definite trough (to minimize toxicity) is required, e.g. as with *gentamicin*, an increased interval will be preferred.

In some cases, there may be an accessible clinical parameter such as blood pressure, blood glucose or clotting time, which will enable the more pragmatic approach of therapeutic monitoring and dose titration without recourse to frequent precise calculation and plasma level monitoring.

The situation is different for patients on dialysis, where clearance may be more difficult to estimate. Once again the advice of a renal pharmacy specialist should be sought.

Renal replacement therapy

The main role of renal replacement therapy (RRT) is in end-stage renal disease patients whose GFR has fallen below 5–10 mL/min or in whom other complications are not responding to conservative therapy. Renal replacement therapy involves either the artificial techniques of dialysis or natural replacement with a transplant. Temporary dialysis may also be required in ARF or poisoning.

Renal dialysis

Aim

Renal dialysis attempts to mimic the excretory and to a lesser extent the homeostatic roles of the kidney. Although dialysis cannot restore renal endocrine function, it ameliorates some of the secondary effects of endocrine dysfunction such as hypertension and hyperphosphataemia. Anaemia may also be improved. Many patients on dialysis lead near-normal lives and half of them return to work. There is a reduced quality of life compared with normal or after a transplant, but there are far fewer restrictions compared with conservative treatment in the later stages of CRF.

When the GFR falls below about 10 mL/min, toxic nitrogenous metabolites, potassium, acid and water start to accumulate to a life-threatening degree. Serum creatinine at this stage would probably be above 1000 µmol/L and blood urea more than 30 mmol/L. If there are persistent complications such as neuropathy, pericarditis or refractory hypertension, intervention is made even earlier.

Although there are nowadays few patients for whom transplantation is absolutely contra-indicated, most will have to wait months or years for an organ to become available, and dialysis is essential to keep them alive until then. Many patients have been successfully maintained on dialysis for decades. Nevertheless, their poor general health results in a greater mortality than that of the general population.

Principles

Two general techniques are currently available, namely haemodialysis (HD) and peritoneal dialysis (PD). Ideally these would perform the same functions as the natural kidney where ultrafiltration is followed by reabsorption.

In health filtration involves removal of water and dissolved small molecules via a size-selective semi-permeable membrane (the glomerular basement membrane, GBM) driven by hydrostatic pressure (arterial blood pressure). Reabsorption involves partially selective, sometimes active recouping of useful substances (in the tubules).

These processes cannot be mimicked exactly. Almost all artificial kidneys utilize a membrane analogous to the GBM, but with a different pore size. In HD the membrane is artificial, while in PD the patient's own peritoneal membrane is used. In PD the dialysis approaches equilibrium before the dialysis fluid is changed, whereas in HD fast cycling of fresh dialysis fluid speeds diffusion by continually exposing the blood to maximal concentration gradients. Thus HD is more efficient.

In addition to its principal use in CRF, dialysis is also used in the oliguric phase of ARF and for drug overdose and poisoning. Some conservatively managed early CRF patients may need temporary dialysis during acute-on-chronic exacerbations, after which they may stabilize again and come off it.

Water removal

In both forms of dialysis, water removal is by ultrafiltration. In HD the driving force is hydrostatic, using negative pressure on the dialysate side; in PD water is removed osmotically.

Removal of waste solutes

Essentially dialysis means solute transfer by diffusion through a membrane down a concentration gradient. In renal dialysis a system is set up whereby blood on one side of a suitable membrane is exposed to a dialysis solution on the other. The dialysis solution may contain low concentrations of the substances to be removed, or none at all. Haemodialysis can generate urea clearances of up to 100 mL/min. Yet because it relies on diffusion, clearance is inversely proportional to molecular weight, so that 'middle molecules' are less efficiently removed than small molecules such as urea and creatinine. With high transmembrane flow rates and especially with larger pores, larger solutes may also be drawn across by solvent drag or convection.

Conservation of useful substances

There is no equivalent in dialysis to the subtle processes of natural tubular reabsorption. However, in practice significant electrolyte and nutrient losses are uncommon. Two rather crude substitutes may be used. There can be replacement by dietary supplementation, e.g. of water-soluble vitamins or amino acids; or else the dialysis fluid can be loaded with the desired substances at normal plasma concentrations, thus inhibiting diffusion. The latter technique may be extended by adding substances to the dialysis fluid in excess, to promote net transfer to the patient's circulation, e.g. bicarbonate to combat acidosis, or insulin for diabetics on PD.

Haemodialysis

The early artificial kidneys were cumbersome and inefficient devices the size of a suitcase, which had to be painstakingly disassembled and cleaned between treatments. Modern artificial kidneys are disposable and little larger than the organ they replace, though they have about the same filtration area of 1 m². In some there are multiple thin cellophane films which separate alternate layers of blood and dialysis fluid; in others the blood is pumped through a parallel array of multiple fine, hollow fibres, which are surrounded by dialysis fluid. In each case the dialysis fluids flows countercurrent to the blood.

Basic system and apparatus

A diagram of the basic HD system is given in Figure 14.14 and the apparatus is shown in use in Figure 14.15. The sequence is:

* Arterial blood is directed outside the body and passed through the system by a peristaltic pump
* The blood is anticoagulated with *heparin* and circulated through the artificial kidney.
* A countercurrent of haemodialysis fluid runs against the blood.
* A small negative pressure is applied to the blood.
* Blood is returned to a vein and the dialysate is discarded.

Apart from the artificial kidney itself, the function of most of the HD apparatus is the

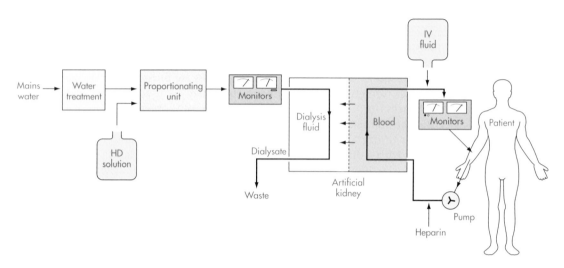

Figure 14.14 Block diagram of the essential elements in a haemodialysis circuit (not to scale).

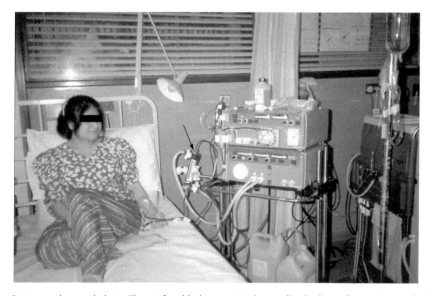

Figure 14.15 Patient on haemodialysis. The artificial kidney unit is the small cylinder in the centre, just below the lamp (arrow). The cabinet beside it is the monitoring and proportionating unit. (Reproduced with permission from Dr JR Curtis, Renal Unit, Charing Cross and Westminster Hospital, London.)

maintenance of a safe extracorporeal blood circulation and the preparation of a suitably purified dialysis fluid. The blood circuit is heparinized using an infusion pump at a rate sufficient to prevent clotting within the appa-ratus, but which ensures the heparin is inacti-vated naturally by the time blood is returned to the patient. Rarely, *protamine* may be needed as an antidote, or *epoprostenol* may be used if the patient has bleeding problems. Up to

500 mL/min of blood may be removed from the patient and this must be returned free of air bubbles and clots and at the correct pressure and temperature. Physiological saline is flushed through the blood circuit beforehand to prime it and afterwards to return as much blood as possible to the patient. This also facilitates a top-up infusion if an overshoot in ultrafiltration has caused fluid depletion.

Vascular access

The patient is usually connected to the HD apparatus via a SC arteriovenous fistula in the arm. This is an artifical connection constructed surgically between an artery and a vein in the wrist area (Figure 14.16(a)). After a few weeks, the fistula is mature and the vein becomes 'arterialized': it swells and its wall becomes thickened, which facilitates repeated puncture for both access and return.

For temporary dialysis, or during the few weeks while a fistula matures, either a temporary IV line (jugular or subclavian catheter) or, less comonly nowadays, an external shunt (Figure 14.16(b)) is used. Fistulae last for several years before becoming unusable, when a different site needs to be fashioned. Shunts, although quick to set up, last less than a year and are very inconvenient.

Dialysis fluid

The 100–200 L of dialysis fluid needed for each treatment are prepared automatically in the proportionating unit using concentrated dialysis solution. This is diluted as required with mains water that has been thoroughly purified. Ion exchange or reverse osmosis remove potentially dangerous cations. Aluminium and calcium are the main problems long term: the former causes encephalopathy ('dialysis dementia') and complicates osteodystrophy, while calcium can cause acute neurological problems during dialysis. Various environmental toxins and pyrogens are adsorbed onto carbon, and ultaviolet radiation is used as a microbicide. Flow rates of up to 800 mL/min mean that up to 150 L of water may be needed for a single treatment. The blood circuit has to be scrupulously sterile, and most of it is disposable.

The ionic composition of the dialysis fluid is adjusted individually to normalize each patient's plasma, i.e. low in those ions to be removed, high in those to be taken up. Usually it is equimolar in Na^+ and Mg^{2+}, K^+ is between 0–3 mmol/L, Ca^{2+} is variable and alkali is supplied as lactate or acetate, bicarbonate being incompatible with Ca^{2+} and Mg^{2+}. For diabetics, glucose is sometimes added to prevent hypoglycaemia.

Routine therapy

Most patients need 3–6 h of HD two to three times each week, depending on their fluid and electrolyte retention between treatments, which itself partly depends on residual urine output. Dialysis requirement is usually monitored by weight gain, and progress of HD is followed measuring dialysate outflow. Ideally the patient should not gain more than 1500 g between treatments, i.e. 1.5 L of fluid, to avoid cardiovascular

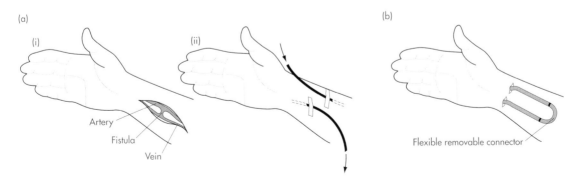

Figure 14.16 Types of vascular access used for haemodialysis. (a) Arteriovenous fistula showing (i) surgery involved and (ii) needles inserted for treatment. (b) Arteriovenous external shunt closed off between treatments.

and pulmonary problems. Moreover, removing more than this in 4–6 h can cause temporary fluid or electrolyte imbalance, the so-called 'disequilibrium syndrome' (involving weakness, hypotension, dizziness or cramps) because plasma concentrations change far more rapidly than in extravascular sites.

Dialysis may be carried out overnight, thus maximizing the utilization of dialysis facilities, although in UK hospitals it is more usually done during the day. Many patients continue full or part-time work. Patients can also make temporary arrangements with dialysis units in holiday areas. Once patients are stabilized, dialysis equipment may be set up in their homes. This depends on whether the patient and carers can cope physically, intellectually and psychologically, and also on logistical factors, such as water supply, whether there is a spare room (some patients have Portakabins erected in their garden) and whether there is someone to help them cope with any problems that may arise while dialysing.

Most CRF dietary restrictions on potassium, phosphate, etc. still need to be observed by patients on HD, and daily fluid intake must not exceed 500 mL plus urine output. Advice and counselling from a dietician is important. Antihypertensive treatment is frequently continued, although the hypertension may improve. Vitamins B complex and C are required to compensate for losses of these water-soluble substances to the dialysate, as are iron and folate for the blood losses incurred. *Epoetin* and osteodystrophy treatments need to be continued.

Problems

Acute problems include fluid or electrolyte imbalance resulting from the rapid changes causing cramps, hypotension, headaches, etc. and ischaemia distal to the access site, e.g. in the hand. Immediately after treatment some patients need an oral sodium supplement for cramps caused by electrolyte deficiency The main chronic problems are related to the vascular access and include thrombosis, local or systemic infection, haemorrhage, phlebitis and haemolysis, etc.

Patients do very well on HD and feel better than they did in the later stages of CRF before starting dialysis, and it is used by about three quarters of all dialysis patients. The quality of life is reduced on account of regular disruption and dependence on machinery, but some patients still prefer this to the continuous commitment of PD.

Haemofiltration

Drawbacks to the conventional HD system include complex apparatus and poor clearance of 'middle molecules'. The intermittent nature of the treatment can impose high haemodynamic stresses, especially in ARF. Several alternatives have been developed that are particularly useful for short-term dialysis, e.g. in ARF or cases of poisoning.

In continuous arteriovenous haemofiltration (CAVH) no dialysis fluid is used. The system operates more like a plasma exchange, with large quantities of fluid (up to 20 L per day) being removed in an artificial kidney with a more permeable membrane. Crystalloids follow by convection, rather than diffusion as in haemodialysis. Fluid and electrolytes (without unwanted toxins) are replaced continuously via the return line, the volume replaced depending on how much fluid needs to be lost. Where urea levels are high, e.g. in the hypercatabolic states of severe ARF, a blood pump and negative pressure are used, which also improves the removal of 'middle molecules'. Alternatively, there may be additional intermittent haemodialysis.

The newer technique of continuous arteriovenous haemodiafiltration (CAV-HD) represents a compromise. Dialysis fluid and a more porous dialyser unit are used and a pump may not be required. Fluid removal is controlled by the dialysis fluid flow rate, which is generally much slower than in normal HD. In haemoperfusion a sterile activated charcoal column is put in the blood circuit rather than an artificial kidney. This is sometimes useful in poisoning treatment. In continuous venovenous haemofiltration a single dual-lumen IV catheter is used and a pump added to the circuit.

Peritoneal dialysis

This process is far simpler mechanically. Up to 2.5 L of sterile dialysis fluid are run directly into the patient's peritoneal cavity under gravity via an indwelling silastic catheter, over about 10 min (Figure 14.17). Dialysis then takes place between the blood in peritoneal capillaries and the dialysis fluid in the peritoneum. The dialysing interface is composed of the vascular basement membranes and the peritoneal membranes, both of which are semi-permeable. The process is thus analogous to the formation of tissue fluid or ascites. The entire fluid volume, including excess water and dialysed substances, is then drained out again under gravity, often by simply putting the empty dialysis fluid bag on the floor below the patient.

PD fluid comes ready-made and sterile, and is similar in composition to diluted HD fluid but with little potassium, clearances being lower than in HD. Because a hydrostatic pressure gradient cannot be set up in the peritoneum to promote water removal, different concentrations of glucose are added (1.36–4%) to effect different rates of removal osmotically. The system is relatively cheap to set up and maintain and requires far simpler equipment and fewer specialized staff when used in hospital.

There are several different ways of organizing and scheduling PD.

Intermittent peritoneal dialysis

In its conventional hospital-based form this method involves multiple hourly fill–drain cycles with short dwell times, repeated 24–48 times over 1–2 days. Because the rate of diffusion of molecules (equivalent to their clearance) declines as their concentration in the peritoneal dialysate increases, a 30-min contact time within the peritoneum is optimal.

Intermittent peritoneal dialysis (IPD) is only about one-fifth as efficient as HD, with urea clearance of about 20 mL/min. The cycle must be repeated, two or three times weekly, using 50–100 L of PD fluid each time. Perhaps surprisingly, it is not overly uncomfortable for most patients, although they are physically restricted for long periods. However, IPD is rarely used nowadays except in patients awaiting some other management, in those for whom all other methods have failed, and in those with some residual renal function when the inefficiency of IPD is less of a problem.

Continuous ambulatory peritoneal dialysis

Originally devised to exploit the simplicity of PD but free the patient of its restrictions, continuous

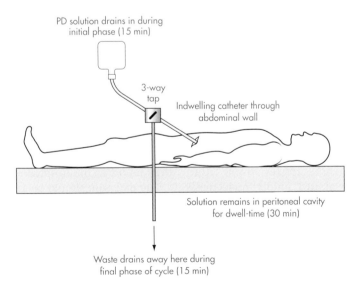

PD solution drains in during initial phase (15 min)

3-way tap

Indwelling catheter through abdominal wall

Solution remains in peritoneal cavity for dwell-time (30 min)

Waste drains away here during final phase of cycle (15 min)

Figure 14.17 Peritoneal dialysis (PD). The diagram shows the basic elements of the system. (Reproduced with permission from Greene R, Harris N (1985) *Chemist Drugg* **224**: 1614.)

ambulatory peritoneal dialysis (CAPD) yielded unexpected additional benefits and is now the most popular form of dialysis in the UK (about 40–50% of cases). Instead of the frequent fluid changes being made during several specified periods in the week, the patient carries the fluid in their abdomen continuously, day and night, while living an otherwise almost normal life. The solution is changed two to five times daily, the longest dwell being overnight.

PD fluid is run in from a soft plastic bag, and the line is then closed. After 4–6 h the dialysate is drained out and fresh fluid run in. The changeover takes 30–40 min, and the patient needs training in aseptic technique. CAPD is not suitable for all: some cannot cope emotionally or intellectually, while others have manipulative difficulties, e.g. the aged or arthritic; others do not appreciate the need for strict asepsis. On the other hand, some patients are even able to judge the right glucose concentration to use each time to extract more or less fluid as required.

To reduce the chances of infection the 'disconnect-flush before fill' system is practised. The intraperitoneal catheter terminates externally as a Y-tube, both arms of which can be sealed. At changeover both an empty and the new bag are connected. The dialysate is first drained off, flushing away potential contamination from the connection procedure; new fluid is then run in.

Successful patients achieve a steady continuous clearance of water, electrolytes and uraemic toxins with stable if somewhat higher than normal blood levels, so the process resembles normal renal function more closely than other forms of dialysis. There is little of the peaking and troughing of electrolyte levels characteristic of both HD and IPD. In addition, the use of a natural membrane and longer dwell time improves the removal of 'middle molecules'. Thus there is a more stable fluid and electrolyte balance and consistently lower levels of toxins, and consequently patients feel very much better. Moreover, there are few dietary restrictions, the main remaining modification being an increased protein intake to compensate for losses across the peritoneum. Water-soluble vitamins are given as usual.

Automated peritoneal dialysis

This technique is increasingly used where CAPD has failed to provide control or where it produces unacceptable daytime restrictions for patients. Automated peritoneal dialysis (APD) involves automation of intermittent PD, with a machine to switch between bags and control the tap. It can be used easily at home, and when run overnight causes less discomfort because the patient is recumbent. The more rapid cycling compared with CAPD means that night-time exchanges may provide sufficient control and obviate the necessity for the patient to dialyse during the day, or else only require a few daytime cycles. Thus, APD is preferred by many patients and now is used by about one-quarter of PD patients in the UK.

Problems

Contra-indications. Patients with respiratory or abdominal disease present difficulties. Diaphragm movement is impeded by the fluid-filled abdomen, and this possibly impairs respiration. Fistula formation might be encouraged in IBD, with consequent peritonitis, and hernias may be aggravated. Gut surgery can leave fibrous adhesions which reduce the effective membrane area.

Peritonitis. Infections from contamination during bag switching are unfortunately common: a CAPD patient experiences one such episode on average every 2–3 years. It is less frequent in hospital-based PD. Usually, a commensal Gram-positive skin organism (*Staphylococcus epidermidis*) is implicated, but enterococcal infection (*Streptococcus faecalis*) suggestive of an intestinal fistula may occur and is far more serious. Infection may be painless and is usually detected when the dialysate becomes cloudy or takes far longer than usual to drain. CAPD patients must then report to the hospital immediately.

The dialysate should be sampled for culturing and sensitivity testing before antibiotics are given, but blind therapy must be started promptly to minimize the development of peritoneal fibrosis. Initial treatment is a cephalosporin plus an aminoglycoside in the dialysis fluid, with one or the other stopped according to sensitivity data. A loading dose, possibly IV, may be needed in severe cases: otherwise most episodes are managed with the patient at home or as an outpatient. Treatment should last 7–10 days, during which normal dialysis may be continued, although at an increased frequency because the inflamed membranes reduce urea clearance.

A less invasive and far cheaper recommendation for mild peritonitis is to perform three rapid exchanges at the first sign of infection and then simply to stop PD for 2 days and allow for natural resolution, though this requires careful supervision in hospital. Exit site or catheter tunnel infections are usually Gram-positive and an antistaphylococcal agent such as *vancomycin* is used.

Apart from the immediate problems of serious infection, each peritonitis episode causes scarring and adhesions that gradually degrade the peritoneal surface area and reduce ultrafiltration efficiency. This may be exacerbated by the continuous exposure of the peritoneum to an abnormal fluid volume.

Hyperglycaemia. The glucose in the dialysis fluid causes hyperglycaemia and obesity, especially in CAPD because there is significant absorption during the long dwell times. This is a particular problem with diabetics. The hyperlipidaemia which all renal patients suffer is exacerbated in PD patients, possibly due to the hyperglycaemia. Another consequence of glucose absorption is a gradual reduction in the osmolarity of the in situ dialysis fluid, which reduces ultrafiltration as each exchange proceeds. Glucose polymers, e.g. *icodextrin*, which exert a significant oncotic pressure in the dialysis fluid but cannot be absorbed, minimise this.

Other problems include:

- Loss of protein and amino acids.
- Blockage of the catheter (which otherwise lasts many months, and is regularly cleared with a heparin flush).
- Local infection around catheter insertion site.
- Sclerosing peritonitis, a rare, potentially fatal complication, possibly associated with dialysis fluid contaminants or additives, e.g. chlorhexidine, acetate.

There is a high drop-out rate from CAPD, with up to half of patients switching to some other method within 3 years, and few lasting 10 years. In the UK many would regard CAPD as the treatment of second choice (after transplantation) for ESRD, and intensive efforts are being made into improving its success rate because of the quality of life it permits and its economic benefits. Up to 50% of dialysis patients are on CAPD and most of the remainder on HD. However, the position is different in the rest of Europe; e.g. in Scandinavia, only 30–40% choose CAPD, the majority preferring HD. There may be economic reasons for this.

Drug therapy in PD

Many drugs can, like antibiotics, be given safely and effectively by the intraperitoneal route in CAPD fluid. The most notable example is insulin for diabetics with ESRD, and very smooth diabetic control can be achieved in this way. Further information may be obtained in the References and further reading section.

Comparison of dialysis types

The 10-year survival rate for both methods is about 75%, with CAPD patients achieving a slightly better rate. Table 14.21 summarizes important features of the two main types of dialysis, and compares their relative advantages and disadvantages.

Transplantation

For the vast majority of ESRD patients a renal transplant is the best possible treatment. In Europe as a whole about 30% of patients receive replacement kidneys, but there are regional differences. The UK, with 30 kidney donations per million population annually, has the lowest rate.

The shortage of organs is still the major impediment to improving these figures, the situation having been exacerbated by seat-belt legislation which has reduced road traffic fatalities. In addition, certain ethnic groups may have cultural or religious objections. On the other hand, as tissue matching and immunosuppressive regimens improve and surgical experience grows, so the survival rate, especially

Table 14.21   Comparison of haemodialysis and peritoneal dialysis

Haemodialysis	Peritoneal dialysis
Complex, expensive	Simple
Special staff (hospital dialysis)	No special staff needed, but patient needs training
Can be done at home, but detailed training and home modification involved	Can be done at home (APD), but storage facilities needed
Needs another person	Complete independence possible; less social and employment disruption Patient motivation more critical Back-up support services required
Patient tied to machine during treatment but free at other times	Patient must change 2–5 times every day (CAPD) but mobile
Fluctuating biochemical parameters	Stable biochemical parameters
Patient's condition varies between treatments and takes time to recover after each	Consistent well-being
Poor removal of 'middle molecules'	Good metabolic control and removal of 'middle molecules'
Vascular access complications	Can be used in patients with vascular problems Serious infective complications Back-up fistula/shunt may be needed for CAPD failure
Can be used for long periods (if vascular access maintained)	CAPD often only possible for a few years
More effective in acute renal failure	Difficult for diabetics

APD, automated peritoneal dialysis; CAPD, continuous ambulatory peritoneal dialysis.

of non-related or unmatched living grafts improves, and the admission criteria to transplant programmes have been relaxed.

Patients who formerly would not have been grafted owing to age or an underlying disease that predisposed them to renewed renal damage, e.g. diabetes, hypertension, arterial disease, are now considered. There remain few absolute contra-indications; these include extensive neoplastic disease, serious infection, and the inability to withstand major surgery or immunosuppression, e.g. otherwise immunocompromised patients.

A successful graft is an almost complete cure: all fluid, electrolyte and toxaemic complications are reversed, and in time the anaemia and even the bone disease resolve. There may be some residual hypertension but the only significant disadvantage is the lifelong immunosuppression that is needed, with its attendant risks, and the inconvenience of regular monitoring.

Organ donation

Live donors

Using live donors is convenient and allows ample preoperative preparation. It also results in improved graft survival because of the reduced time that the organ spends disconnected from a blood supply (cold ischaemic time). Donors are carefully screened for renal disease or relevant risk factors, e.g. hypertension, and for general and psychological health. The loss of a kidney does not adversely affect an otherwise healthy person, and the operative risk is low (mortality about 1/3000). Their remaining kidney hypertrophies, giving an eventual GFR of about two-thirds the pre-donation level. Long-term follow-up of donors has shown no significantly increased risk of renal disease or hypertension, nor any reduction of life expectancy.

Related donors are preferred. Obviously the ideal of an identical twin is rarely achieved; failing that, other siblings are preferred. However, genetically unrelated spouse donors are being increasingly used, with surprising success. Anonymous organ donation for profit is not permitted in most countries. In the future there may be transplants from other species such as pigs (xenotransplantation). One experimental approach is to modify animals genetically to make their tissues immunologically better tolerated by the human immune system.

Increasingly, diabetic patients are being offered simultaneous renal and pancreatic transplantation (see Chapter 9).

Cadaveric donation

About 75% of donations are cadaveric. The preference is for 'beating heart' donors, such as brain-damaged patients taken off life-support systems, and only 10% of cadaveric kidneys come from non-heart beating donors, e.g. road traffic accidents. At 25%, the UK has a relatively low proportion of living donors to cadaveric, the highest being Norway with 45%. The criteria applied in this controversial area are affected by ethical, cultural, ethnic and religious considerations that are outside the scope of this book. However, it should be noted that rigorous rules for determining brain death are now applied, which effectively eliminate the risk of error.

Graft matching

All ESRD patients approaching end-stage are tissue-typed and registered centrally. When a kidney becomes available, several closely matched potential recipients are urgently called to their local renal unit and a direct cross-match is done. All other things being equal, the patient with the best match is then immediately prepared for surgery.

Histocompatibility

Two important immunological criteria affect the risk of rejection. Blood group (ABO) compatibility operates as in blood transfusion, i.e. group O is a universal donor, etc. More complex is HLA compatibility (see Chapter 2). Class II HLA-D antigens seem to be the more important in transplantation.

The intensity of an immune response and thus the likelihood of rejection depends on the degree of HLA similarity between donor and recipient; e.g. they may have the same HLA-A and HLA-B antigens (both Class I), but may differ in HLA-DR. Children have a mixture of their parents' HLA genes. Identical (monozygotic) twins will have identical genes, as occasionally may two siblings by chance. The more distant the relationship, the less compatibility there is likely to be.

In discussing the outcome of transplantation it is usual to refer to graft survival, because if a graft fails the patient is simply returned to the dialysis programme. Grafts from an identical twin (isografts) have the best chance of survival. Survival figures for grafts are better for live donations than from cadaveric (Table 14.18). The longer a graft survives the lower the incidence of rejection; at the best centres the 10-year graft survival rate with well-matched kidneys can reach 70%, although the average is about 50%.

Immunosuppressant drugs can keep rejection at bay at the cost of potential myelosuppression, infection and other chronic iatrogenic complications. Improvements here have brought about gradually increasing graft survival. Better matching reduces not only the chance of rejection but also the immunosuppressant doses required, which itself improves patient survival.

Cross-matching

HLA-A, B, and C can be typed at any time using specific antisera and the patient's or donor's blood. For HLA-D, it is necessary to mix recipient lymphocytes and potential donor serum directly, from which donor lymphocytes must be deleted by a cytotoxic drug so that only the recipient's lymphocytes can respond to any incompatibility. Because typing takes 5 days, it is not practicable for cadaveric donors. The D subgroup called DR (D-related), currently the best predictor of graft tolerance, is detectable serologically, providing faster, more accurate matching.

Nevertheless, even completely HLA-mismatched grafts are sometimes successful and the paramount significance of HLA matching is disputed. Blood group compatibility, general health, previous transfusions and effective immunosuppression seem to be equally important in determining graft survival. Graft survival rates from cadavers and living unrelated donors are fast approaching those from living related donors.

The 'transfusion effect' is an immune tolerance that seems to be induced in ESRD patients. A wide variety of antigens are present in the pooled blood of the numerous transfusions usually received by ESRD patients during the course of their illness. Theoretically these would be expected to stimulate the production of multiple antibodies, some of which could – and sometimes do – reject a subsequent graft. However, a significant overall graft-sparing effect results from transfusions given in the months before grafting.

A final direct cross-matching of recipient serum and donor lymphocytes is performed just before surgery to check if there are any pre-existing cytotoxic serum antibodies which would cause an immediate rejection. Such antibodies could have arisen from previous blood transfusions, transplants or pregnancy.

Surgical procedure

The operation is not complex surgically, compared for example to heart transplanation (Figure 14.18). The donor organ is removed along with lengths of renal artery, renal vein and ureter. For living donors this can now be done laparoscopically ('keyhole surgery') to minimize trauma and improve post-operative recovery. It is placed extraperitoneally in an iliac fossa, where it can easily be felt and biopsied after operation. This also preserves the peritoneum should further dialysis be necessary. The graft's renal artery and vein are connected to major local abdominal vessels and the ureter is implanted into the recipient's bladder. The bladder connection may occasionally cause subsequent problems, but the operation has few complications and a low risk.

The original kidneys are usually conserved even if the patient is anuric, unless there is strong evidence of renal hypertension, stones (a

focus of infection) or a tumour. This preserves and utilizes any remaining function – especially important should the graft fail. Equally important, it helps maintain the haematocrit as some erythropoietin is still secreted even when the GFR is minimal. Bilateral nephrectomy introduces further operative risk for no improvement in graft or patient survival.

Kidneys are implanted as soon as possible after removal from the donor. This is easy to arrange with a living donor using adjoining operating theatres, and this contributes to the success of this type of transplant. Cadaveric kidneys are perfused with specially formulated organ preservation solution at 5°C immediately after removal to preserve their viability during transportation.

The ischaemic period after donor organ removal causes a variable degree of ATN that may manifest as ARF in the recipient for up to about 10 days after transplantation. During this time the patient may need to continue on dialysis, depending on their urine output and blood chemistry. The sooner the organ is implanted the less serious this episode is, and up to 75% of recipients start producing urine within a few days.

Rejection

A kidney graft may be rejected at any time, although the longer it survives the less likely this becomes. Moreover, most rejection episodes can be controlled. About half of patients undergo at least one epispode and a patient may undergo several episodes yet still ultimately retain the graft. However, if it cannot be saved the patient is returned to dialysis and to the transplant waiting list. The failed graft neeed not be removed unless it is a focus of infection or chronic inflammation; otherwise, further surgery can be avoided by allowing it to become fibrosed and eventually atrophy.

There are three main types of rejection:

Hyperacute or immediate rejection. This is caused by either pre-existing plasma antibodies attaching to the graft and initiating an immune response, or by ABO mismatch. It occurs within days or even hours, as soon as the organ becomes adequately perfused, and results in

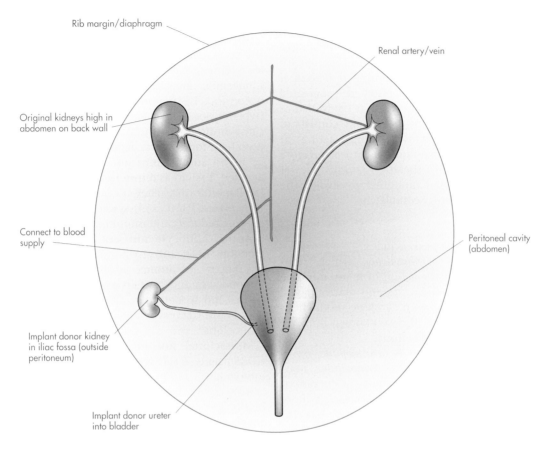

Rib margin/diaphragm

Renal artery/vein

Original kidneys high in abdomen on back wall

Connect to blood supply

Peritoneal cavity (abdomen)

Implant donor kidney in iliac fossa (outside peritoneum)

Implant donor ureter into bladder

Figure 14.18   Renal transplantation.

renal vascular thrombosis and loss of the graft. Fortunately rare, this condition is untreatable because the antibodies are already formed, although plasmapheresis has been tried.

Acute rejection.   This is the most common form. It can occur at any time, but usually in the first fortnight. It is a normal T cell-mediated response to HLA antigens involving primary sensitization, lymphocyte proliferation and subsequent attack. The resulting vascular and tubular damage initially causes non-specific symptoms such as fever and tenderness over the graft. If the organ has started functioning there will be a decline in renal function, with oliguria and a rise in serum creatinine.

There are problems in diagnosing acute rejection. If it occurs during the period of ATN that often follows cadaveric grafting, reduced renal function cannot be identified. Furthermore, a similar picture could be caused by a recurrence of the primary disease, by post-operative infection or obstruction, or by nephrotoxicity especially from *ciclosporin*. Consequently, most such episodes are treated by default as if they were rejection while efforts are made to identify other causes.

Chronic rejection.   This may occur at any time after the first few months, and partly involves immune-complex deposition within the glomeruli and renal vessels resembling chronic glomerulonephritis. Now referred to as chronic allograft nephropathy, it is relentless and usually irreversible, resulting in loss of the graft.

Prevention and treatment of rejection

Immunosuppressant therapy is started immediately before grafting, gradually reduced over 2–6 months to a maintenance dose and, except for isografts (HLA-identical), is continued lifelong. If there is an acute rejection episode it is increased temporararily until the rejection is controlled or the graft is lost. Treatment generally consists of combination therapy with drugs acting at different sites in the immune process (Figure 14.19). Combined therapy permits lower individual doses, but monotherapy avoids the toxicity of some drugs completely.

Prevention

The range of drugs used includes:

Corticosteroids (*prednisolone*), which non-specifically inhibit the action of many immune cells, including lymphocytes and macrophages, partly by interfering with cytokine production. The main drawback is the well-known range of dose-related steroid side-effects.

Anti-proliferative agents (*azathioprine, mycophenolate mofetil, sirolimus*). *Azathioprine* non-specifically depresses cellular proliferation, including immune cells; *mycophenolate* is more specific for lymphocytes, more effective but also more expensive. *Sirolimus* is also more specific and is not nephrotoxic, making it a good substitute if a calcineurin inhibitor is not tolerated. The main adverse effect of all antiproliferatives is some degree of bone marrow depression through inhibition of haematological precursors.

Calcineurin inhibitors (*ciclosporin, tacrolimus*) inhibit activation of lymphocytes targeted against specific antigens, and thus do not depress the bone marrow. They have potentially serious long-term adverse effects, including hyperlipidaemia, hepatotoxicity, lymphoma and, unfortunately, nephrotoxicity that results in hypertension. *Tacrolimus* is diabetogenic and can cause cardiomyopathy, so monitoring is required. Both have formulation dependant bioavailability so brand and formulation changes should be avoided. Toxicity is minimized by careful plasma level monitoring. They are metabolized by the cytochrome P450 (3A4) system so interact with enzyme inducers and inhibitors.

Anti-lymphocyte antisera (anti-lymphocyte globulin, ALG; anti-thymocyte globulin, ATG), are raised in animal hosts against human lymphocytes and contain a wide range of antibodies and so are polyclonal and non-specific. OKT3 (anti-CD3) also targets lymphocytes but is monoclonal.

Monoclonal anti-interleukin agents (anti-CD25 agents: *basiliximab, daclizumab*) block the interleukin-2 receptor (IL-2R), interfering with activated lymphocyte action. These agents are highly specific and appear to have few serious adverse effects. They are recommended by NICE for anti-rejection induction.

Treatment regimens vary widely between centres. A typical combination used in the UK is:

• *Prednisolone*, used high-dose for 'induction' immediately before implantation (1 g *methyl-*

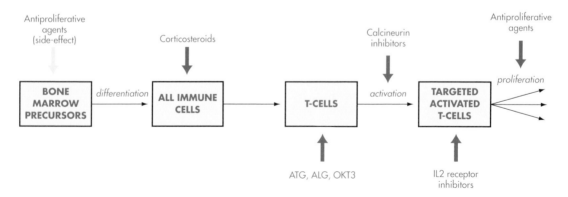

Figure 14.19 Rejection immunosuppression. Simplified diagram of different sites of action of anti-rejection agents, emphasizing advantages of combination therapy. ATG, anti-thymocyte globulin; ALG, anti-lymphocyte globulin; IL2, interleukin-2.

prednisolone IV) and then at moderate doses following implantation (e.g. 20–30 mg *prednisolone* oral daily) for 1–3 months then tailed off to a maintenance level (5–10 mg daily).

- *Azathioprine*, initiated post-operatively at a maintenance dose.
- *Tacrolimus*, also started post-operatively and carefully monitored.

Following a rejection episode the regimen would be changed (rescue or salvage therapy), substituting *mycophenolate* and/or *siroliumus*. The development of numerous alternatives has now made it feasible to tailor regimens for particular patients or situations, which can improve survival or minimize adverse effects, or both, starting with the most suitable drugs. For example, start with the second-line agents for a high risk patient such as a re-transplant; avoid nephrotoxic drugs following implantation with an organ exposed to warm ischaemia; use steroids and *tacrolimus* only with caution if latent diabetes is suspected.

Management of rejection

The standard response to suspected rejection is to increase the steroid dose substantially, e.g. IV *methylprednisolone* 1 g daily for 3 days. There is no point in raising antiproliferative dosage as the cells doing the damage are already in the blood, and calcineurin inhibitors cannot be increased because the dose being used was probably maximal before rejection, so that raising it would cause unacceptable toxicity. The episode will usually be aborted within a few days and normal prophylactic doses can be resumed.

Should steroids fail other immunotherapeutic regimens are used, e.g ATG, ALG, OKT3.

Other post-transplant complications

Successfully transplanted patients are still not entirely problem-free, owing mainly to their immunosuppressant therapy. They need regular renal, liver and blood screening and must be monitored for infective or haematological complications throughout the rest of their lives.

Many patients still have hypertension: contributory factors may include iatrogenic disease (e.g. steroid-induced fluid retention or *ciclosporin*

nephrotoxicity), an imperfectly functioning graft and the influence of the original, diseased kidneys. A slightly increased risk of malignancy (lymphoma and skin) is associated with long-term cytotoxic therapy. Vascular disease is common. Dyslipidaemia due to steroids and calcineurin inhibitors and hypertension lead to atherosclerotic complications, mainly IHD and stroke, which are a major cause of death. The increased incidence of peptic ulcer may be related to steroids, as may osteoporosis and osteonecrosis. Hepatic disease may result from treatment with both *azathioprine* and *ciclosporin*.

Immunosuppression from cytotoxic drug-induced bone marrow suppression and steroids predispose to infections, especially cytomegalovirus, *Pneumocystis*, reactivated TB and bacterial urinary-tract infections. Patients are often put on a combination of antimicrobials for several months post-operatively, including antivirals *co-trimoxazole*, *isoniazid*, and antifungal lozenges.

Important renal diseases

In this final section some of the more important renal diseases, many of which may be the underlying cause of ARF or CRF, are considered.

Obstructive uropathy

Obstruction can occur anywhere from the renal pelvis to the urethra and may be either unilateral or bilateral (Figure 14.20). Certain forms produce acute symptoms; bilateral obstruction, if untreated, may lead to CRF. Drugs have little role in the management of these conditions.

Pathology

The effect of obstruction depends on the site. Obstruction in the ureter or above, e.g. a stone or calculus, causes fluid accumulation in the renal pelvis (hydronephrosis) and a rise in tubular hydrostatic pressure. The increased tubular back pressure reduces the GFR but filtrate continues to be produced for some time, even following

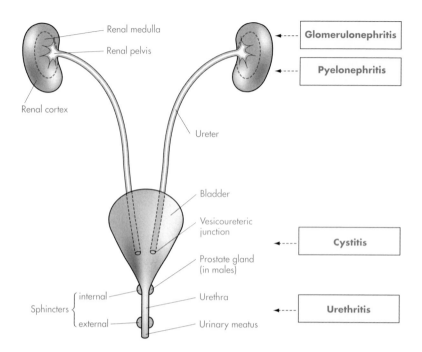

Figure 14.20   Urinary tract showing sites of major renal disease.

complete obstruction. The resulting increase in intrarenal pressure causes dilatation and gross damage owing to compression of renal tissue within the tough renal capsule. The prolonged urinary stasis which follows can promote secondary effects such as urinary-tract infection, because organisms are not regularly flushed out; stasis can also promote stone formation.

If the obstruction is relieved promptly, there may be a complete restoration of renal function. There usually follows a massive and prolonged diuresis, which can be fatally dehydrating: a urine output of up to 50 L in 24 h has been reported. Such losses suggest delayed tubular recovery (compare this with the polyuric phase of ARF, p. 901) in addition to the simple clearance of accumulated fluid. Because post-renal failure is potentially reversible, a patient presenting with sudden oliguria or anuria must always be investigated for possible obstruction. Although a comparatively rare cause of CRF, obstruction is one of the few causes that are preventable.

Chronic partial obstruction leads to chronic renal inflammation, scarring and possible infec-

tion. Such obstruction is often a result of congenital incompetence of the valve mechanism between the ureter and the bladder (the vesicoureteric junction; Figure 14.20), Vesicoureteric reflux leading to reflux nephropathy usually starts in infancy, and may stabilize or progress slowly to CRF in adulthood.

In bladder outflow obstruction, e.g. prostatic hypertrophy, urinary retention may be accommodated by bladder distension, with little serious rise in intrarenal pressure.

Aetiology

The commonest causes of obstruction are listed in Table 14.22. In the West, the most frequent causes are gynaecological problems in women, prostatic hypertrophy in men, and stones in both.

Renal calculi (urolithiasis)

The lifetime prevalence of renal stones is about 10% in males and 5% in females, although not all cases are symptomatic. The causes are poorly

Table 14.22   Causes of renal obstruction

Cause	Example	
Renal calculi	Calcium oxalate	70%
	Calcium-magnesium-ammonium phosphate	10–20%
	Calcium phosphate	10%
	Uric acid	5%
	Cystine	3%
Neuromuscular	Spasm, neurogenic bladder	
Structural	Congenital obstruction (e.g. pelvi-ureteric)	
	Urinary-tract tumour	
	Urethral stricture following infection	
	Prostatic enlargement	
	Abdominal mass (tumour, pregnancy)	
Iatrogenic	Anticholinergic drugs (spasm)	
	Sulphonamides (crystalluria)	
	Antineoplastic therapy (urate nephrolithiasis)	

understood. Calcium oxalate stones, the most common type, may result from hypercalciuria (high urinary calcium) or excessive gastrointestinal absorption of oxalate (hyperoxaluria). Stone formation is encouraged by an alkaline urine, e.g. from renal tubular acidosis, and hyperuricosuria, e.g. in hyperuricaemia or gout (Chapter 12). Conversely, hyperuricaemia together with an acid urine predisposes to urate stones. In urinary infections caused by urease-producing organisms, especially *Proteus* spp., the urinary alkalinity and ammonium content cause co-precipitation of mixed phosphate stones (calcium, magnesium and ammonium). In cystinuria, an inherited metabolic disorder, the reduced tubular reabsorption of cystine results in high urinary levels and cystine stone formation.

Clinical features and investigation

Symptoms depend on whether the lesion is above or below the bladder outlet. In the latter case, dysuria, hesitancy, frequency, terminal dribbling or bladder distension and discomfort occur. Above-bladder obstruction usually causes renal colic (sudden severe and debilitating unilateral loin pain due to ureteric spasm) often associated with haematuria and complete ureteric obstruction. Colic is also caused by the movement of stones in the ureter.

The urine flow disturbance will also depend on the degree and site of obstruction and whether it is bilateral. Paradoxically, polyuria may occur, owing to tubular damage. Chronic reflux nephropathy, caused by bladder contents being refluxed into the renal pelvis, may result in hypertension and recurrent renal infection (pyelonephritis).

Investigation ranges from simple examination and analysis of the urine to sophisticated imaging and biopsy.

Management

Whereas surgery used to be common in treating obstruction, conservative management is increasingly used, owing to the growing appreciation that renal function may be preserved or restored, and to the development of techniques of percutaneous intrarenal manipulation. Surgical repair may be essential in some cases, e.g. a congenital defect, but nephrectomy is now quite rare.

Small stones (especially cystine) may be passed in the urine if output is encouraged by ample fluid intake (more than 3 L daily), especially overnight. Antispasmodics such as *propantheline* (contra-indicated in bladder outflow obstruction) or catheterization may also assist the passage of stones. *Penicillamine* will help to dissolve cystine stones. Reducing urinary urate levels with *allopurinol* may help. Alkalinization of the urine, e.g. with *potassium citrate* mixture, will also reduce hypercalciuria and in turn the formation of both urate and cystine stones. Urinary acidification, e.g. with *ammonium chloride*, will minimize phosphate stone production.

For oxalate stones, sodium restriction and thiazides are used both to reduce urinary calcium (thiazides promote tubular reabsorption of calcium) and to increase urine flow. It is important not to reduce dietary calcium in an attempt to treat hypercalciuria, because, paradoxically, this tends to increase future stone formation and also cause loss of calcium from bones.

Nephrostomy may permit extraction of larger pelvic stones and drainage in hydronephrosis. Stones may be ultrasonically disrupted by extra-corporeal shock-wave lithotripsy (ESWL) and the fragments passed out in the urine. Fibre-optic ureteroscopy, which requires general anaesthetic, may be required. Open surgery is rarely necessary.

In reflux nephropathy prompt treatment of infections and adequate control of hypertension are likely to prevent progression. Surgery is rarely indicated, except for reconstruction of a congenitally abnormal vesicoureteric junction.

Renal colic is treated with either *pethidine* or, increasingly, an NSAID (*diclofenac*), which reduces ureteric spasm in addition to its analgesic effect. IV fluids are used to promote urine flow, especially as the patient is likely to be extremely nauseous.

In all methods employing treatments to encourage urine flow, it is of course important to ensure initially that there is not complete obstruction.

Infection

As with obstruction, there is a significant difference between infections of the lower and upper renal systems. Lower urinary-tract infection (e.g. urethritis, cystitis) causes discomfort, inconvenience and not a little pain, but is essentially benign if restricted to a single attack at that site. Conversely, infection of the kidney (upper urinary-tract infection or pyelonephritis) is always serious and has systemic complications. It may even lead to CRF: indeed, chronic pyelonephritis accounts for some 10% of all ESRD.

However, urinary-tract infection and pyelonephritis are not completely distinct. Most kidney infections are presumed to have ascended from asymptomatic, untreated or inadequately treated urinary-tract infection, and this retrograde infection is encouraged by the urinary stasis, which can result from obstruction. Repeated or serious urinary-tract infection can itself lead to obstruction by causing ureteric fibrosis and stricture (narrowing). The pathological spectrum, from asymptomatic bacteriuria to what is still termed chronic pyelonephritis, is illustrated in Figure 14.21.

Because pyelonephritis causes inflammatory damage there is also some pathological similarity to such conditions as nephrotoxicity, analgesic nephropathy, reflux nephropathy and the renal manifestations of connective tissue disorders, e.g. SLE. The generic term interstitial nephritis is often preferred.

Urinary-tract infection

Because of the close pathogenetic links between urinary-tract infection, reflux nephropathy, obstruction and pyelonephritis, some of the general features of urinary-tract infection are discussed here so as to present a complete picture of renal system infections. Full details of urinary-tract infections, especially their investigation and management, are given in Chapter 8.

Aetiology and pathology

Urine is normally sterile. The faecal commensal *Escherichia coli* is responsible for acute infection in 75% of those cases where a urinary organism is identified. Less common pathogens include staphylococci, faecal streptococci, *Proteus* and *Klebsiella*. Non-specific urethritis (i.e. non-gonococcal) is usually caused by *Chlamydia* spp.

Women. Even with the strictest hygiene, urinary-tract contamination with skin commen-

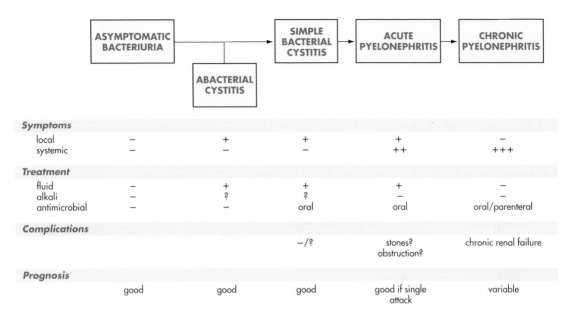

	ASYMPTOMATIC BACTERIURIA	ABACTERIAL CYSTITIS	SIMPLE BACTERIAL CYSTITIS	ACUTE PYELONEPHRITIS	CHRONIC PYELONEPHRITIS
Symptoms					
local	−	+	+	+	−
systemic	−	−	−	++	+++
Treatment					
fluid	−	+	+	+	−
alkali	−	?	?	−	−
antimicrobial	−	−	oral	oral	oral/parenteral
Complications			−/?	stones? obstruction?	chronic renal failure
Prognosis		good	good	good if single attack	variable
	good				

Figure 14.21   Spectrum of renal tract infection. −, absent (symptom) or useless (treatment), +, minor (symptom) or useful (treatment); ++, moderate; +++, substantial; ?, uncertain.

sals or faecal organisms is difficult to avoid in women. This is due to the anatomical proximity of the urethral and anal openings, and the relatively short urethra. Simple urinary-tract infection is far more common among women than men.

The route of infection may be anus–vagina–vulva–urethra. Vaginal secretions, urine and the urinary tract all normally have protective antimicrobial properties, e.g. mucosal IgA, locally acidic pH, frequent flow. Thus, recurrent infection suggests a breakdown in these defence mechanisms, e.g. obstruction, or a protected focus of infection, e.g. infected stones. Persisting vaginal organisms may be introduced into the urethra mechanically, especially during intercourse – hence the rather quaint but now distinctly anachronistic term 'honeymoon cystitis'. Urinary-tract infection is more common among postmenopausal women owing possibly to a loss of protection afforded by oestrogens.

Although bacteriuria is found in about 5% of adult women, few of these suffer symptoms. Such asymptomatic or covert bacteriuria generally does not require treatment except during pregnancy, where there is a 30% chance of progression to acute pyelonephritis due to intra-abdominal ureteric compression. On the other hand, no organism can be found in up to 50% of women who do have symptoms of cystitis; this is known as abacterial cystitis (or 'urethral syndrome').

Men.   Infection in males is much rarer and always requires investigation. Sexually transmitted non-specific urethritis is the most common cause in young men and chronic bacterial prostatitis in older men.

Both sexes.   In the elderly of either sex the prevalence of urinary-tract infection may rise to 30% and this is a particular problem in institutions. Catheterization alone carries a risk of infection variously estimated at between 2% and 20%. In diabetics, reduced host defence and glycosuria predispose to urinary bacterial growth.

Clinical features and course
The hallmark of acute urethritis/cystitis is an intense burning sensation on micturition, to which the simple term dysuria fails to do justice. The condition may be exacerbated by a more acid urine resulting from local bacterial metabolism. Urinary frequency is common and there

may be suprapubic pain or discomfort. Pyuria, purulent discharge or even haematuria may also occur but, although alarming and requiring investigation, are not necessarily sinister. There are no systemic signs. The elderly commonly present with acute confusion, fever, malaise or anorexia but few specific urinary symptoms, making it easy to miss during examination. It is also difficult to spot in young children if not suspected.

Urinary-tract infection is usually self-limiting within a few days, especially if fluid intake is promptly increased substantially. It may have no complications in the absence of any other renal abnormality. However, recurrence is common owing either to infection with a different organism, or to relapse or re-infection with the same organism. The latter situation suggests the presence of a complicating factor that is preventing complete eradication.

Investigation

Two things must be determined: (i) which organism is responsible; and (ii) are there any underlying causes or correctable complications? The collection of urine samples and the indications for further investigation are discussed in Chapter 8.

Management

In the management of urinary-tract infection the aims are to:

• reduce the risk of renal damage.
• provide symptomatic relief.
• render the urine sterile.
• provide prophylactic therapy.

The first of these is achieved by prompt attention and full investigation when appropriate. General measures include increasing the fluid intake substantially to promote urine flow, and providing advice on hygiene. For women, advice includes front-to-back wiping after defaecation (although the role of this has been disputed), and micturition before and after coitus. Frequent recurrence or relapse in the absence of obstructive or other correctable complications may require prophylactic therapy. For details of treatment, see Chapter 8.

Acute pyelonephritis

Like lower urinary-tract infection, most cases of acute pyelonephritis (APN) occur in women. *E. coli* is the usual culprit, but *Proteus*, *Staphylococcus* and *Pseudomonas* are found more commonly than in simple urinary-tract infection. Tubular inflammation causes polyuria and a dilute urine but severe cases may progress to acute oliguric renal failure.

Clinical features

An acute onset of severe loin pain is accompanied by systemic features such as fever, nausea and vomiting. There may also be lower urinary-tract infection symptoms of cystitis and urethritis (Figure 14.20). Rarely, if both kidneys are affected, tubular oedema and inflammatory exudate may cause intrarenal obstruction with acute post-renal failure.

Management

Prompt appropriate oral antimicrobial therapy and an increased fluid intake are always indicated. The same agents are used as in urinary-tract infection. However, close attention to microbiological results is vital because of the greater likelihood of unusual or resistant organisms and the importance of characterizing recurrence as either relapse, i.e. the same organism, or re-infection possibly with another.

Most patients have a single attack of APN and recover completely, but recurrent attacks or persistent asymptomatic bacteriuria require further investigation. If the recurrence is a relapse with the same organism, either the antimicrobial therapy was inadequate or there may be obstructive/reflux abnormalities. Frequent re-infection with different organisms or strains suggests that the host defences are defective, and that prophylactic antimicrobial therapy should be considered. This can be continuous low-dose therapy, or intermittent 5-day full-dose courses at the onset of symptoms, which the patient can be instructed to initiate.

Reflux nephropathy (chronic pyelonephritis)

Definition
The term chronic pyelonephritis has traditionally been used to describe a condition diagnosed radiologically where one or both kidneys appear irregular, shrunken and scarred. However, because evidence is accumulating of a strong association with reflux or infection, the term reflux nephropathy is now preferred. Although most cases do not progress to renal failure, it can be extremely difficult to treat, and renal scarring is present in up to 20% of patients starting dialysis.

Pathogenesis
The relative contributions of chronic infection and sterile reflux (causing simple pressure damage) are still uncertain. Many patients have neither bacteriuria nor a history of urinary-tract infection, and although urinary-tract infection and APN are far more common in women, reflux nephropathy shows equal sex distribution. One form may result from vesicoureteric reflux starting in the very young, and this has a poorer prognosis because it may be silent or undiagnosed for long periods. In adults, recurrent urinary-tract infection or APN may be responsible.

Bacterial reflux nephropathy commonly involves more virulent Gram-negative organisms, including *Pseudomonas*, and persistent infection with relapses is common. In contrast to the urinary tract the renal pelvis seems to have no natural antibacterial defences (presumably evolution never anticipated organisms there). There may even be factors that encourage the microbial persistence, so complete eradication is difficult.

Clinical features and investigation
The condition may be asymptomatic or may present as proteinuria, hypertension or recurrent urinary-tract infection. Rarely, the first indication may be symptoms of incipient renal failure such as polyuria or nocturia, because the renal damage is primarily tubular. Early reflux damage may initiate the hypertension–renal failure vicious cycle, and sometimes a history of related childhood illnesses such as enuresis or cystitis may be traced. Diagnosis and investigation involve urography, urine microbiology and renal function tests.

Management
In the absence of renal impairment, all that may be required is regular monitoring of blood pressure, urine microbiology and renal function. Infective episodes must be treated promptly as for APN, and appropriate antimicrobial prophylaxis may be indicated if bacteriuria cannot be eliminated. In children, surgery to correct reflux may be necessary.

Course and prognosis
Most patients have stable disease, especially if their BP and bacteriuria are managed successfully. Recurrent infective exacerbations carry a poorer prognosis, but only about 1% of patients progress to CRF.

Glomerular disease

Glomerular disease invariably affects both kidneys. Glomeruli seem especially sensitive to inflammatory immune damage, and most forms of glomerular disease involve immunological mechanisms. Glomerulonephritis (GN) is the single most important cause of CRF.

Classification

For such a small and apparently simple structure the glomerulus presents inordinate pathological complexity. Descriptions of glomerular disease have a long history in medicine, and understanding of the condition is confounded by the numerous methods of classification. Moreover, increasingly sophisticated microscopy and immunological techniques continue to identify new criteria and subgroups. Thus, in addition to simple clinical and aetiological classes there are histopathological and immunopathological groupings (Table 14.23).

There is no consistent correlation between these different methods of classification and much overlap. No single classification provides an unequivocal guide to management, and usually each aspect needs to be specified when considering a particular patient. Thus, for example, diabetes is usually associated with chronically progressive glomerulosclerosis and a poor outcome. On the other hand, acute post-infective nephritis showing diffuse proliferative change has an excellent prognosis with minimal treatment being required.

Presenting syndromes

The histopathological classification is becoming the standard among nephrologists but glomerular disease remains perplexing for the non-specialist. It is best tackled by first understanding that there are four main ways in which it may present, ranging in severity from asymptomatic proteinuria through nephritic syndrome and nephrotic syndrome to irreversible renal failure. This is illustrated in Figure 14.22, although this scheme must not be taken to imply an inevitable or direct progression. Each syndrome can have various aetiologies and outcomes, so the likely cause should be identified if possible and the pathology described. It is then possible to decide treatment and judge prognosis.

The clinical features and management options for these syndromes will be summarized in general terms, including a brief description of the main varieties of nephritic syndrome as commonly classified by prognostic categories. The syndrome of chronic renal failure was described above.

Table 14.23   Classification of glomerular disease

Type of classification	Examples
Aetiological – describes cause	**Primary (only the kidney affected)** • idiopathic (i.e. unknown) • post-infective (e.g. post-streptococcal) • iatrogenic (e.g. gold, NSAID) • allergic (e.g. most iatrogenic causes) **Secondary (systemic disease)** • hypertension • diabetic nephropathy • connective tissue disease (e.g. SLE, PAN) • autoimmune (e.g. Goodpasture's disease)
Prognostic – describes course	Acute Rapidly progressive Chronic
Immunological – describes mechanism	Immune complex (type III hypersensitivity) Autoimmune (anti-GBM antibodies) IgA nephropathy
Histopathological – describes damage	Minimal change Membranous Proliferative Glomerulosclerosis

GBM, glomerular basement membrane; IgA, immunoglobulin A; PAN, polyarteritis nodosa; SLE, systemic lupus erythematosus.

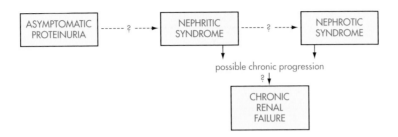

Figure 14.22   Spectrum of glomerular disease. Each syndrome can arise independently and progression is not inevitable.

Asymptomatic proteinuria

Normal urine contains only trace amounts of protein, usually less than 100 mg excreted over 24 h. Most plasma proteins are too large for filtration; smaller ones such as microglobulin are filtered to some extent, but most is reabsorbed in the tubules. Proteinuria means the presence of more than 500 mg protein in 24 h. If these are smaller proteins it implies a tubular defect, i.e. a failure of reabsorption (a 'tubular pattern').

Albumin is larger, and its presence in significant amount suggests a 'glomerular pattern', i.e. a failure of filtration. Thus it is more correctly called albuminuria. Albumin is usually discovered as an incidental finding during a general medical examination or during investigation of some other disease. Albumin loss below about 2 g/24 h may be benign, but such patients are always investigated and regularly monitored for the possible development of conditions such as glomerulonephritis, diabetes and hypertension. A medication history is also important. Intermittent proteinuria is quite a common normal finding after exercise or after prolonged standing or walking.

Microalbuminuria (<200 mg albumin per 24 h) is a prognostic marker of the possible development of nephropathy in diabetes. Urine dipsticks can currently detect this level of proteinuria. Microscopic haematuria may be benign. Even macroscopic haematuria need not be a sinister sign although it is obviously very alarming. Of course, both conditions also require thorough investigation.

Nephritic syndrome

Definition
The hallmarks of nephritis are renal impairment with oliguria, sodium and fluid retention, peripheral oedema, mild to moderate proteinuria and possibly haematuria. Urinary RBC 'casts' are diagnostic; these are clumps of cells that have been shaped by the tubular lumen. Frequently there are no further complications, but hypertension, hypertensive encephalopathy and pulmonary oedema may occur. Serum creatinine is moderately elevated, but only rarely does oliguric ARF supervene. The pathophysiological basis of these features is illustrated in Figure 14.23.

Aetiology and pathogenesis
Acute nephritis following a non-renal streptococcal infection, e.g. streptococcal sore throat, is the most common form although other infections may be responsible, e.g. malaria, bacterial endocarditis. Drug reactions and connective tissue disorders, e.g. SLE and Wegener's granulomatosis, are other possible causes.

Most cases are extra-renal in origin, involving immune complex (IC) deposition on the GBM. These complexes may be Ig plus, for example, streptococcal antigen or a drug acting as a hapten. In connective tissue disorder, antinuclear antibodies may be involved. Why some patients react in this way, and why the ICs are deposited in the glomeruli rather than being cleared by the reticuloendothelial system as usual, is not known. Low plasma complement

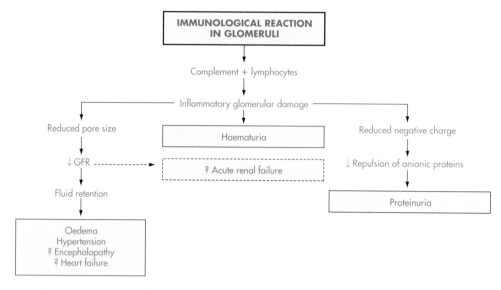

Figure 14.23   Pathogenesis and clinical features of nephritic syndrome. GFR, glomerular filtration rate.

levels may be implicated, although this may be effect rather than cause, complement having been precipitated on the GBM.

Course and prognosis

Usually nephritis runs an acute florid course with excellent recovery, especially in children. Some older patients may have benign persistent or intermittent proteinuria for many months or years. A significant number progress slowly to CRF and a few follow a rapidly progressive decline.

Management

The aims of management are to:

- identify any specific cause (e.g. infection) and treat that,
- institute simple symptomatic and supportive measures until the patient recovers.

The range of therapies used include the following (see Table 14.24), although the precise combinations that are effective will depend on precise histological assessment following biopsy.

Immunosuppression. This can include corticosteroids, often in combination with antiproliferatives such as *cyclophosphamide, azathioprine,*

mycophenolate mofetil, sirolimus and *ciclosporin.* Surprisingly, it is not universally effective.

Plasma exchange (plasmapheresis). The aim of this is to remove circulating auto-antibodies and ICs from the blood. Whole blood is removed and centrifuged: the supernatant plasma, containing the harmful immune products, is discarded and the cellular components are then re-injected. Fluid, electrolytes and albumin must also be administered to compensate for losses.

Renoprotection. As discussed above when consdering CRF, protein restriction needs to be used with caution, for fear of malnutrition. ACEIs, possibly in combination with ARAs, offer reduced progression and blood pressure control.

In addition, antihypertensive agents, antimicrobials, diuretics, fluid restriction and dietary protein manipulation may be necessary, as appropriate.

Common presentations

Acute glomerulonephritis. This is the classic post-streptococcal form usually seen in children or young adults. A very abrupt and severe renal inflammatory response might develop for

Table 14.24   Management of nephritic syndrome

Target symptom/feature	Management	Comment
Glomerular inflammation	Steroids, antiproliferatives, ciclosporin, sirolimus	Not always indicated; particularly useful for disease secondary to systemic disease
	Plasmapheresis	Particularly in immune-complex disease
Proteinuria	–	Protein supplementation not usually required
Uraemia	Protein restriction	Rare
Disease progression	ACEI/ARA	May be used in combination
Fluid retention, oedema	Na/water restriction Loop diuretic Dialysis	As for acute renal failure (Table 14.15) Monitor fluid balance and blood pressure
Hypertension	Antihypertensive therapy	
Infection	Antibiotics	e.g. penicillin in post-streptococcal nephritis

ACEI, angiotensin-converting enzyme inhibitor; ARA, angiotensin receptor antagonist.

example a few weeks after a severe throat infection. Disease severity usually correlates with the patient's titre of ASO. In children particularly, the prognosis is excellent with resolution in a week or less, and only supportive therapy is required. Anti-inflammatory therapy is usually ineffective.

Rapidly progressive glomerulonephritis. In about 1% of patients who develop acute GN there is rapid progression to acute oliguric failure. If this occurs the outlook is poor, with progression to ESRD within 2 years. Progressive GN may be associated with the presence of anti-GBM auto-antibodies (e.g. Goodpasture's disease), or arise in association with vasculitic connective tissue diseases (e.g. polyarteritis nodosa, PAN). The renal damage caused by malignant hypertension usually presents as a rapidly progressive GN although in this case the damage is not immunological.

Treatment and prognosis depend on the aetiology. For the connective tissue diseases early aggressive immunosuppressive therapy with cytotoxic drugs and steroids may induce a remission or retard progression. In idiopathic forms or in Goodpasture's disease this is rarely successful, but plasmapheresis may be helpful. Nevertheless, eventual progression to CRF and renal replace-

ment therapy is common. Following transplantation a recurrence of the disease is still possible, but the tendency nowadays is to transplant anyway.

Chronic glomerulonephritis. About 10% of GN patients, usually adults, progress to chronic illness. It is this slowly progressive, late-presenting form of GN that is the most common cause of CRF. Invariably there are co-existent hypertension and proteinuria. The cause of chronic GN is usually unknown. Diabetic nephropathy could be considered to be one form of the condition, although strictly speaking this is glomerular sclerosis rather than inflammation, and nephrotic syndrome is a more common presentation.

Specific treatment is rarely possible and the patient must enter a renal replacement programme. Certain forms of chronic GN with less glomerular damage ('membranous' and 'minimal change' GN) may respond to immunosuppressant therapy, but this is still controversial.

Nephrotic syndrome

The nephrotic syndrome can occur in association with many forms of nephritis or may arise independently. It is defined by the symptom triad:

- Heavy proteinuria.
- Hypoalbuminaemia.
- Gross pitting oedema.

The hallmark of nephrotic syndrome is extensive urinary protein loss associated with hypoproteinaemia sufficient to cause severe generalized oedema. The liver can synthesize albumin up to a maximum of about 15 g/24 h in an attempt to maintain plasma albumin levels, but paradoxically proteinuria no greater than 4–6 g/24 h may be sufficient to cause nephrotic syndrome. Thus there is probably another avenue of protein loss involved. This is may be an increase in the renal tubular catabolism of albumin, such that measurement of urinary protein loss underestimates the total deficit. These combined losses exceed hepatic capacity to synthesize protein and lead to progressive hypoproteinaemia, regardless of dietary protein intake (Figure 14.24).

Aetiology

The nephrotic syndrome may be a complication or progression of GN or it may present de novo. Specific aetiologies include diabetes, drugs (e.g. *penicillamine, captopril*, heavy metals) and infections (e.g. malaria, endocarditis).

Pathophysiology

The apparently paradoxical combination of a reduced GFR with a 'leak' sufficient to pass albumin molecules of molecular weight >60 kDa may arise because the reduced plasma volume causes a mild pre-renal impairment of filtration, while changes in the GBM electrostatic charge allow smaller proteins, that are normally repelled, to pass through. In mixed nephritic-nephrotic syndromes there is also some glomerular obstruction. The phenomenon of proteinuria is still not understood.

The oedema forms by a quite different mechanism to that of simple nephritis or heart failure. In the latter cases there is redistribution of the raised total body water with increased volumes in all compartments, plasma hypervolaemia causing hypertension and tissue hypervolaemia causing the oedema. By contrast, in nephrotic syndrome there is a reduced plasma volume and often hypotension. The hypovolaemia results from the reduced plasma oncotic pressure brought about by the hypoproteinaemia, which permits a loss of plasma water to the extravascular compartment (Figure 14.23).

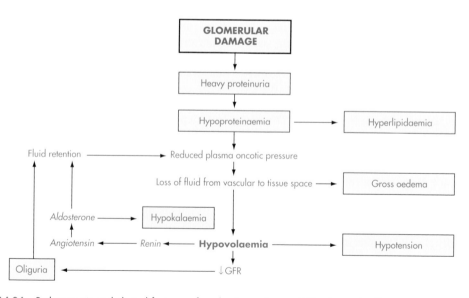

Figure 14.24   Pathogenesis and clinical features of nephrotic syndrome. GFR, glomerular filtration rate.

In nephrotic syndrome the RAAS acts to restore BP by increasing renal sodium and water reabsorption. However, blood volume cannot be expanded while plasma protein is low because the resultant low plasma oncotic pressure permits renally retained fluid to pass straight to the tissue. This exacerbates the oedema and causes further fluid and electrolyte retention. This vicious cycle may result in gross oedema, and the presence of over 20 L of oedema fluid has been reported. Nevertheless, many patients are not overtly hypotensive, possibly owing to the direct vasoconstrictor action of persistently raised angiotensin levels. Postural hypotension is usual, however. This classical account of the pathophysiology of oedema in nephrotic syndrome has been challenged and may not represent the whole picture.

Course and prognosis

The prognosis will depend on the age of the patient and the underlying lesion. In children the cause is usually acute GN and the outlook is good, with an 80% remission rate. In adults the underlying pathology is more likely to be a chronic progressive disease and the average remission rate is nearer 20–30%.

Clinical features

The clinical picture is usually very distinctive. Nephrotic syndrome may have an acute or insidious onset and resembles acute GN, except that the oedema is usually greater, including pulmonary oedema and ascites, and the patient is not hypertensive and may be hypotensive. The patient is usually very ill, weak, anorexic and oliguric. A common unexplained finding is hyperlipidaemia, possibly related to disordered protein metabolism (an attempt to synthesize new amino acids). High aldosterone levels often cause hypokalaemia.

Management

The aims of management are:

- To investigate and treat the cause (e.g. an underlying disease).
- To correct haemodynamic and metabolic abnormalities.
- To reduce glomerular inflammation.

Table 14.25 summarizes the treatment options. The effectiveness of immunosuppressant therapy, initially high-dose steroids, will depend on the cause, but in general steroid therapy is more beneficial than in simple GN. Patients who relapse after steroid withdrawal, i.e. are steroid-dependent, may benefit from cytotoxic drugs.

Reversal of the hypoproteinaemia must usually await resolution of the glomerular damage, but high-protein diets are traditional. The principal clinical problems are oedema and sodium and fluid retention. Salt and water restriction and loop diuretics are used and high doses may be needed, e.g. 50 mg *furosemide*. Care must be taken not to exacerbate hypovolaemia and precipitate pre-renal failure by too rapid a diuresis; thus the use of diuretics may be delayed

Table 14.25   Management of nephrotic syndrome

Target symptom/feature	Management	Comment
Glomerular inflammation	Steroids, cytotoxics, plasmapheresis	Often useful, especially in children
Proteinuria	Protein supplementation (>100 g/day)	Often given, efficacy unproven
Fluid retention, oedema	Na/water restriction Diuretic: spironolactone, thiazide, high-dose loop	Care! Despite hypotension, patient has hypovolaemia and hypokalaemia
Low plasma oncotic pressure	Albumin, mannitol infusion	Albumin effect short-lived
Hypokalaemia	Spironolactone, amiloride	

until there is a recovery in urine output. This can be prevented by subsequent infusion of a plasma expander such as salt-free albumin. Hypokalaemia, which would be exacerbated by loop diuretics, can be treated with high-dose *spironolactone* and potassium supplements.

Polycystic disease

Adult polycystic disease is the most common inherited renal disease. Both kidneys become enlarged up to two or three times normal size, owing to the development of many fluid-filled, inert cysts. These gradually crush adjacent renal structures.

The more common autosomal dominant form has a prevalence of 1/1000. The age of onset and progression are highly variable. Progression to end-stage renal failure usually occurs within 10–20 years of diagnosis, so patients who first present late in life may avoid this. Nevertheless, 10% of ESRD patients have polycystic disease. In the rarer recessive form, onset and rapid progression to renal failure occur in childhood.

Clinical features are similar to those of other forms of RF. Hypertension is common, there may be loin or lumbar pain, and haematuria if a cyst ruptures. Diagnosis is based on ultrasound imaging.

There is no specific treatment beyond the standard procedures for CRF; control of BP will slow progress. Regular screening of siblings and offspring is important.

References and further reading

Aronson J K (2003). Drugs and renal insufficiency. *Medicine* 31(7): 103–109.

Ashley C (2001). Acute renal failure. *Pharm J* 266: 625–628.

Ashley C (2004). Renal failure; how drugs can damage the kidney. *Hosp Pharm* 11: 48–53.

Ashley C (2004). Renal failure; options for renal replacement therapy. *Hosp Pharm* 11: 54–62.

Chadban S J, Atkins R C (2005). Seminar: Glomerulonephritis. *Lancet* 365: 1797–1806.

Eaton D C (2004). *Vander's Renal Physiology*. New York: Appleton Lange.

Hilton R (2006). Acute renal failure. *BMJ* 333: 786–790.

Gokal R, Mallick N P (1999). Peritoneal dialysis. *Lancet* 353: 823–828.

Lee M A (2003). Transplantation: Drug aspects of immunosuppression. *Hosp Pharm* 10: 201–207.

Mallick N P, Gokal R (1999). Haemodialysis. *Lancet* 353: 737–742.

Marshall W J, Bangert S K (2004). *Illustrated Textbook of Clinical Chemistry*, 5th edn. London: Mosby.

Meguid El Nahas A, Bello A K (2005). Chronic kidney disease: the global challenge. *Lancet* 365: 331–340.

Morlidge C, Richards T (2001). Managing chronic renal disease. *Pharm J* 266: 655–657.

Parmar M S (2002). Chronic renal disease. *BMJ* 325: 85–90.

Sexton J (2003). Drug use in the renally impaired adult. *Pharm J* 271: 744–746.

Sexton J, Vincent M (2004). Managing anaemia in renal failure. *Pharm J* 273: 603–606.

Sexton J, Vincent M (2005). Remedying calcium and phosphate problems in chronic kidney disease. *Pharm J* 274: 561–564.

Tompson C R V, Plant W D (1997). *Key Topics in Renal Medicine*. Oxford: Bios Scientific Publishers.

UK Renal Pharmacy Group (2003). *Renal Drug Handbook*, 2nd edn. Oxford: Radcliffe Medical Press.

Internet resources

http://www.dh.gov.uk/PolicyAndGuidance/HealthAnd SocialCareTopics/Renal/fs/en
http://www.renalreg.com/reports
http://www.uktransplant.org.uk

Index

Drug names are in **bold** type. Page numbers in *italics* refer to tables or figures.

methyldopa 232
  haemolytic anaemia 40, 43
  stomatherapy and *137*
methyl phenyl tetrahydropyridine
  (MPTP) 428
methylprednisolone
  parenteral 321
  pulsed high doses, rheumatoid
    arthritis 779
  relative potency to other
    corticosteroids *320*
  renal transplant rejection 929
methylxanthines *see* aminophylline;
  theophylline
methysergide 503
  cluster headache 504
meticillin-resistant *Staphylococcus aureus*
  (MRSA) 541, 542
  antibiotics 530
  pneumonia 560
metoclopramide 435
  antispasmodics, interaction *105*
  gastro-oesophageal reflux 86
  for iatrogenic vomiting 110, 692
  migraine 499
metolazone, heart failure 206
metoprolol, heart failure 201
metronidazole 528
  activity spectrum *516*
  amoebiasis 570
  diarrhoea 571
  Helicobacter pylori therapy 89
  inflammatory bowel disease 122
  rosacea 863
MHC molecules 45
mianserin 395, 396, *397*, 398
micelles 75
microalbuminuria 937
  angiotensin converting enzyme
    inhibitors 603
microangiopathy, diabetes mellitus
  599, 600
microbiology, laboratory investigations
  538
microcirculation, inflammation 46
micro-enemas, constipation 128
microfold cells, small intestine 74
microfractures, bony 755
microorganisms, classification 514–15
microscopic colitis 114
microsomal mixed function enzymes
  160–1
  antibiotics and 547
  anti-epileptic drugs inducing 451
  rifamycins on 530
microvascular complications, diabetes
  mellitus 598
micturition, abnormalities 882
midazolam, epilepsy 453
midstream urine samples, clean-catch
  577
migraine 491, *494*, 495–503
  management 498–503
migrainous neuralgia (cluster headache)
  492, 494, 503–4
miliary tuberculosis 573
milk, bismuth chelate and 104
milk-alkali syndrome 93
milrinone, heart failure 205
mind-body problem 371
minimal-change glomerulonephritis
  939

minimum bactericidal concentration,
  antibiotics 515
minimum inhibitory concentration,
  antibiotics 515
minocycline 527
  acne 862
  rosacea 863
minor depression 389
minor tranquillizers 381
minoxidil 232
  hair growth 817
mirtazapine 395, *397*
miscarriages, antiphospholipid
  syndrome 736
mismatching, ventilation/perfusion 278
misoprostol 106
  NSAIDs with 777
mitosis 657
mitotic spindle inhibitors *682*
mixed affective disorder *377, 379*
mixed agonist-antagonists, opioid
  receptors 469, 475
mixed connective tissue disease 798
mixing, insulin formulations 625
mizolastine 831
moclobemide 401
modes of treatment, defined 8
modified-release preparations
  analgesics 466
  morphine 470
  stomatherapy and *137*
molecular size 18
  glomerular filtration 873
moles *821, 824*
mometasone 320
  asthma *306*
  relative potency to other
    corticosteroids *320*
monitoring
  anti-epileptic drugs 447
  antimicrobials, use 547
  asthma 289
  defined 8
  diabetes mellitus 626, 628–9
  lithium 407
  myocardial infarction 260
  shock 62
monoamine oxidase B inhibitors 431,
  432, 433–4, 437
monoamine oxidase inhibitors 400–1,
  402–3
  antidiabetic drugs and 617
  anxiety disorders 385
  biochemistry 388
  pethidine and 472
monobactams 525
monoclonal antibodies 25, 33
  vs tumour necrosis factor alpha 750
monoctanoin 152
monocytes 28–9
  normal blood count *708*
monoethylfumaric acid, psoriasis 849
monosaccharide intolerance 114
monotherapy, epilepsy 446
monounsaturated fatty acids 239, 603
montelukast 51
  asthma 304
mood
  affect *vs* 386
  antipsychotic drugs on *417*
Moraxella catarrhalis, antibiotic
  sensitivities *516*

morbidity, defined 4
'morning dipping' *see* nocturnal attacks,
  asthma
morning stiffness
  osteoarthritis 757
  polymyalgia rheumatica 806
  rheumatoid arthritis 765
morphine *465*, 470
  adverse effects 476–8
  antihistamines and 480
  diverticular disease and 125
  liver and 159
  local anaesthesia with 482
  palliative care 509–10
  pharmacokinetics *471*
  pulmonary oedema 345–6
  receptor selectivity *468, 469*
  renal failure 510
  spinal analgesia 487
  in surgery 507
mortality
  angina pectoris 251
  asthma 294, 297
  cancer 647
  COPD 327–8
  defined 6–7
  diabetes mellitus 592
  epilepsy 444
  heart failure 197
  hypertension 212, 220
  meningococcal infection 551
  myocardial infarction 259
  Parkinson's disease 429
  pneumonia 559
  tuberculosis 571
motility stimulants 86, *127*, 129
  see also domperidone; metoclopramide
motion sickness 109
mourning 386
mouthpieces, nebulizers 359
mouth ulcers, chemotherapy *691*
mouthwashes, Sjögren's syndrome
  802
movement disorders
  dopamine 435
  see also extrapyramidal syndromes;
    Parkinson's disease
moxifloxacin 529, 530
moxonidine 232
M phase 658, 660–1
mucinous exudate 49
mucolytics 338
mucopurulent exudate 49
mucosa, gastrointestinal 72
mucosal anaesthetics, stomach *94*
mucosal protectants
  gastro-oesophageal reflux 86
  peptic ulcer 104
  see also bismuth chelate
mucositis, chemotherapy *691*
mucous cells (stomach) 73
mucous glands, airways 273
mucus
  antibiotic penetration 543
  COPD 328
  cystic fibrosis 341
multimodal therapy, cancer 676–7
multiple drug resistance
  cytotoxic chemotherapy 687
  Gram-negative organisms,
    polymyxins 531
  tuberculosis 576